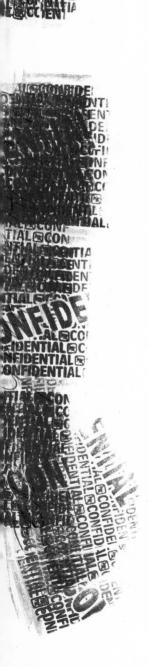

VOLUME ONE

ACKERMAN'S

SURGICAL PATHOLOGY

VOLUME ONE

ACKERMAN'S

SURGICAL PATHOLOGY

JUAN ROSAI, M.D.

Professor and Director of Anatomic Pathology,
Department of Pathology,
Yale University School of Medicine,
New Haven, Connecticut

SEVENTH EDITION

with 2184 illustrations and two 4-color plates

The C. V. Mosby Company

ST. LOUIS • TORONTO • WASHINGTON, D.C.   1989

MOSBY

A TRADITION OF PUBLISHING EXCELLENCE

Editor: George Stamathis
Developmental Editor: Elaine Steinborn
Assistant Editors: Laurel J. Fuller, Jo Salway
Project Manager: Carlotta Seely
Senior Production Editor: Helen C. Hudlin
Production Editors: Radhika Rao Gupta, Cindy Miller
Book and Cover Design: Gail Morey Hudson
Production: Jeanne Genz

SEVENTH EDITION (two volumes)

Copyright © 1989 by The C.V. Mosby Company

Previous editions copyrighted 1953, 1959, 1964, 1968, 1974, 1981

Printed in the United States of America

The C.V. Mosby Company
11830 Westline Industrial Drive, St. Louis, Missouri 63146

Library of Congress Cataloging in Publication Data

Ackerman, Lauren Vedder, 1905-
  Includes bibliographies and index.
    1. Pathology, Surgical.   I. Rosai, Juan, 1940-
II. Title. III. Title: Surgical pathology.   [DNLM:
1. Pathology, Surgical.   WO 142 A182s]
RD57.A2   1989   617'.07   88-13322
ISBN 0-8016-4176-4

GW/VH/VH 9 8 7 6 5 4 3 2 1

To
the memory of my father
EZIO ROSAI
(1908-1977)

Preface to seventh edition

Eight years have elapsed since the previous edition of this book was published, a longer interval than between any of the other editions. These have been years in which the pace of publications in the field has increased almost exponentially, fueled not only by novel observations derived from application of newer techniques and by fresh mental approaches to old problems but also by an exuberant and not always beneficial proliferation of pathology journals and monographs. The incorporation of the best of this new material has necessitated rather drastic changes throughout the book, with many of the chapters being entirely rewritten. The format employed to describe the major tumor types has also been modified. In order to further emphasize the clinicopathologic correlations that have been a major feature of the book from its very inception, clinical and epidemiologic data, gross and microscopic features, other microscopic types, patterns of spread and metastases, therapy, and prognosis have been discussed in separate sections. In the section on prognosis, a detailed listing of the clinical and pathologic parameters of possible prognostic significance have been tabulated for easier reference. A selection from the massive amount of new information about immunocytochemical observations of diagnostic and histogenetic interest has been incorporated in the respective chapters. In addition, a chapter on special techniques in surgical pathology has been added, which incorporates a catalogue with the most important markers currently used in the surgical pathology laboratory. The other major technologic advance that has occurred in the field is represented by the progressive computerization of the surgical pathology laboratory. A section on this subject has been written by Dr. Jon Morrow, Director of Diagnostic Pathology Computer Services at Yale University and a leading expert in the field.

Other changes in format include a new chapter on diseases of the pituitary gland (discussed before as part of the diseases of the central nervous system) and one on diseases of the ear, which was altogether lacking.

As in previous editions, most of the book has been written by one individual, hoping that whatever may be missing as a result has been compensated for by a uniformity of thought and style and the constant attempt to preserve as much as possible the direct and practical approach given to this work by its begetter, Dr. Lauren V. Ackerman. There are, however, areas that could not have been covered adequately without the help of specialists. I was fortunate to have the collaboration of Dr. Kenneth W. Barwick, Director of Gastrointestinal Pathology at Yale University, for the section on medical diseases of the liver; Dr. Richard D. Brunning, Director of Hematopathology at the University of Minnesota, for the section on diseases of bone marrow; and Dr. Michael Kashgarian, Director of Renal and Ultrastructural Pathology at Yale University, for the section on medical diseases of the kidney. In addition, many of the contributions to the text and illustrative material made in the previous edition by Drs. Hector A. Rodriguez-Martinez, Richard K. Sibley, Morton E. Smith, and Robert A. Vickers remain in the present one.

I wish to express my gratitude to Dr. Vincent T. Marchesi, Chairman of the Pathology Department of Yale University for his support for this project and to my colleagues in Anatomic Pathology for assuming a large portion of my service work in the division while I was engaged in this task.

My wife, Maria Luisa Carcangiu, joined me in this effort from the very beginning by making countless suggestions during the preparation, critically reviewing the entire manuscript, selecting and organizing the bibliographic material, and personally choosing most of the material for the new illustrations. Thanking her for the time and energy she spent in this endeavor—while sacrificing her own interests in the meanwhile—would be almost inappropriate. Suffice it to say that this book is hers as much as it is mine.

My good friend, Dr. Jose Costa, Chairman of the Pathology Department at the University of Lausanne, Switzerland, gave me unlimited access to the superb collection of gross photographs filed in his Institute. His generosity is deeply appreciated, as well as that of many other colleagues who have shared their material with me in one form or another over the course of the years; they are too many to be acknowledged individually, but I wish here to thank all of them for their trust and courtesy.

Finally, I want to express my appreciation to Andrea Scafariello and Andrea Feldman for typing most of the manuscript and to Robert L. Specht for producing most of the new illustrative material.

Juan Rosai, M.D.

New Haven, Connecticut

Preface to first edition

This book can be only an introduction to the vast field of surgical pathology: the pathology of the living. It does not pretend to replace in any way the textbooks to general pathology, its purpose being merely to supplement them, assuming that the reader has a background in or access to those texts. The contents are not as complete as they might be because emphasis has been placed on the common rather than the rare lesions and are, to a great extent, based on the author's personal experiences.

This book has been written for the medical student as well as for those physicians who are daily intimately concerned with surgical pathology. This must of necessity include not only the surgeon and the pathologist, but also those physicians in other fields who are affected by its decisions, such as the radiologist and the internist. Gross pathology has been stressed throughout with an attempt to correlate the gross findings with the clinical observations. The many illustrations have been selected as typical of the various surgical conditions, although in a few instances the author has been unable to resist showing some of the more interesting rare lesions he has encountered. Concluding each chapter there is a bibliography listing those references which are not only relatively recent and readily available, but also those which will lead the reader to a more detailed knowledge of the subject.

Dr. Zola K. Cooper, Assistant Professor of Pathology and Surgical Pathology, has written one of the sections on Skin, and Dr. David E. Smith, Assistant Professor of Pathology and Surgical Pathology, has written the chapter on Central Nervous System. Both of these members of the Department are particularly well qualified for their respective roles because of their background and present responsibilities in these fields. Their efforts on my behalf are most gratefully acknowledged.

Many members of the Surgical Staff at Barnes Hospital have given much help both knowingly and unwittingly. I am particularly grateful to Dr. Charles L Eckert, Associate Professor of Surgery, for letting me bother him rather constantly with my questions and for giving freely of his experience. Dr. Richard Johnson, who succeeded me as Pathologist at the Ellis Fischel State Cancer Hospital, agreeably made available all the material there, and Dr. Franz Leidler, Pathologist at the Veterans Hospital, has been most cooperative.

Thanks must be given to Dr. H.R. McCarroll, Assistant Professor of Orthopedics, for constructively criticizing the chapter on Bone and Joint, and to Dr. C.A. Waldron for helping me with the chapters related to the Oral Cavity. Among other faculty friends and colleagues who were especially helpful, I would like to mention Dr. Carl E. Lischer, Dr. Eugene M. Bricker, Dr. Heinz Haffner, Dr. Thomas H. Burford, Dr. Carl A. Moyer, Dr. Evarts A. Graham, Dr. Robert Elman, Dr. Edward H. Reinhard, Dr. J. Albert Key, Dr. Glover H. Copher, Dr. Margaret G. Smith, and Dr. Robert A. Moore.

Mr. Cramer K. Lewis, of our Department of Illustration, has been very patient with my demands, and his efforts and skill have been invaluable. Miss Marion Murphy, in charge of our Medical Library, and her associates gave untiringly of their time.

Because of recent advances in anesthesia, antibiotics, and pre- and postoperative care, modern surgery permits the radical excision of portions or all of various organs. There is a need today for contemplative surgeons, men with a rich background in the fundamental sciences, whether chemistry, physiology, or pathology. The modern surgeon should not ask himself, "Can I get away with this operation?" but rather, "What does the future hold for this patient?" It is hoped that this book may contribute in some small fashion toward the acquisition of this attitude.

Lauren V. Ackerman, M.D.

St. Louis, Missouri

Contents

Appendixes

VOLUME ONE

ACKERMAN'S

SURGICAL PATHOLOGY

1 Introduction

HISTORICAL PERSPECTIVE

Surgical pathology has come a long way since the time that Velpeau, famous professor of clinical surgery at the Paris Faculty, stated in his work on diseases of the breast published in 1853: "The intervention of the microscope is not at all necessary to decide whether such and such a tumor, which has been removed, is or is not of cancerous nature."* In the 1870s, Carl Ruge and his associate Johann Veit, of the University of Berlin, introduced the surgical biopsy as an essential diagnostic tool. Despite the inevitable controversies that followed, Friedrich von Esmarch, professor of surgery at Kiel and a leading military surgeon, presented forceful arguments at the German Surgical Congress of 1889 on the need to establish a microscopic diagnosis before operating in suspected cases of malignant tumors requiring extensive mutilating procedures. Shortly thereafter, the freezing microtome was introduced, and the frozen section procedure hastened the acceptance of this recommendation. In this country, the specialty of surgical pathology was conceived and developed by surgeons and gynecologists. It is said that William S. Halsted was the first American surgeon to create a division of surgical pathology in his department. Joseph Colt Bloodgood is credited as being the first full-fledged American surgical pathologist.[14] Many individuals contributed to consolidate the specialty of surgical pathology in North America during the first half of this century, but special recognition is due to Arthur Purdy Stout of Columbia-Presbyterian Hospital in New York City; James Ewing and his successor Fred Stewart of Memorial Hospital, also in New York City; Pierre Masson of the University of Montreal; and Lauren V. Ackerman of Barnes Hospital in St. Louis, Missouri[2,10,16,19] (Fig. 1-1).

SURGICAL PATHOLOGY AND THE PATHOLOGIST

A department of pathology in a large medical center should have a division of surgical pathology closely affili-

*From Velpeau AALM: Traité des maladies du sein et de la région mammaire. Paris, 1853. Translated into English by Henry M: A treatise on the diseases of the breast and mammary region. London, 1856, pp. 479-480.

ated with the clinical and surgical departments. Surgical pathology implies surgery, but the modern surgical pathologist is closely affiliated with many branches of medicine. This includes all the surgical specialties, internal medicine, dermatology, neurology, diagnostic radiology, radiation therapy, and medical oncology. Although the study of radiology deals with shadows and the study of pathology with substance, the correlation of those shadows with the gross substance strengthens the diagnostic skill of the radiologists, explains errors in radiologic interpretation, and instills humility rather than dogmatism. The radiotherapist and medical oncologist, too, can learn much from the study of surgical pathology, particularly the correlation between sensitivity to therapy and microscopic tumor types and the effects of therapy on normal tissue. Furthermore, explanations for the success or failure of therapy may become apparent by the study of surgical specimens.

The surgical pathologist has the unique opportunity of bridging the gap between the beginning of disease and its end stages, and he should take advantage of this circumstance. He can do this only after a solid foundation of study at the autopsy table, where the ravages of cancer and other diseases are all too clear. With this background, he can then correlate the initial stages of disease seen in specimens from living patients in the surgical pathology laboratory and make fundamental contributions to knowledge. With the integration of clinical findings, pathologic anatomy is still a living science.

By the very nature of the material submitted to him, the surgical pathologist is bound to make some mistakes. He sees the earliest subtle and sometimes bewildering changes in Hodgkin's disease. He may not recognize that the minimal granulomatous response in a lymph node is really a peripheral manifestation of histoplasmosis. The necessity of follow-up on the patient in whom the diagnosis is not certain is mandatory. Time is often a better diagnostician.

The surgical pathologist not only must know his own field thoroughly, but he also must have a rich background in clinical medicine. He needs to understand the clinicians' needs and respond to them accordingly. He must be in a position to advise the clinicians about the biopsy or the excised material he receives. It is not sufficient for him to say whether a lesion is benign or malignant. He must be able to tell the surgeon the extent of the disease, the adequacy of the excision, and other pertinent information. He should also be able to comment on whether additional therapy may be necessary and give information on the prognosis of the disease. He should communicate with clinicians constantly, informally, and through interdepartmental conferences. The ever-increasing complexity of medicine has led to the unavoidable development of subspecialization within surgical pathology. There is no question that in some cases clinicians are best served by pathologists who have special

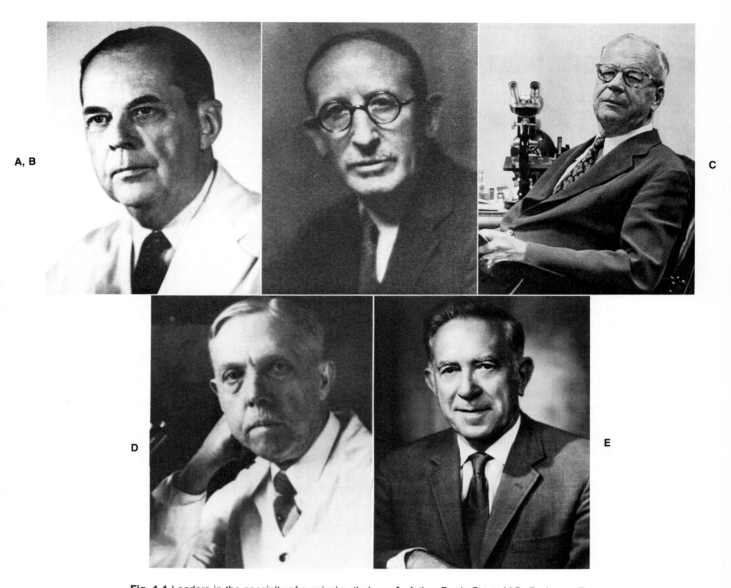

Fig. 1-1 Leaders in the specialty of surgical pathology. **A,** Arthur Purdy Stout, M.D. **B,** James Ewing, M.D. **C,** Fred Stewart, M.D. **D,** Pierre Masson, M.D. **E,** Lauren V. Ackerman, M.D. (**A** from Lattes R: Am J Surg Pathol **10**(Suppl 1):4-5, 1986; **B** from Stewart F: Arch Pathol **36**:325-330, copyright 1943, American Medical Association; **C** from Stout AP: Cancer **14**:frontispiece, 1961; **D** from Masson P: Human tumors. Histology, diagnosis and technique, ed. 2. Detroit, 1970, Wayne State University Press, copyright Librairie MALOINE S.A.)

expertise in certain areas and fully understand the clinical implications of their pathologic findings. Hematopathology, nephropathology, neuropathology, and dermatopathology are prime examples of such subspecialties.

SURGICAL PATHOLOGY AND THE NONPATHOLOGIST

By its very nature, surgical pathology depends heavily on the input of clinicians and surgeons who are fully aware of the potentials and limitations of the specialty. They should know that a microscopic diagnosis is a subjective evaluation that only acquires full meaning when the pathologist is fully cognizant of the essential clinical data, surgical findings, and type of surgery. The requisition slip for pathologic study should ideally be completed by a physician familiar with the case; too often the task is delegated to a medical student, a nurse, or the surgery resident who was requested to perform the biopsy. A conversation between the surgeon and the pathologist the evening before a contemplated frozen section may facilitate matters for both the next morning.

One of the best ways for a clinician to acquire a feeling of what the specialty is and how it can be best used is for him to have a full-time rotation in surgical pathology during his residency years. Ideally, this rotation should be of 6 months' duration; if this is not feasible, a minimum of 2 to 3 months should be required. We have found this practice invaluable in establishing a mutually beneficial rapport between surgeons and pathologists.

A good surgeon has not only technical dexterity (a fairly common commodity), but also, more importantly, good judgment and a personal concern for his patient's welfare. The surgeon with a prepared mind and a clear concept of the pathology of disease invariably is the one with good judgment. Without this background of knowledge, he will not recognize specific pathologic alterations at surgery nor will he have a clear concept of the limitations of his knowledge, and therefore he will not know when to call the pathologist to help him. Without this basic knowledge, he may improve his technical ability but never his judgment. One might say that with him his ignorance is refined rather than his knowledge broadened.

It is unfortunate that in some specialized areas of pathology (especially gynecology, dermatology, and gastrointestinal pathology), a conflict still persists in some quarters as to who should be interpreting the microscopic slides and in which department the laboratory should be located. There are some rare persons who are not trained pathologists but who have made fundamental contributions to pathology in their respective fields of interest; however, there are many reasons why it is inadvisable for clinicians to become their own pathologists. Although it is mandatory for them to have some knowledge of pathology, it is difficult, if not impossible, to be both a competent clinician and a skillful pathologist, just as it is not rational for the surgical pathologist to believe himself capable of performing operations as a sideline. An additional reason is that an objective evaluation of the slide is compromised because of the conscious or unconscious tendency that we all have to agree with ourselves. Since the situation created is one of self-referral, there is an economic incentive to perform more, rather than fewer, microscopic examinations. The situation is comparable to the practice of radiology by nonradiologists, where it has been shown that the nonradiologist physician who owns an x-ray machine uses an average of twice as many x-ray examinations as do colleagues who refer patients to radiologists.[5]

There is a fundamental unity to the morphologic patterns of disease in the human body that can be appreciated only by being familiar with those patterns as they occur in different organ systems. Only by understanding the pathology of disease as a whole can the manifestation of that disease in a given organ be fully comprehended. This is the main reason why a clinician cannot hope to deal adequately with some small branch of surgical pathology. Disease does not cooperate with him by remaining neatly confined to an anatomic system.

It is encouraging to see that the trend in the United States—with the outstanding exception of dermatopathology where financial considerations have unfortunately become the overriding factor—is decidedly toward a restitution to the pathology departments of what logically belongs to them. Medicine has become too complex to be handled with the approach of the Renaissance man. The days in which the gynecologist examined the patient, looked at the x-ray films, performed the surgery, examined the surgical specimen microscopically, and administered radiation therapy are over.

As far as pathology is concerned, the process is likely to be accelerated by the economic factors that are playing an increasingly important role in shaping the practice of medicine. Modern academic surgical pathology can no longer be performed in a laboratory equipped with a tissue processor, a paraffin oven, a set of reagents, and a microscope. It requires facilities for electron microscopy, enzyme histochemistry, immunohistochemistry, tissue culture, and molecular biology techniques. To have these expensive and complicated facilities duplicated within each of the major clinical and surgical departments of a medical center is financially absurd, a fact that has not escaped the attention of hospital administrators and third-party payers. An additional reason why the pathologist interpreting microscopic slides should not belong to a clinical department is that only by remaining independent can he have the unbiased approach necessary for the performance of his functions. He should be in a position to discuss freely with the clinician the indications for the performance of a biopsy, a frozen section, or a surgical procedure. Tissue committees and the important quality control function that they fulfill depend largely on the pathologist's prerogative, free of any interference, to present facts and question procedures.

At this point, it is only fair to mention that many of the problems alluded to are of our own making. One of the main reasons why clinicians began to act as pathologists and set up pathology minilaboratories in their own departments was because many departments of pathology were unable or unwilling to provide the services that clinicians rightfully demanded. In the past, the diagnosis of tissue removed from a living patient often was delegated to a resident, and reports emanating from the department of pathology not only were delayed, but also often indicated only whether the tissue was benign or malignant. These circumstances sometimes forced clinicians to direct some branch of surgical pathology. Under these conditions, the clinician's diagnoses and recommendations were better than those of the experienced but disinterested pathologist. Fortunately, the situation has changed radically. There is, however, no room for complacency. It is the duty of the current generation of pathologists to improve on the quality and quantity of the services provided by continually adapting to the ever-increasing complexity of their task.

SURGICAL PATHOLOGY REPORT

The delivery of a specimen in the surgical pathology laboratory initiates a complex series of events that culminates in the issuance of the final report. A flow chart describing the mechanism for handling the surgical pathology cases in our laboratory is shown in Fig. 1-2.

The surgical pathology report is an important medical document that should describe, as thoroughly and concisely as possible, all the relevant gross and microscopic features

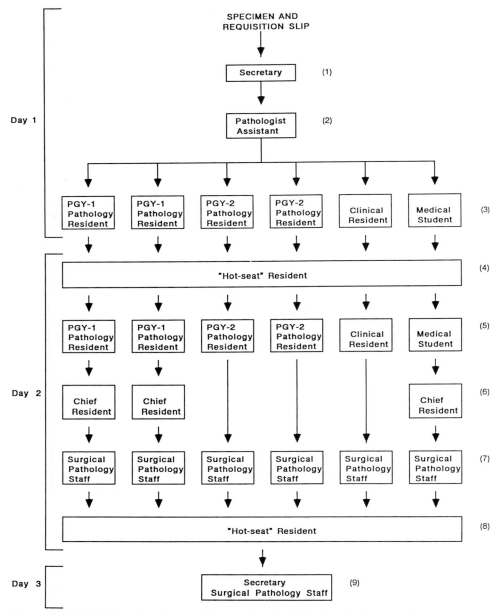

Fig. 1-2 Surgical pathology flow chart outlining the flow of activities from the time a specimen is received in the surgical pathology laboratory to the time the final report is issued. *(1)*, Check for accuracy of data. Enter into the computer; check patient name and hospital number; search for previous pathology material; and assign SP number. *(2)*, Check for completeness of clinical information. Make imprints, deep-freeze, fix for electron microscopy, etc., according to instructions. *(3)*, Perform gross dissection and dictation. Take gross photographs, photocopies, and x-rays if indicated. Take sections for microscopy and enter block identification into computer. *(4)*, Enter provisional diagnosis in "hot-seat" book. Ask for additional embedding, recuts, or special staining, as indicated. Notify clinicians directly in selected cases. *(5)*, Examine microscopic slides. Write microscopic description if indicated. *(6)*, Check microscopic slides and description. *(7)*, Check slides (only selected material in cases already seen by chief resident). *(8)*, Compare provisional and final diagnoses. Notify clinician immediately in cases of discrepancy. *(9)*, Type report into computer. Code diagnosis according to SNOMED. Sign report. Deliver to clinical chart clinician and medical records.

of a case but should also interpret their significance for the clinician. It should be prompt, accurate, and brief. The pathologist should avoid unnecessary histologic jargon that is of no consequence to the case and concentrate on the aspects that bear a relation to therapy and prognosis. To quote Richard Reed: "A competent [pathologist] is not simply a storage site for microscopic verbiage. It is not enough to be able to recite by rote the microscopic findings once the clinical diagnosis is established. The ability to offer clinical differential diagnoses from the interpretation of microscopic findings is the mark of the mature [surgical] pathologist. In addition, he may record data that are prognostically significant or offer suggestions for pertinent clinical tests. The ability to recognize cytologic and histologic features is simply a beginning. The ability to integrate microscopic findings into a meaningful interpretation is the distinguishing characteristic of a pathologist and is the art of pathology."*

The usual surgical pathology report is comprised of five major parts. The first, designated as "History," contains the essential clinical data known to the pathologist at the time he dictates a description of the gross specimen(s), such as sex and age of the patient, symptoms, surgical findings, and type of surgery. If a frozen section has been performed, the information regarding the organ biopsied, the diagnosis given, and the names of the pathologist(s) who performed the procedure should be included as part of the history. This portion of the report should also list previous biopsies on the same patient, if any had been taken. We insist on having a "History" section in all of our reports, no matter how brief, because it gives the reader of the report, whether a clinician or another pathologist, an immediate orientation to the nature of the problem that led to that particular operation in the context of the whole disease.

The second part of the report, known as "Gross," contains the gross description of the specimen(s). This should be precise and thorough, because once the gross specimen is discarded, this description remains the only document by which the gross features of the case can be evaluated. It should indicate how the various specimens were identified by the surgeon and whether they were received fresh or fixed, intact or open. The specimens should be described in a logical sequential fashion, with a clear description of gross abnormalities and their location. Lengthy anatomic descriptions of normal structures should be avoided. Size, color, and location of all lesions should be recorded. The metric system is to be used for all measurements. It is advisable to give specific dimensions and descriptions rather than to provide comparisons with common objects such as fruits or vegetables. The weight of the whole specimen, and sometimes the weight of the individual organs or lesions in a specimen, should be recorded whenever indicated. It is important to be accurate, factual, and noncommittal in the gross description, avoiding subjective interpretations as much as possible. Azzopardi[3] rightly commented that the contents of a mammary cyst are better described as amber,

brownish, greenish, opaque, or white rather than "bloodstained," "pus," or "milky" because the reason for the color of a secretion is often unknown. This sensible advice should be applied to other lesions as well. We prefer to identify the various sections taken by using letters of the English alphabet sequentially (rather than the first letter of the specimen or some other code), and we list this identification at the end of the gross description rather than after each specimen. The "gross" portion of the report is concluded by noting whether or not all of the tissue was submitted for microscopic examination and by including the name of the pathologist who performed the gross examination.

The third part of the report is termed "Microscopic." It should be short and to the point. The surgeon usually is not too interested in whether the nucleoli are acidophilic, basophilic, or amphophilic but rather what that means, if anything; if another pathologist is keen on this point, he probably will like to examine the slide himself.

The fourth and most important part of the report is the "Diagnosis." Each specimen received should have a separate diagnosis or diagnoses. Our practice is to divide each diagnosis into two parts, separated by a dash. The first lists the organ, specific site in that organ, and operation; the second gives the morphologic diagnosis (example: Bone, femur, biopsy—Osteosarcoma). This is useful for coding purposes and, again, it provides the reader with all the essential information on that particular specimen in a single entry. The SNOMED code should follow.

The fifth part, applicable to only some cases, is a "Note" or "Comment." In it, the pathologist may mention the differential diagnosis, give the reasons for this diagnostic interpretation, make some prognostic and therapeutic considerations about the entity, and include selected references. Copies of the pathology report are sent to medical records, the treating physician, station, or clinic, and the tumor registry; of the two copies that remain in the laboratory, one is used for coding purposes and the other is filed and eventually bound or microfilmed.

It is medically and legally important that the diagnoses and comments made by the pathologist on a given case be documented as clearly as possible in a written form in the clinical chart via the pathology report. This should be done because sometimes there is a remarkable discrepancy between the diagnostic considerations given verbally by the pathologist to the clinician and the paraphrasing of these considerations by the clinician in the chart. Each remark of importance given verbally should be incorporated into the final pathology report. At the time of a frozen section, the diagnosis given verbally to the surgeon should be transcribed in an appropriate form and a copy of such form incorporated immediately into the chart. Another copy should remain in the laboratory and be filed with the frozen section slides. If the frozen sections are performed by several individuals on a rotation basis, it is important for a senior pathologist to review the material periodically to ensure that the quality of the sections and the agreement between the frozen section diagnosis and the final diagnosis remains at an acceptable level. These periodic reviews are useful also in pointing out patterns of use and misuse of the procedure by the various departments and their individual members.

*From Reed RJ: New concepts in surgical pathology of the skin. New York, 1976, John Wiley & Sons, Inc. (Wiley Series in Surgical Pathology, Hartmann W, ed).

When an urgent decision needs to be made on the basis of a pathologic finding, the clinician should not have to wait for that information to reach him by routine typewritten report. Computer print-outs, available to stations and clinics minutes after the pathologist has examined the slides and has fed the basic information into a terminal located in the laboratory, are being increasingly used; we have found them very effective in shortening the communication gap. However, no technologic advance can replace the time-honored practice of two medical specialists discussing immediately after the facts are known, how to best treat a patient.

Perhaps it should be stated again that a crucial aspect of the work of the surgical pathologist is the timing of his work. Whether this is counted in minutes, as in a frozen section procedure, or in hours or days, as in a routinely processed specimen, it is essential to keep it at a minimum. The pathologist who spends minutes enraptured in the examination of a frozen section and shares his excitement with his colleagues should remember that there is somebody else who is spending those same minutes under somewhat different circumstances and in a different frame of mind. The same applies to the surgical pathologist who is earnestly attempting to subclassify an obviously benign sweat gland tumor into one of the innumerable subcategories that have been described. This is a laudable academic exercise and one that may have some clinical implications. However, it would be advisable for him also to think in practical terms; before this process is completed and an authoritative final diagnosis made, he should consider calling the clinician to inform him that the lesion is a benign sweat gland tumor (or a benign adnexal tumor, for that matter), that no further surgery is necessary, that in all likelihood the patient is cured, and that additional studies to classify the lesion precisely are in progress.

SLIDE REVIEW AND CONSULTATION

A very fortunate aspect of pathology (although some may regard it as a curse) is the fact that the material on which the diagnosis is made—i.e., the microscopic slide—is of a permanent nature and can be evaluated by different observers or by the same observer at different times. This feature should be used by the pathologist to the maximum. All slides and paraffin blocks should be stored indefinitely. Whenever a specimen is received in the laboratory, the files should be searched for previous material on the same patient. If such material is present and is conceivably related to the present illness, the slides and the report should be reviewed. It is mandatory also for the pathologist to review the outside slides of a patient who is referred to his institution with a microscopic diagnosis made elsewhere before therapy is begun. Whether the slides have been requested by the clinician or the pathology department is immaterial, but eventually they should be examined by the pathologist and a formal report should be issued, a copy of which should be sent to the referring pathologist. Pathologists should not object to this practice since it is not instituted to question their diagnosis but rather to ensure uniformity of diagnosis and nomenclature in a given institution, to allow comparisons with subsequent material in the same patient, and to enable this material to be presented at interdepartmental conferences. Whenever possible, the slides should remain in the institution that requested them, because the need for review or comparison may arise later. I have never understood the insistence of some pathologists that the slides be returned to them, knowing that they have a paraffin block from which fifty or more identical sections can easily be obtained at a relatively low cost. If only one slide shows the diagnostic area, or if the specimen is a cytologic preparation, that is a different matter.

Consultation with other pathologists in difficult and controversial cases has become an increasingly popular practice. When done for the right reasons and in the proper fashion, it is a healthy practice that benefits the referring pathologist, the consultant, and the patient. In order to obtain maximum benefit from this procedure, some basic rules need to be observed.[18] It is important for the referring pathologist to review the clinical history carefully (which should have been done anyway to begin with) and provide all the pertinent information to the consultant, together with a description of the gross findings, *all* the relevant slides, and his interpretation of the lesion. If the need for special stains is anticipated, he should include a set of unstained slides or a paraffin block. Presumably, he will inform the consultant of any subsequent developments on the case, especially those that have a bearing on the diagnosis and evolution; he may do so spontaneously or when so requested by the consultant. The consultant should be as expeditious and careful with these cases as he is with his own material. The medical and legal implications of his diagnoses are of no less importance than those made in his own institution. He also should keep in mind that the case does not become his property just because he was asked to express an opinion on it.

LIMITATIONS OF HISTOLOGIC DIAGNOSIS

It is as important for the surgical pathologist to know the limitations of his specialty as it is for him to be aware of its strength and potential contributions. This fact has been expressed in a most perceptive and amusing way by Dr. Oscar N. Rambo in an article entitled "The limitations of histologic diagnosis." Excerpts from this essay follow.

Pathologists are physicians and human beings. They have as great a capacity for error and susceptibility to subjective distractions as other practitioners of the art of medicine. Because of certain nineteenth century dogmas and because the teaching of pathology used to be relegated primarily to the long-forgotten preclinical phase, pathologists traditionally have been regarded to be more scientific than many of their colleagues. A mystic perversion of this assumption prevails among those clinicians who believe that the pathologist, given only a piece of a patient's tissue, has all of the other ingredients necessary to produce a statement of absolute truth at the end of his report. More dangerous to mankind is a pathologist with the same concept. . . .

Incomplete communication between the clinician and pathologist may make diagnosis difficult or impossible. To perform intelligently, a consultant must know all the facts that have any bearing on the case. To render a diagnosis from an inherently puzzling bit of tissue with only vague knowledge of its source and no concept of the clinical problem is as fool-hardy as to undertake an appendectomy on the basis of hearsay evidence that the patient has a pain in his belly.

As an off-duty exercise, pathologists frequently like to play games with slides as 'pure unknowns.' Sometimes with their brains and microscopes they can give a remarkably accurate reconstruction of the disease process, pronounce the exact diagnosis and flush with pride at the awed applause of those gathered around the optical altar. And sometimes they can be absolutely wrong. Showmanship has no place in life and death diagnosis. . . .

Much of the effort expended in carefully executing a diagnostic biopsy procedure is wasted if the pathologist is regarded as a technician rather than a consultant. In many instances, the physician who will have to interpret the slide can offer valuable advice about the clinical nature of a lesion and where best to sample it if he is [invited] to examine the patient before or during surgery. With historical background, physical findings and precise orientation of anatomic relationships, the [pathologist] can block the tissue in the plane that will give the most meaningful sections. . . .

Most physicians are taught that the best biopsy is a cleanly excised, uncrushed wedge that includes a junction between normal and neoplastic tissue. The edge of an ulcerating squamous carcinoma may be indistinguishable from pseudoepitheliomatous hyperplasia; the junction between colonic mucosa and a well differentiated exophytic carcinoma may be sharp, dramatic and unmistakable, but if the biopsy is inadequate in depth or breadth, the pathologist is obliged to append a note stating that he cannot determine *from the tissue submitted* whether the process is a cancer or a polyp. The normal margin must not be obtained at the expense of representative tumor. Worst of all are expanding soft tissue neoplasms. Junction biopsies may include only a pseudocapsule that can be hard, typically 'fish flesh' and grossly more malignant in character than the tumor beneath. Such a barrier found in the retroperitoneum or deep muscle groups of an extremity may achieve a thickness of one centimeter or more. . . .

. . . While it may not always be technically feasible to obtain bigger, better, or multiple biopsies, there are many occasions in which the advantages of a significant increase in the sample of tumor outweigh the risk to the patient. Adequate volume of tissue permits a choice of fixatives, histochemical studies, bioassay or tissue culture. In some instances, one of the specialized examinations may break a morphologic deadlock. . . .

Before a biopsy specimen is delivered to the laboratory, it may be so damaged that the slides prepared from it are worthless. In place of a diagnosis the pathologist must write, 'Tissue unsatisfactory for interpretation.' A more serious consequence of damage is failure to recognize subtle artefactual changes in cells. False positive, false negative and incorrect histogenetic interpretations have resulted from avoidable mishandling of biopsy fragments. . . .

The complaint of withholding information may also be lodged against the pathologist. The unsophisticated recipient of a pathologist's written consultation will seek out the usually brief, bald diagnostic statement, accept it as the truth and proceed on his definitive therapeutic way. In the majority of instances, the diagnosis is the 'truth,' assuming certain minimum standards of professional competence and permitting considerable philosophic license with the word. But the appearance of a sample of tumors and diseases difficult to classify may be thoroughly misleading when considered out of context.

There are ways in which the pathologist can and should indicate doubts and alternative possibilities when he suspects that the tissue

submitted to him may tell only part of the story of the patient's disease or may be a false representation. Retreat to the smug assertion, 'I can see only what is in the tissues you gave me,' has been forced on pathologists by colleagues who have sought miracles of extrapolation from inadequate biopsies. Differential diagnoses of tissue have been discouraged by the myth of objectivity, the dogma that pathologists have the final word, and the thundering denunciations of pathologists' speculations by physicians who want a single, solid answer, right or wrong. . . .

With full knowledge of the relativity of the term, we use [the term] 'inexperience' with deliberate intent. Neither pride nor pressure should force a pathologist to make a decision about a disease process that he does not recognize. The nearest approximation or look-alike in his experience may be entirely unrelated. A mismatch may result in mutilation or death of the patient.

Recognition of one's limitations is as great an asset as the sharpest diagnostic eye. There is a chain of command for handling serious and unfamiliar problems. Colleagues immediately available may offer a rapid solution from past experience or from lack of obsessive preconception. The community may be polled. Among the members may be one who has perfect and documented recall of an entity not previously encountered. Such a survey may yield only confusion, but from it one can usually salvage a list of experts with series of entities, ones that may come to the average pathologist only once or twice in his lifetime.

While it is true that world renowned experts are human and fallible and that there is an almost irreducible percentage of undiagnosable tumors, it is every physician's obligation to submit his insoluble problems to the highest court of appeal. Such a presentation should be made only after thorough deliberation and must be accompanied by all pertinent clinical data. A complete historical review and serial roentgen studies of a bone tumor may be more important diagnostically than a biopsy. It is sportsmanlike and of great educational value to the pathologist [seeking a second opinion] to submit his own report even if it ends with several speculative diagnoses, each preceded by a question mark.*

BIOPSY

Interpreting biopsies is one of the most important duties of the surgical pathologist. In incisional biopsies, only a portion of the lesion is sampled and therefore the procedure is strictly of a diagnostic nature. In excisional biopsies, the entire lesion is removed, usually with a rim of normal tissue, and therefore the procedure serves both a diagnostic and a therapeutic function. The decision whether to perform an incisional or an excisional biopsy depends primarily on the size of the lesion; the smaller it is, the more logical to take it out completely when first encountered. For large lesions, particularly those of deep soft tissues, an incisional biopsy is usually preferable because of the fact that the type and extent of excision varies considerably depending on the tumor type.

Biopsies are also classified according to the instrument used to obtain them: cold knife, cautery, needle, or endoscope. Of these, the one usually least suitable for microscopic interpretation is that obtained with a cautery, because this instrument chars and distorts the tissue and prevents proper staining.

Some general rules for the biopsy procedure are listed

*From Rambo ON: The limitations of histologic diagnosis. Prog Radiat Ther **2**:215-224, 1962. Reprinted by permission of Grune & Stratton, Inc., and the author.

below. The fact that they are so obvious makes it particularly bothersome that they are so often violated or ignored.

1 The larger the lesion, the more numerous the biopsies that should be taken from it because of the variability in pattern that may exist and the fact that the diagnostic areas may be present only focally.

2 In ulcerated tumors, biopsy of the central ulcerated area may show only necrosis and inflammation. The most informative biopsy is likely to be one taken from the periphery that includes both normal and diseased tissue; however, the biopsy should not be so peripheral that only normal tissue is obtained.

3 The biopsy should be deep enough that the relationship between tumor and stroma can be properly assessed. Epithelia involved by carcinoma have a tendency to detach from the underlying stroma. This should be avoided whenever possible by careful handling of the tissue.

4 Deeply seated lesions are sometimes accompanied by a prominent peripheral tissue reaction, which may be characterized by chronic inflammation, hyperemia, fibrosis, calcification, and metaplastic bone formation. If the biopsy is too peripheral, this may be the only tissue obtained. Similarly, in a mass of lymph nodes, a deep-seated node may show involvement by a malignant tumor, whereas a superficial node may show only nonspecific hyperplasia.

5 When several fragments of tissue are obtained, they should *all* be sent to the pathology department and *all* of them submitted for microscopic examination. Sometimes the smaller or grossly less impressive fragment is the only one that contains the diagnostic elements.

6 Crushing or squeezing of the tissue with forceps at the time of performance of the biopsy by the surgeon, at the time of the gross examination by the pathologists, or at the time of embedding by the histotechnologist should be carefully avoided. The artifacts resulting from it often render a biopsy impossible to interpret.

7 Once the biopsy is obtained, it should be placed *immediately* into a container with adequate volume of fixative. The temptation on the part of the surgeon or the pathologist to turn it around, wash it, or scrape the surface should be resisted, since it will not provide any information of diagnostic significance but rather will create artifacts.

FROZEN SECTION

The frozen section is one of the most important and difficult procedures that the pathologist performs during his practice. It requires experience, knowledge of clinical medicine and pathology, the capacity to make quick decisions under pressure, good judgment, an attitude that is conservative but not excessively so, and a keen awareness of the limitations of the method. It follows from these requirements that the responsibility for frozen section diagnosis should fall on a well-trained pathologist whose main activity is in the division of surgical pathology and who knows well the surgeon requesting the procedure. Exceptions aside, the pathologist who is primarily engaged in basic research and who rotates through surgical pathology once a week "to keep in touch" is ill-equipped to take the main responsibility for this delicate task.

It is unfortunate that a procedure that is time-consuming, costly, and sometimes stressful is so often misused by some surgeons to satisfy their curiosity, to compensate for deficiencies in recognizing normal anatomic structures, or as a mechanism to communicate the results immediately to the patient's relatives. Frozen sections represent a good source of income to the department and excellent training for the residents who participate in them, but when unnecessary they increase the medical bill needlessly and sometimes hamper a proper pathologic evaluation of the specimen. There is a very simple question that the surgeon should ask himself in deciding whether a frozen section should be done or not: will the result of the frozen section examination influence in any way the surgical procedure? If the answer is no, the procedure is not indicated.[1,12] By using this criterion, we have estimated that almost half of the frozen sections done in some hospitals could have been avoided.[8] The three legitimate purposes of a frozen section are (1) to establish the presence and nature of a lesion, (2) to determine the adequacy of surgical margins, and (3) to establish whether the tissue obtained contains diagnosable material (even if the exact diagnosis cannot be made on the frozen sample) or whether additional sampling is indicated.[4,15,17] Sometimes a pathologist cannot reach a decision on the basis of the frozen section. When this is the case, he need not be apologetic. He should state this fact just as affirmatively as when he makes a diagnosis of carcinoma. Sometimes he can add that, according to his evaluation, the tissue removed is representative of the lesion but that the definitive diagnosis will have to wait for the permanent sections. The surgeon will then have to decide, depending on the nature of the case, whether to give the pathologist additional tissue for frozen section or whether to close the incision and wait for the permanent sections.

The indications and limitations of frozen section diagnosis vary from organ to organ and have been detailed in the respective chapters.

The overall accuracy of this procedure has been tested and proved on numerous occasions (Table 1-1).[1,7,8,9b,12,13b] It should also be realized that, since the aim of the frozen section procedure is to influence the course of the operation, advising the surgeon on what to do next may be more useful than providing him with a very specific pathologic diagnosis.

To carry out the task effectively, the pathologist should be thoroughly briefed on the patient's clinical history; ideally the surgeon and the pathologist should have discussed the case beforehand. The pathologist should be prepared to advise the surgeon as to the best area to biopsy. He should also be skillful in selecting from the specimen received the portion to be examined microscopically. The cryostat is now routinely used because of the technical excellence of the sections obtained.[17] Freezing the tissue in isopentane (methylbutane) cooled with liquid nitrogen or with an electronic device (Fig. 1-3) saves valuable time and results in fewer artifacts than when the tissue is frozen on the cryostat stage. Although all kinds of quick stains have been devised for frozen section use, we prefer hematoxylin-eosin because of

Table 1-1 Frozen section diagnosis in 2240 consecutive cases at Barnes Hospital, St. Louis, Missouri*

Organ	Cases	Benign lesions	Malignant lesions	False positives	False negatives	Diagnosis deferred
Breast	639	437	202	0	3 (0.5%)	6 (0.9%)
Soft tissues	298	135	163	1 (0.3%)	1 (0.3%)	7 (2.3%)
Gastrointestinal tract	251	192	59	0	3 (1.2%)	6 (2.4%)
Lymph nodes	232	108	124	0	1 (0.4%)	0
Lung	169	49	120	2 (1.2%)	0	0
Thyroid gland	112	100	12	0	0	5 (4.4%)
Central nervous system	112	18	94	1 (0.9%)	2 (1.8%)	4 (3.6%)
Bone and joints	79	42	37	0	1 (1.3%)	5 (6.3%)
Liver and gallbladder	73	29	44	0	0	1 (1.4%)
Pancreas and bile ducts	45	22	23	0	2 (4.4%)	0
Parathyroid glands	44	44	0	0	0	0
Skin	51	18	33	0	0	0
Miscellaneous	135	73	62	1 (0.7%)	0	4 (3.0%)
Total	2240	1267	973	5 (0.2%)	13 (0.6%)	38 (1.7%)

Adapted from Elsner B: La biopsia por congelación: su valor asistencial y en la educación médica del patólogo. Prensa Med Arg **55**:1741-1749, 1968.
*Ear, nose and throat and gynecologic cases excluded.

the quality of the preparations and the better correlation that this allows with the permanent sections.

A most peculiar variation of the frozen section technique is that incorporated in the concept of Mohs' surgery, as applied to skin tumors.[13a,21] In this procedure, the tumor is removed with a scalpel angled 45° to the skin, divided into quadrants, color coded, oriented *en face,* and sectioned in the cryostat horizontally across the bottom. The slides are then examined "by the Mohs' surgeon serving as his or her own pathologist," the areas of neoplasm are mapped, and immediate re-excision is carried out if indicated. The difficulties of interpreting sections oriented in this fashion are rarely addressed by the proponents of this technique, and the rationale given for "the Mohs' surgeon serving as pathologist" is less than credible. Suffice it to say that, after having seen this procedure in practice a few times, we remain highly skeptical of its scientific validity.

DIAGNOSTIC CYTOLOGY

Diagnostic cytology is now an established technique that no department of pathology can do without. In the past, the procedure was sometimes discredited because poorly trained pathologists, gynecologists, and technicians handled the material and made definitive diagnoses that proved to be incorrect. There is no longer any question that the procedure, when performed by well-trained, experienced individuals, offers an extremely high degree of reliability. Under these circumstances, a positive cytologic diagnosis of malignancy should be given the same weight as one obtained from a surgical biopsy. The cytologist will make a certain number of false negative diagnoses depending on the source of the material, but false positive diagnoses should practically never occur, for they will in themselves invalidate the method.

At present, the procedure has come under a different type of attack by some clinicians and even the lay press. The claim, sometimes justified, is that in some institutions—particularly some private institutions—cytologic examinations are being carried out by poorly supervised cytotechnologists under heavy time constraints because of economic incentives, the emphasis being on the number of tests performed rather than on the quality of the procedure. Obviously, it behooves the pathologist to maintain or restore the professional and scientific quality of this procedure if cytology is to remain an integral component of the practice of pathology.

In writing the cytology reports, we have made it our policy whenever possible to use the same terminology as that used for the microscopic sections instead of employing the original grading system of Papanicolaou. A cytologic diagnosis of "squamous cell carcinoma" rendered on a sputum specimen gives the surgeon a better idea about the nature of a

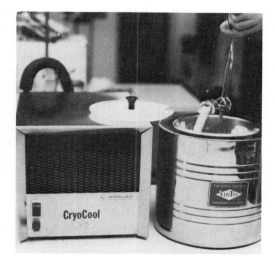

Fig. 1-3 The specimen for frozen section is placed in the cryostat chuck and immersed in isopentane cooled by an electronic device. Freezing of tissue is almost instantaneous.

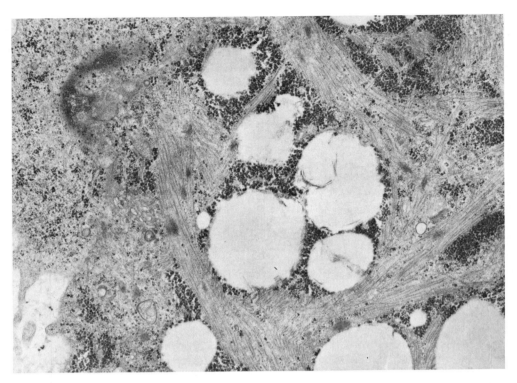

Fig. 1-4 Metastatic alveolar rhabdomyosarcoma to lungs and pleura in 14-year-old girl. Electron microscopy of pleural fluid shows well-preserved neoplastic cells containing large quantities of glycogen and lipid; thick and thin microfilaments also may be noted. (×16,850.)

pulmonary mass than one of "cytology grade IV." We report cases in which we cannot be certain whether the cells present are malignant or not as "suspicious" and ask for additional material.

In most organs, a determined effort should be made to substantiate the cytologic diagnosis by a conventional biopsy procedure before decisive treatment is carried out. For instance, if a diagnosis of cancer is obtained from a cervical smear, irradiation or surgical treatment should not be started until a positive formal biopsy is at hand. For some organs, the approach may be quite different. For instance, a positive bronchial cytology in a patient with a pulmonary shadow justifies the administration of definitive therapy (surgery, radiation therapy, or chemotherapy), even if the bronchoscopic biopsy is negative.

Exfoliative cytology is of little value for lesions that are readily accessible to incisional biopsy, such as the skin or the oral cavity. Neither does it seem advisable to use this time-consuming method as a screening procedure for asymptomatic patients except under special circumstances. The value of cervicovaginal cytology for the screening of cervical carcinoma has been demonstrated beyond doubt, but this is perhaps the only screening technique based on cytology that has proved its worth in terms of human lives saved when related to the cost of the program. The results so far obtained in the screening for other cancers in high-risk populations—such as gastric cytology in patients with pernicious anemia, bronchial cytology in heavy smokers,

and nipple aspiration cytology in older women—are less than encouraging.

In recent years, the technique of aspiration cytology performed with a fine needle (OD 0.6 to 0.9 mm) ("fine needle aspiration") has gained wide popularity, especially for lesions of breast, thyroid, salivary glands, lung, and prostate.[9,9c,11,22,23] There is no question that the procedure is, in most instances, inexpensive, safe, quick, and—when performed by experienced workers—quite accurate. However, like any other technique, it has definite limitations that its overenthusiastic champions sometimes choose to ignore.[9a]

It is not often realized that many of the special stains that are routinely used for tissue sections can also be very useful for the evaluation of cytologic material. This includes stains for glycogen, melanin, fat, and, most importantly, mucin. Cytologic material is also suitable for examination with immunocytochemical and electron microscopic techniques (Figs. 1-4 and 1-5). The indications and limitations of this method are discussed further in the individual chapters.

LEGAL ASPECTS OF SURGICAL PATHOLOGY

The surgical pathologist has not remained immune to the wave of medicolegal actions that is sweeping the country. The most common reasons for surgical pathologists being brought to trial are the claims that (1) a mistaken diagnosis was made on the basis of misinterpretation of the slide; (2) an important lesion or feature present in the specimen was missed, either because of oversight or through failure of

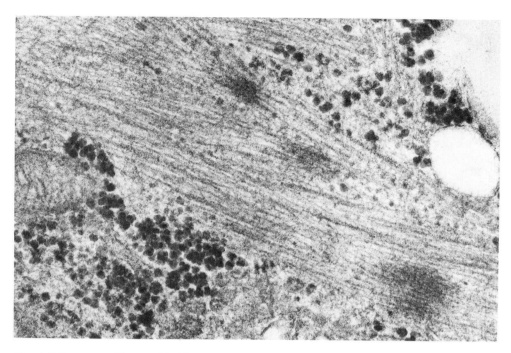

Fig. 1-5 Same case illustrated in Fig. 1-4. Note thick and thin microfilaments diagnostic of rhabdo-myosarcoma, with Z-band formations. (×80,500.)

sampling; or (3) the pathologic diagnosis failed to give the surgeon a clear idea about the nature or extent of the lesion because of poor wording or omissions in the report. A corollary of these claims is that the alleged error or omission resulted in physical, emotional, and/or financial damage to the patient and that such an error or omission was below the standards for the practice of pathology in that particular community at that particular time. On occasion, the pathologist is blamed for not having sought an outside opinion when confronted with an unusually difficult or unusual entity. Although internal and external consultations are desirable under those circumstances and sometimes prove very useful, there is no professional rule that binds the pathologist to such action, and therefore it would seem inappropriate to institute a penalty if such an action is not carried out. A certified and well-qualified pathologist should be given the prerogative—like any other member of the medical profession—to decide if, when, and with whom to consult.

Not infrequently, an incorrect diagnosis is made because the sample provided by the surgeon is inadequate. When this is the case, the pathologist has the right and duty to state this fact in the report, which may read: "The appearance is consistent with actinic keratosis, but invasive squamous cell carcinoma cannot be ruled out because of the superficial nature of the biopsy." It is also true that sometimes the inadequacy of examination is attributable to the pathologist for not having thoroughly studied the material submitted to the laboratory, as when he selects for micro-scopic examination an inadequate number of fragments from a specimen of transurethral resection.

Resolution of the latter claim is sometimes difficult, because there is very little in the way of guidelines on how to process biopsies and surgical specimens. The Appendix in this book is included in an attempt to remedy such deficiency.

A less common claim, but one worth remembering, deals with the instance in which the pathologist has made the right microscopic diagnosis but supposedly has advised the wrong therapeutic procedure. It is within the province of the surgical pathologist to make general considerations about the natural history and possible therapeutic approaches on a case, based on previous experience and review of the literature. Such considerations are generally welcome and often specifically requested by the therapist, especially when the slides are sent to an outside pathology consultant. However, the pathologist should always keep in mind the fact that the microscopic appearance of the tumor is only one of many criteria on which the final therapeutic decision should be based.[13] It is part of the pathologist's duty to explain the probable behavior of a tumor if not treated at all or if treated with different modalities.[20] He is also entitled to list the several therapeutic options and even indicate his personal preference *on the basis of the information furnished by the inquirer*. However, it is prudent for him to leave the final decision to the person responsible for taking and implementing it—i.e., the therapist.

REFERENCES

1 Ackerman LV, Ramirez GA: Indications for and limitations of frozen section diagnosis. A review of 1269 consecutive frozen section diagnoses. Br J Surg **46**:336-350, 1959.

2 Azar HA: Arthur Purdy Stout (1885-1967). The man and the surgical pathologist. Am J Surg Pathol **8**:301-307, 1984.

3 Azzopardi JG: Problems in breast pathology. In Bennington JL (consulting ed): Major problems in pathology, vol. 11. Philadelphia, 1979, W.B. Saunders Co., pp. 1-2.

4 Byers RM, Bland, KI, Borlase B, Luna M: The prognostic and therapeutic value of frozen section determinations in the surgical treatment of squamous carcinoma of the head and neck. Am J Surg **136**:525-528, 1978.

5 Childs AW, Hunter ED: Patterns of primary medical care. Use of diagnostic x-ray by physicians. Berkeley, Calif., 1970, Institute of Business and Economic Research, University of California.

6 Collins VP, Ivarsson B: Tumor classification by electron microscopy of fine needle aspiration biopsy material. Acta Pathol Microbiol Immunol Scand [A] **89**:103-105, 1981.

7 Dankwa EK, Davies JD: Frozen section diagnosis. An audit. J Clin Pathol **38**:1235-1240, 1985.

8 Dehner LP, Rosai J: Frozen section examination in surgical pathology. A retrospective study of one year experience, comprising 778 cases. Minn Med **60**:83-94, 1977.

9 Hajdu SI, Melamed MR: The diagnostic value of aspiration smears. Am J Clin Pathol **59**:350-356, 1973.

9a Hajdu SI, Melamed MR: Limitations of aspiration cytology in the diagnosis of primary neoplasms. Acta Cytol [Baltimore] **28**:337-345, 1984.

9b Holaday WJ, Assor D: Ten thousand consecutive frozen sections. A retrospective study focusing on accuracy and quality control. Am J Clin Pathol **61**:769-777, 1974.

9c Koss LG: Aspiration biopsy. A tool in surgical pathology. Am J Surg Pathol **12**:43-53, 1988.

10 Lattes R: Arthur Purdy Stout and his times. With a history of the laboratory of surgical pathology at the College of Physicians and Surgeons of Columbia University. Am J Surg Pathol **10**[Suppl 1]:4-13, 1986.

11 Lever JV, Trott PA, Webb AJ: Fine needle aspiration cytology. J Clin Pathol **38**:1-11, 1985.

12 Nakazawa H, Rosen P, Lane N, Lattes R: Frozen section experience in 3000 cases. Am J Clin Pathol **49**:41-51, 1968.

13 Pack GT: Functions and dysfunctions of the surgical pathologist. Surgery **52**:752-755, 1962.

13a Roenigk RK: Mohs' micrographic surgery. Mayo Clin Proc **63**:175-183, 1988.

13b Rogers C, Klatt EC, Chandrasoma P: Accuracy of frozen-section diagnosis in a teaching hospital. Arch Pathol Lab Med **111**:514-517, 1987.

14 Rosen G: Beginnings of surgical biopsy. Am J Surg Pathol **1**:361-364, 1977.

15 Schmidt WA: Principles and techniques of surgical pathology. Menlo Park, Calif., 1983, Addison-Wesley Publishing Co.

16 Seemayer TA: The life and legacy of Professor Pierre Masson. Am J Surg Pathol **7**:179-183, 1983.

17 Silva EG, Kraemer BB: Intraoperative pathologic diagnosis. Frozen section and other techniques. Baltimore, 1987, Williams & Wilkins.

18 Sissons HA: On seeking a second opinion. J Clin Pathol **31**:1121-1124, 1978.

19 Stewart TW: Obituaries. James Ewing, M.D., 1866-1943. Arch Pathol **36**:325-330, 1943.

20 Stout AP: Mesenchymal tumors of the soft tissues. Trans Coll Physicians Phila **31**:91-97, 1963.

21 Swanson NA, Grekin RC, Baker SR: Mohs surgery. Techniques, indications, and applications in head and neck surgery. Head Neck Surg **6**:683-692, 1983.

22 Tao L-C, Sanders DE, McLoughlin MJ, Weisbrod GL, Ho C-S: Current concepts in fine needle aspiration biopsy cytology. Hum Pathol **11**:94-96, 1980.

23 Wied GL, Koss LG: Aspiration biopsy cytology. Acta Cytol [Baltimore] **28**:195-197, 1984.

2 Gross techniques in surgical pathology

INTRODUCTION

The routine work associated with a surgical pathology specimen includes gross and microscopic examination. Of the two, the latter is unquestionably the more popular, perhaps because it is esthetically more pleasing, is not associated with any particular odor, and does not involve any manual work other than moving the slide across the microscope, keeping it in focus, and changing objectives. The smaller the specimen, the less significant the gross examination appears to be. Some view it merely as a purely technical step, analogous to tissue processing. It has been stated that autopsy pathology is *gross pathology,* whereas surgical pathology is *histopathology.*

It is unfortunate that this is the prevailing attitude among pathologists. As Chandler Smith stated in his essay "In praise of the gross examination," it is the gross aspect that shows the size, form, and nature of the process so that it can be understood both in a structural sense and in a clinical context.[32]

For some specimens, such as cardiac valves, a careful gross examination and description are infinitely superior to the examination of a random microscopic section. In many cases, an inadequate gross dissection and sampling will invalidate the microscopic interpretation. The dissection, gross description, and selection of sections for microscopic study is a crucial part of the pathologic examination, and one that often cannot be remedied if omitted or done poorly at the time of the initial work-up. If the microscopic description is inadequate, the slide can be reviewed and the problem corrected; if the dimensions of the specimen are not recorded, the key sections not taken, and the proper special studies not performed at the time of the initial gross examination, the chances of acquiring this information may be lost forever.

Complicated specimens demand experience and knowledge in order to be dissected, described, and sampled adequately. There exists a curious reticence among residents and junior pathologists in consulting with a senior staff member about the proper handling of difficult gross specimens, whereas no inhibition is noticeable when the same individuals are confronted with a difficult microscopic slide. This is unfortunate because sometimes the reason the slide is so difficult to interpret is because of an inadequate sampling of the gross specimen.

SURGICAL PATHOLOGY GROSS ROOM

The size and features of the surgical pathology gross room depend on the number of specimens, number of staff pathologists and residents, and the type of institution. The gross room described in the following paragraphs is modeled after a large laboratory in an academic institution, but many of the requirements also apply to laboratories in small hospitals.

First of all, the room should be large enough to permit the simultaneous work of all the pathologists assigned to gross activities; it should be well illuminated and properly ventilated. We have been appalled at the number of pathology departments throughout the country that have woefully inadequate gross room facilities, some merely consisting of a table, a chair, a cutting board, a sink, and a shelf cornered between a cryostat and a secretarial desk.

Each dissection area should contain the following:

1 A cutting board placed inside a metal box designed in such a fashion that all the fluids will flow directly into the sink
2 Shelves for specimen containers
3 Ready access to a sink with hot and cold water
4 Ready access to formalin
5 Dictation equipment, preferably actuated by pedal
6 Box of instruments including heavy and small scissors, different-sized smooth and toothed forceps, a malleable probe, a scapel handle, disposable blades, a long knife, and pins for attaching specimens to a cork surface
7 Box with cassettes and labels

In addition, the gross room should contain the following central equipment:

1 A large formalin container—a very convenient arrangement consists of the suspension of a large container from the ceiling, with formalin pumped into it with a mechanical pump and the fixative delivered to the individual dissection areas by a tubing system ending in faucets (Fig. 2-1)
2 Containers with other fixatives, with instructions on how to mix them at the time of use
3 Photographic facilities for black and white, color, Polaroid photographs, and photocopies (Fig. 2-2)
4 A self-contained x-ray unit (such as Faxitron) (Fig. 2-2)
5 Large refrigerator or, even better, a small cold room kept at 4° C adjacent to the gross room
6 Small refrigerator (for electron microscopy fixatives, photographic film, etc.)
7 Freezer

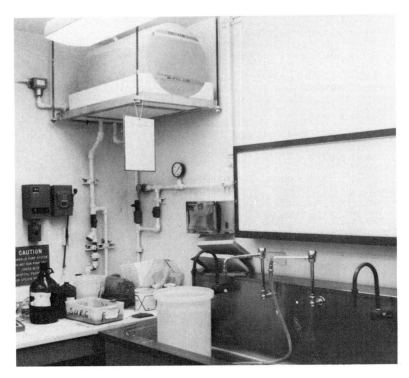

Fig. 2-1 Large formalin tank suspended from ceiling that delivers formalin to individual faucets in each sink. The formalin is pumped into the tank by a mechanical pump system. The large sink in the foreground is used for the dissection of large specimens.

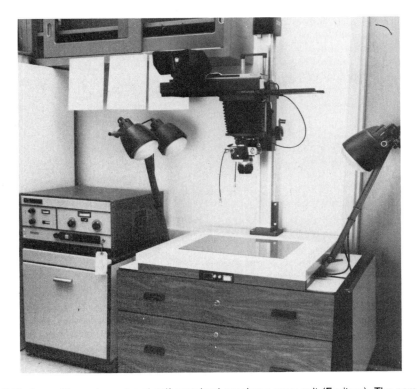

Fig. 2-2 Photographic equipment and self-contained specimen x-ray unit (Faxitron). The same photographic stand is used for a camera loaded with quick-developing black and white film (Polaroid) and a camera loaded with 35 mm color film.

8 Band saw—preferably those designed for use in butcher shops rather than those used by carpenters

9 Balances—one of large capacity for regular specimens and a delicate balance for small specimens, such as parathyroid glands

10 Electrically driven, commercial meat cutter—results in excellent cross sections of solid specimens for demonstration and photographic purposes

11 Dissecting microscope

12 X-ray viewbox

13 Large sink for the dissection of large specimens (such as amputations) (see Fig. 2-1)

14 Central table for multiple use (for placing cassettes to be sent to the histology laboratory, for showing specimens to visitors, for gross conference, etc.)

INITIAL HANDLING OF SPECIMENS

The best arrangement is to have the surgical pathology laboratory in close proximity to the operating room and to have specimens other than small biopsies submitted to the laboratory in a fresh state immediately after resection. They should be transported in a glass, plastic, or metal container or in a plastic bag without addition of any fluids. It is better to avoid using gauzes, which tend to produce desiccation. If a delay is anticipated in the transport of the specimen to surgical pathology or in the handling of that specimen in the laboratory, it is advisable to place the container in a refrigerator at 4° C to slow down autolysis. Most small biopsies (needle biopsies, incisional biopsies, endoscopic biopsies) should be placed in fixative immediately after obtaining them.

Specimens received in the fresh state should be examined as soon as possible, and a determination should be made on the basis of clinical information and gross appearance (and frozen section examination, if necessary) whether special procedures (see following list) other than routine gross and microscopic examination are necessary or desirable. Specific instructions for these procedures are included in the Appendix.

Biochemical extractions
Chemical analysis (stones, etc.)
Chromosomal analysis
Cultures—bacterial, fungal, viral
Electron microscopy*
Examination with dissecting microscope
Formaldehyde vapor-induced fluorescence[6]
Histochemical stains[23]
Hormone receptor assays
Immunohistochemical stains[20,22,34]
Imprints (touch preparations)
Photographs—color transparencies, black and white prints, Polaroid prints, photocopies
Plastic embedding for light microscopy (1 μm sections)[3,5,33]
Roentgenograms
Special fixatives (other than routine formalin)
Cell marker studies
Tissue culture[11]

---

*See references 2, 4, 17, 21, 25, and 29.

The pathologist should always keep in mind the fact that formalin fixation, paraffin embedding, and microscopic examination of hematoxylin-eosin sections is only one way of performing a pathologic study of a specimen. It is usually the most important, but it is often insufficient and sometimes woefully inadequate. With the present sophistication in the study of lymphoproliferative diseases, a "routine" study of these specimens can hardly be regarded as adequate without the performance of imprints, special fixations, surface marker studies, and sometimes, electron microscopy.[18] It is the pathologist's responsibility to think beyond his basic task—to be aware of newer techniques and apply them consistently to his cases. We have found it extremely useful to have a "surgical pathologist assistant" especially trained to perform the technical aspects of these studies in a consistent fashion under the direction and supervision of the surgical pathologist.[14] This assistant should also be proficient in gross photography and roentgenographic techniques, injection of specimens, cutting and staining for frozen sections, and other technical tasks. Having this important collaborator not only frees the surgical pathologist for other activities but also ensures a consistency and continuity in the performance of these tests that are otherwise very difficult to attain. Ideally, a small room should be made available adjacent to the gross room for the assistant to carry out these special tasks, particularly those regarding the processing of tissues for special studies.

FIXATION

Of the many fixatives that have been proposed, *10% buffered formalin* remains the best compromise under most circumstances. It is inexpensive, the tissue can remain in it for prolonged periods without deterioration, and it is compatible with most special stains. "Pure" formalin is a concentrated (40%) solution of the gas formaldehyde in water. Thus a 10% formalin solution represents a 4% solution of the gas. If the final dilution is maintained in a range between 8% and 12%, no noticeable differences will be noted. However, once the concentration of formalin drops below 5%, the quality of the preparation will suffer. This may happen, unknowingly, in places where "pure formalin" is adulterated by diluting it with water. Rodriguez-Martinez et al.[27] have devised a simple-to-follow formula for checking on the final dilution of the fixative and correcting it if necessary by measuring the specific gravity of the fluid (Table 2-1).

Zenker's is an excellent fixative, one of the best that has ever been devised for light microscopic work, but it is expensive, requires careful disposal of the mercury, and necessitates meticulous attention to fixation times and washing procedures to remove the precipitates of mercury. We use this fixative or sublimate sodium acetate formalin ("B-5") for biopsies of kidney, bone marrow, lymph node, and testicle.

Bouin's fixative has been especially recommended for testicular biopsies, but we have found that Zenker's fluid results in almost identical preparations.

Carnoy's fixative is a mixture that contains chloroform. Thus, at the some time that it fixes the tissues, it dissolves most of the fat. We have found this property useful for the identification of lymph nodes in radical resection specimens.

Table 2-1 Formula for the preparation of 10% formalin on the basis of a solution of formaldehyde of unknown concentration

Density of "pure" formalin	Percentage of formaldehyde	Milliliters of formalin	Milliliters of water
		necessary to prepare 10% formalin	
1.090	40.00	10.00	90.00
1.086	39.00	10.25	89.75
1.083	38.00	10.56	89.44
1.080	37.00	10.84	89.16
1.075	35.15	11.37	88.63
1.070	33.30	12.00	88.00
1.065	31.45	12.70	87.30
1.060	29.60	13.35	86.65
1.055	27.75	14.40	85.60
1.050	25.90	15.44	84.56
1.045	24.05	16.62	83.38
1.040	22.20	18.00	82.00
1.035	20.35	19.61	80.39
1.030	18.50	21.65	78.35
1.025	14.80	27.00	73.00
1.020	12.95	30.92	69.08
1.015	11.10	36.10	63.90
1.012	9.25	43.24	56.74
1.010	7.40	54.00	46.00
1.0085	5.55	72.07	27.93
1.0065	4.00	100.00	0.00

Translated from Rodriguez-Martinez HA, Santos-Estrada L, Rosales MM, Cruz-Ortiz H: Formol o formalina al diez por ciento? Patologia (Mexico) **9**:233-231, 1971.

A fixative suitable for both light and electron microscopic examination ("universal fixative") is also available. It is made of a mixture of 4% commercial paraformaldehyde and 1% glutaraldehyde in a neutral buffer.[19] It is a convenient fixative to use, but it represents a second poor choice to the alternative of fixing the tissue immediately after it is excised in the corresponding fixatives for light and electron microscopy.

The volume of fixative should be at least ten times that of the tissue. The container should have an opening large enough so that the tissue can be removed easily after it has hardened by the fixation. The fixative should surround the specimen on all sides. Large specimens that float on a fixative should be covered by a thick layer of gauze. In cases of large, flat, heavy specimens that rest on the bottom of the containers, the gauze should be placed between the container bottom and the specimen.

The fixation can be carried out at room temperature or, in the case of large specimens, at 4° C (see following discussion). Tissue should not be frozen once it has been placed in the fixative solution, for a peculiar ice crystal distortion will result.[30] The freezing point of a 10% formalin solution is − 3° C.

The speed of fixation of the most used fixative (10% buffered formalin) is about 1 mm/hr. Therefore, a fixation time of several hours is needed for most specimens. A shortening of the fixation time can be achieved by the use of a commercial microwave oven (which induces an almost instantaneous fixation by controlled heating at 63-65° C)[38] or by fixing the specimen in a large beaker containing fixative kept at about 60° C and in continuous motion by the action of a heater-rotor. These devices do not induce artifacts such as those seen after boiling the tissues in formalin. They are not recommended for small biopsies but can be used quite effectively for most routine surgical specimens.[16]

GENERAL PRINCIPLES OF GROSS EXAMINATION

Proper identification and orientation of the specimen is always important and may be imperative for the adequate pathologic evaluation of a case. An unlabeled specimen should never be processed; if the biopsy is received in the laboratory with identification, the physician who performed the procedure or, in his absence, one of the assistants should be called to identify and label the specimen. A properly completed surgical pathology requisition form containing the patient's identification, age, and sex, essential clinical data, operation, surgical findings, and tissue submitted should accompany every specimen. If such history is unavailable, the physician or one of his assistants should be contacted and asked to provide it. If this cannot be obtained for one reason or another, the pathologist has the prerogative and obligation, as a medical consultant, to review the chart and even examine the patient personally before rendering an opinion on a slide in which such information is essential.

If there are difficulties with orientation of the specimen, the surgeon should be contacted and cooperation requested in identifying the position, anatomic landmarks, surgical margins, and any other structure of significance.

Careful search and examination of *all* the material submitted is in order. Even the underside of the cover should be searched for tissue fragments. Surgeons should be instructed to submit to the pathology laboratory *all* the material that they have removed, not selected portions from it. The specimen, especially if small, should be handled on a clean cutting board, using spotless, clean instruments. The problem of contamination of a specimen with a fragment from another (the "floater" or "cutting board metastasis") is one of the major catastrophes that can occur in the pathology laboratory because it can lead to irreparable mistakes.

Even if the pathologist is not a surgeon or an anatomist, he should have some knowledge of normal anatomy, the extent of most operations, and the number and types of structures to be expected in a given procedure. The first step is a general inspection of the specimen, with identification of all of its normal and abnormal components. He should place the specimen on the cutting board, in an anatomic position, and record at this point the following information (to be dictated later): (1) type of specimen, (2) structures included, (3) dimensions, (4) weight, (5) shape, and (6) color. This is also the time to identify the surgical margins in order to preserve them in subsequent steps and eventually study them microscopically. The pathologist should keep in mind that in many surgical excisions, the surgeon already knows the microscopic diagnosis of the lesion, and he is now interested in other information, such as extent of the lesion, invasion of neighboring structures, presence of tumor at the surgical margins, vascular invasion, and lymph node metastases. If a surgical margin is involved by tumor, he wants to know where this surgical margin is located. The accumulation of these data requires careful and sometime tedious, but always rewarding, work.

Before the dissection of the specimen is begun, the advisability of taking gross photographs of the external surface should be considered. This is fine, yet it should be remembered that for most specimens the external appearance is merely that of a nondescript mass, whereas a properly made cross section will demonstrate the important gross features of the lesion.

Three situations may arise during dissection of a surgical specimen:

1 It may be necessary to separate each one of its main components in the fresh state, such as in a radical neck dissection.

2 It may be necessary to remove only some components (such as the regional lymph nodes) and leave the rest of the specimen as a single piece.

3 It may be better to fix the entire specimen as a block. This can be achieved in several ways depending on the size, shape, and presence or absence of a cavity in the specimen. Small specimens without particularly thick areas are simply placed in a fixative at room temperature. Larger specimens that cannot be satisfactorily injected (such as a radical resection of a soft tissue tumor or a nephrectomy specimen) are better fixed overnight in a refrigerator at 4° C to slow down the autolytic process. Hollow specimens are either opened fresh or else fixed simultaneously from the outside and the inside. The latter is achieved either by injecting the cavity with formalin by syringe or catheter or by packing the cavity with gauze or cotton impregnated with formalin. Cystic lesions (such as ovarian cystadenomas) can be injected with formalin after the original fluid has been removed. Multilocular cysts require in-

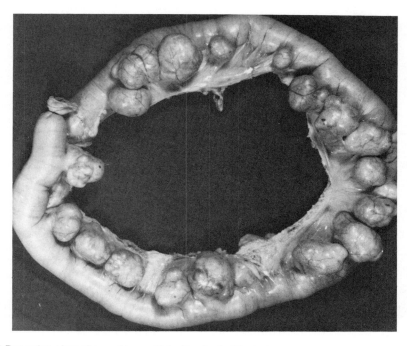

Fig. 2-3 Resection of small bowel for multiple diverticula. The lesions are effectively shown by injecting the lumen with formalin and tying both ends.

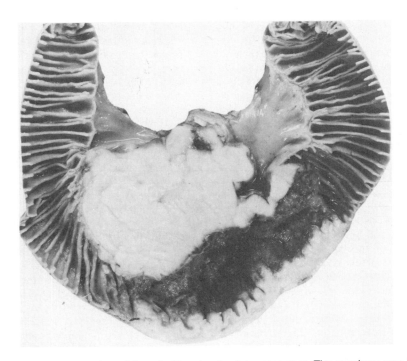

Fig. 2-4 Leiomyosarcoma of small bowel with extension into mesentery. The specimen was injected with formalin, fixed overnight, and then cut in two symmetric halves with scissors and knife.

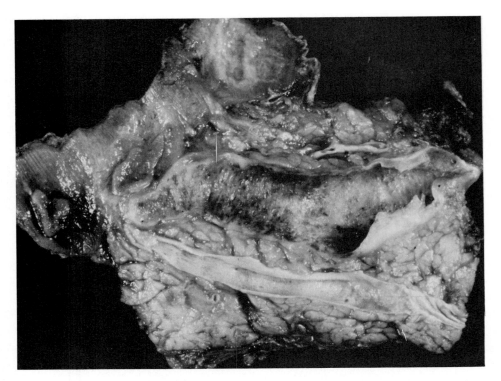

Fig. 2-5 Specimen from Whipple's operation. Both common bile duct and main pancreatic ducts have been injected with formalin prior to opening, in order to show to better advantage dilatation produced by ampullary tumor (not shown in this cut).

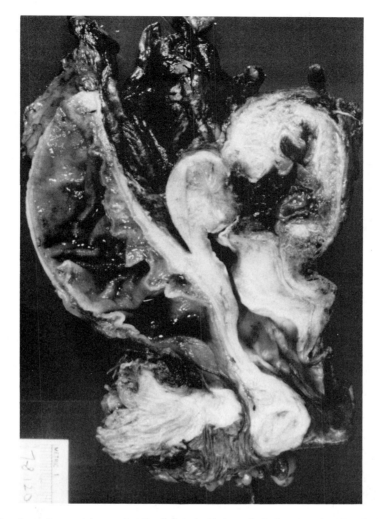

Fig. 2-6 Specimen from pelvic exenteration inflated with formalin before opening. Cervical carcinoma that has recurred following radiation therapy is present. Tumor has resulted in large vesicovaginal fistula.

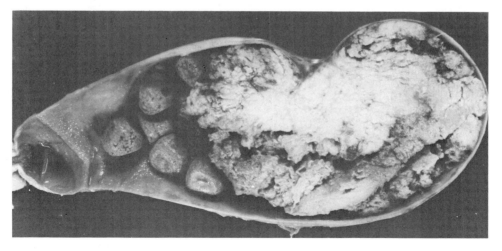

Fig. 2-7 Gallbladder with carcinoma and lithiasis. The bile was extracted and replaced with formalin; the specimen was kept submerged in formalin overnight at 4° C.

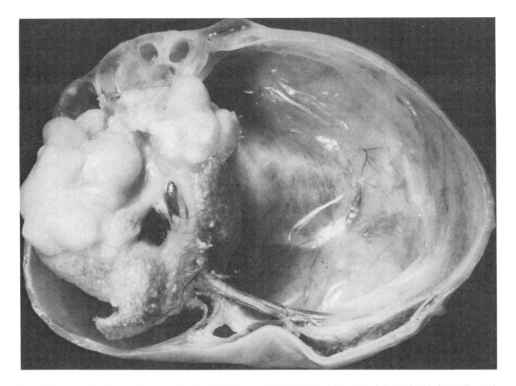

Fig. 2-8 Cystic teratoma of ovary sectioned after the individual cavities were injected with formalin and fixed overnight.

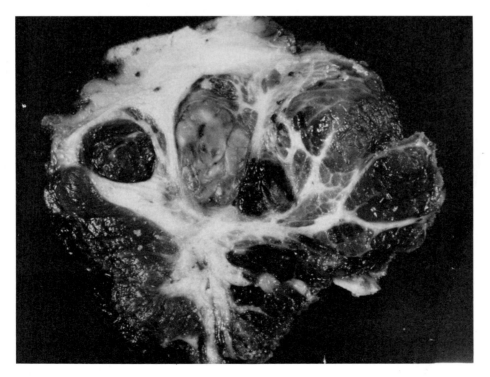

Fig. 2-9 Giant cell tumor of fibula recurrent in soft tissue. Specimen has been frozen prior to cutting, in order to preserve anatomic relationships of tumor with surrounding structures.

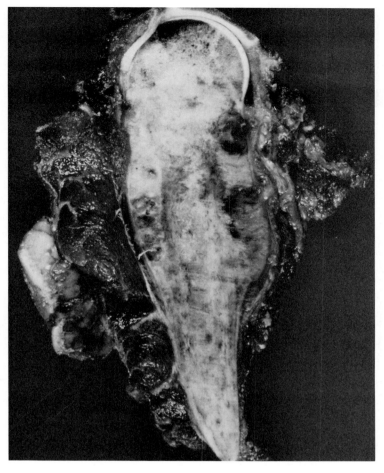

Fig. 2-10 Large osteosarcoma of humerus with soft tissue extension, cut sagittally after freezing.

dividual injection of the larger cavities, combined with fixation of the specimen block at 4° C (Figs. 2-3 to 2-10).

Specimens that contain both soft tissues and bone are handled in a different fashion depending on the site and type of pathology present. One alternative is to freeze the entire fresh specimen and then prepare parallel slices with the band saw while the specimen is still frozen. Washing these slices with tap water results in excellent specimens for photography and demonstration purposes. Another method, which is employed when the bony structures are not involved by tumor, consists in carefully dissecting out the bone in order to process the remaining soft tissue as a single specimen (Fig. 2-11).

As a general rule, when a specimen is sliced, and assuming that several of the slices show similar features, it is advisable to leave one of the best slices intact for possible photography, gross demonstration, or display as a museum specimen. Under no circumstances should *any portion* of a specimen be discarded before the case is signed out. Ac-

tually, it is advisable to save the wet tissue for a minimum of 2 or 3 months, but sometimes the shortage of space prevents implementing this practice. A questionnaire revealed a wide variation in the length of time different laboratories throughout the country keep the wet tissues.[26] This ranged anywhere from less than a month (25.6% of the laboratories) to an indefinite period (3.3%). A uniform national guideline seems necessary, but it seems to us that a length of 2 or 3 months is quite reasonable. We firmly believe that paraffin blocks, microscopic slides, and reports should be kept permanently.

SPECIMEN PHOTOGRAPHY

Documentation of the gross features of a surgical specimen is best achieved by taking one or several gross photographs of the lesion, either in the form of color transparencies or black and white prints. This is far superior to drawings made by the pathologist or to the use of predesigned diagrams. In the system we use, the same stand and illumination serve for a Polaroid MP-4 camera loaded with

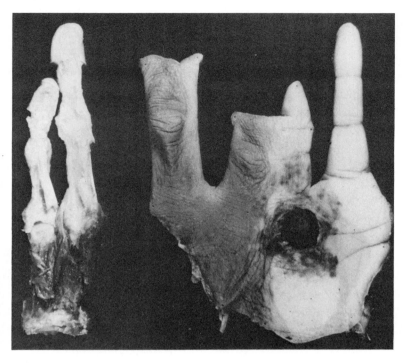

Fig. 2-11 Partial resection of hand and fingers for malignant melanoma. After removing the bony structures, the skin and soft tissues are pinned down on a corkboard as a piece, fixed overnight, and then sectioned.

black and white film and for a 35 mm Nikon F camera with a Micro-Nikkor-P.C. Auto 1:3.5, f:55 mm, loaded with color film. Whenever the possibility of publication exists, a black and white photograph of the specimen should be taken, preferably by a professional photographer. The policy of making black and white prints from color slides is rarely successful and should be discouraged.

Listed below are some hints that we have found useful in obtaining gross photographs that show the lesion at its best advantage and that are also esthetically pleasing.[8a,13]

1 A common mistake is to take a photograph of the external surface of the intact tumor (which is often meaningless, other than providing some information on overall size and configuration) but forgetting to take a photograph of the cut surface, which is usually much more informative.

2 Some consideration should be given to what is the best view of the lesion before the picture is taken. If a specimen is cut in two, it is better to photograph one-half rather than both halves of a partially cut specimen.

3 Preparation and trimming of the specimen is important. This includes the removal of fat and other unnecessary tissue around the lesion, the opening of ducts and vessels, and trimming of fat around the latter structures.

4 The background should be spotlessly clean, kept to a minimum, have no texture, and be illuminated. For color photographs, a gray-toned neutral intensity color is preferable (we use a light blue). Use of drapes, sponges, and gauzes is to be discouraged.

5 Rulers should be used only when reference to size is important. They should be as unobtrusive as possible, always in the metric system, without advertisements or other distractions, clean, clearly legible, and placed in such a way as to allow a quick determination of the measurements of the lesion. They should be of adequate size and be kept in focus by raising or lowering them according to the height of the specimen (Fig. 2-12).

6 Knife marks in the cut surface should be avoided by using sharp instruments and by cutting the specimens with a continuous slow motion of the hand.

7 The specimen should be properly oriented, centered, and framed. A common mistake is to use only half or less of the frame of a photograph. Increase in magnification improves the resolution of detail in the specimen without the loss of any important information.

8 Whenever possible, normal structures should be included in the photograph to serve as a frame of reference for the lesion.

9 Objects such as hands, forceps, probes, scissors, and paper clips are distracting and should generally be avoided.

10 Specimen identification by the use of labels on top of the lesion are distracting. It is better to write the pathology number on the frame than to include it in the projected photograph.

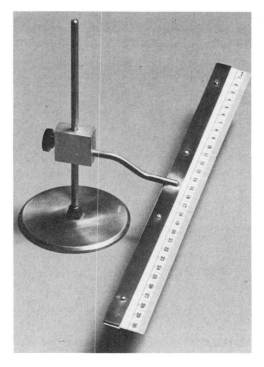

Fig. 2-12 Ruler used for gross photography which may be kept in fous regardless of the height of the specimen by being raised or lowered.

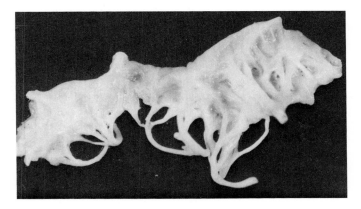

Fig. 2-13 Polaroid photograph of tricuspid valve removed from 24-year-old man with transposition of great vessels. This photograph and the specimen roentgenogram shown in Fig. 2-14 are incorporated in the report and usually provide more information than the microscopic description.

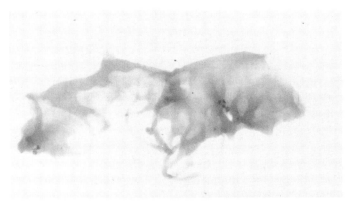

Fig. 2-14 Same case as shown in Fig. 2-13. Specimen roentgenogram taken with Faxitron.

11 Reflective glare (specular reflections) should be avoided by proper placing of the illumination system, by turning off the room lights, by blotting the cut section of the specimen with a gauze, and, if necessary, by the use of diffusion screens.[8a]

12 The proper exposure can be determined with a light meter by trial and error. It is always advisable to take several photographs of a lesion with slightly different exposures.

13 For specimens of substantial height, the lens aperture should be as small as possible (f-stop of 16 or greater) to increase the depth of field.

Because indefinite storage of gross specimens is inconvenient, the gross photograph often remains, together with the gross description, the best permanent documentation of the gross features of a lesion. We routinely take Polaroid black and white prints of all pertinent specimens and attach them to the surgical pathology report (Fig. 2-13), in some cases together with the specimen roentgenogram (Fig. 2-14). Also, we mark the sites of the sections taken for histology on these photographs or in reproductions of the specimen obtained with a Xerox copier or similar duplicating machine.

SPECIMEN ROENTGENOGRAPHY

Roentgenographic examination of surgical specimens sometimes provides important information. Specimens particularly suitable for this type of examination include bone lesions, calcified soft tissue masses, breast biopsies and excisions (especially if they had been studied by mammography), cardiac valves, and lymph node groups in which a lymphangiogram had been taken[10] (Fig. 2-14). Areas of calcification (particularly important in breast biopsies) can be detected even in the paraffin blocks if the casettes are made of plastic or some other radiolucent material.[36] Radiopaque foreign bodies (such as metal clips) can be spotted easily. Radiologic-pathologic correlations can be made by perfusing radiopaque material within the lumina of ducts or vessels, radiographing the specimen, and comparing the results with both the clinical roentgenograms and the gross specimen. Some people have found specimen x-rays useful for locating lymph nodes in radical resection specimens.[1,12,35] Others have used them to perform a microradiographic analysis of bone.[7] Traditionally, these studies were done by taking the specimen to the radiology department. The availability of a self-contained, fully shielded x-ray machine especially divided for pathology specimens (Faxitron*) has greatly facilitated the procedure by allowing the pathologist to take his own roentgenograms in the gross room[9] (Fig. 2-12). It is estimated that more than one fourth of the pathology departments in the United States currently own a Faxitron machine.

LYMPH NODE DISSECTION

Careful dissection of lymph nodes is one of the most important components in the gross evaluation of a radical operation for cancer. The first step consists in dissecting the node-containing fat from the organ in the fresh state, using forceps and sharp scissors. In the gastrointestinal tract and other sites, most of the nodes are found in very close proximity to the muscular wall of the organ, so that dissection of fat should be done in such a way as to expose the muscular surface clean. More than once we have seen a resident searching fruitlessly for nodes in an enormous piece of omentum from a gastrectomy specimen without realizing that he had left all of the nodes attached to the lesser and greater curvature of the stomach when he separated the organs. If the number of nodes found in a given specimen is substantially lower than that expected for that operation, it may be advisable to consult with a senior pathologist or the surgeon before proceeding further. Sometimes the explanation is that the nodes exhibit adipose metaplasia (i.e., they are infiltrated by fat except for a thin peripheral semilunar rim) and are therefore difficult to identify grossly.

The individual nodes may be searched for in the fat in the fresh state or after overnight fixation. If the latter course

---

*Radiographic Inspection System Model 43805, Hewlett-Packard, McMinnville Division, McMinnville, Oregon.

is taken, it is advantageous to fix the specimen in Carnoy's solution, which somewhat clears the specimen by the action of the chloroform at the same time that it fixes it. One should be gentle with the nodes at the time of the dissection; it is too easy to crush them with the forceps and scissors, especially if they are dissected before fixation. Complicated clearing techniques have been devised for maximum recovery of lymph nodes,[8] the yield is certainly impressive, but we are not convinced that the extra time, effort, and money that need to be expended are justified from a practical standpoint.

The lymph nodes should be separated and labeled in groups according to the type of specimen (see Appendix). In some operations, such as radical hysterectomy, this is already done by the surgeon. *All* lymph nodes are to be submitted for histologic examination.

SAMPLING FOR HISTOLOGIC EXAMINATION

Tissues submitted for histology must not be more than 3 mm thick and not larger than the dimensions of the cassette used; otherwise they will not be adequately infiltrated by paraffin. Adipose tissue must be cut even thinner. Overfilling of the cassette should be avoided, or the tissue will not be infiltrated. Suture material, metal clips, and other foreign bodies should be removed from the tissues before putting them in cassettes or the microtome knives will be damaged. Metal clips are especially common in staging laparotomy and lymphadenectomy specimens and can be difficult to detect by plain inspection. If the presence of clips is suspected in a specimen, this can be checked by taking a roentgenogram in the gross room with the Faxitron. This can even be done with the tissue inside the cassette if the latter is made of a nonradiopaque material. Similarly, discrete areas of calcification or ossification should be taken out, or else the specimen should be decalcified. Fragments of tissue that are small enough to go through the cassette perforations must be wrapped in thin paper (such as tea bag paper) or else placed between small porous cushions the size of the cassette (available from the cassette manufacturers). If the fragments are very small, it is advisable to stain them with hematoxylin or Mercurochrome before putting them in the cassette to facilitate their identification by the histotechnologist.

Most specimens from solid tissues are cut in the form of pieces measuring 10 to 15 mm on the sides and 2 to 3 mm in thickness; the histotechnologist will orient them in a flat position in the paraffin block so it will not matter which side is sectioned. However, if one side shows a given feature better than the opposite side, the pathologist can indicate this with India ink on the side *opposite* the one to be cut. Many specimens (in general, those having a luminal side) need to be embedded on edge. If a section of a gallbladder, large bowel, or similar organ is properly taken, the histotechnologist should have no problem in orienting the specimen properly. Additional insurance for proper orientation is provided by including in the cassette a paper tag labeled "on edge." In general, better preparations will be obtained in organs covered by folded mucosa (stomach, bowel, etc.) if the sections are taken perpendicular rather than parallel

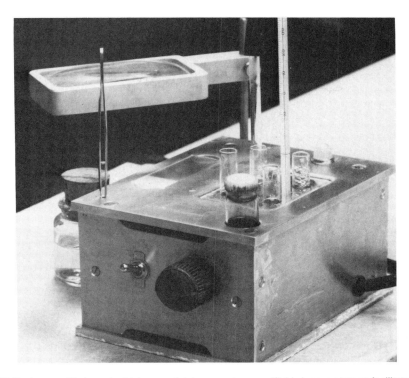

Fig. 2-15 Device used to keep test tubes containing agar in a semifluid viscous state to facilitate proper embedding of specimen. The device also is equipped with rheostat, thermometer, holder for fine forceps, enlarging lens, and hematoxylin bottle (for painting small specimens).

to the mucosal folds. For smaller specimens (cervical biopsies, peroral small bowel biopsies, etc.), orientation is more difficult but just as important. In these cases, the pathologist can help the histotechnologist by showing him the specimen before putting it in the cassette, by embedding it in paraffin himself, or by surrounding it with a material that will keep it in the desired position during the processing steps. We use for this purpose a solution of 3% agar in distilled water, kept in a viscous fluid state at 60° C (Fig. 2-15). The specimen is kept on edge with small forceps on top of a glass slide while 1 or 2 drops of the agar solution are applied to it. Once this solidifies (it should take less than a minute), it is detached from the slide with a sharp blade and transferred to the cassette. Further description of this technique is given in Appendix A.

To assure adequate sampling, multiple microscopic sections ("various levels" or VL) should be requested for some specimens at the time the gross description is dictated. This includes biopsies from the respiratory tract, gastrointestinal tract, bladder, lymph nodes, and bone marrow, all needle and punch biopsies, and, in general, all specimens measuring 3 mm or less.

A question frequently asked is how much of the tissue received should be submitted for microscopic examination. The cryptic reply of a particularly experienced and astute surgical pathologist was "just enough." What he meant, of course, was that there are no all-encompassing rules; the nature of the case, appearance of the gross specimen, ex-

perience, and common sense should dictate how much is enough. For instance, one cassette is plenty for a case of herniated intervertebral disk submitted in numerous fragments, unless the pathologist has a special interest in the pathology of the nucleus pulposus. In general, all tissue usually should be submitted in a diagnostic endometrial curettage. However, if the procedure was done for incomplete abortion and gross examination shows obvious products of conception, one representative section is more than adequate. The main problem is posed by specimens such as prostatic transurethral resections in patients without clinical suspicion of carcinoma. There is no question that the more fragments submitted, the more incidental carcinomas will be found.[15] However, it is impractical and probably not justified to process all the prostatic fragments received regardless of the total amount. The guidelines that we have developed for these specimens are described in Appendix A.

Knowledge of the precise site from which sections were taken for microscopic examination is of great importance, especially when determining whether tumor is present at the surgical margins. This can be achieved by marking these sites and their corresponding numbers or letters in predesigned picture protocols, in a simple drawing of the specimen made at the time of gross examination, or in an instant (Polaroid) photograph taken before sectioning. A quicker, highly informative, and accurate alternative, which we are now using routinely, is a reproduction of the gross specimen

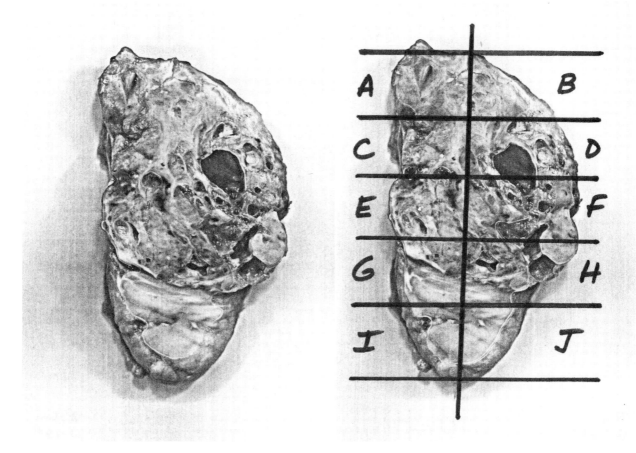

Fig. 2-16 Photocopy of cut surface of a testis with germ cell tumor (teratocarcinoma plus seminoma). Site of sections taken for histology has been indicated in copy on the right.

with a Xerox copier or similar duplicating machine located in the gross room (Figs. 2-16 and 2-17).

The determination of surgical margins is helped by painting them with India ink or a similar pigment before sectioning. This can be done on either the fresh specimen or after fixation by gently wiping the surgical margins with gauze and carefully covering the entire surgical surface with India ink using a cotton swab stick. It is especially important for the epithelial margins of the specimen to be marked carefully with the ink.

Identification of the tissues submitted for histology and other pertinent information should be provided to the his-

totechnologists in a separate form at the time of the gross examination.

Failure to perform these relatively simple steps is responsible for a large proportion of the poor and sometimes uninterpretable microscopic slides being produced. Part of the problem arises from the fact that in most pathology training programs, at least in the United States, no exposure is given to basic histology techniques, such as embedding, cutting, and staining. We have found that even a 1- or 2-day learning session in the histology laboratory by the trainee just before his rotation in the gross room is very effective in avoiding many of these problems.

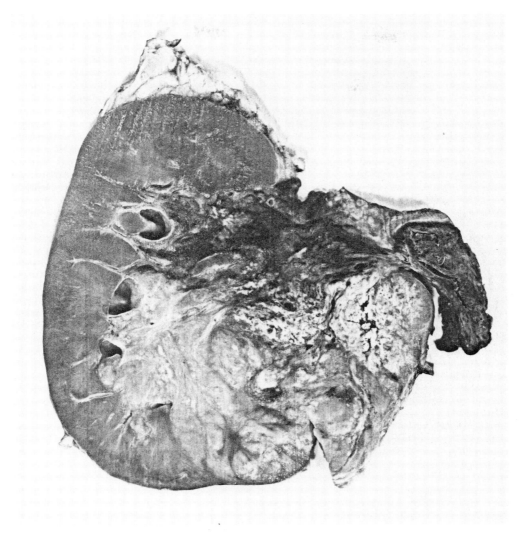

Fig. 2-17 Photocopy of cut surface of a kidney extensively involved by small cell carcinoma. There is extension into the renal vein.

GUIDELINES FOR HANDLING THE MOST COMMON AND IMPORTANT SURGICAL SPECIMENS

In order to achieve a certain consistency in the way the specimens are handled in the gross room, it is important for a manual of procedures to be available to the person performing the gross examination to assist him in dissecting the specimen, describing it, taking the appropriate sections for microscopic examination, and performing whatever other additional tasks may be required depending on the nature of the case.[24,28,31,37] These can be made available in the form of a printed manual, in a microfiche format, or in computer-readable form, with either the manual, microfiche reader, or computer terminal placed by the side of the dissecting area (Fig. 2-18).

These devices can be of great utility to pathology residents and other beginners, as long as one recognizes that they have not been designed to replace entirely the time-honored system of the seasoned practitioner transmitting to the apprentice, with his own words and hands, the secrets of the trade.

Some of these guidelines for handling of the most common and important surgical specimens (procedure, description, and sections for histology) are given in the Appendix.

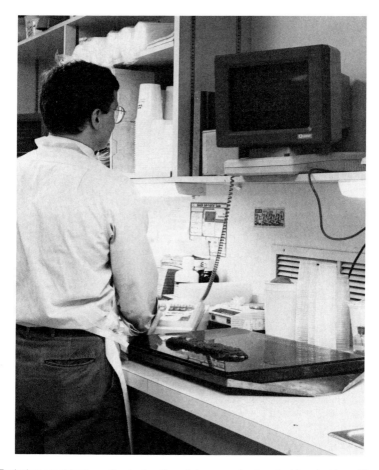

Fig. 2-18 Pathology resident reading instructions into computer terminal located in cutting station on procedure for describing, dissecting, and sampling for histology a gross sepcimen

REFERENCES

1 Andersen J, Jensen J: Lymph node identification. Specimen radiography of tissue predominated by fat. Am J Clin Pathol **68:**511-512, 1977.

2 Bencosme SA, Tsutsumi V: A fast method for processing biologic material for electron microscopy. Lab Invest **23:**447-450, 1970.

3 Burns WA, Bretschneider AM, Morrison AB: Embedding in large plastic blocks. Diagnostic light and potential electron microscopy on the same block. Arch Pathol Lab Med **103:**177-179, 1979.

4 Carr I, Toner PG: Rapid electron microscopy in oncology. J Clin Pathol **30:**13-15, 1977.

5 Chang SC: Hematoxylin-eosin staining of plastic-embedded tissue sections. Arch Pathol **93:**344-351, 1972.

6 DeLellis RA: Formaldehyde-induced fluorescence technique for the demonstration of biogenic amines in diagnostic histopathology. Cancer **28:**1704-1710, 1971.

7 Dunn EJ, Beows DW, Rothert SW, Greer RB: Microradiography of bone, a new use for the versatile Faxitron [letter]. Arch Pathol **99:**62, 1975.

8 Durkin K, Haagensen CD: An improved technique for the study of lymph nodes in surgical specimens. Ann Surg **191:**419-429, 1980.

8a Edwards WD: Photography of medical specimens. Experiences from teaching cardiovascular pathology. Mayo Clin Proc **63:**42-57, 1988.

9 Fingerhut AG: A self-contained radiographic unit. Radiology **90:**1030, 1968.

10 Fornasier VL: Fine detail radiography in the examination of tissue. Hum Pathol **6:**623-631, 1975.

11 Ioachim HL: Tissue culture of human tumors. Its use and prospects. Pathol Annu **5:**217-256, 1970.

12 Jensen J, Anderson J: Lymph node identification in carcinoma of the colon and rectum. Value of tissue specimen radiography. Acta Pathol Microbiol Scand [A] **86:**205-209, 1978.

13 Kent TH, Reynolds JAM: Recognition of quality photographs of gross specimens. Audiovisual teaching set. Iowa City, Iowa, 1978, Department of Pathology, University of Iowa.

14 Kenney TD, Broda KR: The pathologist's assistant. Hum Pathol **5:**503-505, 1974.

15 Lefer LG, Rosier RP: Increased prevalence of prostatic carcinoma due to more thorough microscopical examination [letter]. N Engl J Med **296:**109, 1977.

16 Leong AS-Y, Daymon ME, Milios J: Microwave irradiation as a form of fixation for light and electron microscopy. J Pathol **146:**313-321, 1985.

17 Mackay B, Osborne BM: The contribution of electron microscopy to the diagnosis of tumors. Pathobiol Annu **8:**359-405, 1978.

18 Margolis IB, Organ CH Jr: To improve the yield of biopsy of the lymph nodes. Surg Gynecol Obstet **147:**376-378, 1978.

19 McDowell EM, Trump BF: Histologic fixatives suitable for diagnostic light and electron microscopy. Arch Pathol Lab Med **100:**405-414, 1976.

20 Mesa-Tejada R, Pascal RR, Fenoglio CM: Immunoperoxidase. A sensitive immunohistochemical technique as a "special stain" in the diagnostic pathology laboratory. Hum Pathol **8:**313-320, 1977.

21 Morales AR: Electron microscopy of human tumors. In Fenoglio CM, Wolff M

(eds): Progress in surgical pathology, vol I. New York, 1980, Masson Publishing USA, Inc.

22 Mukai K, Rosai J: Applications of immunoperoxidase techniques in surgical pathology. In Fenoglio CM, Wolff M (eds): Progress in surgical pathology, vol I. New York, 1980, Masson Publishing USA, Inc.

23 Niemi M, Korhonen LK: Histochemical methods in diagnostic pathology. Int Pathol **13:**11-28, 1972.

24 Pierson KK: Principles of prosection. A guide for the anatomic pathologist. New York, 1980, John Wiley & Sons.

25 Regezi JA, Batsakis JC: Diagnostic electron microscopy of head and neck tumors. Arch Pathol Lab Med **102:**8-14, 1978.

26 Ring AM: How long to keep records and specimens. Med Lab Observer, pp. 97-102, Jan 1977.

27 Rodriguez-Martinez HA, Santos-Estrada L, Rosales MM, Cruz-Ortiz H: Formol o formalina al diez por ciento? Patologia [Mexico] **9:**223-231, 1971.

28 Rosai J: Manual of surgical pathology gross room procedures. Minneapolis, 1981, University of Minnesota Press.

29 Rosai J, Rodriguez HA: Application of electron microscopy to the differential diagnosis of tumors. Am J Clin Pathol **50:**555-562, 1968.

30 Rosen Y, Ahuja SC: Ice crystal distortion of formalin-fixed tissues following freezing. Am J Surg Pathol **1:**179-181, 1977.

31 Schmidt WA: Principles and techniques of surgical pathology. Menlo Park, Calif., 1983, Addison-Wesley Publishing Co.

32 Smith JC: In praise of the gross examination. Hum Pathol **5:**505-506, 1974.

33 Snodgress AB, Dorsey CH, Bailey GWH, Dickson LG: Conventional histopathologic staining methods compatible with Epon-embedded, osmicated tissue. Lab Invest **26:**329-337, 1972.

34 Taylor CR: Immunoperoxidase techniques. Arch Pathol Lab Med **102:**113-121, 1978.

35 Wilkinson EJ: Lymph-node identification by specimen radiography and xerography [letter]. Am J Clin Pathol **70:**308-309, 1978.

36 Wilkinson EJ, Gnadt JT, Milbrath J, Clowry LJ: Breast biopsy evaluation by paraffin-block radiography. Arch Pathol Lab Med **102:**470-473, 1978.

37 Wilson RR: Methods in morbid anatomy. New York, 1972, Appleton-Century-Crofts.

38 Zimmerman GR, Raney JA: Fast fixation of surgical pathology specimens. Lab Med **3:**29-30, 1972.

3 Special techniques in surgical pathology

The mainstay of surgical pathology is (and is likely to remain for a long time) the examination of the specimens following fixation in formalin, embedding in paraffin, and staining with hematoxylin-eosin. This technique has proved one of the most durable in medicine and has remained essentially unchanged—except for some time-saving technical modifications—for over half a century. This may be due in part to a certain resistance to change that has been attributed to the practitioners of pathology, but I believe the real reason is that the technique works extremely well. It is certainly far from ideal; Masson, a master of histological techniques, regarded formalin as a poor fixative and hematoxylin-eosin as a poor stain.[2] Yet it is difficult to argue with success. The technique, imperfect as it is, offers considerable advantages: it is relatively quick, inexpensive, suitable for most situations, and comparatively easy to master. Most importantly, it allows an accurate microscopic diagnosis of the large majority of specimens sent to the laboratory. However, it simply cannot answer all the questions that a case poses at the plain diagnostic level and is clearly insufficient when one engages in an etiologic, histogenetic, or pathogenetic quest. As a consequence, the pathologist has always searched for additional techniques to probe those questions. Colloquially, these techniques have been referred to as "special," simply because they are applied only under special circumstances. Most of them have gone (or are going) through three distinct phases: an initial phase of unrestrained enthusiasm followed by a phase of equally unrestrained criticism, the matter eventually settling into a situation in which the techniques are accepted as useful aids only when applied to selected situations and always referring back to conventional morphology as the standard by which they should be interpreted. As Gonzalez-Crussi[1] wisely stated, "however sophisticated and 'modern,' a novel diagnostic technique ought to be suspect if it does violence to a universally agreed upon diagnosis arrived at by more traditional means."

The special techniques that have been found most helpful in diagnostic pathology over the years are discussed in this chapter.

SPECIAL STAINS

Of the extensive battery of "special" stains listed in texts dealing with histological techniques, the surgical pathologist will find a relatively small minority to be of real diagnostic utility. This is especially true since the advent of immunohistochemistry, which has rendered many of them obsolete. Those most commonly used at present in our laboratory are the following:

1 *PAS* (Periodic acid–Schiff). This is an extremely useful and esthetically pleasing technique, to the point that in a few institutions it is used as the standard stain in place of hematoxylin-eosin. Substances containing vicinal glycol groups or their amino or alkylamino derivatives are oxidized by periodic acid to form dialdehydes, which combine with Schiff's reagent to form an insoluble magenta compound. This stain therefore demonstrates glycogen (in a specific fashion, when used with a diastase-digested control) and neutral mucosubstances, outlines basement membranes and reticulin, and makes evident most types of fungi and parasites. It is also the stain of choice for the demonstration of the intracytoplasmic crystals in alveolar soft part sarcoma.

2 *Stains for micro-organisms.* These include techniques for Gram-positive and Gram-negative bacteria, acid-fast mycobacteria, fungi, and parasites. The Gram stain allows the separation of bacteria into those that retain the crystal violet–iodine complex (Gram positive) and those that are decolorized by alcohol or acetone treatment and counterstained by either safranin or fuchsin.[2b] Acid fastness depends on the high lipid content (mycolic acids and long-chain fatty acids) in the cell walls of mycobacteria, which confer on the cell the ability to complex basic dyes (such as carbolfuchsin) and to retain them following strong decoloration with acid-alcohol. The techniques in this group most used in our laboratory are Brown and Brenn (as a modification of the Gram stain), Ziehl-Neelsen (for acid-fast organisms), Grocott's hexamine-silver (for fungi and *Pneumocystis*), PAS (for fungi, amebae, and *Trichomonas*) and Dieterle or one of its modifications (for *Campylobacter*, *Legionella*, syphilis, and Lyme's disease).

3 *Argentaffin and argyrophilic stains.* The argentaffin reaction depends on the presence of a substance in the tissue, often of the phenolic group (such as catecholamines or indolamines), which reduces silver (and other metallic) salts[13,14]; we generally use the Fontana-Masson technique in paraffin-embedded material.[12] In the argyrophilic reaction, an extraneous reducing agent such as hydroquinone or formalin is added; we generally employ the unmodified Grime-

lius' technique and prefer to use it in Bouin's fixed material whenever available. Others have found the Churukian-Schenk's modification to give better results.[12]

4 *Amyloid stains*. We have found stain with Congo Red followed by examination with both standard and polarized light the most reliable and practical technique to detect amyloid. The stain does not have chemical specificity, being dependent upon an arrangement of the molecule in an antiparallel beta-pleated sheet. It should be noted that nonamyloid-related green birefringence can occur as a result of excess dye retained in the tissue and other technical factors.[3]

5 *Reticulin stains*. The traditional use of reticulin stains in tumor pathology (such as Gomori's, Wilder's, and Gordon and Sweet's) has been in separating epithelial from nonepithelial neoplasms, and various mesenchymal neoplasms from each other. In general, foci of carcinoma have reticulin fibers around the tumor nests but not between the individual cells, whereas in most sarcomas and large cell lymphomas the silver-positive material separates single cells. The striking contrast between the two patterns can be readily appreciated by comparing the epithelial and mesenchymal components of a synovial sarcoma. In tumors of endothelial cells the reticulin fibers are seen on the outside of the neoplastic population, whereas the reverse is true in tumors of pericytes or vascular smooth muscle cells. In typical cases of fibrosarcoma the reticulin fibers wrap individual cells completely, whereas in typical cases of malignant schwannoma the reticulum fibers run in parallel to the spindle tumor cells without surrounding them at the poles. Unfortunately, these patterns are well formed in classic cases of these respective entities, i.e., those which are already easily diagnosable with hematoxylin-eosin techniques. In the controversial cases, reticulin stains are likely to provide results that are far from conclusive, to the point that we have found them of extremely limited utility. We agree wholeheartedly with Azzopardi when he stated that ''reticulin silver impregnations are virtually valueless in the differentiation of certain sarcomatoid carcinomas from true sarcomas,'' and that ''reticulin impregnations may be deceptive and merely serve to 'confirm' an erroneous diagnosis of sarcoma.''[2a] It should also be pointed out that reticulum stains demonstrate not only reticular fibers but also basement membrane, a feature that is particularly noticeable in smooth muscle tumors.

6 *Trichrome stains*. The main value of this group of stains is in the evaluation of the type and amount of extracellular material. The three tissue structures demonstrated by the three component dyes are nuclei, cytoplasm, and extracellular collagen.[9] It is not generally realized that the only component of all trichrome stains having some degree of specificity is that staining the collagen fibers; the rest is background nonspecific staining.[10] The often-used statement that a trichrome stain "proved" the smooth muscle nature of a tumor is therefore inaccurate.

7 *PTAH* (Phosphotungstic acid–hematoxylin). This particular variant of trichrome stain has been traditionally used for the demonstration of intracytoplasmic filaments, such as those in muscle and glial cells. It has been largely superseded by the immunohistochemical reactions for the specific microfilaments being searched for. Foraker[6] once made the witty and somewhat irreverent remark that a "special stain" he found most useful as a junior faculty member was a procedure known as the "slow PTAH." This took a week to complete, i.e., enough time for the professor to come back to look at the case.

8 Stains for *hemosiderin* (Perls), *melanin* (Fontana-Masson), and *calcium* (von Kossa).

9 Stains for *neutral lipids*. Oil red O is the one most commonly employed. A limitation of fat stains is the fact that they cannot be performed in paraffin-embedded material because of the solubilizing properties of xylene and other clearing material used. In tumor pathology, the utility of fat stains is minimal and largely limited to the distinction between fibroma and thecoma in the ovary, support for the diagnosis of renal cell carcinoma and sebaceous gland tumors of skin, and identification of lipid-rich carcinoma in various organs. Despite ingrained notions to the contrary, fat stains are of no significance for the diagnosis of liposarcoma; many liposarcomas contain little or no stainable fat, whereas several types of nonadipose tissue neoplasms can contain considerable amounts.

10 *Mucin stains*. The combination of Alcian blue and PAS is probably the best "pan-mucin" stain, since it demonstrates mucosubstances of neutral, slightly acidic, and highly acidic types.[5] Several stains are available for the specific demonstration of highly acidic mucins. These include Alcian blue performed at pH 1.0, colloidal iron, high iron-diamine, and the classic Mayer's mucicarmine. At the risk of sounding old-fashioned, we prefer the latter stain despite the empiric nature upon which it is built.[7]

11 *Giemsa*. The best and most spectacular results with Giemsa and other Romanovsky-type stains are obtained with alcohol-fixed smears.[8] However, reasonably good preparations can also be achieved in paraffin-embedded material. The technique is most useful for the demonstrations of various lymphoreticular elements (including mast cells) and micro-organisms.

12 *Elastic fibers*. Weigert-type techniques are reasonably specific for elastin and are regarded by many as the method of choice. However, the VVG (Verhoeff–van Gieson) stain is more popular because it is quick and outlines the elastic fibers with a strong black color. Both techniques are usually set against the esthetically pleasant trichrome background provided by van Gieson's stain.

13 *Myelin stains*. Luxol fast blue is the nonimmunohistochemical method of choice for the demonstration of myelin. It is based on the strong affinity of the copper phthalocyanin dye for phospholipids and choline bases.

14 *Formaldehyde-induced fluorescence*. This is a very

special type of technique, remarkably sensitive for the demonstration of catecholamines and indolamines but requiring rather costly and cumbersome equipment as originally described. A modified version as applied to touch preparations has made it much more accessible to the practicing pathologist.[4,11] It is based on the principle that biogenic amines subjected to formaldehyde vapors produced by heating the polymer paraformaldehyde form highly fluorescent derivatives.

ENZYME HISTOCHEMISTRY

After a period of enthusiasm in the 1950s and 1960s for the use of enzyme histochemical techniques in pathology,[21] the technique fell in general disuse as far as diagnostic applications were concerned. This was due to the complexity of the techniques, the need for fresh material, and the relative nonspecificity of most of the reactions. At the present time, the enzyme histochemical methods most commonly used for diagnostic purposes are those for skeletal muscle–related enzymes (for the study of myopathies), acetylcholinesterase (for the diagnosis of Hirschprung's disease), and chloroacetate esterase (for the identification of cells of the myeloid series and mast cells). The latter, known as *Leder's technique*, benefits from the fact that chloroacetate esterase is one of the few enzymes that resists the effects of paraffin processing[19] (Plate I, *A*). Another enzyme that can be demonstrated following routine fixation and embedding is acid phosphatase (Plate I, *B*).[18a]

Recently, a plastic embedding technique following paraformaldehyde fixation has been described that combines preservation of various enzymes with excellent morphologic detail.[15,16,17,18] Another enzyme histochemical technique is the DOPA reaction for cells of the melanocytic series. It depends on the presence of the enzyme tyrosinase and requires the use of fresh tissue. A modified version of the technique allows the demonstration of the precipitation product in paraffin-embedded material.[20]

It should also be noted that enzymes, being of protein nature and therefore immunogenic, can also be demonstrated with immunohistochemical techniques in formalin-fixed, paraffin-embedded material even when no longer enzymatically active.[22]

TISSUE CULTURE

The pioneer work of Margaret Murray, Arthur Purdy Stout, and Luciano Ozzello at Columbia-Presbyterian Hospital in New York City showed that some histogenetic clues could be obtained from the examination of primary cultures of human tumors such as thymoma, synovial sarcoma, and hemangiopericytoma.[29] The concepts of the existence of fibrous mesothelioma and fibrous histiocytoma were to a large extent based on tissue culture observations by these investigators.[30,33]

The rationale for diagnostic application of tissue culture in human tumors is based on the observation that tumor cells can express features of differentiation in vitro that are not exhibited or not appreciable in vivo.[25,27] The classic and often quoted example is neuroblastoma, which is seen to grow neurites within 24 hours of having been placed in a suitable culture medium.[28] Another spectacular example is amelanotic melanoma, which sometimes becomes deeply pigmented in vitro.[24] In some instances, this differentiation or maturation has been induced in the culture system by the addition of an exogenous agent, such as cyclic AMP.[26] A recent and exciting development along these lines is the neural differentiation that has been obtained in Ewing's sarcoma—one of the histogenetically most challenging human neoplasms—by the addition of AMP or TPA to the medium.[23] Indeed, at the present time the most useful application of short-term tissue culture techniques is in the differential diagnosis of small round cell tumors, including Ewing's sarcoma.[23a]

It should also be apparent that cells grown in culture can be studied with any of the modern morphologic tools, such as immunohistochemistry, electron microscopy, and ultrastructural immunohistochemistry.[31,32]

Despite these substantial contributions, it should be stated that at a practical, strictly diagnostic level the utility of tissue culture techniques remains very limited, to the point that it is difficult to justify maintaining such operations in a laboratory of surgical pathology. On the other hand, those diagnostic pathologists who have access to tissue culture facilities that have been set up elsewhere in their department for primarily investigative purposes will find it interesting and occasionally useful to have some tumors evaluated by this technique.

QUANTITATIVE METHODS (HISTOMETRY)

Objective measurement of microscopic features has often been advocated as a method to make more reproducible and "scientific" the practice of histopathology, but so far the procedure has found practical application in only a few fields. Traditionally the measurements have been made from photographs, projected images, or by the use of eyepiece graticles. Currently, semiautomatic or fully automated image analyzers are employed. Most contributions connected with this technique have been in the evaluation of nonneoplastic diseases of skeletal muscle, peripheral nerve, small bowel, and bone.[34,35] More recently, the method has also been applied to immunocytochemical stains, such as those done for hormone receptors.[34a]

X-RAY MICROANALYSIS

X-ray microanalysis is based on the principle that when a target atom in a specimen is struck by an electron beam, electron displacement to a higher energy state (orbital shell) and subsequent return will occur. The x-ray photon characteristic for the particular atom is measured, converted to digital form, and expressed in an x-ray spectrogram that allows for identification of elements 11 through 99, i.e., most of the periodic table.[37] It is preferable to use tissue fixed directly in glutaraldehyde, but material can also be processed following formalin-fixation, retrieved from the paraffin block, or even retrieved from the original hematoxylin-eosin slide by the use of the "pop-off" technique.[36] The examination is performed with either a transmission electron microscope or a scanning electron microscope coupled with an x-ray detector of the energy dispersive type. Currently, the main use of x-ray microanalysis is in the determination of the nature of crystalline (usually foreign) material observed in surgical pathology specimens.[37]

ELECTRON MICROSCOPY

The main applications of electron microscopy to diagnostic pathology are in the fields of tumor pathology and renal pathology.[38,39,41,42-56,58] The latter aspect is discussed in Chapter 17. In tumor pathology, ultrastructural examinations have proved very useful in determining the histogenesis (or differentiation) of various tumors but unfortunately have not shown consistent differences between reactive conditions, benign tumors, and malignant tumors of the same cell type. Lesions of controversial nature in which electron microscopy has provided crucial information and sometimes settled the histogenetic issue include granular cell tumor, schwannoma, histiocytosis X, spindle cell (sarcomatoid) carcinoma, mesothelioma, spindle cell thymoma, carcinoid tumors and small cell carcinomas of various sites, spermatocytic seminoma of testis and other germ cell tumors, and several others. At the present time, the role of diagnostic electron microscopy has diminished considerably as a result of the advent of immunohistochemistry and other techniques. However, it remains a powerful tool that can be of great utility to the diagnostic pathologist if used selectively and intelligently, with full knowledge of its potential contributions and limitations. The pathologist confronted with a tumor that he finds undiagnosable by light microscopy who sends a sample for electron microscopic study in the hope that some feature of diagnostic significance will be found is likely to be disappointed by the results. The best chance for electron microscopy to be of utility is when the pathologist has already formulated a definite differential diagnosis between two or three entities at the light microscopic level and examines the tissue ultrastructurally searching *specifically* for the markers to be expected in each of those entities. I believe that this technique is used at its full potential only when the electron microscopic study is carried out by an individual experienced in anatomic pathology who has studied personally the light microscopic preparations of the case, has concluded that electron microscopy is indicated and for what reasons, has examined himself the thick sections, and has sat down at the electron microscope in order to select the proper photographic fields. Diagnostic electron microscopy observations become fully informative only when closely correlated with the light microscopic features, just as the latter acquire their full significance only when paired with the gross pathology and the clinical features of the case.

The limitations of electron microscopy can be summarized as follows:

1 Sampling, wherein only a small proportion of the neoplasm can be studied
2 Paucity of truly specific ultrastructural features, since the number of organelles or other structures that are exclusive of a cell or tissue type is very small
3 Possible misinterpretation of entrapped non-neoplastic elements as belonging to the tumor. Admittedly, this possibility exists with any technique, but it is particularly noticeable with electron microscopy because of the difficulties in evaluating spatial relationships in a small tissue sample

The greatest diagnostic potential of electron microscopy has been realized in the following instances:

1 Identification of a tumor as of (neuro)endocrine nature through the detection of dense-core granules of so-called neurosecretory type
2 Assessment of the nature of tumor cells with granular cytoplasm (oncocytes, granular cells, endocrine cells)
3 Identification of glandular and squamous differentiation in tumors of various types
4 Identification of a tumor as of melanocytic nature through the detection of melanosomes
5 Identification of a lesion as belonging to the histiocytosis X group of conditions through the detection of Birbenck's granules
6 Identification of steroid-producing cells from adrenal cortex and gonads through the detection of abundant smooth endoplasmic reticulum and mitochondria with tubulovesicular cristae
7 Identification of a tumor as of endothelial cell nature through the detection of Weibel-Palade bodies
8 Identification of skeletal and smooth muscle cells through the detection of the respective systems of cytoplasmic filaments
9 Identification of Schwann cells through the detection of mesoaxons and other features
10 Identification of alveolar soft sarcoma through the detection of the characteristic membrane-bound crystals

The main diagnostic situations in which electron microscopy is likely to offer information of diagnostic utility are the following:

1 Differential diagnosis between carcinoma, melanoma, and sarcoma
2 Differential diagnosis between adenocarcinoma and mesothelioma
3 Differential diagnosis of anterior mediastinal tumors between thymoma, thymic carcinoid, malignant lymphoma, and seminoma
4 Differential diagnosis of small round cell tumors between Ewing's sarcoma, embryonal rhabdomyosarcoma, malignant lymphoma, and neuroectodermal tumors
5 Differential diagnosis of spindle cell tumors of soft tissues
6 Differential diagnosis between endocrine and nonendocrine tumors

Undoubtedly, the best ultrastructural evaluation is made when a small sample of fresh material is fixed, immediately after removal, in glutaraldehyde or some other suitable fixative. Failure to follow this practice will result in a number of artifacts that no subsequent procedure can eliminate. Fortunately, some of the structures on which the diagnosis depends (such as desmosomes, dense-core granules, or melanosomes) may still be identifiable despite the artifacts present. Therefore it is worthwhile in many instances to retrieve material originally processed for routine light microscopic study.[54] Tissue fixed in buffered formaldehyde gives better results than tissue exposed to highly acidic fixatives such as Bouin's, Zenker's, or B-5. It is advisable to select the sample from the very periphery of the fragments, which is likely to be better fixed than the

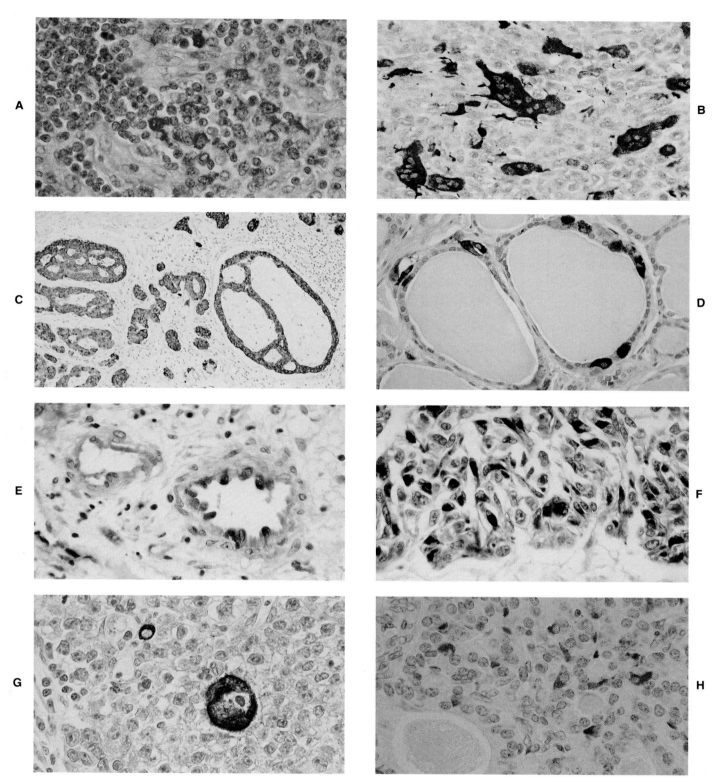

Plate I A, Lymph node involved by systemic mastocytosis. The myeloid precursors stain an intense red color (Leder's chloroacetate esterase). **B,** Specimen from giant cell tumor of bone fixed in formalin and embedded in paraffin. The osteoclasts show strong acid phosphatase activity (Duray's technique). **C,** Carcinoid tumor of stomach (chromogranin). **D,** C-cell hyperplasia of thyroid (calcitonin). **E,** Histiocytoid (epithelioid) hemangioendothelioma of bone (FVIII—related antigen). **F,** Malignant astrocytoma (GFAP). **G,** Seminoma with trophoblast-like giant cells (hCG). **H,** Strumal carcinoid of ovary with scattered insulin-reactive cells (insulin).

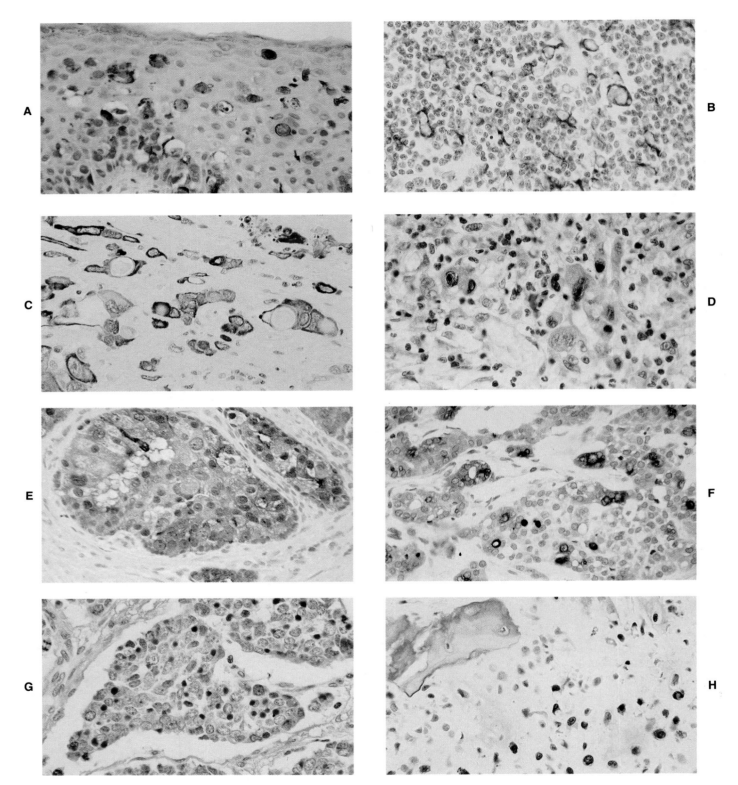

Plate II A, Paget's disease of breast (EMA). **B,** Thymoma with lymphocyte predominance (keratin). **C,** Anaplastic carcinoma of pancreas (keratin). **D,** Viral colitis in an immunosuppressed patient (CMV). **E,** Prostatic adenocarcinoma of large duct type (prostatic acid phosphatase). **F,** Poorly differentiated (insular) carcinoma of thyroid (thyroglobulin). **G,** Merkel cell tumor of skin (neurofilaments). **H,** Chondrosarcoma of bone. There is both cytoplasmic and nuclear staining for S-100 protein.

rest. If wet formalin-fixed material is unavailable, tissue may still be retrieved from the paraffin block, even if the number and magnitude of artifacts will be considerably greater.[57]

Finally, tissue can be obtained even from the hematoxylin-eosin stained section itself, a procedure which can be very useful if the structure in question is present only focally.[40] It should also be remembered that cytologic preparations can also benefit from ultrastructural examination.[49a]

An issue often raised in these increasingly cost-conscious times is whether it is advisable for a pathology laboratory to have an electron microscopic facility fully devoted to diagnostic work, in view of the high cost of the operation. In my opinion, such a facility is a necessity in all academic institutions and in private laboratories handling a large volume of material. Most other places are probably better served by sending their problem cases to large electron microscopic laboratories that perform referral work or, even better, to an expert consultant who can determine whether electron microscopy or some other special technique is truly needed to solve the diagnostic quandary.

IMMUNOHISTOCHEMISTRY

Briefly stated, immunohistochemistry is the application of immunologic principles and techniques to the study of cells and tissues. The original method, devised by Coons, consisted of labeling with a fluorescent probe an antibody raised in rabbits and searching for it (and therefore for the antigen against which the antibody was directed) in tissue sections examined under a fluorescent microscope following incubation. The technical improvements that supervened in subsequent years have been responsible for these methods becoming a staple of the histopathology laboratory.

Several procedures are available, the two most commonly used at present being the peroxidase-antiperoxidase immune complex method and the biotin-avidin immunoenzymatic technique (Figs. 3-1 and 3-2). In the latter procedure, the high affinity of avidin for biotin is used to couple the peroxidase label to the primary antibody.[107,178]

There is probably no other technique that has so revolutionized the field during the past 50 years as the immunohistochemical technique.[144] The advantages are obvious: remarkable sensitivity and specificity, applicability to routinely processed material (even if stored for long periods) and accurate correlation with the traditional morphologic parameters. It is compatible with most of the fixatives currently in use[108a] and is feasible even in material that has been decalcified[148] or in previously stained microscopic sections.[156] It can also be adapted to cytologic preparations[75a,88a,123,190a] and to electron microscopy.[170a] It can be used in conjunction with conventional techniques (such as silver staining) in the same section. It has replaced and rendered obsolete many of the conventional special stains and—to some extent—many of the diagnostic applications of electron microscopy. However, like any other technique, it presents potential pitfalls that need to be acknowledged by the pathologist interpreting the reaction, in order to prevent the technique being misleading rather than helpful.[122] Many of these pitfalls can be avoided by scrupulous technique, periodic checking of the antibody activity, and proper use of positive and negative controls. An ingenious method

for antibody testing—the ''sausage tissue block''—that allows the simultaneous evaluation of over one hundred different tissue samples on a single slide with one drop of antibody has been devised by Battifora.[64]

False negative results can occur when:

1 An antibody is inappropriate, denatured, or used at the wrong concentration.
2 There is loss of antigen through autolysis and/or diffusion. This factor plays a much larger role with some antigens (such as factor VIII–related antigen) than with others (such as actin). It should be remembered that most antigens continue to leak out after fixation; therefore, it is always preferable to perform the stains using the original paraffin block than tissue left in formalin for long periods.
3 Presence of antigen is at a density below the level of detection with the reagents and techniques used, either because of minimal production or excessive release.

Because of the existence of all these factors, an apparently negative immunohistochemical result should not be used to rule out a diagnosis even in the presence of a positive built-in control, especially if such a diagnosis is strongly suggested by the clinical and morphologic features.

False positive results, which are even more dangerous, can result from a variety of causes:

1 Cross-reactivity of the antibody with antigens different from the one being searched for
2 Nonspecific binding of the antibody to the tissue[72]
3 Presence of endogenous peroxidase in—or avidity for the avidin-biotin complex by—some cellular elements
4 Entrapment of normal tissues by the tumor cells. This problem, which also exists in hematoxylin-eosin-stained sections, is amplified through the great sensitivity of the technique. One example of this phenomenon is the entrapment of skeletal muscle by soft tissue tumors, with the resulting misdiagnosis of rhabdomyosarcoma because of positivity for desmin, myoglobin, or some other skeletal muscle marker.[70] Another is the misdiagnosis of malignant lymphoma of thyroid as carcinoma because of the positivity of the entrapped follicular epithelium for thyroglobulin.[171] Still another is the misdiagnosis of Hodgkin's disease or large cell lymphoma of the thymus as malignant thymoma because of the presence of keratin-positive entrapped thymic epithelial cells.[162]

The existence of this phenomenon also makes very difficult the determination of multihormonal secretion in endocrine neoplasms. For instance, the majority of endocrine tumors of the pancreas show positivity for more than one hormone,[143] but the possibility of only one of these hormones representing the neoplastic element and the others expressing the residual non-neoplastic cells should be regarded as an alternative for at least some of the cases. As a matter of fact, the problem of entrapment of normal structures is so subtle and pervasive that it can only be eliminated with certainty if the stain is done in a metastatic site, where entrapped normal tissue from that particular organ would be out of the question.
5 Release of soluble proteins from the cytoplasm of normal cells invaded by the tumor, with subsequent per-

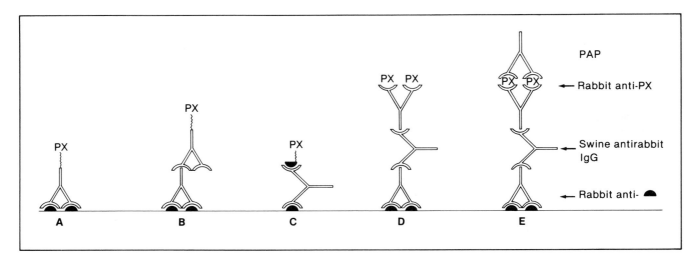

Fig. 3-1 Immunoperoxidase procedures. *A* indicates peroxidase (PX) antibody conjugate, direct; *B,* peroxidase antibody conjugate, indirect; *C,* labeled antigen method; *D,* enzyme bridge procedure; and *E,* peroxidase-antiperoxidase (PAP) immune complex method. Solid semicircle indicates antigen. (From Falini B, Taylor CR: New developments in immunoperoxidase techniques and their application. Arch Pathol Lab Med **107:**105-117, copyright 1983, American Medical Association.)

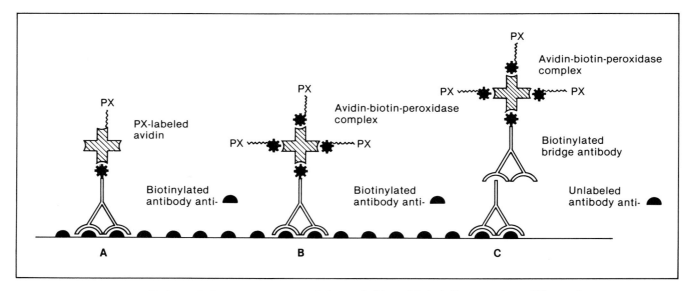

Fig. 3-2 Biotin-avidin immunoenzymatic techniques. Solid semicircle indicates antigen; PX, peroxidase; *, biotin; and shaded open cross, avidin. *A,* biotinylated primary antibody method; *B,* biotinylated peroxidase method; *C,* avidin-biotin-peroxidase complex method. (From Falini B, Taylor CR: New developments in immunoperoxidase techniques and their application. Arch Pathol Lab Med **107:**105-117, copyright 1983, American Medical Association.)

meation of the interstitium and nonspecific absorption (and possibly phagocytosis) by the tumor cells. Perhaps in some cases this phenomenon represents an artifact developed after the removal of the tissue, but in most instances it is probably occurring already in vivo. Immunoglobulins are known to exhibit this phenomenon, which explains the positivity of Reed-Sternberg cells for various light and heavy Ig chains.[139] A marker particularly prone to this artifact (probably because of its great diffusing properties) is thyroglobulin. We have seen in the thyroid gland cases of metastatic clear cell carcinoma from the kidney, malignant lymphoma, and metastatic signet ring carcinoma in which the tumor cells around the trapped thyroid follicles showed strong cytoplasmic staining for thyroglobulin, whereas those located at a greater distance or in other organs were totally negative.[74,171] Still another example of this phenomenon is the malignant tumor growing within blood vessels and picking up factor VIII or other endothelial markers from the adjacent non-neoplastic endothelial cells. This may explain some cases of keratin-positive anaplastic carcinomas of the thyroid with a prominent endovascular component showing an apparent positivity for factor VIII.[138] Still another example of this phenomenon is provided by breast carcinoma that invades the pectoralis muscle, the myoglobin liberated from the injured muscle diffusing into the carcinoma cells and rendering them positive for this skeletal muscle-specific antigen.[90]

There are other factors that have contributed to misinterpretations. We are referring to the apparently anomalous positive stains caused by ectopic antigen expression, by hitherto unrecognized cross reactions, or by the fact that some markers originally claimed to be specific for a certain cell tissue or tumor have proved with increased experience to be shared by other tissues or neoplasms. Examples of this phenomenon are plentiful and include neuron-specific enolase,[89] alpha-1-antitrypsin,[193] S-100 protein (originally claimed to be specific for the central nervous system and now known to be present in a variety of cells, ranging from reticulum cells to chondrocytes), vimentin (originally claimed to be specific for mesenchymal cells but later also detected in neuronal cells and other elements), and epithelial membrane antigen (first thought to be specific for breast, then for breast and skin adnexae, then for epithelial cells in general, and now also demonstrated in several mesenchymal tumors and lymphoreticular neoplasms.[86] Actually, the possibility should always be kept in mind that a marker regarded at the present time as specific for a certain cell type may prove in the future to react with others.

The number of antigens that have been detected with immunohistochemistry in tissue sections is already huge and keeps increasing at a steady rate. Theoretically, any substance that is antigenic and whose antigenicity is at least partially retained in tissue sections can be demonstrated by this technique. With the advent of monoclonal technology, a large number of antibodies have become available for which the antigenic determinant is chemically poorly defined or—in some instances—totally unknown. Although some of these antibodies have proved extremely useful (particularly in the field of hematopathology) one should be particularly careful not to overinterpret the results in terms of presumptive tissue specificity.[98]

The most important diagnostic applications of immunohistochemistry are discussed in the respective chapters. Listed below in alphabetical order for easy reference are most of the antigens that have been applied to surgical pathology problems, whether as diagnostic aids or as histogenetic probes.

Actin. This is an ubiquitous contractile protein responsible for the motility of most cells. It is an extremely useful marker for the identification of smooth muscle cells and for the evaluation of the participation of myoepithelial cells in lesions of breast, salivary glands, and sweat glands.[147] Various isoforms of this protein exist, two of which are specific for smooth muscle and skeletal muscle, respectively.[180b] Antibodies specific for skeletal muscle actin have been used as markers for rhabdomyosarcoma.[83]

Alkaline phosphatase. This group of enzymes consists of membrane-bound glycoproteins that are widely distributed in human tissues. The major isoenzymes are the hepatic, osseous, renal, and placental types. Placental-like alkaline phosphatase reactivity is seen in all types of gonadal and extragonadal germ cell tumors (including intratubular germ cell neoplasia)[67] but is also present in a variety of non-germ cell neoplasms.[194]

Alpha-actinin. This is a constituent protein of sarcomeric muscle, related to Z bands. It has been detected in rhabdomyosarcoma, but its level of sensitivity seems low.[175]

Alpha-fetoprotein. This glycoprotein is a major plasma component of the fetus, the major sources being the liver and the visceral endoderm of the yolk sac. It is one of the major oncofetal antigens. It is invariably present in yolk sac (endodermal sinus) tumors and also in a high proportion of other germ cell tumors.[115]

Alpha-lactalbumin. This is a major protein of human milk, synthesized almost exclusively by mammary tissue. It has been detected in normal, fibrocystic, and neoplastic breast tissue. It is present in breast carcinomas of both ductal and lobular type, at the primary site and in metastases.[78,120a] The only other tumor type in which it has been found is the breast-related hydradenoma papilliferum of vulva.

Alpha-1-ACT. Alpha-1-antichymotrypsin is an acute-phase plasma protease inhibitor (MW 68,000), mainly synthesized in the liver. It shows a high level of homology of DNA sequences with alpha-1-AT. It has been employed, together with the latter, as a marker for histiocytes and reticulum cells. However, it is also found in a large number of other cell types, and as a result its diagnostic utility is rather limited.[120]

Alpha-1-AT. (Alpha-1-antitrypsin; alpha-1-proteinase inhibitor); see under Alpha-1-ACT.

Angiotensin-converting enzyme. This is a membrane-bound enzyme that converts angiotensin I to the biologically active vasopressor angiotensin II and inactivates the depressor substance bradykinin. It is localized in the vascular endothelium of lung and other tissues and in the epithelial cells of the renal proximal tubule and intestinal mucosa. It has also been detected in renal cell carcinoma.[186]

Basement membrane. This extracellular structure can be manufactured by epithelial, smooth muscle, striated muscle, pericytic, endothelial, schwannian, and melanocytic cells. It has a complex structure, the two major components being type IV collagen and laminin (see under individual headings).

BCA-225. This glycoprotein (MW 225,000-250,000) is a glycoprotein isolated from human breast cancer tissue, which cross-reacts with gp52, the envelope glycoprotein of the mouse mammary tumor virus. It is commonly found in breast carcinomas, but only exceptionally in tumors from other sites.[132a]

Blood group antigens. The A, B, and H blood group antigens are glycolipids present in the cell membrane of red blood cells and in many types of epithelial cells, which can be detected with immunohistochemical methods, the red blood cell adherence method, or by the use of lectins (see under Lectin receptors).[94,95] Loss of these isoantigens has been observed in carcinomas of various types.[121,192] Furthermore, a correlation has been found between ABH deletion and tumor aggressiveness.[172]

T (Thompsen-Friedenreich) and Tn antigens are precursor antigens of the MN blood group system. They are masked in most normal adult tissues but are detectable in several types of carcinoma, including breast, large bowel, bladder, and lung.[106b]

CA 125. This is a cell surface glycoprotein originally identified in mucinous epithelial ovarian tumors and recognized by the monoclonal antibody OC 125.[112] It is also expressed by adenocarcinomas of other sites, including cervix, endometrium, gastrointestinal tract, and breast.

Carbonic anhydrase C. Carbonic anhydrase is an ubiquitous metalloprotein enzyme involved in carbon dioxide hydration and, presumably, in the regulation of ionic and acid-base balance. The C isoenzyme, present in the nervous system, has been suggested as a marker for oligodendrocytes and oligodendrogliomas. However, positivity has also been found in astrocytomas, glioblastomas, schwannomas, meningiomas, and other tumors.[161]

Casein. See under EMA.

CEA. Carcino-embryonic antigen is a glycoprotein of heterogeneous composition (MW 200,000) normally detected in the glycocalix of fetal epithelial cells, particularly those of mucin-secreting glandular nature.[99,167] It is detectable only in small amounts in normal adult cells and benign tumors but is present in large quantities in carcinomas, particularly adenocarcinomas of gastrointestinal tract (including pancreas) and lung and in thyroid medullary carcinoma. Because of the fact that it is primarily expressed by fetal tissues and malignant tumors, it is referred to as an oncofetal antigen. Monoclonal antibodies seem to offer a greater degree of tumor specificity than the conventional antisera.[109]

Chromogranin. The chromogranin family is composed of acidic glycoproteins (MW ranging from 20,000 to 100,000) located in the soluble fraction of neurosecretory granules.[126] The most abundant is chromogranin A (MW 75,000).[102] Two others have been named chromogranin B (or secretogranin I) and chromogranin C (or secretogranin II).[126a] Nearly all types of neuroendocrine tumors are reactive, so that chromogranin stain has become the most widely used "pan-endocrine" marker (Plate I, C).

Collagen. Several biochemical types of collagen exist. Collagen type I predominates in dermis, tendons, and bone. Type II is associated with cartilage. Type III is found mainly in fetal skin, scars, and in arterial walls. Collagen type IV is, together with laminin, the major component of the basement membrane[96]; its main application has been in the delineation of the basement membrane surrounding nests of in situ and invasive carcinoma. Type V, the most recently described collagen, has been found to be increased in the desmoplastic stromal reaction induced by carcinomas.[62a]

Creatine kinase. This widely distributed enzyme of contractile or transport systems is composed of two polypeptide subunits, known as B (brain type) and M (muscle type) that combine to form three dimeric enzymes. The MM isoenzyme is abundant in skeletal muscle and has therefore been used as a diagnostic aid in rhabdomyosarcoma.[188,196] However, it is not entirely specific for this tissue type.[188]

Cytokeratins. Cytokeratins or keratins are a family of water-insoluble, intracellular fibrous proteins present in almost all epithelia. Thus they represent an excellent marker for epithelial differentiation regardless of whether the tumor is of endodermal, neuroectodermal, mesenchymal, or germ cell derivation (Plate II, B and C). Some keratins have unexpectedly been found to be expressed by normal and neoplastic myometrial muscle.[71]

Nineteen well-defined subclasses of keratins have been identified on the basis of their molecular weight (MW) (ranging from 40,000 to 68,000) and isoelectric pH value (ranging from 5 to 8). This combination constitutes the so-called keratin catalog, which shows a tissue-specific distribution throughout the epithelia[78b,141] and which can be mapped using a battery of monoclonal antibodies[124] (Fig. 3-3). For scanning purposes, several of these antibodies are combined in the form of "cocktails."

Desmin. This muscle-type intermediate filament (MW 55,000) is found in cells of smooth and striated muscle and allegedly also in myofibroblasts. It is particularly abundant in parenchymal (as opposed to vascular) smooth muscle. Therefore it has been primarily used for the identification of smooth muscle and skeletal muscle tumors.[136]

Desmoplakins. Desmoplakins are membrane-bound structures to which intermediate filaments attach to form specialized cell junctions (desmosomes and related structures). They have been found to contain six major high molecular weight protein components. Two of them, designated respectively as desmoplakin I (MW 250,000) and desmoplakin II (MW 215,000), have been used as markers for the presence of cell junctions, thus providing indirect evidence about the cell type.[140]

EMA. Epithelial membrane antigen is a glycoprotein present in human milk fat globule membranes,[163] probably analogous to the antigen demonstrated with antisera raised against the casein fraction of human milk.[156a] It is an excellent marker for most normal and neoplastic epithelia but is not restricted to them (Plate II, A).[187] It can also be expressed by mesotheliomas, meningiomas, a variety of mesenchymal neoplasms, and even some malignant lymphomas.[168,181] It has also been found to be a marker of normal and neoplastic perineurial cells.[61] There is recent evidence suggesting that monoclonal antibodies raised against various epitopes of human or guinea pig milk fat globule membrane may offer a greter degree of specificity, in the sense of being apparently restricted to epithelial tissues.[100a,106a,197a]

Endorphin. See under Opioid peptides.

Enolases. See under NSE.

Enzymes. All enzymes are proteins and therefore demonstrable immunohistochemically even if their specific activity is no longer present. In addition to those listed individually, enzymes that have been demonstrated with this technique include those of the catecholamine-synthesizing pathway,[111a] those of the steroid hormone–synthesizing pathway, and leukocyte elastase (a serine protease present in cells of the myeloid series).[80a]

Ferritin. Ferritin, together with transferrin and lactoferrin, is a major iron-binding protein. It has been detected immunohistochemically in liver cell carcinoma[78a] and breast carcinoma.[74a,171a]

Fillagrin. Fillagrin is the matrix protein of keratin (MW 50,000), thus named because of its ability to aggregate filaments of keratin into fibers or macrofibrils.[81] It has been used to study disorders of keratinization and various epithelial neoplasms. Its diagnostic utility has not yet been ascertained.

FVIII-related antigen. Factor VIII–related antigen is one of the three functional components of the antihemophiliac factor (factor VIII).[145] It is synthesized in endothelial cells of blood vessels (where it has been located in the Weibel-Palade bodies) and is also found in megakaryocytes, platelets, and mast cells. It is widely used as a nearly specific marker of endothelial cell differentiation (Plate I, E).[145]

Gastricsin. This is an acid protease (MW 35,000) present in the human gastric juice, which is produced in the form of a zymogen (progastricsin), primarily in the stomach but also in the duodenum. A similar enzyme has been found in seminal fluid and in benign and malignant prostatic tissues.[169]

GCDFP-15. Gross cystic disease fluid protein-15, present in the fluid content of fibrocystic disease of the breast, is a marker of apocrine differentiation.[129] It is expressed in normal and neoplastic apocrine glands of skin, in the apocrine metaplasia accompanying fibrocystic disease of breast, and in the rare in situ and invasive apocrine carcinomas of breast.

GFAP. Glial fibrillary acidic protein (MW ranging between 48,000 and 52,000) is one of the five major types of cytoplasmic intermediate filaments.[76,82] It is present in normal, reactive, and neoplastic astrocytes; developing, reactive and neoplastic ependymal cells; and developing and neoplastic oligodendrocytes[161] (Plate I, F). Expression of this marker has also been documented in peripheral nerve tumors and in mixed tumors of salivary glands and sweat glands.

hCG. Human chorionic gonadotropin, which is normally secreted by the syncytiotrophoblast, is composed of two chains. The alpha chain has an aminoacid sequence nearly identical to those of the pituitary glycoprotein hormones FSH, LH, and TSH. The beta chain is hormone-specific.[105] The antibodies prepared against the latter subunit are employed to detect trophoblastic differentiation in germ cell tumors and ectopic hCG production in other neoplasms[105] (Plate I, G).

Hemoglobin. This is a heme-carrying protein specific for cells of the erythroid series, already present at early stages of erythropoiesis.

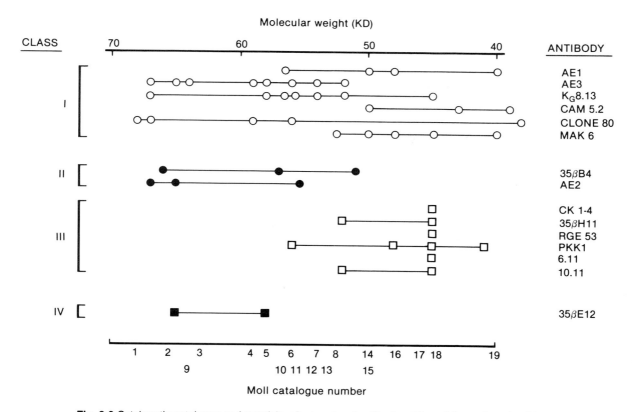

Fig. 3-3 Cytokeratin catalogue and reactivity of monoclonal antibodies. The acidic cytokeratins (Moll's catalogue no. 10 and 12-19) range in molecular weight from 40,000 to 56,500; the basic cytokeratins (Moll's catalogue no. 1-8) range in molecular weight from 53,000 to 67,000. The antibodies have been divided into four classes, based on their pattern of reactivity: *I,* high and low molecular weight cytokeratins present in squamous, ductal, and simple epithelium, broadly reactive; *II,* higher-molecular weight cytokeratins present in squamous epithelium; *III,* lower-molecular weight cytokeratins present in simple and ductal epithelium; *IV,* high molecular weight cytokeratins present in both squamous and ductal epithelium. (From DeLellis RA, Kwan P: Technical considerations in the immunohistochemical demonstration of intermediate filaments. Am J Surg Pathol **12**(Suppl 1):17-23, 1988.)

It represents an excellent marker for the identification of normal, megaloblastic, and dysplastic erythroid cells.[164]

Histaminase. This oxidative deaminating enzyme, also known as diamine oxidase, is present in normal tissues of various types. It has also been detected in certain tumors with endocrine differentiation, such as pulmonary small cell carcinoma[66] and medullary thyroid carcinoma.[132]

HLA. Histocompatibility antigens are membrane-bound glycoproteins that are important in the regulation of the immune response and in resistance or susceptibility to a large number of diseases.[113] They are responsible for the rejection of transplanted organs. Two major categories exist. The first, known as class I antigens (MW 44,000), is formed by antigens coded by HLA-A, -B, and -C loci and is expressed on virtually all nucleated cells. The second category, known as class II antigens, is coded by the HLA-DR locus. They are also known as HLA-DR or Ia-like antigens and are expressed by most types of histiocytes (including connective tissue macrophages), although they are not specific for them (see under Ia-like antigens).

Hormone receptors. Effect of hormones in target organs is mediated by intracellular (largely intranuclear) peptides known as hormone receptors. Monoclonal antibodies for estrogen, progesterone, and androgen receptors are now available.[67a,130] Some of these antibodies have been found to detect receptors in routinely processed

material,[159,180] but fresh-frozen tissue is generally preferable.[131,166,170]

hPL. Human placental lactogen is a placental protein that has been used for the identification of trophoblastic differentiation in germ cell tumors and other neoplasms. Several types of carcinomas of somatic organs (such as lung and stomach) can also express this marker.[106]

Ia-like antigens. These are membrane-bound glycoproteins composed of polypeptides (MW 34,000 and 28,000) that are coded for by genes located in the major histocompatibility complex. They correspond to HLA-DR antigens (see under HLA) and are detected on histiocytes, B lymphocytes, and activated T lymphocytes. They are believed to regulate cell-to-cell interactions leading to immune effector function. Ia-like antigens have also been detected on cells with no apparent immune function, such as epithelial cells of kidney, bowel, bronchi, breast, skin, and vascular endothelium.[154] It has been claimed that they are a marker of malignant transformation, particularly for the melanocytic system.[195]

Immunoglobulins. These proteins produced by plasma cells play a key role in the immune response. Five major types exist, designated as IgG, IgM, IgA, IgD, and IgE. They are constituted by heavy and light polypeptide chains, joined by disulfide bonds. The composition of the heavy chain determines the type of immunoglobulin, and the type of light chain (kappa or lambda) subdivides them into two categories. The usual immunohistochemical method for determining whether a plasma cell population is monotypic or polytypic is to perform a reaction for kappa and lambda light chains.

J chain is a polypeptide around which IgA and IgM molecules polymerize and is produced by immunoglobulin-synthesizing cells. It is present in most B immunoblasts regardless of their class but is absent from mature plasma cells. Its presence in a cell indicates that the immunoglobulin molecule is being synthesized at that site.[108]

IgA molecules present in mucosal membranes are attached to a *secretory component* secreted by the glandular cells (see under Secretory component).

Intermediate filaments. This family of cytoplasmic filaments is so named because their diameter (8 to 10 nm) is intermediate between the diameters of actin (thin) and tubulin (thick). There are five biochemically and immunologically distinct types, which have a remarkable tendency to be expressed in a stable, cell type–specific and differentiation-dependent fashion.* They are respectively named cytokeratin, vimentin, desmin, GFAP, and neurofilaments (see individual headings). Cytokeratins comprise a complex group of about nineteen polypeptides, whereas each of the other four classes consists of a single polypeptide unit. In some fetal and neoplastic tissues, coexpression of two or even three different types of intermediate filaments may occur.[190]

Involucrin. This is a major structural subunit of a protein envelope synthesized by maturing cells (keratinocytes) of human stratified squamous epithelia, visible in electron micrographs as a 10 nm-thick marginal band.[190b] It is absent from basal cells but appears in large amounts as the cells mature. Involucrin has therefore been used as a marker of squamous epithelium and as an expression of suprabasal differentiation.[191]

J-chain. See under Immunoglobulins.

Keratins. See under Cytokeratins.

Lactalbumin. See under Alpha-lactalbumin.

Lactoferrin. See under Ferritin.

Laminin. This structural protein is one of the two major components of the basement membrane, together with type IV collagen. It is therefore present in tumors that produce basement membranes, such as carcinomas, smooth muscle tumors, and tumors of endothelial cells.[134] Laminin is better expressed in blood vessels than lymph vessels, but this feature does not allow a sharp distinction between the two structures.[125]

LCA. Leukocyte common antigen is a major membrane glycoprotein that seems to be restricted to leukocytes and is still identifiable in formalin-fixed, paraffin-embedded material. As a result, it has become the method of choice for the distinction between lymphoid and nonlymphoid neoplasms.[117]

Lectin receptors. Lectins are plant-derived proteins that bind specifically to simple or complex carbohydrate groups acting as lectin receptors. As such, lectins are useful tools to study the glycoprotein and glycolipid structure of the cell surface. These lectin receptors can be localized by standard immunohistochemical methods. Some lectins (such as concanavalin A) seem to have an affinity for cells of the lymphoid system.[185] The lectin of *Ulex europeaus* combines with the H antigen that corresponds to blood group O.[160] It has been found that it binds to endothelial cells regardless of the individual's blood group and has therefore been used as a marker of vessels and vascular neoplasms.[135] Lectins have also been used to map the various segments of the nephron and to correlate the findings with those of renal neoplasms.[189]

Lymphoid and other leukocytic antigens. In addition to leukocyte common antigen, a large variety of lymphoid-related antigens have been described, most of them associated with the cell membranes. These antigens relate both with the subsets of lymphoid cells

(B and T) and their level of functional maturation. These are further discussed in Chapter 21. Interestingly, some of these antigens have been subsequently found to be expressed in nonlymphoid cells. Thus Leu-M1 (an antibody that recognizes hapten X, a carbohydrate moiety linked to the cell membrane protein of myelomonocytic cells) has been seen to react with adenocarcinomas of various sites and found to be of utility in the differential diagnosis with malignant mesothelioma.[165] Leu-7 (a marker for a subset of normal lymphocytes) has been found to react with a variety of neural and neuroendocrine neoplasms and with prostatic adenocarcinomas.[133]

Lysozyme. This bacteriolytic enzyme, also known as muramidase, acts on muramic-acid linkages in bacterial cell walls. It is found in human secretions and in neutrophils, cells of the monocyte-histiocyte series, and some epithelial cells.[73,128] It has often been employed as a histiocytic marker, but it lacks specificity.

Micro-organisms. Immunohistochemical methods for a wide variety of viral, bacterial, spirochaetal, fungal, and parasitic antigens are now available,[142] but the only ones that are used with some frequency for diagnostic purposes are those aimed at detecting viruses such as hepatitis B virus, herpes simplex, cytomegalovirus (Plate II, *D*), and human papilloma virus.[59,93] Recently, an immunohistochemical method for the detection of *Pneumocystis carinii* in sputum has been described.[113a]

Myelin proteins. Myelin basic protein is a myelin-specific protein present both in central and peripheral myelin sheaths. As such, it can be demonstrated in oligodendrocytes and Schwann cells.[161] However, controversy still exists as to whether it represents a reliable marker for oligodendroglioma and peripheral nerve tumors. The same is true for other myelin-related proteins, such as P2 protein and PO protein.[77]

Myoglobin. This oxygen-binding protein is apparently specific for striated (skeletal and myocardial) muscle and is therefore of great utility for the identification of rhabdomyosarcomas and other tumors exhibiting skeletal muscle differentiation.[79,146]

Myosin. Two biochemically distinct forms of this contractile protein exist: smooth muscle-type (nonsarcomeric) and skeletal muscle–type (sarcomeric). Three subtypes of the latter have been described: slow, fast, and fetal. The main use of this marker has been in the identification of skeletal muscle differentiation in tumor.[188]

Neurofilaments. These represent the intermediate filaments of neurons and their processes. They are protein triplets composed of three major subunits (MW 68,000, 150,000, and 200,000), respectively, which are immunochemically distinct.[161] Neurofilaments are expressed in tumors of neuronal origin or displaying neuronal differentiation, such as neuroblastoma, medulloblastoma, and retinoblastoma. Positivity has also been encountered in Merkel's cell tumor of skin, endocrine tumors of the pancreas, carcinoid tumors, parathyroid tumors, and other neoplasms of endocrine nature (Plate II, *G*).

NSE. Enolases are widely distributed glycolytic dimeric enzymes that catalyze the interconversion of 2-phosphoglycerate and phosphoenolpyruvate.[161] The gamma-gamma and alpha-gamma isoenzymes of enolase are preferentially found in neurons and neuroendocrine cells and have therefore been designated as neuron-specific enolases. Positivity is found in the majority of neuroectodermal and neuroendocrine neoplasms, including carcinoid tumors and malignant melanoma. Unfortunately, NSE has also been detected in several other types of normal and neoplastic cells, this obviously limiting their diagnostic usefulness.[158] The best results are obtained with the use of monoclonal antibodies.[176,177] The beta subunit of enolase has been employed as a marker for striated muscle, but it is not specific for it.[111]

Opioid peptides. Alpha-endorphin, met-enkephalin, and dynorphin B production is a feature of neural and neuroendocrine cells. These substances have also been found in a large number of neural

---

*See references 65, 85, 87, 137, 152, 157, and 190c.

and neuroendocrine tumors, including paraganglioma, thyroid medullary carcinoma, and carcinoid tumors. A monoclonal "pan-opioid" antibody has been developed that recognizes the tetrapeptide Tyr-Gly-Gly-Phe, which is the sequence responsible for the pharmacologic activity of all opioid peptides.[69]

Osteonectin. This recently described osteoblast-associated antigen can be employed in the identification of osteosarcoma and other osteoid-forming lesions.[174]

Peptide hormones. A huge number of peptide hormones acting as neuroendocrine mediators has been described, and others are likely to be discovered in the future.[182] Those for which antibodies are available and which have been detected immunohistochemically in normal and neoplastic tissue include: ACTH, ADH (antidiuretic hormone), bombesin, calcitonin (Plate I, *D*), cholecystokinin, enteroglucagon (glycentin), gastrin, GH (growth hormone), glucagon, GRP (gastrin-releasing peptide), insulin (Plate I, *H*), LH, neurotensin, PP (pancreatic polypeptide), prolactin, PTH (parathormone), somatostatin, TSH, P substance, vasopressin, VIP (vasoactive intestinal peptide), Y (NPY) peptide, and YY peptide.

Placental proteins. The placenta is the most active endocrine organ of the human body. Among the many proteins secreted by the trophoblast, the three that have been detected immunohistochemically are hCG (human chorionic gonadotropin), hPL (human placental lactogen), and SP1 (pregnancy-specific beta-1-glycoprotein) (see under individual headings).[68]

Prealbumin. Prealbumin (MW 54,900) is a plasma protein that binds thyroxine and retinol for transport in the blood. It is thought to be produced in the liver but is also present in pancreatic islet cells and their tumors.[123a]

Prostatic acid phosphatase (PAP). This isoenzyme of acid phosphatase is secreted by the normal, hyperplastic, and neoplastic prostatic epithelium (Plate II, *E*). It is a useful marker, but it is not entirely specific for the prostate. Carcinomas of bladder and carcinoid tumors of various sites have also been found to be sometimes reactive for this marker.[179]

Prostate specific antigen (PSA). This poorly defined but highly purified antigen (MW 33,000) has been extracted from prostatic tissue and has been found to have a greater degree of specificity for normal, hyperplastic, and neoplastic prostatic tissue than prostatic acid phosphatase. Therefore it has become the method of choice for the identification of prostatic adenocarcinoma.[151,184]

Renin. This proteolytic enzyme is produced and stored in the granules of the juxtaglomerular cells surrounding the afferent arterioles of renal glomeruli. Renin acts on the basic substrate angiotensinogen to form angiotensin I, which is subsequently changed by a converting enzyme to angiotensin II. Renin has been demonstrated immunohistochemically in the normal kidney,[92] juxtaglomerular cell tumors, in the blood vessels of tumors of lung and other sites,[186a] and—allegedly—in some soft tissue tumors.[88,149]

Retinal S-antigen. This is a protein (MW 50,000) intimately involved in the phototransduction of vision. Together with opsin, it appears to be a good photoreceptor marker.[161] It has been identified in the retinal photoreceptor cells and pinealocytes and in their neoplastic counterparts, i.e., retinoblastoma and pineocytoma. Focal positivity has also been found in medulloblastomas.[161]

S-100 protein. This is an acidic, dimeric calcium-binding protein (MW 21,000) composed of different combinations of alpha and beta subunits and first isolated in the central nervous system. It is present in the nucleus and cytoplasm of glial and Schwann cells, melanocytes, chondrocytes, adipocytes, myoepithelial cells, and other cells, and in the tumors derived from them[153,161] (Plate II, *H*). A quantitative differentiation distribution has been found between alpha and beta forms.[103] The wide expression of this antigen has substantially diminished its diagnostic utility.[105a] Its main use is in the evaluation of tumors presumed to be malignant melanomas.[110]

Secretory component. This glycoprotein is a normal glandular epithelial cell product that combines with dimeric IgA in association with J chain to form intact 11 S secretory IgA molecules.[104] Secretory component is normally present in the epithelial cells lining the various mucosal surfaces and has therefore been employed as a marker for tumors of glandular epithelial origin.[104]

Serotonin. This indolamine, also known as 5-hydroxytryptamine, is widely distributed in neuroendocrine cells and is particularly abundant in Kultschitsky's type cells of the distal small bowel and appendix.[91] Carcinoid tumors and related neuroendocrine neoplasms are usually positive for this marker.

SP-1. Pregnancy-specific B-1-glycoprotein is a recently described placental protein (MW 90,000). Originally thought to be specific for the syncytiotrophoblast, it is now known to be also present in breast carcinomas and a variety of other epithelial malignancies.[114]

Steroid hormones. Estradiol, testosterone, and other steroid hormones have been localized immunohistochemically in normal and neoplastic tissues from gonads and adrenal cortex, despite the considerable loss that occurs during embedding because of the use of organic solvents.[116] The capacity for production of several of these closely related steroids by tumor cells has prevented a close correlation between tumor types and hormonal profile, and has limited the practical utility of this stain.[116]

Surfactant apoprotein. This protein is secreted by type II (granular) pneumocytes in the pulmonary alveoli and is therefore used as a marker for these cells and their tumors. It is found both in cytoplasmic lamellar formations and in intranuclear inclusions.[180a] A related marker found in type II pneumocytes has been named laminoorganel antigen.

Synaptophysin. This is a major glycosylated transmembrane glycoprotein (MW 38,000) that has been isolated from neuronal presynaptic vesicles. It is expressed in normal, reactive, and neoplastic cells of neuroectodermal and neuroendocrine types, including pheochromocytoma, thyroid medullary carcinoma, endocrine pancreatic tumors, and carcinoid tumors.[75,100]

T antigen. See under Blood group antigens.

Tenascin. This is an extracellular matrix glycoprotein that has been found in the early fetal rat mammary gland. It has been claimed that this marker is detectable in the stroma in malignant but not in benign breast tumors.[127b]

Thrombomodulin. This is a newly recognized endothelial cell–associated co-factor that forms a 1:1 stoichiometric complex with thrombin.[197] It has been used as a marker for vascular tumors composed of endothelial cells.[197]

Thymic hormones. Allegedly, alpha-thymosin and other so-called thymic hormones can be detected immunohistochemically in the normal thymus and in thymomas.[173] If these reports are confirmed, these markers could prove very useful in the evaluation of thymic epithelial neoplasms, since no other antigens specific for these cells are currently available.

Thyroglobulin. This is a large glycoprotein (MW 670,000) formed by two identical subunits. It is produced by the thyroid follicular cells and serves as the substratum for iodination and hormonogenesis. It is a specific marker of thyroid differentiation and is widely used in the evaluation of thyroid neoplasms[183] (Plate II, *F*). It has been found to be preferable in this regard than the search for the thyroid hormones T3 and T4.[60]

TPA. Tissue polypeptide antigen is a nonfilamentous protein located in maturing cells (keratinocytes) of human stratified squamous epithelia. As such, it is absent in basal cells and appears in the suprabasal layers.[127] It has been employed as a marker of squamous epithelium.

Transferrin. See under Ferritin.

Tropomyosin. This protein is a molecular subunit of thin filaments.[118,155] It has been used as a marker for rhabdomyosarcoma, but it does not seem to offer any real advantages over the more usual markers of myogenous differentiation.[175]

Tryptase. This neutral protease is the dominant protein component of human mast cells.[80] It has not been found in human eosinophils, basophils, neutrophils, lymphocytes, or monocytes. Therefore it has been employed for the selective staining of mast cells.[80]

Villin. This is an actin bundling and severing protein (MW 95,000) that seems to be restricted in animal tissues to epithelial cells with a brush border. Thus the enterocytes of the intestine and epithelial cells of proximal but not distal tubules of the kidney are strongly positive as are the tumor cells of renal cell carcinoma.[101]

Vimentin. This is one of the five major types of cytoplasmic intermediate filaments (MW 57,000). It is characteristic of cells of mesenchymal nature, such as endothelial cells, fibroblasts, and vascular smooth muscle cells.[119] However, it is not restricted to cells of mesodermal origin but is sometimes also expressed in tumors of epithelial or neural nature, not infrequently in conjunction with keratin and GFAP, respectively.[62]

Viruses. See under Microorganisms.

Z-protein. This protein is normally present in the Z band of striated muscle. It has been detected in cases of rhabdomyosarcoma, but it does not seem to offer particular advantages over the other skeletal muscle markers.[150]

· · ·

This is a long list indeed. Few laboratories will be expected to offer all these techniques, many of which are of only minimal diagnostic value.

The standard surgical pathology laboratory will be well served by acquiring the following selection of antibodies, obviously to be modified according to the type of material handled:

Top choice
    Actin
    Alpha-fetoprotein
    Calcitonin
    Chromogranin
    Desmin
    EMA
    FVIII-related antigen
    GFAP
    hCG
    Immunoglobulins
    Keratin (cocktail)
    LCA
    Myoglobin
    Neurofilaments
    PSA
    S-100 protein
    Vimentin

Desirable
    Alkaline phosphatase (placental)
    Alpha-lactalbumin
    B- and T-cell markers
    CEA
    Leu-M1
    Lysozyme
    Microorganisms (for selected viruses)
    NSE
    PAP
    Peptide hormones (selected ones)
    Synaptophysin
    Thyroglobulin
    Ulex europeaus I lectin

Optional
    All the others

The first choice antibodies should equip the surgical pathologist with the tools needed to tackle the most common diagnostic problems in tumor pathology, including that which epitomizes them all, i.e., the characterization of the undifferentiated or poorly differentiated malignant tumor, whether primary or metastatic.[63,84,97] Antibody panels are used in some laboratories to standardize the immunohistochemical search depending on the nature of the problem.[63] Thus an adenocarcinoma versus mesothelioma panel may consist of stains for keratin, CEA, EMA, and Leu-M1. The preparation of these prepackaged formulas is useful in a well-defined situation such as the one just described, but the number of permutations is so large that it would be impractical and perhaps even undesirable to attempt to devise a list of panels that would cover most eventualities.

FLOW CYTOMETRY

The rapidly expanding field of flow cytometry consists of the simultaneous measurement of several parameters while a suspension of cells flows through a beam of light past stationary detectors.[198,200,202] The instrument focuses hydrodynamically a cell suspension in a sample chamber and passes single cells through a light source, usually a laser. The light scattered at various angles by the cells is registered by detectors and converted to electronic signals, which are then digitized, stored, and analyzed by the computer to produce a histogram (Fig. 3-4). This technique allows the analysis of 5,000 to 10,000 cells per second. Cellular features that can be evaluated with flow cytometry include cell size, cytoplasmic granularity, cell viability, cell cycle time, DNA content, surface marker phenotype, and enzyme content.

The main limitation of flow cytometry is that cells need to be in a single-cell suspension in order to be analyzed. This requirement is easily achieved in blood and other fluids; indeed, flow cytometric analysis of leukemias and lymphomas has become routine in many institutions.[201] Obtaining satisfactory samples from nonhematopoietic solid tumors is more difficult, but suitable techniques have been developed for most. As a matter of fact, flow cytometric DNA analysis can even be performed on nuclear suspensions recovered from thick sections of routine formalin-fixed, paraffin-embedded tissue blocks[199] with results remarkably similar to those obtained using fresh tissues.[200a] (Fig. 3-5). The potential of this technical development for the performance of large scale retrospective studies is obvious.

At present, the main clinical uses of flow cytometry in solid tumors are to (1) support a diagnosis of malignancy when the morphologic changes are equivocal, (2) subclassify lesions of borderline malignancy, (3) provide prognostic information independent of stage and grade, (4) monitor response to therapy, (5) establish the development of tumor relapse, (6) establish the origin of synchronous or metachronous tumors.

Flow cytometric studies have already been performed in a large variety of tumors, particularly carcinomas of urinary bladder and large bowel; these are discussed in the respective chapters.

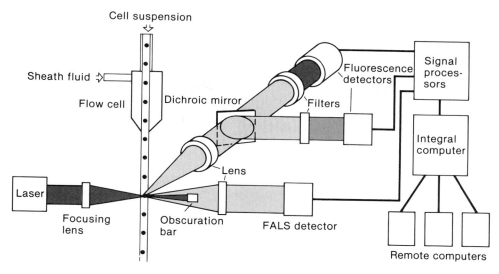

Fig. 3-4 Schematic representation of a modern flow cytometer suitable for clinical work. Stained cells enter the flow chamber where they pass into the center of a stream of sheath fluid in single file. They are then struck by a focused laser beam and emit scattered and fluorescent light, which is separated according to wavelength by appropriate mirrors and filters. An obscuration bar protects the forward angle light scatter (FALS) detector from exposure to the direct laser beam. Only two fluorescence detectors are shown, for sake of simplicity, but a typical instrument has three or four such detectors, one of which can be used to measure laser light scattered perpendicular to the laser beam by the cells. Signals from the detectors pass to amplifying processors and then to the integral (on-board) computer, which digitizes the signals, stores, and displays them. Detailed analysis of the data is often most efficiently done with stand-alone computers. (From Coon JS, Landay AL, Weinstein RS: Biology of disease. Advances in flow cytometry for diagnostic pathology. Lab Invest **57:**453-479, 1987, copyright by U.S. and Canadian Academy of Pathology.)

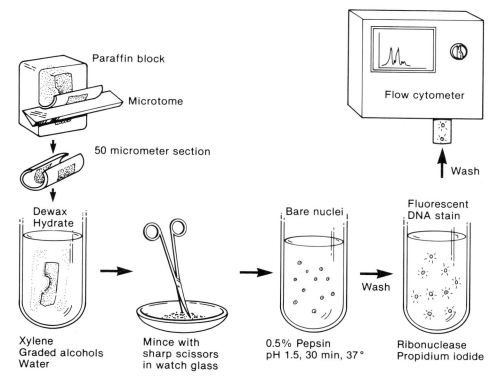

Fig. 3-5 Method of preparing paraffin-embedded tissue for flow cytometry. (From Coon JS, Landay AL, Weinstein RS: Biology of disease. Advances in flow cytometry for diagnostic pathology. Lab Invest **57:**453-479, 1987, copyright by U.S. and Canadian Academy of Pathology.)

NUCLEIC ACIDS HYBRIDIZATION

Hybridization techniques based on the application of recombinant DNA technology represents the latest transfer of basic research methods to diagnostic surgical pathology.[205,208a] The original probes used were nick-translated DNA preparations, but this was soon followed by the use of synthetic oligodeoxyribonucleotides, single stranded cDNA, and single stranded antisense RNA. The labeling of the probes is usually done by the incorporation of radionucleotides, but nonradioactive labeling—particularly with biotin and with bromodeoxyuridine—is being increasingly used[203a,206,209a] (Fig. 3-6). At the present time, the application of this technique to diagnostic pathology has been mainly in the analysis of infections, such as those produced by viruses, *Legionella, Mycoplasma pneumoniae,* and *Mycobacterium avium.*[204a,207,209b,209c] Visualization of mRNA in tumor cells is gaining increasing attention as a means to detect specific gene expression, particularly that encoded by oncogenes and neuroendocrine genes.

Two major techniques are used:

   1 *The transfer method.* In this technique the nucleic acid is isolated, subjected to electrophoresis on a poly-acrylamide gel, blotted to nitrocellulose, hybridized with the probe, and demonstrated with the appropriate label (Fig. 3-7). The procedure used for the hybridization of denatured DNA with a complementary nucleic acid is known as Southern blotting and that used to hybridize RNA to complementary DNA is referred to as Northern blotting.[205]

   2 *In situ hybridization.* This technique allows the visualization of cellular DNA or RNA in tissue sections, single cells, or chromosome preparations.[209] The advantages over the transfer method are that it can be applied to very small samples and in some instances to paraffin-embedded material and that it allows detection of the reaction product in specific cells, subsets of cells, or even subcellular areas. Thus it allows a close correlation between the reaction and the morphologic appearance.[205]

In the case of peptide hormones, the advantage of in situ hybridization over immunohistochemistry is that it demonstrates the amount of specific mRNA present. Instead, immunohistochemical techniques demonstrate the amount of peptide present and are therefore dependent on the degree

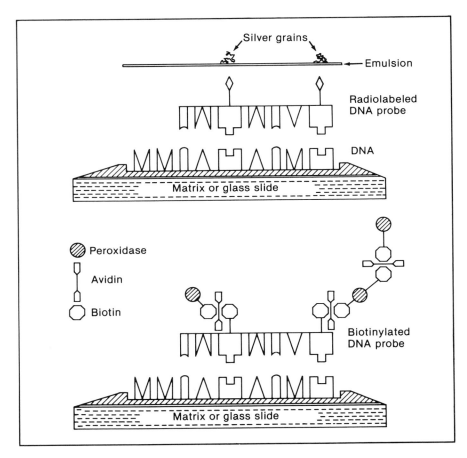

Fig. 3-6 Hybridization procedure. *Top,* Developed by autoradiograph using radiolabeled probe. *Bottom,* Biotin-labeled probe detected by avidin-biotin reaction. (From Fenoglio-Preiser CM, Willman CL: Molecular biology and the pathologist. General principles and applications. Arch Pathol Lab Med **111**:601-619, copyright 1987, American Medical Association.)

of secretion, intracellular degradation, transport, and post-translational processing of the peptide. Incidentally, in situ hybridization can be combined with immunohistochemistry in the same section in order to provide maximum information on the localization of gene products, together with mRNA encoding the specific product.[204]

Another rapidly expanding application of nucleic acids hybridization is in the evaluation of oncogenes. These are pieces of host cellular genomes (protooncogenes or cellular oncogenes) that have been either affected in situ by viral gene insertion or transduced by an RNA/retrovirus.[203,210] Approximately twenty oncogenes have been identified. The functions of the protein products of these oncogenes are closely related to those of proteins involved in normal cell regulatory and cycle activities. The three major groups of oncogenes are (1) those encoding nuclear proteins that probably regulate gene expression; these are known as c-myc, c-myb, and c-fos; (2) those encoding proteins that are bound to the cell membrane and which bind GDP or GTP; these are known as c-ras; and (3) those encoding cytoplasmic protein kinases that transfer phosphate groups from ATP to tyrosine or other aminoacid residues in proteins; these constitute a large group, some representing growth factor receptors (c-erb, c-ros, c-fms, etc.) and others of unknown specificity (c-src, c-abl, c-mos, c-fgr, c-fes, c-raf, c-yes). Whether these products are necessary for neoplastic transformation still needs to be demonstrated, but there is good evidence that they play a role in the transformation process. Information is also accumulating indicating a correlation between the expression of some oncogenes and the aggressiveness of the neoplasm.[203]

The number of potentially useful probes is growing rapidly and therefore we should expect a marked increase in the application of this technique in future years.[208,211]

Another important application of nucleic acid hybridization is the study of gene rearrangements in lymphoid diseases. These rearrangements, which are a normal feature of B and T lymphocytes, are used to determine the monoclonal versus polyclonal nature of a proliferation. They are detected by Southern blotting hybridization techniques and are further discussed in Chapter 21.

OTHER METHODS FOR ANALYSIS OF CELL PROLIFERATION

In addition to flow cytometry, several other methods are available for the evaluation of the degree of cellular proliferation in tumor tissue.

The older and still widely used method is *mitotic count* in routinely processed sections, the standard figure employed being the number of mitoses in a certain number (usually ten) of consecutive "high-power" fields (the combination of $10\times$ eyepiece and $40\times$ objective). The method has found its most useful application in the evaluation of mesenchymal neoplasms, particularly uterine smooth mus-

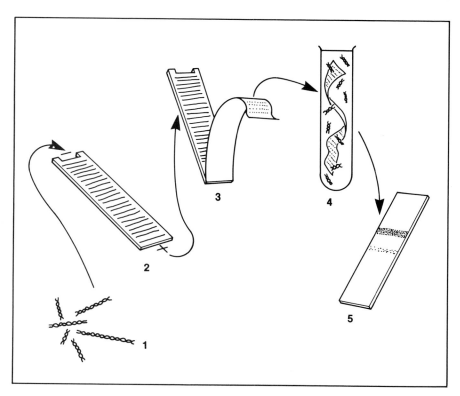

Fig. 3-7 Steps in Southern blot procedure: *(1)*, isolation of DNA; *(2)*, polyacrylamide gel electrophoresis; *(3)*, blotting to nitrocellulose; *(4)*, hybridization with probe; and *(5)*, final product. (From Fenoglio-Preiser CM, Willman CL: Molecular biology and the pathologist. General principles and applications. Arch Pathol Lab Med **111:**601-619, copyright 1987, American Medical Association.)

cle tumors. Despite its apparent objectivity, it is subject to considerable variations depending on the thickness of the section, fields chosen, type of microscope used, delay in fixation time, and—most of all—the observer's variability in the identification of mitotic figures.[214,215,217,225]

Another time-honored method consists in counting nuclei in S (DNA synthesis) phase following in vitro *thymidine labeling*,[221] paraffin embedding, and radioautography. The determination of the TLI (thymidine labeling index) is done by counting 2,000 tumor nuclei.[220] This method has been used extensively in the study of breast carcinoma; it has been found that patients with carcinomas with high TLI have an increased incidence of early recurrence and early death.[222] There is a good correlation between the results obtained with thymidine labeling and flow cytometry[219]; since the latter method offers several important advantages over the former, it is likely to replace it for the study of most neoplasms.

Microspectrophotometric analysis is performed by staining tissue sections obtained from paraffin-embedded material with the Feulgen reaction (which is specific for DNA) and determining the DNA content (expressed in arbitrary units) in a microspectrophotometer using a single wavelength of 560 μm.[227] This tedious technique has been largely replaced by flow cytometry, but it is still being used by some authors.[228]

Cell proliferation can also be investigated with *immunohistochemical techniques* by searching for nuclear antigens related to cell growth and division. Bromodeoxyuridine is a thymidine analogue capable of being incorporated into nuclear DNA during the S-phase and subsequently detectable by the use of monoclonal antibodies.[218] The recently described Ki-67 is a monoclonal antibody that binds to nuclear antigens expressed by cells in the proliferative phases G1, G2, M, and S.[215a,216,219a] Proliferating cell nuclear antigen (PCNA, cyclin) is one of several cycle-related nuclear proteins that is maximally elevated in late G1 and S phases of proliferating cells.[224] Some markers of cell activation can also be detected with more conventional techniques; for instance, nucleolar organizer region–associated proteins, demonstrable with a simple silver technique,[223] have been found to correlate closely to the type and grade of melanocytic, lymphoid, and mammary neoplasms.[212-213b,226]

REFERENCES

1 Gonzalez-Crussi F: Significance of gene rearrangement (Letter to the editor). Am J Surg Pathol 11:491-492, 1987.
2 Masson P: Human tumors. Histology, diagnosis and technique, ed 2. Detroit, 1970, Wayne State University Press.

SPECIAL STAINS

2a Azzopardi JG: Problems in breast pathology. Philadelphia, 1979, W.B. Saunders Co., p. 373.
2b Bottone EJ: The Gram stain. The century-old quintessential rapid diagnostic test. Lab Med 19:288-291, 1988.
3 Carson FL, Kingsley WB: Nonamyloid green birefringence following Congo red staining. Arch Pathol Lab Med 104:333-335, 1980.
4 DeLellis RA: Formaldehyde-induced fluorescence technique for the demonstration of biogenic amines in diagnostic histopathology. Cancer 28:1704-1710, 1971.

5 Filipe MI: Mucins in the human gastrointestinal epithelium. A review. Invest Cell Pathol 2:195-216, 1979.
6 Foraker AG: The "H-and-E fuddy-dud" and the "histochemical snob." Am J Clin Pathol 33:439-440, 1960.
7 Laurén PA, Sorvari TE: Mucicarmine staining in the histochemistry of mucosubstances. Scand J Clin Lab Invest 21(Suppl 101):45-46, 1968.
8 Marshall PN: Romanowsky-type stains in haematology. Histochem J 10:1-29, 1978.
9 Masson P: Some histological methods. Trichrome stainings and their preliminary technique. J Techn Meth 12:75-90, 1929.
10 Puchtler H, Isler H: The effect of phosphomolybdic acid on the stainability of connective tissues in various dyes. J Histochem 6:265-270, 1958.
11 Reynolds CP, German DC, Weinberg AG, Smith RG: Catecholamine fluorescence and tissue culture morphology. Technics in the diagnosis of neuroblastoma. Am J Clin Pathol 75:275-282, 1981.
12 Smith DM Jr, Haggitt RC: A comparative study of generic stains for carcinoid secretory granules. Am J Surg Pathol 7:61-68, 1983.
13 Vialli M: Argentaffinity and argentophilia. I. A critical review about the technique and the possibilities for histochemical research. Acta Histochem 60:103-120, 1977.
14 Vialli M: Argentaffinity and argentophilia. II. The sensitivity of histochemical argentophilic techniques. Acta Histochem 60:211-227, 1977.

ENZYME HISTOCHEMISTRY

15 Beckstead JH: Alkaline phosphatase histochemistry in human germ cell neoplasms. Am J Surg Pathol 7:341-349, 1983.
16 Beckstead JH: The evaluation of human lymph nodes, using plastic sections and enzyme histochemistry. Am J Clin Pathol 80:131-139, 1983.
17 Beckstead JH, Halverson PS, Ries CA, Bainton DF: Enzyme histochemistry and immunohistochemistry on biopsy specimens of pathologic human bone marrow. Blood 57:1088-1098, 1981.
18 Cohen MB, Miller TR, Beckstead JH: Enzyme histochemistry and thyroid neoplasia. Am J Clin Pathol 85:668-673, 1986.
18a Duray PH, Kaplow L: A simplified Azo dye method for the demonstration of acid phosphatase in paraffin embedded tissue. J Histotechnol 7:69-72, 1984.
19 Leder L-D: The chloroacetate esterase reaction. A useful means of histological diagnosis of hematological disorders from paraffin sections of skin. Am J Dermatopathol 1:39-42, 1979.
20 Rodriguez HA, McGavran MH: A modified dopa reaction for the diagnosis and investigation of pigment cells. Am J Clin Pathol 52:219-227, 1969.
21 Sobel HJ: Enzyme cytochemistry for the pathologist. A simple method for the ultrastructural study of tissue alterations with the light microscope. Pathol Annu 3:57-104, 1968.
22 Wick MR, Swanson PE, Manivel JC: Placental-like alkaline phosphatase reactivity in human tumors. An immunohistochemical study of 520 cases. Hum Pathol 18:946-954, 1987.

TISSUE CULTURE

23 Cavazzana AO, Miser JS, Jefferson J, Triche TJ: Experimental evidence for a neural origin of Ewing's sarcoma of bone. Am J Pathol 127:507-518, 1987.
23a Cavazzana AO, Navarro S, Noguera R, Triche TJ: Short term tissue culture in the differential diagnosis of small round cell tumors. Modern Pathol 1988 (In press.)
24 Costa J, Rosai J, Philpott GW: Pigmentation of "amelanotic" melanoma in culture. Arch Pathol 95:371-373, 1973.
25 Gaillard P: Growth and differentiation of explanted tissues. Int Rev Cytol 2:331-401, 1953.
26 Giuffrè L, Schreyer M, Mach J-P, Carrel S: Cyclic AMP induces differentiation in vitro of human melanoma cells. Cancer 61:1132-1141, 1988.
27 Ioachim HL: Tissue culture of human tumors. Its use and prospects. Pathol Annu 5:217-256, 1970.
28 Murray MR, Stout AP: Distinctive characteristics of the sympathicoblastoma cultivated in vitro. A method for prompt diagnosis. Am J Pathol 23:429-441, 1947.
29 Murray MR, Stout AP: The classification and diagnosis of human tumors by tissue culture methods. Tex Rep Biol Med 12:898-915, 1954.
30 Ozzello L, Stout AP, Murray MR: Cultural characteristics of malignant histiocytomas and fibrous xanthomas. Cancer 16:331-344, 1963.
31 Peltonen J, Jaakkola S, Virtanen I, Pelliniemi L: Perineurial cells in culture. An immunocytochemical and electron microscopic study. Lab Invest 57:480-488, 1987.

32 Reynolds CP, German DC, Weinberg AG, Smith RG: Catecholamine fluorescence and tissue culture morphology. Technics in the diagnosis of neuroblastoma. Am J Clin Pathol **75**:275-282, 1981.

33 Stout AP, Murray MR: Localized pleural mesothelioma. Investigation of its characteristics and histogenesis by the method of tissue culture. Arch Pathol **34**:951-964, 1942.

QUANTITATIVE METHODS (HISTOMETRY)

34 Baak JPA, Kurver PHJ, Boon ME: Computer-aided application of quantitative microscopy in diagnostic pathology. Pathol Annu **17**(Pt 2):287-306, 1982.

34a Bacus S, Flowers JL, Press MF, Bacus JW, McCarty KS Jr: The evaluation of estrogen receptor in primary breast carcinoma by computer assisted image analysis. Am J Clin Pathol 1988 (In press.)

35 Beck JS, Anderson JM: Quantitative methods as an aid to diagnosis in histopathology. Rec Adv Histopathol **13**:255-269, 1987.

X-RAY MICROANALYSIS

36 Bretschneider A, Burns W, Morrison A: "Pop-off" technique. The ultrastructure of paraffin-embedded sections. Am J Clin Pathol **76**:450-453, 1981.

37 Terzakis JA: X-ray microanalysis. Problem solving in surgical pathology. Pathol Annu **20**(Pt 2):59-81, 1985.

ELECTRON MICROSCOPY

38 Battifora H, Applebaum EL: Electron microscopy in the diagnosis of head and neck tumors. Head Neck Surg **1**:202-212, 1979.

39 Bonikos DS, Bensch KG, Kempson RL: The contribution of electron microscopy to the differential diagnosis of tumors. Beitr Pathol **158**:417-444, 1976.

40 Bretschneider A, Burns W, Morrison A: "Pop-off" technique. The ultrastructure of paraffin-embedded sections. Am J Clin Pathol **76**:450-453, 1981.

41 Erlandson RA: Diagnostic transmission electron microscopy of human tumors. The interpretation of submicroscopic structures in human neoplastic cells. New York, 1981, Masson Publishing USA, Inc.

42 Erlandson RA: Application of transmission electron microscopy to human tumor diagnosis. An historical perspective. Cancer Invest **5**:487-505, 1987.

43 Fisher C, Ramsay AD, Griffiths M, McDougall J: An assessment of the value of electron microscopy in tumour diagnosis. J Clin Pathol **38**:403-408, 1985.

44 Ghadially FN: Diagnostic electron microscopy of tumours, ed 2. London, 1985, Butterworths.

45 Gyorkey F, Min K-W, Krisko I, Gyorkey, P: The usefulness of electron microscopy in the diagnosis of human tumors. Hum Pathol **6**:421-441, 1975.

46 Hammar S, Bockus D, Remington F: Metastatic tumors of unknown origin. An ultrastructural analysis of 265 cases. Ultrastruct Pathol **11**:209-250, 1987.

47 Harris M: Differential diagnosis of spindle cell tumours by electron microscopy. Personal experience and a review. Histopathology **5**:81-105, 1981.

48 Henderson DW, Papadimitriou JM: Ultrastructural appearances of tumors. A diagnostic atlas, ed 2. New York, 1986, Churchill Livingstone.

49 Johannessen JV (ed): Electron microscopy in human medicine. Vols. I-IIb. London, 1978-1982, McGraw-Hill Book Co.

49a Koss LG: Electron microscopy in cytology. Acta Cytol [Baltimore] **3**:195-196, 1985.

50 Mackay B, Osborne BM: The contribution of electron microscopy to the diagnosis of tumors. In Ioachin IH (ed): Pathobiology annual, vol. 8. New York, 1978, Raven Press, pp. 359-405.

51 Mackay B, Silva EG: Diagnostic electron microscopy in oncology. Pathol Annu **15**:(Pt 2)241-270, 1980.

52 Morales AR: Electron microscopy of human tumors. In Fenoglio CM, Wolff M (eds): Progress in surgical pathology, vol. 1. New York, 1980, Masson Publishing USA, Inc., pp. 51-70.

53 Regezi JA, Batsakis JC: Diagnostic electron microscopy of head and neck tumors. Arch Pathol Lab Med **102**:8-14, 1978.

54 Rosai J, Rodriguez HA: Application of electron microscopy to the differential diagnosis of tumors. Am J Clin Pathol **50**:555-562, 1968.

55 Russo J, Tait L, Russo IH: Current basis for the ultrastructural clinical diagnosis of tumors. A review. J Electron Microsc Tech **2**:305-351, 1985.

56 Trump BF, Jones RT (eds): Diagnostic electron microscopy, vols. 1-4. New York, 1978-1980, 1983, John Wiley & Sons.

57 Wang N-S, Minassian H: The formaldehyde-fixed and paraffin-embedded tissues for diagnostic transmission electron microscopy. A retrospective and prospective study. Hum Pathol **18**:715-727, 1987.

58 Williams MJ, Uzman BG: Uses and contributions of diagnostic electron microscopy in surgical pathology. A study of 20 Veterans Administration hospitals. Hum Pathol **15**:738-745, 1984.

IMMUNOHISTOCHEMISTRY

59 Adams RL, Springall DR, Levene MM: The immunocytochemical detection of herpes simplex virus in cervical smears. A valuable technique for routine use. J Pathol **143**:241-247, 1984.

60 Albores-Saavedra J, Nadji M, Civantos F, Morales AR: Thyroglobulin in carcinoma of the thyroid. Hum Pathol **14**:62-66, 1983.

61 Ariza A, Bilbao JM, Rosai J: Immunohistochemical detection of epithelial membrane antigen in normal perineurial cells and perineurioma. Am J Surg Pathol 1988 (In press.)

62 Azumi N, Battifora H: The distribution of vimentin and keratin in epithelial and nonepithelial neoplasms. A comprehensive immunohistochemical study on formalin- and alcohol-fixed tumors. Am J Clin Pathol **88**:286-296, 1987.

62a Barsky SH, Rao CN, Grotendorst GR, Liotta LA: Increased content of type V collagen in desmoplasia of human breast carcinoma. Am J Pathol **108**:276-283, 1982.

63 Battifora H: Recent progress in the immunohistochemistry of solid tumors. Semin Diagn Pathol **1**:251-271, 1984.

64 Battifora H: The multitumor (sausage) tissue block. Novel method for immunohistochemical antibody testing. Lab Invest **55**:244-248, 1986.

65 Battifora H: Clinical applications of the immunohistochemistry of filamentous proteins. Am J Surg Pathol **12**(Suppl 1):24-42, 1988.

66 Baylin SB, Abeloff MD, Wieman KC, Tomford JW, Ettinger DS: Elevated histaminase (diamine oxidase) activity in small-cell carcinoma of the lung. N Engl J Med **293**:1286-1290, 1975.

67 Beckstead JH: Alkaline phosphatase histochemistry in human germ cell neoplasms. Am J Surg Pathol **7**:341-349, 1983.

67a Bergeron C, Ferenczy A, Shyamala G: Distribution of estrogen receptors in various cell types of normal, hyperplastic, and neoplastic human endometrial tissues. Lab Invest **58**:338-345, 1988.

68 Bohn H, Inaba N, Luben G: New placental proteins and their potential diagnostic significance as tumor markers. Oncodev Biol Med **2**:141-153, 1980.

69 Bostwick DG, Null WE, Holmes D, Weber E, Barchas JD, Bensch KG: Expression of opioid peptides in tumors. N Engl J Med **317**:1439-1443, 1987.

70 Brooks JJ: Immunohistochemistry of soft tissue tumors. Myoglobin as a tumor marker for rhabdomyosarcoma. Cancer **50**:1757-1763, 1982.

71 Brown DC, Theaker JM, Banks PM, Gatter KC, Mason DY: Cytokeratin expression in smooth muscle and smooth muscle tumours. Histopathology **11**:477-486, 1987.

72 Buffa R, Crivelli O, Fiocca R, Fontana P, Solcia E: Complement-mediated unspecific binding of immunoglobulins to some endocrine cells. Histochemistry **63**:15-21, 1979.

73 Burgdorf WHC, Duray P, Rosai J: Immunohistochemical identification of lysozyme in cutaneous lesions of alleged histiocytic nature. Am J Clin Pathol **75**:162-167, 1981.

74 Carcangiu ML, Sibley RK, Rosai J: Clear cell change in primary thyroid tumors. A study of 38 cases. Am J Surg Pathol **9**:705-722, 1985.

74a Charpin C, Lachard A, Pourreau-Schneider N, Jaquemier J, Lavaut MN, Andonian C, Martin PM, Toga M: Localization of lactoferrin and nonspecific cross-reacting antigen in human breast carcinomas. An immunohistochemical study using the avidin-biotin-peroxidase complex method. Cancer **55**:2612-2617, 1985.

75 Chejfec G, Falkmer S, Grimelius L, Jacobsson B, Rodensjö M, Wiedenmann B, Franke WW, Lee I, Gould VE: Synaptophysin. A new marker for pancreatic neuroendocrine tumors. Am J Surg Pathol **11**:241-247, 1987.

75a Chess Q, Hajdu SI: The role of immunoperoxidase staining in diagnostic cytology. Acta Cytol [Baltimore] **30**:1-7, 1985.

76 Clark HB: Immunohistochemistry of nervous system antigens. Diagnostic applications in surgical neuropathology. Semin Diagn Pathol **1**:309-316, 1984.

77 Clark HB, Minesky JJ, Agrawal D, Agrawal HC: Myelin basic protein and P2 protein are not immunohistochemical markers for Schwann cell neoplasms. A comparative study using antisera. Am J Pathol **121**:96-101, 1985.

78 Clayton F, Ordóñez NG, Hanssen GM, Hanssen H: Immunoperoxidase localization of lactalbumin in malignant breast neoplasms. Arch Pathol Lab Med **106**:268-270, 1982.

78a Cohen C, Berson SD, Shulman G, Budgeon LR: Immunohistochemical ferritin in hepatocellular carcinoma. Cancer **53**:1931-1935, 1984.

78b Cooper D, Schermer A, Sun T-T: Classification of human epithelia and their neoplasms using monoclonal antibodies to keratins. Strategies, applications, and limitations. Lab Invest **52**:243-256, 1985.

79 Corson JM, Pinkus GS: Intracellular myoglobin. A specific marker for skeletal muscle differentiation in soft tissue sarcomas. An immunoperoxidase study. Am J Pathol **103**:384-389, 1981.

80 Craig SS, DeBlois G, Schwartz LB: Mast cells in human keloid, small intestine, and lung by an immunoperoxidase technique using a murine monoclonal antibody against tryptase. Am J Pathol **124:**427-435, 1986.

80a Crocker J, Jenkins R, Burnett D: Immunohistochemical demonstration of leucocyte elastase in human tissues. J Clin Pathol **37:**1114-1118, 1984.

81 Dale BA: Filaggrin, the matrix protein of keratin. Am J Dermatopathol **7:**65-68, 1985.

82 De Armond SJ, Eng LF, Rubinstein LJ: The application of glial fibrillary acidic (GFA) protein immunohistochemistry in neurooncology. Pathol Res Pract **168:**374-394, 1980.

83 de Jong ASH, van Kessel-van Vark M, Albus-Lutter ChE, Raamsdonk W, Voûte PA: Skeletal muscle actin as tumor marker in the diagnosis of rhabdomyosarcoma in childhood. Am J Surg Pathol **9:**467-474, 1985.

84 DeLellis RA, Dayal Y: The role of immunohistochemistry in the diagnosis of poorly differentiated malignant neoplasms. Semin Oncol **14:**173-192, 1987.

85 DeLellis RA, Kwan P: Technical considerations in the immunohistochemical demonstration of intermediate filaments. Am J Surg Pathol **12**(Suppl 1):17-23, 1988.

86 Delsol G, Stein H, Pulford KAF, Gatter KC, Erber WN, Zinne K, Mason DY: Human lymphoid cells express epithelial membrane antigen. Implications for diagnosis of human neoplasms. Lancet **2:**1124-1129, 1984.

87 Denk H, Krepler R, Artlieb U, Gabbiani G, Rungger-Brändle E, Leoncini P, Franke WW: Proteins of intermediate filaments. An immunohistochemical and biochemical approach to the classification of soft tissue tumors. Am J Pathol **110:**193-208, 1983.

88 DeSchryver-Kecskemeti K, Kraus FT, Engleman W, Lacy PE: Alveolar soft-part sarcoma. A malignant angioreninoma. Histochemical, immunocytochemical, and electron-microscopic study of four cases. Am J Surg Pathol **6:**5-18, 1982.

88a Domagala W, Lubinski J, Weber K, Osborn M: Intermediate filament typing of tumor cells in fine needle aspirates by means of monoclonal antibodies. Acta Cytol [Baltimore] **30:**214-224, 1986.

89 Dranoff G, Bigner DD: A word of caution in the use of neuron-specific enolase expression in tumor diagnosis. Arch Pathol Lab Med **108:**535, 1984.

90 Eusebi V, Bondi A, Rosai J: Immunohistochemical localization of myoglobin in nonmuscular cells. Am J Surg Pathol **8:**51-55, 1984.

91 Facer P, Polak JM, Jaffe BM, Pearse AGE: Immunocytochemical demonstration of 5-hydroxytryptamine in gastrointestinal endocrine cells. Histochem J **11:**117-121, 1979.

92 Faraggiana T, Gresik E, Tanaka T, Inagami T, Lupo A: Immunohistochemical localization of renin in the human kidney. J Histochem Cytochem **30:**459-465, 1982.

93 Ferenczy A, Braun L, Shah KV: Human papillomavirus (HPV) in condylomatous lesions of cervix. A comparative ultrastructural and immunohistochemical study. Am J Surg Pathol **5:**661-670, 1981.

94 Finan PJ, Wight DG, Lennox ES, Sacks SH, Bleehen NM: Human blood group isoantigen expression in normal and malignant gastric epithelium with anti-A and anti-B monoclonal antibodies. J Natl Canc Inst **70:**679-685, 1983.

95 Flanigan RC, King CT, Clark TD, Cash JB, Greenfield B, Sniecinski IJ, Primus FJ: Immunohistochemical demonstration of blood group antigens in neoplastic and normal human urothelium. A comparison with standard red cell adherence. J Urol **130:**499-503, 1983.

96 Foellmer HG, Madri JA, Furthmayr H: Monoclonal antibodies to type IV collagen. Probes for the study of structure and function of basement membranes. Lab Invest **48:**639-649, 1983.

97 Gatter KC, Alcock C, Heryet A, Pulford KA, Heyderman E, Taylor-Papadimitriou J, Stein H, Mason DY: The differential diagnosis of routinely processed anaplastic tumours using monoclonal antibodies. Am J Clin Pathol **82:**33-43, 1984.

98 Gatter KC, Mason DY: The use of monoclonal antibodies for histopathological diagnosis of human malignancy. Semin Oncol **9:**517-525, 1982.

99 Gold P, Shuster J, Freedman SO: Carcinoembryonic antigen (CEA) in clinical medicine. Historical perspectives, pitfalls and projections. Cancer **42:**1399-1405, 1978.

100 Gould VE: Synaptophysin. A new and promising pan-neuroendocrine marker. Arch Pathol Lab Med **111:**791-794, 1987.

100a Greenwalt DE, Johnson VG, Kuhajda FP, Eggleston JC, Mather IH: Localization of a membrane glycoprotein in benign fibrocystic disease and infiltrating duct carcinomas of the human breast with the use of a monoclonal antibody to guinea pig milk fat globule membrane. Am J Pathol **118:**351-359, 1985.

101 Gröne H-J, Weber K, Helmchen U, Osborn M: Villin. A marker of brush border differentiation and cellular origin in human renal cell carcinoma. Am J Pathol **124:**294-302, 1986.

102 Hagn C, Schmid KW, Fischer-Colbrie R, Winkler H: Chromogranin A, B, and C in human adrenal medulla and endocrine tissues. Lab Invest **55:**405-411, 1986.

103 Haimoto H, Hosoda S, Kato K: Differential distribution of immunoreactive S100-α and S100-β proteins in normal nonnervous human tissues. Lab Invest **57:**489-498, 1987.

104 Harris JP, South MA: Secretory component. A glandular epithelial cell marker. Am J Pathol **105:**47-53, 1981.

105 Heitz PU, von Herbay G, Klöppel G, Komminoth P, Kasper M, Höfler H, Müller K-M, Oberholzer M: The expression of subunits of human chorionic gonadotropin (hCG) by nontrophoblastic, nonendocrine, and endocrine tumors. Am J Clin Pathol **88:**467-472, 1987.

105a Herrera GA, Turbat-Herrera EA, Lott RL: S-100 protein expression by primary and metastatic adenocarcinomas. Am J Clin Pathol **89:**168-176, 1988.

106 Heyderman E, Chapman DV, Richardson TC, Calvert I, Rosen S: Human chorionic gonadotropin and human placental lactogen in extragonadal tumors. Cancer **56:**2674-2682, 1985.

106a Hilkens J, Buijs F, Hilgers J, Hageman Ph, Calafat J, Sonnenberg A, van der Valk M: Monoclonal antibodies against human milk-fat globule membranes detecting differentiation antigens of the mammary gland and its tumors. Int J Cancer **34:**197-206, 1984.

106b Howard DR, Taylor CR: A method for distinguishing benign from malignant breast lesions utilizing antibody present in normal human sera. Cancer **43:**2279-2287, 1979.

107 Hsu SM, Raine L, Fanger H: Use of avidin-biotin peroxidase complex (ABC) in immunoperoxidase techniques. A comparison between ABC and unlabeled antibody (PAP) procedures. J Histochem Cytochem **29:**557-580, 1981.

108 Isaacson P: Immunochemical demonstration of J chain. A marker of B-cell malignancy. J Clin Pathol **32:**802-807, 1979.

108a Jacobsen M, Jacobsen GK: The influence of various fixatives on the immunohistochemical demonstration of a number of plasma proteins and oncofetal proteins in paraffin embedded material. Acta Pathol Microbiol Immunol Scand [A] **92:**461-468, 1984.

109 Jothy S, Brazinsky SA, Chin-A-Loy M, Haggarty A, Krantz MJ, Cheung M, Fuks A: Characterization of monoclonal antibodies to carcinoembryonic antigen with increased tumor specificity. Lab Invest **54:**108-117, 1986.

110 Kahn HJ, Marks A, Thom H, Baumal R: Role of antibody to S100 protein in diagnostic pathology. Am J Clin Pathol **79:**341-347, 1983.

111 Kato K, Ishiguro Y, Ariyoshi Y: Enolase isozymes and disease markers. Distribution of three enolase subunits (α, β and γ) in various human tissues. Dis Markers **1:**213-220, 1983.

111a Kawai K, Takahashi H, Ikuta F, Tanimura K, Honda Y, Yamazaki H: The occurrence of catecholamine neurons in a parietal lobe ganglioglioma. Cancer **60:**1532-1536, 1987.

112 Koelma IA, Nap M, Rodenburg CJ, Fleuren GJ: The value of tumour marker CA 125 in surgical pathology. Histopathology **11:**287-294, 1987.

113 Kostyu D, Amos DB: The major histocompatibility complex. Genetic polymorphism and disease susceptibility. In Stanbury JB, et al. (eds): Metabolic basis of inherited disease, ed 5. New York, 1982, McGraw-Hill Book Co., p. 77.

113a Kovacs JA, Ng VL, Masur H, Leoung G, Hadley WK, Evans G, Lane HC, Ognibene FP, Shelhamer J, Parrillo JE, Gill VJ: Diagnosis of *Pneumocystis carinii* pneumonia. Improved detection in sputum with use of monoclonal antibodies. N Engl J Med **318:**589-593, 1988.

114 Kuhajda FP, Bohn H, Mendelsohn G: Pregnancy-specific beta-1 glycoprotein (SP-1) in breast carcinoma. Pathologic and clinical considerations. Cancer **54:**1392-1396, 1984.

115 Kurman RJ, Ganjei P, Nadji M: Contributions of immunocytochemistry to the diagnosis and study of ovarian neoplasms. Int J Gynecol Pathol **3:**3-26, 1984.

116 Kurman RJ, Goebelsmann U, Taylor CR: Localization of steroid hormones in functional ovarian tumors. In DeLellis RA (ed): Diagnostic immunohistochemistry, New York, 1981, Masson Publishing USA, Inc., pp. 137-148.

117 Kurtin PJ, Pinkus GS: Leukocyte common antigen. A diagnostic discriminant between hematopoietic and nonhematopoietic neoplasms in paraffin sections using monoclonal antibodies. Correlation with immunologic studies and ultrastructural localization. Hum Pathol **16:**353-365, 1985.

118 Lazarides E, Granger BL, Gard DL, O'Connor CM, Breckler J, Price M, Danto SI: Desmin- and vimentin-containing filaments and their role in the assembly of the Z disc in muscle cells. Cold Spring Harbor Symp Quant Biol **46:**351-378, 1982.

119 Leader M, Collins M, Patel J, Henry K: Vimentin. An evaluation of its role as a tumour marker. Histopathology 11:63-72, 1987.

120 Leader M, Patel J, Collins M, Henry K: Anti-α1-antichymotrypsin staining of 194 sarcomas, 38 carcinomas, and 17 malignant melanomas. Its lack of specificity as a tumour marker. Am J Surg Pathol 11:133-139, 1987.

120a Lee AK, DeLellis RA, Rosen PP, Herbert-Stanton T, Tallberg K, Garcia C, Wolfe HJ: Alpha-lactalbumin as an immunohistochemical marker for breast carcinomas. Am J Surg Pathol 8:93-100, 1984.

121 Lee AK, DeLellis RA, Rosen PP, Saigo PE, Gangi MD, Bagin R, Groshen S, Wolfe HJ: ABH blood group isoantigen expression in breast carcinomas. An immunohistochemical evaluation using monoclonal antibodies. Am J Clin Pathol 83:308-319, 1985.

122 Lewis RE Jr, Johnson WW, Cruse JM: Pitfalls and caveats in the methodology for immunoperoxidase staining in surgical pathologic diagnosis. Surv Synth Pathol Res 1:134-152, 1983.

123 Li C-Y, Lazcano-Villareal O, Pierre RV, Yam LT: Immunocytochemical identification of cells in serous effusions. Technical considerations. Am J Clin Pathol 88:696-706, 1987.

123a Liddle C, Reid WA, Kennedy JS, Miller ID, Horne HW: Immunolocalization of prealbumin. Distribution in normal human tissue. J Pathol 146:107-113, 1985.

124 Listrom MB, Dalton LW: Comparison of keratin monoclonal antibodies MAK-6, AE1:AE3, and CAM-5.2. Am J Clin Pathol 88:297-301, 1987.

125 Listrom MB, Fenoglio-Preiser CM: Does laminin immunoreactivity really distinguish between lymphatics and blood vessels? Surg Pathol 1:71-74, 1988.

126 Lloyd RV: Immunohistochemical localization of chromogranin in normal and neoplastic endocrine tissues. Pathol Annu 22(Pt 2):69-90, 1987.

126a Lloyd RV, Cano M, Rosa P, Hille A, Huttner WB: Distribution of chromogranin A and secretogranin I (chromogranin B) in neuroendocrine cells and tumors. Am J Pathol 130:296-304, 1988.

127 Loning Th, Kuhler Ch, Caselitz J, Stegner H-E: Keratin and tissue polypeptide antigen profiles of the cervical mucosa. Int J Gynecol Pathol 2:105-112, 1983.

127a Lundqvist M, Wilander E: A simple procedure for immunocytochemical- and silver-staining of endocrine cells in the same section. Acta Pathol Microbiol Immunol Scand [A] 91:493-494, 1983.

127b Mackie EJ, Chiquet-Ehrismann R, Pearson CA, Inaguma Y, Taya K, Kawarada Y, Sakakura T: Tenascin is a stromal marker for epithelial malignancy in the mammary gland. Proc Natl Acad Sci USA 84:4621-4625, 1987.

128 Mason DY, Taylor CR: The distribution of muramidase (lysozyme) in human tissues. J Clin Pathol 28:124-132, 1975.

129 Mazoujian G, Pinkus GS, Davis S, Haagensen DE Jr: Immunohistochemistry of a gross cystic disease fluid protein (GCDFP-15) of the breast. A marker of apocrine epithelium and breast carcinomas. Am J Pathol 110:105-112, 1983.

130 McCarty KS Jr, McCarty KS Sr: Histochemical approaches to steroid receptor analyses. Semin Diagn Pathol 2:297-308, 1984.

131 McCarty KS Jr, Miller LS, Cox EB, Konrath J, McCarty KS Sr: Estrogen receptor analyses. Correlation of biochemical and immunohistochemical methods using monoclonal antireceptor antibodies. Arch Pathol Lab Med 109:716-721, 1985.

132 Mendelsohn G, Eggleston JC, Weisburger WR, Gann DS, Baylin SB: Calcitonin and histaminase in C-cell hyperplasia and medullary thyroid carcinoma. A light microscopic and immunohistochemical study. Am J Pathol 92:35-52, 1978.

132a Mesa-Tejada R, Palakodety RB, Leon JA, Khatcherian AO, Greaton CJ: Immunocytochemical distribution of a breast carcinoma associated glycoprotein identified by monoclonal antibodies. Am J Pathol 130:305-314, 1988.

133 Michels S, Swanson PE, Robb JA, Wick MR: Leu-7 in small cell neoplasms. An immunohistochemical study with ultrastructural correlations. Cancer 60:2958-2964, 1987.

134 Miettinen M, Foidart J-M, Ekblom P: Immunohistochemical demonstration of laminin, the major glycoprotein of basement membranes, as an aid in the diagnosis of soft tissue tumors. Am J Clin Pathol 79:306-311, 1983.

135 Miettinen M, Holthofer H, Lehto V-P, Miettinen A, Virtanen I: Ulex europaeus I lectin as a marker for tumors derived from endothelial cells. Am J Clin Pathol 79:32-36, 1983.

136 Miettinen M, Lehto V-P, Badley RA, Virtanen I: Alveolar rhabdomyosarcoma. Demonstration of the muscle type of intermediate filament protein, desmin, as a diagnostic aid. Am J Pathol 108:246-251, 1982.

137 Miettinen M, Lehto V-P, Virtanen I: Antibodies to intermediate filament proteins in the diagnosis and classification of human tumors. Ultrastruct Pathol 7:83-107, 1984.

138 Mills SE, Stallings RG, Austin MB: Angiomatoid carcinoma of the thyroid gland. Anaplastic carcinoma with follicular and medullary features mimicking angiosarcoma. Am J Clin Pathol 86:674-678, 1986.

139 Mir R, Kahn LB: Immunohistochemistry of Hodgkin's disease. A study of 20 cases. Cancer 52:2064-2071, 1983.

140 Moll R, Cowin P, Kapprell H-P, Franke WW: Desmosomal proteins. New markers for identification and classification of tumors. Lab Invest 54:4-25, 1986.

141 Moll R, Franke WW, Schiller DL, Geiger B, Krepler R: The catalog of human cytokeratins. Patterns of expression in normal epithelia, tumors and cultured cells. Cell 31:11-24, 1982.

142 Moskowitz LB, Ganjei P, Ziegels-Weissman J, Cleary TJ, Penneys NS, Nadji M: Immunohistologic identification of fungi in systemic and cutaneous mycoses. Arch Pathol Lab Med 110:433-436, 1986.

143 Mukai K, Grotting JC, Greider MH, Rosai J: Retrospective study of 77 pancreatic endocrine tumors using the immunoperoxidase method. Am J Surg Pathol 6:387-399, 1982.

144 Mukai K, Rosai J: Applications of immunoperoxidase techniques in surgical pathology. In Wolff M, Fenoglio CM (eds): Progress in surgical pathology, vol. 1. New York, 1980, Masson Publishing USA, Inc., pp. 15-99.

145 Mukai K, Rosai J, Burgdorf WHC: Localization of factor VIII-related antigen in vascular endothelial cells using an immunoperoxidase method. Am J Surg Pathol 4:273-276, 1980.

146 Mukai K, Rosai J, Hallaway BE: Localization of myoglobin in normal and neoplastic human skeletal muscle cells using an immunoperoxidase method. Am J Surg Pathol 3:373-376, 1979.

147 Mukai K, Schollmeyer JV, Rosai J: Immunohistochemical localization of actin. Applications in surgical pathology. Am J Surg Pathol 5:91-97, 1981.

148 Mukai K, Yoshimura S, Anzai M: Effects of decalcification on immunoperoxidase staining. Am J Surg Pathol 10:413-419, 1986.

149 Mukai M, Iri H, Nakajima T, Hirose S, Torikata C, Kageyama K, Ueno N, Murakami K: Alveolar soft-part sarcoma. A review on its histogenesis and further studies based on electron microscopy, immunohistochemistry, and biochemistry. Am J Surg Pathol 7:679-689, 1983.

150 Mukai M, Iri H, Torikata C, Kageyama K, Morikawa Y, Shimizu K: Immunoperoxidase demonstration of a new muscle protein (Z-protein) in myogenic tumors as a diagnostic aid. Am J Pathol 114:164-170, 1984.

151 Nadji M, Tabei SZ, Castro A, Chu TM, Murphy GP, Wang MC, Morales AR: Prostatic-specific antigen. An immunohistologic marker for prostatic neoplasms. Cancer 48:1229-1232, 1984.

152 Nagle RB: Intermediate filaments. A review of the basic biology. Am J Surg Pathol 12(Suppl 1):4-16, 1988.

153 Nakajima T, Watanabe S, Sato Y, Kameya T, Shimosato Y: An immunoperoxidase study of S-100 protein distribution in normal and neoplastic tissues. Am J Surg Pathol 6:715-727, 1982.

154 Natali PG, deMartino C, Quaranta V, Nicotra R, Frezza F, Pellegrino MA, Ferrone S: Expression of Ia-like antigens in normal human non-lymphoid tissues. Transplantation 31:75-78, 1981.

155 Obinata T, Maruyama K, Sugita H, Kohama K, Ebashi S: Dynamic aspects of structural proteins in vertebrate skeletal muscle. Muscle Nerve 4:456-488, 1981.

156 Ordóñez NG, Brooks T, Thompson S, Batsakis JG: Use of Ulex europaeus agglutinin I in the identification of lymphatic and blood vessel invasion in previously stained microscopic slides. Am J Surg Pathol 11:543-550, 1987.

156a Ormerod MG, Bussolati G, Sloane JP, Steele K, Gugliotta P: Similarities of antisera to casein and epithelial membrane antigen. Virchows Arch [Pathol Anat] 397:327-333, 1982.

157 Osborne M, Weber K: Tumor diagnosis by intermediate filament typing. Lab Invest 48:372-394, 1983.

158 Pahlman S, Esscher T, Nilsson K: Expression of γ-subunit of enolase, neuron-specific enolase, in human non-neuroendocrine tumors and derived cell lines. Lab Invest 54:554-560, 1986.

159 Pascal RR, Santeusanio G, Sarrell D, Johnson CE: Immunohistologic detection of estrogen receptors in paraffin-embedded breast cancers. Correlation with cytosol measurements. Hum Pathol 17:370-375, 1986.

160 Pereira MEA, Kisalus EC, Gruezo G. Kabat EA: Immunohistochemical studies on the combining site of the blood group H-specific lectin I from Ulex europaeus seeds. Arch Biochem Biophys 185:108-115, 1978.

161 Perentes E, Rubinstein LJ: Recent applications of immunoperoxidase histochemistry in human neuro-oncology. An update. Arch Pathol Lab Med 111:796-812, 1987.

162 Perrone T, Frizzera G, Rosai J: Mediastinal diffuse large-cell lymphoma with sclerosis. A clinicopathologic study of 60 cases. Am J Surg Pathol 10:176-191, 1986.

163 Pinkus GS, Kurtin PJ: Epithelial membrane antigen. A diagnostic discriminant in surgical pathology. Immunohistochemical profile in epithelial, mesenchymal, and hematopoietic neoplasms using paraffin sections and monoclonal antibodies. Hum Pathol 16:929-940, 1985.

164 Pinkus GS, Said JW: Intracellular hemoglobin. A specific marker for erythroid cells in paraffin sections. An immunoperoxidase study of normal, megaloblastic, and dysplastic erythropoiesis, including erythroleukemia and other myeloproliferative disorders. Am J Pathol 102:308-313, 1971.

165 Pinkus GS, Said JW: Leu-M1 immunoreactivity in nonhematopoietic neoplasms and myeloproliferative disorders. An immunoperoxidase study of paraffin sections. Am J Clin Pathol 85:278-282, 1986.

166 Press MF, Greene GL: An immunocytochemical method for demonstrating estrogen receptor in human uterus using monoclonal antibodies to human estrophilin. Lab Invest 50:480-486, 1984.

167 Primus FJ, Clark CA, Goldenberg DM: Immunohistochemical detection of carcinoembryonic antigen. In DeLellis RA (ed): Diagnostic immunohistochemistry. New York, 1981, Masson Publishing USA, Inc. p. 263-276.

168 Rabkin MS, Kjeldsberg CR: Epithelial membrane antigen staining patterns of histiocytic lesions. Arch Pathol Lab Med 111:337-338, 1987.

169 Reid WA, Liddle CN, Svasti J, Kay J: Gastricsin in the benign and malignant prostate. J Clin Pathol 38:639-643, 1985.

170 Reiner A, Spona J, Reiner G, Schemper M, Kolb R, Kwasny W, Függer R, Jakesz R, Holzner JH: Estrogen receptor analysis on biopsies and fine-needle aspirates from human breast carcinoma. Correlation of biochemical and immunohistochemical methods using monoclonal antireceptor antibodies. Am J Pathol 125:443-449, 1986.

170a Rooney N, Day C, Gray T, Underwood JCE: Electron microscopic localization of cell-surface markers in tissue sections using monoclonal and gold-conjugated antibodies. J Pathol 148:29-34, 1986.

171 Rosai J, Carcangiu ML: Pitfalls in the diagnosis of thyroid neoplasms. Pathol Res Pract 182:169-179, 1987.

171a Rossiello R, Carriero MV, Giordano GG: Distribution of ferritin, transferrin and lactoferrin in breast carcinoma tissue. J Clin Pathol 37:51-55, 1984.

172 Sadoughi N, Mlsna J, Guinan P, Rubenstone A: Prognostic value of cell surface antigens using immunoperoxidase methods in bladder carcinoma. Urology 20:143-146, 1982.

173 Savino W, Manganella G, Verley J-M, Wolff A, Berrih S, Levasseur P, Binet J-P, Dardenne M, Bach J-F: Thymoma epithelial cells secrete thymic hormone but do not express class II antigens of the major histocompatibility complex. J Clin Invest 76:1140-1146, 1985.

174 Schulz A, Jundt G, Berghäuser K-H, Gehron-Robey P, Termine JD: Immunohistochemical study of osteonectin in various types of osteosarcoma. Am J Pathol, 1988 (In press.)

175 Scupham R, Gilbert EF, Wilde J, Wiedrich TA: Immunohistochemical studies of rhabdomyosarcoma. Arch Pathol Lab Med 110:818-821, 1986.

176 Seshi B, Bell CE Jr: Preparation and characterization of monoclonal antibodies to human neuron-specific enolase. Hybridoma 4:13-25, 1985.

177 Seshi B, True L, Carter D, Rosai J: Immunohistochemical characterization of a set of monoclonal antibodies to human neuron-specific enolase. Am J Pathol 131:258-269, 1988.

178 Sheibani K, Tubbs RR: Enzyme immunohistochemistry. Technical aspects. Semin Diagn Pathol 1:235-250, 1984.

179 Shevchuk MM, Romas NA, Ng PY, Tannenbaum M, Olsson CA: Acid phosphatase localization in prostatic carcinoma. A comparison of monoclonal antibody to heteroantisera. Cancer 52:1642-1646, 1983.

180 Shintaku IP, Said JW: Detection of estrogen receptors with monoclonal antibodies in routinely processed formalin-fixed paraffin sections of breast carcinoma. Use of DNase pretreatment to enhance sensitivity of the reaction. Am J Clin Pathol 87:161-167, 1987.

180a Singh G, Katyal SL: Surfactant apoprotein immunohistochemistry. In DeLellis RA (ed): Advances in immunohistochemistry, New York, Masson Publishing USA, Inc., pp. 263-275.

180b Skalli O, Gabbiani G, Babai F, Seemayer TA, Pizzolato G, Schürch W: Intermediate filament proteins and actin isoforms as markers for soft tissue tumor differentiation and origin. II. Rhabdomyosarcomas. Am J Pathol 130:515-531, 1988.

181 Sloane JP, Ormerod MG: Distribution of epithelial membrane antigen in normal and neoplastic tissues and its value in diagnostic tumor pathology. Cancer 47:1786-1795, 1981.

182 Solcia E, Capella C, Buffa R, Usellini L, Fiocca R, Sessa F, Tortora O: The contribution of immunohistochemistry to the diagnosis of neuroendocrine tumors. Semin Diagn Pathol 1:285-296, 1984.

183 Stanta G, Carcangiu ML, Rosai J: The biochemical and immunohistochemical profile of thyroid neoplasia. Pathol Annu 23 (Pt 1): 129-157, 1988.

184 Stein BS, Vangore S, Petersen RO, Kendall AR: Immunoperoxidase localization of prostate-specific antigen. Am J Surg Pathol 6:553-557, 1982.

185 Strauchen JA: Lectin receptors as markers of lymphoid cells. I. Demonstration in tissue section by peroxidase technique. Am J Pathol 116:297-304, 1984.

186 Takada Y, Hiwada K, Yokoyama M, Ochi K, Takeuchi M, Kokubu T: Angiotensin converting enzyme. A possible histologic indicator for human renal cell carcinoma. Cancer 56:130-133, 1985.

186a Taylor GM, Cook HT, Sheffield EA, Hanson C, Peart WS: Renin in blood vessels in human pulmonary tumors. An immunohistochemical and biochemical study. Am J Pathol 130:543-551, 1988.

187 Thomas P, Battifora H: Keratins versus epithelial membrane antigen in tumor diagnosis. An immunohistochemical comparison of five monoclonal antibodies. Hum Pathol 18:728-734, 1987.

188 Tsokos M, Howard R, Costa J: Immunohistochemical study of alveolar and embryonal rhabdomyosarcoma. Lab Invest 48:148-155, 1983.

189 Ulrich W, Horvat R, Krisch K: Lectin histochemistry of kidney tumours and its pathomorphological relevance. Histopathology 9:1037-1050, 1985.

190 Van Muijen GNP, Ruiter DJ, Warnaar SO: Coexpression of intermediate filament polypeptides in human fetal and adult tissues. Lab Invest 57:359-369, 1987.

190a Walts AE, Said JW: Specific tumor markers in diagnostic cytology. Immunoperoxidase studies of carcinoembryonic antigen, lysozyme and other tissue antigens in effusions, washes and aspirates. Acta Cytol [Baltimore] 27:408-416, 1983.

190b Walts AE, Said JW, Siegel MB, Banks-Schlegel S: Involucrin, a marker of squamous and urothelial differentiation. An immunohistochemical study on its distribution in normal and neoplastic tissues. J Pathol 145:329-340, 1985.

190c Wang E, Fischman D, Liem RKH, Sun T-T (eds): Intermediate filaments. Ann NY Acad Sci 455:1-829, 1985.

191 Warhol MJ, Antonioli DA, Pinkus GS, Burke L, Rice RH: Immunoperoxidase staining for involucrin. A potential diagnostic aid in cervicovaginal pathology. Hum Pathol 13:1095-1099, 1982.

192 Weinstein RS, Coon J, Alroy J, Davidsohn I: Tissue-associated blood group antigens in human tumors. In DeLellis RA (ed): Diagnostic immunohistochemistry, New York, 1981, Masson Publishing USA, Inc., pp. 239-261.

193 Weiss LM, Trela MJ, Cleary ML, Turner RR, Warnke RA, Sklar J: Frequent immunoglobulin and T-cell receptor gene rearrangements in "histiocytic" neoplasms. Am J Pathol 121:369-373, 1985.

193a Wells CA, Taylor SM, Cuello AC: Argentaffin and argyrophil reactions and serotonin content of endocrine tumours. J Clin Pathol 38:49-53, 1985.

194 Wick MR, Swanson PE, Manivel JC: Placental-like alkaline phosphatase reactivity in human tumors. An immunohistochemical study of 520 cases. Hum Pathol 18:946-954, 1987.

195 Wilson BS, Herzig MA, Lloyd RV: Immunoperoxidase staining for Ia-like antigens in paraffin-embedded tissues from human melanoma and lung carcinoma. Am J Pathol 115:102-116, 1984.

196 Wold LE, Li C-Y, Homburger HA: Localization of the B and M polypeptide subunits of creatine kinase in normal and neoplastic human tissues by an immunoperoxidase technic. Am J Clin Pathol 75:327-332, 1981.

197 Yonezawa S, Maruyama I, Sakae K, Igata A, Majerus PW, Sato E: Thrombomodulin as a marker for vascular tumors. Comparative study with factor VIII and Ulex europaeus I lectin. Am J Clin Pathol 88:405-411, 1987.

197a Zotter S, Lossnitzer A, Kunze K-D, Müller M, Hilkens J, Hilgers J, Hageman P: Epithelial markers for paraffin-embeded human tissues. Immunohistochemistry with monoclonal antibodies against milk fat globule antigens. Virchows Arch [Pathol Anat] 406:237-251, 1985.

FLOW CYTOMETRY

198 Braylan RC: Flow cytometry. Arch Pathol Lab Med 107:1-6, 1983.

199 Coon JS, Landay AL, Weinstein RS: Flow cytometric analysis of paraffin embedded tumors. Implications for diagnostic pathology. Hum Pathol 17:435-437, 1986.

200 Coon JS, Landay AL, Weinstein RS: Biology of disease. Advances in flow cytometry for diagnostic pathology. Lab Invest 57:453-479, 1987.

200a Frierson HF Jr: Flow cytometric analysis of ploidy in solid neoplasms. Comparison of fresh tissues with formalin-fixed paraffin-embedded specimens. Hum Pathol 19:290-294, 1988.

201 Krause JR, Penchansky L, Contis L, Kaplan SS: Flow cytometry in the diagnosis of acute leukemia. Am J Clin Pathol 89:341-346, 1988.

202 Lovett EJ III, Schnitzer B, Keren DF, Flint A, Hudson JL, McClatchey KD: Application of flow cytometry to diagnostic pathology. Lab Invest 50:115-140, 1984.

NUCLEIC ACIDS HYBRIDIZATION

203 Bartow SA: Oncogenes and surgical pathology. Semin Diagn Pathol **4:**194-199, 1987.

203a Crum CP, Nuovo G, Friedman D, Silverstein SJ: A comparison of biotin and isotope-labeled ribonucleic acid probes for in situ detection of HPV-16 ribonucleic acid in genital precancers. Lab Invest **58:**354-359, 1988.

204 DeLellis RA, Wolfe HJ: New techniques in gene product analysis. Arch Pathol Lab Med **111:**620-627, 1987.

204a Enns RK: DNA probes. An overview and comparison with current methods. Lab Med **19:**295-300, 1988.

205 Fenoglio-Preiser CM, Willman CL: Molecular biology and the pathologist. General principles and applications. Arch Pathol Lab Med **111:**601-619, 1987.

206 Grody WW, Cheng L, Lewin KJ: Application of in situ DNA hybridization technology to diagnostic surgical pathology. Pathol Annu **22**(Pt 2):151-175, 1987.

207 Grody WW, Cheng L, Lewin KJ: In situ viral DNA hybridization in diagnostic surgical pathology. Hum Pathol **18:**535-543, 1987.

208 Höfler H: What's new in "in situ hybridization." Pathol Res Pract **182:**421-430, 1987.

208a Lambert WC: Beyond hybridomas. Cell identification by in situ nucleic acid hybridization. Am J Dermatopathol **10:**144-154, 1988.

209 Lloyd RV: Use of molecular probes in the study of endocrine diseases. Hum Pathol **18:**1199-1211, 1987.

209a Masih AS, Linder J, Shaw BW Jr, Wood RP, Donovan JP, White R, Markin RS: Rapid identification of cytomegalovirus in liver allograft biopsies by in situ hybridization. Am J Surg Pathol **12:**362-367, 1988.

209b Niedobitek G, Finn T, Herbst H, Bornhoft G, Gerdes J, Stein H: Detection of viral DNA by in situ hybridization using bromodeoxyuridine-labeled DNA probes. Am J Pathol **131:**1-4, 1988.

209c Pfaller MA: Laboratory diagnosis of infections due to *Legionella* species. Practical application of DNA in the clinical microbiology laboratory. Lab Med **19:**301-304, 1988.

210 Sherr CJ, Douglass EC: Oncogenes and cytogenic anomalies in tumor cells. In Finegold M (ed): Pathology of neoplasia in children and adolescents. Philadelphia, 1986, W.B. Saunders Co., pp. 18-30.

211 Sklar J: DNA hybridization in diagnostic pathology. Hum Pathol **16:**654-658, 1985.

OTHER METHODS FOR ANALYSIS OF CELL PROLIFERATION

212 Crocker J, Nar P: Nucleolar organizer regions in lymphomas. J Pathol **151:**111-118, 1987.

213 Crocker J, Skilbeck N: Nucleolar organizer regions in melanotic lesions of the skin. A quantitative study. J Clin Pathol **40:**885-889, 1987.

213a Derenzini M, Betts CM, Ceccarelli C, Eusebi V: Ultrastructural organization of nucleoli in benign naevi and malignant melanomas. Virchows Arch [Cell Pathol] **52:**343-352, 1986.

213b Derenzini M, Romagnoli T, Mingazzini P, Marinozzi V: Interphasic nucleolar organizer region distribution as a diagnostic parameter to differentiate benign from malignant epithelial tumors of human intestine. Virchows Arch [Cell Pathol] **54:**334-340, 1988.

214 Donhuijsen K: Mitosis counts. Reproducibility and significance in grading of malignancy. Hum Pathol **17:**1122-1125, 1986.

215 Ellis PSJ, Chir B, Whitehead R: Mitosis counting. A need for reappraisal. Hum Pathol **12:**3-4, 1981.

215a Gerdes J: An immunohistological method for estimating cell growth fractions in rapid histopathological diagnosis during surgery. Int J Cancer **35:**169-171, 1985.

216 Gerdes J, Lemke H, Baisch H, Wacker HH, Schwab U, Stein H: Cell cycle analysis of a cell proliferation-associated human nuclear antigen defined by the monoclonal antibody Ki-67. J Immunol **133:**1710-1715, 1984.

217 Graem N, Helweg-Larsen K: Mitotic activity and delay in fixation of tumour tissue. The influence of delay in fixation on mitotic activity of a human osteogenic sarcoma grown in athymic nude mice. Acta Pathol Microbiol Scand [A] **87:**375-378, 1979.

218 Gratzner HG: Monoclonal antibody to 5-bromo- and 5-iododeoxyuridine. A new reagent for detection of DNA replication. Science **218:**474-475, 1982.

219 McDivitt RW, Stone KR, Craig RB, Meyer JS: A comparison of human breast cancer cell kinetics measured by flow cytometry and thymidine labeling. Lab Invest **52:**287-291, 1985.

219a McGurrin JF, Doria M Jr, Dawson PJ, Karrison T, Stein HO, Franklin WA: Assessment of tumor cell kinetics by immunohistochemistry in carcinoma of breast. Cancer **59:**1744-1750, 1987.

220 Meyer JS: Cell proliferation in normal human breast ducts, fibroadenomas, and other ductal hyperplasias measured by nuclear labeling with tritiated thymidine. Effects of menstrual phase, age, and oral contraceptive hormones. Hum Pathol **8:**67-81, 1977.

221 Meyer JS, Connor RE: In vitro labeling of solid tissues with tritiated thymidine for autoradiographic detection of S-phase nuclei. Stain Technol **52:**185-195, 1977.

222 Meyer JS, Friedman E, McCrate MM, Bauer WC: Prediction of early course of breast carcinoma by thymidine labeling. Cancer **51:**1879-1886, 1983.

223 Ploton D, Menager M, Jeannesson P, Himber G, Pigeon F, Adnet J-J: Improvement in the staining and in the visualization of the argyrophilic proteins of the nucleolar organizer region at the optical level. Histochem J **18:**5-14, 1986.

224 Robbins BA, de la Vega D, Ogata K, Tan EM, Nakamura RM: Immunohistochemical detection of proliferating cell nuclear antigen in solid human malignancies. Arch Pathol Lab Med **111:**841-845, 1987.

225 Silverberg SG: Reproducibility of the mitosis count in the histologic diagnosis of smooth muscle tumors of the uterus. Hum Pathol **7:**451-454, 1976.

226 Smith R, Crocker J: Evaluation of nucleolar organizer region-associated proteins in breast malignancy. Histopathology **12:**113-125, 1988.

227 Swift H, Rasch E: Microspectrophotometry with visible light. In Orster G, Pollister AW: Physical techniques in biological research—cells and tissue, vol. 3. New York, 1966, Academic Press, pp. 354-400.

228 Talerman A, Fu YS, Okagaki T: Spermatocytic seminoma. Ultrastructural and microspectrophotometric observations. Lab Invest **51:**343-349, 1984.

4 Skin

Dermatoses
Tumors and tumorlike conditions

Dermatoses

INTRODUCTION TO DERMATOPATHOLOGY

The entities described in this section are a select group taken from the large number of diseases that affect the skin. They have been chosen to encompass the types of nonneoplastic material generally seen in surgical pathology laboratories. Many of the infrequently biopsied, histologically nonspecific, and rare dermatoses are excluded. Their characteristics are described in texts devoted wholly to dermatopathology and in the dermatologic literature.[1-9]

Isolated morphologic analysis has distinct limitations. These are even more evident in the evaluation of the reactive processes associated with diseases of the skin than in certain other organs. It is imperative that the clinical differential diagnosis be correlated with the gross and microscopic observations in order to render a clinically meaningful diagnosis.

Skin biopsies are often small and have minimal gross changes. Ideally, the lesion should be examined by the pathologist on the patient, but in lieu of this an accurate clinical description and differential diagnosis should accompany each biopsy. All biopsies should be taken from grossly characteristic areas. It is a waste of time and money to biopsy ruptured bullae, secondarily infected or heavily scratched areas, or the incipient or involuting lesion. Multiple biopsies may be advisable when the lesions present differing forms and stages. Formalin, 10% buffered, is an adequate and available fixative. Bouin's and Zenker's fixatives may be used but have no unique merits. Incisional and punch biopsies can be kept from curling during fixation by placing them on a piece of file card prior to immersion. When the specimen is 0.3 mm or less in diameter, it is best processed into paraffin in one piece. It may then be sampled at various levels in the block. This prevents loss of tissue during the facing-up of the block and allows more adequate sampling. These technical niceties prevent delays, mishaps, and some mistakes.

NORMAL HISTOLOGY

The integument is formed by the epidermis and dermis. Within the dermis are the adnexa, the eccrine and apocrine sweat glands, sebaceous glands, and hair follicles. The regional variations in distribution of the adnexa and the character of the epidermis should be remembered.

The *epidermis* is formed by several layers of cells that differentiate to form the outer protective layer of keratin. Alterations in the pattern and process of keratinization are often produced by disease. All of the epidermal cells are derived from the layer of basal cells. These basal cells are set upon, interdigitate with, and are attached to a basement membrane by hemidesmosomes. The dermoepidermal junction is thrown into undulating folds of interlocking ridges of epidermis, *rete ridges*, and dermal papillae. Thus the undersurface of the epidermis seen in whole mounts presents an anastomosing and reticulated pattern of ridges and valleys. The pattern and size of these ridges vary from area to area. With age, they diminish in size, and the dermoepidermal junction becomes flattened.

The basal cells have a moderately basophilic cytoplasm in which, in contrast to the other epidermal cells, melanin pigment is present. As the cells differentiate, they enter the *stratum spinosum*, lose most of the melanin pigment, and become amphophilic and then eosinophilic. This correlates with the intracytoplasmic accumulation of filaments, which are the precursors of keratin, and a diminution of ribosomes. The cells of the epidermis are attached to each other by focal specializations of their walls called desmosomes. When the cells are separated, as a result of fixation and dehydration or intercellular edema, these areas of attachment are seen via the light microscope as fine spiny bridges. The epidermal cells are not a syncytium, and true intercellular bridges do not exist. Destruction of these attachments causes the cells to lose their cohesiveness. This process, termed *acantholysis,* is seen in pemphigus vulgaris and in some other diseases.

Above the stratum spinosum is a layer of cells containing basophilic keratohyaline granules, the *granular layer*. Immediately above the granular layer, without transition forms, the *stratum corneum* begins. It is formed by flattened eosinophilic ghosts of cells that lack nuclei, keratohyaline granules, and other cytoplasmic organelles. Abnormal keratinization may be manifest by *hyperkeratosis,* in which the stratum corneum is thickened, usually in association with a more prominent granular layer, or by *parakeratosis,* in which the cells of the stratum corneum retain their nuclei and the granular layer is diminished or absent.

Certain descriptive terms are applied to alterations in the pattern of the epidermis. It may become *atrophic* or thinned with age or disease. It may be thickened, and as it proliferates the rete ridges extend deeper into the dermis. This is *acanthosis.* Excessive acanthosis produces a disorganized pattern at the dermoepidermal junction and is termed *pseudoepitheliomatous hyperplasia.* Outward overgrowth of the epidermis accompanied by elongation of the dermal papillae is *papillomatosis.* A degenerative process in which the basal cells become vacuolated, separated, and disorganized is called *liquefactive or hydropic degeneration.* Various combinations of these changes are seen in the dermatoses, and this descriptive jargon allows succinct communication.

Melanocytes are discussed on p. 116.

The *dermis* supports and nourishes the epidermis and adnexa. It contains a sizable vascular plexus and network of sensory and vasomotor nerves that play significant roles in the homeostasis of the organism.[15] The dermis is divided into a superficial papillary layer and a deep reticular layer. Both contain interwoven bands of collagen and elastic fibers bathed in ground substance.[11] Two vascular plexuses are found, one at the junction of the dermis and subcutis and the other in the papillary layer. From the superficial vascular plexus capillary loops extend into the dermal papillae. The details of the anatomic complexities, regional variations, and neurogenic control of the vessels of the skin may be found in the works of Horstman[12] and Winkelmann.[17]

With age, and more so in areas exposed to sunlight, the collagen and elastica undergo structural and tinctorial changes called basophilic degeneration of the collagen and senile elastosis, respectively[14,16] (Fig. 4-1). These changes should not be attributed to some suspect disease and should be differentiated from pathologic connective tissue changes.

The dermis is the site of inflammatory reactions. In normal skin, a few fibrocytes, macrophages, mast cells, and lymphocytes are present. The perivascular and periadnexal spaces and the papillary layer of the dermis are the usual sites in which inflammatory cells aggregate. Certain dermatoses, such as lichen planus and chronic discoid lupus erythematosus, have distinct patterns of inflammatory reaction. Others, such as urticaria pigmentosa, have a specific cellular population. Changes in the nerves, visible in sections stained with hematoxylin-eosin, are infrequent but when present are of note (see Leprosy, p. 58).

The epidermal adnexa are seldom the sites of primary changes. However, diagnostic changes do occur: heterotopias as in nevus sebaceous of Jadassohn, in which apocrine glands are found in the scalp; pigmentation of eccrine gland basement membranes in argyria and hemochromatosis; atrophy, as in scleroderma; duct obstruction with subsequent retention, as in the various forms of miliaria[13]; and deposition of aggregates of granules of mucoprotein in the eccrine gland cells in myxedematous patients.[10]

INFLAMMATORY DISEASES OF KNOWN ETIOLOGY
Viral diseases

The histologically commonly seen viral lesions are warts. However, vesiculobullous lesions caused by herpes simplex and herpes zoster and the varicelliform eruption following vaccination of atopic individuals may occasionally be biopsied. These lesions are formed by ballooning and reticular degeneration of the epidermal cells. The fine points of differentiation were described in the classic work by Ebert and Otsuka.[18] The viruses of herpes, vaccinia, and warts can be detected in the vesicular fluid or tissue by electron microscopy, immunohistochemistry, or in situ hybridization.

Warts

Warts are cutaneous lesions caused by one of the several human papilloma viruses, which are members of the papova group.[23,24,27] Several variants of warts occur.[21] *Verruca vul-*

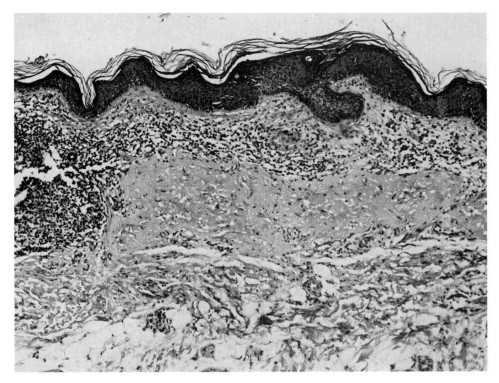

Fig. 4-1 Collagen is clumped and smudged and stains pale blue in this skin from face of 65-year old woman. Mild lymphocytic infiltrate surrounds the area of "basophilic degeneration."

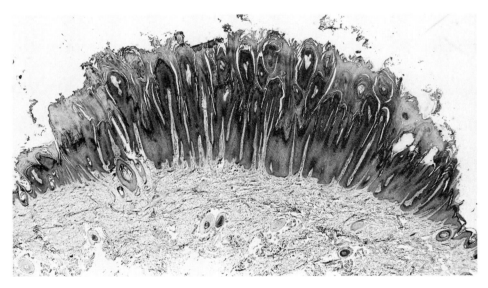

Fig. 4-2 Verruca vulgaris of hand.

garis (generally associated with HPV-2) usually occurs on the hands. It is an elevated, hard, rough, flesh-colored lesion. The top may be peeled off, leaving a pink granular surface. *Verruca plantaris* occurs on the sole of the foot and is covered by a callus. It is often painful. *Verruca plana* (usually associated with HPV-10) is, as its name indicates, a flatter lesion usually seen in crops or clusters on the face and hands. *Condyloma acuminatum* or "venereal wart" (usually caused by HPV-6) occurs around the anus and vulva, on the glans penis, and sometimes in other mucosal membranes such as the oral cavity.

The histologic characteristics of these lesions are those

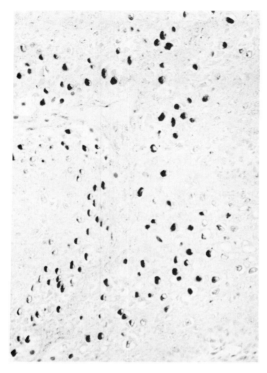

Fig. 4-3 Immunoperoxidase demonstration of papovavirus in nuclei of lesion of verruca vulgaris. (Courtesy Dr. J. Costa, Lausanne, Switzerland.)

of focal epidermal hyperplasia manifest by hyperkeratosis and parakeratosis, varying degrees of acanthosis, and papillomatosis (Fig. 4-2). A trichilemmal type of keratinization may be present.[25] Papillomatosis does not occur in verruca plana. Distinct vacuolization of the cells in the upper portion of the stratum spinosum is a feature in early lesions. These vacuolated cells have pyknotic nuclei and may be seen in the lower portions of the thickened stratum corneum. In condyloma acuminatum, acanthosis may be florid, and tangential cuts can show isolated nests of squamous cells surrounded by inflamed dermis. Care should be taken not to overdiagnose such lesions as squamous carcinoma. Older verrucae may not show the microscopic changes that allow their recognition and appear simply as papillomas or keratoses. Flat warts undergoing involution exhibit marked mononuclear dermal and intraepidermal inflammation, associated with degenerative epidermal changes.[19,20,23] Occasionally, benign or malignant skin tumors of various types are seen in conjunction with the features of verruca vulgaris, suggesting the existence of a causal relationship.[21,26] The viral nuclear inclusions are basophilic, Feulgen-positive, and DNase resistant. They can be demonstrated in formalin-fixed, paraffin-embedded sections with an immunoperoxidase technique[24] (Fig. 4-3). The eosinophilic cytoplasmic masses are not viral but rather accumulations of tonofilaments.

Molluscum contagiosum

Molluscum contagiosum is a skin disease characterized by small, firm, usually multiple nodules that, when fully

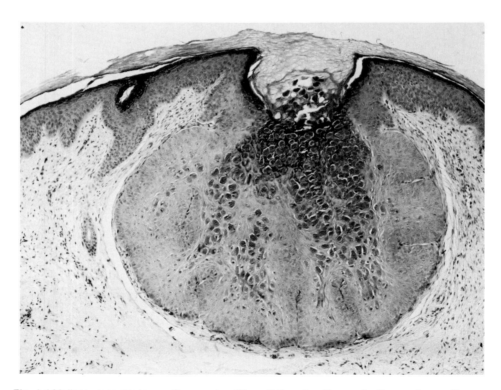

Fig. 4-4 Molluscum contagiosum. Progressive differentiation of molluscum bodies can be readily seen.

developed, have central cores from which white keratinous material can be expressed. The microscopic picture is characteristic (Fig. 4-4). The dermis is indented by a sharply delimited and lobulated mass of proliferating epithelium. As the cells differentiate within the mass, their cytoplasm gradually is filled by a faintly granular eosinophilic inclusion that displaces the nucleus and enlarges the cells. These molluscum bodies are formed of viral particles that are similar in size and mode of formation to the poxviruses.[30] Reed and Parkinson[29] studied the histogenesis of molluscum contagiosum and concluded that the lesion arises on the basis of follicular neogenesis. They found areas of hair bulb differentiation at the periphery, occasionally associated with areas of sebaceous gland differentiation. However, the disease can also appear in places where there are no hair follicles, such as the palms, indicating that the epidermis itself may be affected.[28]

Herpes zoster

A painful disease, herpes zoster is caused by the same virus that causes chickenpox (varicella). It may vary from relatively benign pruritic lesions on the trunk, usually unilateral and in the distribution of a single dermatone, to severe involvement of the first division of the trigeminal nerve with herpetic keratitis and corneal ulceration.[32] Postherpetic neuralgia is the unpleasant sequela. Patients with leukemia and malignant lymphoma develop herpes zoster more frequently.[31]

Bacterial diseases
Hidradenitis suppurativa

Hidradenitis suppurativa is caused by bacterial infection in and about apocrine sweat glands, usually in the axilla but occasionally involving the perineum.[33] Anaerobic organisms are the most important pathogens. Abscesses, sinuses, and perianal fistulas occur with subsequent scarring (Figs. 4-5 and 4-6). The process tends toward chronicity, and in refractory cases excision of the involved skin may be required.[35] Shelley and Cahn[36] suggested that the follicles into which the apocrine glands open are plugged by keratin and that infection develops following stasis. The end stages are similar to those of severe acne vulgaris and the more chronic disfiguring lesions of acne aggregata seu conglobata, in which squamous carcinoma may eventuate.[34]

Tuberculosis and atypical mycobacteriosis

Cutaneous tuberculosis is an uncommon disease in the United States. It has various clinical and morphologic forms depending on the mode of entry and whether it is a primary or secondary infection.[39-41]

Lupus vulgaris is a reactivation type of tuberculosis. It generally involves the face, and the lesions are formed of red patches in which small, firm nodules reside. When pressed with a glass slide (diascopy), these nodules have a pale tan color. Typically, noncaseous tubercles are found in the dermis. Acid-fast bacilli are difficult to demonstrate but may be found. Cultures are recommended. Ulceration of

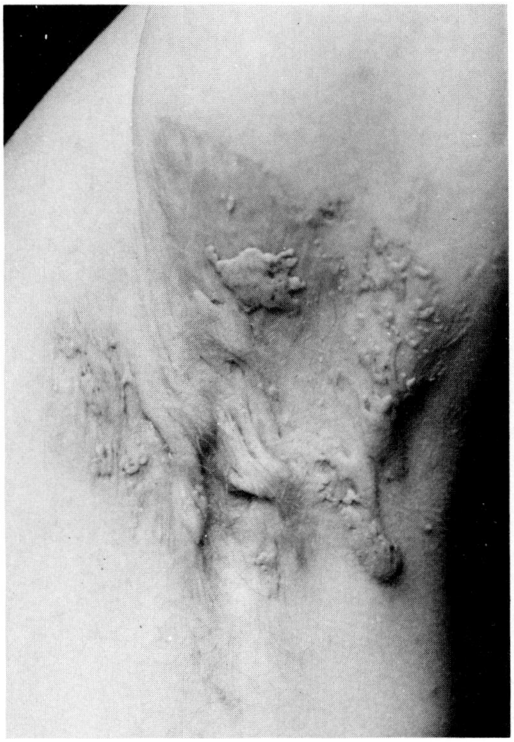

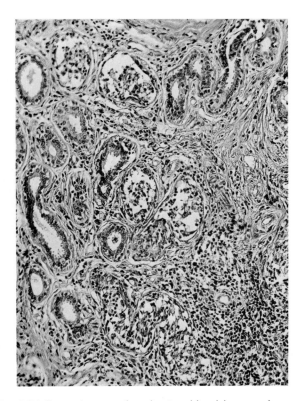

Fig. 4-5 Hidradenitis suppurativa of axilla showing nodules, sinuses, and scars.

Fig. 4-6 Inflammatory reaction about and involving apocrine sweat glands in a case of hidradenitis suppurativa.

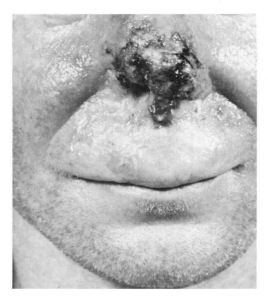

Fig. 4-7 Patient had lupus vulgaris of skin of nose for many years and eventually developed epidermoid carcinoma.

the skin may occur. In long-standing cases, frank squamous carcinoma may arise in conjunction with lupus vulgaris (Figs. 4-7 and 4-8).

Atypical mycobacteria can also affect the skin and result in a variety of lesions, including ulceration, abscesses, granulomas, diffuse histiocytic reactions, panniculitis, and rheumatoid-like nodules.[37,41,42] *M. kansasii, M. marinum,* and *M. ulcerans* are the organisms most commonly implicated.[38,43]

Leprosy

In most regions of the United States, leprosy is a rarity. However, the pathologist should consider it in the differential diagnosis of dermal granulomas[44] and histiocytic tumors.[45] In lepromatous leprosy the lepra cells, filled with acid-fast bacilli, are plentiful (Fig. 4-9), but in tuberculoid and indeterminate leprosy bacilli are very scanty. A diagnosis of leprosy should be suspected whenever the granulomas or the lymphocytic infiltration is located in and around the cutaneous nerves. Subcutaneous nodules are seen only in the lepromatous form and sometimes are designated as erythema nodosum leprorum.

Malakoplakia

A few cutaneous examples of this disease have been reported, the histiocytes having the typical Michaelis-Guttman bodies and sometimes containing identifiable Gram-negative organisms.[46]

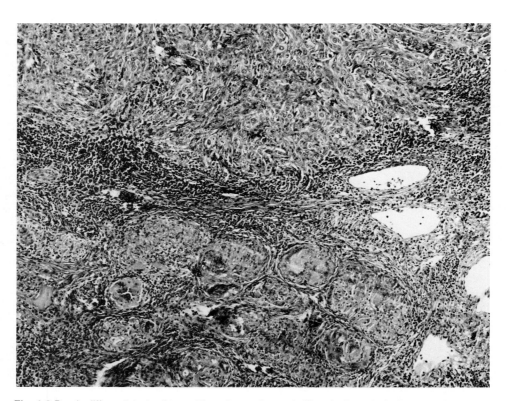

Fig. 4-8 Poorly differentiated epidermoid carcinoma (upper half) and tuberculosis (lower half) in biopsy taken from patient shown in Fig. 4-7.

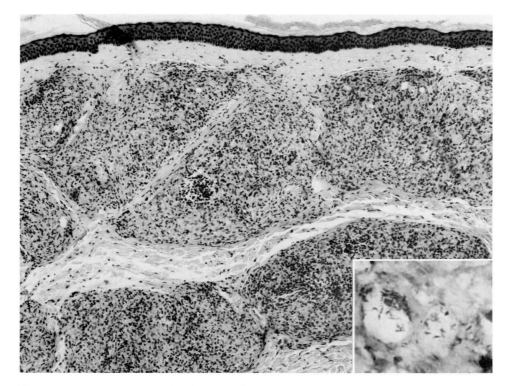

Fig. 4-9 Lepromatous leprosy wherein lepra cells are plentiful in dermis. **Inset** shows acid-fast bacilli in lepra cells stained with Fite-Faraco technique.

Spirochetal diseases

Syphilis

The cutaneous lesions of secondary syphilis are of maculopapular type and can be confused clinically with drug eruption, lichen planus, psoriasis, and other dermatoses. The microscopic appearance can be nonspecific, especially in the macular lesions. The late papular lesions are more likely to exhibit the distinctive microscopic appearance of a dense perivascular or diffuse infiltrate predominantly or exclusively composed of plasma cells.[47] Noncaseating granulomas may also be present.

Lyme disease

Lyme disease, a multisystem disorder caused by the spirochete *Borrelia burgdorferi*, may be manifest in the skin as erythema chronicum migrans, acrodermatitis chronica atrophicans, and perhaps also as cutaneous lymphoid hyperplasia. In the early stages, the predominant microscopic finding is a superficial and deep perivascular infiltrate largely composed of lymphocytes but also containing plasma cells and/or eosinophils (Fig. 4-10). Spirochetes can be demonstrated with the Warthin-Starry silver stain.[49]

It has been recently suggested that some cases of morphea and lichen sclerosus et atrophicus may also be caused by borrelial organisms.[48]

Fungal diseases

Tinea (dermatophytoses)

In the dermatophytoses, the fungal spores and hyphae are found in the stratum corneum and in or about hair shafts.[50]

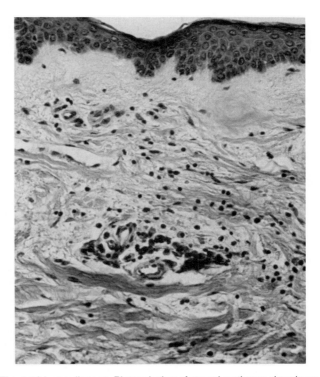

Fig. 4-10 Lyme disease. Picture is that of stage I erythema chronicum migrans showing intact epidermis, unaltered collagen, perivascular lymphocytes, and scattered plasma cells. (Courtesy Dr. P. Duray, Philadelphia, PA.)

Mild epidermal changes such as focal intercellular edema and varying amounts of dermal inflammation may be seen. The fungal elements are readily seen in sections stained by the periodic acid–Schiff or Gomori's methenamine silver methods. Occasionally, atypical clinical forms of tinea are biopsied, and the fungi are readily missed if not sought. Bacterial folliculitis and perifolliculitis may be superimposed on tinea of the scalp and beard. These lesions are known as *kerion celsi* and *sycosis barbae* respectively, and may, on occasion, be mistaken for infected tumors. Histologically, cellulitis, abscesses, pseudoepitheliomatus hyperplasia, and a few fungi in the hair follicles and adjacent tissues are seen.

It should be kept in mind that dermatophytes can be found superimposed in an inflammatory or neoplastic lesion of the skin. We have seen cases of mycosis fungoides that were missed originally because the atypical dermal infiltrate was attributed to the fungi seen in the horny layer.

North American blastomycosis

Isolated cutaneous blastomycosis is an uncommon lesion. Usually the skin lesion is secondary to pulmonary involvement, which may be subclinical.[52] The causative organism, *Blastomyces dermatitidis*, is a spheric, double-contoured 12 μm ± 4 μm yeast. It reproduces by budding, and this characteristic allows its identification in sections. The skin lesions are slowly enlarging verrucous plaques in which numerous small abscesses are present (Fig. 4-11). Microscopically, they are characterized by marked pseudoepitheliomatous hyperplasia and a mixed granulomatous and acute polymorphonuclear infiltrate[51] (Fig. 4-12). The organism is generally found in giant cells. Smears and cultures are recommended diagnostic adjuncts.

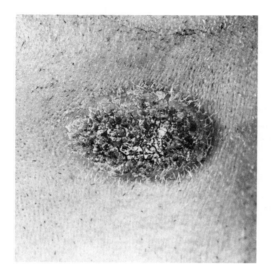

Fig. 4-11 Verrucous plaque of blastomycosis on neck.

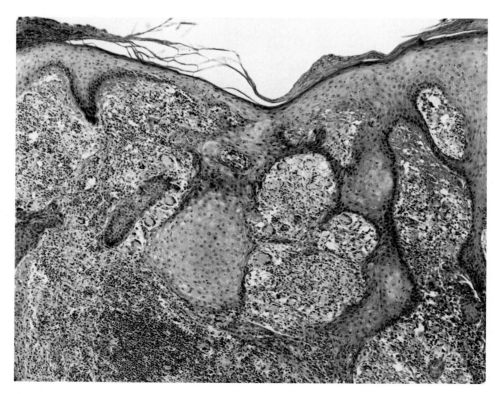

Fig. 4-12 Mixed granulomatous and acute inflammatory reaction of blastomycosis and pseudoepitheliomatosus hyperplasia of epidermis.

Chromoblastomycosis

An indolent cutaneous disease, chromoblastomycosis is usually misdiagnosed clinically as carcinoma and excised[54,56] (Fig. 4-13). Morphologically, identical fungi may be found in small subcutaneous abscesses.[55] Hematogenous dissemination occurs very rarely.[53] The spores are brown, hence their name, and the tissue reaction is similar to that seen in blastomycosis (Fig. 4-14). These fungi, closely related species of *Phialophora* and *Fonsecaëa* and

Cladosporium, multiply by cross wall formation and splitting. Their color, cross walls, and lack of budding differentiate them from *Blastomyces dermatitidis*.

Other granulomatous diseases
Sarcoidosis

Sarcoidosis affects the skin as well as the lymph nodes and viscera. Sarcoid-like reactions may develop in lymph nodes draining sites of carcinomas and in nonspecific inflammatory processes. Granulomas with a microscopically identical appearance can also appear in the skin in conjunction with malignant lymphoma and as a reaction to zirconium, beryllium, and in a variety of infectious diseases, including syphilis; however, the existence of a distinct clinical syndrome, both systemic and dermatologic, designated as sarcoidosis is currently accepted.[57,60] It is discussed here, despite the fact that its etiology is unknown, because of its morphologic similarities with infectious granulomatous diseases.

Impaired immune responses—including anergy to delayed hypersensitivity skin tests, reduced phytohemagglutinin-induced blast transformation, and overactivity of B-cells, as manifested by elevated serum levels of immunoglobulins and circulating immunocomplexes—are suggestive of the possibility that sarcoidosis is an immune-mediated disease.[62] Clinically, the cutaneous manifestations of the disease vary a great deal from case to case. They can be single or multiple and can range from macules to large plaques and nodules. Their basic microscopic appearance,

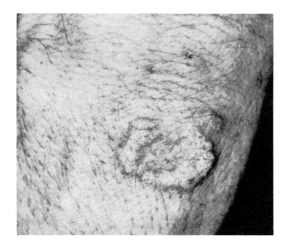

Fig. 4-13 Chromoblastomycosis on forearm.

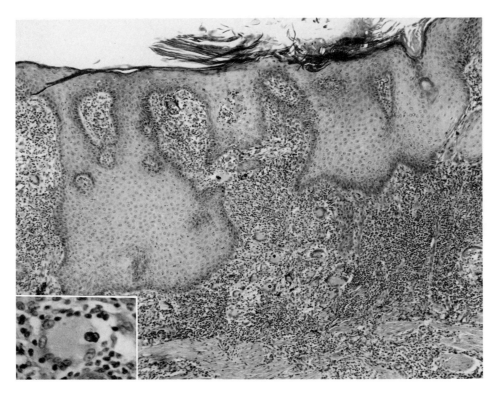

Fig. 4-14 Chromoblastomyces can be seen in giant cells surrounded by granulomatous reaction and acanthosis. **Inset** shows cross wall.

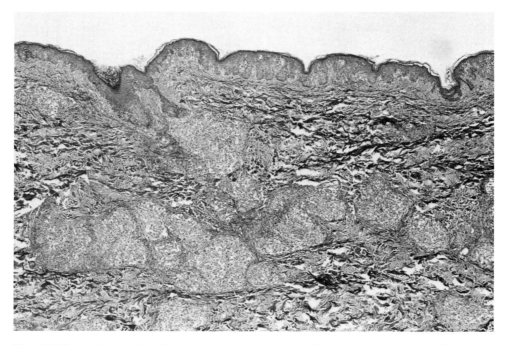

Fig. 4-15 Sarcoidosis of skin. Numerous coalescing noncaseating granulomas are seen throughout the deep dermis and surrounding skin adnexae.

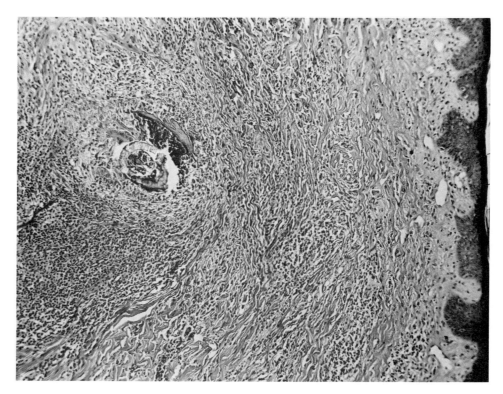

Fig. 4-16 Tick bite in which portion of head of tick was found surrounded by pronounced inflammatory reaction.

however, is similar. The dermis is infiltrated by nests and clusters of noncaseating epithelioid tubercles all but devoid of associated inflammatory cells. Langhans' giant cells are few (Fig. 4-15). The often-mentioned asteroids, seen in giant cells, and the calcified Schaumann bodies are uncommon and nonspecific. The Kveim test was often used in the past to confirm a clinical impression of sarcoidosis, but its popularity as a diagnostic tool has declined. Sterilized brei of sarcoid tissue, usually spleen, is injected intradermally, and 6 weeks later the area is biopsied.[61] The presence of a typical sarcoidal reaction is considered a positive test. Israel and Goldstein[59] deal with the pitfalls and details of this test. When the antigen is potent, the test is reliable, and very few false positive results are found. However, foreign body and nonspecific inflammatory reactions do occur following injections of the Kveim antigen. Hurley and Shelley[58] reported the formation of sarcoid granulomas in five of fifty normal individuals following the inoculation of PPD. Thus the reaction must be typical and the clinical findings consistent for the diagnosis of a positive Kveim test.

Foreign body reaction

Silica, talc, exogenous lipids, zirconium, and beryllium induce granulomatous reactions within the dermis.[64,66-68] Residual particles of talc, silica, and lipids are demonstrable in tissue by routine or polariscopic microscopy. Beryllium, previously a component of the phosphorus in fluorescent lights, induces a distinct necrotizing and granulomatous reaction.[65] Shelley and Hurley[68] described the allergic origin of the zirconium deodorant granulomas. Insect bites may, on occasion, cause inflammatory and granulomatous reactions that can be mistaken for lymphomas[63] (Fig. 4-16).

INFLAMMATORY DISEASES OF UNKNOWN ETIOLOGY
Psoriasis

Psoriasis is one of the commoner dermatoses. Estimates of its incidence vary between 0.5% and 1.5% of the population.[72] It is a chronic, bilaterally symmetric, nonpruritic lesion formed by erythematous plaques covered by fine silvery scales.[74] Typically, it involves the extensor surfaces such as the elbows, the knees, the back, and the scalp. Generalized lesions also occur (Fig. 4-17). Biochemical, histochemical, enzymatic, epidemiologic, and ultrastructural studies have failed so far to determine its cause.[71] The morphologic characteristics are those of incomplete keratinization manifested as parakeratosis, which is thought to result from a markedly shortened turnover time.[78] Keratinocytic differentiation is maintained despite the increased basal cell proliferation.[75]

Acanthosis in which there is a regular elongation of the rete ridges, seen as pegs in two dimensions, is prominent. Above the tips of the dermal papillae, the layer of epidermal cells is distinctly thinned—"suprapapillary thinning." Within the dermal papillae, the capillaries are prominent. Transmigration of polymorphonuclear leukocytes through the reactive epidermis into the parakeratotic scale results in the formation of Munro microabscesses[73] (Fig. 4-18). When these subcorneal abscesses are particularly prominent, the disease is designated as pustular psoriasis, a condition that may be pathogenetically related to subcorneal pustular dermatosis.[76]

Typical psoriasis is seldom biopsied. The atypical cases often are and they create diagnostic difficulties. These difficulties are caused by the fact that irritated epidermis—

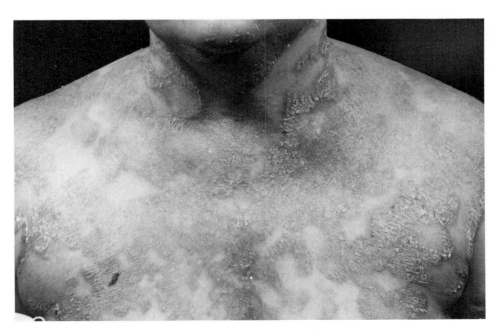

Fig. 4-17 Generalized psoriasis.

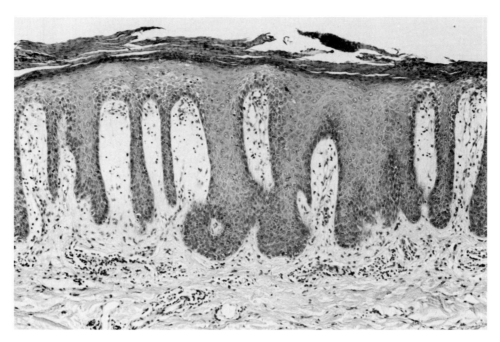

Fig. 4-18 Biopsy of psoriasis showing regular acanthosis, parakeratosis, Munro abscesses, and capillary dilatation. Suprapapillary edema is apparent.

either from lichen simplex chronicus, florid seborrheic dermatitis, pityriasis rubra pilaris, mycosis fungoides, or other causes—can develop comparable morphologic changes, which are often referred to as psoriasiform.[70,77] This also applies to the skin lesions of Reiter's syndrome.[69] Certain fine points of differentiation, such as the extent of suprapapillary thinning, the regularity of the acanthosis, and the lack of hyperkeratosis, may be used but are not absolute. Again, synthesis of all the information is required.

Exfoliative dermatitis and erythroderma

Exfoliative dermatitis and erythroderma can be seen secondary to a variety of disorders, including drug reaction, allergic contact dermatitis, psoriasis, pityriasis rubra pilaris, and various malignancies. The dermatopathic lymphadenitis (lipomelanotic reticulosis) associated with these skin diseases should not be confused with malignant lymphoma. Usually, the histologic changes in the skin are nonspecific and need to be distinguished from those of Sézary's syndrome and erythrodermic mycosis fungoides.[79-81]

Lichen planus

Lichen planus is a pruritic, violaceous, subacute to chronic, papulosquamous dermatitis of unknown etiology.[85a,93] It usually involves the flexor surfaces of the arms and the legs (Fig. 4-19) but occurs elsewhere as well.[82] Lesions may be confined to the oral mucosa,[83] or they may precede or accompany the skin changes. Histologically, the well-developed lesions are rather distinct (Fig. 4-20). The epidermis is hyperkeratotic, the granular layer is prominent, and the hyperplastic epithelium forms irregular acanthotic

pegs. The papillary dermis is heavily infiltrated by lymphocytes and histiocytes that form a band-like infiltrate that involves and destroys the dermoepidermal junction. Eosinophilic PAS-positive round or oval formations (colloid, hyaline, or Civatte bodies) are often seen in the basal layer and sometimes also in the upper dermis and malpighian layer. They show strong immunoreactivity for immunoglobulins and keratin, the latter supporting the interpretation that they represent degenerated keratinocytes.[87] Immunoglobulin deposition is also present along the dermo-epidermal junction. The lymphocytes present in the dermis are almost entirely of T-cell type.[85]

On occasion subepidermal cleavage occurs with the formation of bullae. The border of the inflammatory infiltrate is sharply delimited so that the reticular dermis is uninflamed. The oral lesions are readily mistaken for leukoplakia. Histologically, the absence of atypia and dyskeratotic cells in oral lichen planus assists in differentiating it from leukoplakia. Clinicopathologic variants of lichen planus include bullous, hypertrophic, atrophic, and follicular (lichen planopilaris) forms.[91]

A morphologic pattern akin to that of lichen planus and designated as lichenoid dermatitis or lichenoid tissue reaction can be seen in a variety of conditions, such as drug eruptions, lichenoid actinic keratosis (also known as lichen planus–like keratosis, benign lichenoid keratosis, and solitary lichen planus[86,89]) lupus erythematosus, acute graft-versus-host reaction, and several other conditions.[90,92,93a] The appearance of the lichenoid inflammatory process resembles a delayed hypersensitive reaction and is thought to represent a cell-mediated rejection reaction.[84]

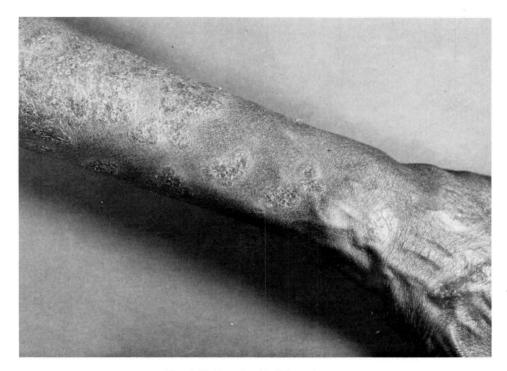

Fig. 4-19 Hypertrophic lichen planus.

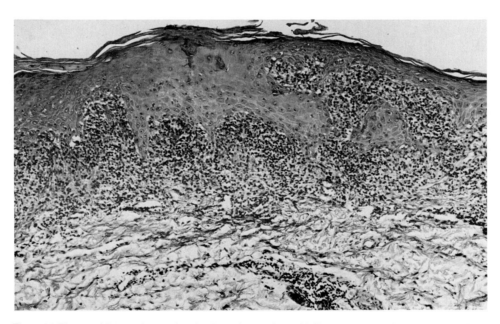

Fig. 4-20 Biopsy of lichen planus showing hyperkeratosis and infiltrate that hugs irregularly acanthotic epidermis.

Graft-versus-host disease

Graft-versus-host disease is one of the most important causes of morbidity and mortality following bone marrow transplantation. The early stages are characterized microscopically by vacuolation of the basal layer, spongiosis, and individual cell necrosis, associated with mononuclear cell infiltration of the upper dermis (Fig. 4-21). Sometimes these epidermal changes occur in the absence of an inflammatory infiltrate.[94] The amount of inflammation seems to be the most important prognostic determinator.[95] In the chronic stage of graft-versus-host disease, the microscopic appearance resembles scleroderma[96] (Fig. 4-22). Granular or linear

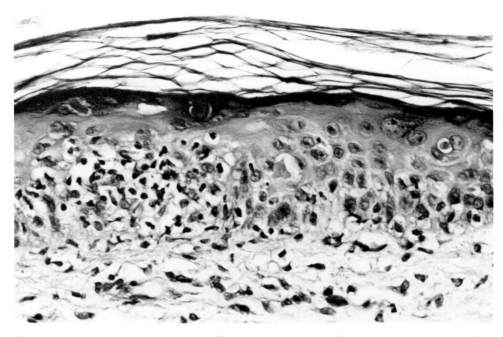

Fig. 4-21 Early graft-versus-host reaction. Biopsy was taken at day 32 post−bone marrow transplant. There is bandlike inflammatory infiltrate hugging epidermis, accompanied by individual cell necrosis of keratinocytes. (Courtesy Dr. D.C. Snover, Minneapolis, MN.)

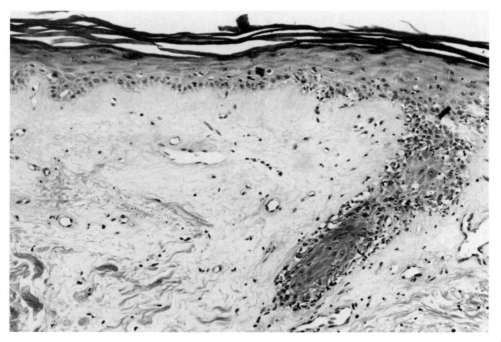

Fig. 4-22 Graft-versus-host reaction in a late stage. This skin biopsy was taken at day 822 post-transplant. Diffuse fibrosis of dermis results in a scleroderma-like appearance. (Courtesy Dr. D.C. Snover, Minneapolis, MN.)

deposition of IgM in the basement membrane zone is often present, particularly in the chronic form.

Vasculitis

There is a large group of cutaneous diseases in which the basic alteration is an inflammatory change in the wall of the dermal and/or subcutaneous vessels; i.e., a vasculitis.[97,110] The mechanism is in all likelihood immune-mediated for the majority of them, through the action of immune complexes.[111,113] The disease can be restricted to the skin or also involve internal organs; if restricted to the skin, it may be generalized or localized to a single focus. The vessels involved may be the capillaries of the papillary dermis, arterioles and venules of the deep dermis and subcutaneous tissue, or deep-seated medium-sized vessels. Red cell extravasation is a constant feature.

The inflammatory infiltrate can be predominantly neutrophilic (usually accompanied by leukocytoclasis), lymphocytic, or granulomatous. Necrotizing changes (usually of fibrinoid type) of the vessel wall may be present or absent.

Taking into account all of the foregoing features, morphologic classifications of cutaneous vasculitides have been proposed that correlate well with a variety of clinical conditions.[101,104,117] Lymphocytic non-necrotizing vasculitis involving small superficial vessels is seen in drug eruption, erythema multiforme, Mucha-Habermann disease, some viral infections,[102] collagen-vascular diseases, the group of diseases known as pigmented purpuric dermatosis, and several other conditions. Neutrophilic vasculitis of small vessels accompanied by fibrinoid necrosis and leukocytoclasis (leukocytoclastic or allergic vasculitis) usually presents as purpuric palpable lesions, most commonly on the lower part of the legs. Systemic involvement, particularly of the kidneys, is found frequently (Henoch-Schönlein purpura). Presence of systemic disease is more likely when the vasculitis extends deeply into the reticular dermis or subcutaneous fat,[116] but in general the morphologic features of the systemic and the purely cutaneous form are the same.[107]

Direct immunofluorescence often shows granular deposits of immunoglobulins, complement, and fibrin in and about vessel walls.[106] Etiologic agents include infections, foreign proteins, chemicals, drugs, and a variety of diseases.[98] Henoch-Schönlein purpura, hypocomplementemic vasculitis, and the vasculitis of essential mixed cryoglobulinemia represent distinct subtypes of leukocytoclastic vasculitis.[114,115]

Granuloma faciale (described in the following section) and erythema elevatum diutinum represent two localized types of non-necrotizing vasculitis involving vessels slightly larger than capillaries. In malignant atrophic papulosis (Degos' disease), the main change is an ischemic infarct of the skin resulting from intimal proliferation of a deep-seated arteriole.[99,112] In segmented hyalinizing vasculitis (atrophic blanche of Milian), the dermal capillaries show focal endothelial proliferation, marked thickening of the wall by PAS-positive eosinophilic hyaline material, and eventually occlusion of the lumen by a fibrin thrombus.[105]

Involvement of larger vessels, often accompanied by necrotizing changes, is seen in allergic granulomatosis of Churg and Strauss,[100,103] polyarteritis nodosa (systemic or limited to the skin), giant cell arteritis, and Wegener's granulomatosis. Prominent vascular involvement without any necrotizing changes is also seen in the cutaneous lesions of lymphomatoid granulomatosis[108,109] (see Chapter 7; Lung).

Granuloma faciale

Granuloma faciale occurs on the face of adults.[120] It is a thickened, purplish patch, which clinically is often confused with infected nevus, tumor, or sarcoid. For this reason, it is often excised or biopsied and acquaintance with its histologic appearance is helpful. The epidermis is unaltered, except in unusual circumstances, and is separated from the zone of dermal inflammation by a narrow band of uninvolved dermis (Fig. 4-23). The inflammatory reaction is formed by lymphocytes, histiocytes, and large numbers of eosinophils. The latter may be concentrated about the vessels and a mild to moderate vasculitis observed.[119] Granuloma faciale differs from the tumor stage of mycosis fungoides by the lack of epidermal involvement (Pautrier microabscesses) and of atypical lymphoid cells. Infected insect bites may have considerable eosinophilic infiltrate but seldom occur on the face.[118]

Erythema nodosum

The painful, red, subcutaneous lesions that characterize erythema nodosum occur on the anterior surface of the legs. They involute within a few days or weeks, leaving slightly depressed pigmented areas. They do not ulcerate as do the lesions of erythema induratum. The pathogenesis is in all likelihood immune-mediated, but the precise mechanism is unknown. In a British population with erythema nodosum, 45% of the patients had antecedent streptococcal infections, 6% had tuberculosis, 36% had sarcoid, and 13% had a variety of lesions.[126] Some cases are associated with chronic ulcerative colitis.[123a] In the endemic areas of the United States, coccidioidomycosis is a common antecedent.

Histologically, the junction of the dermis and the subcutis is inflamed. An inflammatory infiltrate extends along the fibrous septa between the fat and about the vessels of the dermis (Fig. 4-24). The composition depends largely on the age of the lesion. It may be predominantly neutrophilic, lymphocytic, or histiocytic, with isolated giant cells or noncaseating granulomas.[122,128] Varying degrees of vasculitis, chiefly of veins, may be seen.

Other nodular lesions of the leg that are probably the result of antigen-antibody precipitates with ensuing vasculitis are nodular vasculitis[123] (Fig. 4-25) and subacute nodular migratory panniculitis.[124] A common feature of these panniculitides, some of which are associated with collagen-vascular diseases, is their predominantly *septal* distribution.[121,127] In contrast, the panniculitis of Weber-Christian disease has a predominantly *lobular* distribution.[125]

Granuloma annulare

Granuloma annulare occurs most frequently on the dorsum of the hands and arms as circinate or grouped clusters of pink nodules with slight central depressions. Occasionally, the disease may be generalized. No associated symptoms or diseases are known.[135] Histologically, the key com-

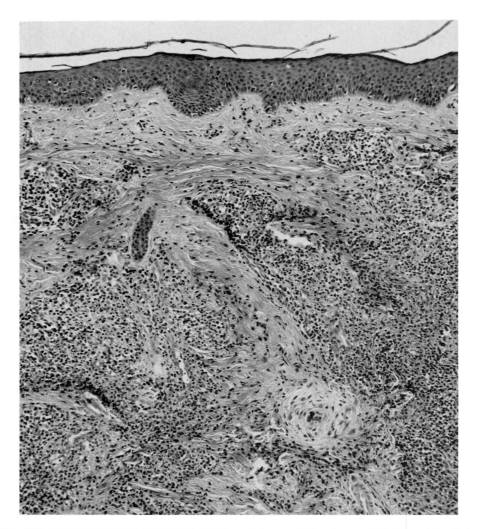

Fig. 4-23 Mixed infiltrate of granuloma faciale is well demarcated and separated from epidermis by narrow band of uninvolved dermis.

ponent of the lesion is the so-called necrobiotic granuloma or palisading granuloma.[130a] This is characterized by a well-demarcated zone of disintegrating collagen mixed with cell debris that is found in the mid-dermis surrounded by a cuff of radially oriented fibroblasts mixed with lymphocytes and histiocytes (Fig. 4-26). Occasional foreign body giant cells and foci of vasculitis may be found, and mucin is present in the areas of altered collagen. In many lesions, the abnormal collagen is not so distinctly demarcated, and multiple sections are necessary to arrive at a specific diagnosis.

The subcutaneous nodules of rheumatoid arthritis and rheumatic fever are histologically similar.[136]

Isolated, large, rather deep, necrobiotic nodules are sometimes seen on the extremities and occiput in children.[130,131] They have been referred to as deep, subcutaneous or giant granuloma annulare and as pseudorheumatoid nodules.[132,133] These children *do not develop rheumatic or rheumatoid disease*, and prolonged prophylaxis is not indicated. Occasionally, siblings may be affected.[129]

Granuloma annulare needs to be distinguished from a peculiar erythematous or brownish annular infiltrate sometimes encountered in the faces of elderly people and variously designated as actinic granuloma, Miescher's granuloma, and annular elastolytic giant cell granuloma.[134] Presence of elastic fibers in the giant cells, as seen by light and electron microscopy, is one of its most important distinguishing features.[137]

Necrobiosis lipoidica

Necrobiosis lipoidica typically presents as atrophic, yellow, depressed plaques involving the legs of diabetic patients; however, it can also occur in other sites and in the absence of clinical diabetes.[138,139,141] Microscopically, ill-defined areas of disintegrating dermal collagen are seen surrounded by a lymphohistiocytic infiltrate often arranged in a palisading fashion. Thickening of the blood vessel wall is usually prominent. In contrast with granuloma annulare, stains for mucin and immunoreactivity for lysozyme tend to be negative.[142] A disease somewhat similar to necrobiosis lipoidica but occurring in the head, neck, and trunk of pa-

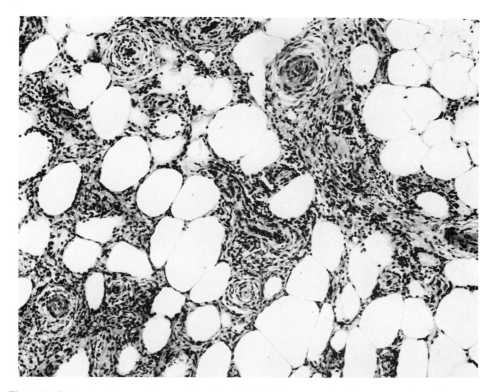

Fig. 4-24 Subacute inflammatory reaction almost limited to connective tissue septa in erythema nodosum.

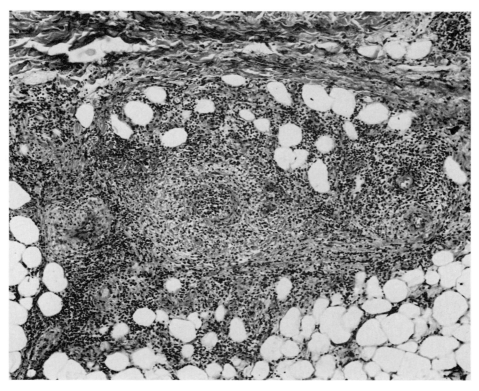

Fig. 4-25 Obliterative vasculitis within subcutis from thigh of woman with nodular vasculitis.

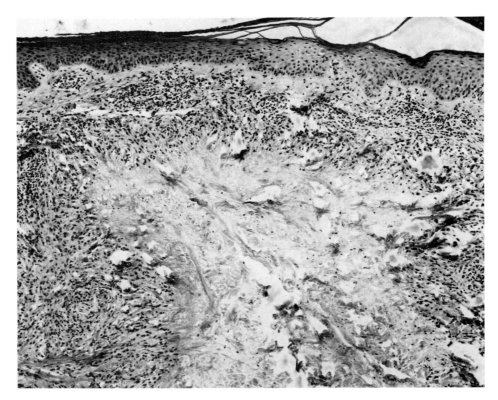

Fig. 4-26 Granuloma annulare showing central core of altered collagen surrounded by zone of radially oriented histiocytes and lymphocytes.

tients with paraproteinemia was recently described as necrobiotic xanthogranuloma.[140]

Weber-Christian disease

The changes seen in Weber-Christian disease are acute to subacute inflammation of the subcutaneous adipose tissue with necrosis of fat cells (Fig. 4-27) and resolution by macrophagic ingestion and subsequent fibrosis. The distribution of the inflammation is lobular rather than septal. The lesions are tender and usually accompanied by malaise and remittent fever.[143,145] In contrast, the lipogranulomatosis subcutanea of Rothman and Makai has no associated systemic symptoms and does not appear in crops.[144] Changes similar to those of Weber-Christian disease can be seen as a complication of alpha-1-antitrypsin deficiency,[145a] chronic pancreatitis, and pancreatic carcinoma. A clue to the diagnosis of the latter two conditions is the presence of large foci of fat necrosis containing the "ghosts" of the fat cells and the thick "shadows" of their walls.

Urticaria pigmentosa

Urticaria pigmentosa usually has its onset during childhood, but on occasions it may make its first appearance in adults.[148] The brown macules may be diffusely distributed (Fig. 4-28) or, less frequently, may be single.[151] When the lesions are stroked, the skin urticates because of the release of histamine.

A systemic form of mastocytosis exists, characterized by involvement of spleen, liver, bone marrow, and lymph nodes, with or without cutaneous lesions.[146,147,153,155] This systemic form runs a malignant clinical course and on occasion it is accompanied by circulating mast cells. In general, it is not possible on morphologic grounds to distinguish urticaria pigmentosa with systemic involvement from that having skin disease only,[157] but some prediction along these lines is possible by the use of a pH-dependent toluidine blue stain.[152] The diagnosis of urticaria pigmentosa in a skin biopsy can be easily missed unless the cytologic features of mast cells in sections stained with hematoxylin-eosin are remembered.[154] Some of the cells have large, pale nuclei, distinct cytoplasmic boundaries, and a faintly granular cytoplasm (Fig. 4-29). Others are elongated and closely simulate fibroblasts or perithelial cells. In sections stained with toluidine blue or Giemsa, the metachromatic granules are obvious.[149] Eosinophils usually are mixed with the mast cells in the dermis. Mast cell tumors of the skin are common in the dog[156] and also occur in the cat and ox.[150]

Lupus erythematosus

Chronic discoid lupus erythematosus and systemic lupus erythematosus represent distinct and almost uniformly separable entities. Some authors accept the existence of an intermediate form known as subacute cutaneous lupus erythematosus.[158] Chronic discoid lupus erythematosus is a

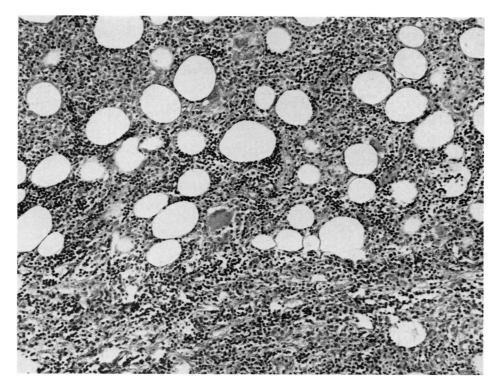

Fig. 4-27 Weber-Christian disease in which destruction of fat cells and inflammatory infiltrate with giant cells are apparent.

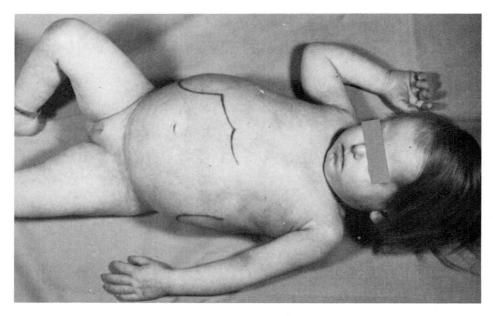

Fig. 4-28 Generalized, faint brown, macular rash and outlines of enlarged liver and spleen in infant with systemic mastocytosis.

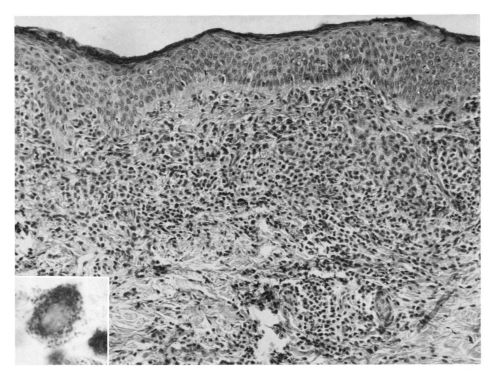

Fig. 4-29 Biopsy from child illustrated in Fig. 4-28 showing dermis heavily infiltrated with mast cells. **Inset** shows mast cell's granules stained metachromatically with toluidine blue.

relatively common condition with a distinct preference for women, presenting as delimited erythematous to hyperkeratotic to atrophic patches on the face, neck, scalp, and, less frequently, the arms and trunk[159b,165] (Fig. 4-30). Sunlight may cause exacerbations. Histologically, the lesions are characterized by predominantly follicular hyperkeratosis, epidermal atrophy with liquefactive degeneration of the basal layer, and a distinct, patchy, periadnexal lymphocytic infiltrate (Fig. 4-31). The changes seen in biopsies reflect the stage and type of lesion sampled. None of the changes is pathognomonic. Polymorphous light eruption and lymphocytic infiltration of the skin may be difficult to distinguish from chronic discoid lupus erythematosus.[163,168] Chronic discoid lupus erythematosus very rarely progresses to the acute disease.[159a,162]

Systemic lupus erythematosus is an "auto-immune" malady in which antibodies to homologous and heterologous deoxyribonucleic acid have been demonstrated. It manifests a protean symptomatology usually characterized by fatigue, fever, arthritis, various cutaneous lesions of which the erythematous bimalar "butterfly" blush is most common, signs of renal involvement, lymphadenopathy, and panserositis.[167] The typical, but not always present, dermal histologic picture is fibrinoid necrosis at the dermoepidermal junction accompanied by atrophy and liquefactive degeneration of the epidermis[160] (Fig. 4-32). Occasionally, lesions of lupus erythematosus appear as verrucous, hyperkeratotic lesions on the upper extremities resembling keratoacanthomas or hypertrophic lichen planus.[166] The systemic lesions have

been described often, but no better than in the original paper by Klemperer et al.[164]

Direct immunofluorescence will show the presence of immunoglobulins (usually IgG and IgM) and so-called membrane attack complex (C5b, C6, C7, C8, and C9) in about 90% of the specimens obtained from clinically involved skin of patients with either systemic or chronic discoid lupus erythematosus.[159] The deposition consists of coalescing clumps along the dermoepidermal junction, resulting in the formation of an irregular band, a finding that is of great diagnostic importance but not entirely specific for this entity.[169] Clinically uninvolved areas will show deposition of immunoglobulins in about half of the patients with systemic lupus erythematosus but no deposition of the membrane attack complex.[159,161] With few exceptions, direct immunofluorescence is negative in the lesions of polymorphous light eruption and lymphocytic infiltration.

Dermatomyositis

Dermatomyositis is an inflammatory disorder affecting skeletal muscle and skin, characterized clinically by proximal, symmetric muscle weakness and cutaneous lesions. Microscopically, the skin changes may be those of a nonspecific chronic dermatitis or may acquire features very similar to those of systemic lupus erythematosus.[171,172] Biopsies of the afflicted muscles show distinct myositis with necrosis of myofibers, fragmentation, phagocytosis, and some sarcolemmal nuclear proliferation. In the later stages, fibrosis, fat infiltration, and fascicular atrophy appear.[170]

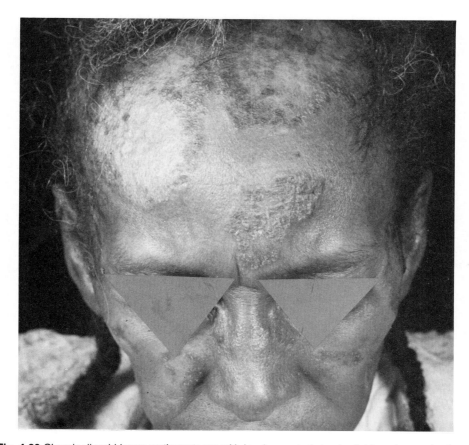

Fig. 4-30 Chronic discoid lupus erythematosus with involvement of cheeks, bridge of nose, forehead, and scalp.

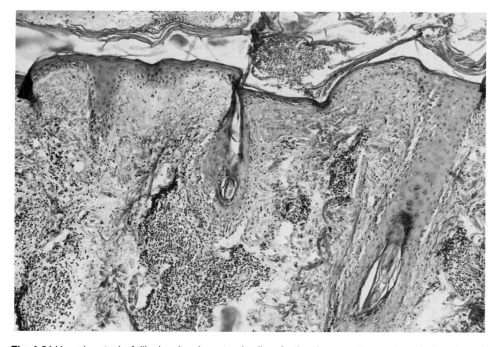

Fig. 4-31 Hyperkeratosis, follicular plugging, atrophy, liquefactive degeneration, and patchy lymphocytic infiltrate of chronic discoid lupus erythematosus.

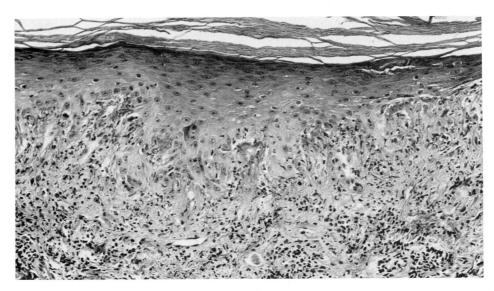

Fig. 4-32 Subacute lupus erythematosus in which fibrinoid necrosis at dermoepidermal junction and some inflammatory reactions are present.

Williams[173] reviewed the experience of many regarding the incidence or coincidence of adenocarcinoma with dermatomyositis. He found that 15% of the patients have neoplasms of the stomach, breast, ovary, lung, and colon. Remissions have occurred following resection of the neoplasm. Thus careful investigation of adults with dermatomyositis for undetected carcinoma is certainly worthwhile. However, in the majority none will be found, and the etiology remains obscure. Corticosteroid therapy is beneficial.

In long-standing dermatomyositis and in lupus erythematosus, acrodermatitis atrophicans, and mycosis fungoides, a secondary change called poikiloderma atrophicans vasculare may appear. The histologic changes are generally those of the associated disease.

Scleroderma

Scleroderma is manifest in two distinct forms: localized scleroderma or morphea[173a,175,188] and systemic scleroderma, in which the skin, particularly of the face, the upper trunk, hands, and arms (acrosclerosis) (Fig. 4-33), the esophagus, the heart, and the lungs are diseased. Most patients are adults, but the disease can also present in childhood.[185a]

Sometimes visceral disease typical of systemic scleroderma occurs in the absence of cutaneous involvement. A few cases of morphea have been associated with generalized or systemic disease. The etiology and pathogenesis are unknown.[187] Systemic sclerosis is often classified as one of the "collagen diseases." The dominant change is an increase in the amount of collagen. This is, morphologically, ultrastructurally, and biochemically indistinguishable from normal collagen.[177,178] The relative proportions and distribution of type I and type III collagens are closely similar to those found in the normal dermis.[181] Thus the histologic diagnosis depends on the evaluation of increments in the amount and distribution of collagen. The "smudging," "homogenization," and variable tinctorial changes seen in sections stained with hematoxylin-eosin do not necessarily indicate structural changes in the collagen. In fact, some care should be exercised not to confuse the changes of senile elastosis and basophilic degeneration of collagen and the normally thicker dermis of the fingers with scleroderma.[185] The dermis, particularly the papillary portion, becomes a dense feltwork of closely woven collagen bundles (Fig. 4-34). The sclerosis may extend in depth to encircle the secretory coils of the eccrine sweat glands. Concomitantly, the epidermis becomes atrophic. Varying amounts of mild and nonspecific inflammatory reaction may be seen in the dermis, more so at the advancing edge of a patch of morphea. The inflammatory infiltrate and vascular damage are particularly pronounced in the early stages of the disease, suggesting that the fibrosis may represent a secondary phenomenon, that is, a post-inflammatory sclerosis.[176,179] Direct immunofluorescence studies are almost uniformly negative. Dystrophic calcification may occur in scleroderma, and in some patients the dominant pattern is that of acrosclerosis preceded by, or associated with, Raynaud's phenomenon.

Scleroderma needs to be distinguished from eosinophilic fasciitis (Shulman's disease), a condition characterized clinically by swelling, tenderness, and stiffness of an extremity, often involving the lower forearm and sometimes associated with carpal tunnel syndrome.[174,180,183] The most important difference on histologic grounds is that in the latter condition there is marked inflammation and thickening of the deep fascia (with or without eosinophils), whereas in scleroderma this structure tends to show minimal or no abnormalities.[182] What the relationship between these two entities is, if any, remains controversial.[184,186]

VESICULOBULLOUS DISEASES

The key morphologic features in the microscopic evaluation of vesiculobullous lesions are the level of the plane of separation and the type of cellular change seen, partic-

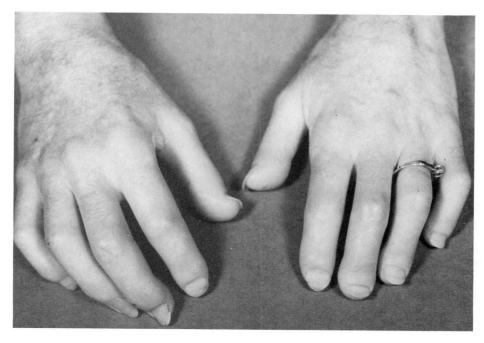

Fig. 4-33 Shiny, tense skin of fingers in well-developed scleroderma.

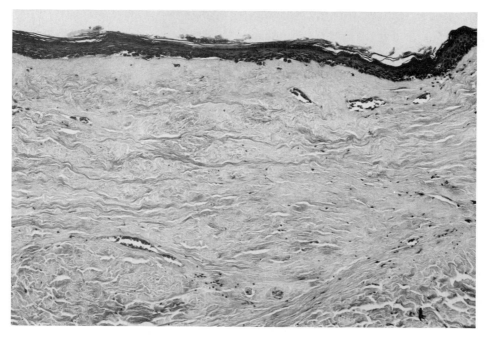

Fig. 4-34 Distinct increase in amount of dermal collagen, epidermal atrophy, and slight hyperkeratosis in patch of localized scleroderma (morphea).

ularly the presence or absence of acantholysis.[201] Vesicles and bullae (large vesicles) are divided according to their location into subepidermal and intraepidermal categories, which in turn may be suprabasal or subcorneal. In making this distinction, one should be aware of the fact that a bulla that was originally subepidermal can become intra-

epidermal because of regrowth of epithelium across its base, a process that can be very rapid. Actually, large intraepidermal bullae unassociated with acantholytic changes should be suspected of being healed subepidermal bullae. Biopsying early lesions (less than 24 hours old) minimizes this problem.

Subepidermal bullae occur in dermatitis herpetiformis, bullous pemphigoid, erythema multiforme, porphyria cutanea tarda, epidermolysis bullosa, and cicatricial pemphigoid[194,212] (Fig. 4-35). They can also be seen as a secondary event in any dermatosis associated with liquefactive degeneration of the basal layer, such as lupus erythematosus and lichen planus. Occasionally, two of these diseases are seen to coexist.[210] The differential diagnosis should be made on the basis of the combined clinical, microscopic, and immunohistochemical findings.[200] Some of these disorders are easily recognizable on clinical grounds. This is particularly true of dermatitis herpetiformis because of its symmetric

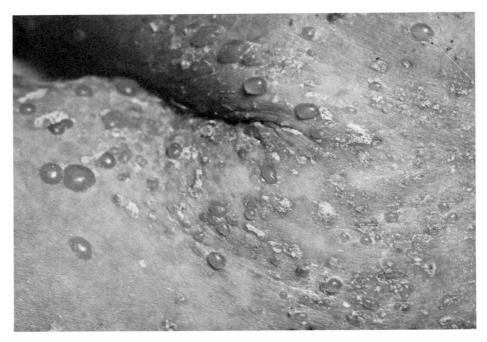

Fig. 4-35 Bullae of dermatitis herpetiformis on anterior portion of chest and upper arm. Previous lesions have ruptured, causing changes between intact blisters.

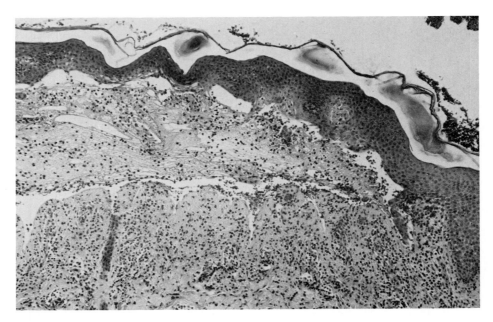

Fig. 4-36 Subepidermal bulla from patient with dermatitis herpetiformis. Many of the inflammatory cells are eosinophilic leukocytes. Junction with intact skin is at right.

distribution, intense pruritus, frequent association with gluten-sensitive enteropathy, and its response to sulfapyridine and diaxone.[202]

Microscopically, a distinction between these various subepidermal processes is not always possible[200]; however, careful evaluation of a set of criteria as seen in routinely stained sections results in a 90% concordance with the clinical diagnosis[206,208] (Tables 4-1 and 4-2). The most consistent histologic features of *bullous pemphigoid* are festooning of the dermal papillae, absence of adjacent microabscesses, and a unilocular blister with a mild dermal infiltrate. The most useful criterion for the diagnosis of *dermatitis herpetiformis* is the presence of papillary microabscesses forming a multilocular subepidermal bulla. Eosinophils tend to be particularly numerous in this condition (Fig. 4-36). The most characteristic features of bullous *erythema multiforme* are subepidermal edema, the presence of basement membrane in the roof of the bulla, abundant nuclear dust in the dermis, and occasional vasculitis, epidermal spongiosis, and epidermal necrosis. It should be realized that a wide spectrum of histologic changes exists in erythema multiforme, ranging from a predominantly dermal disturbance to a necrotizing epidermal reaction similar to the adult type of toxic epidermal necrolysis.[191] Thus the bullae of erythema multiforme can be subepidermal, with the basal lamina at the top of the blister (as a result of dermal edema), or dermo-epidermal, with the basal lamina at the floor of the bulla (as a result of epidermal damage).[204]

Somewhat similar considerations apply to the group of over twelve genetically determined disorders collectively known as *epidermolysis bullosa,* in which the site of cleavage can be in the dermis (dermolytic form), at the dermoepidermal junction (junctional form), or in the epidermis (epidermolytic form).

Immunofluorescent studies in bullous diseases have been shown to be of considerable diagnostic value, especially in distinguishing bullous pemphigoid from dermatitis herpetiformis.[197,203] In the former, there is in vivo subepidermal linear binding of IgG and complement with an occasional mixture of IgA and IgM; there are also circulating antibodies that bind to the basement zone of normal skin or mucous membrane in 70% of the patients.[195] In dermatitis herpetiformis, there are no circulating antibodies and the in vivo immunofluorescent pattern is that of subepidermal granular binding of IgA, mainly at the tips of dermal papillae. The presence of these antibodies is better demonstrated by immunofluorescence on snap-frozen tissue, but positive results can also be obtained in most cases by immunoperoxidase on paraffin-embedded material.[214]

Among the **intraepidermal bullous dermatoses** are *pemphigus vulgaris* and a variant thereof, *pemphigus vegetans*. In these diseases, the cleavage plane is just above the

Table 4-1 Main clinical differences among the three major subepidermal bullous dermatoses

Criteria	Bullous pemphigoid (BP)	Dermatitis herpetiformis (DH)	Bullous erythema multiforme (BEM)
Distribution	Generalized	Grouped on extensor surfaces	Generalized, often with mucosal involvement
Appearance of lesions	Large, tense bullae, often haemorrhagic, with erosions	Small papules, papulovesicles and vesicles with small excoriations	Polymorphous, erythematous, urticarial, with blisters and characteristic target lesions
Pruritus	Variable	Extreme pruritus	Not a feature
Healing stages	Scars and pigmentation	Small hyper- and depigmented lesions	No residual lesions
Age	Majority older age group	Younger age group	Any age
Therapeutic response	Favourable response to small dosage corticosteroids	Favourable response to dapsone	Self-limited cause

From Saxe N, Kahn LB: Subepidermal bullous disease. A correlated clinico-pathologic study of 51 cases. J Cutan Pathol **3**:88-94, 1976; © by Munksgaard International Publishers Ltd., Copenhagen, Denmark.

Table 4-2 Main pathologic differences among the three major subepidermal bullous dermatoses

Criteria	Bullous pemphigoid (BP)	Dermatitis herpetiformis (DH)	Bullous erythema multiforme (BEM)
Festooning of dermal papillae	Always present	May be present	Absent
Microabscesses	Absent	Present	Absent
Architecture of bulla	Unilocular	Multilocular	Variable
Basement membrane	In floor	In floor	In roof
Dermal inflammatory infiltrate	Usually mild	Usually mild	Severe, extends beyond bulla, nuclear dust present
Overlying epidermis	Shows necrosis rarely	No diagnostic features	Often shows necrosis

From Saxe N, Kahn LB: Subepidermal bullous disease. A correlated clinico-pathologic study of 51 cases. J Cutan Pathol **3**:88-94, 1976; © by Munksgaard International Publishers Ltd., Copenhagen, Denmark.

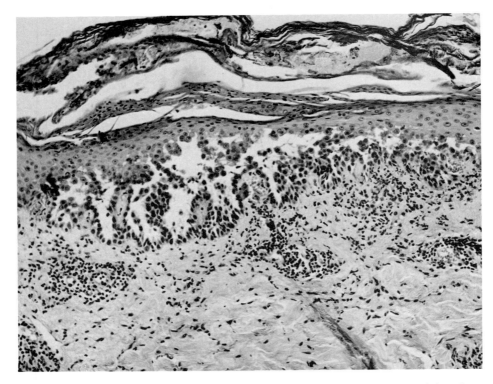

Fig. 4-37 Pemphigus vulgaris in which characteristic suprabasal bulla and dark acantholytic cells can be seen.

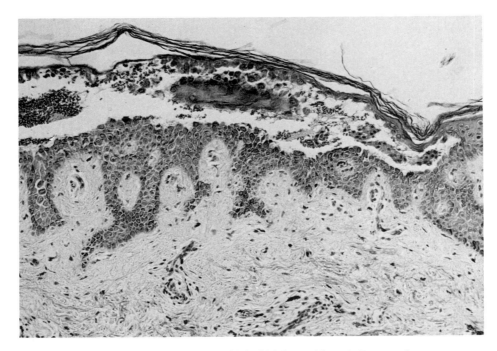

Fig. 4-38 Pemphigus foliaceus with its high intraepidermal cleavage plane.

basal layer and is caused by acantholysis (Fig. 4-37). In contrast, the separation in *pemphigus foliaceus*[205] and *pemphigus erythematosus*[198] is in or just below the granular layer (Fig. 4-38). Indirect immunofluorescent stains performed with sera of patients with pemphigus demonstrate the presence of antiepithelial auto-antibodies in most cases, although the test may be negative in the early stages.[192,213] In addition, immunoglobulins can be detected in over 90% of the cases in the epidermal intercellular spaces by a direct immunofluorescence technique.[195,211] These autoantibodies are thought to play an important role in the pathogenesis of pemphigus vulgaris,[194a] as suggested by the fact that the disease can be passively transferred to laboratory animals.[190] Judd and Lever[199] believe that, despite earlier reports, indirect immunofluorescence is unreliable for evaluating the status of the disease or for gauging therapy in patients with pemphigus.

Acantholysis can be seen in several other dermatologic conditions, such as familial benign pemphigus (Hailey-Hailey disease), viral vesicles, the pemphigus-like lesions induced by D-penicillamine,[207] actinic keratosis and the type of epidermoid carcinoma arising from it (adenoid or pseudoglandular), Darier's disease, warty dyskeratoma, and transient acantholytic dermatosis (Grover's disease). The latter is characterized by transient edematous and excoriated papules and vesicles located predominantly on the trunk, thought to be the result of heat and sweating.[196] According to Chalet et al.,[193] the most important clue to the diagnosis is the association of acantholysis and spongiosis. In addition, focal acantholytic dyskeratotic changes (sometimes limited to a single rete ridge) can be found in association with a variety of localized lesions, such as dermatofibroma, basal cell carcinoma, melanocytic nevus, and malignant melanoma.[189,215]

In *subcorneal pustular dermatosis*,[209] the vesicles are just beneath the keratin layer, as they are in *impetigo contagiosa*. Another subcorneal vesicular lesion that has been mistaken clinically for junctional nevus is the blood blister, in which the erythrocytes are trapped beneath the thick stratum corneum of the toes or fingers.

DEGENERATIVE AND MISCELLANEOUS DISEASES
Lichen sclerosus et atrophicus

Lichen sclerosus et atrophicus occurs most often on the upper trunk and neck, flexor surface of the wrist, and the anogenital areas. When this disease is located in the vulva it is sometimes designated as kraurosis and when in the glans penis as balanitis xerotica obliterans.[216,217] The disease occurs most commonly in women, often at or around menopause, and its etiology is unknown. Atrophy and hyperkeratosis of the epidermis are associated with complete obliteration of the structure of the upper dermis. It is replaced by an edematous, hypocellular, faintly staining band beneath which a moderate chronic inflammatory infiltrate appears (Fig. 4-39). In older lesions, some hyalinization and angiectasia occur in this band.

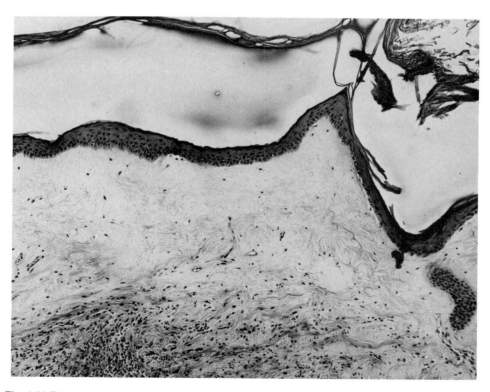

Fig. 4-39 Edematous hypocellular band of upper dermis, epidermal atrophy, and hyperkeratosis typical of lichen sclerosus et atrophicus. Keratin is artifactually lifted from epidermis.

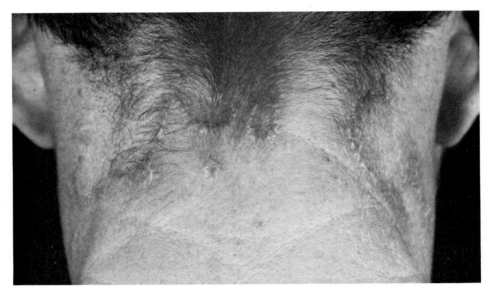

Fig. 4-40 Serpiginous line of papules just within hairline on nape characteristic of elastosis perforans.

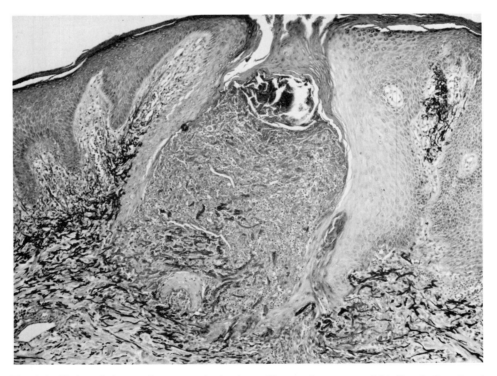

Fig. 4-41 Skeins of abnormally coarse elastica in papillae can be seen on right. Penetrating strands can be seen entering follicle that is plugged with necrotic debris. (Verhoeff–van Gieson.)

Lichen sclerosus et atrophicus should be clearly distinguished from localized scleroderma (morphea).[218] It should also be separated from the hyperplastic mucosal lesions accompanied by various degrees of atypia ("leukoplakia").

Elastosis perforans

In elastosis perforans, clumps and strands of abnormally coarse elastic fibers penetrate the epidermis and produce a

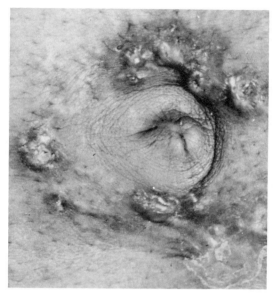

Fig. 4-42 Nodules and plaques about umbilicus in patient with pseudoxanthoma elasticum.

focal epidermal hyperplasia.[219,220,222,225] The common site is the back of the neck in adolescent boys (Fig. 4-40). The altered elastica in the papillary dermis is easily missed, and recognition usually requires elastic tissue stains (Fig. 4-41).

Elastosis perforans needs to be distinguished from other perforating dermatoses, such as reactive perforating collagenosis, perforating folliculitis, and Kyrle's disease.[223,223a,224] The nosologic identity of the latter two disorders and their relationship to each other remains controversial. A high proportion of them are seen in patients with chronic renal failure and diabetes mellitus.[221,226]

Pseudoxanthoma elasticum

The dermal changes in pseudoxanthoma elasticum are manifestations of a generalized disorder of connective tissue.[228] Angioid streaks in the retina and degenerative changes in arteries leading to occlusion or rupture are described. Yellow streaks and plaques of the skin, particularly in areas of creases such as the neck, axillae, and groin, account for the name *pseudoxanthoma* (Fig. 4-42). Histologically, the mid and lower dermis contain clumps and strands of altered, faintly basophilic connective tissue that stain intensely with aldehyde fuchsin and Verhoeff's elastic tissue stain (Fig. 4-43). This tinctorial reaction suggests that the abnormality is, in fact, one of the elastic fibers.[227] The exact nature of the defect remains unknown.

Cutaneous mucinoses

Pretibial myxedema is characterized by nodular lesions that occur on the legs of patients who are or have been thyrotoxic.[231] The lesions may become quite large. The accumulation of mucopolysaccharides in the dermis is similar

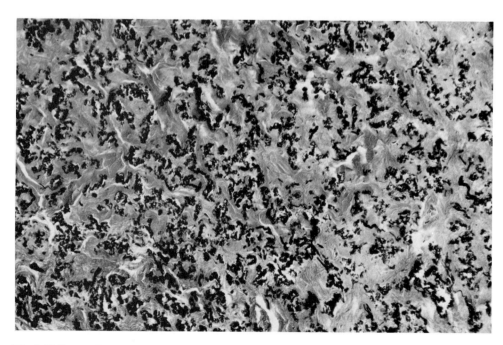

Fig. 4-43 Coarse, fragmented, and calcified pieces of elastica in pseudoxanthoma elasticum. (Verhoeff's elastic tissue stain.)

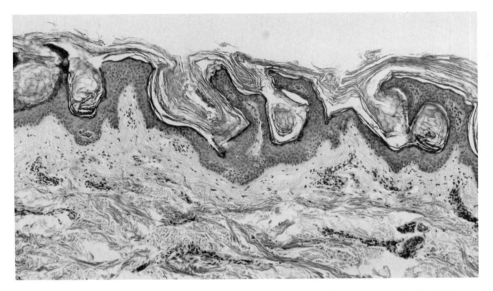

Fig. 4-44 Biopsy from axilla showing papillomatosus and hyperkeratosis of acanthosis nigricans.

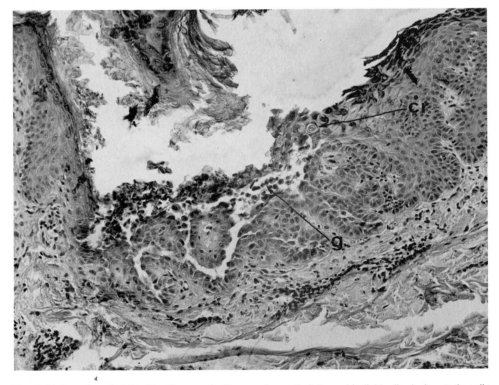

Fig. 4-45 Suprabasal cleft with villous projections and acantholytic and individually dyskeratotic cells of Darier's disease. **cr,** Corp ronds. **g,** Grains.

to that in the orbital tissues, which is caused by excess TSH secretion by the pituitary gland.[229] Histologically, the dermal collagen is separated by aggregates of faintly basophilic material that stains with mucicarmine and with Hale's colloidal iron reaction for acid mucopolysaccharides and that is PAS-positive and diastase resistant.

Other conditions associated with the deposition of large amounts of acid mucopolysaccharides in the dermis are the generalized myxedema of hypothyroidism, papular mucinosis (lichen myxedematosus), myxoid cyst, cutaneous focal mucinosis, and follicular mucinosis.[230,233-236] The latter condition is a reaction pattern of follicular epithelium that is particularly prominent in alopecia mucinosa but that can also be seen in a variety of other diseases, including mycosis fungoides.[232] Cutaneous myxoid nodules are an important component of a recently described syndrome that also includes cardiac myxomas, spotty hyperpigmentation, and endocrine hyperactivity.[229a]

Acanthosis nigricans

Acanthosis nigricans manifests clinically as brown, velvety plaques most often found in the axillae, back of the neck, and other flexural areas. Two major forms exist, one associated with internal malignant neoplasms (particularly of the gastrointestinal tract) and the other with a heterogeneous group of disorders having as common denominator the presence of tissue resistance to insulin.[237,238] The latter form includes diabetes, obesity, and Cushing's syndrome. Microscopically, the changes are similar in both types and are characterized by papillomatosis and hyperkeratosis (rather than by acanthosis and hyperpigmentation, as suggested by the name) (Fig. 4-44). In the cases associated with malignancy, the disease may be the result of production of epidermal growth factors by the tumor cells.[239]

Darier's disease

The keratotic and papular lesions of Darier's disease (an autosomal dominant genodermatosis) are characterized histologically by suprabasal clefts in which acantholytic cells called *grains* are found. The dermal papillae covered by a layer of basal cells form small villi at the base of the lesion. In addition, within the epidermis large individually dyskeratotic cells called *corps ronds* are found (Fig. 4-45). When the lesions are closely spaced, the skin assumes a verrucous appearance. The oral mucosa and hairless skin may be involved, showing that the disease is not limited to the hair follicle as suggested by the name *keratosis follicularis*. Warty dyskeratoma, an isolated follicular lesion, is histologically similar but unrelated to Darier's disease (see p. 112).

REFERENCES
INTRODUCTION TO DERMATOPATHOLOGY

1 Ackerman AB: Histologic diagnosis of inflammatory skin disease. A method by pattern analysis. Philadelphia, 1978, Lea & Febiger.

1a Demis DJ: Clinical dermatology. Philadelphia, 1985, Harper & Row.

2 Fitzpatrick TB, Freedberg IM: Dermatology in general medicine, ed. 3. New York, 1987, McGraw-Hill Book Co.

3 Gans O: Histologie der Hautkrankheiten. Berlin, 1928, Julius Springer, vols. I and II.

4 Kimming J, Jannes M: Color atlas of dermatology. Philadelphia, 1966, W.B. Saunders Co.

5 Lever WF, Schaumburg-Lever G: Histopathology of the skin, ed. 6. Philadelphia, 1983, J.B. Lippincott Co.

6 Lynch PJ, Epstein S (eds): Burckhardt's atlas and manual of dermatology and venereology, ed. 3. Baltimore, 1977, The Williams & Wilkins Co.

7 Mehregan AH: Pinkus' guide to dermatohistopathology, ed. 4. Norwalk, 1986, Appleton-Century-Crofts.

8 Montgomery H: Dermatopathology. New York, 1967, Hoeber Medical Division, Harper & Row, Publishers, vols. I and II.

9 Rook A, Wilkinson DS, Ebling FJG, Champion RH, Burton JL: Textbook of dermatology, ed. 4. Oxford, England, 1986, Blackwell Scientific Publications.

NORMAL HISTOLOGY

10 Dobson RL, Abele DC: Cytologic changes in the eccrine sweat gland in hypothyroidism. A preliminary report. J Invest Dermatol 37:457-458, 1961.

11 Gersh I, Catchpole HR: The nature of ground substance of connective tissue. Perspect Biol Med 3:282-319, 1960.

12 Horstman E: Die Haut. In Möllendorff WV (ed): Handbuch der microskopichen Anatomie des Menschen, vol. 3, part 3. Berlin, 1957, Springer-Verlag, pp. 1-488.

13 Loewenthal LJA: The pathogenesis of miliaria. Arch Dermatol 84:2-17, 1961.

14 Lund HZ, Sommerville RL: Basophilic degeneration of the cutis. Am J Clin Pathol 27:183-190, 1957.

15 Montagna W, Parakkal PF: The structure and function of the skin, ed. 3. New York, 1974, Academic Press, Inc.

16 Sams WM Jr, Smith JG Jr: The histochemistry of chronically sun-damaged skin. J Invest Dermatol 37:447-453, 1961.

17 Winkelmann RK: Cutaneous vascular patterns. In Montagna W, Ellis RA (eds): Advances in biology of the skin. Vol. 2. The blood vessels and circulation of blood in the skin. New York, 1961, Pergamon Press, Inc.

INFLAMMATORY DISEASES OF KNOWN ETIOLOGY
Viral diseases

18 Ebert MH, Otsuka M: Virus diseases of skin, with special reference to elementary and inclusion bodies. Arch Dermatol 48:635-649, 1943.

Warts

19 Aiba S, Rokugo M, Tagami H: Immunohistologic analysis of the phenomenon of spontaneous regression of numerous flat warts. Cancer 58:1246-1251, 1986.

20 Berman A, Winkelmann RK: Flat warts undergoing involution. Histopathological findings. Arch Dermatol 113:1219-1221, 1977.

21 Brownstein MH: The benign acanthomas. J Cutan Pathol 12:172-188, 1985.

22 Dvoretzky I, Lowy DR: Infections by human papillomavirus (warts). Am J Dermatopathol 4:85-89, 1982.

23 Iwatsuki K, Tagami H, Takigawa M, Yamada M: Plane warts under spontaneous regression. Immunopathologic study on cellular constituents leading to the inflammatory reaction. Arch Dermatol 122:655-659, 1986.

24 Jenson AB, Sommer S, Payling-Wright C, Pass F, Link CC Jr, Lancaster WD: Human papillomavirus. Frequency and distribution in plantar and common warts. Lab Invest 47:491-497, 1982.

25 Kimura S, Komatsu T, Ohyama K: Common and plantar warts with trichilemmal keratinization-like keratinizing process. A possible existence of pseudo-trichilemmal keratinization. J Cutan Pathol 9:391-395, 1982.

26 Phillips ME, Ackerman AB: "Benign" and "malignant" neoplasms associated with verrucae vulgaris. Am J Dermatopathol 4:61-84, 1982.

27 Rowson KEK, Mahy BWJ: Human papova (wart) virus. Bacteriol Rev 31:110-131, 1967.

Molluscum contagiosum

28 Legrain A, Pierard GE: Molluscum contagiosum may affect primarily the epidermis without involving hair follicles. Am J Dermatopathol 7:131-132, 1985.

29 Reed RJ, Parkinson RP: The histogenesis of molluscum contagiosum. Am J Surg Pathol 1:161-166, 1977.

30 Sutton JS, Burnett JW: Ultrastructural changes in dermal and epidermal cells of skin infected with molluscum contagiosum virus. J Ultrastruct Res 26:177-196, 1969.

Herpes zoster

31 Merselis JG, Kaye D, Hook EW: Disseminated herpes zoster. Report of 17 cases. Arch Intern Med 113:679-686, 1964.

32 Molin I: Aspects of the natural history of herpes zoster. Acta Derm Venereol [Stockh] 48:569-583, 1969.

Bacterial diseases
Hidradenitis suppurativa

33 Brunsting HA: Hidradenitis suppurativa. Abscess of the apocrine sweat glands. A study of the clinical and pathologic features with a report of 23 cases and a review of the literature. Arch Dermatol **39:**108-119, 1939.

34 Dillon JS, Spjut HJ: Acne aggregata seu conglobata. Ann Surg **195:**451-455, 1964.

35 Masson JK: Surgical treatment for hidradenitis suppurativa. Surg Clin North Am **49:**1043-1052, 1969.

36 Shelley WB, Cahn MM: The pathogenesis of hidradenitis suppurativa in man. Arch Dermatol **72:**562-569, 1955.

Tuberculosis and atypical mycobacteriosis

37 Beyt BE Jr, Ortbals DW, Santa Cruz DJ, Kobayaski GS, Eisen AZ, Medoff G: Cutaneous mycobacteriosis. Analysis of 34 cases with a new classification of the disease. Medicine [Baltimore] **60:**95-109, 1980.

38 Hayman J, McQueen A: The pathology of *Mycobacterium ulcerans* infection. Pathology **17:**594-600, 1985.

39 Montgomery H: Histopathology of various types of cutaneous tuberculosis. Arch Dermatol **35:**698-715, 1937.

40 Russell B: Tuberculosis of the skin. Practitioner **180:**553-563, 1958.

41 Santa Cruz DJ, Strayer DS: The histologic spectrum of the cutaneous mycobacterioses. Hum Pathol **13:**485-495, 1982.

42 Saxe N: Mycobacterial skin infections. J Cutan Pathol **12:**300-312, 1985.

43 Travis WD, Travis LB, Roberts GD, Su DW, Weiland LW: The histopathologic spectrum in *Mycobacterium marinum* infection. Arch Pathol Lab Med **109:**1109-1113, 1985.

Leprosy

44 Binford CH: Leprosy as a diagnostic problem in surgical pathology. South Med J **51:**200-207, 1958.

45 Mansfield RE: Histoid leprosy. Arch Pathol **87:**580-585, 1969.

Malakoplakia

46 Nieland ML, Silverman AR, Borochovitz D, Saferstein HL: Cutaneous malakoplakia. Am J Dermatopathol **3:**287-291, 1981.

Spirochetal diseases
Syphilis

47 Alessi E, Innocenti M, Ragusa G: Secondary syphilis. Clinical morphology and histopathology. Am J Dermatopathol **5:**11-17, 1983.

Lyme disease

48 Aberer E, Stanek G: Histological evidence for spirochetal origin of morphea and lichen sclerosus et atrophicans. Am J Dermatopathol **9:**374-379, 1987.

49 Berger BW, Clemmensen OJ, Ackerman AB: Lyme disease is a spirochetosis. A review of the disease and evidence for its cause. Am J Dermatopathol **5:**111-124, 1983.

Fungal diseases
Tinea (dermatophytoses)

50 Graham JH, Johnson WC, Burgoon CF, Helwig EB: Tinea capitis. Arch Dermatol **89:**528-543, 1964.

North American blastomycosis

51 Baker RD: Tissue reaction in human blastomycosis. Am J Pathol **18:**479-497, 1942.

52 Harrell ER, Curtis AC: North American blastomycosis. Am J Med **27:**750-766, 1959.

Chromoblastomycosis

53 Azulay RD, Serruya J: Hematogenous dissemination in chromoblastomycosis. Arch Dermatol **95:**57-60, 1966.

54 French AJ, Russell SR: Chromoblastomycosis. Arch Dermatol **67:**129-134, 1953.

55 Kempson RL, Sternberg WH: Chronic subcutaneous abscesses caused by pigmented fungi, a lesion distinguishable from cutaneous chromoblastomycosis. Am J Clin Pathol **39:**598-606, 1963.

56 Moore M, Cooper ZK, Weiss RS: Chromomycosis (chromoblastomycosis). JAMA **122:**1237-1243, 1943.

Other granulomatous diseases
Sarcoidosis

57 Cronin E: Skin changes in sarcoidosis. Postgrad Med J **46:**507-509, 1970.

58 Hurley HJ, Shelley WB: Sarcoid granulomas with intradermal tuberculin in normal human skin. Arch Dermatol **82:**65-72, 1960.

59 Israel HL, Goldstein RA: Relations of Kveim-antigen reaction to lymphadenopathy. N Engl J Med **284:**345-349, 1971.

60 Maycock RL, Bertrand P, Morrison CE, Scott JH: Manifestations of sarcoidosis. Am J Med **35:**67-89, 1963.

61 Siltzbach LE: The Kveim test in sarcoidosis. JAMA **178:**476-482, 1961.

62 Thomas PD, Hunninghake GW: Current concepts of the pathogenesis of sarcoidosis. Am Rev Respir Dis **135:**747-760, 1987.

Foreign body reaction

63 Allen AC: Persistent "insect bites" (dermal eosinophilic granulomas) simulating lymphoblastomas, histiocytoses, and squamous cell carcinomas. Am J Pathol **24:**367-387, 1948.

64 Epstein E: Silica granuloma of the skin. Arch Dermatol **71:**24-35, 1955.

65 Helwig EB: Chemical (beryllium) granulomas of the skin. Milit Surg **109:**540-558, 1951.

66 Newcomer VD, Graham JH, Schaffert RR, Kaplan L: Sclerosing lipogranuloma resulting from exogenous lipids. Arch Dermatol **73:**361-371, 1956.

67 Shelley WB, Hurley HJ: The allergic origin of zirconium deodorant granulomas. Br J Dermatol **70:**75-101, 1958.

68 Shelley WB, Hurley HJ: The pathogenesis of silica granulomas in man. A nonallergic colloidal phenomenon. J Invest Dermatol **34:**107-123, 1960.

INFLAMMATORY DISEASES OF UNKNOWN ETIOLOGY
Psoriasis

69 Albert J, Crone RI: Keratosis blenorrhagica (Reiter's disease?) and its treatment. Arch Dermatol **79:**581-586, 1959.

70 Barr RJ, Young EM Jr: Psoriasiform and related papulosquamous disorders. J Cutan Pathol **12:**412-425, 1985.

71 Champion RH: Psoriasis. Br Med J [Clin Res] **292:**1693-1969, 1986.

72 Farber EM, McClintock RP: A current review of psoriasis. Calif Med **108:**440-457, 1968.

73 Helwig EB: Pathology of psoriasis. Ann NY Acad Sci **73:**924-935, 1958.

74 Fox BJ, Odom RB: Papulosquamous diseases. A review. J Am Acad Dermatol **12:**597-624, 1985.

75 Leigh IM, Pulford KA, Ramaekers FCS, Lane EB: Psoriasis. Maintenance of an intact monolayer basal cell differentiation compartment in spite of hyperproliferation. Br J Dermatol **113:**53-64, 1985.

76 Sanchez NP, Perry HO, Muller SA, Winkelmann RK: Subcorneal pustular dermatosis and pustular psoriasis. A clinicopathologic correlation. Arch Dermatol **119:**715-721, 1983.

77 Soeprono FF: Histologic criteria for the diagnosis of pityriasis rubra pilaris. Am J Dermatopathol **8:**277-283, 1986.

78 Weinstein GD, van Scott EJ: Autoradiographic analysis of turnover times of normal and psoriatic epidermis. J Invest Dermatol **45:**257-262, 1965.

Exfoliative dermatitis and erythroderma

79 Abrahams I, McCarthy JT, Sanders SL: One hundred and one cases of exfoliative dermatitis. Arch Dermatol **87:**96-101, 1963.

80 Nicolis GD, Helwig EB: Exfoliative dermatitis. Arch Dermatol **108:**788-797, 1973.

81 Sentis HJ, Willemze R, Scheffer E: Histopathologic studies in Sezary syndrome and erythrodermic mycosis fungoides. A comparison with benign forms of erythroderma. Am Acad Dermatol **15:**1217-1226, 1986.

Lichen planus

82 Altman J, Perry HO: The variations and course of lichen planus. Arch Dermatol **84:**179-191, 1961.

83 Andreasen JO: Oral lichen planus. A histologic evaluation of 97 cases. Oral Surg **25:**158-166, 1968.

84 Berman A, Herszenson S, Winkelmann RK: The involuting lichenoid plaque. Arch Dermatol **118:**93-96, 1982.

85 DePanfilis G, Manara G, Sansoni P, Allegra F: T-cell infiltrate in lichen planus. Demonstration of activated lymphocytes using monoclonal antibodies. J Cutan Pathol **10:**52-58, 1983.

85a Fox, BJ, Odom RB: Papulosquamous disease. A review. J Am Acad Dermatol **12:**597-624, 1985.

86 Frigy AF, Cooper PH: Benign lichenoid keratosis. Am J Clin Pathol **83:**439-443, 1985.

87 Gomes MA, Staquet MJ, Thivolet J: Staining of colloid bodies by keratin antisera in lichen planus. Am J Dermatopathol 3:341-347, 1981.

88 Johnson WC: Necrobiotic granulomas. J Cutan Pathol 12:289-299, 1984.

89 Lumpkin LR, Helwig EB: Solitary lichen planus. Arch Dermatol 93:54-55, 1966.

90 Pinkus H: Lichenoid tissue reactions. Arch Dermatol 107:840-846, 1973.

91 Ragaz A, Ackerman AB: Evolution, maturation, and regression of lesions of lichen planus. New observations and correlations of clinical and histologic findings. Am J Dermatopathol 3:5-25, 1981.

92 Sale GE, Lerner KG, Barker EA, Shulman HM, Thomas ED: The skin biopsy in the diagnosis of acute graft-versus-host disease in man. Am J Pathol 89:621-635, 1977.

93 Scully C, El-Kom M: Lichen planus. Review and update on pathogenesis. J Oral Pathol 14:431-458, 1985.

93a Weedon D: The lichenoid tissue reaction. J Cutan Pathol 12:279-281, 1985.

Graft-versus-host disease

94 Elliott CJ, Sloane JP, Sanderson KV, Vincent M, Shepherd V, Powles R: The histological diagnosis of cutaneous graft versus host disease. Relationship of skin changes to marrow purging and other clinical variables. Histopathology 11:145-155, 1987.

95 Hymes SR, Farmer ER, Lewis PG, Tutschka PJ, Santos GW: Cutaneous graft-versus-host reaction. Prognostic features seen by light microscopy. J Am Acad Dermatol 12:468-474, 1985.

96 Spielvogel RL, Goltz RW, Kersey JH: Scleroderma-like changes in chronic graft vs host disease. Arch Dermatol 113:1424-1428, 1977.

Vasculitis

97 Ackerman AB, Jones RE Jr: Making chronic nonspecific dermatitis specific. How to make precise diagnoses of superficial perivascular dermatitides devoid of epidermal involvement. Am J Dermatopathol 7:307-323, 1985.

98 af Ekenstam E, Callen JP: Cutaneous leukocytoclastic vasculitis. Clinical and laboratory features of 82 patients seen in private practice. Arch Dermatol 120:484-489, 1984.

99 Black MM, Wilson Jones E: Malignant atrophic papulosis (Degos syndrome). Br J Dermatol 85:290-292, 1971.

100 Chumbley LC, Harrison EG Jr, DeRemee RA: Allergic granulomatosis and angiitis (Churg-Strauss syndrome). Report and analysis of 30 cases. Mayo Clin Proc 52:477-484, 1977.

101 Copeman PWM, Ryan TJ: The problems of classification of cutaneous angiitis with reference to histopathology and pathogenesis. Br J Dermatol 82:2-14, 1970.

102 Curtis JL, Egbert BM: Cutaneous cytomegalovirus vasculitis. An unusual clinical presentation of a common opportunistic pathogen. Hum Pathol 13:1138-1141, 1982.

103 Finan MC, Winkelmann RK: The cutaneous extravascular necrotizing granuloma (Churg-Strauss granuloma) and systemic disease. A review of 27 cases. Medicine [Baltimore] 62:142-157, 1983.

104 Gilliam JN, Smiley JD: Cutaneous necrotizing vasculitis and related disorders. Ann Surg 37:328-339, 1976.

105 Gray HR, Graham JH, Johnson W, Burgoon CF Jr: Atrophie blanche. Periodic painful ulcers of the lower extremities. Arch Dermatol 93:187-193, 1966.

106 Harrist TJ, Mihm MC Jr: The diagnostic use of direct and indirect immunofluorescence techniques in dermatologic disease. Hum Pathol 10:625-653, 1979.

107 Hodge SJ, Callen JP, Ekenstam E: Cutaneous leukocytoclastic vasculitis. Correlation of histopathological changes with clinical severity and course. J Cutan Pathol 14:279-284, 1987.

108 James WD, Odom RB, Katzenstein A-LA: Cutaneous manifestations of lymphomatoid granulomatosis. Report of 44 cases and a review of the literature. Arch Dermatol 117:196-202, 1981.

109 Kessler S, Lund HZ, Leonard DD: Cutaneous lesions of lymphomatoid granulomatosis. Comparison with lymphomatoid papulosis. Am J Dermatopathol 3:115-127, 1981.

110 Lie JT: The classification and diagnosis of vasculitis in large and medium-sized blood vessels. Pathol Annu 22(Pt 1):125-162, 1987.

111 Mackel SE, Jordon RE: Leukocytoclastic vasculitis. A cutaneous expression of immune complex disease. Arch Dermatol 118:296-301, 1982.

112 Molenaar WM, Rosman JB, Donker AJM, Houthoff HJ: The pathology and pathogenesis of malignant atrophic papulosis (Degos' disease). A case study with reference to other vascular disorders. Pathol Res Pract 182:98-106, 1987.

113 Ryan TJ: Cutaneous vasculitis. J Cutan Pathol 12:381-387, 1985.

114 Sams WM Jr, Claman HN, Kohler PF, McIntosh RM, Small P, Mass MF: Human necrotizing vasculitis. Immunoglobulins and complement in vessel walls of cutaneous lesions and normal skin. J Invest Dermatol 64:441-445, 1975.

115 Sams WM Jr, Thorne EG, Small P, Mass MF, McIntosh RM, Stanford RE: Leukocytoclastic vasculitis. Arch Dermatol 112:219-226, 1976.

116 Sanchez NP, Van Hale HM, Su WPD: Clinical and histopathologic spectrum of necrotizing vasculitis. Report of findings in 101 cases. Arch Dermatol 121:220-224, 1985.

117 Winkelmann RK, Ditto WB: Cutaneous and visceral syndromes of necrotizing or "allergic" angiitis. A study of 38 cases. Medicine [Baltimore] 43:59-89, 1964.

Granuloma faciale

118 Allen AC: Persistent "insect bites" (dermal eosinophilic granulomas) simulating lymphoblastomas, histiocytoses, and squamous cell carcinomas. Am J Pathol 24:367-387, 1948.

119 Johnson WC, Higdon RS, Helwig EB: Granuloma faciale. Arch Dermatol 79:42-52, 1959.

120 Pedace FJ, Perry HO: Granuloma faciale. Arch Dermatol 94:387-395, 1966.

Erythema nodosum

121 Black MM: Panniculitis. J Cutan Pathol 12:366-380, 1985.

122 Förström L, Winkelmann RK: Acute panniculitis. A clinical and pathologic study of 34 cases. Arch Dermatol 113:909-917, 1977.

123 Irgang S: Nodular vasculitis. Arch Dermatol 74:245-249, 1956.

123a Mir-Madjlessi SH, Taylor JS, Farmer RG: Clinical course and evolution of erythema nodosum and pyoderma gangrenosum in chronic ulcerative colitis. A study of 42 patients. Am J Gastroenterol 80:615-620, 1985.

124 Perry HO, Winkelmann RK: Subacute nodular migratory panniculitis. Arch Dermatol 89:170-179, 1964.

125 Reed RJ, Clark WH, Mihm MC: Disorders of the panniculus adiposus. Hum Pathol 4:219-229, 1973.

126 Vesey CMR, Wilkinson DS: Erythema nodosum. A study of 70 cases. Br J Dermatol 71:139-155, 1959.

127 Winkelmann RK: Panniculitis in connective tissue disease. Arch Dermatol 119:336-344, 1983.

128 Winkelmann RK, Förström L: New observations on the histopathology of erythema nodosum. J Invest Dermatol 65:441-446, 1975.

Granuloma annulare

129 Arner S, Aspegren N: Familial granuloma annulare. Acta Derm Venereol [Stockh] 48:253-254, 1968.

130 Beatty EC: Rheumatic-like nodules occurring in nonrheumatic children. Arch Pathol 68:154-159, 1959.

130a Johnson WC: Necrobiotic granulomas. J Cutan Pathol 12:289-299, 1984.

131 Mesara BW, Brody GL, Oberman HA: "Pseudorheumatoid" subcutaneous nodules. Am J Clin Pathol 45:684-691, 1966.

132 Patterson JW: Rheumatoid nodule and subcutaneous granuloma annulare. A comparative histologic study. Am J Dermatopathol 10:1-8, 1988.

133 Rubin M, Lynch FW: Subcutaneous granuloma annulare. Comment on familial granuloma annulare. Arch Dermatol 93:416-429, 1966.

134 Schwarz TH, Lindlbauer R, Gschnait F: Annular elastolytic giant cell granuloma. J Cutan Pathol 10:321-326, 1983.

135 Wells RS, Smith MA: The natural history of granuloma annulare. Br J Dermatol 75:199-205, 1963.

136 Wood MG, Beerman H: Necrobiosis lipoidica, granuloma annulare and rheumatoid nodule. J Invest Dermatol 34:139-147, 1960.

137 Yanagihara M, Kato F, Mori S: Extra- and intra-cellular digestion of elastic fibers by macrophages in annular elastolytic giant cell granuloma. An ultrastructural study. J Cutan Pathol 14:303-308, 1987.

Necrobiosis lipoidica

138 Bauer M, Levan NE: Diabetic dermangiopathy. A spectrum including pigmented pretibial patches and necrobiosis lipoidica diabeticorum. Br J Dermatol 83:528-535, 1970.

139 Fisher ER, Danowski TS: Histologic, histochemical, and electron microscopic features of the shin spots of diabetes mellitus. Am J Clin Pathol 50:547-554, 1968.

140 Holden CA, Winkelmann RK, Wilson Jones E: Necrobiotic xanthogranuloma. A report of four cases. Br J Dermatol 114:241-250, 1986.

141 Muller SA, Winkelmann RK: Necrobiosis lipoidica diabeticorum. Histopathologic study of 98 cases. Arch Dermatol 94:1-10, 1966.

142 Padilla RS, Mukai K, Dahl MV, Burgdorf WH, Rosai J: Differential staining pattern of lysozyme in palisading granulomas. An immunoperoxidase study. J Am Acad Dermatol 8:634-638, 1983.

Weber-Christian disease

143 Christian HA: Relapsing febrile nodular nonsuppurative panniculitis. Arch Intern Med **42:**338-341, 1928.

144 Laymon CW, Peterson WC Jr: Lipogranulomatosis subcutanea (Rothmann-Makai). An appraisal. Arch Dermatol **90:**288-292, 1964.

145 Lever WF: Nodular nonsuppurative panniculitis (Weber-Christian disease). Arch Dermatol **59:**31-35, 1949.

145a Su WPD, Smith KC, Pittelkow MR, Winkelmann RK: α1-antitrypsin deficiency panniculitis. A histopathologic study of four cases. Am J Dermatopathol **9:**483-490, 1987.

Urticaria pigmentosa

146 Berlin C: Urticaria pigmentosa as a systemic disease. Arch Dermatol **71:**703-712, 1955.

147 Brunning RD, McKenna RW, Rosai J, Parkin JL, Risdall R: Systemic mastocytosis. Extracutaneous manifestations. Am J Surg Pathol **7:**425-438, 1983.

148 Caplan RM: The natural course of urticaria pigmentosa. Analysis and follow-up of 112 cases. Arch Dermatol **87:**144-157, 1963.

149 Drennan JM: The mast cells in urticaria pigmentosa. J Pathol Bacteriol **63:**513-520, 1951.

150 Head KW: Cutaneous mast cell tumors in the dog, cat, and ox. Br J Dermatol **70:**390-408, 1958.

151 Johnson WC, Helwig EB: Solitary mastocytosis (urticaria pigmentosa). Arch Dermatol **84:**806-815, 1961.

152 Klatt EC, Lukes RJ, Meyer PR: Benign and malignant mast cell proliferations. Diagnosis and separation using a pH-dependent toluidine blue stain in tissue section. Cancer **51:**1119-1124, 1983.

153 Lennert K, Parkaresch MR: Mast cells and mast cell neoplasia. A review. Histopathology **3:**349-365, 1979.

154 Mihm MC, Clark WH, Reed RJ, Caruso MG: Mast cell infiltrates of the skin and the mastocytosis syndrome. Hum Pathol **4:**231-239, 1973.

155 Nickel WR: Urticaria pigmentosa. Arch Dermatol **76:**476-498, 1957.

156 Nielsen SW, Cole CR: Canine mastocytoma. A report of one hundred cases. Am J Vet Res **19:**417-432, 1958.

157 Travis WD, Li C-Y, Su WPD: Adult-onset urticaria pigmentosa and systemic mast cell disease. Am J Clin Pathol **84:**710-714, 1985.

Lupus erythematosus

158 Bangert JL, Freeman RG, Sontheimer RD, Gilliam JN: Subacute cutaneous lupus erythematosus and discoid lupus erythematosus. Comparative histopathologic findings. Arch Dermatol **120:**332-337, 1984.

159 Biesecker G, Lavin L, Ziskind M, Koffler D: Cutaneous localization of the membrane attack complex in discoid and systemic lupus erythematosus. N Engl J Med **306:**264-270, 1982.

159a Callen JP: Systemic lupus erythematosus in patients with chronic cutaneous (discoid) lupus erythematosus. Clinical and laboratory findings in seventeen patients. J Am Acad Dermatol **12:**278-288, 1985.

159b Clark SK: Cutaneous lupus erythematosus. Recognition of its many forms. Postgrad Med **79:**195-203, 1986.

160 Clark WH, Reed RJ, Mihm MC: Lupus erythematosus. Histopathology of cutaneous lesions. Hum Pathol **4:**157-163, 1973.

161 Harrist TJ, Mihm MC Jr: The diagnostic use of direct and indirect immunofluorescence techniques in dermatologic disease. Hum Pathol **10:**625-653, 1979.

162 Harvey AM, Schulman LE, Tumulty PA, Conley CL, Schoenrich EH: Systemic lupus erythematosus. Review of the literature and clinical analysis of 138 cases. Medicine [Baltimore] **33:**291-437, 1954.

163 Jessner M, Kanof NB: Lymphocytic infiltration of the skin. Arch Dermatol **68:**447-449, 1953.

164 Klemperer P, Pollack AD, Baehr G: Pathology of disseminated lupus erythematosus. Arch Pathol **32:**569-631, 1941.

165 Tuffanelli DL: Lupus erythematosus. Arch Dermatol **106:**553-566, 1972.

166 Uitto J, Santa-Cruz DJ, Zeisen A, Leone P: Verrucous lesions in patients with discoid lupus erythematosus. Br J Dermatol **98:**507-520, 1978.

167 Wechsler HL: Lupus erythematosus. A clinician's coign of vantage. Arch Dermatol **119:**877-882, 1983.

168 Willemze R, Verneer BJ, Meijer CJ: Immunohistochemical studies in lymphocytic infiltration of skin (Jessner) and discoid lupus erythematosus. A comparative study. J Am Acad Dermatol **11:**832-840, 1984.

169 Wojnarowska F, Bhogal B, Black MM: The significance of an IgM band at the dermoepidermal junction. J Cutan Pathol **13:**359-362, 1986.

Dermatomyositis

170 Adams RD: Diseases of muscle. A study in pathology, ed. 3. Hagerstown, Md., 1975, Medical Department, Harper & Row, Publishers, Inc., pp. 337-365.

171 Golitz LE: Collagen diseases. J Cutan Pathol **12:**358-365, 1985.

172 Janis JF, Winkelmann RK: Histopathology of the skin in dermatomyositis. Arch Dermatol **97:**640-649, 1968.

173 Williams RC Jr: Dermatomyositis and malignancy. A review of the literature. Ann Intern Med **50:**1174-1181, 1959.

Scleroderma

173a Asboe-Hansen G: Scleroderma. J Am Acad Dermatol **17:**102-108, 1987.

174 Barnes L, Rodnan GP, Medsger TA Jr, Short D: Eosinophilic fasciitis. A pathologic study of twenty cases. Am J Pathol **96:**493-518, 1979.

175 Christianson HB, Dorsey CS, O'Leary PA, Kierland RR: Localized scleroderma. A clinical study of 235 cases. Arch Dermatol **74:**629-639, 1956.

176 Doyle JA, Connolly SM, Winkelmann RK: Cutaneous and subcutaneous inflammatory sclerosis syndromes. Arch Dermatol **118:**886-890, 1982.

177 Fisher ER, Rodnan GP: Pathological observations concerning the cutaneous lesion of progressive systemic sclerosis. An electron microscopic histochemical and immunohistochemical study. Arthritis Rheum **3:**536-545, 1960.

178 Fleischmajer R: The collagen in scleroderma. Arch Dermatol **89:**437-441, 1964.

179 Fleischmajer R, Perlish JS, Duncan M: Scleroderma. A model for fibrosis. Arch Dermatol **119:**957-962, 1983.

180 Jones HR Jr, Beetham WP Jr, Silverman ML, Margles SW: Eosinophilic fasciitis and the carpal tunnel syndrome. J Neurol Neurosurg Psychiatry **49:**324-327, 1986.

181 Lovell CR, Nicholls AC, Duance VC, Bailey AJ: Characterization of dermal collagen in systemic sclerosis. Br J Dermatol **100:**359-369, 1979.

182 Michet CJ Jr, Doyle JA, Ginsburg WW: Eosinophilic fasciitis. Report of 15 cases. Mayo Clin Proc **56:**27-34, 1981.

183 Moutsopoulos HM, Webber BL, Pavlidis NA, Fostiropoulos G, Goules D, Shulman LE: Diffuse fasciitis with eosinophilia. A clinicopathologic study. Am J Med **68:**701-709, 1980.

184 Person JR, Su WPD: Subcutaneous morphea. A clinical study of sixteen cases. Br J Dermatol **100:**371-380, 1979.

185 Reed RJ, Clark WH, Mihm MC: The cutaneous collagenoses. Hum Pathol **4:**165-186, 1973.

185a Singsen BH: Scleroderma in childhood. Pediatr Clin North Am **33:**1119-1139, 1986.

186 Su WPD, Person JR: Morphea profunda. A new concept and a histopathologic study of 23 cases. Am J Dermatopathol **3:**251-260, 1981.

187 Winkelmann RK: Classification and pathogenesis of scleroderma. Mayo Clin Proc **46:**83-91, 1971.

188 Young EM Jr, Barr RJ: Sclerosing dermatoses. J Cutan Pathol **12:**426-441, 1985.

VESICULOBULLOUS DISEASES

189 Ackerman AB: Focal acantholytic dyskeratosis. Arch Dermatol **106:**702-706, 1972.

190 Anhalt GJ, Labib RS, Voorhees JJ, Beals TF, Diaz LA: Induction of pemphigus in neonatal mice by passive transfer of IgG from patients with the disease. N Engl J Med **306:**1189-1196, 1982.

191 Bedi TR, Pinkus H: Histopathological spectrum of erythema multiforme. Br J Dermatol **95:**243-250, 1976.

192 Beutner EH, Chorzelski TP, Jordan RE: Autosensitization in pemphigus and bullous pemphigoid. Springfield, Ill., 1970, Charles C Thomas, Publisher.

193 Chalet M, Grover R, Ackerman AB: Transient acantholytic dermatosis. A re-evaluation. Arch Dermatol **113:**431-435, 1977.

194 Farmer ER: Subepidermal bullous diseases. J Cutan Pathol **12:**316-321, 1985.

194a Flowers FP, Sherertz EF: Immunologic disorders of the skin and mucous membranes. Med Clin North Am **69:**657-673, 1985.

195 Harrist TJ, Mihm MC Jr: The diagnostic use of direct and indirect immunofluorescence techniques in dermatologic disease. Hum Pathol **10:**625-653, 1979.

196 Hu C-H, Michel B, Farber EM: Transient acantholytic dermatosis (Grover's disease). A skin disorder related to heat and sweating. Arch Dermatol **121:**1439-1441, 1985.

197 Jablonska S (with Working and Organizing Committee): Cooperative study. Uses for immunofluorescence tests of skin and sera. Utilization of immunofluorescence in the diagnosis of bullous diseases, lupus erythematosus and certain other dermatoses. Arch Dermatol **111:**371-381, 1975.

198 Jordon RE: Commentary. Pemphigus erythematosus. A unique member of the pemphigus group. Arch Dermatol **118:**742, 1982.

199 Judd KP, Lever WF: Correlation of antibodies in skin and serum with disease severity in pemphigus. Arch Dermatol 115:428-432, 1979.

200 Lazaro-Medina A, Robbins TO, Bystryn J-C, Ackerman AB: Limitations in the diagnosis of vesiculobullous diseases. Am J Dermatopathol 5:7-10, 1983.

201 Lever WF: Pemphigus and pemphigoid. Springfield, Ill., 1965, Charles C Thomas, Publisher.

202 Lyell A: Dermatitis herpetiformis enteropathy. Br J Dermatol 81:228-229, 1968.

203 Maize JC, Provost TT: Value of immunofluorescent techniques in studies of bullous disease. Am J Dermatopathol 5:67-72, 1983.

204 Orfanos CE, Schaumburg-Lever G, Lever WF: Dermal and epidermal types of erythema multiforme. A histopathologic study of 24 cases. Arch Dermatol 109:682-688, 1974.

205 Perry HO, Brunsting LA: Pemphigus foliaceus. Further observations. Arch Dermatol 91:10-23, 1965.

206 Piérard J, Whimster I: The histological diagnosis of dermatitis herpetiformis, bullous pemphigoid and erythema multiforme. Br J Dermatol 73:253-266, 1961.

207 Santa Cruz DJ, Prioleau PG, Marcus MD, Uitto J: Pemphigus-like lesions induced by D-penicillamine. Analysis of clinical, histopathological, and immunofluorescence features in 34 cases. Am J Dermatopathol 3:85-92, 1981.

208 Saxe N, Kahn LB: Subepidermal bullous disease. A correlated clinico-pathologic study of 51 cases. J Cutan Pathol 3:88-94, 1976.

209 Sneddon IB, Wilkinson DS: Subcorneal pustular dermatosis. Br J Dermatol 68:385-394, 1956.

210 Stoll DM, King LE Jr: Association of bullous pemphigoid with systemic lupus erythematosus. Arch Dermatol 120:362-366, 1984.

211 Thivolet J, Faure M: Immunohistochemistry in cutaneous pathology. J Cutan Pathol 10:1-32, 1983.

212 Tollman MM: Dermatitis herpetiformis. Arch Dermatol 77:462-465, 1968.

213 Tuffanelli DL: Clinical importance of autoantibodies in pemphigus. Arch Dermatol 118:844-845, 1982.

214 Turbitt ML, Mackie RM, Young H, Campbell I: The use of paraffin-processed tissue and the immunoperoxidase technique in the diagnosis of bullous diseases, lupus erythematosus and vasculitis. Br J Dermatol 106:411-418, 1982.

215 Waldo ED, Ackerman AB: Epidermolytic hyperkeratosis and focal acantholytic dyskeratosis. A unified concept. Pathol Annu 13:149-175, 1978.

DEGENERATIVE AND MISCELLANEOUS DISEASES
Lichen sclerosus et atrophicus

216 Barker LP, Gross P: Lichen sclerosus et atrophicus of the female genitalia. Arch Dermatol 85:362-373, 1962.

217 Montgomery H, Hill WR: Lichen sclerosus et atrophicus. Arch Dermatol 42:755-779, 1940.

218 Patterson JAK, Ackerman AB: Lichen sclerosus et atrophicus is not related to morphea. A clinical and histologic study of 24 patients in whom both conditions were reputed to be present simultaneously. Am J Dermatopathol 6:323-335, 1984.

Elastosis perforans

219 Golitz L: Follicular and perforating disorders. J Cutan Pathol 12:282-288, 1985.

220 Hitch JM, Lund HZ: Elastosis perforans serpiginosa. Arch Dermatol 79:407-421, 1959.

221 Hood AF, Hardegen GL, Zarate AR, Nigra TP, Gelfand MC: Kyrle's disease in patients with chronic renal failure. Arch Dermatol 118:85-88, 1982.

222 Mehregan AH: Elastosis perforans serpiginosa. Arch Dermatol 97:381-393, 1968.

223 Millard PR, Young E, Harrison DE, Wojnarowska F: Reactive perforating collagenosis. Light, ultrastructural and immunohistological studies. Histopathology 10:1047-1056, 1986.

223a Patterson JW: The perforating disorders. J Am Acad Dermatol 10:561-581, 1984.

224 Poliak SC, Lebwohl MG, Parris A, Prioleau PG: Reactive perforating collagenosis associated with diabetes mellitus. N Engl J Med 306:81-84, 1982.

225 Reed RJ, Clark WH, Mihm MC: The cutaneous elastoses. Hum Pathol 4:187-199, 1973.

226 White CR Jr, Heskel NS, Pokorny DJ: Perforating folliculitis of hemodialysis. Am J Dermatopathol 4:109-116, 1982.

Pseudoxanthoma elasticum

227 Graham Smith J Jr, Davidson EA, Clark RD: Dermal elastica in actinic elastosis and pseudoxanthoma elastica. Nature [London] 195:716-717, 1962.

228 Robertson MG, Schroder JS: Pseudoxanthoma elasticum. A systemic disorder. Am J Med 27:433-442, 1959.

Cutaneous mucinoses

229 Beierwaltes WH, Bollet AJ: Mucopolysaccharide content of skin in patients with pretibial myxedema. J Clin Invest 38:945-948, 1959.

229a Carney JA, Headington JT, Su WPD: Cutaneous nyxomas. A major component of the complex of myxomas, spotty pigmentation, and endocrine overactivity. Arch Dermatol 122:790-798, 1986.

230 Farmer ER, Hambrick GW Jr, Shulman LE: Papular mucinosis. A clinicopathologic study of four patients. Arch Dermatol 118:9-13, 1982.

231 Gabrilove JL, Ludwig AW: The histogenesis of myxedema. J Clin Endocrinol Metab 17:925-932, 1957.

232 Hempstead RW, Ackerman AB: Follicular mucinosis. A reaction pattern in follicular epithelium. Am J Dermatopathol 7:245-257, 1985.

233 Johnson WC, Graham JH, Helwig EB: Cutaneous myxoid cyst. A clinicopathological and histochemical study. JAMA 191:109-114, 1965.

234 Johnson WC, Helwig EB: Cutaneous focal mucinosis. A clinicopathological and histochemical study. Arch Dermatol 93:13-20, 1966.

235 Reed RJ, Clark WH, Mihm MC: The cutaneous mucinoses. Hum Pathol 4:201-205, 1973.

236 Steigleder GK, Küchmeister B: Cutaneous mucinous deposits. J Cutan Pathol 12:334-347, 1985.

Acanthosis nigricans

237 Brown J, Winkelmann RK: Acanthosis nigricans. A study of 90 cases. Medicine [Baltimore] 47:33-51, 1968.

238 Curth HO: Cancer associated with acanthosis nigricans. Arch Surg 47:517-522, 1943.

239 Ellis DL, Kafka SP, Chow JC, Nanney LB, Inman WH, McCadden ME, King LE Jr: Melanoma, growth factors, acanthosis nigricans, the sign of Leser-Trélat, and multiple acrochordons. A possible role for alpha-transforming growth factor in cutaneous paraneoplastic syndromes. N Engl J Med 317:1582-1587, 1987.

Tumors and tumorlike conditions

Epidermis
  Seborrheic keratosis
  Achrochordon
  Actinic keratosis
  Cutaneous horn
  Bowen's disease
  Epidermoid (squamous cell) carcinoma
    General features
    Microscopic features
    Other microscopic types
    Treatment
    Prognosis
  Pseudoepitheliomatous hyperplasia
  Basal cell carcinoma
    General features
    Microscopic features
    Other microscopic types
    Spread and metastases
    Treatment
Skin adnexae
  Eccrine sweat gland
    Poroma
    Acrospiroma
    Syringoma
    Chondroid syringoma (mixed tumor)
    Eccrine cylindroma
    Eccrine spiradenoma
    Papillary syringadenoma
    Papillary eccrine adenoma
    Aggressive digital papillary adenoma
    Clear cell acanthoma
    Intraepidermal epithelioma
    Sweat gland carcinoma
    Extramammary Paget's disease
  Apocrine sweat gland
  Sebaceous gland
    Senile sebaceous hyperplasia
    Nevus sebaceus of Jadassohn
    Sebaceous adenoma
    Sebaceous carcinoma
  Hair follicle
    Inverted follicular keratosis
    Trichoepithelioma
    Trichilemmoma
    Trichofolliculoma
    Keratoacanthoma
    Keratinous cyst
    Other cutaneous cysts
    Isolated follicular keratosis (warty dyskeratoma)
    Pilar tumor (proliferating trichilemmal cyst)
    Pilomatrixoma

Melanocytes
  Nevi
    Junctional, intradermal, and compound nevi
    Blue and cellular blue nevi
    Spitz nevus
    Other nevi
    Treatment
    Active and dysplastic nevi
  Malignant melanoma
    General features
    Clinical appearance and clinicopathologic types
    Microscopic features
    Biopsy and frozen section
    Regression
    Atypical in situ melanocytic lesions
    Spread and metastases
    Treatment
    Prognosis
  Pigmentation in other skin tumors
Neuroendocrine cells
  Merkel cell tumor
  Other neuroendocrine tumors
Dermis
  Fibroblastic tumors and tumorlike conditions
  Fibrohistiocytic tumors and tumorlike conditions
    Benign fibrous histiocytoma
    Atypical fibroxanthoma
    Dermatofibrosarcoma protuberans
    Malignant fibrous histiocytoma
    Xanthoma
    Juvenile xanthogranuloma (nevoxanthoendothelioma)
    Other histiocytic proliferations
  Smooth muscle tumors
  Peripheral nerve tumors
  Vascular tumors and tumorlike conditions
    Hemangioma
    Lymphangioma
    Lobular capillary hemangioma
    Masson's hemangioma
    Histiocytoid hemangioma
    Kaposi's sarcoma
    Angiosarcoma
  Lymphoid tumors and tumorlike conditions
    Cutaneous lymphoid hyperplasia
    Lymphomatoid papulosis
  Mycosis fungoides and related T-cell lymphomas
    Lymph nodes in mycosis fungoides
    Other malignant lymphomas
    Leukemia
  Other primary tumors and tumorlike conditions
  Metastatic carcinoma

The skin is, contrary to the ubiquitous simplistic concept, a remarkably heterogeneous organ. The tumors (hamartomatous, reactive, and neoplastic) that occur in the skin are more numerous than those produced by any other organ. For example, the eccrine sweat gland alone gives rise to ten or more histologically distinct adenomas. This diversity, combined with a body of descriptive data (clinical, histologic, histochemical, and ultrastructural) amassed over the past century and dispersed in varying literatures, produces confusion, chiefly in the area of nomenclature. Within the limits inherent in this book, it is impossible to pursue finite segmentation, interesting and accurate as it may be. The more common lesions will be discussed in some detail and pertinent references provided for the rare lesions.

EPIDERMIS
Seborrheic keratosis

Seborrheic keratoses are common, benign, pigmented, basal, and keratinocytic proliferations occurring chiefly on the trunk of adults. They may be single or multiple. The

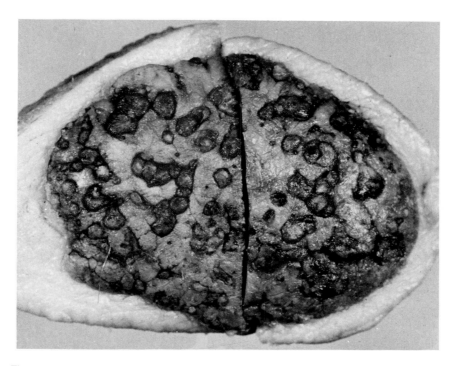

Fig. 4-46 Large, deeply pigmented, sharply circumscribed, elevated, seborrheic keratosis.

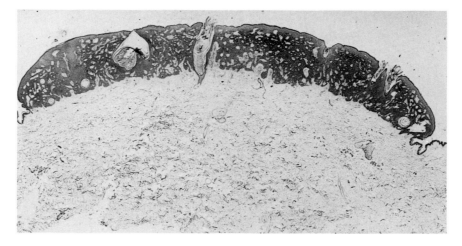

Fig. 4-47 Seborrheic keratosis projecting above level of epidermis. Cysts represent sections of hyperkeratotic follicles.

sudden appearance of, or increase in number and size of, seborrheic keratoses in association with internal malignant disease is known as the Leser-Trélat sign.[1]

Grossly, the lesions of seborrheic keratosis protrude above the surface of the skin, are soft, and vary in color from tan to black. The single, heavily pigmented seborrheic keratosis may be confused clinically with malignant melanoma (Fig. 4-46).

Microscopically, the number of epidermal basal cells is greatly increased, presumably as result of a maturation defect. The acanthotic pattern is the most frequent, in which a thick layer of basal cells is seen interspersed with pseudohorny cysts (Fig. 4-47). Some of these cells contain melanin, as the result of transfer from neighboring melanocytes (see p. 136). Other microscopic patterns of seborrheic keratosis are the hyperkeratotic and the adenoid.

In irritated seborrheic keratosis, squamous metaplasia is pronounced; this should not be misdiagnosed as basosquamous carcinoma. Exceptionally, bowenoid changes develop in lesions otherwise typical of seborrheic keratosis; the clinical significance of this finding has yet to be determined.[2] The multiple, small, seborrheic keratoses are readily treated by superficial curettage or freezing.[3]

Achrochordon

Achrochordon is the preferred name for a common and inconsequential skin lesion also known as fibroepithelial papilloma, fibroepithelial polyp, fibroma molle, and skin tag. As these various names indicate, it is a polypoid lesion composed of varying amounts of stroma covered by a papillomatous epidermis. It is probably not a specific entity, but a pattern of growth that may result from seborrheic keratosis, warts, and perhaps other benign processes.

A distinctive variant of this exophytic fibroepithelial process is represented by the *acquired (digital) fibrokeratoma*, characterized by collagenous protrusions covered by hyperkeratotic epidermis, usually occurring around interphalangeal joints but sometimes in other sites.[4]

Actinic keratosis

In that portion of the epidermis exposed to sunlight, chiefly that of the near ultraviolet spectrum, a sequence of atrophic, dysplastic, and eventually hyperplastic changes known as actinic or solar keratosis may develop (Fig. 4-48). The term "senile" keratosis often is inappropriate. Histologically, actinic keratoses involve the interfollicular epidermis, sparing the follicular apparatus and the intraepidermal portion of the sweat duct.[6] The stratum corneum is replaced by a parakeratotic scale. Excessive production and accumulation of this scale lead to the formation of cutaneous horns. The granular layer is generally absent except at and about the follicular orifices. The malphigian layer shows disorderly maturation as well as individually dysplastic and dyskeratotic cells (Fig. 4-49). On occasion, suprabasal acantholysis produces vesicles reminiscent of those seen in pemphigus vulgaris. Foci of basal cell proliferation resembling basal cell carcinoma may occur. Not infrequently, the basal melanocytes participate in

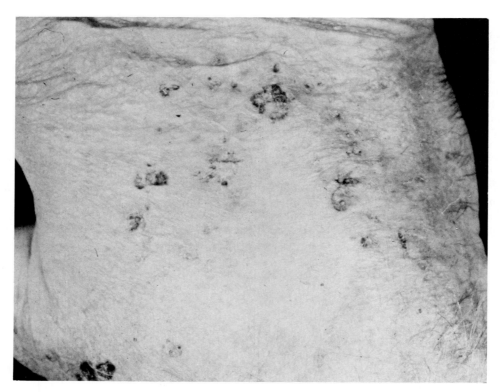

Fig. 4-48 Actinic (senile) keratoses on back of hand. Central area had been previously excised and grafted.

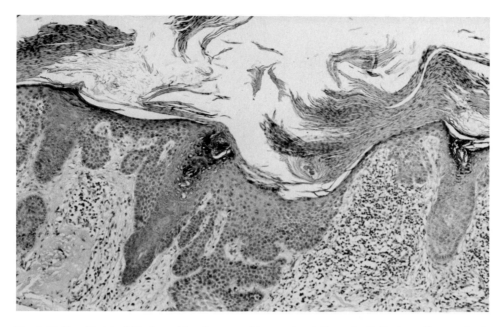

Fig. 4-49 Atrophic interfollicular epidermis covered by parakeratotic scale. Follicular orifices maintain their granular layer and orthokeratosis. Slight atypia is evident in areas of acanthotic hyperplasia in this actinic keratosis.

the proliferation and atypia, resulting in a combination of actinic keratosis and actinic melanosis. Such cases appear clinically as heavily pigmented lesions.[5] The papillary dermis is often chronically inflamed, and basophilic degenerative changes are prominent in the collagen. In florid forms of actinic keratosis, the atypical epithelial proliferation produces irregularly elongated acanthotic ridges, and this process extends down the external root sheaths of the hair follicles.

Actinic keratoses may be treated by a variety of methods—freezing, superficial curettage, application of antineoplastic chemotherapeutic agents, and surgical excision.[7] Excision is, in fact, unnecessarily radical therapy except for the more florid and infiltrative types and those not responding to topical 5-fluorouracil.

Cutaneous horn

Cutaneous horn (cornu cutaneum) is a clinical term for a protruding skin lesion largely composed of keratin and resembling the shape of a horn. This clinical appearance can result from a variety of diseases; therefore cutaneous horn should not be used as a pathologic term. Most cases are caused by actinic keratosis, but others may be the result of verruca, seborrheic keratosis, inverted follicular keratosis, or epidermoid carcinoma. The keratin formed is usually of epidermal type, but occasionally it has trichilemmal-like features. When this is the case, the lesion has been referred to as trichilemmal keratosis, verrucous trichilemmal tumor, and trichilemmal horn.[8,9]

Bowen's disease

The condition described by Bowen[10] consists clinically of indolent, scaly, erythematous plaques occurring predom-

inantly on skin unexposed to sunlight (Fig. 4-50). Histologically, the lesions show a variety of atypical epithelial changes, such as cytoplasmic vacuolization, nuclear hyperchromasia, multinucleated keratinocytes, individual cell dyskeratosis, and increased number of mitoses, including atypical forms (Fig. 4-51). The maturation pattern is markedly altered, but some surface flattening and keratinization are almost always present. In its fully developed stage, Bowen's disease can be regarded as a carcinoma in situ of the skin or as a form of squamous intraepidermal neoplasia, a concept supported by the presence of distinct aneuploidy in flow cytometric studies.[13] It should be emphasized that the diagnosis of Bowen's disease is a clinicopathologic one. Lesions showing similar microscopic changes but located in sun-exposed areas and having the clinical appearance of actinic keratosis should not be diagnosed as Bowen's disease but rather as a variant of actinic keratosis (appropriately called bowenoid type).

Some studies[11,12] have shown an apparent increase in the incidence of visceral cancer in patients with Bowen's disease, but others have failed to document such an association. Since arsenic is capable of inducing hyperplastic and dysplastic epidermal changes that may lead to the development of invasive epidermoid carcinoma, this element has been looked for in lesions of Bowen's disease. So far, this search has proved inconclusive.

Epidermoid (squamous cell) carcinoma
General features

The large majority of epidermoid carcinomas of the skin are actinic induced. The incidence of this tumor is directly related with the amount of exposure to the sun and the lack of pigmentation of the skin. Blond, blue-eyed, fair-skinned

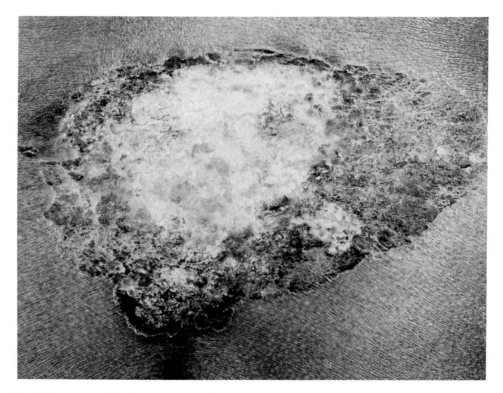

Fig. 4-50 Large patch of carcinoma in situ, located on small of back, that conforms to syndrome originally described by Bowen.

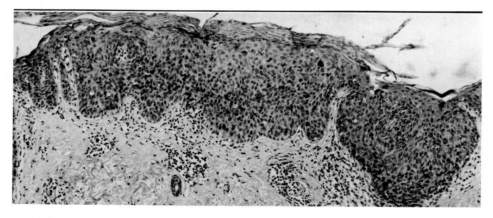

Fig. 4-51 Parakeratotic scale overlies dysplastic and atypical keratinocytes that involve full thickness of epidermis. This is carcinoma in situ.

persons living in Texas have a higher incidence of skin cancer than do their counterparts in Minnesota. Epidermoid carcinoma in black people is a rare disease. In urban populations, frankly invasive squamous carcinoma is uncommon, whereas in rural populations it is common.[26] Nearly all of these actinic-induced tumors are preceded and accompanied by lesions of actinic keratosis.

Epidermoid carcinomas of the skin can also be seen as a complication of:

1 Xeroderma pigmentosum, a genetically determined condition characterized by a diminished capacity of DNA repair following ultraviolet light irradiation.[16,18] These patients may also develop basal cell carcinomas and malignant melanomas.
2 Epidermodysplasia verruciformis, a generalized virally-induced dermatosis.
3 Cutaneous scars of various types: from burns (Marjolin's ulcer), x-rays, epidermolysis bullosa, chronic

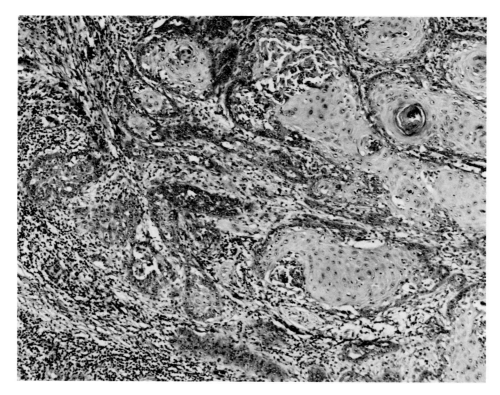

Fig. 4-52 Moderately to well-differentiated invasive epidermoid carcinoma that arose on forehead of 77-year-old man.

osteomyelitic sinuses, necrobiosis lipoidica, acne aggregata seu conglobata, or hidradenitis suppurativa.[14,15,19,22,24]

4 Chemical exposure: arsenic, coal tars, soot, and a variety of oils and distillation products.

5 Renal transplantation: in these patients the carcinomas are often associated with severe actinic keratosis or, less commonly, widespread warts.[23]

6 PUVA-treated psoriatic patients, in whom the risk is dose dependent.[25]

7 Ichthyosis,[21] epidermal nevus,[20] and congenital lymphedema.[17] Only a few cases have been reported in each of these disorders.

Microscopic features

Over 80% of epidermoid carcinomas are well differentiated and, as such, produce large amounts of keratin (Fig. 4-52). Intercellular bridges can be found with ease in most cases. Immunohistochemically, there is positivity for high molecular–weight keratin, involucrin (a precursor of the cross-linked envelope protein of the stratum corneum) and epithelial membrane antigen, and often also for CEA and basement membrane components, such as laminin and type IV collagen.[27,28,30]

Invasion of the dermis is a sine qua non for the diagnosis, but this remains a very subjective evalution. A lesion interpreted by some as florid actinic keratosis may be interpreted by others as a superficially invasive epidermoid carcinoma.[29] This is a reflection of the fact that actinic ker-

atosis and epidermoid carcinoma are part of a continuous spectrum. Fortunately, the issue is of no great practical importance, since the treatment and prognosis for the borderline lesions are essentially the same.

Other microscopic types

Spindle cell epidermoid carcinomas occur, particularly in the lip (see Fig. 5-20). The differential diagnosis includes malignant melanoma and atypical fibroxanthoma. Continuity of tumor cells with the basal layer of the epidermis, foci of clearcut squamous change, and keratin immunoreactivity are the most important distinguishing features.[32,34]

Adenoid (pseudoglandular) epidermoid carcinoma results from acantholysis, i.e., lack of cell cohesiveness caused by a desmosomal defect (Fig. 4-53). Nearly all cases occur in sun-exposed areas, and many are associated with actinic keratosis and with acantholysis. The differential diagnosis includes primary or metastatic adenocarcinoma and true *adenosquamous carcinoma* of the skin, a rare aggressive neoplasm that exhibits squamous differentiation and mucin production.[37]

Verrucous carcinoma is an extremely well-differentiated type of epidermoid carcinoma, also known as carcinoma or epithelioma cuniculatum.[31,36] It appears as an ulcerated, fungating, and polypoid mass with openings of sinus tracts onto the skin surface. Most cases are located in the sole of the foot. Local invasion is the rule and extension to bone is frequent, but nodal metastases are exceptional.[33,35] It is re-

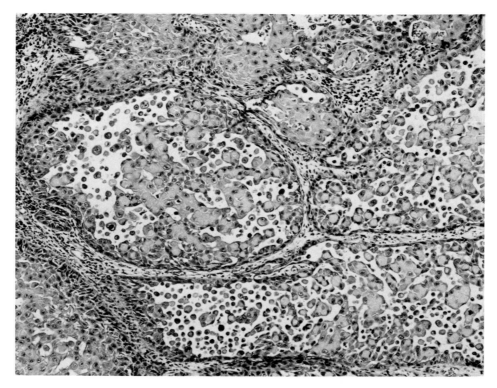

Fig. 4-53 False glands caused by acantholylsis produce adenoid variant of epidermoid carcinoma.

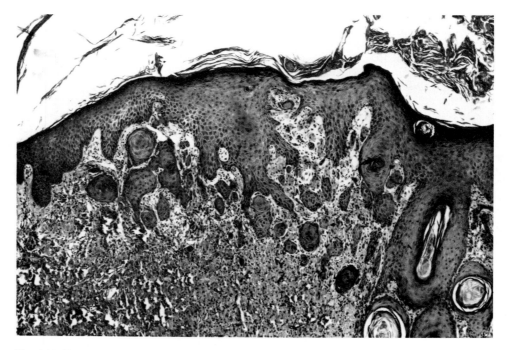

Fig. 4-54 Pseudoepitheliomatous hyperplasia. In this particular case, changes were due to granular cell tumor. Downgrowth proliferation of squamous epithelium into dermis simulates appearance of squamous cell carcinoma.

garded as the cutaneous counterpart of the more common verrucous carcinoma of the oral cavity and other mucosal membranes.

Treatment

Complete excision is the treatment of choice for epidermoid carcinoma.[38] Careful pathologic examination, including marking of the surgical margins with India ink or silver nitrate, allows identification of those cases in which the tumor has been transected.

Prognosis

The overall prognosis of epidermoid carcinoma is excellent, particularly for the actinic-induced tumors. Superficially invasive cancers (less than 1.5 cm) metastasize only occasionally.[41] Even in lesions larger than 2 cm with unequivocal invasion into the reticular dermis, the incidence of regional lymph node metastases is less than 5%. The best prognostic determinators are level of dermal invasion and vertical tumor thickness.[39,40] In a recent series, all tumors that recurred were 4 mm or more thick and involved the deep half of the dermis or deeper; all tumors that proved fatal were at least 1 cm in maximum thickness, and most extended into the subcutaneous fat or beyond.[39]

Pseudoepitheliomatous hyperplasia

At sites of trauma, chronic irritation, and ulcers, the reparative hyperplasia of the epidermis may produce seemingly invasive tongues of epithelial cells. This abnormality, known as pseudoepitheliomatous hyperplasia, can also be caused by mycotic infections (particularly North American blastomycosis), bromoderma, pyoderma vegetans, tuberculosis, syphilis, granular cell tumor, and melanocytic lesions (particularly Spitz nevi).[42] The epithelial proliferation is generally associated with a dermal fibrocytic and vascular proliferation and a definite acute to subacute inflammatory infiltrate. Characteristically, the proliferating strands of epithelium are thin, markedly elongated, anastomosing, and heavily infiltrated by inflammatory cells (Fig. 4-54). Clear separation of pseudoepitheliomatous hyperplasia from epidermoid carcinoma is not always easy. The absence of atypical epithelial cells and the presence of the inflammatory reaction, as well as the history, are helpful in distinguishing these false cancers from the real ones. Conservatism is warranted in doubtful cases.

Basal cell carcinoma
General features

Basal cell carcinoma derives its name from the cytologic similarity of the tumor cells to the normal basal cells of the epidermis and the hair follicle. It is the most frequent form of skin cancer and occurs predominantly on the sun-exposed skin in direct proportion to the number of pilosebaceous units present therein.[45] Fair-skinned, blue-eyed persons engaged in outdoor occupations suffer a higher incidence of these tumors.[44] Synchronous and metachronous tumors are frequent.[50] Exceptionally, children and young adults are affected.[48,49]

Basal cell carcinomas may also develop in sunlight-protected skin,[47] in nevus sebaceous of Jadassohn, in the lower leg in association with chronic venous stasis,[43] and following arsenic ingestion, x-ray exposure, skin injury, chicken pox scars, tattoos, hair transplantation scars, and immune suppression.[46]

The clinical appearance of basal cell carcinoma is as variable as its histologic patterns. Nodular, ulcerative, superficial, erythematous, multicentric, and sclerosing or morphea-like forms occur.

Microscopic features

Basal cell carcinomas arise from basally located cells of the epidermis and pilosebaceous units and differentiate incompletely in the direction of adnexal (particularly pilar) structures.[52] Epidermal attachment is present in nearly all cases. The tumors may have solid, cystic, adenoid, keratotic, pigmented, infiltrating, and sclerosing (morphea-like) patterns[56] (Figs. 4-55 to 4-57). The keratotic pattern represents an expression of differentiation toward hair follicles, has no clinical significance, and should be distinguished from so-called basosquamous carcinoma (see following discussion).

The nests of basal cell carcinoma show prominent palisading and are surrounded by a typical loose stroma, which contains myofibroblasts and often exhibits mucinous change.[57] Cleft-like retraction spaces, some of artifactual nature and some resulting from the accumulation of stromal mucin, are often seen between the epithelial nests and the stroma.[55] Stromal amyloid deposition is not infrequent, and is sometimes accompanied by the presence of immunoglobulins.[53,63] Mitotic activity, atypia, and giant cell formation have no prognostic significance. Perineurial or endoneurial invasion are rarely present.[54]

Immunohistochemically, the cells of basal cell carcinoma are positive for keratin (particularly low molecular weight type[60,62]) but usually negative for EMA, CEA, and involucrin.[51,58] The basement membrane that surrounds the tumor nests reacts with antibodies against laminin, types IV and V collagen, and bullous pemphigoid antigen.[61] The latter antigen, in contrast to epidermoid carcinoma, is faint and discontinuous.[59]

The differential diagnosis of basal cell carcinoma includes the areas of highly organoid basaloid proliferation sometimes seen on top of dermatofibromas and the more atypical foci of basaloid proliferation that may be found in association with actinic keratosis and Bowen's disease (see respective discussions).

Other microscopic types

Superficial basal cell carcinoma arises in skin with sparse, fine hairs and whose epidermis is thin, such as that of the trunk. It grows chiefly in a lateral direction, beneath a relatively flat epidermis and exhibits a high recurrence rate.[70,74]

Basosquamous (metatypical) carcinoma has the general configuration of a basal cell carcinoma, but it also contains atypical squamous cells (Fig. 4-58). This variant is more aggressive than the conventional basal cell carcinoma; a high proportion of the metastasizing basal cell tumors belong to this type, which should be distinguished from the keratotic form of basal cell carcinoma.[66,72]

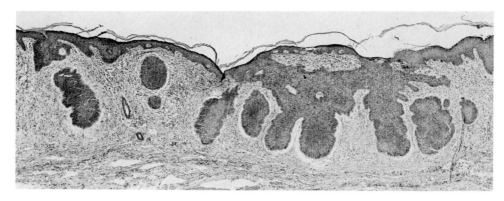

Fig. 4-55 Example of superficial multicentric type of basal cell carcinoma.

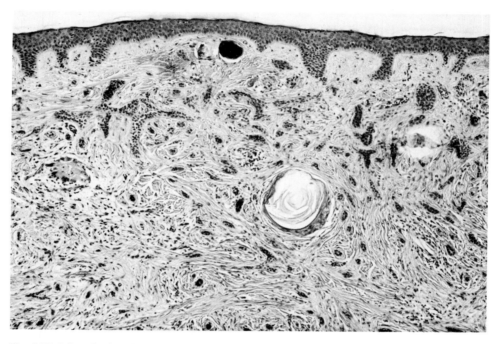

Fig. 4-56 Sclerosing basal cell carcinoma with distinct desmoplastic response. Focal keratotic differentiation forms nests of squamous debris.

Granular basal cell carcinoma contains tumor cells with cytoplasmic granules analogous in every way to those seen in granular cell tumor of the dermis and other locations.[65] No clinical significance is ascribed to this variety.

Clear cell basal cell carcinoma contains clear cells with prominent cytoplasmic vacuoles; some of these cells may even have a signet ring configuration.[64]

Fibroepithelial tumor (Pinkus' tumor; fibroepithelioma) is a polypoid variant of basal cell carcinoma, often occurring on the back, in which the stroma is very abundant[67] (Fig. 4-59).

The *basal cell nevus syndrome* (Gorlin's syndrome) is characterized by multiple basal cell carcinomas, palmar pits, calcification of dura, keratinous cysts of the jaws, skeletal anomalies, and occasional abnormalities of the central ner-

vous system, mesentery, and endocrine organs.[68,69] Microscopically, the basal cell carcinomas exhibit a broader spectrum of subtypes than the sporadic tumors.[71] The syndrome should be suspected when basal cell cancers are seen in young persons who have multiple tumors, many of which are of the superficial multicentric type and in which osteoid is an occasional finding.[73]

Spread and metastases

Growth of basal cell carcinoma is slow and indolent. However, if untreated, the tumor may invade the subcutaneous fat, skeletal muscle, and bone ("ulcus rodens"). Tumors of the face may invade skull, nares, orbit, or temporal bone via the auditory canal. They can thus reach the central nervous system and produce a lethal meningitis. Micro-

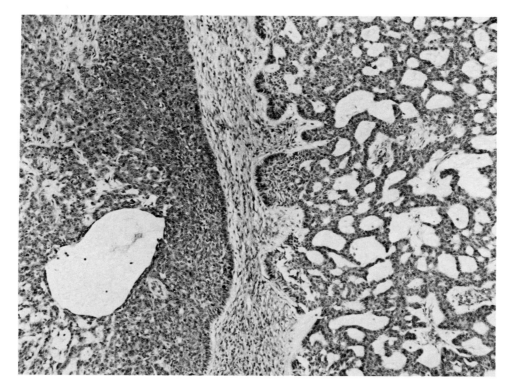

Fig. 4-57 Basal cell carcinoma with both soild (left) and adenoid (right) cystic areas.

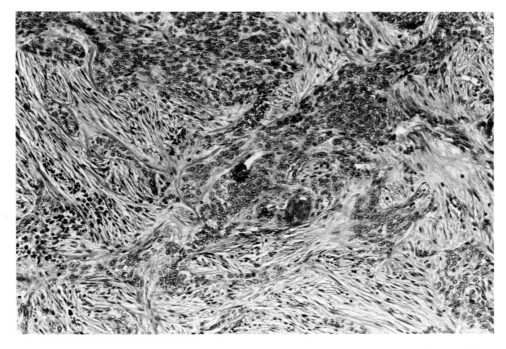

Fig. 4-58 Metatypical basal cell carcinoma. Overall architecture and cytologic composition are those of basal cell carcinoma, but there are foci of squamoid differentiation, increased degree of nuclear atypicality, and extremely dense desmoplastic tissue reaction.

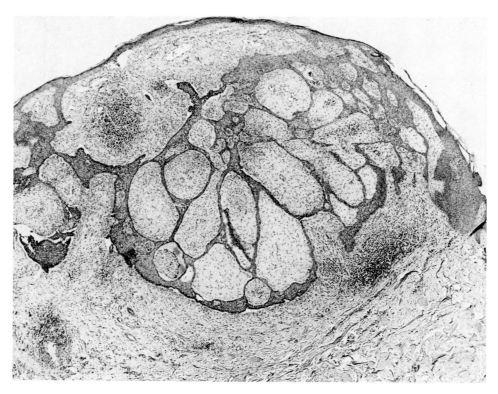

Fig. 4-59 Fibroepithelial tumor of Pinkus, a variant of basal cell carcinoma.

scopically, the locally more aggressive tumors tend to show loss of peripheral palisading and a dense, fibrous stroma rather than a loose stroma.[75] In terms of location, local recurrence is more common in tumors of the nasolabial fold, inner canthus, and postauricular region.[76]

Distant metastases are extraordinarily rare, but over 100 cases have been reported.[78] About 60% to 75% of these metastases involved the regional lymph nodes, and the others affected organs such as lung, bone, and liver. Metastases in basal cell carcinoma are more likely in the basosquamous types, in those with perineurial spread, and in tumors located on sunlight-protected skin.[77]

Treatment

Excision, curettage and desiccation, irradiation, and caustic pastes used appropriately cure almost all these tumors. In instances wherein basal cell carcinoma extends to the margin of surgical excision (an occurrence of approximately 5% in large series), only one third show evidence of recrudescence over the ensuing 2 to 5 years.[79] Thus immediate reexcision is not indicated. Careful follow-up is sufficient.

SKIN ADNEXAE

All of the adnexa are derived from the same primitive ectodermal cell as the epidermis, and thus it is not surprising that adnexal tumors have certain similar histologic appearances and cytologic features. Readily recognizable homogeneous groups can be identified and separated, and their structure, cytochemistry, and immunohistochemistry can be correlated with those of the analogous adnexa or even with a subdivision thereof.

Eccrine sweat gland

The three major divisions of the eccrine sweat gland are the intraepidermal portion of the duct (acrosyringium), the dermal portion of the same duct (syrinx), and the secretory coil. Useful immunohistochemical markers are EMA, CEA, the enzyme carbonic anhydrase, and pregnancy-specific–β1-glycoprotein (SP1) for the secretory and duct lining cells, and actin and S-100 protein for the myoepithelial cells.[82,84-86,88] Antibodies against an apocrine epithelial antigen are also available, but their specificity remains to be demonstrated.[81]

Tumors of sweat gland derivation constitute a numerous and complex group of interrelated lesions.[80,83,87]

Poroma

Eccrine poroma occurs chiefly on the palms and soles but has been reported in many other sites.[89,91,92]

Poromas often show a moat and hillock pattern and histologically are characterized by a sharp junction between the proliferating, nonpigmented, basal type of keratinocytes and the adjacent epidermis (Fig. 4-60). Within these cords and nests, ducts and ductlike structures may be formed. The tumor may be purely intraepidermal or purely intradermal (also referred to as dermal duct tumor) or, more commonly, may involve both areas.

Purely intraepidermal poromas have been described in the past as hydroacanthoma simplex.[93,94] Heavily pigmented

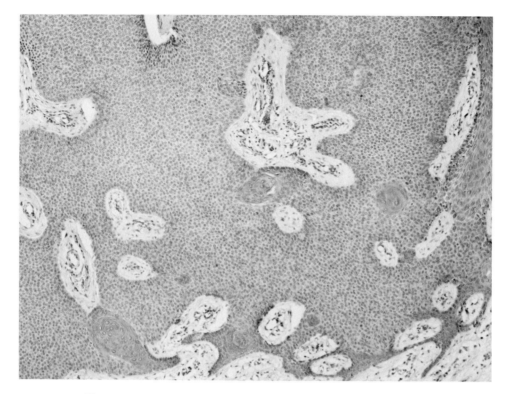

Fig. 4-60 Eccrine poroma showing most of features described in text.

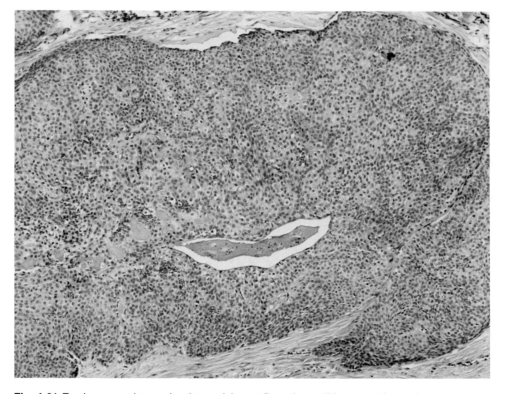

Fig. 4-61 Eccrine acrospiroma showing nodular configuration, solid pattern of growth, and clear cell changes.

variants of this tumor have also been reported. Ultrastructural and histochemical studies show that the predominant cell has features similar to those of the acrosyringium.[90] The dermis beneath often shows a distinct proliferation of reactive vessels and some inflammation. These lesions are to be distinguished from basal cell carcinoma and seborrheic keratoses.

Acrospiroma

Eccrine acrospiroma, also known as solid-cystic hidradenoma, arises from the distal excretory duct.[97] It forms nodules with occasional cystic foci high in the dermis (Fig. 4-61). Some of the proliferating cells are cytologically similar to those of the poroma. Others have an abundant clear cytoplasm (hence the synonym, clear cell hidradenoma), and still others exhibit prominent squamous metaplasia.[96] Johnson and Helwig[95] regard eccrine poroma as a morphologic variant of eccrine acrospiroma.

Syringoma

Syringomas are generally multiple, yellowish, papulonodular lesions that occur chiefly on the neck and face (particularly lower eyelids) of women. Other forms are vulvar syringoma, acral syringoma (limited to the dorsal proximal and middle phalanges of the hand), and eruptive syringoma (appearing in crops in young patients and affecting the anterior half of the body, including neck, shoulder, chest, and anterior surfaces of arms). Microscopically, these tumors are formed by clusters of small ducts lined by two-cell-thick epithelium, occasionally with comma-shaped extensions (Fig. 4-62). A clear cell variety has been described, resulting from intracellular accumulation of glycogen.[98] The ultrastructural[99] and histochemical[100] findings indicate that these lesions arise from eccrine and not apocrine derivatives.

Chondroid syringoma (mixed tumor)

Chondroid syringomas are benign, nodular, nonulcerated tumors that occur predominantly on the face, head, and neck but also on the extremities and trunk.[104,106] Histologically, immunohistochemically, and ultrastructurally, their appearance is comparable to that of mixed tumors of salivary gland origin[102,103,107] (Fig. 4-63). This includes the presence of cells with an abundant hyaline cytoplasm.[105] Immunohistochemically, the inner layer cells express cytokeratin, CEA, and EMA; the outer cell layers are positive for vimentin, S-100 protein, NSE, and—sometimes—glial fibrillary acidic protein.[101] Despite the occasionally atypical appearance of the cartilaginous component, the overwhelming majority of these tumors are benign.

Eccrine cylindroma

Classically, cylindroma of the skin has been described as a large, multicentric tumor of the scalp (turban tumor). In fact, the majority of these slowly growing adenomas are solitary and small, and approximately 10% occur on sites other than the head and neck.[109] Exceptionally, they are seen in association with microscopically identical tumors in the major salivary glands.[112] Microscopically, the heavy accumulation of basement membrane material around and within

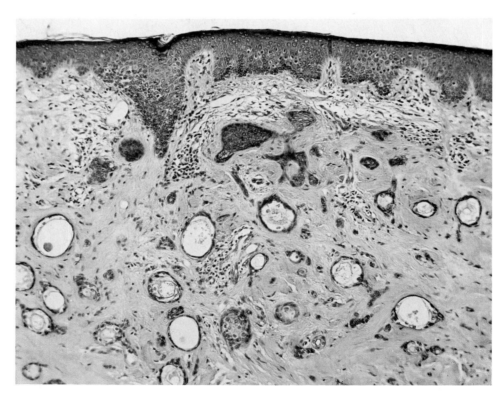

Fig. 4-62 Multiple ducts and cysts of syringoma.

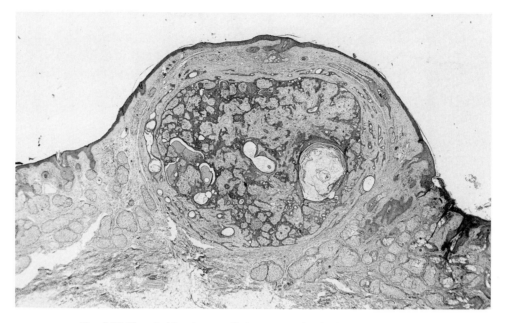

Fig. 4-63 Chondroid syringoma that arose on cheek of 77-year-old man.

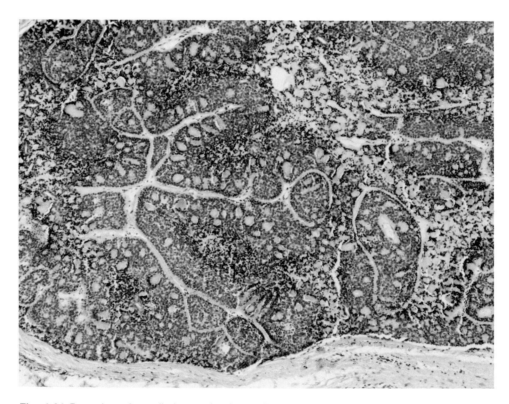

Fig. 4-64 Dermal eccrine cylindroma showing perilobular and intralobular deposition of basement membrane material.

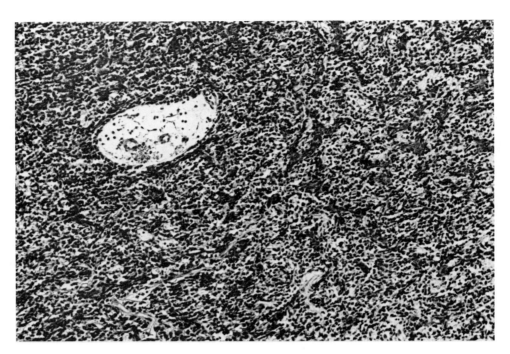

Fig. 4-65 Eccrine spiradenoma. Tumor is extremely cellular and composed of two cell types. There is a perivascular space that is reminiscent of those seen in thymoma.

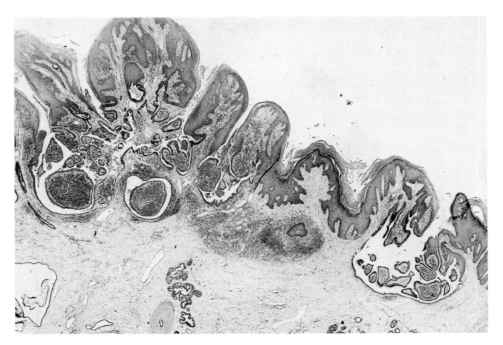

Fig. 4-66 At bases of epidermal papillae are clefts and glands lined by eccrine epithelium. Chronic, lymphocytic, and plasmocellular inflammatory infiltrate is not uncommon in papillary syringadenomas.

the tumor lobules is the most important distinguishing feature (Fig. 4-64). The ultrastructural and immunohistochemical features support an origin from the intradermal coiled duct region of eccrine sweat glands.[108,111] Sometimes, features of cylindroma and eccrine spiradenoma coexist in the same lesion.[110]

Eccrine spiradenoma

Eccrine spiradenomas are sharply delimited, lobular adenomas that can occur almost anywhere in the body and can be extremely painful.[116] They originate from the lower portion of the eccrine duct and are microscopically very cellular[114,117,118] (Fig. 4-65). The scanty cytoplasm and prominent nuclei may lead the unwary to an erroneous diagnosis of malignancy. We have seen them confused with synovial sarcoma and with metastatic carcinoma. They can also be confused with vascular tumors because of their high degree of vascularity.[113] Ultrastructurally, they contain an admixture of epithelial and myoepithelial cells.[115]

Papillary syringadenoma

Papillary syringadenomas are verrucous, moist tumors that occur chiefly on the scalp, neck, and face but may be found elsewhere on the skin. They are seen from childhood to senescence, and often there is a history of slow growth or of a recent change in a "birthmark." Microscopically, a glandular papillary proliferation connected to the skin surface is seen (Fig. 4-66). Dense plasma cell infiltration is common. These plasma cells are predominantly of the IgG and IgA class.[120,121] Juxtaposed nevus sebaceus was found

in one third and basal cell carcinoma in one tenth of the patients reported by Helwig and Hackney.[119]

Papillary eccrine adenoma

Rulon and Helwig[122] reported fourteen cases of a distinctive sweat gland tumor, most often located on the distal extremities of blacks, that they designated *papillary eccrine adenoma.* Microscopically, tubular structures resembling eccrine ducts are seen; many are dilated and exhibit intraluminal papillomatosis (Fig. 4-67). One lesion recurred, but none metastasized.

Aggressive digital papillary adenoma

Another sweat gland neoplasm with a marked predilection for the digits is aggressive digital papillary adenoma.[123] Microscopically, tubuloalveolar and ductal structures alternate with areas of papillary projections protruding into cystic lumina (Fig. 4-68). The appearance is somewhat reminiscent of carcinoma of the breast. Local recurrence is common.[123] A malignant counterpart of this tumor—recognized by its poor glandular differentiation and by necrosis, cellular atypia, and invasiveness—metastasizes in a high proportion of cases, particularly to the lung.[123]

Clear cell acanthoma

Degos' *clear cell acanthoma*[124,126] is a distinct intraepithelial tumor composed of clear, glycogen-filled keratinocytes associated with dermal inflammation (Fig. 4-69). It is seen almost invariably in the leg of females, is occasionally multiple, and is thought to arise from intraepidermal

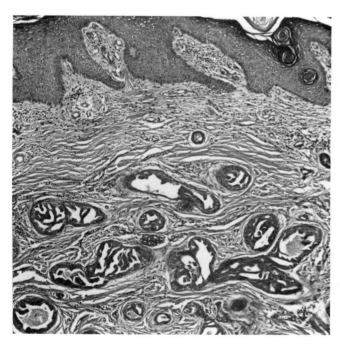

Fig. 4-67 Papillary eccrine adenoma. Tubular formations with micropapillary projections are growing in the dermis, covered by a slightly hyperplastic epidermis.

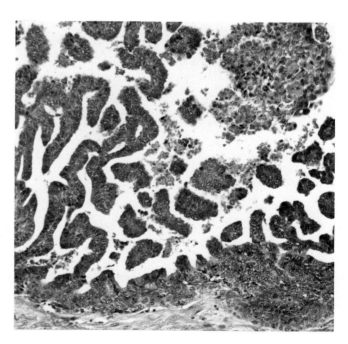

Fig. 4-68 Aggressive digital papillary adenoma. Cellular tumor with numerous papillary projections is present in the dermis. There is focal necrosis in the lumen. Appearance is reminiscent of intraductal carcinoma of breast. (Courtesy Dr. D. Santa Cruz, St. Louis, MO.)

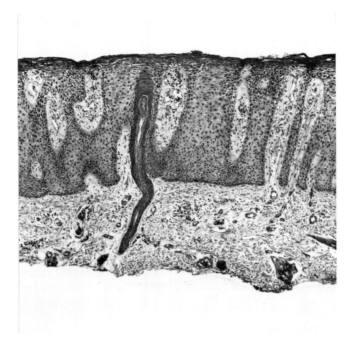

Fig. 4-69 Clear cell acanthoma. There is lengthening of malphigian layer, which is formed by enlarged clear keratinocytes. Mild chronic inflammatory infiltrate is present in the dermis. (Courtesy Dr. D. Santa Cruz, St. Louis, MO.)

eccrine ducts. Similar cytologic changes ("pale cell acanthosis") can be seen focally in seborrheic keratosis and several other skin disorders as an expression of a reaction pattern of epidermal epithelium.[125]

Intraepidermal epithelioma

The lesion previously known as **intraepithelial epithelioma** of Borst-Jadassohn is probably composed of an heterogeneous group of disorders, the two most common being irritated seborrheic keratosis and eccrine poroma (and related intraepidermal sweat gland tumors).[127,128]

Sweat gland carcinoma

Identification of adenocarcinomas arising from eccrine glands is difficult. These are rare tumors and comprise a minute fraction of sweat gland neoplasms[143] (Figs. 4-70 to 4-74). Most occur in adults, but they have also been reported in children.[130] Those with well-developed ductal differentiation simulate metastatic carcinoma, particularly from the breast,[150] those with large clear cells resemble metastatic renal cell carcinoma,[134] and those with prominent basaloid formations may be confused with basal cell carcinoma.[141] Some sweat gland carcinomas retain morphologic features that allow them to be recognized as the malignant counterparts of the various types of sweat gland adenomas.[129,135] Of these, malignant poroma (porocarcinoma) is the most frequent.[136,141,147] Most cases occur in the lower extremities, like their benign counterparts.[149] Other varieties include malignant chondroid syringoma, malignant syringoma (syringoid eccrine carcinoma), and malignant acrospiro-

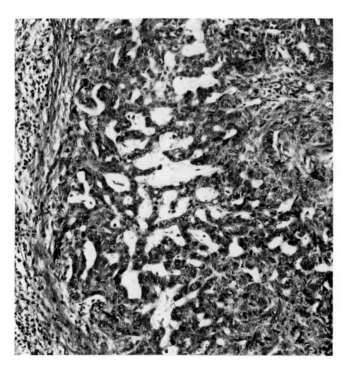

Fig. 4-70 Sweat gland carcinoma. This tumor has trabecular configuration and a pushing pattern of growth.

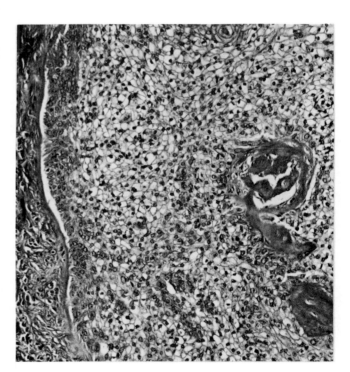

Fig. 4-71 Sweat gland carcinoma composed of large clear cells. This tumor could be viewed as malignant counterpart of eccrine acrospiroma. In other areas, there was pronounced cellular atypia.

ma.[138,139,141] Eccrine acrospiroma and cylindroma can undergo malignant transformation, manifesting clinically as enlargement of a cutaneous nodule of long standing.[132,140,152]

Several other distinctive types of sweat gland carcinoma occur. One is *mucinous (adenocystic) carcinoma*, often appearing in the scalp of elderly patients.[142,146] Its microscopic appearance resembles mucinous carcinoma of the breast by virtue of the presence of clusters of tumor cells floating in lakes of mucin. This tumor should be distinguished from the even rarer primary *adenoid cystic carcinoma* of the skin, a tumor morphologically equivalent to the salivary gland neoplasm that bears that name.[131,151]

Another variant of sweat gland carcinoma, originally designated as microcystic adnexal carcinoma and recently renamed *sclerosing sweat duct carcinoma*, appears as a slow-growing, indurated nodule or plaque, usually on the face.[133,137] The upper lip is a particularly common location. Microscopically, the tumor shares several features with benign syringoma. Cords and nests of uniform keratinocytes, keratin-containing cysts, and foci of ductal differentiation are present (Fig. 4-74, *B*). The stroma has a dense, collagenous quality. The tumor has invasive properties, sometimes extending into the subcutaneous fat and/or perineurial spaces.[133] Recurrence is common, but metastases are extremely rare. *Lymphoepithelial tumor of the skin* is a recently redescribed tumor in which large epithelial tumor cells are intimately admixed with lymphocytes[145]; it remains to be determined whether this tumor is of sweat gland or pilosebaceous differentiation.

Nearly all sweat gland carcinomas exhibit immunoreac-

tivity for CEA, cytokeratin, and EMA, like their benign counterparts.[144, 148]

Extramammary Paget's disease

Extramammary Paget's disease results from the presence in the epidermis of malignant epithelial cells with signs of glandular differentiation. Concomitant involvement of eccrine glands and/or hair follicles is present nearly always, whereas dermal invasion is seen in about one quarter of the cases.[156] Cases limited to the epidermis are explained by postulating an origin from the intraepidermal portion of the sweat glands or from primitive basal cells with the capacity to differentiate toward glandular elements.[155] The latter hypothesis would explain the occasional occurrence of lesions combining the features of Paget's disease and Bowen's disease.[164]

The labia majora, scrotum, and perineum are the most frequent sites, with adjacent areas following. The lesions are grossly circinate, annular, erythematous, and eczematoid plaques. Histologically, large, pale, vacuolated cells are seen concentrated just above the basal layer (Fig. 4-75). They may form nests and extend into the stratum spinosum. Electron microscopic examination shows that Paget's cells are not altered keratinocytes or melanocytes, but rather cells with glandular differentiation.[153,157,158] In contrast to Paget's disease of the breast, the extramammary form is consistently positive for mucin stains. Immunohistochemically, the tumor cells show reactivity for epithelial membrane antigen, CEA, and the type of low molecular weight cytokeratin present in simple epithelia.[154,161,162,164a] Positivity of some of

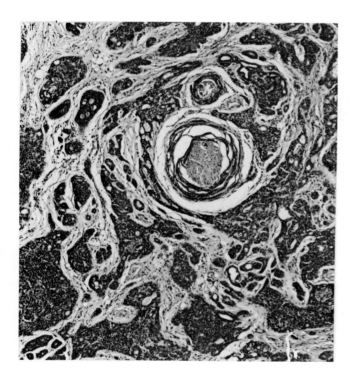

Fig. 4-72 Sweat gland carcinoma with adenoid cystic features, including prominent perineural invasion.

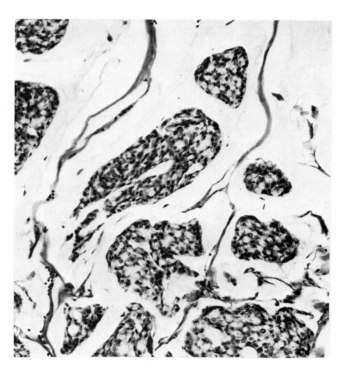

Fig. 4-73 Sweat gland carcinoma of adenocystic type. Clusters of carcinoma cells are floating in a sea of mucin, appearance being reminiscent of that seen in mucinous carcinoma of breast.

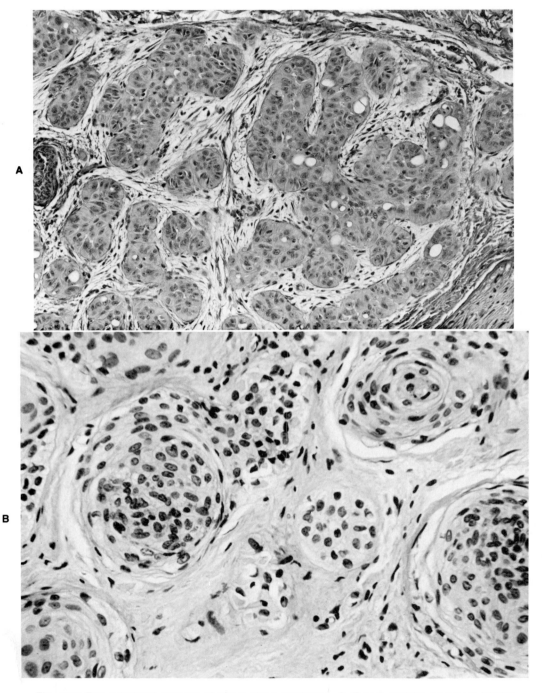

Fig. 4-74 Two additional patterns of sweat gland carcinoma. **A,** Tumor exhibits prominent lobular configuration, which is important clue to the diagnosis. **B,** Sweat gland carcinoma of sclerosing type composed of nests of keratinocytes in a whorling pattern. This tumor was located in skin of upper lip in a 28-year-old woman.

these lesions for GCDFP-15 (a marker of apocrine epithelium) and the pattern of lectin-binding sites suggest an origin from (or differentiation toward) apocrine rather than eccrine sweat glands.[160,163,165,166]

Adequate surgical excision is the treatment of choice. The differential diagnosis of extramammary Paget's disease includes Bowen's disease, junctional nevi, malignant melanoma, and the recently described *clear cell papulosis*.[159] We have seen several cases in which the cleftlike separation between the malignant cells and the overlying keratinocytes resulted in an acantholytic effect that was confused with pemphigus vulgaris.

Apocrine sweat gland

Apocrine sweat glands are concentrated in the axillae, groin, and perineum, but they also occur in small numbers on the face and elsewhere. A useful immunohistochemical marker of apocrine differentiation is gross cystic disease fluid protein (GCDFP-15).[167a]

It is possible that some of the sweat gland tumors already described, particularly papillary syringadenoma, cylindroma, and chondroid syringoma, exhibit apocrine differentiation[167a]; as a matter of fact, the existence of eccrine and apocrine forms of the latter has been proposed. However, tumors composed exclusively of apocrine glands are extremely rare. *Cystadenomas* are discussed on p. 112.

Tubular apocrine adenomas have been described by Landry and Winkelmann.[167]

Papillary hydradenoma and *ceruminous adenoma* have been traditionally regarded as tumors of apocrine glands. They are discussed in Chapter 19 (Vulva) and 31 (Ear), respectively.

Sebaceous gland
Senile sebaceous hyperplasia

The most common nodular lesion of the sebaceous glands is due to hyperplasia. It occurs chiefly on the nose and cheeks of elderly persons, hence the name senile sebaceous nevus or, preferably, senile sebaceous hyperplasia[168] (Fig. 4-76).

Nevus sebaceus of Jadassohn

Nevus sebaceus of Jadassohn is a distinct clinicopathologic type of epithelial nevus.[170] It is composed of a hamartomatous conglomerate of large sebaceous glands associated with heterotopic apocrine glands, defective hair follicles, acanthosis, and papillomatosis (Fig. 4-77). The lesions occur on the scalp and face, are present from infancy, and gradually enlarge.[169,171] Basal cell carcinomas, a variety of adnexal tumors, and, very rarely, epidermoid carcinomas can arise within this lesion.[173]

Epithelial nevi without an adnexal component are generically referred to as *epidermal nevi.* They are characterized microscopically by hyperkeratosis, papillomatosis, and acanthosis and are sharply demarcated from the adjacent skin. Several clinicopathologic varieties exist.[172]

Sebaceous adenoma

Sebaceous adenoma presents as a nodular lobulated growth with generative cells at the periphery and cells showing varying degrees of sebaceous differentiation toward the center.[174] Although well differentiated, it lacks the distinctly organoid quality of senile sebaceous hyperplasia. It should be realized that the so-called sebaceous adenoma occurring on the face of patients with the tuberous sclerosis syndrome

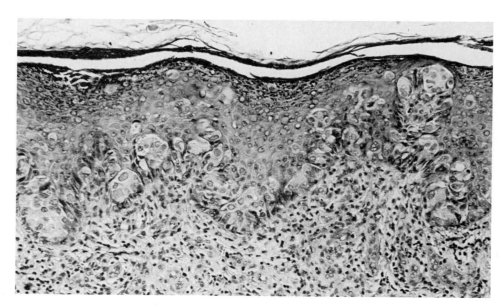

Fig. 4-75 Paget's cells, individual and in clusters, are present just above basal layer and farther up in epidermis in this lesion from scrotum. There was no dermal component. Patient has had no recrudescence in 9 years following surgical excision.

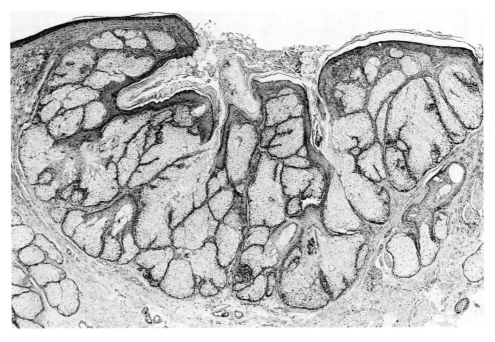

Fig. 4-76 Example of senile sebaceous hyperplasia in glands about two follicular orifices.

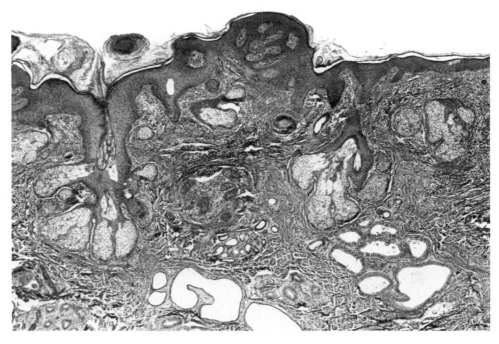

Fig. 4-77 Nevus sebaceous of Jadassohn. There is acanthosis, papillomatosis, increasing number of sebaceous glands, dilatation of eccrine sweat glands, and ectopic appearance of apocrine sweat glands.

is not a sebaceous neoplasm at all but a fibrovascular hamartoma accompanied by a mild degree of sebaceous hyperplasia.

Sebaceous carcinoma

Bonafide sebaceous carcinoma is extremely rare.[181] Those occurring in the eyelids, in caruncles, and in the orbit are much more aggressive than those located elsewhere in the skin.[183] Some of the cases have followed irradiation therapy to the area.[179] Microscopically, sebaceous carcinomas exhibit, together with evidence of sebaceous differentiation, prominent atypia, increased mitotic activity, and invasive features (Fig. 4-78). Immunoreactivity for keratin and cytokeratin, EMA, and Leu-M1 is present; CEA and S-100 protein are absent.[181a] Carcinoma should be distinguished from the various related types of basal cell tumors with sebaceous differentiation (basal cell epithelioma, sebaceoma, superficial epithelioma with sebaceous differentiation[177,182]) and from epidermoid carcinomas accompanied by hydropic changes in the tumor cells.[180]

Sebaceous carcinoma may be seen as a component of *Muir-Torre's syndrome*.[178] In this condition, multiple cutaneous tumors exhibiting varying degrees of sebaceous and hair follicle differentiation occur in association with multiple internal malignancies.[175,176]

Hair follicle

A myriad of neoplasms, hamartomas, and cysts can develop from the hair follicle. In an exhaustive review of the subject, Headington[184] listed twenty-six entries, and some additional ones have been described since.[185,186,187] Only the most common ones will be described here.

Inverted follicular keratosis

The lesions of inverted follicular keratosis occur mostly on the face of elderly patients, the eyelid being a preferred location. Clinically, they present as a papule or nodule, practically always single, usually projecting from the surface. Microscopically, the most distinctive feature is the presence of squamous eddies[190] (Fig. 4-79). They usually have a papillomatous, as well as an acanthotic inverted, component. In contrast to keratoacanthoma, the borders are sharply outlined and inflammation is usually lacking.[188]

The histogenesis and pathogenesis are controversial. Some view it as a unique keratotic lesion of the infundibular portion of the hair follicle (hence the name),[189] whereas others regard it as an irritated form of seborrheic keratosis or verruca vulgaris.[191]

Trichoepithelioma

Trichoepitheliomas are hair follicle tumors of long standing.[193] They are often multiple, do not ulcerate, and histologically have a stromal element surrounding abortive pilar differentiation (Fig. 4-80). The main differential diagnosis is with basal cell carcinoma; the most helpful features are the frond-like arrangement of the basaloid cells, the presence of epithelial tracts comprised of two or more layers of basaloid cells, and the formation of papillary mesenchymal

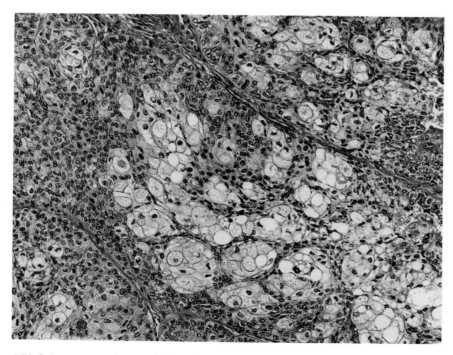

Fig. 4-78 Sebaceous carcinoma of skin. Clearcut evidence of sebaceous differentiation is seen in center of tumor lobules.

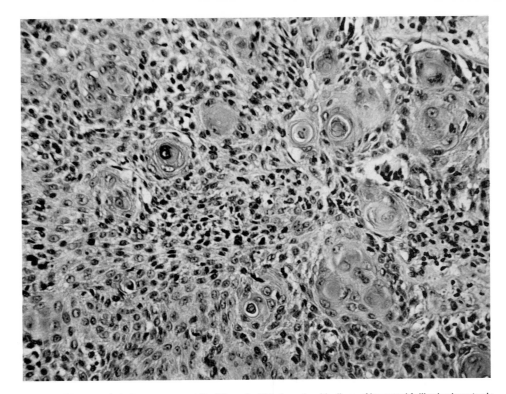

Fig. 4-79 Characteristic "squamous eddies" found within basal epithelium of inverted follicular keratosis.

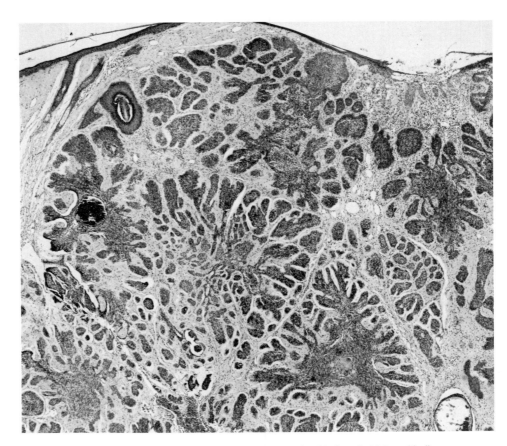

Fig. 4-80 Stromal component and segmentation of epithelium in trichoepithelioma.

bodies, which represent attempts to form the papillary mesenchyme responsible for hair follicle induction.[191a] A variant of this tumor, appropriately known as *desmoplastic trichoepithelioma*, is accompanied by extensive fibrous proliferation that surrounds and distorts the epithelial islands.[192] In contrast with the conventional form, this variant is usually single. Detailed criteria for the distinction between this lesion and the morphea-like form of basal cell carcinoma were described by Takei et al.[194]

Trichilemmoma

Trichilemmoma is a benign solid tumor that presents as a lobular formation or platelike growth of glycogen-rich clear cells often surrounded by a palisading, sometimes exhibiting central keratinization. Multiple trichilemmomas are associated with acral keratoses, papillomas of the oral mucosa, and, occasionally, tumors of the breast, thyroid, and gastrointestinal tract—a condition known as *Cowden's disease* or multiple hamartoma syndrome.[195,196] A rare malignant counterpart of this tumor has been described as *trichilemmal carcinoma*.[196a]

Trichofolliculoma

Trichofolliculomas are solitary, nodular, highly organoid hamartomatous lesions that should be distinguished from trichoepitheliomas and basal cell carcinomas.[198] Their characteristic dilated central follicle is surrounded by proliferating epithelium showing various stages of pilar formation. The occurrence of multiple fibrofolliculomas in association with trichodiscomas (another type of benign hair follicle tumor) and acrochordons (fibroepithelial polyps) constitutes a recently described syndrome.[197]

Keratoacanthoma

Keratoacanthoma typically presents as a dome-shaped lesion with a central crater filled with keratin. It occurs in males three or four times more frequently than in females. When compared with conventional epidermoid carcinoma of the skin, keratoacanthoma is seen to occur in a somewhat younger population in a similar but not identical distribution.[208]

The most important microscopic feature is the architecture of the lesion as seen on cross section: overhanging edges, keratin-filled crater, and hemispheric shape (Fig. 4-81). Cytologic criteria are of little use in the differential diagnosis with squamous cell carcinoma.[200] Most of the epithelium is well differentiated, with abundant ground-glass cytoplasm, but nuclear abnormalities and mitotic activity can be prominent. The growing edge is usually of the pushing type, a feature accentuated by the heavy rim of inflammatory cells, in which eosinophils may be prominent. However, in some instances there is extension into the underlying skeletal muscle, perineurial invasion, or even blood vessel invasion.[201,204] It should be noted that eosinophilic infiltration can also occur in epidermoid carcinoma and may actually be more frequent in it.[205] Recently, it has been suggested that immunohistochemical staining for filaggrin (a histidine-rich protein normally present in the granular and horny layers of the epidermis) may be useful in the differential diagnosis between keratoacanthoma and epidermoid carcinoma because filag-

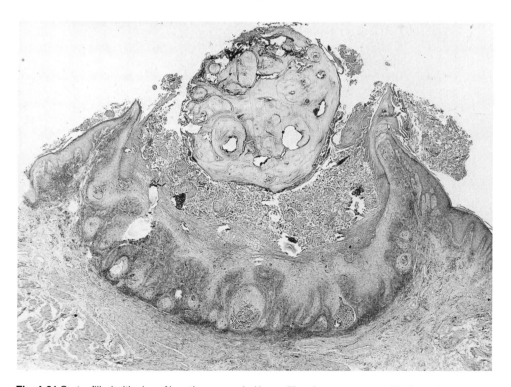

Fig. 4-81 Crater filled with plug of keratin surrounded by proliferating squamous epithelium characteristic of keratoacanthoma.

grin is always present in the former but only exceptionally in the latter.[203]

Keratoacanthoma is thought to represent a proliferation of the infundibular portion of hair follicles rather than of the epidermis. In its most typical form, it arises from previously normal skin, grows rapidly for 4 to 6 weeks, and then undergoes spontaneous regression over the following 4 to 6 weeks to leave a slightly depressed, annular scar.[209] This natural history and the type of nuclear changes sometimes present have suggested a viral etiology. However, many variations exist. Some lesions grow slowly, some lesions do not regress spontaneously, and some lesions (referred to as *actinic keratoacanthomas*) are seen in sun-exposed skin in association with typical changes of actinic keratosis.[207] Perhaps keratoacanthoma is a pattern of proliferation of the infundibular epithelium rather than a specific entity. Some have been reported in association with inflammatory dermatoses, congenital skin lesions, genetic diseases, scars, and actinic keratoses. Some patients have numerous eruptive lesions (Gryzbowski type), and others have multiple ulcerating tumors with atypical distribution (Ferguson-Smith type).[202] Some keratoacanthomas may actually represent highly differentiated epidermoid carcinomas. This would explain the fact that, occasionally, lesions with the characteristic clinical and microscopic features of keratoacanthoma have been found to grow to huge sizes and/or to metastasize to regional lymph nodes, particularly when the patient's immunity is impaired.[206]

Yet another variant of this process is so-called subungual keratoacanthoma, thought to arise from the nail matrix, which presents as a rapidly growing mass in the tip of a finger or toe, often associated with a lytic cup-shaped defect of the distal phalanx.[199]

Keratinous cyst

Keratinous cysts have been known for many years as sebaceous cysts, a misnomer born of a mistaken gross interpretation of the cyst content and perpetuated by uncritical repetition.[211,215]

Two types of keratinous cysts occur, with occasional hybrid forms. The most common (90%), known as *epidermal* or *epidermoid type*, is lined by cornified epithelium, has a distinct granular layer, and contains lamellated keratin without calcification (Fig. 4-82). Although some of these cysts (particularly those located in the fingers) result from traumatic inclusion of epidermis—hence the term, epidermal inclusion cyst—the majority probably arise from the infundibular portion of hair follicles, a possibility supported by the fact that amino acid analysis of the content shows reduction of cystine and presence of citrulline.[214] A few of these cysts exhibit seborrheic keratosis–like changes in their wall.[216]

The second type of keratinous cyst is the *pilar* or *trichilemmal* type.[212,213,215] It occurs almost exclusively in the scalp and is microscopically characterized by a trichilemmal type of keratinization, i.e., sudden keratinization without the formation of a granular layer and an uneven borderline between the keratinized and nonkeratinized cells (Fig. 4-83). The keratin inside the cyst is not lamellated, some of the nuclei are retained, and focal calcification is frequent.

Ultrastructural and immunohistochemical studies also support a trichilemmal derivation for this lesion.[210] In amino acid analysis, the trichilemmal cyst content is low in sulfur-containing amino acids and thus distinct from hair cortex.[214]

Other cutaneous cysts

Several other varieties of cutaneous cysts occur. Although some of them are not of hair follicle derivation, they are listed here for comparison purposes.

1 *Dermoid cyst.* These are microscopically similar in most respects to keratinous cysts of the epidermal type except for the fact that they contain hair adnexae in their wall opening into the cavity. Most of them are found in the face of children along lines of embryonic closure.

2 *Steatocystoma.* This is lined by a thin layer of stratified squamous epithelium resembling the ductal portion of a sebaceous gland; lobules of sebaceous glands and small hair follicles are present. It may occur as a solitary lesion[217] or in the more common multiple form known as *steatocystoma multiplex.*[220]

3 *Hydrocystoma* (solitary or multiple, usually on the face), and *apocrine cystadenoma*. Both of these are lined by a layer of sweat duct–like epithelium, which in the latter lesion has apocrine features.[221]

4 *Cutaneous ciliated cyst (cystadenoma).* This is usually seen in the extremities of females and is thought by some to be of müllerian derivation.[219]

5 *Vellus hair cyst.* This presents as small multiple eruptive cysts over the chest wall and extremities of young individuals. It is lined by a layer of flattened, follicular sheath epithelium and contains numerous vellous hairs and soft keratinous material.[218]

6 *Pigmented follicular cyst.* This is a hyperpigmented lesion with epidermoid keratinization, which contains laminated keratin, many pigmented hair shafts, and some growing hair follicles.[222]

7 *So-called bronchogenic cyst.* This is usually discovered at birth or soon thereafter in the suprasternal notch.[219a] The lining is made up of pseudostratified columnar ciliated epithelium. Despite its name, the lesion is probably of branchial cleft derivation rather than of bronchial origin.[222a]

Isolated follicular keratosis (warty dyskeratoma)

Isolated follicular keratosis is a small papulonodular lesion usually occurring in sun-exposed skin and characterized microscopically by a peculiar follicular acantholysis and dyskeratosis reminiscent of that seen in Darier's disease (Fig. 4-84). It does not represent an isolated manifestation of Darier's disease (which is not a follicular process); it may instead be pathogenetically related to actinic keratosis.[223]

Pilar tumor (proliferating trichilemmal cyst)

This lesion represents the neoplastic counterpart of the pilar (trichilemmal) cyst, and it therefore exhibits the same predilection for the scalp and base of neck of women.[225-227,229] All types of transitional forms can be found between the ordinary pilar cyst and the full-blown pilar

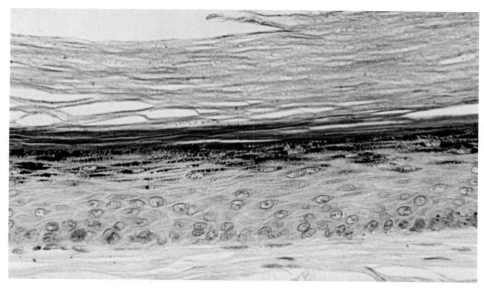

Fig. 4-82 Lining of keratinous cyst of epidermal type that has distinct granular layer.

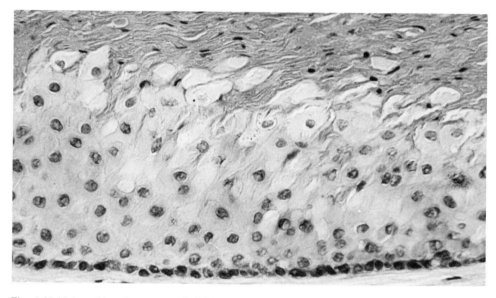

Fig. 4-83 Lining of keratinous cyst of trichilemmal type that cornifies without granular layer. Pallor of cells just beneath keratin is not due to fat.

tumor, and sometimes the two lesions coexist in the same individual. Pilar tumor can reach huge proportions[230] (Fig. 4-85). In the past, some of these lesions have been misinterpreted as epidermoid carcinomas arising from sebaceous cysts (Fig. 4-86).

Microscopically, pilar tumors have a predominantly solid appearance and pushing borders. Occasionally, they open into the skin surface. Interlacing bands of squamous epithelium exhibiting trichilemmal-type keratinization are characteristic (Fig. 4-87). Nuclear atypia may be prominent, and some irregularities at the interphase between epithelium

and stroma can be observed, but the behavior is generally benign. Several instances of local recurrence have been reported, but metastases are exceptionally rare.[225,228,231] The few well-documented instances of metastases have occurred in tumors with clearcut malignant microscopic features.[224]

Pilomatrixoma

Pilomatrixoma (pilomatricoma), formerly known as calcified epithelioma of Malherbe, is a nodular, subepidermal benign tumor arising from the hair matrix. It occurs predominantly in children and young adults, and most of the

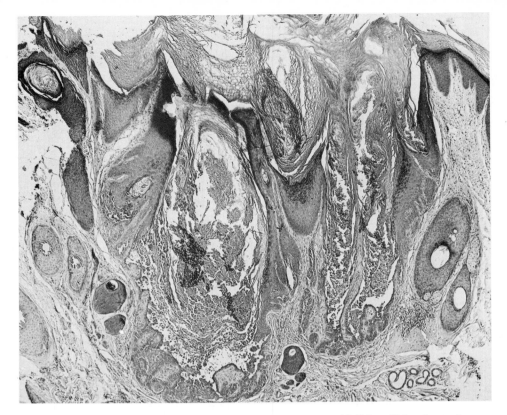

Fig. 4-84 Dysplastic and acantholytic process involving lower part of follicle, which, when cut appropriately, produces diagnostic picture of isolated follicular keratosis.

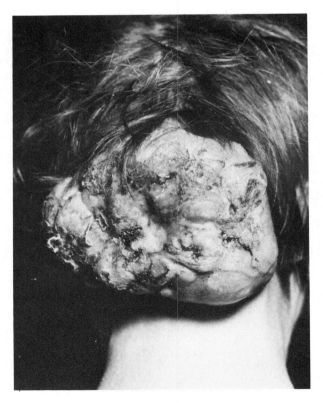

Fig. 4-85 Pilar tumor of 5 years' duration in scalp of 52-year-old woman. It recurred following local removal, but reexcision was apparently curative. Patient has been followed for 6 years. (From Dabska M: Giant hair matrix tumor. Cancer **28:**701-706, 1971.)

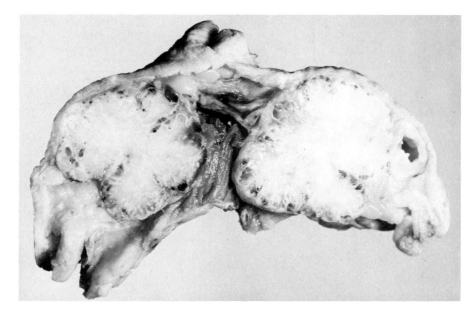

Fig. 4-86 Transected pilar tumor. This is not epidermoid carcinoma arising in keratinous cyst.

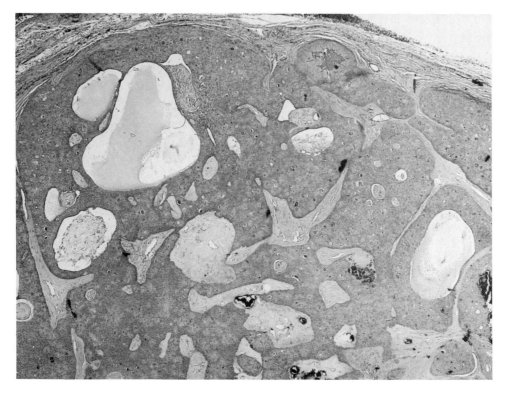

Fig. 4-87 Interlacing proliferating epithelium in pilar tumor with microscopic features that characterize it as follicular in type.

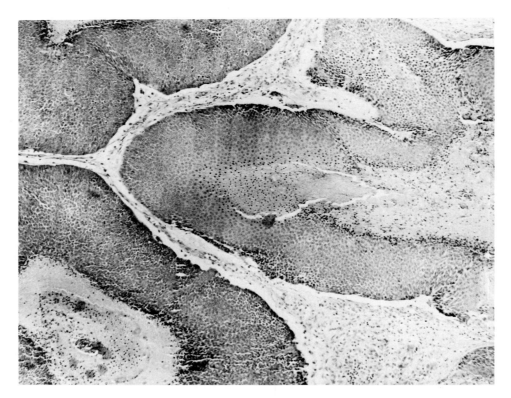

Fig. 4-88 In this pilomatrixoma, basal cells keratinize, as does cortex of hair without granular layer, and produce "ghost" cells.

cases are located on the head, neck, and upper extremities.[232] Microscopically, it is composed of solid nests of small basaloid cells that may lead to a mistaken diagnosis of basal cell carcinoma, particularly on cytologic examination.[237] The key feature is the fact that these basaloid cells undergo abrupt keratinization, leading to the formation of "ghost" and "shadow" cells (Fig. 4-88). Foreign body reaction, calcification, and ossification are common secondary events. The histochemical and ultrastructural features are in keeping with an origin from the hair matrix.[234,236] It should be remarked that focal features of hair matrix differentiation can sometimes be seen in lesions other than pilomatrixoma.[235]

An extremely rare malignant counterpart of this tumor has been designated malignant pilomatrixoma or pilomatrix carcinoma.[233,238]

MELANOCYTES

Melanocytes are neuroectodermally derived cells located in the basal layer of skin, skin adnexae, and some mucosal membranes; their function is to produce an insoluble pigment known as *melanin* and to transfer this product through the process of cytocrinia to the adjacent epithelial cells. The neuroectodermal origin of melanocytes, proposed many years ago by Masson and others,[244] has been proved by a variety of techniques, among which the chick-quail chimera model of LeDouarin is the most elegant and convincing.[243] Normal melanocytes with scant pigment appear as clear

cells in routinely stained sections, but other intraepidermal clear cells are of keratinocytic nature.[239] Melanocytes are generally positive for melanin (silver) stains, DOPA reaction, S-100 protein, and vimentin; the intensity of these reactions shows marked variability, possibly depending on the functional status of the cell.[240,245,246] Stains for keratin, neurofilament, or glial fibrillary acidic protein are negative.[245] Monoclonal antibodies allegedly specific for subpopulations of melanocytes have recently been developed.[242] Ultrastructurally, all stages in the production of melanin from the premelanosome to the mature melanin granule are seen.

The term *melanocyte* should be reserved for the mature melanin-forming cell. Its immature counterpart is the *melanoblast*. Dermal macrophages with phagocytosed melanin are *melanophages*. The *melanophore* is a melanin-containing "contractile cell" found in amphibians.[241]

Nevi

The word nevus (L. *naevus*, birthmark) can be properly applied to any circumscribed growth of the skin of congenital origin. However, it is usually used as a synonym for mole (L. *moles*, a shapeless mass) to designate a localized benign abnormality of the melanocytic system, which is usually acquired, in the sense that it becomes clinically apparent after the first year of life. Most of them will appear between the second and sixth years, and nearly all will have become manifest by the age of 20. They follow a rather predictable evolution, which only rarely is upset by some dramatic event, such as spontaneous resolution, activation, or malignant transformation. The adjectives *melanocytic* (which we prefer), *nevocellular*, and *pigmented* refer specifically to this type of nevus.

Every person has a variable number of nevi, the average being between twenty and thirty.[248] Their distribution is not the same as that of malignant melanoma. They are much more common in the skin of the head, neck, and trunk, whereas a high percentage of malignant melanomas occur in the lower extremities.

Nevi of every conceivable size, shape, and degree of pigmentation occur, and they may be more or less hairy. Nevi have been variously classified, but it is most logical to divide them according to the location of the melanocytes inasmuch as their position bears a definite relationship to the likelihood of malignant transformation.

Melanocytic nevi straddle the fence between malformation and neoplasia. Cellular blue nevi and Spitz nevi have morphologic and behavioral features consistent with a true neoplastic process, whereas the usual compound nevus has such a distinctive organoid configuration (with adnexal participation) as to strongly suggest a developmental abnormality, perhaps related to atavistic structures such as the tactile corpuscles of reptiles.[247] Masson suggested that the ordinary compound mole has a dual origin from intraepidermal melanoblasts (some of which become intradermal) and dermal Schwann cells.[249,250] Many ultrastructural, histochemical, immunohistochemical, and experimental studies support his proposal that the cells from the upper portion of compound nevi have melanocytic properties, whereas those in the deep portion have schwannian characteristics.[246a]

Junctional, intradermal, and compound nevi

A *junctional nevus* is one in which the melanocytic proliferation is restricted to the basal portion of the epidermis.

Grossly, it is flat or slightly elevated, nonhairy, and fawn colored (Fig. 4-89). Microscopically, it is characterized by the presence of melanocytic nests on the epidermal side of the dermoepidermal junction (Fig. 4-90). Malignant melanomas may arise from this lesion.

In the ***intradermal nevus,*** all the melanocytes are in the dermis. This is the common adult type of nevus. It may be papillary, pedunculated, or flat, and it is often hairy (Fig. 4-91). Multiplicity of lesions is common. Microscopically, small nests or bundles of melanocytes are seen in the dermis, with no evidence of circumscription (Fig. 4-92). The degree of pigmentation and cellularity varies widely. The lower half of the lesion tends to be less cellular, with spindle cells sometimes arranged in neuroid bundles consistent with their presumed schwannian derivation. Occasionally, a storiform pattern of growth is present in this deep portion, establishing a link with the dermal tumor known as storiform neurofibroma.[251] Multinucleated melanocytes can be seen scattered throughout the lesion, particularly in the upper half. Ultrastructurally and immunohistochemically, the intradermal nevus cells are surrounded by basement membrane components.[256a]

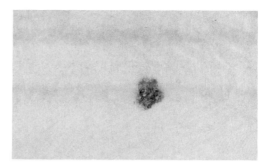

Fig. 4-89 Junctional nevus, nonhairy and fawn colored, on plantar surface of foot.

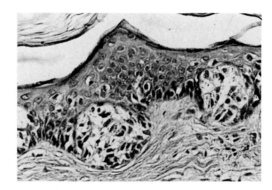

Fig. 4-90 Typical junctional nevus in adult. Note location of cells at dermoepidermal junction.

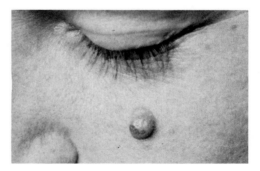

Fig. 4-91 Typical intradermal nevus of skin of cheek.

Morphologic curiosities that have been described in melanocytic nevi include presence of amyloid, bone, elastotic fibers, folliculitis and abscess formation, psammoma bodies, pseudoglandular spaces, permeation of lymphatic vessels, and changes of eczema or focal acantholytic keratosis in the overlying epidermis.[256] Malignant melanomas practically never arise from intradermal nevi.

The ***compound nevus*** combines the features of the junctional and intradermal types. The percentage of nevi with junctional changes decreases as the age of the patient increases.[253,255] The outstanding exceptions are the palms and soles, in which nevi tend to maintain a junctional character throughout life.

Although the overwhelming majority of nevi are located in the skin, they can also be found in any mucosal membrane covered by squamous epithelium (see respective sections). Clusters of benign nevus cells can also be seen in the capsule of a lymph node, the axillary region being the most common location.[252,254] These nests, which do not penetrate into the node itself, should not be confused with malignant melanoma, a mistake particularly likely to occur when found in

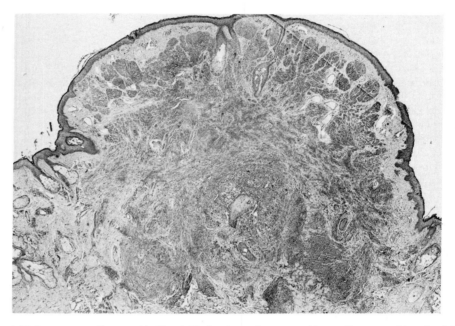

Fig. 4-92 Same nevus illustrated in Fig. 4-91 showing cells arranged in small nests and bundles lying entirely within dermis.

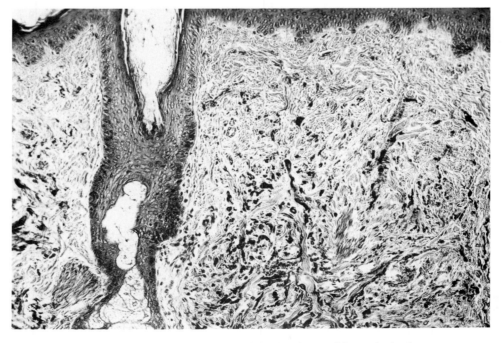

Fig. 4-93 Blue nevus. Note fusiform cells in dermis containing melanin pigment.

specimens from axillary lymphadenectomy performed because of cutaneous melanoma.

Blue and cellular blue nevi

Blue nevus is usually small and located in the head, neck, or upper extremity. Microscopically, it is characterized by an ill-defined dermal proliferation of elongated dermal melanocytes. Melanin pigment is usually abundant (Fig. 4-93). There is a band of uninvolved dermis between the epidermis and the lesion, and junctional activity is consistently absent. When present, either in the form of conventional *theques* or intraepidermal dendritic melanocytes, the

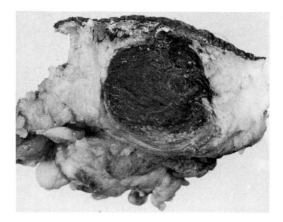

Fig. 4-94 Large cellular blue nevus occurring in buttock of young woman. Note lack of involvement of epidermis and well delimited pushing borders.

lesion is known as compound nevus. Blue nevi are sometimes misdiagnosed as benign fibrous histiocytomas because the pigment present is misinterpreted as hemosiderin. Combined blue and intradermal nevi occur.[261] Blue nevi have also been reported in the hard palate,[259] breast, cervix,[258] prostate,[260] and lymph nodes.[257]

The *cellular blue nevus* is a distinctive variety of blue nevus, often suspected of being malignant because of its size and rather intense pigmentation[262,263] (Fig. 4-94). The most common location is the buttock and sacrococcygeal areas; less common sites include the scalp, face, and dorsa of hands and feet.[263] Microscopically, these lesions are extremely cellular, hence their name. They differ microscopically from malignant melanomas by the absence of junctional activity, epidermal invasion, peripheral inflammation, and necrosis; the presence of pushing margins, biphasic pattern, fasciculation, and neuroid structures; and the relative lack of atypia and mitotic figures[263] (Fig. 4-95).

The behavior of cellular blue nevus is usually benign, but a few cases with local recurrence or involvement of regional lymph nodes have been documented.[263] However, even these patients are usually cured by excision of the primary lesion and involved nodes.

Spitz nevus

Spitz nevus (spindle and/or epithelioid cell nevus) characteristically occurs before puberty, but it may also appear in adult life.[265,267] The most typical presentation is in the form of a raised, pink or red nodule in the skin of the face.

Microscopically, most of these nevi are of the compound type, with a prominent intraepidermal component. About 5% to 10% are junctional, and 20% or more are intradermal.[268] They are composed of spindle cells, epithelioid cells, or an admixture of both.

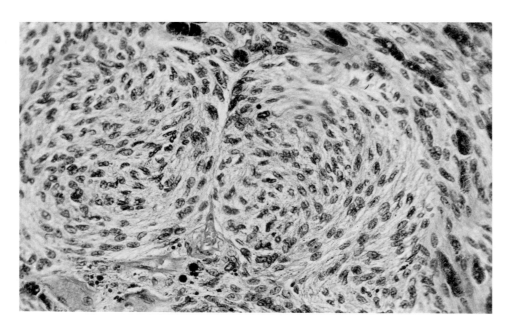

Fig. 4-95 Large cellular blue nevus of buttock with whorl-like areas and fusiform cells producing melanin pigment.

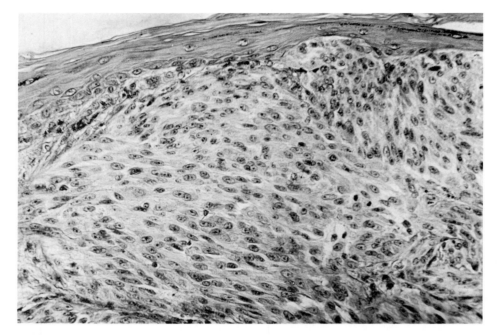

Fig. 4-96 Spitz nevus of spindle-cell type excised from skin of abdomen of 14-year-old child. Cells are spindle shaped and have numerous mitotic figures, abundant cytoplasm, and uniform nuclei.

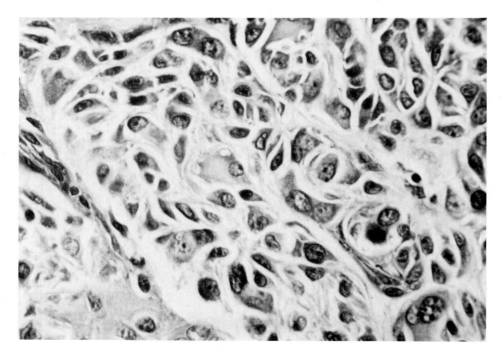

Fig. 4-97 Spitz nevus of epithelioid type occurring in 5-year-old child. The cells are large and polygonal, with abundant acidophilic cytoplasm.

The spindle cell variant is characterized by cigar-shaped cells with large nuclei and prominent nucleoli (Fig. 4-96). The cells of the epithelioid type have similar nuclei and a large, polygonal cytoplasm with distinct borders (Fig. 4-97). A variant of the latter is a multinucleated giant melanocyte containing up to ten or twenty nuclei. Mitoses are found in about half of the cases,[274] but atypical mitoses are exceptional. Pigmentation is usually scanty, but a deeply pigmented variant (often of recent onset and located on the proximal extremities of young adults) exists; this is referred to as *pigmented spindle cell nevus* and is regarded as by some as a separate entity from Spitz nevus.[270,272] Sometimes, Spitz nevi of predominantly dermal location are accompanied by an extensive stromal desmoplasia, which encircles the individual cells and simulates an invasive pattern.[264] This feature is more commonly seen in adults, and this adds to the diagnostic difficulty.[268] Other features occasionally present in Spitz nevi that may lead to a mistaken diagnosis of malignancy are invasion of lymphatic vessels[266] and florid pseudoepitheliomatous hyperplasia[271] (Fig. 4-98).

Features that favor a diagnosis of Spitz nevus over one of malignant melanoma are symmetric shape; sharp lateral demarcation; maturation in depth; arrangement of the spindle cells perpendicularly to the skin surface; presence of tadpole and multinucleated giant cells; lack of upward epidermal spread; presence of telangiectasia, edema, and fi-brosis; presence of eosinophilic hyaline bodies along the dermo-epidermal junction; and lack of ulceration.[269,273] In addition, the cytoplasm of benign epithelioid nevi has a homogeneous acidophilic ground-glass appearance, whereas that of melanoma cells tends to be more irregular in configuration and staining reaction.

The behavior of Spitz nevi is almost uniformly benign. However, a few unquestionable cases of uncontrollable local recurrence and distant metastases in lesions originally diagnosed as Spitz nevi have been documented. On review, some of these lesions have been found to have the features of malignant melanomas, but others are indistinguishable from benign Spitz nevi.[273] Interestingly, some of these "malignant Spitz nevi" have occurred in immunosuppressed patients.

Other nevi

Halo nevus (leukoderma acquisitum centrifugum) is used to describe a melanocytic nevus surrounded by a zone of depigmented skin[280] (Fig. 4-99). It is most commonly found on the trunk of young patients.[288] Microscopically and ultrastructurally it is characterized by a heavy infiltration of the nevus by lymphocytes and histiocytes[278] (Fig. 4-100). The lesion can be confused with melanoma, lymphoma, and dermatitis. It should be mentioned that malignant melanoma may also be surrounded by a halo of depigmented skin. However, in this instance the halo tends to be irregular and the pigmented spot is usually off center.

Balloon nevus is another unusual variety of nevus, identified by the presence of large melanocytes with foamy cytoplasm, perhaps the result of a biochemical alteration in melanin synthesis.[285] Balloon cells also can occur in blue nevi and malignant melanomas.[277]

Congenital nevus differs from the more common acquired variety because of its generally larger size (Fig. 4-101), tendency to involve the reticular dermis and subcutaneous tissue, single cell permeation of dermal collagen bundles, and involvement of skin adnexae, nerves, and vessels.[281,286,287a] However, there are too many exceptions to

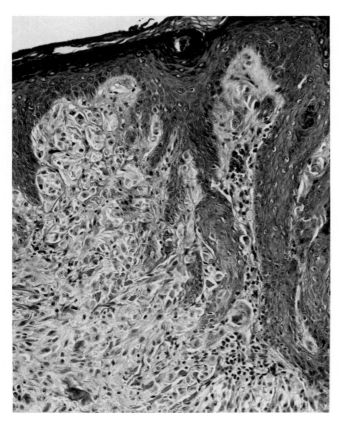

Fig. 4-98 Spitz nevus with pseudoepitheliomatous hyperplasia. This change should not be confused with squamous cell carcinoma.

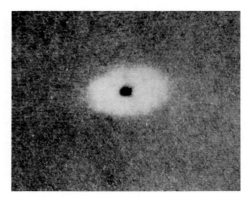

Fig. 4-99 Typical clinical appearance of halo nevus. Heavily pigmented center is surrounded by sharply defined oval area of depigmentation. Pigmented nevus may be situated in center, as here, or be eccentric. (Courtesy Dr. A.W. Kopf, New York, NY.)

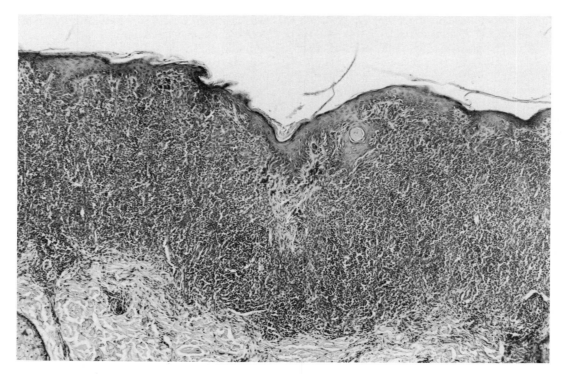

Fig. 4-100 Halo nevus. Intense mononucleated inflammatory infiltrate of bandlike distribution seen in association with melanin-laden macrophages and marked irregularity of dermoepidermal junction. Degenerating melanocytes were identified on higher power examination.

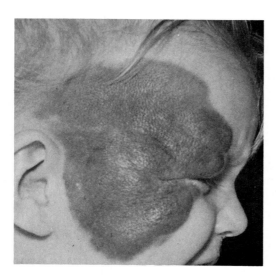

Fig. 4-101 Congenital nevus on skin of face of child. Lesion is elevated, well circumscribed, and uniformly brown.

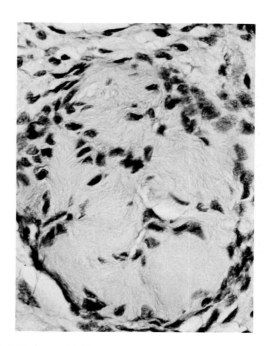

Fig. 4-102 Wagner-Meissner corpuscle in large congenital nevus of posterior wall of chest of infant.

allow for an absolute distinction based on microscopic criteria alone.[284] Neuroid differentiation, such as formation of Wagner-Meissner–like corpuscles, is common (Fig. 4-102). The term *neuronevus* has been applied in the past to congenital (and some acquired) nevi in which this feature was particularly prominent.[282]

When removed a few months after birth, these congenital nevi can show marked intraepidermal melanocytic hyperplasia, simulating the appearance of superficially spreading melanoma.

Giant pigmented (hairy) nevus is a variant of congenital nevus characterized by its extensive size, its surface area being by definition 144 sq cm or larger. It has a tendency to distribute along a dermatome and often has a "bathing trunk" or "garment" configuration. It may involve a whole extremity, the entire scalp, most of the trunk, and even extend into the placenta.[276] It is sometimes associated with meningeal or cerebral melanosis.[287] It may give rise to malignant melanoma of the skin or central nervous system and to related malignant neuroectodermal tumors[279,283] (Fig. 4-103). Whether the smaller congenital nevi are also subject to an increased risk of malignant transformation has not yet been established with certainty.[275,281]

Treatment

Since every adult has, on the average, ten to twenty nevi, it is obvious that specific indications are needed for their removal, other than those dictated by cosmetic considerations. The presence of a junctional component per se is not an indication; most plantar and palmar nevi are junctional,

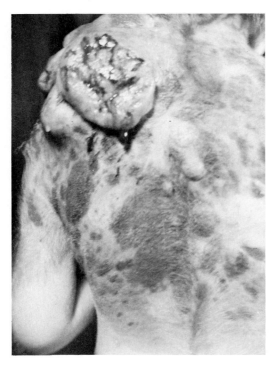

Fig. 4-103 Malignant ulcerating neurogenous tumor arising in giant pigmented (hairy) nevus in child.

but they are too common and the possibility of malignant transformation too remote to warrant routine removal.[292,293] Definite indications for excision include appearance of a pigmented lesion in an adult, chronic mechanical irritation of a nevus, or the appearance of any of the following changes in a pre-existing nevus: deepening of pigmentation or spread of the pigment beyond the gross confines of the lesion, appearance of flat areas of depigmentation within the nevus, appearance of a red inflamed zone around the nevus, rapid growth, ulceration, itching, oozing of serum, or bleeding with trivial trauma.[290]

Removal of a nevus should be carried out with a cold knife rather than a cautery, in order to prevent the distortion of tissue and peculiar staining reactions associated with the latter. Incomplete removal may result in local recurrence. The recurrent lesion often shows junctional activity, even if this feature was not present in the original excision.[289] This, plus the nuclear enlargement and nucleolar prominence that often accompany these recurrences, has sometimes resulted in a mistaken diagnosis of malignant melanoma.[291]

Active and dysplastic nevi

The term *active nevus* has been applied to benign melanocytic nevi that show prominence of the junctional component and hyperplasia of individual basal melanocytes, often associated with increased overall cellularity and dermal inflammatory infiltrate. Activation of nevi, thus defined, has been reported as a result of sunlight exposure,[300] in pregnancy,[298] in association with malignant melanoma elsewhere in the skin,[303] in recurrent nevi,[301] and sometimes for no obvious reason.

Exceptionally, myriads of eruptive nevi with the microscopic signs of "activation" will appear in an adult unassociated with any recognizable cause.[296]

Dysplastic nevus is a recently introduced and highly controversial concept, which seems to blend or at least exhibit some morphologic similarities with activation of nevi. In its better defined form, it occurs as a genetically determined syndrome in families prone to develop malignant melanoma (dysplastic nevus syndrome or B-K mole syndrome).[299,302] The nevi are clinically atypical, with an irregular outline and a variegated appearance; they appear in adolescence and continue to develop in adult life. Microscopically, most dysplastic nevi are compound nevi exhibiting basal melanocytic hyperplasia with some degree of atypia. These melanocytes may be spindle shaped[302] (often arranged horizontally to the skin surface) or epithelioid. The papillary dermis shows a lymphocytic infiltrate, together with lamellar and concentric fibroplasia.[295,297] Ultrastructurally, melanosomal alterations occur.[302a]

Although the importance of having identified a familial syndrome with a predisposition toward melanoma cannot be overemphasized, the application of this concept to the solitary pigmented lesions remains questionable, both in terms of morphologic criteria and biologic significance. On the basis of present evidence, we think that solitary melanocytic nevi with "dysplastic" features should be regarded as benign and handled as such for all practical purposes. Thus we agree wholeheartedly with Ackerman et al.[294] when they stated that "use of the term dysplastic nevus is unfortunate, because it conveys a sinister connotation to what may be a rather conventional melanocytic lesion." Furthermore, we believe that many of the lesions now being reported as dysplastic nevi in patients with malignant melanoma are of the same type as those previously interpreted by us as representing activation of nevi in this population.[303]

Malignant melanoma
General features

The large majority of melanomas are associated with sunlight exposure. Therefore most are found in the head and neck area and on the lower extremities, the latter location being particularly common in females.[309,323] Rare but well-known locations of cutaneous melanomas are the subungual region ("melanotic whitlow")[316,320] and the palms and soles[312] (Fig. 4-104).

Whites, particularly those of fair complexion, red hair, and tendency to burn or develop freckles after exposure to sunlight,[307] are particularly susceptible to the development of melanomas. The few melanomas developing in blacks tend to occur in the palms and soles.

The overwhelming majority of melanomas arise after puberty. However, there is no longer any question that they can also occur in children.[305,317] These melanomas have the same microscopic pattern as those in adults and therefore can be distinguished in most cases on morphologic grounds from Spitz nevi.[310,313,314]

Malignant melanomas can present as multiple primary tumors.[311,322] In a series of 712 patients with melanomas,

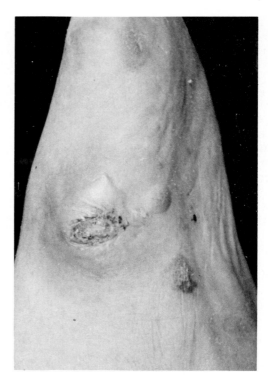

Fig. 4-104 Malignant melanoma of foot, relatively nonpigmented. Such lesions can be misinterpreted for long periods as a benign process.

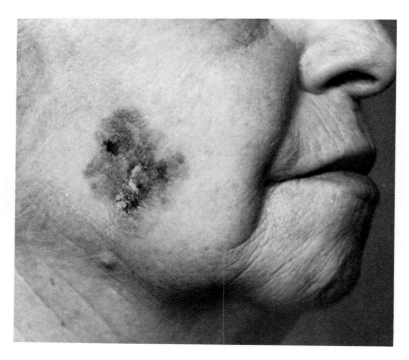

Fig. 4-105 Hutchinson's freckle that had been present for many years in 67-year-old woman. Raised area in center represents invasive melanoma.

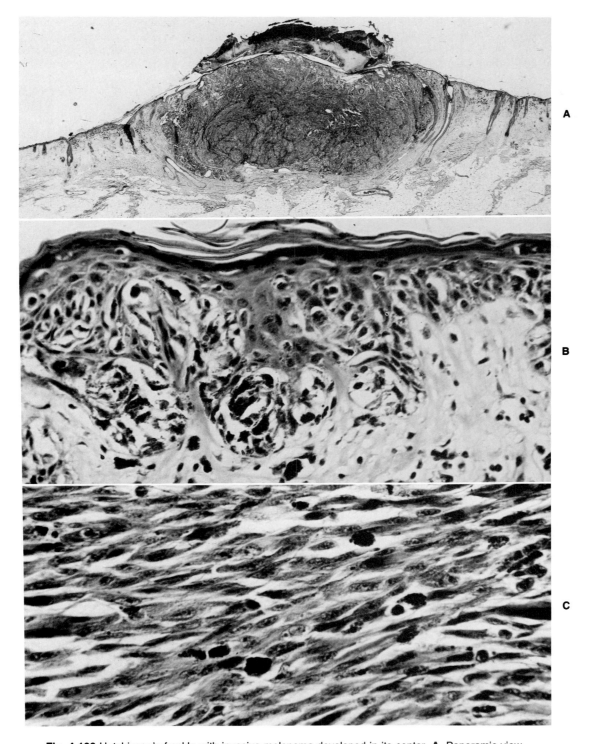

Fig. 4-106 Hutchinson's freckle with invasive melanoma developed in its center. **A,** Panoramic view, showing large central nodule of invasive tumor. **B,** High-power view of Hutchinson's freckle. Atypical melanocytes, isolated or forming *theques,* are present along basal layer. Numerous melanin-containing macrophages can be seen in dermis. **C,** High-power view of invasive melanoma. Tumor cells are spindle shaped and contain abundant melanin, as is often case with melanomas arising in Hutchinson's freckle.

thirty-eight (5.3%) had more than one primary melanoma: twenty-four had two primary lesions, eleven had three, two had four, and one had eight.[315] The prognosis was more dependent on the type and stage of the largest lesion than on the number of primary lesions. Multiple primary melanomas should be distinguished from the phenomenon of nevus activation in patients with melanomas.[321]

The existence of hereditary forms of malignant melanoma has been known for a long time.[304] Reimer et al.[318] have described in members of melanoma-prone families the presence of atypical melanocytic lesions ("dysplastic nevi") that serve as a cutaneous marker of those at high risk (see p. 123).

Melanoma can be associated with generalized melanosis[308,319] and with lesions resembling vitiligo.[306] Melanin, dopa, and a variety of metabolites can be detected in the urine.[324]

Clinical appearance and clinicopathologic types

For the purposes of clinical and microscopic description, it is useful to divide melanomas into four categories by following the criteria championed by Clark et al.[328,329,342] in the United States and McGovern[336,337,339,340] in Australia, even acknowledging the fact that the clinicopathologic or prognostic differences among them are not as sharp as originally claimed.[325,349] These categories are: melanoma arising in Hutchinson's freckle, superficially spreading melanoma, nodular melanoma, and acral lentiginous melanoma. A high degree of accuracy in the differential diagnosis among these types is possible on the basis of location and gross appearance.[343,344]

Hutchinson's freckle (lentigo maligna) typically occurs in the sun-exposed areas of elderly white persons (Fig. 4-105), most commonly on the cheek.[338,353] It is a flat, slowly growing lesion, its color varying from tan to black.[330] Microscopically, it is characterized by a proliferation of atypical melanocytes in the basal layer, distributed individually as well as in nests (Fig. 4-106). Retraction of the cytoplasm and pleomorphism are prominent. Hutchinson's freckle is an actinically induced atypia of melanocytes; as such, it could be regarded as the melanocytic analog of actinic keratosis. As a matter of fact, both components may coexist in the same lesion. A more descriptive term for Hutchinson's freckle, which also may be applied to histologically similar lesions that do not quite fit this clinical picture, is *actinic melanosis*.

The proliferation of atypical basal melanocytes in the deep portion of the rete ridges can simulate invasion, especially in a tangential section. It is advisable to be very conservative in the evaluation of this lesion, just as in actinic keratosis. If no clear-cut dermal infiltration can be demonstrated despite the examination of multiple sections, it is better not to classify the lesion as a melanoma.

The malignant melanoma that develops on the basis of Hutchinson's freckle is often of the spindle-cell type and is endowed with a low degree of aggressiveness. Of eighty-five cases studied by Wayte and Helwig,[353] forty-five were thought to contain an invasive melanoma in the center of the lesion, but the criteria might have been somewhat liberal. In any event, of the eighty-five cases, only three patients

died of the tumor; a fourth developed lymph node metastases but remained well after resection of the involved nodes. Another type of melanoma that can develop on the basis of Hutchinson's freckle has a much more aggressive behavior. It has been called *desmoplastic melanoma* by Conley et al.[331] As the name indicates, it is associated with an extensive degree of fibrosis, and the tumor cells have a spindle configuration; this combination results in an appearance reminiscent of atypical fibroxanthoma. As a matter of fact, it has been suggested that the bulk of the tumor is indeed of fibrohistiocytic nature.[332] We favor the interpretation that the atypical cells are histiocytoid or sarcomatoid melanocytes, and some ultrastructural evidence backs this assumption.[352] The distinction from atypical fibroxanthoma, which can be extremely difficult, is made on the basis of lesser degree of pleomorphism, vascularity, and inflammation, and the presence of ill-defined borders, deep invasion, and, most of all, a lesion with the features of Hutchinson's freckle in the overlying epidermis. All four of the cases reported by Labrecque et al.[332] recurred locally, and three gave rise to distant metastases. Desmoplastic melanoma also can be seen in connection with other pigmented lesions.[351]

Superficial spreading melanoma is the most common form of melanoma. It also has been called premalignant melanosis or pagetoid melanoma[336] and can occur anywhere on the body surface. It has a variegated appearance, the colors including hues of tan, brown, black, blue, pink, and white. According to Mihm et al.,[344] the telltale color of early superficially spreading melanoma is most frequently a shade of blue admixed with tan, brown, or dark brown. The surface is slightly elevated and the margins barely palpable (Fig. 4-107). The white areas correspond to areas of spontaneous regression. They are related to tumor size but not to the level of invasion or prognosis.[341] Pink and blue areas also correspond to areas of tumor regression, associ-

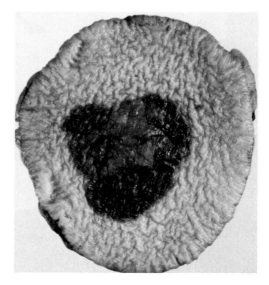

Fig. 4-107 Superficial spreading malignant melanoma with invasive focus in center.

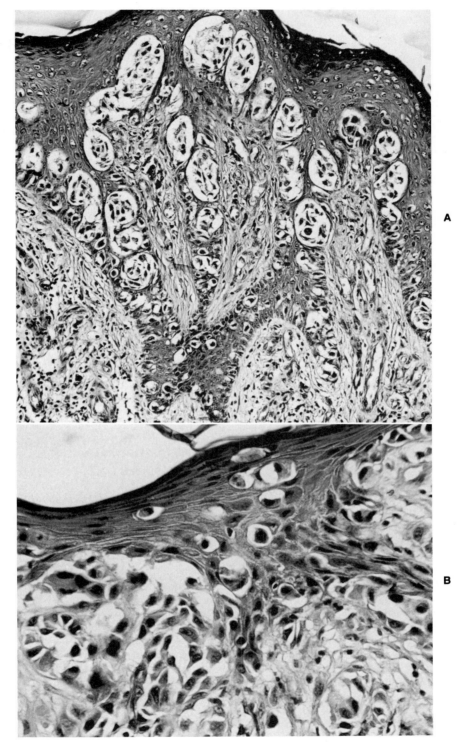

Fig. 4-108 Malignant melanoma of superficial spreading type. **A,** Marked proliferation of clear cells in well-defined nests resembles appearance of Paget's disease. **B,** Tumor cells have epithelioid appearance and permeate malpighian layers throughout.

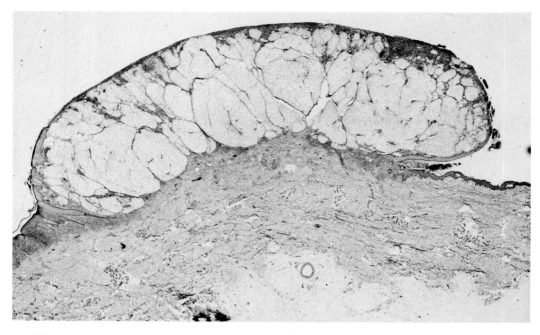

Fig. 4-109 Balloon cell melanoma involving skin of right shoulder of 50-year-old man. Low-power view showing polypoid tumor with only superficial dermal invasion. (Slide contributed by Dr. W.A. Gardner, Jr., Durham, NC.)

ated with dermal fibrosis and accumulation of melanin-laden macrophages. The borders of the lesion are irregular and usually include a prominent indentation or notch. Deep invasion generally is accompanied by the appearance of an elevated nodule on the surface. Microscopically, the noninvasive areas are composed of uniform atypical melanocytes with nest formation and pagetoid appearance (Fig. 4-108).

Nodular melanoma can present as a smooth nodule covered by normal epidermis, as an elevated blue-black plaque, or as a polypoid, frequently ulcerated mass.[335] A lateral flat component is not seen clinically or microscopically. This type of melanoma affects all body surfaces, is usually of short duration, and occurs in a younger age group than either of the foregoing two categories.

(Acral) lentiginous melanoma has a radial (intraepidermal) component of lentiginous type, which is similar in many respects to that seen in Hutchinson's freckle.[326,334,347,350] In contrast to the latter, however, the intraepidermal melanocytes tend to be bizarre, the involved epidermis is markedly hyperplastic rather than atrophic, and the papillary dermis in this region is widened and inflamed. Tumors with these features have been seen on the palms, soles, subungual areas, mucocutaneous junction of the oral and nasal cavities, and the anus.[346] This type of melanoma is more common in blacks and Orientals.[345,348]

• • •

The clinical differential diagnosis of malignant melanoma includes a wide variety of lesions, particularly those containing melanin or hemosiderin pigment: benign nevi of various types, benign fibrous histiocytoma, inflamed or thrombosed hemangioma, pigmented seborrheic keratosis, and pigmented basal cell carcinoma.[327,333] Conversely, malignant melanomas that are amelanotic or covered by a thick layer of keratin can simulate a pyogenic granuloma or a callus, respectively.

Microscopic features

The typical example of malignant melanoma is easily identified microscopically because of its junctional activity, prominent melanin pigmentation, deep invasion of the surrounding tissue, and many abnormal mitotic figures. Alas, this is not always the case. As a matter of fact, malignant melanoma is notorious for the great microscopic variability that it may exhibit.[372] The cells can be epithelioid, spindle shaped, or extremely bizarre. Their size can be so small as to simulate a lymphocytic lymphoma or as large as that of a pleomorphic soft tissue sarcoma. The cytoplasm can be eosinophilic, basophilic, foamy, of signet-ring type, or completely clear (balloon cell melanoma)[367,382a] (Figs. 4-109 and 4-110). Melanin can be abundant, scanty, or absent. The pattern of growth may be pseudoglandular, peritheliomatous, trabecular, or verrucous (pseudonevoid).[370,372] The tumor can be accompanied by marked fibroblastic response, myxoid changes,[355] or by pseudoepitheliomatous hyperplasia of the overlying epidermis. Occasionally, formations suggesting differentiation toward Schwann's cells, tactile corpuscles, ganglion cells, other neuroid structures, and fetal cartilage are observed.[381,385] Additional variations include the already mentioned desmoplastic melanoma,[363,382] the perhaps related neurotropic or neurosarcomatous mel-

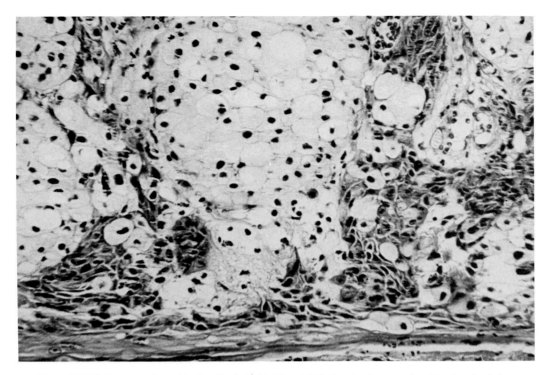

Fig. 4-110 High-power view of lesion illustrated in Fig. 4-109 showing tumor cells with abundant clear cytoplasm and well-defined cell membranes. (Slide contributed by Dr. W.A. Gardner, Jr., Durham, NC.)

anoma,[360,386] and the controversial minimal deviation melanoma.[379] As a result of all these variations, malignant melanoma can simulate carcinoma, various types of sarcoma, malignant lymphoma, and several other disorders (Figs. 4-111 and 4-112).

Nearly all malignant melanomas exhibit an intraepidermal component ("junctional activity") during their initial phase. Therefore a melanoma lying entirely within the dermis should be strongly suspected of being metastatic.[354] However, some well-documented cases of primary intradermal melanoma exist, the possible explanations for their occurrence being total regression of the intraepidermal component or origin from an intradermal nevus.

At a practical level, there are two major problems that a pathologist confronted with such a tumor faces. The first is how to identify as malignant melanoma an obviously malignant tumor when melanin formation is not apparent in routine sections. Features suggestive of melanoma in hematoxylin-eosin sections are cells with abundant acidophilic, finely granular cytoplasm, pseudonuclear inclusions, combination of epithelial and spindle-cell patterns of growth, fascicular arrangement of tumor cells, and pseudoalveolar arrangement.

Stains for melanin should always be obtained in these lesions; they may show finely dispersed positive granules that were not apparent in hematoxylin-eosin sections. The dopa reaction can be useful, but this technique requires fresh tissue. Perhaps an immunocytochemical reaction can be developed for the identification of dopa-oxidase that can be performed in routinely fixed material. Electron microscopy can demonstrate melanosomes and the less diagnostic premelanosomes[362] (Figs. 4-113 and 4-114). Melanin precursors in the cytoplasm of the tumor cells can be detected by formaldehyde-induced fluorescence, both in touch preparations and freeze-dried sections.[361,369,374] Some malignant melanomas that are amelanotic in vivo can produce large amounts of melanin when placed in a tissue culture system.[359]

The technique that has proved most practical in the identification of melanoma has been the immunohistochemical detection of S-100 protein[365,375,383] (Fig. 4-115). Although this marker is far from being specific for melanoma, it is negative in most of the tumors that enter in the differential diagnosis and is therefore of great utility. Positivity for vimentin is also obtained regularly.[356] Some tumor cells also react for alpha-1-antichymotrypsin.[371] It remains to be seen whether any of the recently developed monoclonal antibodies against "melanoma-specific antigens" will offer a greater degree of sensitivity and specificity.[364,366,376-378,384,384a] S-100 protein stain has also been used to detect metastatic malignant melanoma in lymph nodes, but we doubt whether its routine use for this purpose is warranted.[357]

The other important diagnostic problem is the decision about whether a skin lesion of obvious melanocytic nature is benign or malignant. Benign lesions most commonly overdiagnosed as melanomas are Spitz nevi (especially the desmoplastic type of pure epithelioid nevus), irritated nevi, halo nevi, activated nevi in patients with malignant melanomas, and nevi that have recurred following incomplete excision.[358] Conversely, the type of melanoma that is more likely to be underdiagnosed as benign is a level I or level II superficially spreading type. We have found the criteria listed below the most useful for the identification of early malignant melanoma.[380] Unfortunately, none of them is pathognomonic. The diagnosis of melanoma can only be made on the basis of a combination of features.

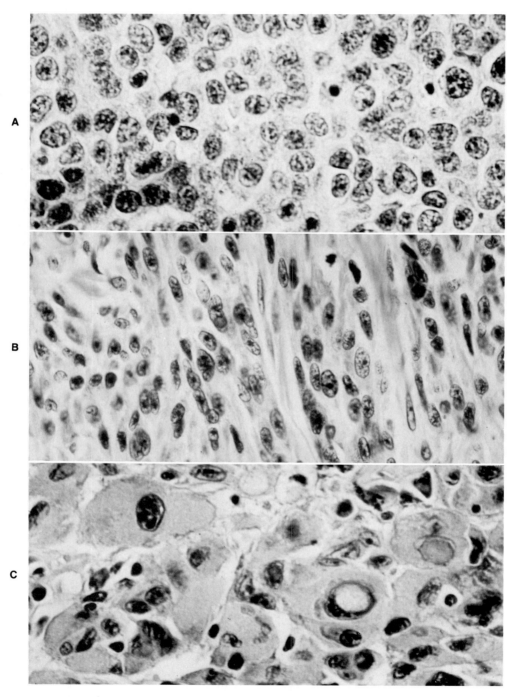

A

B

C

Fig. 4-111 Different malignant melanomas at same magnification demonstrating wide range of microscopic variations. Tumor shown in **A** resembles malignant lymphoma. Fusiform cells of tumor shown in **B** resemble those of fibrosarcoma. Great variation of tumor cells and giant forms shown in **C** suggest pleomorphic sarcoma.

1 Poor circumscription (lack of cohesiveness) of the intraepidermal melanocytic component. The nests are not so sharply defined as those of benign lesions, and the individual cells within the nests are separated from each other.

2 Lateral extension of individual melanocytes. Benign lesions usually exhibit a sharp cutoff, whereas in most malignant lesions there is a trailing off of atypical melanocytes spreading from the center of the lesion.

3 Extension of melanocytes, individually and in nests, throughout the malpighian layer and within adnexal epithelium. This phenomenon of transepidermal migration results in a pagetoid appearance of the lesion, hence the term "pagetoid melanoma" that is sometimes used. The melanin pigment can reach the horny layer, a process known as pigmented parakeratosis; this is very rare in benign nevi although it appears with some frequency in some variants of benign lentigo.

4 Size variation, shape variation, and confluence of melanocytic nests.

5 Lack of maturation of dermal melanocytes.

6 Melanocytic atypia, evidenced by prominence of nuclei and nucleoli and increase of the nucleocytoplasmic ratio.

7 Presence of mitoses in melanocytes. Most benign nevi have a very small number of mitotic figures, although some spindle and epithelioid cell nevi may contain many. The presence of atypical mitoses is a strong indication that the lesion is malignant. The same is true for the presence of mitoses in the *dermal* component of melanocytic lesions other than Spitz nevi. Some benign and malignant melanocytic lesions are associated with marked hyperplasia of the epidermis; in these cases, one should be careful to distinguish mitoses in keratinocytes from mitoses in melanocytes.

8 Melanocytes with an abundant clear cytoplasm having a finely dispersed ("dusty") chromatin. This has been interpreted as a sign of degeneration.

9 Necrosis of individual melanocytes. This phenomenon should be distinguished from the eosinophilic hyaline bodies seen most often in Spitz nevi.

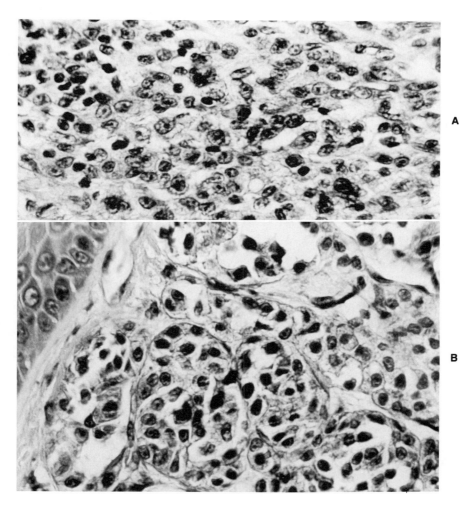

Fig. 4-112 A, Undifferentiated nonpigmented malignant melanoma metastatic to scalp in 17-year-old girl. **B,** Primary tumor contained areas similar to those shown in **A.** Its true character is indicated by nevoid pattern seen in this section taken near surface.

10 Dermal infiltrate of chronic inflammatory cells, mainly lymphocytes. This is particularly prominent in the early lesions and tends to have a bandlike distribution instead of the patchy appearance usually seen in irritated nevi.

So far, no reliable ultrastructural or immunohistochemical differences between benign and malignant melanocytic lesions have been described. At the ultrastructural level, malignant melanomas have a greater tendency for abnormal melanosome formation than the benign lesion, but there is a great degree of overlap.[373] The melanosomes in Hutchinson's freckle–melanoma tend to be ellipsoidal, resembling those of normal melanocytes, whereas those of superficial spreading and nodular melanoma are most often spheroidal and abnormal in appearance.[368]

Biopsy and frozen section

There is no evidence that incisional biopsy of a malignant melanoma increases the probability of spread. Comparison of patients on whom incisional biopsy was done and those

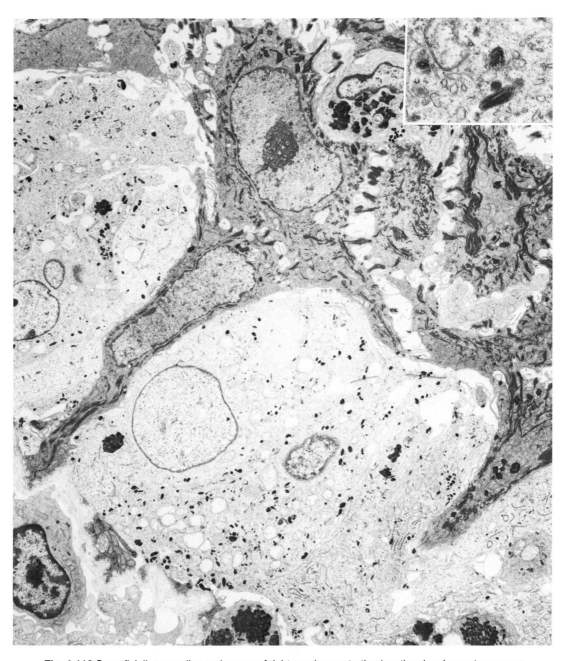

Fig. 4-113 Superficially spreading melanoma of right ear demonstrating junctional melanocytes among keratinocytes. **Inset,** Stage 3 melanosomes present in neoplastic cells. (×3,850; **inset** ×25,270.)

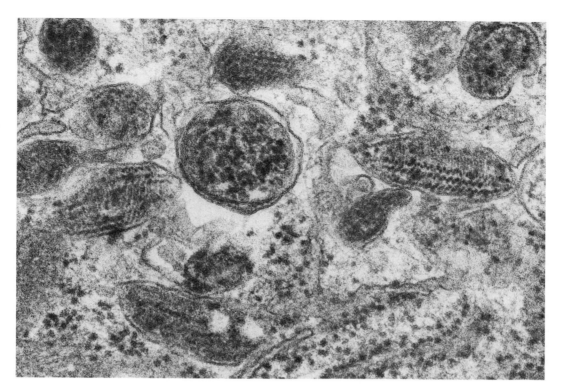

Fig. 4-114 Metastatic melanoma of lung in 60-year-old man with superficial spreading type of malignant melanoma of skin. Note presence of stage 2 and stage 3 melanosomes with characteristic lattice arrangement. (×81,000.)

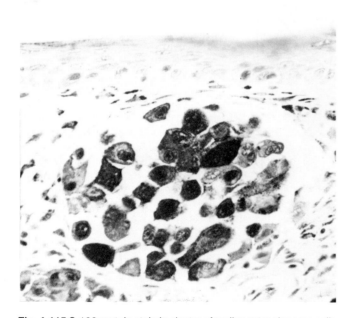

Fig. 4-115 S-100 protein stain in cluster of malignant melanoma cells located beneath epidermis. Strong nuclear and cytoplasmic positivity is present.

who had excision without biopsy have shown no differences in survival rate.[388] Primary adequate excision in the form of excisional biopsy should be done if the lesion is located in an area in which no deformity will result.[391] However, if the lesion is of such a size and in such a location that radical excision implies disfigurement or disability, then careful incisional biopsy is indicated.

In experienced hands, the diagnosis of malignant melanoma by frozen section is reliable.[387,389,392] However, one can hardly justify its routine use on practical grounds.[390]

Regression

Partial regression is a common feature in melanoma, particularly in the Hutchinson's freckle type. Total regression is much less common, but numerous cases in which the primary tumor regressed completely after giving rise to nodal and distant metastases have been documented.[396] This phenomenon may also explain some apparent discrepancies between expected and observed prognosis based on tumor thickness,[394] and also the fact that in 5% to 15% of patients with metastatic melanoma the primary tumor is never found.[393]

Clinically, the spontaneous regression of melanoma is often heralded by the sudden onset of an irregular halo around the tumor. Microscopically, the early stage of regression is characterized by a dense infiltrate of lymphocytes similar to that seen in spontaneously disappearing nevi. This change may be partial or complete. In the late stage, vascular scar tissue with a variable number of melanin-laden macrophages is present. McGovern[395] described seven distinctive clinical patterns resulting from this process and pointed out that only melanomas with an intraepidermal component have been found to undergo spontaneous regression.

Atypical in situ melanocytic lesions

One of the most controversial aspects in the pathology of the melanocytic system is the evaluation and nomenclature of atypical melanocytic lesions that are limited to the epidermis. Such changes may be seen at the periphery of an obvious malignant melanoma,[398,399] in the epidermal component of a compound nevus, or as an isolated finding. Terms such as atypical (intraepidermal, premalignant) melanocytic hyperplasia, melanocytic dysplasia, premalignant melanosis, and melanoma in situ have been used for this process, depending on location, some variations in morphologic appearance, and—most of all—observer's bias.[397-399] In a broad sense, Hutchinson's freckle and dysplastic nevi also fall into this category. In general, we have avoided the term malignant melanoma in situ for lesions of this sort in order to prevent unnecessary surgical procedures and undue concern on the part of the patient. We believe that descriptive names such as *atypical melanocytic hyperplasia* or equivalent terms such as intraepithelial atypical melanocytic proliferation and intraepithelial melanocytic neoplasia identify the nature of the process while avoiding the many undesirable consequences of the word "malignant."[399a]

Spread and metastases

Malignant melanoma spreads by growing along the dermoepidermal junction (horizontal or radial growth phase) and later by invading the dermis and eventually the subcutis and deeper structures (vertical growth phase). The depth of invasion can be quantified and is of great prognostic significance (see Prognosis). Metastases in regional lymph nodes are common even if the nodes appear clinically negative. Detection of metastases in lymph nodes can be increased by serially sectioning the nodes or by staining them for S-100 protein, but neither technique seems particularly practical or useful.[402] Distant metastases occur most often in the liver, lungs, gastrointestinal tract, bone, and central nervous system but can occur anywhere. At autopsy, metastases to the heart are found in one half of the patients. A certain pattern in the distribution of these metastases, related to the embryologic origin of the organs involved, has been noted.[400] Cutaneous metastases are also common. Many of them are located close to the tumor ("satellite nodules"), suggesting a lymphatic rather than a blood vessel mechanism. Cutaneous and subcutaneous metastases located between the site of the primary tumor and the regional lymph node are sometimes referred to as "in-transit metastases." Both satellite nodules and in-transit metastases are usually indicators of disseminated systemic disease.[403] Cutaneous metastases from melanoma can be difficult to distinguish from a primary lesion because the metastases may develop a secondary intraepidermal component ("epidermotropic" metastases). A useful differential feature is the fact that in metastatic carcinoma with secondary intraepithelial spread, the dermal component is much wider than the epidermal one, whereas the opposite is generally true for the primary lesion.[401]

The behavior of malignant melanoma is very unpredictable. Deaths from metastatic melanoma have been documented 15 years or more after the initial therapy.[404] Conversely, some patients with widespread satellite nodules in one extremity may survive for many years without evidence of tumor spread beyond that extremity. Immunologic factors probably play an important although still ill-understood role in the evolution of this neoplasm.

Treatment

The treatment of choice of most malignant melanomas is wide excision of the primary lesion. A margin of 2 to 3 cm or perhaps even 1 cm is probably sufficient for the average-sized tumor, even if some surgeons in the past have recommended a margin of 5 cm.[406,411] Balch et al.[407] recommended a margin of 2 cm for thin melanomas (less than 0.76 mm in thickness) and a margin of 3 to 5 cm for thicker lesions, but even this proposal has been questioned in view of the fact that survival in melanoma is unrelated to the width of the margins, irrespectively of the width of the tumor.[405,408,417] Removal of the underlying fascia, once considered a must, has fallen into discredit in recent years.[416] Distal lymph stasis can be a serious consequence of the procedure, especially in lesions located below the knee. If the regional lymph nodes are clinically considered to be involved, a radical lymph node dissection should be performed. In the cases in which melanoma is in proximity to a lymph node group, excision of the tumor with in-continuity lymphadenectomy is probably warranted regardless of the clinical appearance of the nodes. However, this can be applied only to a very small percentage of melanomas. Routine removal of clinically negative lymph nodes is a very controversial subject. Some authors are in favor of the procedure based on the finding of microscopic foci of malignant melanoma in almost a fourth of clinically negative nodes.[412] However, most series fail to show an improvement of survival in the patients so treated.[410,413-415] A prospective randomized study of stage I melanoma of the limbs showed no differences in survival between the patients who had regional node dissection at the time of the original excision and those who had it only when clinically detectable metastases appeared.[419,420] An alternative to surgery for Hutchinson's freckle is represented by radiation therapy; Dancuart et al.[409] have reported very good results with this technique. Unfortunately, radiation therapy, chemotherapy, and immunotherapy have proved so far generally ineffective in invasive or metastatic melanoma.[418]

Prognosis

The death rate for malignant melanoma is still unacceptably high if one considers the fact that this lesion is diagnosable at a stage when it can be cured in nearly every instance. In a series of nearly 3,000 patients with melanoma in Norway, the overall 5-year relative survival rate was about 60%.[442]

There are many clinical and pathologic factors that have

been studied in regard to their influence in prognosis. They are the following:

1 *Disease stage.* This is by far the most important prognostic parameter. In one large series, the 10-year survival rate was almost 70% for localized disease and less than 20% for metastatic disease.[442]

2 *Depth of invasion.* This is the second most important prognostic determinator. The depth of invasion can be determined by using the level system of Clark or by actually measuring the thickness of the melanoma in the section by inserting a micrometer in the microscope eyepiece (microstage system). Clark divides melanomas into five levels of invasion according to the following scheme:

  I Intraepidermal (in situ)
 II In the papillary dermis
III Filling the papillary dermis and stopping at the interphase between the papillary and reticular dermis
 IV In the reticular dermis
  V In the subcutaneous fat

A direct relationship exists between the level of invasion and the incidence of lymph node metastases and, therefore, the prognosis. In one series, regional node metastases were present in 32% of the patients with level III invasion, 67% with level IV, and 66% with level V[439]; patients with level I and level II did not undergo node dissection, but none of them had clinical evidence of metastases. In the series of Wanebo et al.,[457,458] the 5-year disease-free survival after surgery was 100% in patients with level II invasion, 88% in those with level III, 66% in those with level IV, and 15% in those with level V.
The microstage system assigns the melanomas to low, intermediate, and high-risk categories depending on whether their depth is less than 0.76 mm, between 0.76 and 1.5 mm, or greater than 1.5 mm, respectively.[424] The 5-year disease-free survival is 98% for the first group, 44% to 63% for the third, and somewhere in between for the second.[421,423,426,458] In one series, the 3-year actuarial incidence of subsequent regional metastases in patients initially treated by wide local excision of the melanoma was 0% for lesions less than 0.76 mm, 25% for 0.76 to 1.50 mm lesions, 51% for 1.50 to 3.99 mm lesions, and 62% for lesions over 4 mm in thickness.[421] It should be emphasized, however, that "thin" melanomas (less than 0.76 mm) can still result in metastases and death.[447,460]
Superficially, it would seem that the methods are comparable, yet they examine different parameters. In Clark's level system, what is being evaluated is the ability of the tumor cells to invade the dermis. For instance, a large and rather thick melanoma may stop at the bottom of the papillary dermis with very sharp margins (level III), whereas a smaller and thinner melanoma can be seen freely invading the reticular dermis. The microstage system defines the *amount* of invasive tumor present in the section. There is actually little correlation between the two methods,

and a lively controversy has arisen over which is the better of the two.[424,425] Thickness seems to be emerging as the most important determinant,[441,455] but until this fact is established with certainty, it is probably wise for the pathologist to measure and establish the level of invasion in all cases. Both methods present problems of interpretation. A common problem with the level system is the assignment of a higher level than the real one because of the failure to recognize that a seemingly deep collection of malignant melanocytes actually may be attached to a pilosebaceous unit or that a melanoma can expand massively the papillary dermis but still be limited to this layer. Another difficulty is the fact that in some parts of the body the boundary between papillary and reticular dermis is a very indistinct one. A potential problem to keep in mind with the microstage method is that with tangential cutting of a lesion, a marked artificial increase of the tumor thickness will result. Another factor to keep in mind is that the measured thickness is a function of the number of sections examined.[454]

3 *Shape of the lesion.* This feature, as determined clinically, is closely related to the tumor thickness as evaluated by the Breslow system. Thus prognosis is related to the maximum tumor elevation and is worse for polypoid than for dome-shaped lesions.[435,444] This is not because of the polypoid shape itself but rather the greater tumor thickness usually associated with these lesions.[450]

4 *Sex.* In one large series,[442] the 5-year survival rate was 50.5% for males and 70.5% for females. This improved survival for females results from a variety of factors, such as location and depth of invasion.[448]

5 *Effect of pregnancy.* This remains a controversial subject. Isolated case reports have strongly suggested an adverse effect, but several large studies showed no statistical differences in prognosis.[449,459] Perhaps part of the difficulty resides in the fact that this alleged influence may be dependent on the stage of the melanoma. Shiu et al.[453] found no statistical difference in stage I disease but a significantly lower survival rate in pregnant patients (29%) with stage II lesions as compared with nonparous (51%) or nulliparous (55%) patients.

6 *Anatomic location.* Rogers et al.[451] have defined as high risk sites the following: scalp, mandibular area, midline of trunk, upper medial thighs, hands, feet, popliteal fossae, and genitalia.

7 *Size.* The diameter of the melanoma has no independent prognostic significance once this parameter has been corrected for tumor thickness.

8 *Clinicopathologic type.* Early articles describing the three major types of malignant melanoma claimed a better prognosis for melanoma arising in Hutchinson's freckle, a worse prognosis for nodular melanoma, and an intermediate prognosis for superficially spreading melanoma.[428,429] More recent studies have shown that once depth of invasion is entered into the equation, most of these differences are erased. The behavior of acral lentiginous melanoma is particularly aggressive, but again this may be the consequence of its propensity for deep invasion: in the series of Coleman et al.,[431] the average 3-year survival rate was 11%.

9 *Cytologic features*. Whether the melanoma cells are spindle, epithelioid, or any other shape seems to bear no direct relationship to the prognosis.[430,445]

10 *Degree of pigmentation*. This feature does not seem to influence prognosis.[430]

11 *Mitotic activity*. Although controversy exists, most authors have shown a relationship between mitotic activity and prognosis independently from other parameters.[456]

12 *Plasma cells*. Presence of plasma cells within the inflammatory infiltrate is associated with poor prognosis, but seems to be dependent on other microscopic parameters.[442a]

13 *Ulceration*. Presence of ulceration is said to be an adverse prognostic finding, even when the tumor is matched with nonulcerated lesions by thickness, type, and stage.[422,446,452]

14 *Regression*. It has been claimed that the presence of focal areas of regression in a malignant melanoma may modify the significance of the level or thickness of the residual tumor. This may explain why relatively superficial melanomas exhibiting focal regression are associated with an incidence of lymph node metastases higher than that expected on the basis of these determinations.[436] However, more recent studies have failed to confirm this claim.[432,440,443] Parenthetically, the prognosis of patients with metastatic malignant melanoma and unknown (presumably regressed) primary is the same as for patients with an overt primary malignancy.[427]

15 *Staining pattern*. No consistent relationships have been detected between any histochemical or immunohistochemical staining patterns in melanoma and prognosis.[437]

16 *Microscopic satellites*. Presence of microscopic satellites, defined as tumor nests over 50 μm in diameter separate from the main tumor mass, show a high association with regional lymph node metastases and therefore with prognosis.[438]

17 *Pre-existing benign nevus*. In one large series, the prognosis of melanoma was significantly better when the tumor had histologic evidence of a coexisting acquired melanocytic nevus.[434]

18 *Cell kinetics*. Preliminary observations suggest that determination of cell kinetics through 3H-thymidine labeling index may provide information of diagnostic significance.[433]

Pigmentation in other skin tumors

Several epithelial neoplasms may become deeply pigmented because of an increased activity of melanocytes or increased retention of pigment in the epithelial cells. The most striking example is *melanoacanthoma*, in which dendritic melanocytes and keratinocytes participate in the formation of the neoplasm.[461] Other lesions that may be heavily pigmented are seborrheic keratosis, acrochordon, dermatosis papulosa nigra, actinic keratosis, Bowen's disease and bowenoid papulosis, basal cell carcinoma, and some adnexal tumors (particularly trichoepithelioma, pilomatrixoma, and eccrine poroma). In pigmented basal cell carcinoma, both participation of dendritic melanocytes and retention of pigment in the epithelial cells occur.

NEUROENDOCRINE CELLS
Merkel cell tumor

Merkel cell tumor is the currently preferred term for a distinctive cutaneous malignancy originally described as trabecular carcinoma[479,480] and also known as small cell carcinoma, endocrine carcinoma, and neuroendocrine carcinoma of the skin.[477] It occurs in adults and elderly individuals, the face and extremities being the most common location.[470,473] Clinically, it appears as a nodular, sometimes ulcerated lesion with a reddish or violaceous hue. Microscopically, the monotonous nature of the dermal round cell infiltrate is responsible for the frequent misdiagnosis as malignant lymphoma[475,483] (Fig. 4-116). The second most common pattern is trabecular, but it is rare for this to be a prominent feature. The overlying epidermis is usually uninvolved. The diagnosis of Merkel cell tumor can be made on the basis of the cytologic features as seen in a good hematoxylin and eosin–stained slide (Fig. 4-116, *inset*).

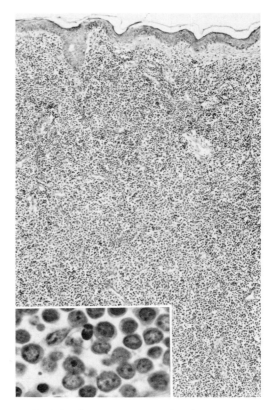

Fig. 4-116 Merkel cell tumor of skin. Light microscopic appearance is that of round cell tumor diffusely invading dermis. **Inset** shows finely granular, dusty chromatin and small nucleoli.

The cytoplasm is scanty but visible as a thin acidophilic rim; the nuclei are round, vesicular, with a typically fine granular ("dusty") chromatin and multiple nucleoli. Mitotic figures and fragmented nuclei ("apoptosis") are plentiful. The stroma may contain proliferated vessels with plump endothelial cells.

Merkel cell carcinoma can be seen in association with in situ or invasive epidermoid carcinoma, with duct-like structures and with basal cell carcinoma-like areas, suggesting that it originates from a multipotential stem cell of ectodermal derivation.[465] The tumor cells are argyrophilic with the Grimelius reaction (especially if the tissue had been fixed in Bouin's) and when examined ultrastructurally they are seen to contain dense-core neurosecretory granules (sometimes arranged immediately beneath the cell membrane) and tightly packed perinuclear intermediate filaments[463,475,476] (Fig. 4-117). Filament-rich cytoplasmic spikes similar to those seen in normal Merkel's cells have been detected in a few cases.[474,481] Immunohistochemically, positivity for low molecular weight keratin, neurofilament, and neuron-specific enolase is usually obtained[462,466,467,469,484] (see Color plate II, *G*). In addition, a few cases have shown focal

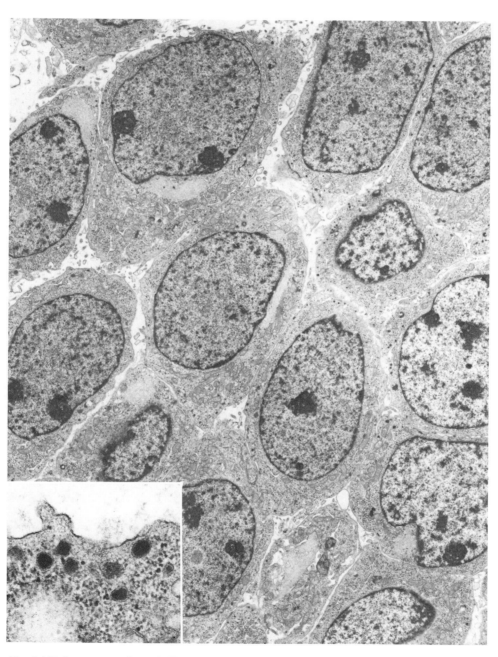

Fig. 4-117 Same tumor shown in Fig. 4-116. Ultrastructurally, neurosecretory-type granules are seen in periphery of cytoplasm beneath cell membrane. (×4,400; **inset,** ×41,100.)

reactivity for vasoactive intestinal peptide, pancreatic poly-peptide, calcitonin, substance P, somatostatin, ACTH, and other peptide hormones.[468,472,478]

Merkel cell tumor is an aggressive neoplasm. Regional nodal metastases are common, and distant metastases also occur, particularly to the lungs, liver, and bones.[464,482] The recommended initial treatment is wide resection of the primary site and regional lymph node dissection.[471]

Other neuroendocrine tumors

Sometimes, tumors with an appearance identical to pulmonary *small cell carcinoma* are found in the skin. They probably represent morphologic variants of Merkel's cell tumor, but the possibility of a metastasis from an internal organ should always be ruled out.[487] Most cases reported as *peripheral neuroblastomas* of skin also fit into the category of Merkel cell tumor; others are clearly different and of unquestionable neural derivation.[485] *Carcinoid tumors* of both insular and trabecular types, allegedly primary in the skin, have also been reported.[486,488,489]

DERMIS

Most of the mesenchymal tumors that may involve the dermis are discussed in the chapter on soft tissues. Only those showing exclusive or preferential involvement of the skin are included here.

Fibroblastic tumors and tumorlike conditions

Keloid is an abnormal pattern of dermal reaction to injury, seen most commonly in black persons. It can be separated on morphologic grounds from a *hyperplastic scar* on the basis of the formation of wide acidophilic bands of collagen, with fibroblasts and myofibroblasts running parallel between them[490] (Fig. 4-118). This distinction is useful in estimating the probability of recrudescence, which is much higher for keloids than for hypertrophic scars. In keloids that have been injected with steroids, pools of mucinous material can be found.[492] The myofibroblasts present in these lesions are immunoreactive for vimentin, nonmuscle myosin, and fibronectin.[491]

Fibrohistiocytic tumors and tumorlike conditions
Benign fibrous histiocytoma

Benign fibrous histiocytoma (also known as subepidermal nodular fibrosis, dermatofibroma, histiocytoma, and sclerosing hemangioma) refers to a spectrum of firm, nodular, nonencapsulated, often pigmented lesions that occur chiefly on the extremities.[493] Clinically, they may be single or multiple and have a flat polypoid or depressed shape. Most of them are less than 1 cm in diameter, but some can reach huge proportions. When heavily pigmented, they may be confused clinically with nevi, malignant melanoma, Kaposi's sarcoma, and other vascular tumors. On transection,

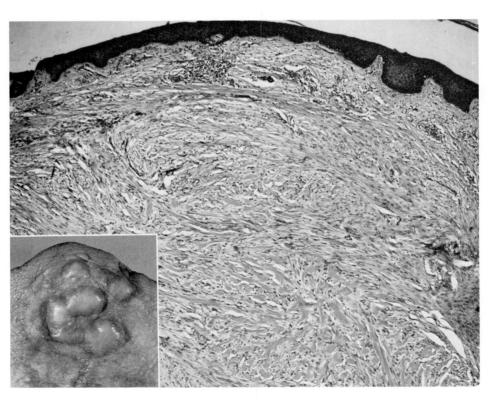

Fig. 4-118 Keloid characterized by coarse collagen bundles traversing dermis in a haphazard fashion.
Inset shows the clinical appearance of the lesion.

they are usually solid, rather well circumscribed but not encapsulated, the color ranging from white to yellow to dark brown, depending on the relative amounts of fibrous tissue, fat, and hemosiderin (Fig. 4-119). Microscopically, there is a cellular fibroblastic proliferation with varying amounts of collagen deposition, admixed with a variable number of macrophages, most of which contain fat (thereby acquiring a foamy appearance) or hemosiderin. Some of these histiocytes are multinucleated and may acquire the features of Touton's giant cells. This fibrohistiocytic proliferation is set in a fine vascular network (Fig. 4-120). Focal storiform features may be seen, but they are rarely as well developed

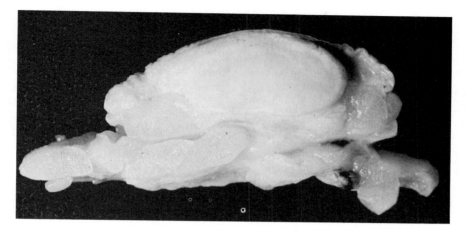

Fig. 4-119 Transected lesion of benign fibrous histiocytoma. Epidermis was not involved, and lesion was bright yellow.

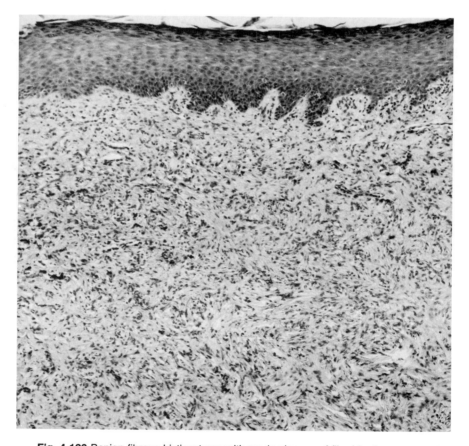

Fig. 4-120 Benign fibrous histiocytoma with predominance of fibroblastic component.

as in dermatofibrosarcoma protuberans. The lesions blend imperceptibly into the adjacent dermis. The overlying epidermis can be normal, atrophic, or acanthotic or even exhibit changes similar to and sometimes indistinguishable from those of basal cell carcinoma.[496,500] These have been interpreted as indicating induction of pilar epithelium by the tumor.[495]

Morphologic variations include prominent palisading similar to that seen in peripheral nerve tumors,[501] marked focal cellular atypia ("monster cells"),[498,502] and presence of large cystic changes filled with blood. These variants do not have prognostic significance. The latter lesion, referred to as *hemorrhagic, aneurysmal,* or *angiomatoid,* should be distinguished from the angiomatoid malignant fibrous histiocytoma, seen in deeper sites in younger patients (see Chapter 25).[499]

Immunohistochemically, the proliferating spindle cells of this lesion are positive for vimentin but usually negative for lysozyme and other histiocytic markers; these results raise questions about their alleged histiocytic nature.[494,497] They have also been found to be reactive for factor XIIIa, a proenzyme known to be present in dermal fixed connective tissue cells.[494a]

The behavior of this lesion is benign; local recurrence is rare even if the excision contains little normal tissue around the lesion.

Atypical fibroxanthoma

Atypical fibroxanthomas are nodular, sometimes ulcerated tumors that typically occur on the sun-exposed skin of elderly persons and are often regarded clinically as carcinomas[506,508,509] (Fig. 4-121). Similar lesions have been reported at sites of irradiation damage.[503,512] Others have been seen in sun-protected areas of younger individuals. Histologically, the tumor is often polypoid and ulcerated (Fig. 4-122). Bizarre tumor cells are seen scattered within a fibrocytic stroma with varying amounts of inflammation (Fig. 4-123). Mitoses are plentiful, some of them being atypical. A helpful point to remember is that the scattered tumor cells have a very abnormal appearance, but that the background in which they are situated has an inflammatory or reactive appearance. The overlying epidermis may be normal, atrophic, hyperplastic, or ulcerated, but by definition it should not show continuity with the tumor. Immunohistochemically, the tumor cells show reactivity for vimentin, alpha-1-antitrypsin, alpha-1-antichymotrypsin, and cathepsin-B, and negativity for keratin, EMA, S-100 protein, and desmin.[512a]

Despite the bizarre microscopic features that suggest a high-grade lesion, atypical fibroxanthomas are relatively indolent lesions that are usually cured by local excision.[504] However, some cases have resulted in local recurrence, and

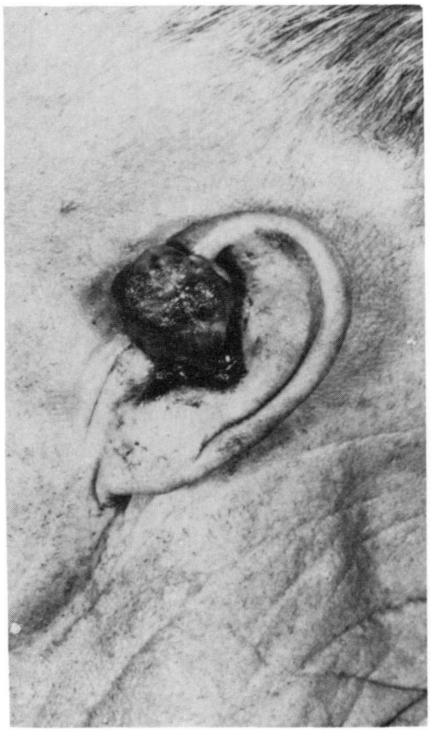

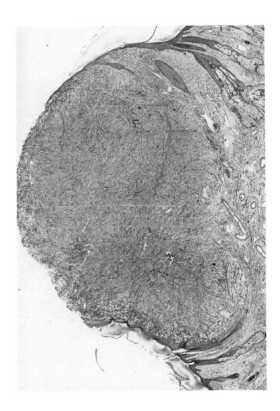

Fig. 4-121 Atypical fibroxanthoma arising on ear. (From Kempson R., McGavran MH: Atypical fibroxanthomas of the skin. Cancer **17:**1463-1471, 1964.)

Fig. 4-122 Low-power view of atypical fibroxanthoma showing its delimitation and cellularity. (From Kempson RL, McGavran MH: Atypical fibroxanthomas of the skin. Cancer **17:**1463-1471, 1964.)

a few have metastasized.[507] Factors that portend aggressive behavior and possible metastases in atypical fibroxanthoma are previous recurrence, vascular invasion, deep invasion, tumor necrosis, and perhaps immunosuppression.[507]

The currently favored view is that these lesions represent yet another clinicopathologic manifestation of fibrous histiocytoma, based on morphologic, ultrastructural, and immunohistochemical criteria.[511] However, we do not believe that the matter of histogenesis has been entirely settled. Some unquestionable squamous cell carcinomas and malignant melanomas (of the so-called desmoplastic variety) exhibit in their deep portions a pattern of growth that is indistinguishable from that of atypical fibroxanthoma.[510] This being the case, one cannot help wondering whether at least some of the tumors presently designated as atypical fibroxanthomas may not actually be carcinomas or melanomas in disguise. Evans and Smith[505] favored this point of view and therefore used for them the noncommittal term *sarcoma-like tumors* of the skin. They made the interesting observation that the prognosis was not significantly different whether there was a definite component of squamous cell carcinoma or not.

Dermatofibrosarcoma protuberans

Dermatofibrosarcomas protuberans are slow-growing, nodular, polypoid neoplasms that are found almost exclusively in the dermis, from which they often invade the subcutaneous tissue (Fig. 4-124). As a group, they are much larger than benign fibrous histiocytomas; however, the diagnosis of dermatofibrosarcoma protuberans should never be made or ruled out on the basis of size alone. Microscopically, the appearance of radial whorls of spindle cells producing the storiform or cartwheel pattern is characteristic although not pathognomonic (Fig. 4-125). Other features of diagnostic importance are the high cellularity, monomorphic appearance, moderate-to-high mitotic activity, lack or inconspicuousness of foamy or hemosiderin-laden macrophages and/or multinucleated giant cells, and entrapment of isolated fat cells when the subcutis is infiltrated. Myxoid features can be present focally and exceptionally be the dominant feature of the tumor.[514]

It has been postulated that dermatofibrosarcomas are of histiocytic origin and that they belong to the group of fibrous histiocytomas.[516] The issue, however, is far from settled. The occasional occurrence of histologically identical tumors containing melanin (see discussion following) suggests that at least some of them may be of peripheral nerve origin.[515]

The natural history of dermatofibrosarcoma protuberans is characterized by an extremely high tendency for local recurrence following limited resection.[517] Very rare instances of metastases to regional nodes and/or internal organs have also been documented.[513]

Pigmented dermatofibrosarcoma protuberans (Bednar's tumor, pigmented storiform neurofibroma) is a neoplasm looking in all respects like an ordinary dermatofibrosarcoma protuberans but containing in addition a variable

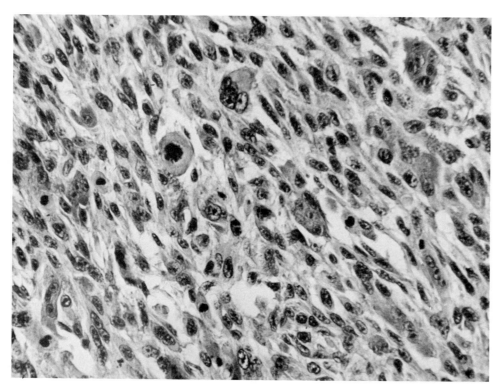

Fig. 4-123 Marked hypercellularity, pleomorphism, and mitotic activity in a typical fibroxanthoma. (From Kempson RL, McGavran MH: Atypical fibroxanthomas of the skin. Cancer **17**:1463-1471, 1964.)

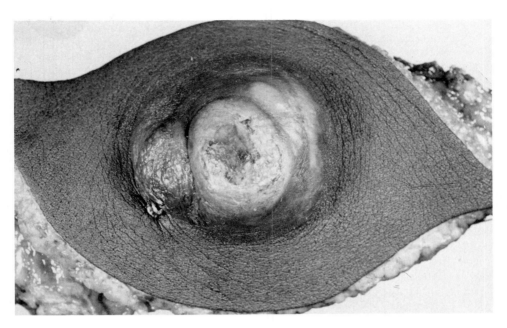

Fig. 4-124 Multinodular dermatofibrosarcoma protuberance from buttock.

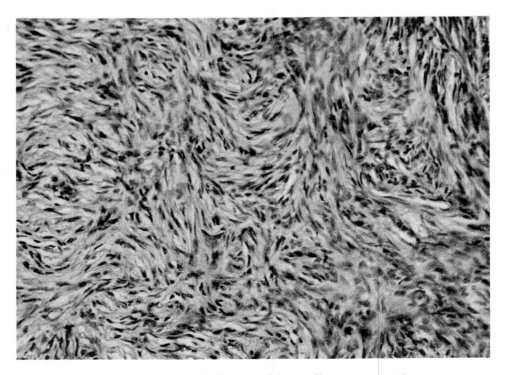

Fig. 4-125 Storiform or cartwheel pattern of dermatofibrosarcoma protuberance.

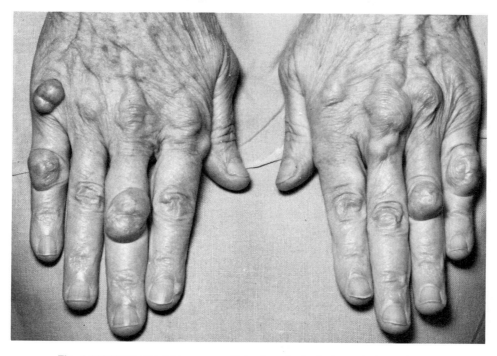

Fig. 4-126 Xanthoma tuberosum multiplex in patient with hypercholesterolemia.

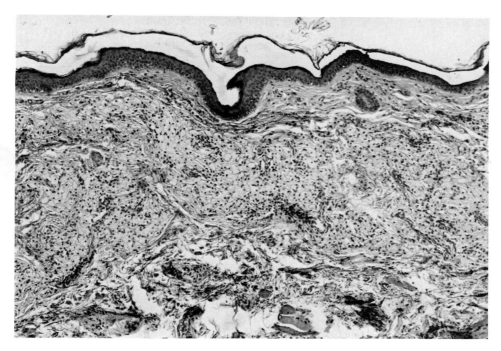

Fig. 4-127 Clusters and sheets of foamy histiocytes within dermis from xanthelasma.

but usually small and patchy population of dendritic cells containing large amounts of melanin pigment. Although this finding obviously raises the possibility of schwannian-melanocytic derivation, the tumor is negative for S-100 protein and other melanocyte-related markers and should not be equated with malignant melanoma, of either conventional, desmoplastic, or soft tissue (clear cell sarcoma) types.

Malignant fibrous histiocytoma

A tumor morphologically analogous to the pleomorphic-storiform type of malignant fibrous histiocytoma of soft tissues occurs in the skin, but its separation from atypical fibroxanthoma and dermatofibrosarcoma protuberans is not clear-cut. Perhaps the term should be restricted to malignant fibrohistiocytic tumors of skin that infiltrate deeply into the subcutis, fascia, or muscle and have considerable necrosis.[518] Some of the reported cases have occurred in chronic ulcers or scars.[519]

Xanthoma

Xanthomas are non-neoplastic nodules resulting from the accumulation of fat-laden histiocytes in the dermis and tendons. They are usually periarticular and few in number, but desseminated forms occur[519a] (Fig. 4-126). They are often associated with hyperlipidemia, either primary (familial) or secondary to diabetes mellitus, hypothyroidism, multiple myeloma, malignant lymphoma, leukemia, and obstructive liver disease. Flat xanthomas of the eyelid, referred to as *xanthelasma*, show a similar microscopic appearance (Fig. 4-127). Only a minority of these patients have hyperlipidemia. In *eruptive xanthoma*, there is an abrupt onset of crops of yellowish papules with erythematous halos on the extensor surfaces. It can be confused with granuloma annulare at the microscopic level.[519b] In *verruciform xanthoma*, there is a papillomatous, verruca-like change of the overlying epidermis[519c] (Fig 4-128).

Juvenile xanthogranuloma (nevoxanthoendothelioma)

The name *nevoxanthoendothelioma* is descriptive in that the lesion occurs in infants and thus is a nevus in the sense of congenital mark (Fig. 4-129). It contains fat-laden histiocytes and Touton giant cells and thus is xanthomatous (Fig. 4-130). Proliferation of small vessels may be seen. A preferable name is *juvenile xanthogranuloma*. Most of the lesions occur in infants and are limited to the skin. However, extradermal involvement can occur.[520-522] Occasionally, glaucoma and amblyopia, caused by involvement of the iris and the ciliary body, are the presenting complaint. Ultrastructural studies have shown a polymorphic population with two dominant cell types. One is histiocytic, and the cells contain fat in areas of regression. The other cell is probably fibrocytic. The uncommon visceral involvement does not, in our opinion, allow classification of this lesion in the "lipoidoses" nor consideration of it as a *forme fruste* of Hand-Schüller-Christian syndrome.

Other histiocytic proliferations

Many other types of histiocytic infiltrates of the skin occur.[525]

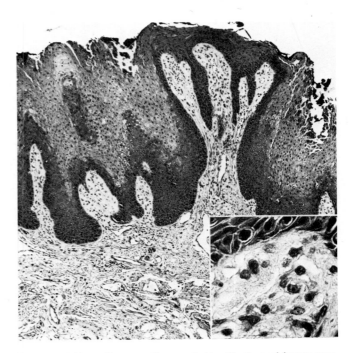

Fig. 4-128 Verruciform xanthoma of skin. Clusters of foamy macrophages are seen occupying rete ridges in between a hyperplastic epidermis with a warty appearance. Foamy appearance of macrophages can be appreciated in **inset.**

Giant cell reticulohistiocytoma can present in a solitary or multicentric form.[524,526]

In *histiocytosis X*, scattered ordinary histiocytes are seen admixed with S-100 positive Langerhans' cells, the latter defining the nature of the disorder (see Chapter 21).

Sinus histiocytosis with massive lymphadenopathy may involve the skin[527] (Fig. 4-131); in most instances the diagnosis is obvious because of the presence of prominent cervical lymphadenopathy, but in a few instances the cutaneous lesions represent the predominant or exclusive manifestation of the disease.

Histioid forms of *leprosy* can be easily confused with fibrous histiocytoma.[523]

Smooth muscle tumors

Leiomyomas of skin can be divided into three distinct types: the genital lesions located in the nipple or scrotum; the multiple superficial nodules of nevoid or hamartomatous type derived from arrectores piloris muscle; and the solitary angioleiomyoma (vascular leiomyoma), which is usually subcutaneous rather than dermal[530,531] (Fig. 4-132). Cutaneous leiomyomas can be very painful. Microscopically, they show intersecting fascicles of smooth muscle, without atypia, mitotic activity, or necrosis.

Leiomyosarcomas are larger, more cellular, mitotically active, and may contain areas of necrosis.[528,529] Some of them exhibit a prominent vascular pattern, suggesting that they may represent the malignant counterpart of vascular leiomyoma.[532] Cutaneous leiomyosarcomas often recur. However, they metastasize only exceptionally if at all, in stark contrast with their subcutaneous counterpart.[529]

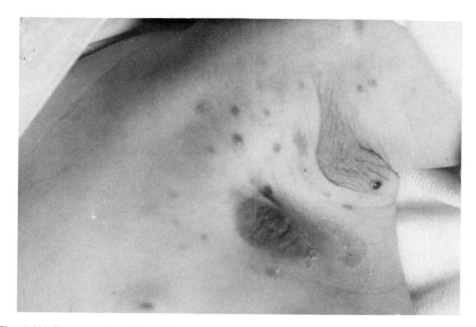

Fig. 4-129 Plaques and nodules of juvenile xanthogranuloma of axillary skin and chest wall in 11-month-old infant.

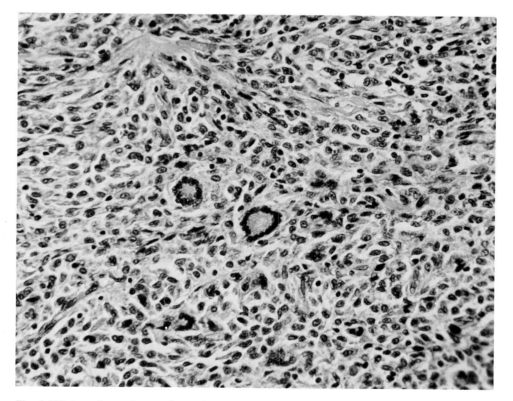

Fig. 4-130 Juvenile xanthogranuloma showing Touton giant cells and fibroblastic and histiocytic proliferation.

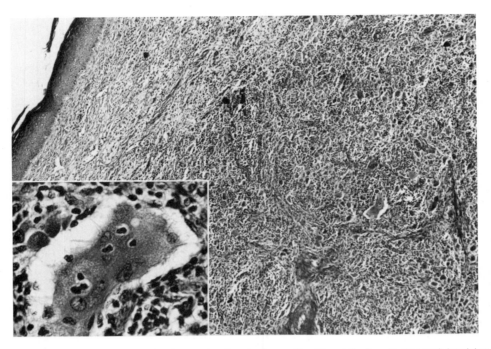

Fig. 4-131 Sinus histiocytosis with massive lymphadenopathy (Rosai-Dorfman's disease) involving skin. There is lymphohistiocytic infiltrate expanding superficial and deep dermis. Histiocyte in **inset** shows abundant cytoplasm containing white blood cells within vacuoles.

Peripheral nerve tumors

Of the various types of peripheral nerve tumors, those with a particular predilection for cutaneous (dermal)—as opposed to subcutaneous or deeper—involvement are *neurofibroma, granular cell tumor, nerve sheath myxoma* (neurothekeoma, cutaneous lobular neuromyxoma)[534,535] (Fig. 4-133), and a controversial type of malignancy that Enzinger and Weiss propose to designate as the *superficial type of malignant epithelioid schwannoma*.[533] The latter entity is probably analogous to neurotropic melanoma (p. 128). Although other forms of malignant schwannoma are usually located in the deep soft tissue, cutaneous examples have been described in patients with or without Recklinghausen's disease.[532a]

Most of these peripheral nerve tumors are further discussed in Chapter 25.

Vascular tumors and tumorlike conditions

A large variety of tumors and ectasias arising from blood and lymph vessels of the skin exists.[536,536a] Most of these lesions are discussed in Chapter 25. Only those features pertaining to their cutaneous location will be mentioned in this section.

Hemangioma

The more distinctive types of benign blood vessel tumors of skin are capillary hemangioma, benign hemangioendothelioma, cavernous hemangioma, angiokeratomas of various types,[538] verrucous hemangioma,[539] acral arteriovenous tumor,[537] and glomus tumor. The hemangiomas associated with Maffucci's syndrome, blue rubber-bleb nevus, and Kasabach-Merritt syndrome are of the cavernous type.

Spider angioma, venous lake, capillary aneurysm, angioma serpiginosum, and the lesion of hereditary hemorrhagic telangiectasia are not true neoplasms but rather telangiectatic processes of either hamartomatous or acquired nature.[540] This is also probably true for some of the lesions in the former category.

Lymphangioma

Cutaneous lymphangiomas usually present in infancy, the majority being present by the age of 5 years.[542] Sites of predilection are the neck, axilla, breasts, chest, buttocks, and thighs. The lesions are divided into superficial (lymphangioma circumscriptum), deep (lymphangioma cavernosum), and cystic (cystic hygroma) varieties. Recurrence developed in 25% of the patients reviewed by Flanagan and Helwig.[541] This might be caused by the presence of large muscular-coated lymphatic cisterns lying deep in the subcutis and feeding the superficial vesicles.[544]

A peculiar variant of lymphangioma, described as *acquired progressive lymphangioma*, presents as a bruiselike lesion and simulates angiosarcoma because of the presence of anastomosing vascular channels. However, atypia of endothelial cells is totally absent.[543]

Lobular capillary hemangioma

Lobular capillary hemangioma is the term we prefer for the benign vascular proliferation that in its most usual and typical form is referred to as pyogenic granuloma (granu-

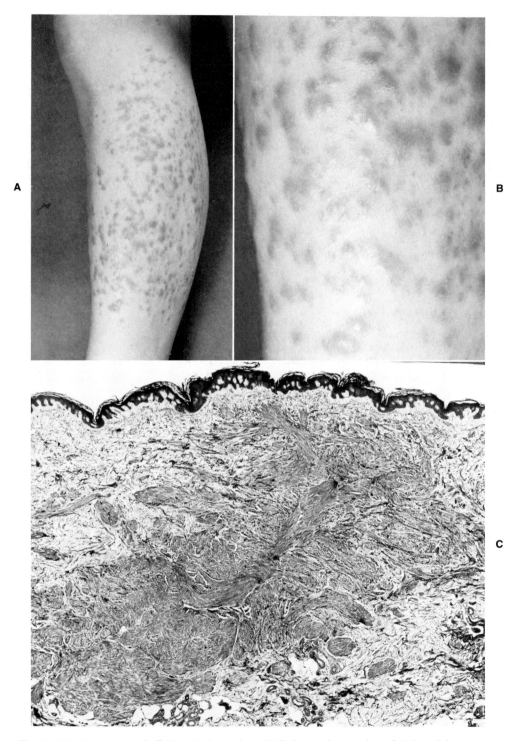

Fig. 4-132 Leiomyomas. **A,** Patient had noted gradually increasing number of pink nodules on one leg over period of 20 years. **B,** Closer view of lesions illustrated in **A** showing single and confluent dermal nodules which, when pressed, caused severe pain. **C,** Biopsy from lesions illustrated in **A** and **B** showing unencapsulated nodules of hyperplastic smooth muscle. (**C,** Masson trichrome.)

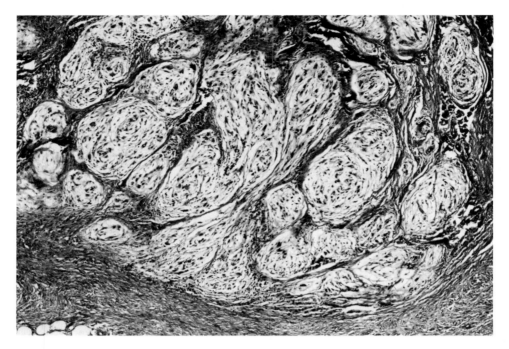

Fig. 4-133 Neurothekeoma of skin. Neuroid bundles with myxoid appearance are separated by fibrous stroma. Some degree of pleomorphism is present.

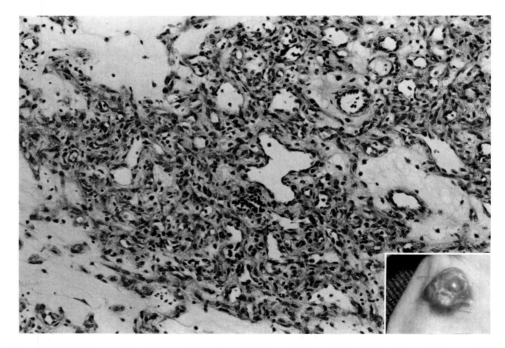

Fig. 4-134 Lobular capillary hemangioma (so-called pyogenic granuloma) showing typical vascular lobule with a central branching vessel. Lobule is surrounded by edematous and slightly inflamed tissue. **Inset** shows clinical appearance of lesion, which was located at the base of a finger.

loma pyogenicum). Clinically, it presents as a rapidly grow-ing polypoid red mass, surrounded by a collarete of thick-ened epidermis. The fingers are the most common location. Microscopically, there is vascular proliferation, edema, in-flammation, and epidermal ulceration at the top, acanthosis and hyperkeratosis at the sides. The most distinctive feature is the so-called *vascular lobule*, a central branching vessel usually devoid of red blood cells, surrounded by a highly cellular proliferation of endothelial cells[547] (Fig. 4-134). High cellularity and abundant mitotic activity may be pres-ent and are not indicative of an aggressive behavior. The lesion is self-limited, and spontaneous regression may be complete. Excision is usually curative, although some ex-amples located on the trunk may recur as multiple satel-lites.[551] Lobular capillary hemangioma can also occur in a disseminated form,[548] develop within port-wine stains,[550] be located in the deep dermis or subcutaneous tissue,[546] or present as a polypoid mass within a vein.[545] Deeply seated lesions usually lack the edema and inflammation seen in the more superficial examples.

We view *acquired tufted angioma* and the *angioblas-toma* described in the Orient as disorders closely related to lobular capillary hemangioma.[549]

Masson's hemangioma

Masson's hemangioma (vegetant intravascular heman-gioendothelioma; Masson's pseudoangiosarcoma; intravas-cular papillary endothelial hyperplasia) is probably the result of an exuberant organization and recanalization of a throm-bus. It may develop in a previously normal vessel as a result of trauma or it may superimpose itself on a pyogenic gran-uloma or cavernous hemangioma.[552,553] It is characterized microscopically by a papillary proliferation of endothelial cells (which are plump but lack atypia) located entirely within the lumen of a dilated vessel.

Histiocytoid hemangioma

Histiocytoid hemangioma (epithelioid hemangioma, an-giolymphoid hyperplasia with eosinophilia) presents clini-cally as inflammatory-looking nodules, the head and neck (particularly the periauricular region) being the preferred location.[555,557,559] Despite earlier claims to the contrary, this disease seems to be different from Kimura's disease as seen in the Orient.[556,561] Microscopically, a central area of pro-liferated blood vessels is infiltrated and surrounded by a heavy inflammatory infiltrate rich in eosinophils and con-taining lymphoid follicles with germinal centers. The most characteristic feature is the peculiar histiocytoid or epithe-lioid appearance of the endothelial cells (Fig. 4-135). Some-times the inflammatory infiltrate is nil or absent.[554] Tumors with similar appearing endothelial cells can occur in other sites, such as soft tissue, large vessels, and bone,[560] some-times in combination with skin lesions.[558]

Kaposi's sarcoma

In its classic form, Kaposi's sarcoma is infrequent in the United States but relatively common in some regions of the Mediterranean basin and even more so in equatorial Africa, where it comprises 10% of all malignant tumors.[562] The incidence of Kaposi's sarcoma in this country has increased

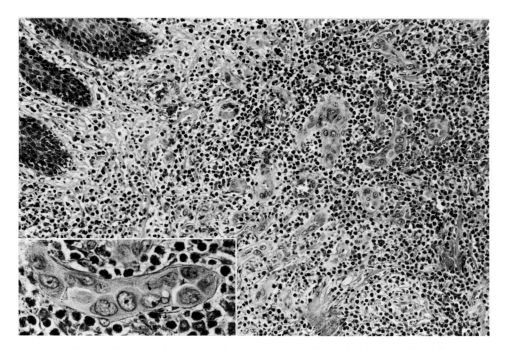

Fig. 4-135 Histiocytoid hemangioma (so-called angiolymphoid hyperplasia with eosinophilia). Heavy inflammatory infiltrate rich in eosinophils is seen surrounding blood vessels lined by very plump en-dothelial cells. Histiocytoid or epithelioid appearance of endothelial cells is better seen in the **inset.**

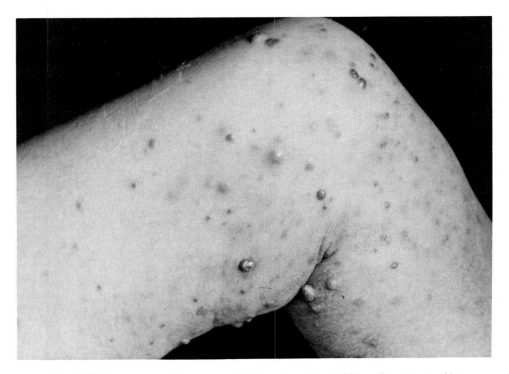

Fig. 4-136 Numerous nodules, some virtually pedunculated, of Kaposi's sarcoma of leg.

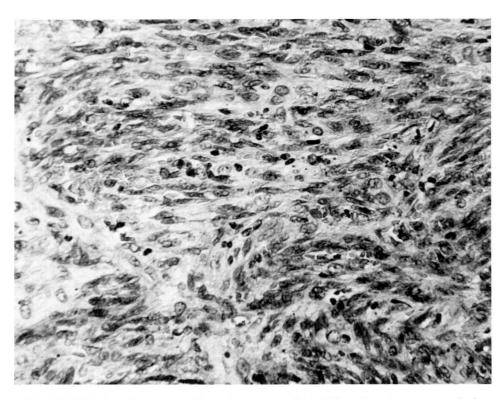

Fig. 4-137 Spindle-cell elements of Kaposi's sarcoma within which erythrocytes are enmeshed.

in recent years several hundredfold through its occurrence in the AIDS population and, to a lesser degree, in persons with other forms of immunosuppression, such as organ transplant recipients.[563,572,583] An association with the systemic form of Castleman's disease and with angioimmunoblastic lymphadenopathy (two disorders of the immune system) has also been reported.[569,587] In AIDS, Kaposi's sarcoma is predominantly a feature of the homosexual population, but it has also been seen in heterosexual drug users.[570]

In classic Kaposi's sarcoma, the disease manifests itself by multiple blue dermal plaques or nodules starting on the feet and legs (Fig. 4-136). These nodules progress up the extremity and occasionally assume a pedunculated appearance reminiscent of pyogenic granuloma. By angiographic techniques, clinically inapparent subcutaneous nodules can be identified. Temporary control is effected by irradiation, chemotherapy, or, if the lesion is sharply delimited, excision. The course of Kaposi's sarcoma is variable although usually prolonged. Some elderly persons die of intercurrent disease. An increased incidence of malignant tumors, particularly of lymphoid type, has been documented.[580] In patients in whom the disease runs its full course, widespread visceral involvement may be found. Lymph nodes and the gastrointestinal tract are the organs most commonly involved. Visceral involvement can precede the development of skin lesions or occur in their absence.[585] Other clinical forms of Kaposi's sarcoma have been described in the African cases.[586] In the AIDS population, the lesions of Kaposi's sarcoma have a more erratic distribution, a wider variety of clinical appearance, and a more rapidly aggressive clinical course.[588]

Microscopically, the most typical feature of Kaposi's sarcoma is the presence of spindle cells forming slits containing red blood cells (Fig. 4-137). Mitotic activity is only moderate, and pleomorphism is usually absent. Admixed in this lesion are lymphocytes, hemosiderin-laden macrophages, and other inflammatory cells. Variously sized hyaline bodies, which are PAS-positive, are often seen in the cytoplasm of the proliferating cells and sometimes extracellularly. In early lesions, the spindle proliferation may be limited to the papillary dermis and to the vascular plexus surrounding the secretory coil of sweat glands.[578] Histochemical and ultrastructural studies show that this tumor is derived from vasoformative mesenchyme with multipotential capabilities[576,582] (Fig. 4-138). It has been suggested that the spindle cells of this lesion are endothelial, of either blood vessel or lymph vessel origin. Indeed, FVIII-related antigen and other endothelial markers have been detected in at least some of the cases.[568,571,581a] However, the results of the many immunohistochemical and ultrastructural studies that have been performed on this disorder have given confusing and often contradictory results.* At this point, it should be said that the precise histogenesis of Kaposi's sarcoma still remains to be determined, even if an origin from or differentiation towards an activated (histiocytoid) type of endothelial cell appears the most likely.[567,577] It should be realized that not all of the vascular lesions of the skin present in

AIDS patients have the morphologic features of Kaposi's sarcoma. Some exhibit anastomosing vascular channels resembling those of angiosarcoma; others are composed of plump (histiocytoid or epithelioid) cells[566a]; others are solid and undifferentiated[581]; still others have an angiomatous appearance with a somewhat lobular configuration. It seems likely that all these morphologic forms of AIDS-related vascular proliferation are pathogenetically and histogenetically related. However, the startling suggestion has recently been made that the AIDS-related vascular lesions with a histiocytoid (epithelioid) appearance[566a] are associated with the cat scratch bacillus.[572a]

Benign lesions that can be microscopically confused with Kaposi's sarcoma include arteriovenous malformations, acroangiodermatitis, lobular capillary hemangioma, pigmented purpuric dermatosis, and the predominantly vascular or hemorrhagic forms of benign fibrous histiocytoma[565,573,584] (see p. 140).

Angiosarcoma

Angiosarcoma (malignant hemangioendothelioma) of the skin is almost exclusively restricted to the head and neck of elderly persons, if the varieties associated with long-standing lymphedema or radiation therapy are excluded.[589,590,592,593,597-599] It characteristically presents as a violaceous flat lesion of ill-defined margins, on which elevated nodules may develop.[595] Microscopically, three distinct patterns are seen, singly or in combination: undifferentiated foci, indistinguishable from carcinoma or malignant melanoma; freely anastomosing channels lined by atypical endothelial cells, surrounding skin adnexa and dissecting dermal collagen fibers; and areas resembling Kaposi's sarcoma[600] (Fig. 4-139). The tumor cells have ultrastructural and immunohistochemical features of endothelial cells, although these can be lost in the poorly differentiated tumors.[594,596]

Angiosarcoma is a slow-growing but highly aggressive neoplasm that stubbornly recurs following surgery or radiation therapy to involve extensive areas of the scalp and face and eventually metastasizes to regional lymph nodes, lung, and other organs.[599,600] Any vascular lesion of the skin diagnosed as angiosarcoma in a young patient or not located in the head and neck should be immediately suspected of being something else and, more often than not, a benign process.[591]

Lymphoid tumors and tumorlike conditions
Cutaneous lymphoid hyperplasia

Cutaneous lymphoid hyperplasia (also known as lymphoplasia, lymphadenoma, lymphocytoma benigna cutis, and Spiegler-Fendt sarcoid) occurs predominantly in the face of women as livid nodules or plaques, usually solitary.[603] It probably represents a response to trauma, insect bites, and other undetermined stimuli.[602] Microscopically, an infiltrate predominantly composed of lymphocytes and histiocytes is present in the dermis[606] (Fig. 4-140). The morphologic and immunoarchitectural features of the lesion are very similar to those of reactive lymph nodes.[609]

Features that favor a diagnosis of lymphoid hyperplasia over one of malignant lymphoma are the following: multiplicity of cell types, including plasma cells and eosino-

---

*See references 564, 566, 566b, 574, 575, and 579.

phils; formation of lymphoid follicles, with or without germinal centers; phagocytosis of nuclear debris; vascular proliferation; predominantly perivascular or periadnexal distribution of the infiltrate; and prominent epidermal hyperplasia. If these features are present, extension of the process into the reticular dermis or even the subcutaneous fat should not cause undue concern. The lesions respond to antibiotics or low doses of x-ray therapy.

Jessner's lymphocytic infiltration of the skin is reported by many as a clinicopathologic variant of cutaneous lym-

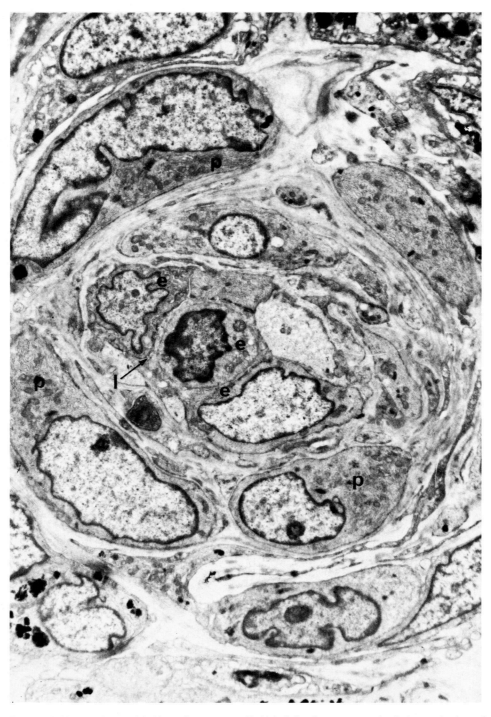

Fig. 4-138 Abnormal vessel in Kaposi's sarcoma. Endothelial cells, *e,* are markedly hyperplastic and have reduced lumen, *l,* to fine slit. Perithelial cells, *p,* are prominent. Pigmented macrophages surround vessel. (Uranyl acetate–lead citrate; ×4,200.)

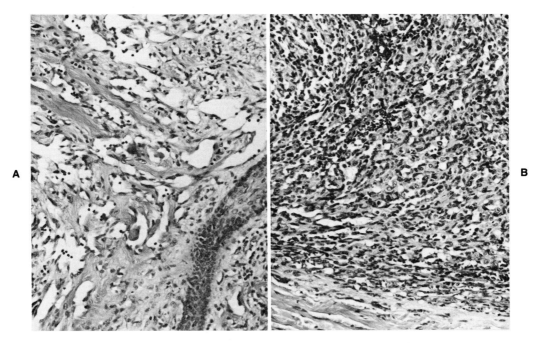

Fig. 4-139 Angiosarcoma of the skin. **A,** Tumor is well differentiated and shows freely anastomosing vascular channels lined by only moderately atypical endothelial cells. **B,** Tumor is poorly differentiated and difficult to distinguish from other malignant neoplasms of the skin.

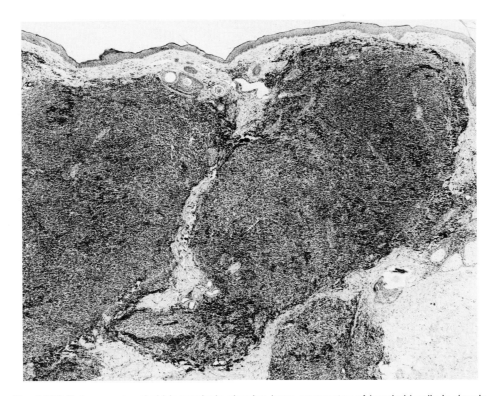

Fig. 4-140 Cutaneous lymphoid hyperplasia showing large aggregates of lymphoid cells in dermis. This is not malignant lymphoma of skin.

phoid hyperplasia, although controversy about its nature persists.[608]

Other clinically benign lymphocytic infiltrates that can simulate microscopically malignant lymphoma are related to molluscum contagiosum,[601] syphilis,[604] nodular scabies,[607] and actinic reticuloid.[605]

Lymphomatoid papulosis

Lymphomatoid papulosis is a self-healing, recurrent papular eruption with a generally benign clinical course but a set of microscopic features that resemble malignant lymphoma.[615] A polymorphic dermal infiltrate is usually located superficially; it sometimes exhibits a distinct perivascular distribution. This infiltrate contains scattered, markedly atypical lymphoid cells, many of them having convoluted nuclei and some resembling Reed-Sternberg cells[610,616,619] (Fig. 4-141). Their phenotype is that of activated helper T-cells, and some express Hodgkin's disease–associated antigens, such as Ki-1.[612,614,620] The nature of this disorder remains controversial; some view it as a variant of pityriasis lichenoides acuta (Mucha-Habermann disease), others as a specific dermatosis, and still others as a lymphoproliferative disease related to malignant lymphoma. The fact that in 10% to 20% of the cases an association with, or evolution into, malignant lymphoma (including mycosis fungoides) has occurred[611,617] and the recent demonstration of a clonal T-cell population by gene rearrangement techniques[613,618] would seem to support the latter view.

Mycosis fungoides and related T-cell lymphomas

Mycosis fungoides is a distinct clinicopathologic type or T-cell malignant lymphoma[651] (Fig. 4-142). It has various manners of presentation and progression, most identified by eponymic designations.[622,623] The simplest classification is in three stages: premycotic, mycotic, and tumorous. In the premycotic stage, the skin is erythematous, scaly, and pruritic. Clinical variations characterized by solitary, follicular, granulomatous, pustular, bullous, hyperkeratotic, verrucous, and hypopigmented forms exist.[625,647a] Large plaque parapsoriasis is a clinically defined entity that is known to "convert" to mycosis fungoides in a small percentage of cases; whether these lesions were malignant from the beginning or not remains a moot point. At this stage, the microscopic features are usually those of a chronic nonspecific dermatitis associated with psoriasiform changes in the epidermis. In the mycotic stage, infiltrative plaques appear, and biopsies show a polymorphous inflammatory infiltrate in the dermis that contains small numbers of frankly atypical lymphoid cells. These cells may invade the epidermis to form Pautrier microabscesses[656] (Fig. 4-143). In the tumorous stage, infiltrates of atypical lymphoid cells predominate. The characteristic cell of mycosis fungoides is a small or medium-sized lymphocyte with cerebroid nucleus. This refers to the highly irregular contour of the thick nuclear membrane, which results in an appearance somewhat reminiscent of brain convolutions. Thin, well-prepared sections are necessary to identify this feature.[626] These cerebroid cells

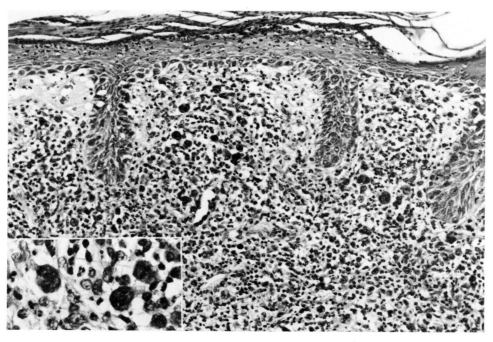

Fig. 4-141 Lymphomatoid papulosis. The dermis contains heavy inflammatory infiltrate with highly bizarre and sometimes multinucleated lymphoid cells, which are highlighted in the **inset.** (Courtesy Dr. D. Santa Cruz, St. Louis, MO.)

represent a neoplastic proliferation of T-cells; their phenotype is usually that of helper T-cells, but sometimes it is suppressor/cytotoxic or aberrant.[621,652] In advanced stages of the disease, they may express Leu-M1 antigen.[664] Although the presence of these cells is necessary to make a diagnosis of mycosis fungoides, they are not pathognomonic of the disease. Scattered cells with these nuclear features can be seen in other lymphomas and in some types of acute and chronic dermatitis.[636,637,640]

A more accurate evaluation of these cells can be achieved by determining ultrastructurally the value of the nuclear contour index, but this is unlikely to become useful at the practical level.[643,646,658] Similar considerations apply to the in situ study of T-cell subpopulations.[630,631,650]

The course of mycosis fungoides is usually protracted over a period of years. Clinical signs associated with poor prognosis are presence of generalized plaques or tumors, diffuse erythema, and presence of lymphadenopathy.[639,641] A definite correlation exists between the histologic findings and the clinical course.[654,662] In about one half to two thirds of patients with mycosis fungoides of the skin, involvement of lymph nodes and internal viscera occurs. In most instances, the internal disease is still recognizable as mycosis fungoides by the polymorphism of the infiltrate and, most importantly, the cerebroid nuclei of the tumor cells.[649,653] In other cases, the internal malignancy has features of other types of malignant lymphoma, including Hodgkin's disease.[629,657,659] The internal infiltrates of mycosis fungoides can be found in the lymph nodes, lung, spleen, liver,[645] kidney, bone marrow, central nervous system, and practically every other organ.[624,644,653,655] The neoplastic cells selectively involve the T-cell–dependent regions of the lymph node and spleen. The disease can even present as a primary extracutaneous lesion, either in the lymph nodes or in internal organs.[644,663]

Sepsis is a frequent terminal complication. The forms of therapy for disease limited to the skin include total-skin electron beam irradiation, topical chemotherapy, and PUVA.[635,638,642,661]

Sézary's syndrome is a variant of mycosis fungoides characterized clinically by infiltrative erythroderma with pruritus, lymphadenopathy, and the presence of large or small cerebroid cells (Sézary's cells) in the peripheral blood.[627] PAS-positive cytoplasmic granules are present in their cytoplasm. The distinction between mycosis fungoides and Sézary's syndrome is an artificial one because circulating cerebroid cells of the same phenotype are found in about 20% of the patients with mycosis fungoides.[628,632]

Woringer-Kolopp disease (pagetoid reticulosis) is another T-cell cutaneous disorder, which is characterized morphologically by a monomorphic *intraepidermal* infiltrate of cells with cerebroid nuclei, indistinguishable from those of the usual mycosis fungoides and Sézary syndrome.[633,634,648] The lesion presents clinically as a solitary erythematosquamous patch, and the evolution is extremely slow.

Other forms of T-cell lymphoma that lack the clinicopathologic features of mycosis fungoides can develop in the skin.[647,660]

Lymph nodes in mycosis fungoides

Lymphadenopathy is common in patients with mycosis fungoides. The pathologic changes may be those of dermatopathic lymphadenitis, involvement by mycosis fungoides, or both.[665,668] The distinction between these processes can be extremely difficult to make. Preservation or distortion of the nodal architecture and the number of atypical lymphoid cells in T-cell–dependent paracortical areas are the two most important prognostic features.[666, 667] Immunophenotyping and determination of clonal rearrangement of T-cell receptor genes may offer a more sensitive and reliable means to make the distinction[669,670] (see Chapter 21).

Other malignant lymphomas

Malignant lymphoma other than mycosis fungoides presenting as skin nodules in adults may represent an expression of generalized disease or may be the only manifestation of the tumor.[681] For those with initial skin involvement, the head and neck are the most common sites.[674] Many of these lymphomas are of follicular center type and therefore of B-cell nature.[694] In contrast to the T-cell lymphomas, these tumors tend to be nodular, nonpruritic, and nonulcerative.[684] Microscopically, the pattern

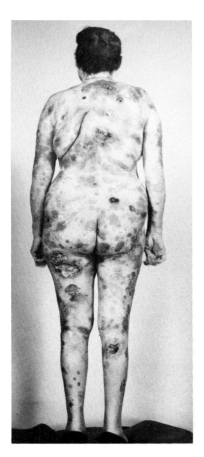

Fig. 4-142 Mycosis fungoides showing both infiltrative plaques and nodules, some ulcerated, over virtually entire body.

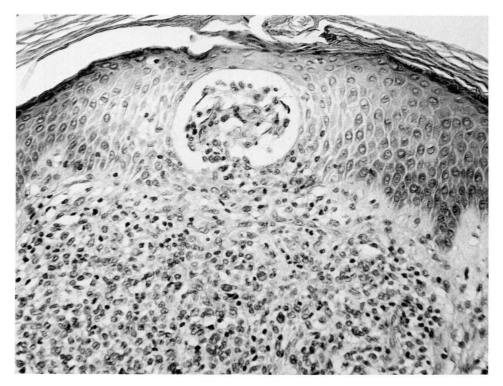

Fig. 4-143 Dermal infiltrate of atypical lymphoid cells extending focally into epidermis, forming Pautrier's abscess.

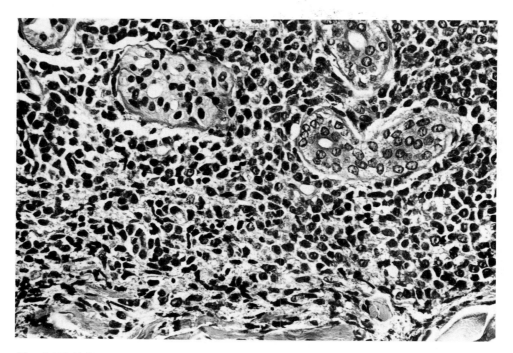

Fig. 4-144 Malignant lymphoma of skin predominantly composed of small cleaved cells. Tumor is surrounding and beginning to infiltrate sweat glands of region.

of growth may be nodular or diffuse.[679] The majority are of large or mixed cell type.[671,674]

Important features for microscopic recognition include: surrounding and destruction of cutaneous structures by the infiltrate; blood vessel involvement, with fragmentation or destruction of the vessel wall; and linear arrays (Indian file arrangement) of abnormal cells along the collagen fibers (Fig. 4-144). The lymphomas most difficult to identify microscopically are those composed of well-differentiated lymphocytes; in many cases, only a noncommittal diagnosis of "cutaneous lymphocytic infiltrate" or "small lymphocytic proliferation" can be made, with an indication for the clinician to investigate the possibility of lymphoma further.[676,677] Cell marker analysis has provided evidence that the majority of these proliferations are clonal and therefore presumably neoplastic, but it has not improved a great deal our ability to predict the clinical outcome. It is well to remember that the majority of these diffuse, small lymphocytic lesions, whether polyclonal or monoclonal, are characterized by a benign clinical course and long survival with only minimal therapeutic intervention.[683]

Occasionally, the cutaneous lymphomatous infiltrate is accompanied by a florid sarcoidlike granulomatous reaction.[682,688] Some cases of T-cell lymphoma have been accompanied by panniculitis.[672]

In a series of twenty-five cases reported by Long et al.,[685] 88% subsequently developed extracutaneous lymphoma, the interval ranging from 6 months to 5 years (mean duration of 21 months).

Cutaneous lymphomas in children are very rare.[679a] The predominant type is *lymphoblastic lymphoma.*[695]

Hodgkin's disease of the skin presents in most instances as papules and nodules forming distally to involved lymph nodes; they are an indication of stage IV disease and probably result from retrograde lymphatic spread.[691,692] A few well-documented cases of primary Hodgkin's disease of the skin have been reported,[692] but many of the cases published in the past under this rubric were examples of lymphomatoid papulosis.

Plasmacytoma may exceptionally present in the form of localized cutaneous disease.[686]

Malignant histiocytosis involves the skin in about 13% of the cases, and in some instances the skin lesions may be the first sign of the disease.[675] It seems likely that the cases originally described as *regressing atypical histiocytosis* and characterized by indolent course and regression of individual lesions[678] represent true malignancies of either histiocytic or T-cell derivation.[680,687]

Malignant (systemic, neoplastic) angioendotheliomatosis is a peculiar disorder characterized by multifocal intravascular proliferation of malignant cells[689] (Fig. 4-145). The cutaneous and neurologic manifestations dominate the clinical presentation, but the disease may present initially in the uterine cervix, prostate, nasal cavity, bone, skeletal muscle, or other sites. Although originally regarded as a systemic malignancy of vascular endothelium, immunocytochemical studies have shown that it represents an angiotropic form of malignant lymphoma, usually of B-cell type.[673,690,693]

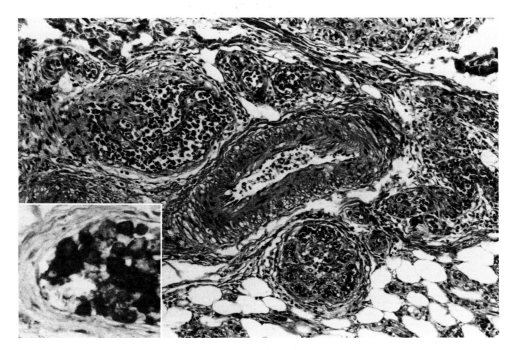

Fig. 4-145 Malignant angioendotheliomatosis. There is packing of dermal and subcutaneous blood vessels by undifferentiated malignant cells, some of which are also present in walls of vessels and in the interstitium. **Inset** shows strong positivity of neoplastic cells for leukocyte common antigen, supporting their lymphoid nature.

Leukemia

Involvement of the skin occurs in about 10% of patients with monocytic leukemia, 8% with chronic lymphocytic leukemia, and 5% with chronic granulocytic leukemia.[696] Most patients have an abnormal blood count at the time of diagnosis, but in some instances the skin lesions are accompanied by a normal peripheral blood ("aleukemic" forms). Granulocytic leukemia of skin is usually a manifestation of recurrence in treated patients or a late development in association with widespread dissemination. Rarely, the disease manifests initially as multiple tumors in the skin; these cases tend to be misdiagnosed as large cell lymphoma.[697]

It is well to remember that a large portion of the skin lesions occurring in leukemic patients are histologically nonspecific inflammatory reactions and are not caused by infiltration by neoplastic cells.

Other primary tumors and tumorlike conditions

Endometriosis can present in women of reproductive age in the umbilicus or groin without antecedent surgery. When present in other cutaneous sites, there is nearly always an associated surgical scar.[702] Microscopically, the combination of endometrial glands and stroma is characteristic; the lesion should not be confused with a sweat gland tumor or, worse, with a metastatic adenocarcinoma. Marked hemorrhage or decidual changes in the stroma may render the recognition difficult.[701]

Benign cystic teratoma exceptionally presents as a skin nodule; the presence of tissue components from all three germinal layers distinguishes it from the more common dermoid cyst (see p. 112).[698]

Meningioma can occur as a skin nodule, either in the scalp or along the vertebral axis, with or without an associated skin defect (see Chapter 28); some of these lesions are congenital and probably of malformative nature.[698a] *Nasal glioma* is a form of glial heterotopia that is seen in neonates at the root of the nose, sometimes immediately beneath the skin (see Chapter 7).

Extraosseous chondromas are usually located in the soft tissues, but a few dermal examples are on record.[700]

Metaplastic synovial cyst is the name proposed for a peculiar postsurgical intradermal cystic formation associated with transepidermal fistulae and lined microscopically by tissue resembling hyperplastic synovium.[699]

Metastatic carcinoma

In males the most common sources of metastatic carcinoma to the skin are lung (25%), large bowel, melanoma, kidney, and epidermoid carcinoma of the oral cavity. In females, breast is by far the most common source (69%), followed by lung, malignant melanoma, kidney, and ovary.[703,704,707] Most cases are multiple and appear as firm, nonulcerated nodules.[706] When solitary, they may be misdiagnosed as primary skin tumors. This is particularly true for renal cell carcinoma, which is often misinterpreted as a sweat gland tumor[705]; presence of dilated sinusoid-type vessels, extravasated red blood cells in the glandular lumina, and nuclear atypia should suggest the correct diagnosis. Occasionally, metastatic signet ring carcinomas from the stomach or other sites elicit a brisk fibroblastic reaction with storiform features, thus closely simulating a dermatofibrosarcoma protuberans.

The most common sites for the skin metastases are chest and abdomen, followed by head and neck; location in the extremities is rare. Those metastases situated in the scalp can be associated with alopecia ("alopecia neoplastica"). The interesting observation has been made that the skin metastases tend to be close to the site of the primary tumor: chest in lung carcinoma, abdominal wall in gastrointestinal tumors, and lower back in renal cell carcinoma.[704]

REFERENCES

EPIDERMIS
Seborrheic keratosis

1 Holdiness MR: The sign of Leser-Trélat. Int J Dermatol **25:**564-572, 1986.
2 Rahbari H: Bowenoid transformation of seborrhoeic verrucae (keratoses). Br J Dermatol **101:**459-463, 1979.
3 Scully JP: Treatment of seborrheic keratosis. JAMA **213:**1498, 1970.

Achrochordon

4 Cooper PH, Mackel SE: Acquired fibrokeratoma of the heel. Arch Dermatol **121:**386-388, 1985.

Actinic keratosis

5 James MP, Wells GC, Whimster IW: Spreading pigmented actinic keratoses. Br J Dermatol **98:**373-379, 1978.
6 Pinkus H: Keratosis senilis. A biologic concept of its pathogenesis and diagnosis based on the study of normal epidermis and 1730 seborrheic and senile keratoses. Am J Clin Pathol **29:**193-207, 1958.
7 Spira M, Freeman R, Arfai P, Gerow FJ, Hardy SB: Clinical comparison of chemical peeling, dermabrasion and 5-FU for senile keratoses. Plast Reconstr Surg **46:**61-66, 1970.

Cutaneous horn

8 Kimura S: Trichilemmal keratosis (horn). A light and electron microscopic study. J Cutan Pathol **10:**59-68, 1983.
9 Nakamura K: Two cases of trichilemmal-like horn. Arch Dermatol **120:**386-387, 1984.

Bowen's disease

10 Bowen JT: Precancerous dermatoses. A study of two cases of chronic atypical epithelial proliferation. J Cutan Dis **30:**241-255, 1912.
11 Callen JP, Headington J: Bowen's and non-Bowen's squamous intradermal neoplasia of the skin. Relationship to internal malignancy. Arch Dermatol **116:**422-426, 1980.
12 Graham JH, Helwig EB: Bowen's disease and its relationship to systemic cancer. Arch Dermatol **80:**133-159, 1959.
13 Newton JA, Camplejohn RS, McGibbon DH: Aneuploidy in Bowen's disease. Br J Dermatol **114:**691-694, 1986.

Epidermoid (squamous cell) carcinoma
General features

14 Alexander SJ: Squamous cell carcinoma in chronic hydradenitis suppurativa. A case report. Cancer **43:**745-748, 1979.
15 Barr LH, Menard JW: Marjolin's ulcer. The LSU experience. Cancer **52:**173-175, 1983.
16 Cleaver JE: Xeroderma pigmentosa. Variants with normal DNA repair and normal sensitivity to ultraviolet light. J Invest Dermatol **58:**124-128, 1972.
17 Epstein JI, Mendelsohn G: Squamous carcinoma of the foot arising in association with long-standing verrucous hyperplasia in a patient with congenital lymphedema. Cancer **54:**943-947, 1984.
18 Friedberg EC: Xeroderma pigmentosum. Recent studies on the DNA repair defects. Arch Pathol Lab Med **102:**3-7, 1978.
19 Johnson LL, Kempson RL: Epidermoid carcinoma in chronic osteomyelitis. Diagnostic problems and management. J Bone Joint Surg [A] **47:**133-145, 1965.
20 Levin A, Amazon K, Rywlin AM: A squamous cell carcinoma that developed in an epidermal nevus. Report of a case and a review of the literature. Am J Dermatopathol **6:**51-55, 1984.

21 Madariaga J, Fromowitz F, Phillips M, Hoover HC Jr: Squamous cell carcinoma in congenital ichthyosis with deafness and keratitis. A case report and review of the literature. Cancer **57:**2026-2029, 1986.

22 Martin H, Strong E, Spiro RH: Radiation-induced skin cancer of the head and neck. Cancer **25:**61-71, 1970.

23 Mullen DL, Silverberg SG, Penn I, Hammond WS: Squamous cell carcinoma of the skin and lip in renal homograft recipients. Cancer **37:**729-734, 1976.

24 Schwartz RA, Birnkrant AP, Rubenstein DJ, Kim U, Burgess GH, Stoll HL Jr, Chai SW, Southwick GJ, Milgrom H: Squamous cell carcinoma in dominant type epidermolysis bullosa dystrophica. Cancer **47:**615-620, 1981.

25 Stern RS, Laird N, Melski J, Parrish JA, Fitzpatrick TB, Bleich HL: Cutaneous squamous-cell carcinoma in patients treated with PUVA. N Engl J Med **310:**1156-1161, 1984.

26 Urbach F: Geographic pathology of skin cancer. In Urbach F (ed): International conference on the biologic effects of ultraviolet radiation (with emphasis on the skin). New York, 1969, Pergamon Press, Inc., pp. 635-650.

Microscopic features

27 Gusterson BA, Clinton S, Gough G: Studies of early invasive and intraepithelial squamous cell carcinomas using an antibody to type IV collagen. Histopathology **10:**161-169, 1986.

28 Heyderman E, Graham RM, Chapman DV, Richardson TC, McKee PH: Epithelial markers in primary skin cancer. An immunoperoxidase study of the distribution of epithelial membrane antigen (EMA) and carcinoembryonic antigen (CEA) in 65 primary skin carcinomas. Histopathology **8:**423-434, 1984.

29 Jones RE Jr (ed): What is the boundary that separates a thick solar keratosis and a thin squamous-cell carcinoma? Am J Dermatopathol **6:**301-306, 1984.

30 Said JW, Sassoon AF, Shintaku IP, Banks-Schlegel S: Involucrin in squamous and basal cell carcinomas of the skin. An immunohistochemical study. J Invest Dermatol **82:**449-452, 1984.

Other microscopic types

31 Brownstein MH, Shapiro L: Verrucous carcinoma of skin. Epithelioma cuniculatum plantare. Cancer **38:**1710-1716, 1976.

32 Eusebi V, Ceccarelli C, Piscioli F, Cristofolini M, Azzopardi JG: Spindle cell tumours of the skin of debatable origin. An immunocytochemical study. J Pathol **144:**189-199, 1984.

33 Kao GF, Graham JH, Helwig EB: Carcinoma cuniculatum (verrucous carcinoma of the skin). A clinicopathologic study of 46 cases with ultrastructural observations. Cancer **49:**2395-2403, 1982.

34 Kuwano H, Hashimoto H, Enjoji M: Atypical fibroxanthoma distinguishable from spindle cell carcinoma in sarcoma-like skin lesions. A clinicopathologic and immunohistochemical study of 21 cases. Cancer **55:**172-180, 1985.

35 McKee PH, Wilkinson JD, Black MM, Whimster IW: Carcinoma (epithelioma) cuniculatum. A clinico-pathological study of nineteen cases and review of the literature. Histopathology **5:**425-436, 1981.

36 Reingold IM, Smith BR, Graham JH: Epithelioma cuniculatum pedis, a variant of squamous cell carcinoma. Am J Clin Pathol **69:**561-565, 1978.

37 Weidner N, Foucar E: Adenosquamous carcinoma of the skin. An aggressive mucin- and gland-forming squamous carcinoma. Arch Dermatol **121:**775-779, 1985.

Treatment

38 Sober AJ: Diagnosis and management of skin cancer. Cancer **51:**2448-2452, 1983.

Prognosis

39 Friedman HI, Cooper PH, Wanebo HJ: Prognostic and therapeutic use of microstaging of cutaneous squamous cell carcinoma of the trunk and extremities. Cancer **56:**1099-1105, 1985.

40 Immerman SC, Scanlon EF, Christ M, Knox KL: Recurrent squamous cell carcinoma of the skin. Cancer **51:**1537-1540, 1983.

41 Lund HZ: How often does squamous cell carcinoma metastasize? Arch Dermatol **92:**635-637, 1965.

Pseudoepitheliomatous hyperplasia

42 Civatte J: Pseudo-carcinomatous hyperplasia. J Cutan Pathol **12:**214-223, 1985.

Basal cell carcinoma
General features

43 Black MM, Walkden VM: Basal cell carcinomatous changes on the lower leg. A possible association with chronic venous stasis. Histopathology **7:**219-227, 1983.

44 Gellin GE, Kopf AW, Garfinkel L: Basal cell epithelioma. A controlled study of associated factors. Arch Dermatol **91:**38-45, 1965.

45 Graham PG, McGavran MH: Basal-cell carcinomas and sebaceous glands. Cancer **17:**803-806, 1964.

46 McGibbon DH: Malignant epidermal tumours. J Cutan Pathol **12:**224-238, 1985.

47 Mehregan AH: Aggressive basal cell epithelioma on sunlight-protected skin. Report of eight cases, one with pulmonary and bone metastases. Am J Dermatopathol **5:**221-229, 1983.

48 Milstone EB, Helwig EB: Basal cell carcinoma in children. Arch Dermatol **108:**523-527, 1973.

49 Rahbari H, Mehregan AH: Basal cell epitheliomas (carcinoma) in children and teenagers. Cancer **49:**350-353, 1982.

50 Robinson JK: Risk of developing another basal cell carcinoma. A 5-year prospective study. Cancer **60:**118-120, 1987.

Microscopic features

51 Heyderman E, Graham RM, Chapman DV, Richardson TC, McKee PH: Epithelial markers in primary skin cancer. An immunoperoxidase study of the distribution of epithelial membrane antigen (EMA) and carcinoembryonic antigen (CEA) in 65 primary skin carcinomas. Histopathology **8:**423-434, 1984.

52 Kint A: Histogenetic study of the basal cell epithelioma. Curr Probl Dermatol **3:**82-123, 1970.

53 Looi LM: Localized amyloidosis in basal cell carcinoma. A pathologic study. Cancer **52:**1833-1836, 1983.

54 Mark GJ: Basal cell carcinoma with intraneural invasion. Cancer **40:**2181-2187, 1977.

55 McArdle JP, Roff BT, Muller HK: Characterization of retraction spaces in basal cell carcinoma using an antibody to type IV collagen. Histopathology **8:**447-455, 1984.

56 McGibbon DH: Malignant epidermal tumours. J Cutan Pathol **12:**224-238, 1985.

57 Nagao S, Nemoto H, Suzuki M, Satoh N, Iijima S: Myofibroblasts in basal cell epithelioma. With special reference to the phagocytic function of myofibroblasts. J Cutan Pathol **13:**261-267, 1986.

58 Said JW, Sassoon AF, Shintaku IP, Banks-Schlegel S: Involucrin in squamous and basal cell carcinomas of the skin. An immunohistochemical study. J Invest Dermatol **82:**449-452, 1984.

59 Stanley JR, Beckwith JB, Fuller RP, Katz SI: A specific antigenic defect of the basement membrane is found in basal cell carcinoma but not in other epidermal tumors. Cancer **50:**1486-1490, 1982.

60 Thomas P, Said JW, Nash G, Banks-Schlegel S: Profiles of keratin proteins in basal and squamous cell carcinomas of the skin. An immunohistochemical study. Lab Invest **50:**36-41, 1984.

61 Van Cauwenberge D, Pierard GE, Foidart JM, Lapiere ChM: Immunohistochemical localization of laminin, type IV and type V collagen in basal cell carcinoma. Br J Dermatol **108:**163-170, 1983.

62 Viac J, Reano A, Thivolet J: Cytokeratins in human basal and squamous cell carcinomas. Biochemical, immunohistological findings and comparisons with normal epithelia. J Cutan Pathol **9:**377-390, 1982.

63 Weedon D, Shand E: Amyloid in basal cell carcinomas. Br J Dermatol **101:**141-146, 1979.

Other microscopic types

64 Barnadas MA, Freeman RG: Clear cell basal cell epithelioma. Light and electron microscopic study of an unusual variant. J Cutan Pathol **15:**1-7, 1988.

65 Barr RJ, Graham JH: Granular cell basal cell carcinoma. A distinct histopathologic entity. Arch Dermatol **115:**1064-1067, 1979.

66 Farmer ER, Helwig EB: Metastatic basal cell carcinoma. A clinicopathologic study of seventeen cases. Cancer **46:**748-757, 1980.

67 Gellin GE, Bender B: Giant premalignant fibroepithelioma. Arch Dermatol **94:**70-73, 1966.

68 Gorlin RJ, Vickers RA, Kelln E, Williamson JJ: The multiple basal-cell nevi syndrome. An analysis of a syndrome consisting of multiple nevoid basal cell carcinoma, jaw cysts, skeletal anomalies, medulloblastoma, and hyporesponsiveness to parathormone. Cancer **18:**89-104, 1965.

69 Howell JB, Anderson DE: The nevoid basal cell carcinoma syndrome. Arch Dermatol **118:**824-826, 1982.

70 Imayama S, Yashima Y, Higuchi R, Urabe H: A new concept of basal cell epitheliomas based on the three-dimensional growth pattern of the superficial multicentric type. Am J Pathol **128:**497-504, 1987.

71 Lindeberg H, Jepsen FL: The nevoid basal cell carcinoma syndrome. Histopathology of the basal cell tumors. J Cutan Pathol **10:**68-73, 1983.

72 Lopes De Faria J: Basal cell carcinoma of the skin with areas of squamous cell carcinoma. A basosquamous cell carcinoma? J Clin Pathol **38:**1273-1277, 1985.

73 Mason JK, Helwig EB, Graham JH: Pathology of the nevoid basal cell carcinoma syndrome. Arch Pathol **79:**401-408, 1965.

74 McGibbon DH: Malignant epidermal tumours. J Cutan Pathol **12:**224-238, 1985.

Spread and metastases

75 Jacobs GH, Rippey JJ, Altini M: Prediction of aggressive behavior in basal cell carcinoma. Cancer **49:**533-537, 1982.

76 McGibbon DH: Malignant epidermal tumours. J Cutan Pathol **12:**224-238, 1985.

77 Mehregan AH: Aggressive basal cell epithelioma on sunlight-protected skin. Report of eight cases, one with pulmonary and bone metastases. Am J Dermatopathol **5:**221-229, 1983.

78 Wermuth BM, Fajardo LF: Metastatic basal cell carcinoma. A review. Arch Pathol **90:**458-462, 1970.

Treatment

79 Gooding CA, White G, Yatsuhashi M: Significance of marginal extension in excised basal cell carcinoma. N Engl J Med **273:**923-924, 1965.

SKIN ADNEXAE
Eccrine sweat gland

80 Cooper PH: Carcinomas of sweat glands. Pathol Annu **22**(Pt 1):83-124, 1987.

81 Kariniemi A-L, Forsman LM, Wahlström T, Andersson LC: Expression of differentiation antigens in benign sweat gland tumours. Br J Dermatol **111:**175-182, 1984.

82 Maiorana A, Nigrisoli E, Papotti M: Immunohistochemical markers of sweat gland tumors. J Cutan Pathol **13:**187-196, 1986.

83 Massa MC, Medenica M: Cutaneous adnexal tumors and cysts. A review. Part II. Tumors with apocrine and eccrine glandular differentiation and miscellaneous cutaneous cysts. Pathol Annu **22**(Pt 1):225-276, 1987.

84 Noda Y, Horike H, Watanabe Y, Mori M: Immunohistochemical identification of epithelial membrane antigen in sweat gland tumours by the use of a monoclonal antibody. Pathol Res Pract **182:**797-804, 1987.

85 Noda Y, Oosumi H, Morishima T, Tsujimura T, Mori M: Immunohistochemical study of carbonic anhydrase in mixed tumours and adenomas of sweat and sebaceous glands. J Cutan Pathol **14:**285-290, 1987.

86 Penneys NS, Nadji M, Morales A: Carcinoembryonic antigen in benign sweat gland tumors. Arch Dermatol **118:**225-227, 1982.

87 Santa Cruz DJ: Sweat gland carcinomas. A comprehensive review. Semin Diagn Pathol **4:**38-74, 1987.

88 Tamaki K, Furue M, Matsukawa A, Ohara K, Mizoguchi M, Hino H: Presence and distribution of carcinoembryonic antigen and lectin-binding sites in benign apocrine sweat gland tumours. Br J Dermatol **113:**565-571, 1985.

Poroma

89 Freeman RG, Knox JM, Spiller WF: Eccrine poroma. Am J Clin Pathol **36:**444-450, 1961.

90 Hashimoto K, Lever WF: Eccrine poroma: histochemical and electron microscopic studies. J Invest Dermatol **43:**237-247, 1964.

91 Okun MR, Ansell HB: Eccrine poroma. Report of three cases, two with an unusual location. Arch Dermatol **88:**561-566, 1963.

92 Pinkus H, Rogin JR, Goldman F: Eccrine poroma. Tumors exhibiting features of the epidermal sweat duct unit. Arch Dermatol **74:**511-521, 1956.

93 Rahbari H: Hidroacanthoma simplex—a review of 15 cases. Br J Dermatol **109:**219-225, 1983.

94 Warner TFCS, Goell WS, Cripps DJJ: Hidroacanthoma simplex. An ultrastructural study. J Cutan Pathol **9:**189-195, 1982.

Acrospiroma

95 Johnson BL Jr, Helwig EB: Eccrine acrospiroma. Cancer **23:**641-657, 1969.

96 Stanley RJ, Sanchez NP, Massa MC, Cooper AJ, Crotty CP, Winkelmann RK: Epidermoid hidradenoma. A clinicopathologic study. J Cutan Pathol **9:**293-302, 1982.

97 Winkelmann RK, Wolff K: Solid-cystic hidradenoma of the skin. Clinical and histopathologic study. Arch Dermatol **97:**651-661, 1968.

Syringoma

98 Feibelman GE, Maize JC: Clear-cell syringoma. A study of conventional and electron microscopy. Am J Dermatopathol **6:**139-150, 1984.

99 Hashimoto K, Gross BG, Lever WF: Syringoma. Histochemical and electron microscopic studies. J Invest Dermatol **46:**150-166, 1966.

100 Winkelmann RK, Gottlieb BF: Syringoma. An enzymatic study. Cancer **16:**665-669, 1963.

Chondroid syringoma (mixed tumor)

101 Angényi ZB, Balogh K, Goeken JA: Immunohistochemical characterization of chondroid syringomas. Am J Pathol (In press).

102 Hirsch P, Helwig EB: Chondroid syringoma. Arch Dermatol **84:**835-847, 1961.

103 Jaworski RC: The ultrastructure of chondroid syringoma (mixed tumor of skin). Ultrastruct Pathol **6:**153-159, 1984.

104 Kunikane H, Ishikura H, Yamaguchi J, Yoshiki T, Itoh T, Aizawa M: Chondroid syringoma (mixed tumor of the skin). A clinicopathological study of 13 cases. Acta Pathol Jpn **37:**615-625, 1987.

105 Mambo NC: Hyaline cells in a benign chondroid syringoma. Report of a case and findings by conventional and electron microscopy. Am J Dermatopathol **6:**265-272, 1984.

106 Stout AP, Gorman JG: Mixed tumors of the skin of the salivary gland type. Cancer **12:**537-543, 1959.

107 Yoneda K, Kitajima Y, Furuta H, Tsuneda Y, Mori S: The distribution of keratin type intermediate-sized filaments in so-called mixed tumour of the skin. Br J Dermatol **109:**393-400, 1983.

Eccrine cylindroma

108 Cotton DWK, Braye SG: Dermal cylindromas originate from the eccrine sweat gland. Br J Dermatol **111:**53-61, 1984.

109 Crain RC, Helwig EB: Dermal cylindroma (dermal eccrine cylindroma). Am J Clin Pathol **35:**504-515, 1961.

110 Goette DK, McConnell MA, Fowler VR: Cylindroma and eccrine spiradenoma coexistent in the same lesion. Arch Dermatol **118:**273-274, 1982.

111 Kallioinen M: Immunoelectron microscope demonstration of the basement membrane components laminin and type IV collagen in the dermal cylindroma. J Pathol **147:**97-102, 1985.

112 Reingold IM, Keasbey LE, Graham JH: Multicentric dermal-type cylindromas of the parotid glands in a patient with florid turban tumor. Cancer **40:**1702-1710, 1977.

Eccrine spiradenoma

113 Cotton DWK, Slater DN, Rooney N, Goepel JR, Mills PM: Giant vascular eccrine spiradenomas. A report of two cases with histology, immunohistology and electron microscopy. Histopathology **10:**1093-1099, 1986.

114 Hashimoto K, Gross BG, Nelson RG, Lever WF: Eccrine spiradenoma. Histochemical and electron microscopic studies. J Invest Dermatol **46:**347-365, 1966.

115 Jitsukawa K, Sueki H, Sato S, Anzai T: Eccrine spiradenoma. An electron microscopic study. Am J Dermatopathol **9:**99-108, 1987.

116 Kersting DW, Helwig EB: Eccrine spiradenoma. Arch Dermatol **73:**199-227, 1956.

117 Mambo NC: Eccrine spiradenoma. Clinical and pathologic study of 49 tumors. J Cutan Pathol **10:**312-320, 1983.

118 Munger BL, Berghorn BM, Helwig EB: A light and electron microscopic study of a case of multiple eccrine spiradenoma. J Invest Dermatol **38:**289-297, 1962.

Papillary syringadenoma

119 Helwig EB, Hackney VC: Syringadenoma papilliferum. Arch Dermatol **71:**361-372, 1955.

120 Mambo NC: Immunohistochemical study of the immunoglobulin classes of the plasma cells in papillary syringadenoma. Virchows Arch [Pathol Anat] **397:**1-6, 1982.

121 Vanatta PR, Bangert JL, Freeman RG: Syringocystadenoma papilliferum. A plasmacytotropic tumor. Am J Surg Pathol **9:**678-683, 1985.

Papillary eccrine adenoma

122 Rulon DB, Helwig EB: Papillary eccrine adenoma. Arch Dermatol **113:**596-598, 1977.

Aggressive digital papillary adenoma

123 Kao GF, Helwig EB, Grahan JH: Aggressive digital papillary adenoma and adenocarcinoma. A clinicopathological study of 57 patients, with histochemical, immunopathological, and ultrastructural observations. J Cutan Pathol **14:**129-146, 1987.

Clear cell acanthoma

124 Brownstein MH, Fernando S, Shapiro L: Clear cell acanthoma. Clinicopathologic analysis of 37 new cases. Am J Clin Pathol **59:**306-311, 1973.

125 Fukushiro S, Takei Y, Ackerman AB: Pale-cell acanthosis. A distinctive histologic pattern of epidermal epithelium. Am J Dermatopathol **7:**515-527, 1985.

126 Landry M, Winkelmann RK: Multiple clear-cell acanthoma and ichthyosis. Arch Dermatol 105:371-383, 1972.

Intraepidermal epithelioma

127 Mehregan AH, Pinkus H: Intraepidermal epithelioma. A critical study. Cancer 17:609-636, 1964.
128 Steffen C, Ackerman AB: Intraepidermal epithelioma of Borst-Jadassohn. Am J Dermatopathol 7:5-24, 1985.

Sweat gland carcinoma

129 Berg JW, McDivitt RW: Pathology of sweat gland carcinoma. Pathol Annu 3:123-144, 1968.
130 Chow CW, Campbell PE, Burry AF: Sweat gland carcinomas in children. Cancer 53:1222-1227, 1984.
131 Cooper PH, Adelson GL, Holthaus WH: Primary cutaneous adenoid cystic carcinoma. Arch Dermatol 120:774-777, 1984.
132 Cooper PH, Frierson HF, Morrison AG: Malignant transformation of eccrine spiradenoma. Arch Dermatol 121:1445-1448, 1985.
133 Cooper PH, Mills SE, Leonard DD, Santa Cruz DJ, Headington JT, Barr RJ, Katz DA: Sclerosing sweat duct (syringomatous) carcinoma. Am J Surg Pathol 9:422-433, 1985.
134 Cooper PH, Robinson CR, Greer KE: Low-grade clear cell eccrine carcinoma. Arch Dermatol 120:1076-1078, 1984.
135 Dissanayake RVP, Salm R: Sweat-gland carcinomas. Prognosis related to histological type. Histopathology 4:445-466, 1980.
136 Eng AM, Reyes C: Porocarcinoma associated with extramammary Paget's disease. J Cutan Pathol 1:249-255, 1974.
137 Goldstein DJ, Barr RJ, Santa Cruz DJ: Microcystic adnexal carcinoma. A distinct clinicopathologic entity. Cancer 50:566-572, 1982.
138 Headington JT, Niederhuber JE, Beals TF: Malignant clear cell acrospiroma. Cancer 41:641-647, 1978.
139 Ishimura E, Iwamoto H, Kobashi Y, Yamabe H, Ichijima K: Malignant chondroid syringoma. Report of a case with widespread metastasis and review of pertinent literature. Cancer 52:1966-1973, 1983.
140 Lin PY, Fatteh SM, Lloyd KM: Malignant transformation in a solitary dermal cylindroma. Arch Pathol Lab Med 111:765-767, 1987.
141 Mehregan AH, Hashimoto K, Rahbari H: Eccrine adenocarcinoma. A clinicopathologic study of 35 cases. Arch Dermatol 119:104-114, 1983.
142 Mendoza S, Helwig EB: Mucinous (adenocystic) carcinoma of the skin. Arch Dermatol 103:68-78, 1971.
143 Miller WL: Sweat gland carcinoma. Am J Clin Pathol 47:767-780, 1967.
144 Penneys NS, Nadji M, Ziegels-Weissman J, Ketabchi M, Morales AR: Carcinoembryonic antigen in sweat-gland carcinomas. Cancer 50:1608-1611, 1982.
145 Santa Cruz DJ, Barr RJ: Lymphoepithelial tumor of the skin. J Cutan Pathol 14:369, 1987.
146 Santa Cruz DJ, Meyers JH, Gnepp DR, Perez BM: Primary mucinous carcinoma of the skin. Br J Dermatol 98:645-653, 1978.
147 Shaw M, McKee PH, Lowe D, Black MM: Malignant eccrine poroma. A study of twenty-seven cases. Br J Dermatol 107:675-680, 1982.
148 Swanson PE, Cherwitz DL, Neumann MP, Wick MR: Eccrine sweat gland carcinoma. An histologic and immunohistochemical study of 32 cases. J Cutan Pathol 14:65-86, 1987.
149 Turner JJ, Maxwell L, Bursle GA: Eccrine porocarcinoma. A case report with light microscopy and ultrastructure. Pathology 14:469-475, 1982.
150 Wick MR, Goellner JR, Wolfe JT III, Su WPD: Adnexal carcinomas of the skin. I. Eccrine carcinomas. Cancer 56:1147-1162, 1985.
151 Wick MR, Swanson PE: Primary adenoid cystic carcinoma of the skin. A clinical, histological, and immunocytochemical comparison with adenoid cystic carcinoma of salivary glands and adenoid basal cell carcinoma. Am J Dermatopathol 8:2-13, 1986.
152 Wick MR, Swanson PE, Kaye VN, Pittelkow MR: Sweat gland carcinoma *ex* eccrine spiradenoma. Am J Dermatopathol 9:90-98, 1987.

Extramammary Paget's disease

153 Fisher ER, Beyer F Jr: Differentiation of neoplastic lesions characterized by large vacuolated intraepidermal (pagetoid) cells. Arch Pathol 67:140-145, 1959.
154 Guldhammer B, Nørgaard T: The differential diagnosis of intraepidermal malignant lesions using immunohistochemistry. Am J Dermatopathol 8:295-301, 1986.
155 Helwig EB, Graham JH: Anogenital (extramammary) Paget's disease. A clinicopathological study. Cancer 16:387-403, 1963.
156 Jones RE Jr, Austin C, Ackerman AB: Extramammary Paget's disease. A critical reexamination. Am J Dermatopathol 1:101-132, 1979.

157 Kariniemi A-L, Ramaekers F, Lehto V-P, Virtanen I: Paget cells express cytokeratins typical of glandular epithelia, Br J Dermatol 112:179-183, 1985.
158 Koss LG, Brockunier A Jr: Ultrastructural aspects of Paget's disease of the vulva. Arch Pathol 87:592-600, 1969.
159 Kuo T-t, Chan H-L, Hsueh S: Clear cell papulosis of the skin. A new entity with histogenetic implications for cutaneous Paget's disease. Am J Surg Pathol 11:827-834, 1987.
160 Merot Y, Mazoujian G, Pinkus G, Momtaz-T K, Murphy GF: Extramammary Paget's disease of the perianal and perineal regions. Evidence of apocrine derivation. Arch Dermatol 121:750-752, 1985.
161 Nadji M: Immunoperoxidase techniques. II. Application to cutaneous neoplasms. Am J Dermatopathol 8:124-129, 1986.
162 Nagle RB, Lucas DO, McDaniel KM, Clark VA, Schmalzel GM: Paget's cells. New evidence linking mammary and extramammary Paget cells to a common cell phenotype. Am J Clin Pathol 83:431-438, 1985.
163 Ordóñez NG, Awalt H, Mackay B: Mammary and extramammary Paget's disease. An immunocytochemical and ultrastructural study. Cancer 59:1173-1183, 1987.
164 Peralta OC, Barr RJ, Romansky SG: Mixed carcinoma in situ. An immunohistochemical study. J Cutan Pathol 10:350-358, 1983.
164a Shah KD, Tabizzadeh SS, Gerber MA: Immunohistochemical distinction of Paget's disease from Bowen's disease and superficial spreading melanoma with the use of monoclonal cytokeratin antibodies. Am J Clin Pathol 88:689-695, 1987.
165 Tamaki K, Hino H, Ohara K, Furue M: Lectin-binding sites in Paget's disease. Br J Dermatol 113:17-24, 1985.
166 Vanstapel M-J, Gatter KC, DeWolf-Peeters C, Millard PR, Desmet VJ, Mason DY: Immunohistochemical study of mammary and extra-mammary Paget's disease. Histopathology 8:1013-1023, 1984.

Apocrine sweat gland

167 Landry M, Winkelmann RK: An unusual tubular apocrine adenoma. Arch Dermatol 105:869-879, 1972.
167a Mazoujian G, Margolis R: Immunohistochemistry of gross cystic disease fluid protein (GCDFP-15) in 65 benign sweat gland tumors of the skin. Am J Dermatopathol 10:28-35, 1988.

Sebaceous gland
Senile sebaceous hyperplasia

168 Mehregan AH: Sebaceous tumors of the skin. J Cutan Pathol 12:196-199, 1985.

Nevus sebaceus of Jadassohn

169 Alessi E, Sala F: Nevus sebaceus. A clinicopathologic study of its evolution. Am J Dermatopathol 8:27-31, 1986.
170 Mehregan AH, Pinkus H: Life history of organoid nevi. Special reference to nevus sebaceus of Jadassohn. Arch Dermatol 91:274-289, 1965.
171 Morioka S: The natural history of *nevus sebaceus*. J Cutan Pathol 12:200-213, 1985.
172 Su WPD: Histopathologic varieties of epidermal nevus. A study of 160 cases. Am J Dermatopathol 4:161-170, 1982.
173 Wilson Jones E, Heyl T: Naevus sebaceus. A report of 140 cases with special regard to the development of secondary malignant tumours. Br J Dermatol 82:99-117, 1970.

Sebaceous adenoma

174 Rulon DB, Helwig EB: Cutaneous sebaceous neoplasms. Cancer 33:82-102, 1974.

Sebaceous carcinoma

175 Burgdorf WHC, Pitha J, Fahmy A: Muir-Torre syndrome. Histologic spectrum of sebaceous proliferation. Am J Dermatopathol 8:202-208, 1986.
176 Finan MC, Connolly SM: Sebaceous gland tumors and systemic disease. A clinicopathologic analysis. Medicine [Baltimore] 63:232-242, 1984.
177 Friedman KJ, Boudreau S, Farmer ER: Superficial epithelioma with sebaceous differentiation. J Cutan Pathol 14:193-197, 1987.
178 Graham R, McKee P, McGibbon D, Heyderman E: Torre-Muir syndrome. An association with isolated sebaceous carcinoma. Cancer 55:2868-2873, 1985.
179 Hood IC, Qizilbash AH, Salama SS, Young JEM, Archibald SD: Sebaceous carcinoma of the face following irradiation. Am J Dermatopathol 8:505-508, 1986.
180 Kuo T: Clear cell carcinoma of the skin. Am J Surg Pathol 4:573-583, 1980.
181 Rulon DB, Helwig EB: Cutaneous sebaceous neoplasms. Cancer 33:82-102, 1974.

181a Swanson PE, Campbell RJ, Wick MR: Sebaceous carcinoma. An immuno-histochemical study of 36 ocular and 5 extraocular neoplasms (abstract). J Cutan Pathol **14:**374, 1987.

182 Troy JL, Ackerman AB: Sebaceoma. A distinctive benign neoplasm of adnexal epithelium differentiating toward sebaceous cells. Am J Dermatopathol **6:**7-13, 1984.

183 Wick MR, Goellner JR, Wolfe JT III, Su WPD: Adnexal carcinomas of the skin. II. Extraocular sebaceous carcinomas. Cancer **56:**1163-1172, 1985.

Hair follicle

184 Headington JT: Tumors of the hair follicle. A review. Am J Pathol **85:**480-505, 1976.

185 Massa MC, Medenica M: Cutaneous adnexal tumors and cysts. A review. Part I. Tumors with hair follicular and sebaceous glandular differentiation and cysts related to different parts of the hair follicle. Pathol Annu **20**(Pt 2):189-233, 1985.

186 Mehregan AH: Hair follicle tumors of the skin. J Cutan Pathol **12:**189-195, 1985.

187 Mehregan AH, Brownstein MH: Pilar sheath acanthoma. Arch Dermatol **114:**1495-1497, 1978.

Inverted follicular keratosis

188 Azzopardi JG, Laurini R: Inverted follicular keratosis. J Clin Pathol **28:**465-471, 1975.

189 Mehregan AH: Inverted follicular keratosis. Arch Dermatol **89:**229-235, 1964.

190 Sim-Davis D, Marks R, Wilson Jones E: The inverted follicular keratosis. A surprising variant of seborrheic wart. Acta Derm Venereol [Stockh] **56:**337-344, 1976.

191 Spielvogel RL, Austin C, Ackerman AB: Inverted follicular keratosis is not a specific keratosis but a verruca vulgaris (or seborrheic keratosis) with squamous eddies. Am J Dermatopathol **5:**427-442, 1983.

Trichoepithelioma

191a Brooke JD, Fitzpatrick JE, Golitz LE: Papillary mesenchymal bodies. A histologic finding useful in differentiating trichoepitheliomas from basal cell carcinoma (abstract). J Cutan Pathol **14:**350, 1987.

192 Brownstein MH, Shapiro L: Desmoplastic trichoepithelioma. Cancer **40:**2979-2986, 1977.

193 Gray HR, Helwig EB: Epithelioma adenoides cysticum and solitary trichoepithelioma. Arch Dermatol **87:**102-114, 1963.

194 Takei Y, Fukushiro S, Ackerman AB: Criteria for histologic differentiation of desmoplastic trichoepithelioma (sclerosing epithelial hamartoma) from morphea-like basal-cell carcinoma. Am J Dermatopathol **7:**207-221, 1985.

Trichilemmoma

195 Brownstein MH, Wolf M, Bikowski JB: Cowden's disease. A cutaneous marker of breast cancer. Cancer **41:**2393-2398, 1978.

196 Carlson GJ, Nivatvongs S, Snover DC: Colorectal polyps in Cowden's disease (multiple hamartoma syndrome). Am J Surg Pathol **8:**763-770, 1984.

196a Swanson PE, Cherwitz DL, Wick MR: Tricholemmal carcinoma. A clinico-pathologic study of 6 cases (abstract). J Cutan Pathol **14:**374, 1987.

Trichofolliculoma

197 Fujita WG, Barr RJ, Headley JL: Multiple fibrofolliculomas with trichodiscomas and acrochordons. Arch Dermatol **117:**32-35, 1981.

198 Gray HR, Helwig EB: Trichofolliculoma. Arch Dermatol **86:**619-625, 1962.

Keratoacanthoma

199 Cramer SF: Subungual keratoacanthoma. A benign bone-eroding neoplasm of the distal phalanx. Am J Clin Pathol **75:**425-429, 1981.

200 Fisher ER, McCoy MM, Wechsler HL: Analysis of histopathologic and electron microscopic determinants of keratoacanthoma and squamous cell carcinoma. Cancer **29:**1387-1397, 1972.

201 Janecka IP, Wolff M, Crikelair F, Cosman B: Aggressive histological features of keratoacanthoma. J Cutan Pathol **4:**342-348, 1978.

202 Kingman J, Callen JP: Keratoacanthoma. A clinical study. Arch Dermatol **120:**736-740, 1984.

203 Klein-Szanto AJP, Barr RJ, Reiners JJ Jr, Mamrack MD: Filaggrin distribution in keratoacanthomas and squamous cell carcinoma. Arch Pathol Lab Med **108:**888-890, 1984.

204 Lapius NA, Helwig EB: Perineurial invasion by keratoacanthoma. Arch Dermatol **116:**791-793, 1980.

205 Lowe D, Fletcher CDM, Shaw MP, McKee PH: Eosinophil infiltration in ker-

atoacanthoma and squamous cell carcinoma of the skin. Histopathology **8:**619-625, 1984.

206 Piscioli F, Boi S, Zumiani G, Cristofolini M: A gigantic, metastasizing keratoacanthoma. Report of a case and discussion on classification. Am J Dermatopathol **6:**123-129, 1984.

207 Reed RJ: Actinic keratoacanthoma. Arch Dermatol **106:**858-864, 1972.

208 Rook A, Champion RH: Keratoacanthoma. Natl Cancer Inst Monogr **10:**257-274, 1963.

209 Rossman RE, Freeman RG, Knox JM: Multiple keratoacanthoma. Arch Dermatol **89:**374-381, 1964.

Keratinous cyst

210 Cotton DWK, Kirkham N, Young BJJ: Immunoperoxidase anti-keratin staining of epidermal and pilar cysts. Br J Dermatol **111:**63-68, 1984.

211 Kligman AM: The myth of the sebaceous cyst. Arch Dermatol **89:**253-256, 1964.

212 Leppard BJ, Sanderson KV: The natural history of trichilemmal cysts. Br J Dermatol **94:**379-390, 1976.

213 McGavran MH, Binnington B: Keratinous cysts of the skin. Arch Dermatol **94:**499-508, 1966.

214 McGavran MH, Orman SK: Unpublished data.

215 Pinkus H: "Sebaceous cysts" are trichilemmal cysts. Arch Dermatol **99:**544-553, 1969.

216 Rahbari H: Epidermoid cysts with seborrheic verruca-like cyst walls. Arch Dermatol **118:**326-328, 1982.

Other cutaneous cysts

217 Brownstein MH: Steatocystoma simplex. A solitary steatocystoma. Arch Dermatol **118:**409-411, 1982.

218 Esterly NB, Fretzin DF, Pinkus H: Eruptive vellus hair cysts. Arch Dermatol **113:**500-503, 1979.

219 Farmer ER, Helwig EB: Cutaneous ciliated cysts. Arch Dermatol **114:**70-73, 1978.

219a Fraga S, Helwig EB, Rosen SM: Bronchogenic cysts in the skin and subcutaneous tissue. Am J Clin Pathol **56:**230-238, 1971.

220 Kligman AM, Kirschbaum JD: Steatocystoma multiplex. A dermoid tumor. J Invest Dermatol **42:**383-387, 1964.

221 Mehregan AH: Apocrine cystadenoma. A clinicopathologic study with special reference to the pigmented variety. Arch Dermatol **90:**274-279, 1964.

222 Mehregan AH, Medenica M: Pigmented follicular cysts. J Cutan Pathol **9:**423-427, 1982.

222a Shareef DS, Salm R: Ectopic vestigial lesions of the neck and shoulders. J Clin Pathol **34:**1155-1162, 1981.

Isolated follicular keratosis (warty dyskeratoma)

223 Graham JH, Helwig EB: Isolated follicular dyskeratosis. Arch Dermatol **77:**377-389, 1958.

Pilar tumor (proliferating trichilemmal cyst)

224 Amaral ALMP, Nascimento AG, Goellner JR: Proliferating pilar (trichilemmal) cyst. Report of two cases, one with carcinomatous transformation and one with distant metastases, Arch Pathol Lab Med **108:**808-810, 1984.

225 Brownstein MH, Arluk DJ: Proliferating trichilemmal cyst. A simulant of squamous cell carcinoma. Cancer **48:**1207-1214, 1981.

226 Dabska M: Giant hair matrix tumor. Cancer **28:**701-706, 1971.

227 Hohnes EJ: Tumors of the lower hair sheath. Cancer **21:**234-248, 1968.

228 Jones EW: Proliferating epidermoid cysts. Arch Dermatol **94:**11-19, 1966.

229 Mann B, Salm R, Azzopardi JG: Pilar tumour. A distinctive type of trichilemmoma. Diagn Histopathol **5:**157-167, 1982.

230 Poiares Baptista A, Garcia E Silva L, Born MC: Proliferating trichilemmal cyst. J Cutan Pathol **10:**178-187, 1983.

231 Reed RJ, Lamar LM: Invasive hair matrix tumors of the scalp. Invasive pilomatrixoma. Arch Dermatol **94:**310-316, 1966.

Pilomatrixoma

232 Forbis RJ, Helwig EB: Pilomatrixoma. Arch Dermatol **83:**606-618, 1961.

233 Gould E, Kurzon R, Kowalczyk AP, Saldana M: Pilomatrix carcinoma with pulmonary metastasis. Report of a case. Cancer **54:**370-372, 1984.

234 Hashimoto K, Nelson RG, Lever WF: Calcifying epithelioma of Malherbe. Histochemical and electron microscopic studies. J Invest Dermatol **46:**391-408, 1966.

235 LeBoit PE, Parslow TG, Choy S-H: Hair matrix differentiation. Occurrence in lesions other than pilomatricoma. Am J Dermatopathol **9:**399-405, 1987.

236 McGavran MH: Ultrastructure of pilomatrixoma (calcifying epithelioma). Cancer **18**:1445-1456, 1965.

237 Solanki P, Ramzy I, Durr N, Henkes D: Pilomatrixoma. Cytologic features with differential diagnostic considerations. Arch Pathol Lab Med **111**:294-297, 1987.

238 Wood MG, Parhizgar B, Beerman H: Malignant pilomatricoma. Arch Dermatol **120**:770-773, 1984.

MELANOCYTES

239 Clark WH Jr, Watson MC, Watson BEM: Two kinds of "clear" cells in the human epidermis. With a report of a modified DOPA reaction for electron microscopy. Am J Pathol **39**:333-344, 1961.

240 Cochran AJ, Wen D-R: S-100 protein as a marker for melanocytic and other tumours. Pathology **17**:340-345, 1985.

241 Fitzpatrick TB, Lerner AB: Terminology of pigment cells. Science **117**:640, 1953.

242 Gown AM, Vogel AM, Hoak D, Gough F, McNutt MA: Monoclonal antibodies specific for melanocytic tumors distinguish subpopulations of melanocytes. Am J Pathol **123**:195-203, 1986.

243 Le Douarin N: Cell migration in early vertebrate development studied in interspecific chimaeras. In Embryogenesis in mammals. Ciba Foundation Symposium. Amsterdam, 1976, Elsevier Excerpta Medica—North Holland, pp. 71-101.

244 Masson P: Pigment cells in man. In Miner RW (ed): The biology of melanomas (special publication). New York, 1948, The New York Academy of Sciences, vol. 4, pp. 15-51, 1948.

245 Miettinen M, Lehto V-P, Virtanen I: Presence of fibroblast-type intermediate filaments (vimentin) and absence of neurofilaments in pigmented nevi and malignant melanomas. J Cutan Pathol **10**:188-192, 1983.

246 Stefansson K, Wollman R, Jerkovic M: S-100 protein in soft-tissue tumors derived from Schwann cells and melanocytes. Am J Pathol **106**:261-268, 1982.

Nevi

246a Kanno J, Matsubara O, Kasuga T: Induction of melanogenesis in Schwann cell and perineural epithelium by 9, 10-dimethyl-1, 2-benzanthracene (DMBA) and 12-o-tetradecanoylphorbol-13-acetate (TPA) in BDF1 mice. Acta Pathol Jpn **37**:1297-1304, 1987.

247 Laidlaw GF, Murray MF: Melanoma studies. Theory of pigmented moles. Their relation to evolution of hair follicles. Am J Pathol **9**:827-838, 1933. Addendum: Theory of pigmented moles. Am J Pathol **10**:319-320, 1934.

248 Mackie RM, English J, Aitchison TC, Fitzsimons CP, Wilson P: The number and distribution of benign pigmented moles (melanocytic naevi) in a healthy British population. Br J Dermatol **113**:167-174, 1985.

249 Masson P: Les naevi pigmentaires, tumeurs nerveuses. Ann Anat Pathol (Paris) **3**:417-453, 657-696, 1926.

250 Masson P: My conception of cellular nevi. Cancer **4**:9-38, 1951.

Junctional, intradermal, and compound nevi

251 Bednár B: Storiform neurofibroma in the core of naevocellular naevi. J Pathol **101**:199-201, 1970.

252 Johnson WT, Helwig EB: Benign nevus cells in the capsule of lymph nodes. Cancer **23**:747-753, 1969.

253 Lund HZ, Stobbe GD: The natural history of the pigmented nevus. Factors of age and anatomic location. Am J Pathol **25**:1117-1155, 1949.

254 Ridolfi RL, Rosen PP, Thaler H: Nevus cell aggregates associated with lymph nodes. Estimated frequency and clinical significance. Cancer **39**:164-171, 1977.

255 Stegmaier OC, Montgomery H: Histopathologic studies of pigmented nevi in children. J Invest Dermatol **20**:51-64, 1953.

256 Weedon D: Unusual features of nevocellular nevi. J Cutan Pathol **9**:284-292, 1982.

256a Yaar M, Woodley DT, Gilchrest BA: Human nevocellular nevus cells are surrounded by basement membrane components. Immunohistologic studies of human nevus cells and melanocytes in vivo and in vitro. Lab Invest **58**:157-162, 1988.

Blue and cellular blue nevi

257 Epstein JI, Erlandson RA, Rosen PP: Nodal blue nevi. A study of three cases. Am J Surg Pathol **8**:907-915, 1984.

258 Goldman RL, Friedman NB: Blue nevus of the uterine cervix. Cancer **20**:210-214, 1967.

259 Harper JC, Waldron CA: Blue nevus of palate. Oral Surg **20**:145-149, 1965.

260 Jao W, Fretzin DF, Christ ML, Prinz LM: Blue nevus of the prostate gland. Arch Pathol **91**:187-192, 1971.

261 Leopold JG, Richards DB: The interrelationship of blue and common naevi. J Pathol Bacteriol **95**:37-46, 1968.

262 Masson P: Neuro-nevi "bleu." Arch De Vecchi Anat Patol **14**:1-28, 1950.

263 Rodriguez H, Ackerman LV: Cellular blue nevus. Cancer **21**:393-405, 1968.

Spitz nevus

264 Barr RJ, Morales RV, Graham JH: Desmoplastic nevus. A distinct histologic variant of mixed spindle cell and epithelioid cell nevus. Cancer **46**:557-564, 1980.

265 Echevarria R, Ackerman LV: Spindle and epithelioid cell nevi in the adult. A clinicopathologic report of 26 cases. Cancer **20**:175-189, 1967.

266 Howat AJ, Variend S: Lymphatic invasion in Spitz nevi. Am J Surg Pathol **9**:125-128, 1985.

267 Kernen JA, Ackerman LV: Spindle cell nevi and epithelioid cell nevi (so-called juvenile melanomas) in children and adults. A clinicopathologic study of 27 cases. Cancer **13**:612-625, 1960.

268 Paniago-Pereira C, Maize JC, Ackerman AB: Nevus of large spindle and/or epithelioid cells (Spitz's nevus). Arch Dermatol **114**:1811-1823, 1978.

269 Peters MS, Goellner JR: Spitz naevi and malignant melanomas of childhood and adolescence. Histopathology **10**:1289-1302, 1986.

270 Sagebiel RW, Chinn EK, Egbert BM: Pigmented spindle cell nevus. Clinical and histologic review of 90 cases. Am J Surg Pathol **8**:645-653, 1984.

271 Scott G, Chen KTK, Rosai J: Pseudoepitheliomatous hyperplasia in Spitz's nevi. A possible source of confusion with squamous cell carcinoma. Am J Dermatopathol (In press.)

272 Smith NP: The pigmented spindle cell tumor of Reed. An underdiagnosed lesion. Semin Diagn Pathol **4**:75-87, 1987.

273 Weedon D: Borderline melanocytic tumors. J Cutan Pathol **12**:266-270, 1985.

274 Weedon D, Little JH: Spindle and epithelioid cell nevi in children and adults. A review of 211 cases of the Spitz nevus. Cancer **40**:217-225, 1977.

Other nevi

275 Alper JC: Congenital nevi. The controversy rages on. Arch Dermatol **121**:734-735, 1985.

276 Demian S, Donnelley W, Monif GRG: Placental involvement in giant pigmented nevi (abstract). Am J Pathol **71**:14a, 1973.

277 Gardner WA Jr, Vazquez MD: Balloon cell melanoma. Arch Pathol **89**:470-472, 1970.

278 Hashimoto K: Ultrastructural studies of halo nevus. Cancer **34**:1653-1666, 1974.

279 Hendrickson MR, Ross JC: Neoplasms arising in congenital giant nevi. Morphologic study of seven cases and a review of the literature. Am J Surg Pathol **5**:109-135, 1981.

280 Kopf AW, Morrill SD, Silberberg I: Broad spectrum of leukoderma acquisitum centrifugum. Arch Dermatol **92**:14-35, 1965.

281 Mark GJ, Mihm MC Jr, Liteplo MG, Reed RJ, Clark WH Jr: Congenital melanocytic nevi of the small and garment type. Clinical, histologic and ultrastructural study. Hum Pathol **4**:395-418, 1973.

282 Masson P: Giant neuro-naevus of the hairy scalp. Ann Surg **93**:218-222, 1931.

283 Reed WB, Becker SW, Becker SW Jr, Nickel WR: Giant pigmented nevi, melanoma, and leptomeningeal melanocytosis. A clinical and histopathological study. Arch Dermatol **91**:100-119, 1965.

284 Rhodes AR, Silverman RA, Harrist TJ, Melski JW: A histologic comparison of congenital and acquired nevomelanocytic nevi. Arch Dermatol **121**:1266-1273, 1985.

285 Schrader WA, Helwig EB: Balloon cell nevi. Cancer **20**:1502-1514, 1967.

286 Silvers DN, Helwig EB: Melanocytic nevi in neonates. J Am Acad Dermatol **4**:166-175, 1981.

287 Slaughter JC, Hordman JM, Kempe LG, Earle KM: Neurocutaneous melanosis and leptomeningeal melanomatosis in children. Arch Pathol **88**:298-304, 1969.

287a Walsh MY, MacKie RM: Histological features of value in differentiating small congenital melanocytic naevi from acquired naevi. Histopathology **12**:145-154, 1988.

288 Wayte DM, Helwig EB: Halo nevi. Cancer **22**:69-90, 1968.

Treatment

289 Cox AJ, Walton RG: The induction of junctional changes in pigmented nevi. Arch Pathol **79**:428-434, 1965.

290 Davis NC, Herron J, McLeon GR: The macroscopic appearance of malignant melanoma of the skin. Med J Aust **2**:883-886, 1966.

291 Kornberg R, Ackerman AB: Pseudomelanoma. Recurrent melanocytic nevus following partial surgical removal. Arch Dermatol **111**:1588-1590, 1975.

292 Mundth ED, Gurainick EA, Raker JW: Malignant melanoma. A clinical study of 427 cases. Ann Surg **162**:15-28, 1965.

293 Wilson FC Jr, Andersonk PC: A dissenting view on the prophylactic removal of plantar and palmar nevi. Cancer 14:102-104, 1961.

Active and dysplastic nevi

294 Ackerman AB, Mihara I: Dysplasia, dysplastic melanocytes, dysplastic nevi, the dysplastic nevus syndrome, and the relation between dysplastic nevi and malignant melanomas. Hum Pathol 16:87-91, 1985.

295 Brodell RT, Santa Cruz DJ: Borderline and atypical melanocytic lesions. Semin Diagn Pathol 2:63-86, 1985.

296 Eady RAJ, Gilkes JJH, Jones EW: Eruptive naevi. Report of two cases, with enzyme histochemical, light and electron microscopical findings. Br J Dermatol 97:267-278, 1977.

297 Elder DE, Green MH, Guerry DP IV, Kraemer KH, Clark WH Jr: The dysplastic nevus syndrome. Our definition. Am J Dermatopathol 4:455-460, 1982.

298 Foucar E, Bentley TJ, Laube DW, Rosai J: A histopathologic evaluation of nevocellular nevi in pregnancy. Arch Dermatol 121:350-354, 1985.

299 Greene MH, Clark WH Jr, Tucker MA, Elder DE, Kraemer KH, Guerry DP IV, Witmer WK, Thompson J, Matozzo I, Fraser MC: Acquired precursors of cutaneous malignant melanoma. The familial dysplastic nevus syndrome. N Engl J Med 312:91-97, 1985.

300 Holman CDJ, Heenan PJ, Caruso V, Glancy RJ, Armstrong BK: Seasonal variation in the junctional component of pigmented naevi. Int J Cancer 31:213-215, 1983.

301 Kornberg R, Ackerman AB: Pseudomelanoma. Recurrent melanocytic nevus following partial surgical removal. Arch Dermatol 111:1588-1590, 1975.

302 Lynch HT, Fusaro RM, Pester J, Lynch JF: Familial atypical multiple mole melanoma (FAMMM) syndrome. Genetic heterogeneity and malignant melanoma. Br J Cancer 42:58-70, 1980.

302a Rhodes AR, Seki Y, Fitzpatrick TB, Stern RS: Melanosomal alterations in dysplastic melanocytic nevi. A quantitative, ultrastructural investigation. Cancer 61:358-369, 1988.

303 Tucker SB, Horstmann JP, Hertel B, Aranha G, Rosai J: Activation of nevi in patients with malignant melanoma. Cancer 46:822-827, 1980.

Malignant melanoma
General features

304 Anderson DE, Smith JL Jr, McBride CM: Hereditary aspects of malignant melanoma. JAMA 200:741-746, 1967.

305 Bader JL, Li FP, Olmstead PM, Strickman NA, Green DM: Childhood malignant melanoma. Incidence and etiology. Am J Pediatr Hematol Oncol 7:341-345, 1985.

306 Balasanov K, Andreev VC, Tchernozemski I: Malignant melanoma and vitiligo. Dermatologica 139:211-219, 1969.

307 Beral V, Evans S, Shaw H, Milton G: Cutaneous factors related to the risk of malignant melanoma. Br J Dermatol 109:165-172, 1983.

308 Eide J: Pathogenesis of generalized melanosis with melanuria and melanoptysis secondary to malignant melanoma. Histopathology 5:285-294, 1981.

309 Gussack GS, Reintgen D, Cox E, Fisher SR, Cole TB, Seigler HF: Cutaneous melanoma of the head and neck. A review of 399 cases. Arch Otolaryngol 109:803-808, 1983.

310 Helwig EB: Malignant melanoma in children. In Neoplasms of the skin and malignant melanoma. Proceedings of the 20th Annual Clinical Conferences on Cancer, Houston, Texas, 1975. Chicago, 1976, Year Book Medical Publishers, Inc. pp. 11-26.

311 Kahn LB, Donaldson RC: Multiple primary melanoma. Case report and study of tumor growth in vitro. Cancer 25:1162-1169, 1970.

312 Kopf AW, Bart RS, Rodríguez-Sains RS, Ackerman AB: Malignant melanoma. New York, 1979, Masson Publishing USA, Inc.

313 Lerman RI, Murray D, O'Hara JM, Booher RH, Foote FW Jr: Malignant melanoma of childhood. A clinicopathologic study and a report of 12 cases. Cancer 25:436-449, 1970.

314 McWhorter HE, Woolner LB: Pigmented nevi, juvenile melanomas, and malignant melanomas in children. Cancer 7:564-585, 1955.

315 Moseley HS, Giuliano AE, Storm FK III, Clark WH, Robinson DS, Morton DL: Multiple primary melanoma. Cancer 43:939-944, 1979.

316 Patterson H, Helwig EB: Subungual malignant melanoma. A clinical-pathologic study. Cancer 46:2074-2087, 1980.

317 Pratt CB, Palmer MK, Thatcher N, Crowther D: Malignant melanoma in children and adolescents. Cancer 47:392-397, 1981.

318 Reimer RR, Clark WH Jr, Greene MH, Ainsworth AM, Fraumeni JF Jr: Precursor lesions in familial melanoma. A new genetic preneoplastic syndrome. JAMA 239:744-746, 1978.

319 Sohn N, Gang H, Gumport SL, Goldstein M, Depisch LM: Generalized melanosis secondary to malignant melanoma. Report of a case with serum and tissue tyrosinase studies. Cancer 24:893-903, 1969.

320 Takematsu H, Obata M, Tomita Y, Kato T, Takahashi M, Abe R: Subungual melanoma. A clinicopathologic study of 16 Japanese cases. Cancer 55:2725-2731, 1985.

321 Tucker SB, Horstmann JP, Hertel B, Aranha G, Rosai J: Activation of nevi in patients with malignant melanoma. Cancer 46:822-827, 1980.

322 Unger SW, Wanebo HJ, Cooper PH: Multiple cutaneous malignant melanomas with features of primary melanoma. Ann Surg 193:245-249, 1981.

323 Urist MM, Balch CM, Soong S-J, Milton GW, Shaw HM, McGovern VJ, Murad TM, McCarthy WH, Maddox WA: Head and neck melanoma in 534 clinical stage I patients. A prognostic factors analysis and results of surgical treatment. Ann Surg 200:769-775, 1984.

324 Voorhess ML: Urinary excretion of DOPA and metabolites by patients with melanoma. Cancer 26:146-149, 1970.

Clinical appearance and clinicopathologic types

325 Ackerman AB, David KM: A unifying concept of malignant melanoma. Biologic aspects. Hum Pathol 17:438-440, 1986.

326 Arrington JH III, Reed RJ, Ichinose H, Krementz ET: Plantar lentiginous melanoma. A distinctive variant of human cutaneous malignant melanoma. Am J Surg Pathol 1:131-143, 1977.

327 Becker SW: Pitfalls in the diagnosis and treatment of melanoma. Arch Dermatol 69:11-30, 1954.

328 Clark WH Jr, Elder DE, Guerry DP IV, Epstein MN, Greene MH, Van Horn M: A study of tumor progression. The precursor lesions of superficial spreading and nodular melanoma. Hum Pathol 15:1147-1165, 1984.

329 Clark WH Jr, Elder DE, Van Horn M: The biologic forms of malignant melanoma. Hum Pathol 17:443-450, 1986.

330 Clark WH Jr, Mihm MC Jr: Lentigo maligna and lentigo-maligna melanoma. Am J Pathol 55:39-67, 1969.

331 Conley J, Lattes R, Orr W: Desmoplastic malignant melanoma (a rare variant of spindle cell melanoma). Cancer 28:914-936, 1971.

332 Labrecque PG, Hu C-H, Winkelmann RK: On the nature of desmoplastic melanoma. Cancer 38:1205-1213, 1976.

333 Levene A: An experience of malignant melanoma. Pathology 17:266-270, 1985.

334 Krementz ET, Reed RJ, Coleman WP III, Sutherland CM, Carter RD, Campbell M: Acral lentiginous melanoma. A clinicopathologic entity. Ann Surg 195:632-645, 1982.

335 Manci EA, Balch CM, Murad TM, Soong S-J: Polypoid melanoma, a virulent variant of the nodular growth pattern. Am J Clin Pathol 75:810-815, 1981.

336 McGovern VJ: The classification of melanoma and its relationship with prognosis. Pathology 2:85-98, 1970.

337 McGovern VJ: Malignant melanoma. Clinical and histological diagnosis. New York, 1976, John Wiley & Sons, Inc.

338 McGovern VJ: The nature of melanoma. A critical review. J Cutan Pathol 9:61-81, 1982.

339 McGovern VJ, Cochran AJ, Van Der Esch EP, Little JH, MacLennan R: The classification of malignant melanoma, its histological reporting and registration. A revision of the 1972 Sydney classification. Pathology 18:12-21, 1986.

340 McGovern VJ, Mihm MC Jr, Bailly C, Booth JC, Clark WH Jr, Cochran AJ, Hardy EG, Hicks JD, Levene A, Lewis MG, Little JH, Milton GW: The classification of malignant melanoma and its histologic reporting. Cancer 32:1446-1457, 1973.

341 McLean DI, Lew RA, Sober AJ, Mihm MC, Fitzpatrick TB: On the prognostic importance of white depressed areas in the primary lesion of superficial spreading melanoma. Cancer 43:157-161, 1979.

342 Mihm MC Jr, Clark WH Jr, From L: The clinical diagnosis, classification and histogenetic concepts of the early stages of cutaneous malignant melanomas. N Engl J Med 284:1078-1082, 1971.

343 Mihm MC Jr, Fitzpatrick TB: Early detection of malignant melanoma. Cancer 37:597-603, 1976.

344 Mihm MC Jr, Fitzpatrick TB, Lane Brown MM, Raker JW, Malt RA, Kaiser JS: Early detection of primary cutaneous malignant melanoma. N Engl J Med 289:989-996, 1973.

345 Mishima Y, Nakanishi T: Acral lentiginous melanoma and its precursor—heterogeneity of palmo-plantar melanomas. Pathology 17:258-265, 1985.

346 Paladugu RR, Winberg CD, Yonemoto RH: Acral lentiginous melanoma. A clinicopathologic study of 36 patients. Cancer 52:161-168, 1983.

347 Scrivner D, Oxenhandler RW, Lopez M, Perez-Mesa C: Plantar lentiginous melanoma. A clinicopathologic study. Cancer 60:2502-2509, 1987.

348 Seiji M, Takahashi M: Acral melanoma in Japan. Hum Pathol 13:607-609, 1982.

349 Søndergaard K: Histological type and biological behavior of primary cutaneous malignant melanoma. 1. An analysis of 1916 cases. Virchows Arch [Pathol Anat] 401:315-331, 1983.

350 Søndergaard K: Histological type and biological behavior of primary cutaneous malignant melanoma. 2. An analysis of 86 cases located on so-called acral regions as plantar, palmar, and sub-/parungual areas. Virchows Arch [Pathol Anat] **401**:333-343, 1983.

351 Valensi QJ: Desmoplastic malignant melanoma. A report on two additional cases. Cancer **39**:286-292, 1977.

352 Valensi QJ: Desmoplastic malignant melanoma. A light and electron microscopic study of two cases. Cancer **43**:1148-1155, 1979.

353 Wayte DM, Helwig EB: Melanotic freckle of Hutchinson. Cancer **21**:893-911, 1968.

Microscopic features

354 Allen AC, Spitz S: Malignant melanoma. A clinicopathological analysis of the criteria for diagnosis and prognosis. Cancer **6**:1-45, 1953.

355 Bhuta S, Mirra JM, Cochran AJ: Myxoid malignant melanoma. A previously undescribed histologic pattern noted in metastatic lesions and a report of four cases. Am J Surg Pathol **10**:203-211, 1986.

356 Caselitz J, Jänner M, Breitbart E, Weber K, Osborn M: Malignant melanomas contain only the vimentin type of intermediate filaments. Virchows Arch [Pathol Anat] **400**:43-51, 1983.

357 Cochran AJ, Wen D-R, Herschman HR: Occult melanoma in lymph nodes detected by antiserum to S-100 protein. Int J Cancer **34**:159-163, 1984.

358 Connors RC, Ackerman AB: Histologic pseudomalignancies of the skin. Arch Dermatol **112**:1767-1780, 1976.

359 Costa J, Rosai J, Philpott GW: Pigmentation of "amelanotic" melanoma in culture. A finding of diagnostic relevance. Arch Pathol **95**:371-373, 1973.

360 DiMaio SM, Mackay B, Smith JL Jr, Dickersin GR: Neurosarcomatous transformation in malignant melanoma. An ultrastructural study. Cancer **50**:2345-2354, 1982.

361 Dunn DR, Barth RF: Identification of melanoma cells by formaldehyde-induced fluorescence. Cancer **33**:701-706, 1974.

362 Erlandson RA: Ultrastructural diagnosis of amelanotic malignant melanoma. Aberrant melanosomes, myelin figures or lysosomes? Ultrastruct Pathol **11**:191-208, 1987.

363 From L, Hanna W, Kahn HJ, Gruss J, Marks A, Baumal R: Origin of the desmoplasia in desmoplastic malignant melanoma. Hum Pathol **14**:1072-1080, 1983.

364 Gatter KC, Ralfkiaer E, Skinner J, Brown D, Heryet A, Pulford KAF, Hou-Jensen K, Mason D: An immunocytochemical study of malignant melanoma and its differential diagnosis from other malignant tumours. J Clin Pathol **38**:1353-1357, 1985.

365 Guldhammer B, Nørgaard T: The differential diagnosis of intraepidermal malignant lesions using immunohistochemistry. Am J Dermatopathol **8**:295-301, 1986.

366 Herlyn M, Clark WH, Rodeck U, Mancianti ML, Jambrosic J, Koprowski H: Biology of tumor progression in human melanocytes. Lab Invest **56**:461-474, 1987.

367 Horton JJ, MacDonald DM: Balloon cell melanoma. A case report. Br J Dermatol **108**:617-619, 1983.

368 Hunter JAA, Zaynoun S, Paterson WD, Bleehen SS, Mackie R, Cochran AJ: Cellular fine structure in the invasive nodules of different histogenetic types of malignant melanoma. Br J Dermatol **98**:255-272, 1978.

369 Inoshita T, Youngberg GA: Fluorescence of melanoma cells. A useful diagnostic tool. Am J Clin Pathol **78**:311-315, 1982.

370 Kuehnl-Petzoldt Ch, Berger H, Wiebelt H: Verrucous-keratotic variations of malignant melanoma. A clinicopathological study. Am J Dermatopathol **4**:403-410, 1982.

371 Leader M, Patel J, Collins M, Henry K: Anti-α1-antichymotrypsin staining of 194 sarcomas, 38 carcinomas, and 17 malignant melanomas. Its lack of specificity as a tumour marker. Am J Surg Pathol **11**:133-139, 1987.

372 Levene A: On the histological diagnosis and prognosis of malignant melanoma. J Clin Pathol **33**:101-124, 1980.

373 Mintzis MM, Silvers DN: Ultrastructural study of superficial spreading melanoma and benign simulants. Cancer **42**:502-511, 1978.

374 Morishima T, Nagashima N, Hanawa S, Fukada E, Kanematsu S, Shibata A: Quick diagnosis of malignant melanoma with the touch-fluorescence method during operation. Cancer **57**:2037-2041, 1986.

375 Nakajima T, Watanabe S, Sato Y, Kameya T, Shimosato Y, Ishihara K: Immunohistochemical demonstration of S 100 protein in malignant melanoma and pigmented nevus, and its diagnostic application. Cancer **50**:912-918, 1982.

376 Nakanishi T, Hashimoto K: The differential reactivity of benign and malignant nevomelanocytic lesions with mouse monoclonal antibody TNKH1. Cancer **59**:1340-1344, 1987.

377 Natali PG, Aguzzi A, Veglia F, Imai K, Burlage RS, Giacomini P, Ferrone S: The impact of monoclonal antibodies on the study of human malignant melanoma. J Cutan Pathol **10**:514-528, 1983.

378 Natali PG, Roberts JT, Difilippo F, Bigotti A, Dent PB, Ferrone S, Liao S-K: Immunohistochemical detection of antigen in human primary and metastatic melanomas by the monoclonal antibody 140.240 and its possible prognostic significance. Cancer **59**:55-63, 1987.

379 Phillips ME, Margolis RJ, Merot Y, Sober AJ, Reed RJ, Muhlbauer JE, Mihm MC Jr: The spectrum of minimal deviation melanoma. A clinicopathologic study of 21 cases. Hum Pathol **17**:796-806, 1986.

380 Price NM, Rywlin AM, Ackerman AB: Histologic criteria for the diagnosis of superficial spreading malignant melanoma. Formulated on the basis of proven metastatic lesions. Cancer **38**:2434-2441, 1976.

381 Reed RJ, Leonard DD: Neurotropic melanoma. A variant of desmoplastic melanoma. Am J Surg Pathol **3**:301-311, 1979.

382 Reiman HM, Goellner JR, Woods JE, Mixter RC: Desmoplastic melanoma of the head and neck. Cancer **60**:2269-2274, 1987.

382a Sheibani K, Battifora H: Signet-ring cell melanoma. A rare morphologic variant of malignant melanoma. Am J Surg Pathol **12**:28-34, 1988.

383 Springall DR, Gu J, Cocchia D, Michetti F, Levene A, Levene MM, Marangos PJ, Bloom SR, Polak JM: The value of S-100 immunostaining as a diagnostic tool in human malignant melanomas. A comparative study using S-100 and neuron-specific enolase antibodies. Virchows Arch [Pathol Anat] **400**:331-343, 1983.

384 Van Duinen SG, Ruiter DJ, Hageman P, Vennegoor C, Dickersin GR, Scheffer E, Rümke P: Immunohistochemical and histochemical tools in the diagnosis of amelanotic melanoma. Cancer **53**:1566-1573, 1984.

384a Vennegoor C, Hageman Ph, Van Nouhuijs H, Ruiter DJ, Calafat J, Ringens PJ, Rumke Ph: A monoclonal antibody specific for cells of the melanocyte lineage. Am J Pathol **130**:179-192, 1988.

385 Wahlström T, Saxen L: Malignant skin tumors of neural crest origin. Cancer **38**:2022-2026, 1976.

386 Warner TFCS, Lloyd RV, Hafez GR, Angevine JM: Immunocytochemistry of neurotropic melanoma. Cancer **53**:254-257, 1984.

Biopsy and frozen section

387 Braun-Falco O, Korting HC, Konz B: Histological and cytological criteria in the diagnosis of malignant melanomas by cryostat sections. Virchows Arch [Pathol Anat] **393**:115-121, 1981.

388 Epstein E, Bragg K, Linden G: Biopsy and prognosis of malignant melanoma. JAMA **208**:1369-1371, 1969.

389 Little JH, Davis NC: Frozen section diagnosis of suspected malignant melanoma of the skin. Cancer **34**:1163-1172, 1974.

390 McGovern VJ, McPeak C, Reed RJ, Sugarbaker EV: Malignant melanoma. A clinical and pathologic symposium. Pathol Annu **17**(Pt 2):361-393, 1982.

391 Rampen FHJ, Kint A, Hunter JAA, Hulsebosch H-J: Primary management of melanoma. Br J Dermatol **111**:431-436, 1984.

392 Shafir R, Hiss J, Tsur H, Bubis JJ: Pitfalls in frozen section diagnosis of malignant melanoma. Cancer **51**:1168-1170, 1983.

Regression

393 Chang P, Knapper WH: Metastatic melanoma of unknown primary. Cancer **49**:1106-1111, 1982.

394 Gromet MA, Epstein WL, Blois MS: The regressing thin malignant melanoma. A distinctive lesion with metastatic potential. Cancer **42**:2282-2292, 1978.

395 McGovern VJ: Spontaneous regression of melanoma. Pathology **7**:91-99, 1975.

396 Smith JL Jr, Stehlin JS Jr: Spontaneous regression of primary malignant melanomas with regional metastases. Cancer **18**:1399-1415, 1965.

Atypical in situ melanocytic lesions

397 Ackerman AB: Malignant melanoma in situ. The flat, curable stage of malignant melanoma. Pathology **17**:298-300, 1985.

398 Cook MG, Robertson I: Melanocytic dysplasia and melanoma. Histopathology **9**:647-658, 1985.

399 McGovern VJ, Shaw HM, Milton GW: Histogenesis of malignant melanoma with an adjacent component of the superficial spreading type. Pathology **17**:251-254, 1985.

399a Rywlin AM: Intraepithelial melanocytic neoplasia (IMN) versus intraepithelial atypical melanocytic proliferation (IAMP). Am J Dermatopathol **10**:92-93, 1988.

Spread and metastases

400 de la Monte SM, Moore GW, Hutchins GM: Patterned distribution of metastases from malignant melanoma in humans. Cancer Res **43**:3427-3433, 1983.

401 Kornberg R, Harris M, Ackerman AB: Epidermotropically metastatic malignant melanoma. Differentiating malignant melanoma metastatic to the epidermis from malignant melanoma primary in the epidermis. Arch Dermatol **114**:67-69, 1978.

402 Reichert CM, Rosenberg SA, Weber BL, Costa J: Malignant melanoma. A search for occult lymph node metastases. Hum Pathol **12**:449-451, 1981.

403 Roses DF, Harris MN, Rigel D, Carrey Z, Friedman R, Kopf AW: Local and in-transit metastases following definitive excision for primary cutaneous malignant melanoma. Ann Surg **198**:65-69, 1983.

404 Steiner A, Wolf C, Pehamberger H, Wolff K: Late metastases of cutaneous malignant melanoma. Br J Dermatol **114**:737-740, 1986.

Treatment

405 Ackerman AB, Scheiner AM: How wide and deep is wide and deep enough? A critique of surgical practice in excisions of primary cutaneous malignant melanoma. Hum Pathol **14**:743-744, 1983.

406 Aitken DR, Clausen K, Klein JP, James AG: The extent of primary melanoma excision. A re-evaluation—how wide is wide? Ann Surg **198**:634-641, 1983.

407 Balch CM, Murad TM, Soong S-J, Ingalls AL, Richards PC, Maddox WA: Tumor thickness as a guide to surgical management of clinical stage I melanoma patients. Cancer **43**:883-888, 1979.

408 Cosimi AB, Sober AJ, Mihm MC, Fitzpatrick TB: Conservative surgical management of superficially invasive cutaneous melanoma. Cancer **53**:1256-1259, 1984.

409 Dancuart F, Harwood AR, Fitzpatrick PJ: The radiotherapy of lentigo maligna and lentigo maligna melanoma of the head and neck. Cancer **45**:2279-2283, 1980.

410 Elder DE, Guerry DP IV, Van Horn M, Hurwitz S, Zehngebot L, Goldman LI, LaRossa D, Hamilton R, Bondi EE, Clark WH Jr: The role of lymph node dissection for clinical stage I malignant melanoma of intermediate thickness (1.51-3.99 mm). Cancer **56**:413-418, 1985.

411 Kelly JW, Sagebiel RW, Calderon W, Murillo L, Dakin RL, Blois MS: The frequency of local recurrence and microsatellites as a guide to reexcision margins for cutaneous malignant melanoma. Ann Surg **200**:759-763, 1984.

412 McNeer G: Malignant melanoma. Surg Gynecol Obstet **120**:343-344, 1965.

413 Sandeman TF: The radical treatment of enlarged lymph nodes in malignant melanoma. Am J Roentgenol Radium Ther Nucl Med **97**:969-979, 1966.

414 Sim FH, Taylor WF, Ivins JC, Pritchard DJ, Soule EH: A prospective randomized study of the efficacy of routine elective lymphadenectomy in management of malignant melanoma. Preliminary results. Cancer **41**:948-956, 1978.

415 Sim FH, Taylor WF, Pritchard DJ, Soule EH: Lymphadenectomy in the management of stage I malignant melanoma. A prospective randomized study. Mayo Clin Proc **61**:697-705, 1986.

416 Stahlin JS Jr: Malignant melanoma. An appraisal. Surgery **64**:1149-1157, 1968.

417 Urist MM, Balch CM, Soong S-J, Shaw HM, Milton GW, Maddox WA: The influence of surgical margins and prognostic factors predicting the risk of local recurrence in 3445 patients with primary cutaneous melanoma. Cancer **55**:1398-1402, 1985.

418 Veronesi U, Adamus J, Aubert C, Bajetta E, Beretta G, Bonadonna G, Bufalino R, Cascinelli N, Cocconi G, Durand J, DeMarsillac J, Ikonopisov RL, Kiss B, Lejeune F, MacKie R, Madej G, Mulder H, Mechl Z, Milton GW, Morabito A, Peter H, Priario J, Paul E, Rumke P, Sertoli R, Tomin R: A randomized trial of adjuvant chemotherapy and immunotherapy in cutaneous melanoma. N Engl J Med **307**:913-916, 1982.

419 Veronesi U, Adamus J, Bandiera DC, Brennhovd IO, Caceres E, Cascinelli N, Claudio F, Ikonopisov RL, Javorski VV, Kirov S, Kulakowski A, Lacour J, Lejeune F, Mechl Z, Morabito A, Rodé I, Sergeev S, van Slooten E, Szczygiel K, Trapeznikov NN, Wagner RI: Stage I melanoma of the limbs. Immediate versus delayed node dissection. Tumori **66**:373-396, 1980.

420 Veronesi U, Adamus J, Bandiera DC, Brennhovd IO, Caceres E, Cascinelli N, Claudio F, Ikonopisov RL, Javorski VV, Kirov S, Kulakowski A, Lacour J, Lejeune F, Mechl Z, Morabito A, Rodé I, Sergeev S, van Slooten E, Szczygiel K, Trapeznikov NN, Wagner RI: Delayed regional lymph node dissection in stage I melanoma of the skin of the lower extremities. Cancer **49**:2420-2430, 1982.

Prognosis

421 Balch CM, Murad TM, Soong S-J, Ingalls AL, Halpern NB, Maddox WA: A multifactorial analysis of melanoma. Prognostic histopathological features comparing Clark's and Breslow's staging methods. Ann Surg **188**:732-742, 1978.

422 Balch CM, Wilkerson JA, Murad TM, Soong S-J, Ingalls AL, Maddox WA: The prognostic significance of ulceration of cutaneous melanoma. Cancer **45**:3012-3017, 1980.

423 Breslow A: Thickness, cross-sectional areas and depth of invasion in the prognosis of malignant melanoma. Ann Surg **172**:902-908, 1970.

424 Breslow A: Tumor thickness, level of invasion and node dissection in stage I cutaneous melanoma. Ann Surg **182**:572-575, 1975.

425 Breslow A: Problems in the measurement of tumor thickness and level of invasion in cutaneous melanoma. Hum Pathol **8**:1-2, 1977.

426 Breslow A, Cascinelli N, van der Esch EP, Morabito A: Stage I melanoma of the limbs. Assessment of prognosis by levels of invasion and maximum thickness. Tumori **64**:273-284, 1978.

427 Chang P, Knapper WH: Metastatic melanoma of unknown primary. Cancer **49**:1106-1111, 1982.

428 Clark WH Jr, From L, Bernardino EA, Mihm MC: The histogenesis and biologic behavior of primary human malignant melanomas of the skin. Cancer Res **29**:705-726, 1969.

429 Clark WH Jr, Goldman LI, Mastrangelo MJ: Human malignant melanoma. Clinical Oncology Monographs. New York, 1979. Grune & Stratton, Inc.

430 Cochran AJ: Histology and prognosis in malignant melanoma. J Pathol **97**:459-468, 1969.

431 Coleman WP, Loria PR, Reed RJ, Krementz ET: Acral lentiginous melanoma. Arch Dermatol **116**:773-776, 1980.

432 Cooper PH, Wanebo HJ, Hagar RW: Regression in thin malignant melanoma. Microscopic diagnosis and prognostic importance. Arch Dermatol **121**:1127-1131, 1985.

433 Costa A, Silvestrini R, Grignolio E, Clemente C, Attili A, Testori A: Cell kinetics as a prognostic tool in patients with metastatic malignant melanoma of the skin. Cancer **60**:2797-2800, 1987.

434 Friedman RJ, Rigel DS, Kopf AW, Lieblich L, Lew R, Harris MN, Roses DF, Gumport SL, Ragaz A, Waldo E, Levine J, Levenstein M, Koenig R, Bart RS, Trau H: Favorable prognosis for malignant melanomas associated with acquired melanocytic nevi. Arch Dermatol **119**:455-462, 1983.

435 Funk W, Schmoeckel CH, Hölzel D, Braun-Falco O: Prognostic classification of malignant melanoma by clinical criteria. Br J Dermatol **111**:129-138, 1984.

436 Gromet MA, Epstein WL, Blois MS: The regressing thin malignant melanoma. A distinctive lesion with metastatic potential. Cancer **42**:2282-2292, 1978.

437 Hagen EC, Vennegoor C, Schlingemann RO, Van Der Velde EA, Ruiter DJ: Correlation of histopathological characteristics with staining patterns in human melanoma assessed by (monoclonal) antibodies reactive on paraffin sections. Histopathology **10**:689-700, 1986.

438 Harrist TJ, Rigel DS, Day CL Jr, Sober AJ, Lew RA, Rhodes AR, Harris MN, Kopf AW, Friedman RJ, Golomb FM, Cosimi AB, Gorstein F, Malt RA, Wood WC, Postel A, Hennessey P, Gumport SL, Roses DF, Mintzis MM, Raker JW, Fitzpatrick TB, Mihm MC Jr: "Microscopic satellites" are more highly associated with regional lymph node metastases than is primary melanoma thickness. Cancer **53**:2183-2187, 1984.

439 Holmes EC, Clark W, Morton DL, Eilber FR, Bochow AJ: Regional lymph node metastases and the level of invasion of primary melanoma. Cancer **37**:199-201, 1976.

440 Kelly JW, Sagebiel RW, Blois MS: Regression in malignant melanoma. A histologic feature without independent prognostic significance. Cancer **56**:2287-2291, 1985.

441 Lee Y-TN: Diagnosis, treatment and prognosis of early melanoma. The importance of depth of microinvasion. Ann Surg **191**:87-97, 1980.

442 Magnus K: Prognosis in malignant melanoma of the skin. Significance of stage of disease, anatomical site, sex, age and period of diagnosis. Cancer **40**:389-397, 1977.

442a Mascaro JM, Molgo M, Castel T, Castro J: Plasma cells within the infiltrate of primary cutaneous malignant melanoma of the skin. A confirmation of its histoprognostic value. Am J Dermatopathol **9**:497-499, 1987.

443 McGovern VJ, Shaw HM, Milton GW: Prognosis in patients with thin malignant melanoma. Influence of regression. Histopathology **7**:673-680, 1983.

444 McGovern VJ, Shaw HM, Milton GW: Prognostic significance of a polypoid configuration in malignant melanoma. Histopathology **7**:663-672, 1983.

445 McGovern VJ, Shaw HM, Milton GW, Farago GA: Prognostic significance of the histological features of malignant melanoma. Histopathology **3**:385-393, 1979.

446 McGovern VJ, Shaw HM, Milton GW, McCarthy WH: Ulceration and prognosis in cutaneous malignant melanoma. Histopathology **6**:399-407, 1982.

447 Naruns PL, Nizze JA, Cochran AJ, Lee MB, Morton DL: Recurrence potential of thin primary melanomas. Cancer **57**:545-548, 1986.

448 O'Doherty CJ, Prescott RJ, White H, McIntyre M, Hunter JAA: Sex differences in presentation of cutaneous malignant melanoma and in survival from stage I disease. Cancer **58**:788-792, 1986.

449 Pack GT, Scharnagel IM: The prognosis for malignant melanoma in the pregnant woman. Cancer **4:**324-334, 1951.

450 Reed KM, Bronstein BR, Mihm MC Jr, Sober AJ: Prognosis for polypoidal melanoma is determined by primary tumor thickness. Cancer **57:**1201-1203, 1986.

451 Rogers GS, Kopf AW, Rigel DS, Friedman RJ, Levine JL, Levenstein M, Bart RS, Mintzis MM: Effect of anatomical location on prognosis in patients with clinical stage I melanoma. Arch Dermatol **119:**644-649, 1983.

452 Shaw HM, Balch CM, Soong S-J, Milton GW, McCarthy WH: Prognostic histopathological factors in malignant melanoma. Pathology **17:**271-274, 1985.

453 Shiu MH, Schottenfeld D, Maclean B, Fortner JG: Adverse effects of pregnancy on melanoma. A reappraisal. Cancer **37:**181-187, 1976.

454 Solomon AR, Ellis CN, Headington JT: An evaluation of vertical growth in thin superficial spreading melanomas by sequential serial microscopic sections. Cancer **52:**2338-2341, 1983.

455 Søndergaard K: Depth of invasion and tumor thickness in primary cutaneous malignant melanoma. A study of 2012 cases. Acta Pathol Microbiol Immunol Scand [A] **93:**49-55, 1985.

456 Van Der Esch EP, Cascinelli N, Preda F, Morabita A, Bufalino R: Stage I melanoma of the skin. Evaluation of prognosis according to histologic characteristics. Cancer **48:**1668-1673, 1981.

457 Wanebo HJ, Fortner JG, Woodruff J, MacLean B, Binkowski E: Selection of the optimum surgical treatment of stage I melanoma by depth of microinvasion. Use of the combined microstage technique (Clark-Breslow). Ann Surg **182:**302-315, 1975.

458 Wanebo HJ, Woodruff J, Fortner JG: Malignant melanoma of the extremities. A clinicopathologic study using levels of invasion (microstage). Cancer **35:**666-676, 1975.

459 White LP, Linden G, Breslow L, Harzfeld L: Studies on melanoma. The effect of pregnancy on survival in human melanoma. JAMA **177:**235-238, 1961.

460 Woods JE, Soule EH, Creagan ET: Metastasis and death in patients with thin melanomas (less than 0.76 mm). Ann Surg **198:**63-64, 1983.

Pigmentation in other skin tumors

461 Mishima Y, Pinkus H: Benign mixed tumor of melanocytes and malpighian cells. Melanoacanthoma. Its relationship to Bloch's benign nonnevoid melanoepithelioma. Arch Dermatol **81:**539-550, 1960.

NEUROENDOCRINE CELLS
Merkel cell tumor

462 Battifora H, Silva EG: The use of antikeratin antibodies in the immunohistochemical distinction between neuroendocrine (Merkel cell) carcinoma of the skin, lymphoma, and oat cell carcinoma. Cancer **58:**1040-1046, 1986.

463 Frigerio B, Capella C, Eusebi V, Tenti P, Azzopardi JG: Merkel cell carcinoma of the skin. The structure and origin of normal Merkel cells. Histopathology **7:**229-249, 1983.

464 Goepfert H, Remmler D, Silva E, Wheeler B: Merkel cell carcinoma (endocrine carcinoma of the skin) of the head and neck. Arch Otolaryngol **110:**707-712, 1984.

465 Gomez LG, DiMaio S, Silva EG, Mackay B: Association between neuroendocrine (Merkel cell) carcinoma and squamous carcinoma of the skin. Am J Surg Pathol **7:**171-177, 1983.

466 Gu J, Polak JM, Tapia FJ, Marangos PJ, Pearse AGE: Neuron-specific enolase in the Merkel cells of mammalian skin. The use of specific antibody as a simple and reliable histologic marker. Am J Pathol **104:**63-68, 1981.

467 Hofler H, Kerl H, Lackinger E, Helleis G, Denk H: The intermediate filament cytoskeleton of cutaneous neuroendocrine carcinoma (Merkel cell tumour). Immunohistochemical and biochemical analyses. Virchows Arch [Pathol Anat] **406:**339-350, 1985.

468 Layfield L, Ulich T, Liao S, Barr R, Cheng L, Lewin KL: Neuroendocrine carcinoma of the skin. An immunohistochemical study of tumor markers and neuroendocrine products. J Cutan Pathol **13:**268-273, 1986.

469 Leff EL, Brooks JSJ, Trojanowski JQ: Expression of neurofilament and neuron-specific enolase in small cell tumors of skin using immunohistochemistry. Cancer **56:**625-631, 1985.

470 Pilotti S, Rilke F, Lombardi L: Neuroendocrine (Merkel cell) carcinoma of the skin. Am J Surg Pathol **6:**243-254, 1982.

471 Raaf JH, Urmacher C, Knapper WK, Shiu MH, Cheng EWK: Trabecular (Merkel cell) carcinoma of the skin. Treatment of primary, recurrent, and metastatic disease. Cancer **57:**178-182, 1986.

472 Sibley RK, Dahl D: Primary neuroendocrine (Merkel cell?) carcinoma of the skin. II. An immunocytochemical study of 21 cases. Am J Surg Pathol **9:**109-116, 1985.

473 Sibley RK, Dehner LP, Rosai J: Primary neuroendocrine (Merkel cell?) carcinoma of the skin. I. A clinicopathologic and ultrastructural study of 43 cases. Am J Surg Pathol **9:**95-108, 1985.

474 Sibley RK, Rosai J, Foucar E, Dehner LP, Bosl G: Neuroendocrine (Merkel cell) carcinoma of the skin. A histologic and ultrastructural study of two cases. Am J Surg Pathol **4:**211-221, 1980.

475 Sidhu GS, Feiner H, Flotte TJ, Mullins JD, Schaefler K, Schultenhover SJ: Merkel cell neoplasms. Histology, electron microscopy, biology, and histogenesis. Am J Dermatopathol **2:**101-119, 1980.

476 Silva E, Mackay B: Neuroendocrine (Merkel cell) carcinomas of the skin. An ultrastructural study of nine cases. Ultrastruct Pathol **2:**1-9, 1981.

477 Silva EG, Mackay B, Goepfert H, Burgess MA, Fields RS: Endocrine carcinoma of the skin (Merkel cell carcinoma). Pathol Annu **19**(Pt 2):1-30, 1984.

478 Silva EG, Ordóñez NG, Lechago J: Immunohistochemical studies in endocrine carcinoma of the skin. Am J Clin Pathol **81:**558-562, 1984.

479 Tang C-K, Toker C: Trabecular carcinoma of the skin. An ultrastructural study. Cancer **42:**2311-2321, 1978.

480 Toker C: Trabecular carcinoma of the skin. Arch Dermatol **105:**107-110, 1972.

481 Warner TFCS, Uno H, Hafez GR, Burgess J, Bolles C, Lloyd RV, Oka M: Merkel cells and Merkel cell tumors. Ultrastructure, immunocytochemistry and review of the literature. Cancer **52:**238-245, 1983.

482 Wick MR, Goellner JR, Scheithauer BW, Thomas JR III, Sanchez NP, Schroeter AL: Primary neuroendocrine carcinomas of the skin (Merkel cell tumors). A clinical, histologic, and ultrastructural study of thirteen cases. Am J Clin Pathol **79:**6-13, 1983.

483 Wick MR, Kaye VN, Sibley RK, Tyler R, Frizzera G: Primary neuroendocrine carcinoma and small-cell malignant lymphoma of the skin. A discriminant immunohistochemical comparison. J Cutan Pathol **13:**347-358, 1986.

484 Wick MR, Scheithauer BW, Kovacs K: Neuron-specific enolase in neuroendocrine tumors of the thymus, bronchus, and skin. Am J Clin Pathol **79:**703-707, 1983.

Other neuroendocrine tumors

485 Argenyi ZB, Bergfeld WF, McMahon JT, Goeken JA, Garewal GS: Primitive neuroectodermal tumor in the skin with features of neuroblastoma in an adult patient. J Cutan Pathol **13:**420-430, 1986.

486 Collina G, Quarto F, Eusebi V: Trabecular carcinoid of the skin with cellular stroma. Am J Dermatopathol (In press.)

487 Gould VE, Moll R, Moll I, Lee I, Franke WW: Neuroendocrine (Merkel) cells of the skin. Hyperplasias, dysplasias, and neoplasms. Lab Invest **52:**334-353, 1985.

488 Smith PA, Chappell RH: Another possible primary carcinoid tumour of skin? Virchows Arch [Pathol Anat] **408:**99-103, 1985.

489 van Dijk C, ten Seldam REJ: A possible primary cutaneous carcinoid. Cancer **36:**1016-1020, 1975.

DERMIS
Fibroblastic tumors and tumorlike conditions

490 Blackburn WR, Cosman B: Histologic basis of keloid and hypertrophic scar differentiation. Clinicopathologic correlation. Arch Pathol **82:**65-71, 1966.

491 Eddy RJ, Petro JA, Tomasek JJ: Evidence for the nonmuscle nature of the "myofibroblast" of granulation tissue and hypertropic scar. An immunofluorescence study. Am J Pathol **130:**252-260, 1988.

492 Santa Cruz DJ, Ulbright TM: Mucin-like changes in keloids. Am J Clin Pathol **75:**18-22, 1981.

Fibrohistiocytic tumors and tumorlike conditions
Benign fibrous histiocytoma

493 Black WC III, McGavran MH, Graham P: Nodular subepidermal fibrosis. Arch Surg **98:**296-300, 1969.

494 Burgdort WHC, Duray P, Rosai J: Immunohistochemical identification of lysozyme in cutaneous lesions of alleged histiocytic nature. Am J Clin Pathol **75:**162-167, 1981.

494a Cerio R, Spaull J, Jones EW: Dermatofibroma. A tumor of dermal dendrocytes? (abstract) J Cutan Pathol **14:**351, 1987.

495 Dalziel K, Marks R: Hair follicle-like change over histiocytomas. Am J Dermatopathol **8:**462-466, 1986.

496 Goette DK, Helwig EB: Basal cell carcinomas and basal cell carcinoma-like changes overlying dermatofibromas. Arch Dermatol **111:**589-592, 1975.

497 Gonzalez BS: Benign fibrous histiocytoma of the skin. An immunohistochemical analysis of 30 cases. Pathol Res Pract **180:**486-489, 1985.

498 Leyva WH, Santa Cruz DJ: Atypical cutaneous fibrous histiocytoma. Am J Dermatopathol **8:**467-471, 1986.

499 Santa Cruz DJ, Kyriakos M: Aneurysmal ("angiomatoid") fibrous histiocytoma of the skin. Cancer **47**:2053-2061, 1981.

500 Schoenfield RJ: Epidermal proliferation overlying histiocytomas. Arch Dermatol **90**:266-270, 1964.

501 Schwob VS, Santa Cruz DJ: Palisading cutaneous fibrous histiocytoma. J Cutan Pathol **13**:403-407, 1986.

502 Tamada S, Ackerman AB: Dermatofibroma with monster cells. Am J Dermatopathol **9**:380-387, 1987.

Atypical fibroxanthoma

503 Bourne RG: Paradoxical fibrosarcoma of skin (pseudosarcoma). A review of 13 cases. Med J Aust **1**:504-510, 1963.

504 Dahl I: Atypical fibroxanthoma of the skin. A clinicopathological study of 57 cases. Acta Pathol Microbiol Scand [A] **84**:183-197, 1976.

505 Evans HL, Smith JL: Spindle cell squamous carcinomas and sarcoma-like tumors of the skin. A comparative study of 38 cases. Cancer **45**:2687-2697, 1980.

506 Fretzin DF, Helwig EB: Atypical fibroxanthoma of the skin. A clinicopathologic study of 140 cases. Cancer **31**:1541-1552, 1973.

507 Helwig EB, May D: Atypical fibroxanthoma of the skin with metastasis. Cancer **57**:368-376, 1986.

508 Hudson AW, Winkelmann RK: Atypical fibroxanthoma of the skin. A reappraisal of 19 cases in which the original diagnosis was spindle-cell squamous carcinoma. Cancer **29**:413-422, 1972.

509 Kempson RL, McGavran MH: Atypical fibroxanthomas of the skin. Cancer **17**:1463-1471, 1964.

510 Kuwano H, Hashimoto H, Enjoji M: Atypical fibroxanthomas distinguishable from spindle cell carcinoma in sarcoma-like skin lesions. A clinicopathologic and immunohistochemical study of 21 cases. Cancer **55**:172-180, 1985.

511 Leong AS-Y, Milios J: Atypical fibroxanthoma of the skin. A clinicopathological and immunohistochemical study and a discussion of its histogenesis. Histopathology **11**:463-475, 1987.

512 Rachmaninoff N, McDonald JR, Cook JC: Sarcoma-like tumors of the skin following irradiation. Am J Clin Pathol **36**:427-437, 1961.

512a Silvis NG, Swanson PE, Manivel JC, Kaye VN, Wick MR: Spindle-cell and pleomorphic neoplasms of the skin. A clinicopathologic and immunohistochemical study of 30 cases, with emphasis on "atypical fibroxanthomas." Am J Dermatopathol **10**:9-19, 1988.

Dermatofibrosarcoma protuberans

513 Adams JT, Saltzstein SL: Metastasizing dermatofibrosarcoma protuberans. Report of two cases. Am Surg **29**:879-886, 1963.

514 Frierson HF, Cooper PH: Myxoid variant of dermatofibrosarcoma protuberans. Am J Surg Pathol **7**:445-450, 1983.

515 Hashimoto K, Brownstein MH, Jakobiec FA: Dermatofibrosarcoma protuberans. A tumor with perineural and endroneural cell features. Arch Dermatol **110**:874-885, 1974.

516 Ozzello L, Hamels J: The histiocytic nature of dermatofibrosarcoma protuberans. Tissue culture and electron microscopic study. Am J Clin Pathol **65**:136-148, 1976.

517 Taylor HB, Helwig EB: Dermatofibrosarcoma protuberans. Cancer **15**:717-725, 1962.

Malignant fibrous histiocytoma

518 Kuwano H, Hashimoto H, Enjoji M: Atypical fibroxanthomas distinguishable from spindle cell carcinoma in sarcoma-like skin lesions. A clinicopathologic and immunohistochemical study of 21 cases. Cancer **55**:172-180, 1985.

519 Routh A, Hickman BT, Johnson WW: Malignant fibrous histiocytoma arising from chronic ulcer. Arch Dermatol **121**:529-531, 1985.

Xanthoma

519a Altman J, Winkelman RI: Xanthoma disseminatum. Arch Dermatol **86**:582-596, 1962.

519b Cooper PH: Eruptive xanthoma. A microscopic simulant of granuloma annulare. J Cutan Pathol **13**:207-215, 1986.

519c Duray PH, Johnston YE: Verruciform xanthoma of the nose in an elderly male. Am J Dermatopathol **8**:237-240, 1986.

Juvenile xanthogranuloma (nevoxanthoendothelioma)

520 Seo IS, Min KW, Mirkin LD: Juvenile xanthogranuloma. Ultrastructural and immunocytochemical studies. Arch Pathol Lab Med **110**:911-915, 1986.

521 Sonoda T, Hashimoto H, Enjoji M: Juvenile xanthogranuloma. Clinicopathologic analysis and immunohistochemical study of 57 patients. Cancer **56**:2280-2286, 1985.

522 Tahan SR, Pastel-Levy C, Bahn A, Mihm MC: Juvenile xanthogranuloma. Characterization of the clinical, histopathologic, and immunohistochemical features as found in 34 cases; evidence of immunologic participation (abstract). J Cutan Pathol **14**:375, 1987.

Other histiocytic proliferations

523 Azulay RD: Histopathology of skin lesions in leprosy. Int J Lepr **39**:244, 1971.

524 Heathcote JG, Guenther LC, Wallace AC: Multicentric reticulohistiocytosis. A report of a case and a review of the pathology. Pathology **17**:601-608, 1985.

525 Mihm MC Jr, Clark WH, Reed RJ: The histiocytic infiltrates of the skin. Hum Pathol **5**:45-54, 1974.

526 Tani M, Hori K, Nakanishi T, Iwasaki T, Ogawa Y, Jimbo T: Multicentric reticulohistiocytosis. Electron microscopic and ultracytochemical studies. Arch Dermatol **117**:495-499, 1981.

527 Thawerani H, Sanchez RL, Rosai J, Dorfman RF: The cutaneous manifestations of sinus histiocytosis with massive lymphadenopathy. Arch Dermatol **114**:191-197, 1978.

Smooth muscle tumors

528 Dahl I, Angervall L: Cutaneous and subcutaneous leiomyosarcoma. A clinicopathologic study of 47 patients. Pathol Europ **9**:307-315, 1974.

529 Fields JP, Helwig EB: Leiomyosarcoma of the skin and subcutaneous tissue. Cancer **47**:156-169, 1981.

530 Hachisuga T, Hashimoto H, Enjoji M: Angioleiomyoma. A clinicopathologic reappraisal of 562 cases. Cancer **54**:126-130, 1984.

531 Montgomery H, Winkelmann RK: Smooth muscle tumors of the skin. Arch Dermatol **79**:32-41, 1959.

532 Varela-Duran J, Oliva H, Rosai J: Vascular leiomyosarcoma. The malignant counterpart of vascular leiomyoma. Cancer **44**:1684-1691, 1979.

Peripheral nerve tumors

532a Dabski K, Reiman HM, Muller SA: Neurofibrosarcoma of the skin. A report of 13 cases (abstract). J Cutan Pathol **14**:354, 1987.

533 Enzinger FM, Weiss SW: Soft tissue tumors. St. Louis, 1983, The C.V. Mosby Co., pp. 644-648.

534 Gallager RL, Helwig EB: Neurothekeoma—a benign cutaneous tumor of neural origin. Am J Clin Pathol **74**:759-764, 1980.

535 Holden CA, Wilson Jones E, MacDonald DM: Cutaneous lobular neuromyxoma. Br J Dermatol **106**:211-215, 1982.

Vascular tumors and tumorlike conditions

536 Johnson WC: Pathology of cutaneous vascular tumors. Int J Dermatol **15**:239-270, 1976.

536a Ryan TJ, Cherry GW: Vascular birthmarks. Pathogenesis and management. New York, 1987, Oxford Press.

Hemangioma

537 Connelly MG, Winkelmann RK: Acral arteriovenous tumor. A clinicopathologic review. Am J Surg Pathol **9**:15-21, 1985.

538 Imperial R, Helwig E: Angiokeratoma. A clinicopathologic study. Arch Dermatol **95**:166-175, 1967.

539 Imperial R, Helwig E: Verrucous hemangioma. A clinico-pathologic study of 21 cases. Arch Dermatol **96**:247-253, 1967.

540 Johnson WC: Pathology of cutaneous vascular tumors. Int J Dermatol **15**:239-270, 1976.

Lymphangioma

541 Flanagan BP, Helwig EB: Cutaneous lymphangioma. Arch Dermatol **113**:24-30, 1977.

542 Peachey R, Whimster I: Lymphangioma of skin. A review of 65 cases. Br J Dermatol **83**:519-527, 1970.

543 Watanabe M, Kishiyama K, Ohkawara A: Acquired progressive lymphangioma. J Am Acad Dermatol **8**:663-667, 1983.

544 Whimster IW: The pathology of lymphangioma circumscriptum. Br J Dermatol **94**:473-486, 1976.

Lobular capillary hemangioma

545 Cooper PH, McAllister HA, Helwig EB: Intravenous pyogenic granuloma. Am J Surg Pathol **3**:221-228, 1979.

546 Cooper PH, Mills SE: Subcutaneous granuloma pyogenicum. Lobular capillary hemangioma. Arch Dermatol **118**:30-33, 1982.

547 Mills SE, Cooper PH, Fechner RE: Lobular capillary hemangioma. The underlying lesion of pyogenic granuloma. A study of 73 cases from the oral and nasal mucous membranes. Am J Surg Pathol **4**:471-479, 1980.

548 Nappi O, Wick MR: Disseminated lobular capillary hemangioma (pyogenic granuloma). A clinicopathologic study of two cases. Am J Dermatopathol 8:379-385, 1986.

549 Padilla RS, Orkin M, Rosai J: Acquired "tufted" angioma (progressive capillary hemangioma). A distinctive clinicopathologic entity related to lobular capillary hemangioma. Am J Dermatopathol 9:292-300, 1987.

550 Swerlick RA, Cooper PH: Pyogenic granuloma (lobular capillary hemangioma) within port-wine stains. J Am Acad Dermatol 8:627-630, 1983.

551 Warner J, Wilson Jones E: Pyogenic granuloma recurring with multiple satellites. A report of 11 cases. Br J Dermatol 80:218-227, 1968.

Masson's hemangioma

552 Clearkin KP, Enzinger FM: Intravascular papillary endothelial hyperplasia. Arch Pathol Lab Med 100:441-444, 1976.

553 Kuo T, Sayers CP, Rosai J: Masson's "vegetant intravascular hemangioendothelioma." A lesion often mistaken for angiosarcoma. Study of seventeen cases located in the skin and soft tissues. Cancer 38:1227-1236, 1976.

Histiocytoid hemangioma

554 Burrall BA, Barr RJ, King F: Cutaneous histiocytoid hemangioma. Arch Dermatol 118:166-170, 1982.

555 Castro C, Winkelmann RK: Angiolymphoid hyperplasia with eosinophilia in the skin. Cancer 34:1696-1705, 1974.

556 Googe PB, Harris NL, Mihm MC Jr: Kimura's disease and angiolymphoid hyperplasia with eosinophilia. Two distinct histopathological entities. J Cutan Pathol 14:263-271, 1987.

557 Olsen TG, Helwig EB: Angiolymphoid hyperplasia with eosinophilia. A clinicopathologic study of 116 patients. J Am Acad Dermatol 12:781-796, 1985.

558 Ose D, Vollmer R, Shelburne J, McComb R, Harrelson J: Histiocytoid hemangioma of the skin and scapula. A case report with electron microscopy and immunohistochemistry. Cancer 51:1656-1662, 1983.

559 Reed RJ, Terazakis N: Subcutaneous angioblastic lymphoid hyperplasia with eosinophilia (Kimura's disease). Cancer 29:489-497, 1972.

560 Rosai J, Gold J, Landy R: The histiocytoid hemangiomas. A unifying concept embracing several previously described entities of skin, soft tissues, large vessels, bone and heart. Hum Pathol 10:707-730, 1979.

561 Urabe A, Tsuneyoshi M, Enjoji M: Epithelioid hemangioma versus Kimura's disease. A comparative clinicopathologic study. Am J Surg Pathol 11:758-766, 1987.

Kaposi's sarcoma

562 Ackerman LV, Murray JF (eds): Symposium on Kaposi's sarcoma. Acta Un Int Cancer 18:312-511, 1962.

563 Akhtar M, Bunuan H, Ali MA, Godwin JT: Kaposi sarcoma in renal transplant recipients. Ultrastructural and immunoperoxidase study of four cases. Cancer 53:258-266, 1984.

564 Beckstead JH, Wood GS, Fletcher V: Evidence for the origin of Kaposi's sarcoma from lymphatic endothelium. Am J Pathol 119:294-300, 1985.

565 Blumenfeld W, Egbert BM, Sagebiel RW: Differential diagnosis of Kaposi's sarcoma. Arch Pathol Lab Med 109:123-127, 1985.

566 Burgdorf WHC, Mukai K, Rosai J: Immunohistochemical identification of factor VIII–related antigen in endothelial cells of cutaneous lesions of alleged vascular nature. Am J Clin Pathol 75:167-171, 1981.

566a Cockerell CJ, Whitlow MA, Webster GF, Friedman-Kien AE: Epithelioid angiomatosis. A distinct vascular disorder in patients with the acquired immunodeficiency syndrome or AIDS-related complex. Lancet 2: 654-656, 1987.

566b Dictor M, Andersson C: Lymphaticovenous differentiation in Kaposi's sarcoma. Cellular phenotypes by stage. Am J Pathol 130:411-417, 1988.

567 Dorfman RF: Kaposi's sarcoma revisited. Hum Pathol 15:1013-1017, 1984.

568 Flotte TJ, Hatcher VA, Friedman-Kien AE: Factor VIII–related antigen in Kaposi's sarcoma in young homosexual men. Arch Dermatol 120:180-182, 1984.

569 Frizzera G, Banks PM, Massarelli G, Rosai J: A systemic lymphoproliferative disorder with morphologic features of Castleman's disease. Pathological findings in 15 patients. Am J Surg Pathol 7:211-231, 1983.

570 Garrett TJ, Lange M, Ashford A, Thomas L: Kaposi's sarcoma in heterosexual intravenous drug users. Cancer 55:1146-1148, 1985.

571 Guarda LG, Silva EG, Ordóñez NG, Smith JL Jr: Factor VIII in Kaposi's sarcoma. Am J Clin Pathol 76:197-200, 1981.

572 Klepp O, Dahl O, Stenwig JT: Association of Kaposi's sarcoma and prior immunosuppressive therapy. A 5-year material of Kaposi's sarcoma in Norway. Cancer 42:2626-2530, 1978.

572a LeBoit P, Berger T, Egbert B, English C, Stoler M, Yen T, Wear D: Atypical cutaneous vascular proliferations in patients with AIDS are associated with the cat scratch disease bacillus (abstract). Lab Invest 58:53A, 1988.

573 Marshall ME, Hatfield ST, Hatfield DR: Arteriovenous malformation simulating Kaposi's sarcoma (pseudo-Kaposi's sarcoma). Arch Dermatol 121:99-101, 1985.

574 McNutt NS, Fletcher V, Conant MA: Early lesions of Kaposi's sarcoma in homosexual men. An ultrastructural comparison with other vascular proliferations in skin. Am J Pathol 111:62-77, 1983.

575 Nadji M, Morales AR, Ziegles-Weissman J, Penneys NS: Kaposi's sarcoma. Immunohistologic evidence for an endothelial origin. Arch Pathol Lab Med 105:274-275, 1981.

576 O'Connell KM: Kaposi's sarcoma. Histopathological study of 159 cases from Malawi. J Clin Pathol 30:687-695, 1977.

577 Russel Jones R, Wilson Jones E: The histogenesis of Kaposi's sarcoma. Am J Dermatopathol 8:369-370, 1986.

578 Ruszczak Zb, Mayer-Da Silva A, Orfanos CE: Kaposi's sarcoma in AIDS. Multicentric angioneoplasia in early skin lesions. Am J Dermatopathol 9:388-398, 1987.

579 Rutgers JL, Wieczorek R, Bonetti F, Kaplan KL, Posnett DN, Friedman-Kien AE, Knowles DM II: The expression of endothelial cell surface antigens by AIDS-associated Kaposi's sarcoma. Evidence for a vascular endothelial cell origin. Am J Pathol 122:493-499, 1986.

580 Safai B, Mike V, Giraldo G, Beth E, Good RA: Association of Kaposi's sarcoma with second primary malignancies. Possible etio-pathogenic implications. Cancer 45:1472-1479, 1980.

581 Schwartz RA, Kardashian JF, McNutt NS, Crain WR, Welch KL, Choy SH: Cutaneous angiosarcoma resembling anaplastic Kaposi's sarcoma in a homosexual man. Cancer 51:721-726, 1983.

581a Scully PA, Steinman HK, Kennedy C, Trueblood K, Frisman DM, Voland JR: AIDS-related Kaposi's sarcoma displays differential expression of endothelial surface antigens. Am J Pathol 130:244-251, 1988.

582 Sterry W, Steigleder G-K, Bodeux E: Kaposi's sarcoma. Venous capillary hemangioblastoma. Arch Dermatol Res 266:253-267, 1979.

583 Stribling J, Weitzner S, Smith GV: Kaposi's sarcoma in renal allograft recipients. Cancer 42:442-446, 1978.

584 Strutton G, Weedon D: Acro-angiodermatitis. A simulant of Kaposi's sarcoma. Am J Dermatopathol 9:85-89, 1987.

585 Sunter JP: Visceral Kaposi's sarcoma. Occurrence in a patient suffering from celiac disease. Arch Pathol Lab Med 102:543-545, 1978.

586 Taylor JF, Templeton AC, Vogel CL, Ziegler JL, Kyalwazi SK: Kaposi's sarcoma in Uganda. A clinicopathological study. Int J Cancer 8:122-135, 1971.

587 Varsano S, Manor Y, Steiner Z, Griffel B, Klajman A: Kaposi's sarcoma and angioimmunoblastic lymphadenopathy. Cancer 54:1582-1585, 1984.

588 Ziegler JL, Templeton AC, Vogel CL: Kaposi's sarcoma. A comparison of classical, endemic, and epidemic forms. Semin Oncol 11:47-52, 1984.

Angiosarcoma

589 Capo V, Ozzello L, Fenoglio CM, Lombardi L, Rilke F: Angiosarcomas arising in edematous extremities, immunostaining for factor VIII-related antigen and ultrastructural features. Hum Pathol 16:144-145, 1985.

590 Chen TKK, Gilbert EF: Angiosarcoma complicating generalized lymphangiectasia. Arch Pathol Lab Med 103:86-88, 1979.

591 Connors RC, Ackerman AB: Histologic pseudomalignancies of the skin. Arch Dermatol 112:1767-1780, 1976.

592 Cooper PH: Angiosarcomas of the skin. Semin Diagn Pathol 4:2-17, 1987.

593 Hodgkinson DJ, Soule EH, Woods JE: Cutaneous angiosarcoma of the head and neck. Cancer 44:1106-1113, 1979.

594 Holden CA, Spaull J, Das AK, McKee PH, Wilson Jones E: The histogenesis of angiosarcoma of the face and scalp. An immunohistochemical and ultrastructural study. Histopathology 11:37-51, 1987.

595 Holden CA, Spittle MF, Wilson Jones E: Angiosarcoma of the face and scalp, prognosis and treatment. Cancer 59:1046-1057, 1987.

596 Leader M, Collins M, Patel J, Henry K: Staining for factor VIII related antigen and Ulex europaeus agglutinin I (UEA-I) in 230 tumours. An assessment of their specificity for angiosarcoma and Kaposi's sarcoma. Histopathology 10:1153-1162, 1986.

597 Maddox JC, Evans HL: Angiosarcoma of skin and soft tissue. A study of forty-four cases. Cancer 48:1907-1921, 1981.

598 Otis CN, Peschel R, McKhann C, Merino M, Duray PH: The rapid onset of cutaneous angiosarcoma after radiotherapy for breast carcinoma. Cancer 57:2130-2134, 1986.

599 Rosai J, Sumner HW, Kostianovsky M, Perez-Mesa C: Angiosarcoma of the skin. A clinicopathologic and fine structural study. Hum Pathol 7:83-109, 1976.

600 Wilson Jones E: Malignant vascular tumours. Clin Exp Dermatol 1:287-312, 1976.

Lymphoid tumors and tumorlike conditions
Cutaneous lymphoid hyperplasia

601 Ackerman AB, Tanski EV: Pseudoleukemia cutis. Report of a case in association with molluscum contagiosum. Cancer 40:813-817, 1977.

602 Caro WA, Helwig EB: Cutaneous lymphoid hyperplasia. Cancer 24:487-502, 1969.

603 Cerio R, MacDonald DM: Benign cutaneous lymphoid infiltrates. J Cutan Pathol 12:442-452, 1985.

604 Cochran REI, Thomson J, Fleming KA, Strong AMM: Histology simulating reticulosis in secondary syphilis. Br J Dermatol 95:251-254, 1976.

605 Ive FA, Magnus IA, Warin RP, Jones EW: "Actinic reticuloid." A chronic dermatosis association with severe photosensitivity and the histological resemblance to lymphoma. Br J Dermatol 81:469-485, 1969.

606 Mach KW, Wilgram GF: Characteristic histopathology of cutaneous lymphoplasia (lymphocytoma). Arch Dermatol 94:26-34, 1966.

607 Thomson J, Cochrane T, Cochran R, McQueen A: Histology simulating reticulosis in persistent nodular scabies. Br J Dermatol 90:421-429, 1974.

608 Willemze R, Dijkstra A, Meijer CJLM: Lymphocytic infiltration of the skin (Jessner). A T-cell lymphoproliferative disease. Br J Dermatol 110:523-529, 1984.

609 Wirt DP, Grogan TM, Jolley CS, Rangel CS, Payne CM, Hansen PC, Lynch PJ, Schuchardt M: The immunoarchitecture of cutaneous pseudolymphoma. Hum Pathol 6:492-510, 1985.

Lymphomatoid papulosis

610 Black MM, Wilson Jones E: Lymphomatoid pityriasis lichenoides. A variant with histologic features simulating a lymphoma. Br J Dermatol 86:329-347, 1972.

611 Chen KTK, Flam MS: Hodgkin's disease complicating lymphomatoid papulosis. Am J Dermatopathol 7:555-561, 1985.

612 Kadin M, Nasu K, Sako D, Said J, Vonderheid E: Lymphomatoid papulosis. A cutaneous proliferation of activated helper T cells expressing Hodgkin's disease–associated antigens. Am J Pathol 119:315-325, 1985.

613 Kadin ME, Vonderheid EC, Sako D, Clayton LK, Olbricht S: Clonal composition of T cells in lymphomatoid papulosis. Am J Pathol 126:13-17, 1987.

614 Ralfkiaer E, Stein H, Wantzin GL, Thomsen K, Ralfkiaer N, Mason DY: Lymphomatoid papulosis. Characterization of skin infiltrates by monoclonal antibodies. Am J Clin Pathol 84:587-593, 1985.

615 Sina B, Burnett JW: Lymphomatoid papulosis. Case reports and literature review. Arch Dermatol 119:189-197, 1983.

616 Valentino LA, Helwig EB: Lymphomatoid papulosis. Arch Pathol 96:409-416, 1973.

617 Wantzin GL, Thomsen K, Brandrup F, Larsen JK: Lymphomatoid papulosis. Development into cutaneous T-cell lymphoma. Arch Dermatol 121:792-794, 1985.

618 Weiss LM, Wood GS, Trela M, Warnke RA, Sklar J: Clonal T-cell populations in lymphomatoid papulosis. Evidence of a lymphoproliferative origin for a clinically benign disease. N Engl J Med 315:475-479, 1986.

619 Willemze R, Meyer CJLM, Van Vloten WA, Scheffer E: The clinical and histological spectrum of lymphomatoid papulosis. Br J Dermatol 107:131-144, 1982.

620 Willemze R, Scheffer E, Ruiter DJ, Van Vloten WA, Meijer CJLM: Immunological, cytochemical, and ultrastructural studies in lymphomatoid papulosis. Br J Dermatol 108:381-394, 1983.

Mycosis fungoides and related T-cell lymphomas

621 Berger CL, Warburton D, Raafat J, LoGerfo P, Edelson RL: Cutaneous T-cell lymphoma. Neoplasm of T cells with helper activity. Blood 53:642-651, 1979.

622 Blasik LG, Newkirk RE, Dimond RL, Clendenning WE: Mycosis fungoides d'emblée. A rare presentation of cutaneous T-cell lymphoma. Cancer 49:742-747, 1982.

623 Block JB, Edgcomb J, Eisen A, Van Scott EJ: Mycosis fungoides. Natural history and aspects of its relationship to other malignant lymphomas. Am J Med 34:228-235, 1963.

624 Bodensteiner DC, Skikne B: Central nervous system involvement in mycosis fungoides. Diagnosis, treatment and literature review. Cancer 50:1181-1184, 1982.

625 Breathnach SM, McKee PH, Smith NP: Hypopigmented mycosis fungoides. Report of five cases with ultrastructural observations. Br J Dermatol 106:643-649, 1982.

626 Brehmer-Andersson E: Mycosis fungoides and its relation to Sezary's syndrome, lymphomatoid papulosis, and primary cutaneous Hodgkin's disease. A clinical, histopathologic and cytologic study of fourteen cases and a critical review of the literature. Acta Derm Venereol [Suppl 75] (Stockh) 56:1-142, 1976.

627 Buechner SA, Winkelmann RK: Sézary syndrome. A clinicopathologic study of 39 cases. Arch Dermatol 119:979-986, 1983.

628 Buechner SA, Winkelmann RK, Banks PM: T cells in cutaneous lesions of Sézary syndrome and T-cell leukemia. Characterization by monoclonal antibodies. Arch Dermatol 119:895-900, 1983.

629 Chan WC, Griem ML, Grozea PN, Freel RJ, Variakojis D: Mycosis fungoides and Hodgkin's disease occurring in the same patient. Report of three cases. Cancer 44:1408-1413, 1979.

630 Chu AC: The use of monoclonal antibodies in the in situ identification of T-cell subpopulations in cutaneous T-cell lymphoma. J Cutan Pathol 10:479-498, 1983.

631 Chu A, Patterson J, Berger C, Vonderheid E, Edelson R: In situ study of T-cell subpopulations in cutaneous T-cell lymphoma. Diagnostic criteria. Cancer 54:2414-2422, 1984.

632 Clendenning WE, Brecher G, Van Scott EJ: Mycosis fungoides. Relationship to malignant cutaneous reticulosis and the Sézary syndrome. Arch Dermatol 89:785-791, 1964.

633 Degreef H, Holvoet C, Van Vloten WA, Desmet V, De Wolf-Peeters C: Woringer-Kolopp disease. An epidermotropic variant of mycosis fungoides. Cancer 38:2154-2165, 1976.

634 Deneau DG, Wood GS, Beckstead J, Hoppe RT, Price N: Woringer-Kolopp disease (pagetoid reticulosis). Four cases with histopathologic, ultrastructural, and immunohistologic observations. Arch Dermatol 120:1045-1051, 1984.

635 Epstein EH Jr, Levin DL, Croft JD Jr, Lutzner MA: Mycosis fungoides. Survival, prognostic features, response to therapy, and autopsy findings. Medicine (Baltimore) 15:61-72, 1972.

636 Fisher ER, Horvat BC, Wechsler HL: Ultrastructural features of mycosis fungoides. Am J Clin Pathol 58:99-110, 1972.

637 Flaxman BA, Zelasny G, Van Scott EJ: Nonspecificity of characteristic cells in mycosis fungoides. Arch Dermatol 104:141-147, 1971.

638 Fuks Z, Bagshaw MA: Total skin electron treatment of mycosis fungoides. Radiology 100:145-150, 1971.

639 Fuks ZY, Bagshaw MA, Farber EM: Prognostic signs and management of the mycosis fungoides. Cancer 32:1385-1395, 1973.

640 Gissner SD, Young I: Mycosis fungoides–like cells. Their presence in a case of pityriasic dermatitis with a comment on their significance as an indicator of primary T-cell dyscrasia. Am J Surg Pathol 2:97-101, 1978.

641 Green SB, Byar DP, Lamberg SI: Prognostic variables in mycosis fungoides. Cancer 47:2671-2677, 1981.

642 Hamminga L, Hermans J, Noordijk EM, Meijer CJLM, Scheffer E, Van Vloten WA: Cutaneous T-cell lymphoma. Clinicopathological relationships, therapy and survival in ninety-two patients. Br J Dermatol 107:145-156, 1982.

643 Hashimoto K, Iwahara K: Immunoelectron microscopy related to T-cell monoclonal surface antigen in mycosis fungoides. Am J Dermatopathol 5:129-134, 1983.

644 Hood AF, Mark GJ, Hunt JV: Laryngeal mycosis fungoides. Cancer 43:1527-1532, 1979.

645 Huberman MS, Bunn PA Jr, Matthews MJ, Ihde DC, Gazdar AF, Cohen MH, Minna JD: Hepatic involvement in the cutaneous T-cell lymphomas. Results of percutaneous biopsy and peritoneoscopy. Cancer 45:1683-1688, 1980.

646 Iwahara K, Hashimoto K: T-cell subsets and nuclear contour index of skin-infiltrating T-cells in cutaneous T-cell lymphoma. Cancer 54:440-446, 1984.

647 Jimbow K, Maeda K, Ito Y, Ishida O, Takami T: Heterogeneity of cutaneous T-cell lymphoma. Phenotypic and ultrastructural characterization of four unusual cases. Cancer 56:2458-2469, 1985.

647a LeBoit PE, Zackheim HS, White CR Jr: Granulomatous variants of cutaneous T-cell lymphoma. The histopathology of granulomatous mycosis fungoides and granulomatous slack skin. Am J Surg Pathol 12:83-95, 1988.

648 Lever WF: Localized mycosis fungoides with prominent epidermotropism. Woringer-Kolopp disease. Arch Dermatol 113:1254-1256, 1977.

649 Long JC, Mihm MC: Mycosis fungoides with extra-cutaneous dissemination. A distinct clinicopathologic entity. Cancer 34:1745-1755, 1974.

650 Nasu K, Said J, Vonderheid E, Olerud J, Sako D, Kadin M: Immunopathology of cutaneous T-cell lymphomas. Am J Pathol 119:436-447, 1985.

651 National Cancer Institute, Division of Cancer Treatment: Proceedings of the workshop on cutaneous T-cell lymphomas (mycosis fungoides and Sézary syndrome). Cancer Treat Rep 63:561-736, 1979.

652 Ralfkiaer E, Wantzin GL, Mason DY, Hou-Jensen K, Stein H, Thomsen K: Phenotypic characterization of lymphocyte subsets in mycosis fungoides. Com-

parison with large plaque parapsoriasis and benign chronic dermatoses. Am J Clin Pathol **84**:610-619, 1985.

653 Rappaport H, Thomas LB: Mycosis fungoides. The pathology of extracutaneous involvement. Cancer **34**:1198-1229, 1974.

654 Reed RJ, Cummings CE: Malignant reticulosis and related conditions of the skin. A reconsideration of mycosis fungoides. Cancer **19**:1231-1247, 1966.

655 Rosai J, Spiro J: Central nervous system involvement by mycosis fungoides. Acta Derm Venereol (Stockh) **48**:482-488, 1968.

656 Sanchez JL, Ackerman A: The patch of mycosis fungoides. Am J Dermatopathol **1**:5-26, 1979.

657 Scheen SR III, Banks PM, Winkelmann RK: Morphologic heterogeneity of malignant lymphomas developing in mycosis fungoides. Mayo Clin Proc **59**:95-106, 1984.

658 Shum DT, Roberts JT, Smout MS, Wells GA, Simon GT: The value of nuclear contour index in the diagnosis of mycosis fungoides. An assessment of current ultrastructural morphometric diagnostic criteria. Cancer **57**:298-304, 1986.

659 Simrell CR, Boccia RV, Longo DL, Jaffe ES: Coexisting Hodgkin's disease and mycosis fungoides. Immunohistochemical proof of its existence. Arch Pathol Lab Med **110**:1029-1034, 1986.

660 Van Der Putte SCJ, Toonstra J, De Weger RA, Van Unnik JAM: Cutaneous T-cell lymphoma, multilobated type. Histopathology **6**:35-54, 1982.

661 Van Scott EJ, Kalmanson JD: Complete remissions of mycosis fungoides lymphoma induced by topical nitrogen mustard (HN2). Control of delayed hypersensitivity in HN2 by desensitization and by induction of specific immunologic tolerance. Cancer **32**:18-30, 1973.

662 Vonderheid EC, Tam DW, Johnson WC, Van Scott EJ, Wallner PE: Prognostic significance of cytomorphology in the cutaneous T-cell lymphomas. Cancer **47**:119-125, 1981.

663 Weisenburger DD, Nathwani BN, Forman SJ, Rappaport H: Noncutaneous peripheral T-cell lymphoma histologically resembling mycosis fungoides. Cancer **49**:1839-1847, 1982.

664 Wieczorek R, Suhrland M, Ramsay D, Reed ML, Knowles DM II: Leu-M1 antigen expression in advanced (tumor) stage mycosis fungoides. Am J Clin Pathol **86**:25-32, 1986.

Lymph nodes in mycosis fungoides

665 Colby TV, Burke JS, Hoppe RT: Lymph node biopsy in mycosis fungoides. Cancer **47**:351-359, 1981.

666 Sausville EA, Worsham GF, Matthews MJ, Makuch RW, Fischmann AB, Schechter GP, Gazdar AF, Bunn PA Jr: Histologic assessment of lymph nodes in mycosis fungoides/Sézary syndrome (cutaneous T-cell lymphoma). Clinical correlations and prognostic import of a new classification system. Hum Pathol **16**:1098-1109, 1985.

667 Schechter GP, Bunn PA, Fischmann AB, Young SW, Fukes Z: Blood and lymph node T-lymphocytes in cutaneous T-cell lymphoma. Evaluation by light microscopy. Cancer Treat Rep **63**:581-586, 1979.

668 Scheffer E, Meijer CJ, van Vloten WA: Dermatopathic lymphadenopathy and lymph node involvement in mycosis fungoides. Cancer **45**:137-148, 1980.

669 Weiss LM, Hu E, Wood GS, Moulds C, Cleary ML, Warnke R, Sklar J: Clonal rearrangements of T-cell receptor genes in mycosis fungoides and dermatopathic lymphadenopathy. N Engl J Med **313**:539-544, 1985.

670 Weiss LM, Wood GS, Warnke RA: Immunophenotypic differences between dermatopathic lymphadenopathy and lymph node involvement in mycosis fungoides. Am J Pathol **120**:179-185, 1985.

Other malignant lymphomas

671 Aozasa K, Inoue A, Yamamura T, Nishida K, Sano S: Cutaneous malignant lymphomas. A clinicopathologic study of thirty-seven cases. Acta Pathol Jpn **35**:1181-1189, 1985.

672 Aronson IK, West DP, Variakojis D, Ronan SG, Iossifides I, Zeitz HJ: Panniculitis associated with cutaneous T-cell lymphoma and cytophagocytic histiocytosis. Br J Dermatol **112**:87-96, 1985.

673 Bhawan J: Angioendotheliomatosis proliferans systemisata. An angiotropic neoplasm of lymphoid origin. Semin Diagn Pathol **4**:18-27, 1987.

674 Burke JS, Hoppe RT, Cibull ML, Dorfman RF: Cutaneous malignant lymphoma. A pathologic study of 50 cases with clinical analysis of 37. Cancer **47**:300-310, 1981.

675 Dodd HJ, Stansfeld AG, Chambers TJ: Cutaneous malignant histiocytosis. A clinicopathological review of five cases. Br J Dermatol **113**:455-461, 1985.

676 Evans HL, Winkelmann RK, Banks PM: Differential diagnosis of malignant and benign cutaneous lymphoid infiltrates. A study of 57 cases in which malignant lymphoma had been diagnosed or suspected in the skin. Cancer **44**:699-717, 1979.

677 Fisher ER, Park EJ, Wechsler HL: Histologic identification of malignant lymphoma cutis. Am J Clin Pathol **65**:149-158, 1976.

678 Flynn KJ, Dehner LP, Gajl-Peczalska KJ, Dahl MV, Ramsay N, Wang N: Regressing atypical histiocytosis. A cutaneous proliferation of atypical neoplastic histiocytes with unexpectedly indolent biologic behavior. Cancer **49**:959-970, 1982.

679 Garcia CF, Weiss LM, Warnke RA, Wood GS: Cutaneous follicular lymphoma. Am J Surg Pathol **10**:454-463, 1986.

679a Grümayer ER, Ladenstein RL, Slavc I, Urban C, Radaszkiewicz T, Bettelheim P, Gadner H: B-cell differentiation pattern of cutaneous lymphomas in infancy and childhood. Cancer **61**:303-308, 1988.

680 Headington JT, Roth MS, Schnitzer B: Regressing atypical histiocytosis. A review and critical appraisal. Semin Diagn Pathol **4**:28-37, 1987.

681 Holbert JM Jr, Chesney TMcC: Malignant lymphoma of the skin. A review of recent advances in diagnosis and classification. J Cutan Pathol **9**:133-168, 1982.

682 Kahn LB, Gordon W, Camp R: Florid sarcoid reaction associated with lymphoma of the skin. Cancer **33**:1117-1122, 1974.

683 Knowles DM II, Jakobiec FA: Cell marker analysis of extranodal lymphoid infiltrates. To what extent does the determination of mono- or polyclonality resolve the diagnostic dilemma of malignant lymphoma vs pseudolymphoma in an extranodal site? Semin Diagn Pathol **2**:163-168, 1985.

684 Krishnan J, Li C-Y, Su WPD: Cutaneous lymphomas. Correlation of histochemical and immunohistochemical characteristics and clinicopathologic features. Am J Clin Pathol **79**:157-165, 1983.

685 Long JC, Mihm MC, Qazi R: Malignant lymphoma of the skin. A clinicopathologic study of lymphoma other than mycosis fungoides diagnosed by skin biopsy. Cancer **38**:1282-1296, 1976.

686 Prost C, Reyes F, Wechsler J, Gaston A, Richard I, Poirier J: High-grade malignant cutaneous plasmacytoma metastatic to the central nervous system. A case report with electron microscopy, immunohistological, and neuropathological studies. Am J Dermatopathol **9**:30-36, 1987.

687 Rilke F, Giardini R, Lombardi L: Recurrent atypical cutaneous histiocytosis. Pathol Annu **20**(Pt 2):29-58, 1985.

688 Saxe N, Kahn LB, King H: Lymphoma of the skin. A comparative clinico-pathologic study of 50 cases including mycosis fungoides and primary and secondary cutaneous lymphoma. J Cutan Pathol **4**:111-122, 1977.

689 Scott PWB, Silvers DN, Helwig EB: Proliferating angioendotheliomatosis. Arch Pathol **99**:323-326, 1975.

690 Sheibani K, Battifora H, Winberg CD, Burke JS, Ben-Ezra J, Ellinger GM, Quigley NJ, Fernandez BB, Morrow D, Rappaport H: Further evidence that "malignant angioendotheliomatosis" is an angiotropic large-cell lymphoma. N Engl J Med **314**:943-948, 1986.

691 Smith JL Jr, Butler JJ: Skin involvement in Hodgkin's disease. Cancer **45**:354-361, 1980.

692 White RW, Patterson JW: Cutaneous involvement in Hodgkin's disease. Cancer **55**:1136-1145, 1985.

693 Wick MR, Mills SE, Scheithauer BW, Cooper PH, Davitz MA, Parkinson K: Reassessment of malignant "angioendotheliomatosis." Evidence in favor of its reclassification as "intravascular lymphomatosis." Am J Surg Pathol **10**:112-123, 1986.

694 Willemze R, Meijer CJLM, Scheffer E, Kluin PM, Van Vloten WA, Toonstra J, Van Der Putte SCJ: Diffuse large cell lymphomas of follicular center cell origin presenting in the skin. A clinicopathologic and immunologic study of 16 patients. Am J Pathol **126**:325-333, 1987.

695 Zaatari GS, Chan WC, Kim TH, Williams DL, Kletzel M: Malignant lymphoma of the skin in children. Cancer **59**:1040-1045, 1987.

Leukemia

696 Greenwood R, Barker DJ, Tring FC, Parapia L, Reid M, Scott CS, Lauder I: Clinical and immunohistological characterization of cutaneous lesions in chronic lymphocytic leukaemia. Br J Dermatol **113**:447-453, 1985.

697 Long JC, Mihm MC: Multiple granulocytic tumors of the skin. Report of six cases of myelogenous leukemia with initial manifestations in the skin. Cancer **39**:2004-2016, 1977.

Other primary tumors and tumorlike conditions

698 Camacho F: Benign cutaneous cystic teratoma. J Cutan Pathol **9**:345-351, 1982.

698a Cooper PH, Sibley DA: Congenital cutaneous meningothelial tumors (abstract). J Cutan Pathol **14**:353, 1987.

699 Gonzalez JG, Ghiselli RW, Santa Cruz DJ: Synovial metaplasia of the skin. Am J Surg Pathol **11**:343-350, 1987.

700 Hsueh S, Santa Cruz DJ: Cartilaginous lesions of the skin and superficial soft tissue. J Cutan Pathol **9**:405-416, 1982.

701 Pellegrini AE: Cutaneous decidualized endometriosis. A pseudomalignancy. Am J Dermatopathol **4:**171-174, 1982.

702 Steck WD, Helwig EB: Cutaneous endometriosis. JAMA **191:**167-170, 1965.

Metastatic carcinoma

703 Brownstein MH, Helwig EB: Metastatic tumors of the skin. Cancer **29:**1298-1307, 1972.

704 Brownstein MH, Helwig EB: Patterns of cutaneous metastases. Arch Dermatol **105:**862-868, 1972.

705 Conner DH, Taylor HB, Helwig EB: Cutaneous metastasis of renal cell carcinoma. Arch Pathol **76:**339-346, 1963.

706 McKee PH: Cutaneous metastases. J Cutan Pathol **12:**239-250, 1985.

707 Reingold IM: Cutaneous metastases from internal carcinoma. Cancer **19:**162-168, 1966.

5 Oral cavity and Oropharynx

The oral cavity is the site of numerous diseases, both congenital and acquired, affecting a large variety of tissues and systems. Only those that occur commonly enough to be of interest to the surgical pathologist are discussed here. For a more thorough discussion of these and the rarer diseases, the reader is referred to the excellent treatise edited by Gorlin and Goldman.[1]

CONGENITAL ABNORMALITIES

Dermoid cysts are seen in the midline of the floor of the mouth. Although present at birth, they may become evident only later on when secondarily inflamed.[6] They are lined by squamous epithelium and contain skin adnexae.[10] *Cysts lined by gastric or intestinal epithelium* have been reported in the tongue and floor of the mouth.[7] Minute *cysts of odontogenic origin* are commonly seen in the alveolar and palatal mucosa of newborn and older infants[4]; they need not be biopsied (see Chapter 6). Nodules of *heterotopic nerve tissue* in the palate or parapharyngeal space, mainly composed of glial elements and ependymal-lined clefts, have been reported[3,13]; in rare cases, a neoplasm may arise from them.[2] *White sponge nevus*, an autosomal dominantly inherited disease, is characterized by large white plaques in the oral mucosa. Microscopically there is striking intracellular edema throughout the malphigian layer.[11] *Fordyce's disease* refers to the presence of normal sebaceous glands inside the oral cavity, a very common occurrence. The entity *lingual thyroid* is discussed in Chapter 9.

Although it does not represent a congenital anomaly, the occurrence of *epithelial nests* in intraoral sensory nerve endings should be mentioned here.[5,9] Their importance relates to the fact that pathologists unaware of their existence might easily confuse them with perineural invasion by epidermoid carcinoma. These formations are normally occurring neuroepithelial structures of alleged receptor function, known by anatomists as the organ of Chievitz, Chievitz's paraparotid organ, and juxtaoral organ[12,14] (Fig. 5-1). They lie deep to the internal pterygoid muscle near the pterygomandibular raphe and are associated with small branches from the buccal nerve. This structure can undergo nodular hyperplasia.[8]

INFLAMMATORY DISEASES

Chronic inflammatory lesions are produced in the oral cavity by ill-fitting dentures, ragged sharp teeth, and poor dental hygiene (Figs. 5-2, 5-3, and 5-4). Removal of the offending agent allows the pathologic process to subside.[20] Microscopically, a combination of hyperplastic epithelium, fibrous tissue, and inflammatory cells in varying proportions is seen. Bhaskar et al.[19] described 341 such cases, all associated with the use of dentures, under the term *inflammatory papillary hyperplasia*; 82.7% of the lesions were located in the palate. Localized overgrowth of the epithelium with or without ulceration is frequent, and it is not rare to see large pseudotumors made up of fibrous tissue and chronic inflammatory cells, among which plasma cells may be prominent.[16] The inflammation distorts the epithelial pegs and may produce areas in which squamous cells are isolated from the overlying epithelium (Fig. 5-5).[15] Lesions in which the fibrous proliferation predominates are sometimes described as *irritation fibromas*. Scattered stellate and multinucleated giant cells can be seen throughout the fibrous tissue, in which case the term *giant cell fibroma* has been used.[25,29]

Tuberculosis is a rare lesion within the oral cavity. It is usually seen on the tongue as a painful ulcer, but it also may occur on the buccal mucosa.[28] It nearly always is associated with advanced pulmonary disease. Microscopically, there are typical tubercles.

Syphilis may produce a gumma in the tongue or palate appearing as a painless indurated mass. Microscopically, there is a granuloma with giant cells, numerous plasma cells, and prominent vascular changes. There seems to be a relationship between syphilis and tongue cancer, although the percentage of patients with such association is no longer as high as old reports indicated. A study of 243 patients with cancer of the tongue revealed that only 15 (6.1%) had a history of syphilis.[26]

Histoplasmosis can occur anywhere in the oral cavity and can closely simulate epidermoid carcinoma on clinical ex-

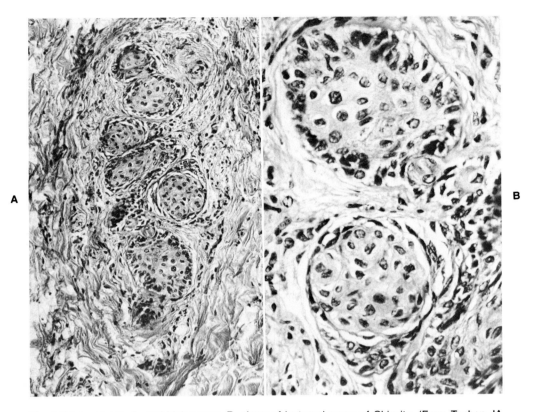

Fig. 5-1 Low-power, **A,** and high-power, **B,** views of juxtaoral organ of Chievitz. (From Tschen JA, Fechner RE: The juxtaoral organ of Chievitz. Am J Surg Pathol **3:**147-150, 1979. Copyrighted by MASSON PUBLISHING USA, Inc., New York.)

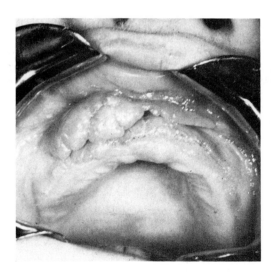

Fig. 5-2 Localized non-neoplastic overgrowth of upper alveolus produced by ill-fitting denture. (Courtesy Dr. C.A. Waldron, Atlanta, GA.)

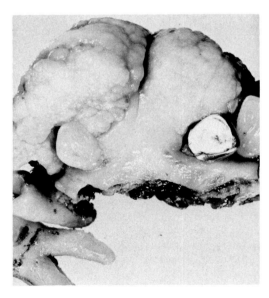

Fig. 5-3 Resected pseudotumor of alveolar process made up of fibrous tissue and chronic inflammatory cells.

amination. Indurated ulcers (Fig. 5-6), nodular lesions, or verrucous masses can be present. The usual microscopic appearance is that of a granuloma, although sometimes only a nonspecific inflammatory reaction is seen (Fig. 5-7). Special stains (Gomori's methenamine-silver or PAS-Gridley) are necessary for the identification of the fungi (Fig. 5-7, inset).[18]

Crohn's disease can involve the oral cavity and pharynx.[31] In a review of 332 cases of Crohn's disease, Croft and Wilkinson[21] found 20 patients (6.1%) with oral ulcers in some stage of the disease. Microscopically, there is edema, dilatation of lymphatic vessels, chronic inflammation, scattered giant cells and, rarely, noncaseating granulomas.[17,30]

Sarcoidosis may affect the oral mucosa, gingiva, tongue, hard palate, and major salivary glands. Random biopsy of the lower lip has been successfully used to confirm a diagnosis of sarcoidosis; in a series of seventy-five consecutive patients, noncaseating granulomas were found by this procedure in 58%.[27]

Melkersson-Rosenthal syndrome is composed of the triad of orofacial swelling, peripheral facial nerve paralysis, and plicated tongue. Cheilitis granulomatosa is probably an abortive variant of this syndrome, the etiology and pathogenesis of which remain obscure.[33] Microscopically, there is a granulomatous inflammation primarily involving the stroma of the lip. The differential diagnosis includes sarcoidosis and Crohn's disease.

Wegener's granulomatosis may manifest in the oral cavity as a red to purple hyperplastic gingiva, which on microscopic examination shows epithelioid histiocytes, giant cells, eosinophils, pseudoepitheliomatous hyperplasia, and—in rare cases—vasculitis.[24] Both this condition and so-called *lethal midline granuloma*, which may present initially as a nonhealing ulcer of the hard palate, are described in more detail in Chapter 7.

Tongue ulceration with eosinophilia (ulcerative eosinophilic granuloma; Riga-Fede disease) may result from crush injury to the tongue muscle, which initiates an in-flammatory response with tissue eosinophilia.[32] Because of its presumed pathogenesis, the lesion is also known as *traumatic granuloma*.[22,34] A probable variant of this condition in which the cellularity and mitotic activity may lead to confusion with a malignant process has been designated *atypical histiocytic granuloma*.[23]

OTHER NON-NEOPLASTIC LESIONS

Fibrous hyperplasia of the gingiva is usually the result of diphenylhydantoin (Dilantin) therapy, but it may also be genetically inherited, idiopathic, or associated with other drugs, such as cyclosporin A.[51] The gingival thickening can be so extreme as to necessitate surgical removal (Fig. 5-8).

Oral submucosal fibrosis, as seen in Indians and Pakistanis, is a reactive process that has a different microscopic appearance.[47] It is thought to be the result of hypersensitivity to chillies. The overlying epithelium is usually atrophic. A relationship with oral carcinoma has been suggested but not yet established with certainty.

Mucous cyst (mucocele), when applied to a lesion of the oral cavity, refers to two different processes. The first and most common is referred to as *extravasation mucocele* and represents a focus of stromal reaction to spillage of mucus from a minor salivary gland. It is often seen in young individuals, the lower lip being the classic location, and the microscopic pattern is that of granulation tissue surrounding one or more spaces containing mucin[44] (Fig. 5-9). An anatomic variant of this process is known as *ranula* when it occurs as a blue-domed cyst in a sublingual location, and as *plunging ranula* when it extends into the neck above the hyoid bone.[45]

The second type, named *retention mucocele*, occurs most often in older patients and in other locations in the oral cavity, such as the floor of the mouth and the inside of the cheek; microscopically, a mucus-filled cyst completely lined by cylindric, cuboidal, or flattened cells is seen.[41] Extravasation mucocele should be distinguished microscopically from *oral focal mucinosis*, the oral counterpart of the most common cutaneous focal mucinosis;[49] this condition is located in sites other than the lip and lacks the granulation tissue wall and inflammatory cells consistently seen in the former.

Necrotizing sialometaplasia is a reactive condition involving minor or—less commonly—major salivary glands; its importance lies in the fact that it can be confused histologically with epidermoid or mucoepidermoid carcinoma.[35,37,38] The disease usually presents as an ulcerating lesion of the hard palate characterized by vascular proliferation, prominent inflammatory infiltrate, and partial necrosis of salivary glands, associated with regeneration and squamous metaplasia of the adjacent duct and acini. Cases also have been described in the nasal cavity, gingiva, lip, hypopharynx, maxillary sinus, and major salivary glands. The morphologic changes are somewhat similar to those seen in this region following radiation therapy. The pathogenesis is probably ischemic, and some cases have been seen as a complication of vasculitis and other primary vascular disorders. The lobular configuration that these lesions present is an important differential sign with epidermoid carcinoma[39] (Fig. 5-10).

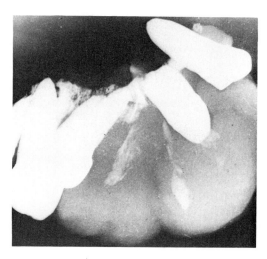

Fig. 5-4 Alveolar process from which pseudotumor shown in Fig. 5-3 was resected, showing extent of soft tissue mass.

Amyloidosis of the tongue is a common microscopic finding in older individuals, but only in a small proportion of cases are the deposits extensive enough to result in diffuse macroglossia or a localized tumor.[50,52]

Malakoplakia has been reported as a unilateral tonsillar lesion.[42]

The oral cavity can also be affected by a variety of primary dermatologic disorders, including *lichen planus*,[36,43] *lupus erythematosus*,[43,48] *pemphigus vulgaris*,[40] and *Mucha-Habermann's disease*.[46]

TUMORS AND TUMORLIKE CONDITIONS OF SURFACE EPITHELIUM
Hyperplasia and dysplasia

Leukoedema presents as a diffuse opalescent lesion of the cheek mucosa that can extend to the lips; microscopically, the only change is vacuolization or intracellular edema of the malpighian cells of a probably degenerative nature.[70]

Focal epithelial hyperplasia (Heck's disease) presents clinically as a well-circumscribed, sessile, pale elevation of the buccal mucosa. Microscopically, the most prominent

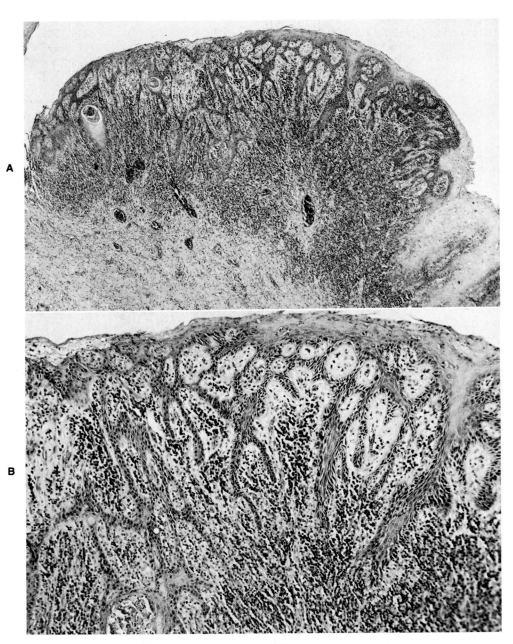

Fig. 5-5 Extreme pseudoepitheliomatous hyperplasia of inflamed gingiva. Long, thin strands of distorted, well-differentiated squamous cells infiltrated by inflammatory cells are present.

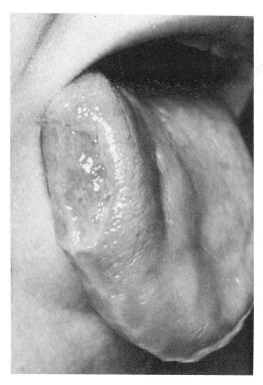

Fig. 5-6 Oral histoplasmosis presenting as indurated ulcer of tongue.

feature is the presence of balloon cells in the malpighian layers. This disorder, which is not related to cancer, is very common among Native Americans and Eskimos.[62]

Leukoplakia is a clinical term.[58,72] It has been defined by Pindborg et al.[63] as a white patch or plaque, not less than 5 mm in diameter, which cannot be removed by rubbing and cannot be classified as any other diagnosable disease (Fig. 5-11). It is more appropriate to diagnose this lesion microscopically as epithelial atrophy or hyperplasia and to grade the atypicality (if any) as mild, moderate, or severe,[55,56,59,60] the implication being that the greater the degree of atypicality or dysplasia, the higher its premalignant potential. Other authors have proposed to designate these lesions as *oral intraepithelial neoplasia (OIN)*, grades I to III, by analogy with the terminology now commonly used in the uterine cervix.[56] Sometimes these dysplastic changes are accompanied by a "lichenoid" histology, i.e., hyperkeratosis, prominent granular layer, irregular basal layer, saw-toothed rete pegs, and band-like inflammatory infiltrate. This change, which has been referred to as *lichenoid dysplasia*, should not be confused with true lichen planus of the oral cavity.[53,61] The dysplastic changes can extend to the ducts of minor salivary glands.[54] Admittedly, standardization of these changes is difficult, and a certain degree of subjectivity exists in this evaluation. Whether morphometry or immunohistochemistry will result in a more accurate assessment remains to be seen.[64,65]

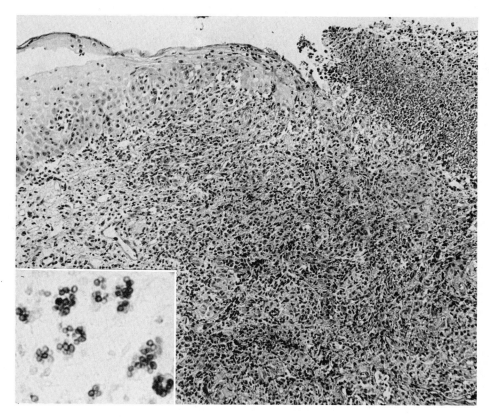

Fig. 5-7 Histoplasmosis of oral cavity. Ulcer shows histiocytic and chronic inflammatory reaction without granulomas. **Inset,** Numerous fungi can be seen with PAS stain.

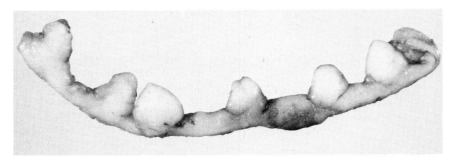

Fig. 5-8 Surgically removed tremendously hypertrophied gingival mucosa caused by Dilantin therapy in 13-year-old girl.

The commonest location of leukoplakia is the buccal gingival gutter.[66] Waldron and Shafer[71] found that the highest incidence of epithelial alterations, ranging from dysplasia to carcinoma in situ, was seen in leukoplakia of the floor of the mouth, particularly in men. This correlates well with the location of epidermoid carcinoma of the oral cavity. Pindborg et al.[63] divide leukoplakia into two types: speckled and homogeneous. Over 60% of the former have superimposed infection by *Candida albicans*.[67] Pindborg et al.[63] followed 248 patients with oral leukoplakia for 1 to 10 years; only 4.4% developed epidermoid carcinoma. Most of these leukoplakias in this group were of the speckled type. In Einhorn and Wersäll's series[57] of 782 patients with a mean follow-up of 11.7 years, the incidence of carcinoma was 2.4% after 10 years and 4% after 20 years. Most other series quote figures ranging from less than 1% to 6%,[68,69] the outstanding exception being a series of 257 cases from San Francisco followed for an average period of 7.2 years in which the incidence of epidermoid carcinoma was 17.5%.[69] It should also be pointed out that some epidermoid carcinomas of the mouth present without any atypia of the adjacent mucosa.[56]

Papillomatous lesions and human papilloma virus (HPV)

In recent times, it has become apparent that the oral cavity can be the site of a variety of HPV-induced lesions, most of which are microscopically and behaviorally analogous to those located in the genital tract.[78] These include *verruca vulgaris*,[75a] *condyloma acuminatum*,[79] *squamous papillomas*,[72a,77] and the oral *condyloma planus* (also known as hairy leukoplakia), recently described in the tongues of homosexual males and characteristically located along the lateral edges.[75,76] An etiologic role for HPV has also been implicated for verrucous carcinoma[74] and epidermoid carcinoma.[73] Not all squamous papillomas of the oral cavity are virally induced. Some may be the result of mechanical irritation, and others are genetically determined, such as those occurring as a component of Cowden's syndrome.[80,81]

Carcinoma in situ

Epidermoid carcinoma in situ can be a precursor of invasive oral cancer (Fig. 5-12). How often this occurs is not known, and neither is the speed of its evolution.[85] In contrast to leukoplakia, the lesions of carcinoma in situ and even those of microinvasive carcinoma often have a red ("erythroplastic") component.[82] Of 158 early asymptomatic epidermoid carcinomas studied by Mashberg et al.,[83] 143 (90.5%) had red components, whereas only 98 (62%) had white components; only four lesions were solely white, and there was no color distinction between invasive and in situ carcinoma. Induration almost guaranteed the presence of invasion. The authors concluded that an erythroplastic (red-velvety) lesion is the earliest visible sign of asymptomatic oral epidermoid carcinoma—invasive or in situ—and that the presence of a white component was not significant in itself.

The microscopic criteria for the diagnosis of carcinoma

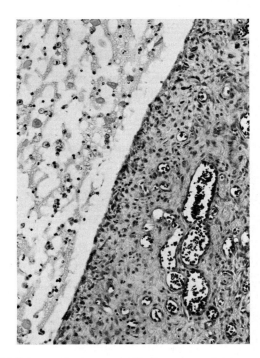

Fig. 5-9 Extravasation mucocele. Cystic space containing mucin and inflammatory cells is surrounded by inflammatory tissue with dilated vessels.

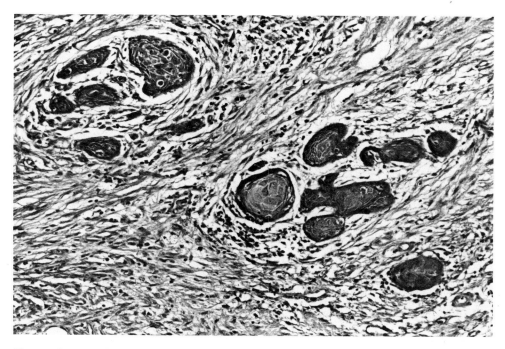

Fig. 5-10 Necrotizing sialometaplasia. Appearance simulates invasive epidermoid carcinoma, but squamous proliferation retains lobular architecture. Lesion is surrounded by cellular and inflammatory stroma.

in situ are essentially the same as for other mucosal membranes, notably the uterine cervix: epithelial disarray with full thickness atypia, no flattening or horizontal elongation of the surface layer, and a basement membrane which appears intact in routinely stained sections. However, immunohistochemical stains for basement membrane components such as type IV collagen and laminin have shown thinning and discontinuity of these markers in severe dysplasia/carcinoma in situ.[84]

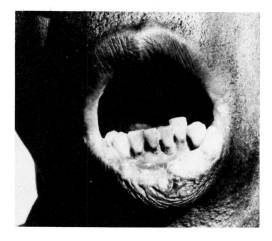

Fig. 5-11 Marked leukoplakia of lower lip in Bantu. (Courtesy Dr. A. Schmaman, Johannesburg, South Africa.)

In the presence of carcinoma in situ in a biopsy, the possibility that the lesion is the peripheral expression of an invasive carcinoma should be considered.

Epidermoid carcinoma
General features

Practically speaking, carcinoma of the oral cavity mucosa is synonymous with epidermoid (squamous cell) carcinoma. Known predisposing factors vary according to the location of the tumor. For carcinoma of the lip, they include sunlight, fair complexion, and—to a lesser extent—smoking and mechanical irritation.[86,88,89] Organ transplant recipients are also at an incrased risk, presumably as a result of immunosuppression.[91]

Oropharyngeal carcinomas have been related to tobacco, alcohol, syphilis, oral sepsis, iron deficiency, oral candidiasis, and Fanconi's anemia.[87,88,93,94] Most cases occur in males over the age of 50, although the relative incidence among women and younger patients seems to be increasing.[90,92] Some cases have been documented in children, particularly in the tongue.[95]

Location

Oropharyngeal carcinoma is classified topographically according to its site of origin as follows: (1) *lip,* including only the vermilion surface and comprising an upper and lower lip joined at the commissures of the mouth (2) *floor of the mouth,* a U-shaped area bounded by the lower gingiva and the oral tongue; (3) *oral tongue,* defined as the portion

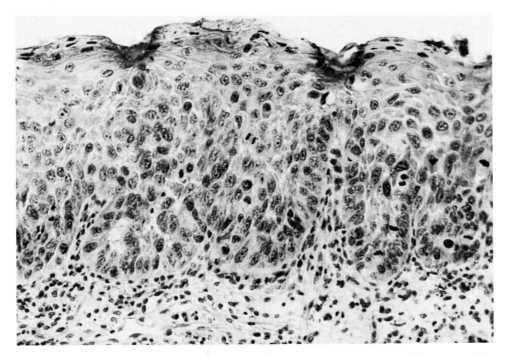

Fig. 5-12 Epidermoid carcinoma in situ of floor of mouth. Note intact basement membrane, complete disorganization of epithelium throughout all layers, and many mitotic figures.

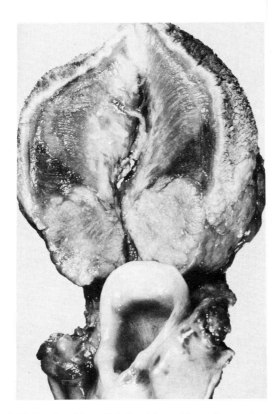

Fig. 5-13 Poorly differentiated epidermoid carcinoma in base of tongue. Patient had cervical node metastases. Primary lesion shown was not discovered clinically because of lack of proper examination. It was only found after death.

of the tongue anterior to the circumvallate papillae; (4) *buccal mucosa,* which covers the inner surface of the cheeks and lips; (5) *gingiva* (alveolar ridge), i.e., the mucosa covering the mandible or maxilla from the gingivobuccal gutter to the origin of the mobile mucosa; (6) *retromolar trigone,* a small triangular surface behind the third molar covering the ascending ramus of the mandible; (7) *hard palate,* a semilunar area located between the upper alveolar ridge and the mucous membrane covering the palatine process of the maxillary bones; (8) *base of the tongue,* bound anteriorly by the circumvallate papillae, laterally by the glossotonsillar sulci, and posteriorly by the epiglottis (Fig. 5-13); (9) *tonsillar area,* which includes the anterior and posterior tonsillar pillars and the tonsillar fossa; (10) *soft palate;* and (11) *pharyngeal walls*[96] (Fig. 5-14).

In a large series from the M.D. Anderson Hospital in Houston, Texas,[100] the location of the tumors within the oral cavity was listed as follows: lip, 45%; tongue, 16%; floor of mouth, 12%; buccal mucosa, 10%; lower gingiva, 12%; upper gingiva and hard palate, 5%. Of the lip tumors, over 90% involve the lower lip. In a careful study of early asymptomatic epidermoid oral cancers, Mashberg and Megers[101] found that the overwhelming majority of carcinomas of the oral cavity proper occur in three locations: floor of the mouth (especially at the papilla at the exit of Wharton's duct), soft palate–anterior pillar–retromolar complex, and ventrolateral aspect of the mobile portion of the tongue (Fig. 5-15). These "high-risk areas" have in common a lining of thin nonkeratinized squamous epithelium, with short or absent rete ridges and a narrow lamina propria.

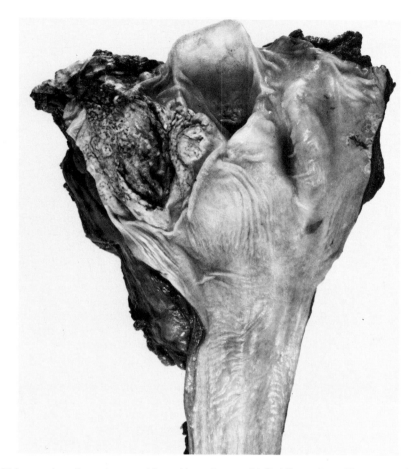

Fig. 5-14 Large ulcerating primary epidermoid carcinoma of left piriform sinus. There was also small carcinoma in right piriform sinus and in situ carcinoma in left vocal cord. (Courtesy Dr. J. Costa, Lausanne, Switzerland.)

Multiplicity of tumors is common.[97,98] Patients with carcinoma of the oral cavity have a hundredfold probability of developing a second primary tumor in the region.[99,102] The chances of this occurrence are particularly high when the carcinoma is associated with dysplastic changes elsewhere in the oral cavity.[102]

Microscopic appearance

Epidermoid carcinomas within the oral cavity are usually moderately or poorly differentiated. Those located at the base of the tongue or in the tonsil tend to be particularly undifferentiated and solid, thereby creating diagnostic confusions with large cell malignant lymphoma. The epithelium adjacent to the invasive cancer often shows carcinoma in situ or atypical (dysplastic) changes.[105] Some variations in the microscopic appearance of this tumor exist. A few epidermoid carcinomas are massively infiltrated with mature eosinophils, a feature that may create diagnostic difficulties and that is said to be associated with an improved prognosis.[103] Other epidermoid carcinomas have an adenoid or pseudoglandular appearance because of acantholysis. Most of these are located in the lip and, like their more common cutaneous counterparts, are associated with and probably induced by actinic radiation; however, a few have been seen in the gingiva or tongue, where an actinic pathogenesis is out of the question.[104]

Biopsy, cytology, and frozen section

Dentists have the best opportunity to discover early lesions of the oral cavity. It is their responsibility to examine the oral cavity carefully and to refer patients with suspicious lesions for proper evaluation and possible biopsy.[106]

The diagnosis is usually obvious in a well-taken sample.[107] A biopsy specimen that is often much more difficult to interpret is the one taken from an abnormal-appearing mucosa some time after irradiation therapy for an invasive epidermoid carcinoma has been completed. Under these circumstances, it is better to refrain from making a diagnosis of carcinoma unless there is definite stromal invasion, because from a cytologic standpoint it is often impossible to distinguish residual carcinoma in situ from radiation atypia. Generally speaking, it is better to wait a minimum of 6 to 8 weeks following completion of the therapy before taking a new biopsy.

Cytologic examination of oral lesions is of no great practical value. In a series of 158 epidermoid carcinomas studied

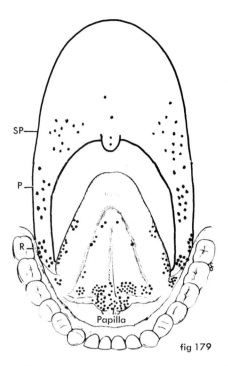

Fig. 5-15 Scattergram indicating site of origin of over 200 asymptomatic early epidermoid carcinomas. Note concentration of lesions around papilla at exit of Wharton's duct, ventrolateral aspect of tongue, lingual aspect of retromolar trigon, *R*, anterior pillar, *P*, and soft palate, *SP*. (Adapted from Mashberg A, Meyers H: Anatomic site and size of 222 early asymptomatic oral squamous cell carcinomas. A continuing prospective study of oral cancer. II. Cancer **37:**2149-2157, 1976.)

by Shklar et al.,[109] there was a false negative incidence of 13.9%. Furthermore, there was not a single case with positive cytology in which the biopsy had failed to reveal the tumor.

The main role of frozen section in oropharyngeal epidermoid carcinoma is in the evaluation of surgical margins. A good correlation has been found between presence or closeness of the tumor at the margin and the probability of local recurrence and mortality.[108]

Spread and metastases

The pattern of direct spread of oropharyngeal carcinoma is dictated by the anatomic features of the primary site.[110] Carcinoma of the lip invades adjacent skin, the orbicular muscle, and—when advanced—the buccal mucosa, the adjacent mandible, and the mental nerve. Tumors of the floor of the mouth penetrate early beneath the mucosa into the sublingual gland, into the midline muscles, and extend towards the gingiva and mandible.[114] Tumors of the oral tongue, which usually arise on the lateral and undersurfaces, tend to remain localized for long periods, but eventually invade the floor of the mouth and root of the tongue, resulting in fixation of the organ. Tumors of the buccal mucosa invade the underlying muscles and may eventually penetrate into the skin. Tumors of gingiva extend quickly into the periosteum, the adjacent buccal mucosa, and the floor of

mouth. Tumors of the hard palate may spread into the underlying bone, but extension into the maxillary antrum is very rare. Tumors of retromolar trigone spread to adjacent buccal mucosa, anterior tonsillar pillar, maxilla, pterygomandibular space, medial pterygoid muscle, and buccinator muscle.

Metastases occur primarily by the lymphatic route, the distribution of lymph node involvement depending on the location of the primary tumor. The more anterior the tumor, the lower the position of the cervical nodal metastasis. Carcinomas of the base of the tongue and oropharynx tend to metastasize to the deep retropharyngeal lymph nodes. Features of the primary tumor associated with the likelihood of nodal metastases in the neck are location (higher for the posterior portion of the tongue and oropharynx, intermediate for the anterior portion of the tongue, and low for the lip, floor of mouth, cheek mucosa, hard palate, and gingiva), poor microscopic differentiation, and depth of invasion.[112,116,116a]

Occasionally, the cervical node metastases from these epidermoid carcinomas undergo cystic degeneration. This, plus the well-differentiated nature of the lesion, has led on occasion to a mistaken diagnosis of branchial cyst with malignant transformation ("branchial carcinoma").[111] The occult primary lesion is often located in the tonsil, particularly its posterior pillar.[113] Another peculiar morphologic pattern that epidermoid carcinoma can exhibit when metastasizing to cervical nodes is that of an extensive foreign body giant cell reaction around clumps of keratin, without viable tumor cells; this is particularly common if the tumor has been previously irradiated.[115]

Treatment

The two pillars of therapy for oropharyngeal carcinoma are surgery and radiation therapy, used either singly or in combination. For most early stage lesions, the results of irradiation and surgery are very similar, so that the final decision as to which to use often depends on factors such as functional and cosmetic results, the patient's general status, and the physician's bias.[117]

Prognosis

The main prognostic determinators in oral cavity cancer are stage of the disease, location, and microscopic grading.[118,122,127] Tumor size does not correlate closely with clinical outcome, except for the very small tumors.[126] Depth of invasion is a better prognostic indicator, at least in some locations.[119,120] Determination of DNA ploidy by flow cytometry correlates with microscopic degree of differentiation and therefore may prove to be of prognostic value.[129]

The overall 5-year survival rates are about 90% for carcinomas of the lower lip[120]; 60% for tumors of the anterior tongue; 40% for tumors of the posterior tongue, floor of mouth, tonsil, gingiva, and hard palate[124]; and 20% to 30% for tumors of the soft palate.[121,123-125,128]

Verrucous carcinoma

Verrucous carcinoma is a variant of well-differentiated epidermoid carcinoma endowed with enough clinical, pathologic, and behavioral peculiarities to justify it being regarded as a specific tumor entity.[130,136,138] The oral cavity

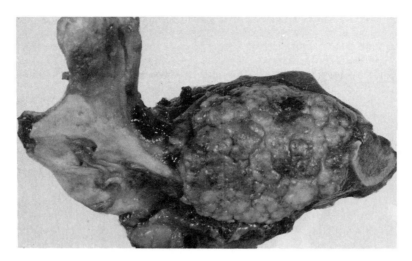

Fig. 5-16 Large verrucous carcinoma of oral cavity invading jaw. (From Ackerman, LV, del Regato JA: Cancer, ed. 4. St. Louis, 1970, The C.V. Mosby Co.)

is its classic location, but this lesion also has been reported in the larynx, nasal cavity, esophagus, penis, anorectal region, vulva, vagina, uterine cervix, and skin (particularly in the sole of the foot). Within the oral cavity, the most common sites are the buccal mucosa and lower gingiva.[134,135] Most patients are elderly males, and there is a close connection with the use of tobacco, especially chewing or snuff dipping.[140] Grossly, it presents as a large, fungating, soft papillary growth that tends to become infected and slowly invades contiguous structures (Fig. 5-16). It may grow through the soft tissues of the cheek, penetrate into the mandible or maxilla, and invade perineurial spaces.[132] Regional lymph node metastases are exceedingly rare, and distant metastases have not been reported.

The microscopic diagnosis of verrucous carcinoma may be difficult because of its well-differentiated character. A superficial biopsy will only show hyperkeratosis, acanthosis, and benign-appearing papillomatosis. Sections of an adequate biopsy show swollen and voluminous rete pegs that extend into the deeper tissues, where their pattern becomes quite complex[131] (Figs. 5-17 and 5-18). The most important differential feature with epidermoid carcinoma is the good cytologic differentiation *throughout* the tumor. In about one fifth of the cases, foci of epidermoid carcinoma occur within a lesion that looks otherwise like a verrucous carcinoma, hence the importance of thorough sampling.[137] These hybrid tumors are said to be associated with a higher recurrence rate.[137]

Resection is the treatment of choice. If surgery is inadequate, the tumor will recur.[130] Radiation therapy is usually not used, since it may alter the nature of the tumor to a highly malignant, rapidly metastasizing, poorly differentiated epidermoid carcinoma.[134] This has occurred in as many as 30% of the cases in some series, the average postirradiation interval being 6 months.

It is likely that most of the cases reported in the past as *oral florid papillomatosis*[141] represent early and noninvasive stages of verrucous carcinoma. Along the same lines, the similar if not identical conditions known as *verrucous*

hyperplasia,[139] *proliferative verrucous leukoplakia,*[133] *verrucous keratosis,* and *leukoplakia verrucosa* can be regarded as precursor lesions of verrucous carcinoma, from which they are distinguished by the fact that the verrucous process is *superficial* to the adjacent squamous epithelium.

Other microscopic types

Carcinomas of surface epithelial origin of types other than epidermoid or verrucous carcinoma are the following:

1 *Adenosquamous carcinoma.* In contrast to adenoid (pseudoglandular) carcinoma, the rare adenosquamous carcinoma shows areas of squamous differentiation mixed with others having true glandular differentiation[145] (Fig. 5-19). Some of these cases may be of minor salivary gland derivation.

2 *Basaloid carcinoma.* In this variant, areas with obvious squamous differentiation are mixed with solid tumor islands that exhibit peripheral palisading and a thick basement membrane.[150] Cystic spaces containing hyaline material are present, resulting in a vague resemblance to adenoid cystic carcinoma. The appearance of this tumor, which is highly malignant, is also reminiscent of some "cloacogenic" carcinomas of the anal canal. It seems likely that the pattern is indicative of an abortive attempt at glandular differentiation. The differential diagnosis includes minor salivary gland tumors and peripheral ameloblastoma (see p. 189).

3 *Spindle cell (sarcomatoid) carcinoma.* This may appear as an ulcerated and infiltrative mass or as a polypoid growth in the lip, tongue, or other portions of the oral cavity. Sometimes the sarcoma-like formation blends with areas of obvious epidermoid carcinoma, is associated with epidermoid carcinomas elsewhere in the oral cavity, or represents the recurrence of what originally was an obvious epidermoid carcinoma[142,146,148] (Fig. 5-20). The appearance of the sarcoma-like component is often reminiscent of malignant fibrous histiocytoma of soft tissues. Hyaline globules may be found in the cytoplasm of the larger tumor

cells. Ultrastructural and immunohistochemical studies may or may not show epithelial markers in these foci.[144,151,152] The nodal and distal metastases of this tumor may be purely carcinomatous, have a mixed appearance as in the primary neoplasm, or—in rare cases—be entirely composed of sarcoma-like elements. The prognosis is closely related to the depth of invasion and is not significantly different from ordinary epidermoid carcinoma of equivalent stage and thickness.[149,151]

4 *Small cell (oat cell) carcinoma.* The appearance is similar to that of the homonymous lung carcinoma.[143] It may be pure or associated with a squamous component, and its behavior is very aggressive.[147]

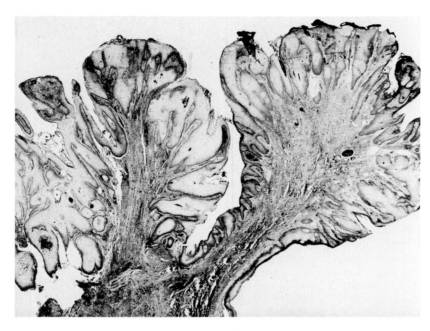

Fig. 5-17 Frondlike growth pattern of verrucous carcinoma.

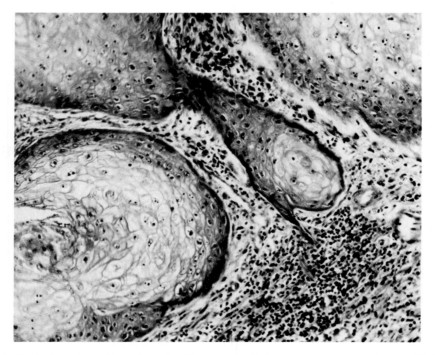

Fig. 5-18 Detailed view of swollen rete ridges of deeply invasive verruous carcinoma with intact basement membrane.

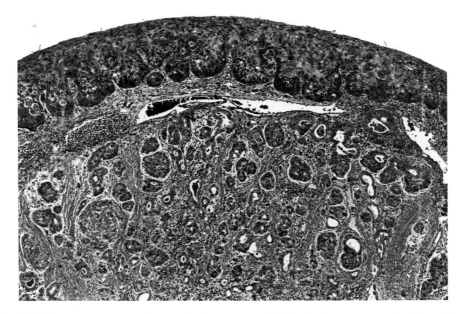

Fig. 5-19 Adenosquamous carcinoma. In situ component with typical appearance of epidermoid carcinoma is associated with invasive component that shows squamous and glandular features.

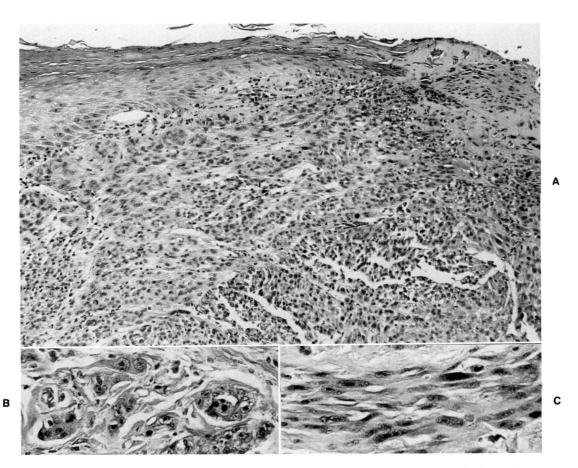

Fig. 5-20 Spindle cell carcinoma of lip. **A,** Panoramic view, showing cellular neoplasm growing beneath attenuated and partially ulcerated epidermis. **B,** In this area, tumor cells have clear-cut epithelial appearance. **C,** In other foci, cellular shape and pattern of growth closely simulate sarcoma. This peculiar variety of epidermoid cell carcinoma, which has strong predilection for involvement of lip, should be clearly separated from atypical fibroxanthoma of skin and from "pseudosarcoma" of upper respiratory and digestive tracts.

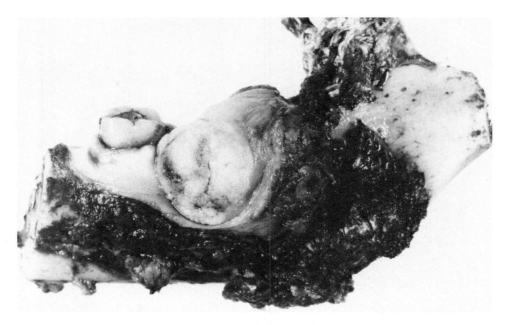

Fig. 5-21 Acinic cell carcinoma arising from minor salivary glands of gingiva. Tumor had invaded bone and had also ulcerated in oral cavity.

TUMORS AND OTHER LESIONS OF MINOR SALIVARY GLANDS

Minor salivary glands, present in practically all structures within the oral cavity, participate in many of the diseases affecting their major counterparts, a feature that can be exploited for diagnostic purposes. Thus biopsy of the lower lip has shown involvement of the minor salivary glands in cases of *cystic fibrosis*[178] and *Sjögren's syndrome*[158,160] and is also being increasingly used to diagnose and stage *chronic graft-versus-host disease*.

Salivary gland choristoma presents as a gingival nodule microscopically composed of disorganized seromucinous salivary gland tissue mixed with sebaceous glands.[156]

Adenomatoid hyperplasia is a term used for a localized hyperplastic process of minor salivary glands appearing clinically as a nodule, usually in the hard palate, but occasionally in the retromolar area.[155]

These glands also can be the site of benign and malignant tumors. The hard palate is the most common location, but the tumors also occur in the soft palate, cheek, tonsil, floor of the mouth, tongue, lip (usually the upper), gingiva, and jaw (Fig. 5-21). It is important to remember that tumors arising in the deep lobe of the parotid gland may present as primary intraoral masses. With a few exceptions, minor salivary gland tumors are morphologically analogous to those located in the major glands[170,177] (see Chapter 12); however, they differ from the latter in their relative incidence and, to some extent, in their natural history.[157]

Benign mixed tumors (pleomorphic adenomas), which constitute over 75% of all parotid neoplasms, make up only about half of the salivary gland tumors of the palate.[161,162,164]

Adenoid cystic carcinoma, mucoepidermoid carcinoma, and *terminal duct carcinoma* comprise the large majority of intraoral malignant salivary gland tumors, in contrast to the more even distribution of tumor types seen in the parotid. The prognosis of adenoid cystic carcinoma is better when the tumor is located in the palate than when present in the parotid or submaxillary gland.[162] The prognostic difference among the various morphologic subtypes of this tumor, which has been noted for the major salivary gland, seems to apply also to this location.[159]

Of the salivary gland tumors located in the lip, about 80% are benign. Among the malignant, adenoid cystic carcinoma and mucoepidermoid carcinoma are the most frequent.[176]

Some types of salivary gland tumors occur predominantly or—in some instances—almost exclusively in the minor salivary glands of the oral cavity. They include the following:

1 *Basal cell adenoma.* This tumor, with a canalicular pattern of growth, has a predilection for the upper lip, where it is sometimes confused with adenoid cystic carcinoma.[164] As discussed in Chapter 12, some authors like to distinguish this tumor from other basal cell adenomas and designate it as canalicular adenoma (Fig. 5-22).

2 *Myoepithelioma.* This lesion, composed of hyaline or plasmacytoid cells, usually involves the hard palate (Fig. 5-23). The differential diagnosis includes plasmacytoma, oncocytoma, and even skeletal muscle neoplasms. Despite its high cellularity and occasional nuclear atypia, the behavior is generally benign[172,175] (see Chapter 12).

3 *Sialadenoma papilliferum.* This lesion is a papillary lesion of the oral cavity, usually located in the hard palate and characterized microscopically by a biphasic composition. An exophytic mass of well-differentiated

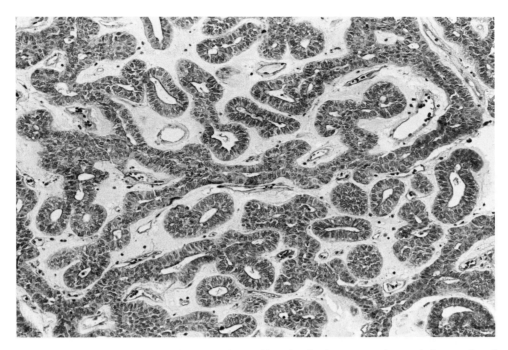

Fig. 5-22 Canalicular carcinoma. This is a form of basal cell adenoma made up of elongated and branching canaliculi separated by hyaline stroma.

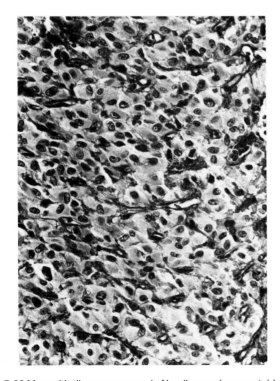

Fig. 5-23 Myoepithelioma composed of hyaline or plasmacytoid cells. Tumor has solid pattern of growth and there is some degree of nuclear pleomorphism.

squamous epithelium is seen covering a glandular component consisting of cleftlike cystic spaces lined by cuboidal or columnar epithelium; some of these glands may contain oncocytic cells, and others may exhibit squamous metaplasia.[165,166] The appearance is reminiscent both of Warthin's tumor of the parotid gland and papillary syringadenoma of skin, both at the light and electron microscopic level[165] (Fig. 5-24).

4 *Inverted ductal papilloma.* This tumor has a pattern of growth similar to that of inverted papilloma of the nasal cavity. It appears clinically as a small submucosal mass in the oral cavity of adults. Microscopically, there are complex invaginations formed by well-differentiated, predominantly squamous epithelium-associated microcysts, occasional mucous cells, and a lining of columnar cells. The behavior is benign.[179]

5 *Syringoma.* This neoplasm has an appearance similar to that of the homonymous skin tumor of sweat gland origin.[171]

6 *Terminal duct carcinoma.* This term has been recently proposed for a low-grade malignant tumor that has also been called *low-grade papillary adenocarcinoma,*[154,174] *polymorphous low-grade adenocarcinoma,*[163,168] and *lobular carcinoma.*[153,167] The palate is the most common location; actually, terminal duct carcinoma is the second most common type of salivary gland carcinoma in this location, following adenoid cystic carcinoma. Microscopically, there is uniformity of cell type but a marked variation in architectural

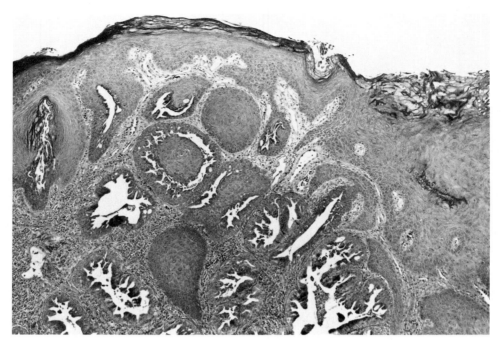

Fig. 5-24 Sialadenoma papilliferum. Glandular proliferation reaching surface epithelium results in complicated microscopic feature that may simulate malignancy. Pattern is somewhat reminiscent of that seen in adenoma of nipple.

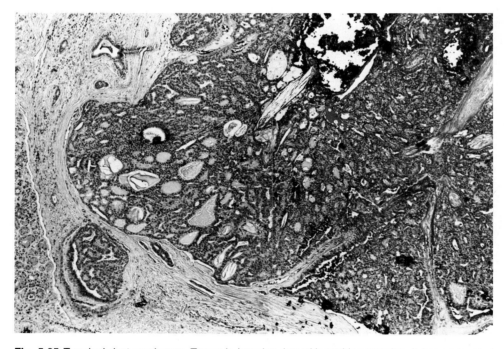

Fig. 5-25 Terminal duct carcinoma. Tumor is invasive, but with pushing margins. It has variegated appearance ranging from solid to microglandular.

patterns, which is responsible for the various names that this tumor has received. Tubular, cribriform, papillary, solid, and fascicular formations may appear, with frequent combinations and transitions (Fig. 5-25). The periphery of the tumor has invasive features, sometimes in an Indian-file pattern, which has led to a strained analogy with invasive lobular carcinoma of the breast.[167] Perineurial invasion is also common. S-100 protein immunoreactivity is present, suggesting an important myoepithelial participation.[173,180] The differential diagnosis includes benign mixed tumor, basal cell adenoma (both of which lack infiltrative features), and adenoid cystic carcinoma, with which terminal duct carcinoma is probably closely related.[168] However, the former lacks the plump and columnar cells of terminal duct carcinoma, as well as its papillary and fascicular growth patterns. The behavior of terminal duct carcinoma is that of a low-grade malignancy. In one series of sixty-nine cases, recurrences developed in 12% and regional lymph node metastases in 10%, but there were no distant metastases, and there was only one tumor-related death.[173]

The treatment for minor salivary gland tumors is primarily surgical. It has been emphasized that the first excision should be the most definitive and comprehensive, and that treatment of recurrent disease is rarely curative.[169] Post-operative irradiation is generally recommended for all high-grade malignancies, including adenoid cystic carcinoma.[169]

TUMORS OF ODONTOGENIC EPITHELIUM

Peripheral ameloblastoma is a tumor of the oral cavity, not involving bone but exhibiting microscopic features of ameloblastic differentiation (Fig. 5-26). As a matter of fact, its appearance is indistinguishable from that of ameloblastoma of the jaw.[181] Most of the reported cases have occurred in the gingiva, and several have been published in the past as basal cell carcinomas. They may arise from remnants of the dental lamina within the gingiva ("rests of Serres") or, more likely, from the surface epithelium. They are relatively innocuous and are generally cured by local excision.[181]

TUMORS OF MELANOCYTES

Ephelis and *lentigo* (melanotic macules) can present as solitary lesions of the lip.[195] They are characterized by hyperpigmentation of the basal layer, associated in the latter with elongation of the rete ridges. The term *melanoacanthoma* has been used when the melanocytic proliferation extends above the basal layer and is found mixed intimately with the keratinocytes.[189,195] Multiple pigmented macules of the lip are one of the components of the Peutz-Jeghers' syndrome (see Chapter 11, Small bowel). The presence of pigmented patches within the oral cavity (usually located in the hard palate or gingiva) is known as *melanosis.*

Melanocytic nevi may involve the lips and, in rare cases, the inside of the oral cavity.[185,186,188] In one series, there were three junctional, thirty compound, thirty-two intramucosal (equivalent of the cutaneous intradermal), and six

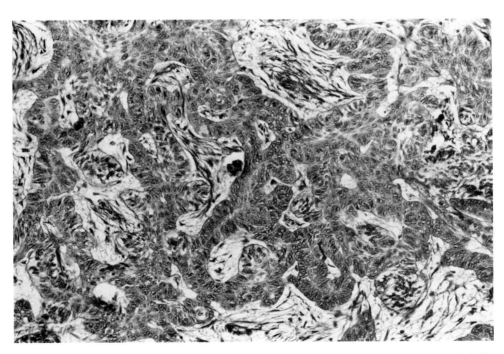

Fig. 5-26 Peripheral ameloblastoma. Intricate basaloid appearance is present, morphologically indistinguishable from that seen in more common intraosseous counterpart.

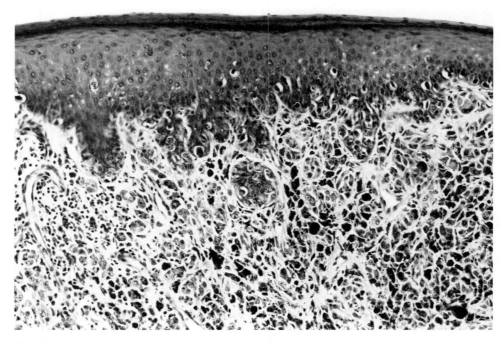

Fig. 5-27 Intraoral malignant melanoma. There is junctional activity associated with extensive invasive component. Tumor has produced large amounts of melanin.

blue nevi.[197] The nevus of Ota may also involve the oral cavity in the region of the palate.[191]

Malignant melanomas of the oral cavity are particularly common in people of Japanese and Black African origin.[196] The palate and gingiva are the most common locations.[183,192] Both pigmented and amelanotic varieties occur[187] (Fig. 5-27). Some of the tumors have desmoplastic features, especially when occurring in the lower lip. Stains for S-100 protein should be done in any undifferentiated or spindle-shaped malignant neoplasm of the oral cavity.

Oral "melanosis" adjacent to the area of invasive tumor is found in about 30% of the cases[196]; in most instances, there is some degree of atypia in this intraepithelial component. Several authors have likened this lesion to Hutchinson's freckle of the skin.[194] Although some morphologic similarities certainly exist, the analogy is probably unwarranted because of the different natural history and genesis of these two lesions. Arrington et al.[182] prefer to regard this as a distinct subtype of melanoma and designate it as (acral) *lentiginous melanoma*.[190] Lymph node and distant metastases are common, and the prognosis is extremely poor.[184,193]

TUMORS AND TUMORLIKE CONDITIONS OF LYMPHOID TISSUE

Benign nodules made of well-differentiated lymphocytes, with or without an admixture of histiocytes, are not uncommon in the oral cavity. They may represent enlarged buccal lymph nodes or hypertrophic buccal tonsils or may be associated with cystic glandular structures ("lymphoepithelial cysts").[200] The most prominent of these benign lymphoid proliferations are designated *lymphoid polyps* or *pseudo-lymphomas*.[211] We have also seen several cases of nodular collections of mature lymphocytes in the hard palate accompanied by florid epimyoepithelial islands of minor salivary gland derivation. Although these patients did not have clinical abnormalities in the major salivary glands, we think that these cases could be regarded as oral cavity counterparts of Mikulicz's disease (see Chapter 12).

Malignant lymphoma most commonly occurs in the Waldeyer's ring, particularly in the palatine and lingual tonsil, but it can also develop in the gingival area, buccal mucosa, or palate (Fig. 5-28). The typical clinical presentation is that of a soft bulky mass covered by normal or ulcerated mucosa. Microscopically, most cases are of B-cell nature and follicular center cell origin, either large cell or poorly differentiated lymphocytic, with a generally diffuse pattern of growth[199,203,205,208,214] (Fig. 5-29). It is common for the lymphocytic tumors to exhibit a peculiar artifact characterized by a marked elongation (streaking) of nuclei.[213] In about 40% of the cases, there is evidence of disease outside the oral cavity, particularly in the cervical lymph nodes and gastrointestinal tract.[205,212] The latter feature suggests that malignant lymphomas of the Waldeyer's ring share some of the characteristics of so-called mucosa-associated lymphoid tissue (MALT) lymphomas.[203] In a series of 225 patients reported by Banfi et al.,[198] lymphangiography revealed retroperitoneal lymph node involvement in one third. As for malignant lymphomas elsewhere, clinical staging and microscopic typing are the two most important prognostic factors.[199]

Plasmacytomas can occur in the soft tissues of the oral cavity, although not so commonly as in the upper air passages.[206] It is important to distinguish them from the more common plasma cell granulomas of reactive nature. The latter are composed of mature plasma cells, have a mixture of other inflammatory cells, and are associated with fibrosis.

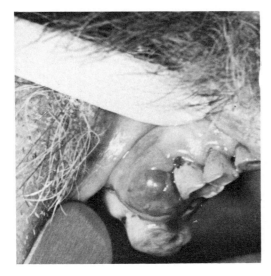

Fig. 5-28 Malignant lymphoma arising from upper alveolus.

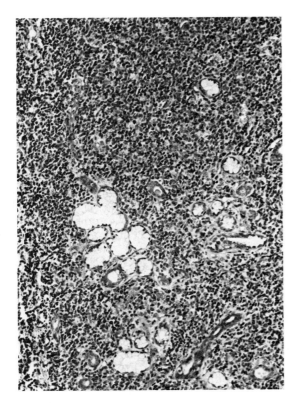

Fig. 5-29 Malignant lymphoma of oral cavity. Tumor is composed of monotonous population of small cleaved cells that are surrounding and distorting normal minor salivary glands of region.

Immunohistochemical staining for immunoglobulin types may help in this differential diagnosis.[210]

Hodgkin's disease and *malignant histiocytosis* presenting initially in the oral cavity are extremely rare, but several reported cases are on record.[201]

Histiocytosis X can involve the oral cavity, either as an isolated focus or as an expression of multisystem disease.[209] The lesions are most often found in the gingiva but also can affect the hard palate.[207]

Leukemia of acute myelocytic or myelomonocytic type is associated with gingival involvement in about 4% of the cases, with or without concomitant skin involvement.[204] In rare cases, oral cavity disease is the first manifestation of granulocytic sarcoma.[202]

OTHER TUMORS AND TUMORLIKE CONDITIONS

So-called *peripheral giant cell granuloma (giant cell epulis)* is seen in all age groups and is more common in females.[229] Maxilla and mandible are affected with equal frequency. A soft-to-firm mass forms in the gingiva, pushes the teeth aside, and may erode the mandible. Microscopically, the lesion shows numerous osteoclast-like giant cells, an active vascular stroma, and—at times—small amounts of neoformed bone (Fig. 5-30). This common lesion is benign and probably of reactive nature.

Granular cell tumor can involve any portion of the oral cavity, the tongue being the most common site. The overlying epithelium often shows florid pseudoepitheliomatous

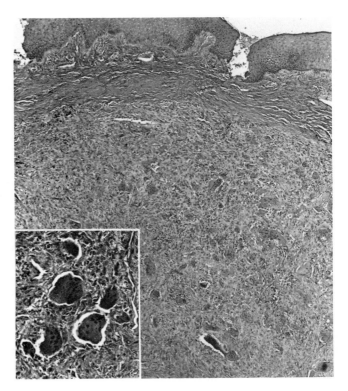

Fig. 5-30 Peripheral giant cell granuloma. Well-circumscribed but not encapsulated nodule composed of fibrohistiocytic cells and multinucleated giant cells is seen beneath epithelium. Osteoclast-like appearance of giant cells can be appreciated in **inset**.

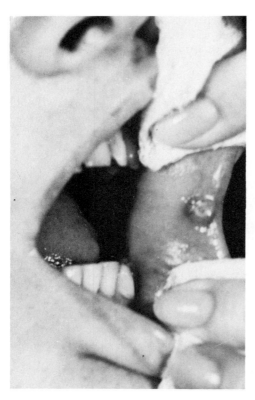

Fig. 5-31 Sharply circumscribed and elevated pyogenic granuloma of buccal mucosa.

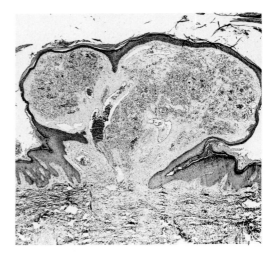

Fig. 5-32 Typical low-power pattern of pyogenic granuloma. Note elevation above lining epithelium and its narrowing at base.

hyperplasia.[224,247,262] An exceptionally rare malignant counterpart of this lesion has also been described.[263] A lesion that is indistinguishable from granular cell tumor by light microscopy is seen occasionally in the gingiva of newborn infants and is called *congenital epulis*.[235] This lesion occurs almost exclusively in females and it behaves in a benign fashion even if incompletely excised.[240] Ultrastructural studies have suggested a mesenchymal (fibroblastic, pericytic, or smooth muscle) rather than an odontogenic origin.[233,239,257,264] Staining for S-100 protein is negative, in contrast to the adult form of this lesion.[241]

Verruciform xanthoma presents in middle-aged persons as a raised, granular, or verrucous lesion of the oral cavity, usually in the gingiva or alveolar ridge.[220,252] Collections of foamy macrophages in the lamina propria are covered by a verrucous and acanthotic epithelium.[251] The lesion is probably a reactive process rather than a true neoplasm.[250]

Benign epithelial proliferations of skin adnexal type are sometimes seen in the oral cavity. These include keratoacanthoma (common in the lip, but occasionally situated intraorally),[225] inverted follicular keratosis (most often in the lower lip),[215] and warty dyskeratoma.[221,231]

Vascular tumors of the oral cavity are largely represented by hemangiomas and lymphangiomas.[218] Most of these are located in the tongue, where they can result in soft cystic masses large enough to interfere with speech and mastication.[242] Microscopically, most of these lesions have mark-

edly dilated ("cavernous") vascular or lymphatic channels. The treatment is surgical.

Another common vascular proliferation of the oral cavity is *pyogenic granuloma* (lobular capillary hemangioma). It appears as an elevated, dark red lesion that may or may not be ulcerated (Fig. 5-31). Large masses of proliferating endothelial cells are separated by an edematous stroma containing inflammatory cells. Characteristically, the covering epithelium almost meets at the base of the lesion (Fig. 5-32). It heals as a residual fibrous mass or fibroepithelial papilloma.[236] An identical lesion occurring during pregnancy has been referred to as granuloma gravidarum or pregnancy tumor.[245]

Other benign vascular tumors that may present intraorally are *glomus tumor*[260] and *histiocytoid (epithelioid) hemangioma,* a disorder also known as *angiolymphoid hyperplasia with eosinophilia*.[254] *Angiosarcoma* is very rare.[219,255] We have seen a case appearing many years after irradiation of a lymphangioma, and a similar case has been reported.[248]

Smooth muscle tumors can also occur in this location.[244,249] Most leiomyomas are located in the tongue, and many are of vascular type. Leiomyosarcomas are more common in the cheek region.

Rhabdomyomas have a special predilection for the oral cavity and neck. Most are seen in adults, and the floor of the mouth is the most common location.[223,227] Both adult and fetal forms have been described. They are usually well-circumscribed and may be multiple[217,228] (Fig. 5-33).

Peripheral nerve tumors of the oral cavity include neurilemoma (often located in the tongue), neurofibroma,[253] and the multiple mucosal neuromas seen as a component of multiple endocrine adenomatosis type III. The individual lesions resemble plexiform neurofibromas and may be found in the lips, tongue, conjunctiva, nasal cavity, and larynx.[230] Malignant schwannomas of the oral cavity, some of which are pigmented, have also been described.[232]

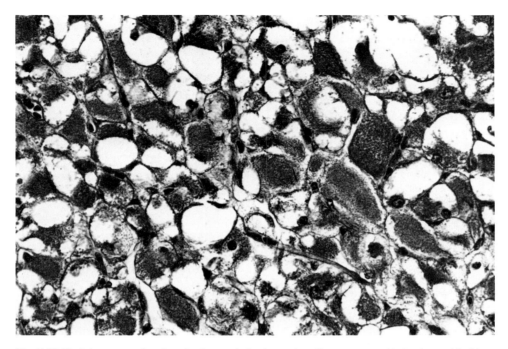

Fig. 5-33 Rhabdomyoma of oral cavity. Large skeletal muscle cells are arranged in haphazard fashion. Some of them contain cross-striations and others exhibit prominent cytoplasmic vacuolization.

Other *benign soft tissue tumors* that have been reported in this location are lipoma (sometimes exhibiting myxoid changes or cartilaginous/osseous metaplasia)[216,222] and angiolipoma.[226]

Synovial sarcomas can occur as primary tumors in the pharynx, tonsil, cheek, tongue, or palate of young adults[246,261]; the main differential diagnosis is with salivary gland tumors, particularly benign mixed tumor.

Kaposi's sarcoma can be accompanied by buccal involvement, and occasionally an oral lesion is the initial manifestation of the disease. In a series of fifty-three AIDS patients with Kaposi's sarcoma, twenty-seven had biopsy-proven oral disease, the palate being the most common site.[243]

Other reported sarcomas of oral cavity include *alveolar soft part sarcoma*,[238] *extraskeletal osteosarcoma*,[256] and *liposarcoma*.[259]

Metastatic tumors may present as primary intraoral masses. The gingiva is the classic location, with or without oral involvement. The lung is the most common site of the primary lesion.[234,237] We have seen metastatic renal cell carcinoma masquerading clinically and microscopically as a pyogenic granuloma. Other sites for the primary tumor include breast, skin (melanoma), prostate, and large bowel.[258,265]

REFERENCES

1 Gorlin RJ, Goldman HM: Thoma's oral pathology, ed. 6. St. Louis, 1970, The C.V. Mosby Co.

CONGENITAL ABNORMALITIES

2 Bossen EH, Hudson WR: Oligodendroglioma arising in heterotopic brain tissue of the soft palate and nasopharynx. Am J Surg Pathol **11:**571-574, 1987.

3 Broniatowski M, Witt WJ, Shah AC, Galloway PG, Abramowsky CR: Glial tissue in the parapharyngeal space. Arch Otolaryngol **107:**638-641, 1981.

4 Cataldo E, Berkman MD: Cysts of the oral mucosa in newborns. Am J Dis Child **116:**44-48, 1968.

5 Dunlap CL, Barker BF: Diagnostic problems in oral pathology. Semin Diagn Pathol **2:**16-30, 1985.

6 Gibson WS Jr, Fenton NA: Congenital sublingual dermoid cyst. Arch Otolaryngol **108:**745-748, 1982.

7 Gorlin RJ, Jirasek JE: Oral cysts containing gastric or intestinal mucosa. An unusual embryological accident or heterotopia. Arch Otolaryngol **91:**594-597, 1970.

8 Leibl W, Pflüger H, Kerjaschki D: A case of nodular hyperplasia of the juxtaoral organ in man. Virchows Arch [Pathol Anat] **371:**389-391, 1976.

9 Lutman GB: Epithelial nests in intraoral sensory nerve endings simulating perineural invasion in patients with oral carcinoma. Am J Clin Pathol **61:**275-284, 1974.

10 Meyer I: Dermoid cysts (dermoids) of the floor of the mouth. Oral Surg Oral Med Oral Pathol **8:**1149-1164, 1955.

11 Simpson HE: White sponge nevus. J Oral Surg **24:**463-466, 1966.

12 Tschen JA, Fechner RE: The juxtaoral organ of Chievitz. Am J Surg Pathol **3:**147-150, 1979.

13 Zarem HA, Gray GF Jr, Morehead D: Heterotopic brain in the nasopharynx and soft palate. Surgery **61:**483-486, 1967.

14 Zenker W, Salzer G: Die histologie des chievitzen organs. Acta Anat [Basel] **44:**286-321, 1961.

INFLAMMATORY DISEASES

15 Ackerman LV, McGavran MH: Proliferating benign and malignant epithelial lesions of the oral cavity. J Oral Surg **16:**400-413, 1958.

16 Barker DS, Lucas RB: Localized fibrous overgrowths of the oral mucosa. Br J Oral Surg **5:**86-92, 1967.

17 Basu MK, Asquith P, Thompson RA, Cooke WT: Oral manifestations of Crohn's disease. Gut 16:249-254, 1975.

18 Bennett DE: Histoplasmosis of the oral cavity and larynx. A clinicopathologic study. Arch Intern Med 120:417-427, 1967.

19 Bhaskar SN, Beasley JD, Cutright DE: Inflammatory papillary hyperplasia of the oral mucosa. Report of 341 cases. J Am Dent Assoc 81:949-952, 1970.

20 Bodine RL: Oral lesions caused by ill-fitting dentures. J Prosthet Dent 21:580-588, 1969.

21 Croft CB, Wilkinson AR: Ulceration of the mouth, pharynx, and larynx in Crohn's disease of the intestine. Br J Surg 59:249-252, 1972.

22 Elzay RP: Traumatic ulcerative granuloma with stromal eosinophilia (Riga-Fede's disease and traumatic eosinophilic granuloma). Oral Surg Oral Med Oral Pathol 55:497-506, 1983.

23 Eversole LR, Leider AS, Jacobsen PL, Kidd PM: Atypical histiocytic granuloma. Light microscopic, ultrastructural, and histochemical findings in an unusual pseudomalignant reactive lesion of the oral cavity. Cancer 55:1722-1729, 1985.

24 Handlers JP, Waterman J, Abrams AM, Melrose RJ: Oral features of Wegener's granulomatosis. Arch Otolaryngol 111:267-270, 1985.

25 Houston GD: The giant cell fibroma. A review of 464 cases. Oral Surg Oral Med Oral Pathol 53:582-586, 1982.

26 Meyer I, Abbey LM: Relationship of syphilis to primary carcinoma of tongue. Oral Surg Oral Med Oral Pathol 30:678-681, 1970.

27 Nessan VJ, Jacoway JR: Biopsy of minor salivary glands in the diagnosis of sarcoidosis. N Engl J Med 301:922-924, 1979.

28 Oppenheim H, Livingston CS, Nixon JW, Miller CD: Streptomycin therapy in oral tuberculosis. Oral Surg Oral Med Oral Pathol 4:1389-1405, 1951.

29 Regezi JA, Courtney RM, Kerr DA: Fibrous lesions of skin and mucous membranes which contain stellate and multinucleated cells. Oral Surg Oral Med Oral Pathol 39:605-614, 1975.

30 Schnitt SJ, Antonioli DA, Jaffe B, Peppercorn MA: Granulomatous inflammation of minor salivary gland ducts. A new oral manifestation of Crohn's disease. Hum Pathol 18:405-407, 1987.

31 Snyder MB, Cawson RA: Oral changes in Crohn's disease. J Oral Surg 34:594-599, 1976.

32 Tang TT, Glicklich M, Hodach AE, Oechler HW, McCreadie SR: Ulcerative eosinophilic granuloma of the tongue. A light- and electron-microscopic study. Am J Clin Pathol 75:420-425, 1981.

33 Worsaae N, Christensen KC, Schiødt M, Reibel J: Melkersson-Rosenthal syndrome and cheilitis granulomatosa. A clinicopathologic study of thirty-three patients with special reference to their oral lesions. Oral Surg Oral Med Oral Pathol 54:404-413, 1982.

34 Wright JM, Rankin KV, Wilson JW: Traumatic granuloma of the tongue. Head Neck Surg 5:363-366, 1983.

OTHER NON-NEOPLASTIC LESIONS

35 Abrams AM, Melrose RJ, Howell FV: Necrotizing sialometaplasia. A disease simulating malignancy. Cancer 32:130-135, 1973.

36 Bouquot JE, Gorlin RJ: Leukoplakia, lichen planus, and other oral keratoses in 23,616 white Americans over the age of 35 years. Oral Surg Oral Med Oral Pathol 61:373-381, 1986.

37 Dunlap CL, Barker BF: Necrotizing sialometaplasia. Report of five additional cases. Oral Surg Oral Med Oral Pathol 37:722-727, 1974.

38 Dunlap CL, Barker BF: Diagnostic problems in oral pathology. Semin Diagn Pathol 2:16-30, 1985.

39 Fechner RE: Necrotizing sialometaplasia. A source of confusion with carcinoma of the palate. Am J Clin Pathol 67:315-317, 1977.

40 Handlers JP, Melrose RJ, Abrams AM, Taylor CR: Immunoperoxidase technique in diagnosis of oral pemphigus vulgaris. An alternative method to immunofluorescence. Oral Surg Oral Med Oral Pathol 54:207-212, 1982.

41 Harrison JD: Salivary mucoceles. Oral Surg Oral Med Oral Pathol 39:268-278, 1975.

42 Kalfayan B, Seager GM: Malakoplakia of palatine tonsil. Am J Clin Pathol 78:390-394, 1982.

43 Konttinen YT, Malmström M, Reitamo S, Tolvanen E, Seppä A, Sirelius K: Oral lesions in lichen planus and systemic lupus erythematosus. A histochemical and immunohistochemical study. Acta Pathol Microbiol Immunol Scand [A] 90:295-299, 1982.

44 Lattanand A, Johnson WC, Graham JH: Mucous cyst (mucocele). A clinicopathologic and histochemical study. Arch Dermatol 101:673-678, 1970.

45 McClatchey KD, Appelblatt NH, Zarbo RJ, Merrel DM: Plunging ranula. Oral Surg Oral Med Oral Pathol 57:408-412, 1984.

46 McDaniel RK, White JW Jr, Edwards PA: Mucha-Habermann's disease with oral lesions. Oral Surg Oral Med Oral Pathol 53:596-601, 1982.

47 Pindborg JJ, Poulsen HE, Zachariah J: Oral epithelial changes in thirty Indians with oral cancer and submucous fibrosis. Cancer 20:1141-1146, 1967.

48 Schiødt M: Oral discoid lupus erythematosus. III. A histopathologic study of sixty-six patients. Oral Surg Oral Med Oral Pathol 57:281-293, 1984.

49 Tomich CE: Oral focal mucinosis. A clinicopathologic and histochemical study of eight cases. Oral Surg Oral Med Oral Pathol 38:714-724, 1974.

50 van der Wal N, Henzen-Logmans S, van der Kwast WAM, van der Waal I: Amyloidosis of the tongue. A clinical and postmortem study. J Oral Pathol 13:632-639, 1984.

51 Wysocki GP, Gretzinger HA, Laupacis A, Ulan RA, Stiller CR: Fibrous hyperplasia of the gingiva. A side effect of cyclosporin A therapy. Oral Surg Oral Med Oral Pathol 55:274-278, 1983.

52 Yamaguchi A, Nasu M, Esaki Y, Shimada H, Yoshiki S: Amyloid deposits in the aged tongue. A postmortem study of 107 individuals over 60 years of age. J Oral Pathol 11:237-244, 1982.

TUMORS AND TUMORLIKE CONDITIONS OF SURFACE EPITHELIUM
Hyperplasia and dysplasia

53 Bánóczy J: Oral leukoplakia and other white lesions of the oral mucosa related to dermatological disorders. J Cutan Pathol 10:238-256, 1983.

54 Browne RM, Potts AJC: Dysplasia in salivary gland ducts in sublingual leukoplakia and erythroplakia. Oral Surg Oral Med Oral Pathol 62:44-48, 1986.

55 Burkhardt A: Advanced methods in the evaluation of premalignant lesions and carcinomas of the oral mucosa. J Oral Pathol 14:751-778, 1985.

56 Crissman JD, Gnepp DR, Goodman ML, Hellquist H, Johns ME: Preinvasive lesions of the upper aerodigestive tract. Histologic definitions and clinical implications. A symposium. Pathol Annu 22(Pt 1):311-352, 1987.

57 Einhorn J, Wersäll J: Incidence of oral carcinoma in patients with leukoplakia of the oral mucosa. Cancer 20:2189-2193, 1967.

58 Fischman SL, Ulmansky M, Sela J, Bab I, Gazit D: Correlative clinico-pathological evaluation of oral premalignancy. J Oral Pathol 11:283-289, 1982.

59 Katz HC, Shear M, Altini M: A critical evaluation of epithelial dysplasia in oral mucosal lesions using the Smith-Pindborg method of standardization. J Oral Pathol 14:476-482, 1985.

60 King OH: Intraoral leukoplakia? Cancer 17:131-136, 1964.

61 Krutchkoff DJ, Eisenberg E: Lichenoid dysplasia. A distinct histopathologic entity. Oral Surg Oral Med Oral Pathol 30:308-315, 1985.

62 Pilgard G: Focal epithelial hyperplasia. Report of nine cases from Sweden and review of the literature. Oral Surg Oral Med Oral Pathol 57:540-543, 1983.

63 Pindborg JJ, Jølst O, Renstrup G, Roed-Petersen B: Studies in oral leukoplakia. A preliminary report on the period prevalence of malignant transformation in leukoplakia based on a follow-up study of 248 patients. J Am Dent Assoc 76:767-771, 1968.

64 Prime SS, Pitigala-Arachchi A, Crane IJ, Rosser TJ, Scully C: The expression of cell surface MHC class I heavy and light chain molecules in pre-malignant and malignant lesions of the oral mucosa. Histopathology 11:81-91, 1987.

65 Reibel J, Clausen H, Dabelsteen E: Staining patterns of human pre-malignant oral epithelium and squamous cell carcinomas by monoclonal anti-keratin antibodies. Acta Pathol Microbiol Immunol Scand [A] 93:323-330, 1985.

66 Renstrup G: Leukoplakia of the oral cavity. A clinical and histopathologic study. Acta Odontol Scand 16:99-111, 1958.

67 Renstrup G: Occurrence of Candida in oral leukoplakias. Acta Pathol Microbiol Scand [B] 78:421-424, 1970.

68 Silverman S Jr, Bhargava K, Mani NJ, Smith LW, Malaowalla AM: Malignant transformation and natural history of oral leukoplakia in 57,518 industrial workers in Gujarat, India. Cancer 38:1790-1795, 1976.

69 Silverman S Jr, Gorsky M, Lozada F: Oral leukoplakia and malignant transformation. A follow-up study of 257 patients. Cancer 53:563-568, 1984.

70 van Wyk CW, Ambrosio SC: Leukoedema. Ultrastructural and histochemical observations. J Oral Pathol 12:319-329, 1983.

71 Waldron CA, Shafer WG: Leukoplakia revisited. A clinicopathologic study of 3256 oral leukoplakias. Cancer 36:1386-1392, 1975.

72 WHO Collaborating Centre for Oral Precancerous Lesions: Definition of leukoplakia and related lesions. An aid to studies on oral precancer. Oral Surg Oral Med Oral Pathol 46:518-539, 1978.

Papillomatous lesions and human papilloma virus (HPV)

72a Abby LJ, Page DG, Sawyer DR: The clinical and histopathologic features of a series of 464 oral squamous cell papillomas. Oral Surg Oral Med Oral Pathol 49:419-428, 1980.

73 de Villiers E-M, Weidauer H, Otto H, zur Hausen H: Papillomavirus DNA in human tongue carcinomas. Int J Cancer 36:575-578, 1985.

74 Eisenberg E, Rosenberg B, Krutchkoff DJ: Verrucous carcinoma. A possible viral pathogenesis. Oral Surg Oral Med Oral Pathol **59**:52-57, 1985.

75 Eversole LR, Jacobsen P, Stone CE, Freckleton V: Oral condyloma planus (hairy leukoplakia) among homosexual men. A clinicopathologic study of thirty-six cases. Oral Surg Oral Med Oral Pathol **61**:249-255, 1986.

75a Eversole LR, Laipis PJ, Greer TL: Human papillomavirus type 2 DNA in oral and labial verruca vulgaris. J Cutan Pathol **14**:319-325, 1987.

76 Greenspan D, Greenspan JS, Conant M, Petersen V, Silverman S Jr, de Souza Y: Oral "hairy" leukoplakia in male homosexuals. Evidence of association with both papillomavirus and a herpes-group virus. Lancet **13**:831-834, 1984.

77 Jenson AB, Lancaster WD, Hartmann D-P, Shaffer EL Jr: Frequency and distribution of papillomavirus structural antigens in verrucae, multiple papillomas, and condylomata of the oral cavity. Am J Pathol **107**:212-218, 1982.

78 Scully C, Prime S, Maitland N: Papillomaviruses. Their possible role in oral disease. Oral Surg Oral Med Oral Pathol **60**:166-174, 1985.

79 Swan RH, McDaniel RK, Dreiman BB, Rome WC: Condyloma acuminatum involving the oral mucosa. Oral Surg Oral Med Oral Pathol **51**:503-508, 1981.

80 Swart JGN, Lekkas C, Allard RHB: Oral manifestations in Cowden's syndrome. Report of four cases. Oral Surg Oral Med Oral Pathol **59**:264-268, 1985.

81 Welch TB, Barker BF, Williams C: Peroxidase-antiperoxidase evaluation of human oral squamous cell papillomas. Oral Surg Oral Med Oral Pathol **61**:603-606, 1986.

Carcinoma in situ

82 Amagasa T, Yokoo E, Sato K, Tanaka N, Shioda S, Takagi M: A study of the clinical characteristics and treatment of oral carcinoma in situ. Oral Surg Oral Med Oral Pathol **60**:50-55, 1985.

83 Mashberg A, Morrissey JB, Garfinkel L: A study of the appearance of early asymptomatic oral squamous cell carcinoma. Cancer **32**:1436-1445, 1973.

84 Sakr WA, Zarbo RJ, Jacobs JR, Crissman JD: Distribution of basement membrane in squamous cell carcinoma of the head and neck. Hum Pathol **18**:1043-1050, 1987.

85 Shafer WG: Oral carcinoma in situ. Oral Surg Oral Med Oral Pathol **39**:227-238, 1975.

Epidermoid carcinoma
General features

86 Anderson DL: Cause and prevention of lip cancer. J Can Dent Assoc **37**:138-142, 1971.

87 Binnie WH, Rankin KV: Epidemiological and diagnostic aspects of oral squamous cell carcinoma. J Oral Pathol **13**:333-341, 1984.

88 Binnie WH, Rankin KV, Mackenzie IC: Etiology of oral squamous cell carcinoma. J Oral Pathol **12**:11-29, 1983.

89 Douglass CW, Gammon MD: Reassessing the epidemiology of lip cancer. Oral Surg Oral Med Oral Pathol **57**:631-642, 1984.

90 Ildstad ST, Tollerud DJ, Bigelow ME, Remensnyder JP: Squamous cell carcinoma of the head and neck at the Massachusetts General Hospital. A comparison of biologic characteristics in men and women. Surgery **99**:7-14, 1986.

91 Mullen DL, Silverberg SG, Penn I, Hammond WS: Squamous cell carcinoma of the skin and lip in renal homograft recipients. Cancer **37**:729-734, 1976.

92 Newman AN, Rice DH, Ossoff RH, Sisson GA: Carcinoma of the tongue in persons younger than 30 years of age. Arch Otolaryngol **109**:302-304, 1983.

93 Reed K, Ravikumar TS, Gifford RRM, Grage TB: The association of Fanconi's anemia and squamous cell carcinoma. Cancer **52**:926-928, 1983.

94 Rich AM, Radden BG: Squamous cell carcinoma of the oral mucosa. A review of 244 cases in Australia. J Oral Pathol **13**:459-471, 1984.

95 Usenius T, Kärjä J, Collan Y: Squamous cell carcinoma of the tongue in children. Cancer **60**:236-239, 1987.

Location

96 Barnes L, Johnson JT: Pathologic and clinical considerations in the evaluation of major head and neck specimens resected for cancer. I. Pathol Annu **21**(Pt 1):173-250, 1986.

97 Byars LT, Anderson R: Multiple cancers of the oral cavity. Am Surg **18**:386-391, 1952.

98 Gluckman JL, Crissman JD, Donegan JO: Multicentric squamous-cell carcinoma of the upper aerodigestive tract. Head Neck Surg **3**:90-96, 1980.

99 Ildstad ST, Bigelow ME, Remensnyder JP: Intra-oral cancer at the Massachusetts General Hospital. Squamous cell carcinoma of the floor of the mouth. Ann Surg **197**:34-41, 1983.

100 MacComb WS, Fletcher GH, Healey JE: Intra-oral cavity. In MacComb WS, Fletcher GH (eds): Cancer of the head and neck. Baltimore, 1967, The Williams & Wilkins Co., pp. 89-151.

101 Mashberg A, Meyers H: Anatomical site and size of 222 early asymptomatic oral squamous cell carcinomas. A continuing prospective study of oral cancer. II. Cancer **37**:2149-2157, 1976.

102 Shibuya H, Amagasa T, Seto K-I, Ishibashi K, Horiuchi J-I, Suzuki S: Leukoplakia-associated multiple carcinomas in patients with tongue carcinoma. Cancer **57**:843-846, 1986.

Microscopic appearance

103 Lowe D, Fletcher CDM: Eosinophilia in squamous cell carcinoma of the oral cavity, external genitalia, and anus—clinical correlations. Histopathology **8**:627-632, 1984.

104 Takagi M, Sakota Y, Takayama S, Ishikawa G: Adenoid squamous cell carcinoma of the oral mucosa. Report of two autopsy cases. Cancer **40**:2250-2255, 1977.

105 Wright A, Shear M: Epithelial dysplasia immediately adjacent to oral squamous cell carcinoma. J Oral Pathol **14**:559-564, 1985.

Biopsy, cytology, and frozen section

106 Bhaskar SN: Oral pathology in the dental office. Survey of 20,575 biopsy specimens. J Am Dent Assoc **76**:761-766, 1968.

107 Giunta J, Meyer I, Shklar G: The accuracy of the oral biopsy in the diagnosis of cancer. Oral Surg Oral Med Oral Pathol **28**:552-556, 1969.

108 Looser KG, Shah JP, Strong EW: The significance of "positive" margins in surgically resected epidermoid carcinomas. Head Neck Surg **1**:107-111, 1978.

109 Shklar G, Cataldo E, Meyer I: Reliability of cytologic smear in diagnosis of oral cancer. A controlled study. Arch Otolaryngol **91**:158-160, 1970.

Spread and metastases

110 Barnes L, Johnson JT: Pathologic and clinical considerations in the evaluation of major head and neck specimens resected for cancer. Part I. Pathol Annu **21**(Pt 1):173-250, 1986.

111 Compagno J, Hyams VJ, Safavian M: Does branchiogenic carcinoma really exist? Arch Pathol Lab Med **100**:311-314, 1976.

112 Frierson HF Jr, Cooper PH: Prognostic factors in squamous cell carcinoma of the lower lip. Hum Pathol **17**:346-354, 1986.

113 Micheau C, Cachin Y, Caillou B: Cystic metastases in the neck revealing occult carcinoma of the tonsil. A report of six cases. Cancer **33**:228-233, 1974.

114 O'Brien CJ, Carter RL, Soo K-C, Barr LC, Hamlyn PJ, Shaw HJ: Invasion of the mandible by squamous carcinomas of the oral cavity and oropharynx. Head Neck Surg **8**:247-256, 1986.

115 Safaii H, Azar HA: Keratin granulomas in irradiated squamous cell carcinoma of various sites. Cancer Res **26**:500-508, 1966.

116 Shear M, Hawkins DM, Farr HW: The prediction of lymph node metastases from oral squamous carcinoma. Cancer **37**:1901-1907, 1976.

116a Yamamoto E, Miyakawa A, Kohama G-I: Mode of invasion and lymph node metastasis in squamous cell carcinoma of the oral cavity. Head Neck Surg **6**:938-947, 1984.

Treatment

117 Perez CA, Purdy JA, Breaux SR, Ogura JH, Von Essen S: Carcinoma of the tonsillar fossa. A nonrandomized comparison of preoperative radiation and surgery or irradiation alone. Long-term results. Cancer **50**:2314-2322, 1982.

Prognosis

118 Anneroth G, Hansen LS, Silverman S Jr: Malignancy grading in oral squamous cell carcinoma. I. Squamous cell carcinoma of the tongue and floor of mouth. Histologic grading in the clinical evaluation. J Oral Pathol **15**:162-168, 1986.

119 Crissman JD, Gluckman J, Whiteley J, Quenelle D: Squamous-cell carcinoma of the floor of the mouth. Head Neck Surg **3**:2-7, 1980.

120 Frierson HF Jr, Cooper PH: Prognostic factors in squamous cell carcinoma of the lower lip. Hum Pathol **17**:346-354, 1986.

121 Givens CD Jr, Johns ME, Cantrell RW: Carcinoma of the tonsil. Analysis of 162 cases. Arch Otolaryngol **107**:730-734, 1981.

122 Grandi C, Alloisio M, Moglia D, Podrecca S, Sala L, Salvatori P, Molinari R: Prognostic significance of lymphatic spread in head and neck carcinomas. Therapeutic implications. Head Neck Surg **8**:67-73, 1985.

123 Ildstad ST, Bigelow ME, Remensnyder JP: Intra-oral cancer at the Massachusetts General Hospital. Squamous cell carcinoma of the floor of the mouth. Ann Surg **197**:34-41, 1983.

124 Ildstad ST, Bigelow ME, Remensnyder JP: Squamous cell carcinoma of the alveolar ridge and palate. A 15-year survey. Ann Surg **199**:445-453, 1984.

125 Marks JE, Smith PG, Sessions DG: Pharyngeal wall cancer. A reappraisal after comparison of treatment methods. Arch Otolaryngol **111**:79-85, 1985.

126 Moore C, Flynn MB, Greenberg RA: Evaluation of size in prognosis of oral cancer. Cancer 58:158-162, 1986.

127 Oreggia F, De Stéfani E, Deneo-Pellegrini H, Olivera L: Carcinoma of the tonsil. A retrospective analysis of prognostic factors. Arch Intern Med 109:305-309, 1983.

128 Rollo J, Rozenbom CV, Thawley S, Korba A, Ogura J, Perez CA, Powers WE, Bauer WC: Squamous carcinoma of the base of the tongue. A clinicopathologic study of 81 cases. Cancer 47:333-342, 1981.

129 Tytor M, Franzén G, Olofsson J: DNA pattern in oral cavity carcinomas in relation to clinical stage and histological grading. Pathol Res Pract 182:202-206, 1987.

Verrucous carcinoma

130 Ackerman LV: Verrucous carcinoma of the oral cavity. Surgery 23:670-678, 1948.

131 Batsakis JG, Hybels R, Crissman JD, Rice DH: The pathology of head and neck tumors. Verrucous carcinoma. Part 15. Head Neck Surg 5:29-38, 1982.

132 Demian SDE, Bushkin FL, Echevarria RA: Perineural invasion and anaplastic transformation of verrucous carcinoma. Cancer 32:395-401, 1973.

133 Hansen LS, Olson JA, Silverman S Jr: Proliferative verrucous leukoplakia. A long-term study of thirty patients. Oral Surg Oral Med Oral Pathol 60:285-298, 1985.

134 Kraus FT, Perez-Mesa C: Verrucous carcinoma. Clinical and pathologic study of 105 cases involving oral cavity, larynx and genitalia. Cancer 19:26-38, 1966.

135 McCoy JM, Waldron CA: Verrucous carcinoma of the oral cavity. A review of forty-nine cases. Oral Surg Oral Med Oral Pathol 52:623-629, 1981.

136 McDonald JS, Crissman JD, Gluckman JL: Verrucous carcinoma of the oral cavity. Head Neck Surg 5:22-28, 1982.

137 Medina JE, Dichtel W, Luna MA: Verrucous-squamous carcinomas of the oral cavity. A clinicopathologic study of 104 cases. Arch Otolaryngol 110:437-440, 1984.

138 Prioleau PG, Santa Cruz DJ, Meyer JS, Bauer WC: Verrucous carcinoma. A light and electron microscopic, autoradiographic, and immunofluorescence study. Cancer 45:2849-2857, 1980.

139 Shear M, Pindborg JJ: Verrucous hyperplasia of the oral mucosa. Cancer 46:1855-1862, 1980.

140 Sundström B, Mörnstad H, Axéll T: Oral carcinomas associated with snuff dipping. Some clinical and histological characteristics of 23 tumours in Swedish males. J Oral Pathol 11:245-251, 1982.

141 Wechsler HL, Risher ER: Oral florid papillomatosis. Clinical, pathological and electron microscopic observations. Arch Dermatol 86:140-152, 1962.

Other microscopic types

142 Batsakis JG, Rice HD, Howard DR: The pathology of head and neck tumors. Spindle cell lesions (sarcomatoid carcinomas, nodular fasciitis, and fibrosarcoma) of the aerodigestive tracts. Part 14. Head Neck Surg 4:499-513, 1982.

143 Baugh RF, Wolf GT, McClatchey KD: Small cell carcinoma of the head and neck. Head Neck Surg 8:343-354, 1986.

144 Ellis GL, Langloss JM, Heffner DK, Hyams VJ: Spindle-cell carcinoma of the aerodigestive tract. An immunohistochemical analysis of 21 cases. Am J Surg Pathol 11:335-342, 1987.

145 Gerughty RM, Hennigar GR, Brown FM: Adenosquamous carcinoma of the nasal, oral and laryngeal cavities. A clinicopathologic survey of ten cases. Cancer 22:1140-1155, 1968.

146 Green GW Jr, Bernier J: Spindle cell squamous carcinoma of the lip. Report of four cases. Oral Surg Oral Med Oral Pathol 12:1008-1016, 1959.

147 Hull MT, Eble JN, Warfel KA: Extrapulmonary oat-cell carcinoma of the tongue. An electron-microscopic study. J Oral Pathol 13:489-496, 1984.

148 Leifer C, Miller AS, Putong PB, Min BH: Spindle-cell carcinoma of the oral mucosa. A light and electron microscopic study of apparent sarcomatous metastasis to cervical lymph nodes. Cancer 34:597-605, 1974.

149 Leventon GS, Evans HL: Sarcomatoid squamous cell carcinoma of the mucous membranes of the head and neck. A clinicopathologic study of 20 cases. Cancer 48:994-1003, 1981.

150 Wain SL, Kier R, Vollmer RT, Bossen EH: Basaloid-squamous carcinoma of the tongue, hypopharynx, and larynx. Report of 10 cases. Hum Pathol 17:1158-1166, 1986.

151 Weidner N: Sarcomatoid carcinoma of the upper aerodigestive tract. Semin Diagn Pathol 4:157-168, 1987.

152 Zarbo RJ, Crissman JD, Venkat H, Weiss MA: Spindle-cell carcinoma of the upper aerodigestive tract mucosa. An immunohistologic and ultrastructural study of 18 biphasic tumors and comparison with seven monophasic spindle-cell tumors. Am J Surg Pathol 10:741-753, 1986.

TUMORS AND OTHER LESIONS OF MINOR SALIVARY GLANDS

153 Aberle AM, Abrams AM, Bowe R, Melrose RJ, Handlers JP: Lobular (polymorphous low-grade) carcinoma of minor salivary glands. A clinicopathologic study of twenty cases. Oral Surg Oral Med Oral Pathol 60:387-395, 1985.

154 Allen MS Jr, Fitz-Hugh GS, Marsh WL Jr: Low-grade papillary adenocarcinoma of the palate. Cancer 33:153-158, 1974.

155 Arafat A, Brannon RB, Ellis GL: Adenomatoid hyperplasia of mucous salivary glands. Oral Surg Oral Med Oral Pathol 52:51-55, 1981.

156 Brannon RB, Houston GD, Wampler HW: Gingival salivary gland choristoma. Oral Surg Oral Med Oral Pathol 61:185-188, 1986.

157 Chaudhry AP, Vickers RA, Gorlin RJ: Intraoral minor salivary gland tumors. An analysis of 1414 cases. Oral Surg Oral Med Oral Pathol 14:1194-1226, 1961.

158 Chisholm DM, Mason DK: Labial salivary gland biopsy in Sjögren's disease. J Clin Pathol 21:656-660, 1968.

159 Chomette G, Auriol M, Tranbaloc P, Vaillant JM: Adenoid cystic carcinoma of minor salivary glands. Analysis of 86 cases. Clinico-pathological, histoenzymological and ultrastructural studies. Virchows Arch [Pathol Anat] 395:289-301, 1982.

160 Chomette G, Auriol M, Van Cat N, Szpirglas H, Tranbaloc P, Vaillant JM: Biopsie des glandes salivaires labiales dans le syndrome de Gougerot-Sjögren. Étude clinico-pathologique, histoenzymologique et ultrastructurale. Virchows Arch [Pathol Anat] 392:339-354, 1981.

161 Coates HLC, Devine KD, DeSanto LW, Weiland LH: Glandular tumors of the palate. Surg Gynecol Obstet 140:589-593, 1975.

162 Eneroth C-M: Incidence and prognosis of salivary-gland tumors at different sites. A study of parotid, submandibular and palatal tumors in 2632 patients. Acta Otolaryngol [Stockh] 263:174-178, 1970.

163 Evans HL, Batsakis JG: Polymorphous low-grade adenocarcinoma of minor salivary glands. A study of 14 cases of a distinctive neoplasm. Cancer 53:935-942, 1984.

164 Eveson JW, Cawson RA: Tumours of the minor (oropharyngeal) salivary gland. A demographic study of 336 cases. J Oral Pathol 14:500-509, 1985.

165 Fantasia JE, Nocco CE, Lally ET: Ultrastructure of sialadenoma papilliferum. Arch Pathol Lab Med 110:523-527, 1986.

166 Freedman PD, Lumerman H: Sialadenoma papilliferum. Report of 2 cases. Oral Surg Oral Med Oral Pathol 45:88-94, 1978.

167 Freedman PD, Lumerman H: Lobular carcinoma of intraoral minor salivary gland origin. Report of twelve cases. Oral Surg Oral Med Oral Pathol 56:157-165, 1983.

168 Frierson HF Jr, Mills SE, Garland TA: Terminal duct carcinoma of minor salivary glands. A nonpapillary subtype of polymorphous low-grade adenocarcinoma. Am J Clin Pathol 84:8-14, 1985.

169 Gates GA: Malignant neoplasms of the minor salivary glands. N Engl J Med 306:718-722, 1982.

170 Isacsson G, Shear M: Intraoral salivary gland tumors. A retrospective study of 201 cases. J Oral Pathol 12:57-62, 1983.

171 Johnston CA, Toker C: Syringomatous tumors of minor salivary gland origin. Hum Pathol 13:182-184, 1982.

172 Lomax-Smith JD, Azzopardi JG: The hyaline cell. A distinctive feature of "mixed" salivary tumors. Histopathology 2:77-92, 1978.

173 Luna MA, Batsakis JG, Ordóñez NG, Mackay B, Tortoledo ME: Salivary gland adenocarcinomas. A clinicopathologic analysis of three distinctive types. Semin Diagn Pathol 4:117-135, 1987.

174 Mills SE, Garland TA, Allen MS Jr: Low-grade papillary adenocarcinoma of palatal salivary gland origin. Am J Surg Pathol 8:367-374, 1984.

175 Nesland JM, Olafsson J, Sobrinho-Simões M: Plasmacytoid myoepithelioma of the palate. A case report with ultrastructural findings and review of the literature. J Oral Pathol 10:14-21, 1981.

176 Owens OT, Calcaterra TC: Salivary gland tumors of the lip. Arch Otolaryngol 108:45-47, 1982.

177 Regezi JA, Lloyd RV, Zarbo RJ, McClatchey KD: Minor salivary gland tumors. A histologic and immunohistochemical study. Cancer 55:108-115, 1985.

178 Warwick WJ, Bernard B, Meskin LH: The involvement of the labial mucous salivary gland in patients with cystic fibrosis. Pediatrics 34:621-638, 1964.

179 White DK, Miller AS, McDaniel RK, Rothman BN: Inverted ductal papilloma. A distinctive lesion of minor salivary gland. Cancer 49:519-524, 1982.

180 Zarbo RJ, Regezi JA, Batsakis JG: S-100 protein in salivary gland tumors. An immunohistochemical study of 129 cases. Head Neck Surg 8:268-275, 1986.

TUMORS OF ODONTOGENIC EPITHELIUM

181 Gardner DG: Peripheral ameloblastoma. A study of 21 cases, including 5 reported as basal cell carcinoma of the gingiva. Cancer 39:1625-1633, 1977.

TUMORS OF MELANOCYTES

182 Arrington JH III, Reed RJ, Ichinose H, Krementz ET: Plantar lentiginous melanoma. A distinctive variant of human cutaneous malignant melanoma. Am J Surg Pathol **1**:131-143, 1977.

183 Batsakis JG, Regezi JA, Solomon AR, Rice DH: The pathology of head and neck tumors. Mucosal melanomas. Part 13. Head Neck Surg **4**:404-418, 1982.

184 Berthelsen A, Andersen AP, Jensen TS, Hansen HS: Melanomas of the mucosa in the oral cavity and the upper respiratory passages. Cancer **54**:907-912, 1984.

185 Buchner A, Hansen LS: Pigmented nevi of the oral mucosa. A clinicopathologic study of 32 new cases and review of 75 cases from the literature. Part I. Oral Surg Oral Med Oral Pathol **48**:131-142, 1979.

186 Buchner A, Hansen LS: Pigmented nevi of the oral mucosa. A clinicopathologic study of 32 new cases and review of 75 cases from the literature. Part II. Oral Surg Oral Med Oral Pathol **49**:55-62, 1980.

187 Chaudhry AP, Hampel A, Gorlin RJ: Primary malignant melanoma of the oral cavity. A review of 105 cases. Cancer **11**:923-928, 1958.

188 Devildos LR, Langlois CC: Intramucosal cellular nevi. Oral Surg Oral Med Oral Pathol **52**:162-166, 1981.

189 Goode RK, Crawford BE, Callihan MD, Neville BW: Oral melanoacanthoma. Review of the literature and report of ten cases. Oral Surg Oral Med Oral Pathol **56**:622-628, 1983.

190 McDonald JS, Miller RL, Wagner W, Giammara B: Acral lentiginous melanoma of the oral cavity. Head Neck Surg **5**:257-262, 1983.

191 Page DG, Svirsky JA, Kaugars GE: Nevus of Ota with associated palatal involvement. Oral Surg Oral Med Oral Pathol **59**:282-284, 1985.

192 Panje WR, Moran WJ: Melanoma of the upper aerodigestive tract. A review of 21 cases. Head Neck Surg **8**:309-312, 1986.

193 Rapini RP, Golitz LE, Greer RO Jr, Krekorian EA, Poulson T: Primary malignant melanoma of the oral cavity. A review of 177 cases. Cancer **55**:1543-1551, 1985.

194 Robinson L, Hukill P: Hutchinson's melanotic freckle in oral mucous membrane. Cancer **26**:297-302, 1976.

195 Sexton FM, Maize JC: Melanotic macules and melanoacanthomas of the lip. A comparative study with census of the basal melanocyte population. Am J Dermatopathol **9**:438-444, 1987.

196 Takagi M, Ishikawa G, Mori W: Primary malignant melanoma of the oral cavity in Japan. With special reference to mucosal melanosis. Cancer **34**:358-370, 1974.

197 Tradahl JN, Sprague WG: Benign and malignant melanocytic lesions of the oral mucosa. An analysis of 135 cases. Cancer **25**:812-823, 1970.

TUMORS AND TUMORLIKE CONDITIONS OF LYMPHOID TISSUE

198 Banfi A, Bonadonna G, Carnevali G, Molinari R, Monfardini R, Salvini E: Lymphoreticular sarcomas with primary involvement of Waldeyer's ring. Clinical evaluation of 225 cases. Cancer **26**:341-351, 1970.

199 Barton JH, Osborne BM, Butler JJ, Meoz RT, Kong J, Fuller LM, Sullivan JA: Non-Hodgkin's lymphoma of the tonsil. A clinicopathologic study of 65 cases. Cancer **53**:86-95, 1984.

200 Bernier JL, Bhaskar SN: Lymphoepithelial lesions of salivary glands. Histogenesis and classification based on 186 cases. Cancer **11**:1156-1179, 1958.

201 Cannon ML, Cooley RO, Gonzalez-Crussi F, Labokta R: Oral manifestations of malignant histiocytosis (histiocytic medullary reticulosis). Oral Surg Oral Med Oral Pathol **54**:180-186, 1982.

202 Castella A, Davey FR, Elbadawi A, Gordon GB: Granulocytic sarcoma of the hard palate. Report of the first case. Hum Pathol **15**:1190-1192, 1984.

203 Chan JKC, Ng CS, Lo STH: Immunohistological characterization of malignant lymphomas of the Waldeyer's ring other than the nasopharynx. Histopathology **11**:885-899, 1987.

204 Dreizen S, McCredie KB, Keating MJ, Luna MA: Malignant gingival and skin "infiltrates" in adult leukemia. Oral Surg Oral Med Oral Pathol **55**:572-579, 1983.

205 Eisenbud L, Sciubba J, Mir R, Sachs SA: Oral presentations in non-Hodgkin's lymphoma. A review of thirty-one cases. Part I. Data analysis. Oral Surg Oral Med Oral Pathol **56**:151-156, 1983.

206 Ewing MR, Foote FW Jr: Plasma-cell tumors of the mouth and upper air passages. Cancer **5**:499-513, 1952.

207 Gorsky M, Silverman S Jr, Lozada F, Kushner J: Histiocytosis X. Occurrence and oral involvement in six adolescent and adult patients. Oral Surg Oral Med Oral Pathol **55**:24-29, 1983.

208 Handlers JP, Howell RE, Abrams AM, Melrose RJ: Extranodal oral lymphoma. Part I. A morphologic and immunoperoxidase study of 34 cases. Oral Surg Oral Med Oral Pathol **61**:362-367, 1986.

209 Harman KS: Histiocytosis X. A review of 114 cases with oral involvement. Oral Surg Oral Med Oral Pathol **49**:38-54, 1980.

210 Regezi JA, Zarbo RJ, Keren DF: Plasma cell lesions of the head and neck. Immunofluorescent determination of clonality from formalin-fixed, paraffin-embedded tissue. Oral Surg Oral Med Oral Pathol **56**:616-621, 1983.

211 Saltzstein SL: Extranodal malignant lymphomas and pseudolymphomas. Pathol Annu **4**:159-164, 1969.

212 Saul SH, Kapadia SB: Primary lymphoma of Waldeyer's ring. Clinicopathologic study of 68 cases. Cancer **56**:157-166, 1985.

213 Tomich CE, Shafer WG: Lymphoproliferative disease of the hard palate. A clinicopathologic entity. A study of twenty-one cases. Oral Surg Oral Med Oral Pathol **39**:754-768, 1975.

214 Yamanaka N, Harabuchi Y, Sambe S, Shido F, Matsuda F, Kataura A, Ishii Y, Kikuchi K: Non-Hodgkin's lymphoma of Waldeyer's ring and nasal cavity. Clinical and immunologic aspects. Cancer **56**:768-776, 1985.

OTHER TUMORS AND TUMORLIKE CONDITIONS

215 Adrian JC: Inverted follicular keratosis of the lip. Oral Surg Oral Med Oral Pathol **57**:625-630, 1984.

216 Allard RHB, Blok P, van der Kwast WAM, van der Waal I: Oral lipomas with osseous and chondrous metaplasia. Report of two cases. J Oral Pathol **11**:18-25, 1982.

217 Assor D, Thomas JR: Multifocal rhabdomyoma. Report of a case. Arch Otolaryngol **90**:489-491, 1969.

218 Batsakis JG, Rice DH: The pathology of head and neck tumors. Vasoformative tumors. Part 9A. Head Neck Surg **3**:231-239, 1981.

219 Batsakis JG, Rice DH: The pathology of head and neck tumors. Vasoformative tumors. Part 9B. Head Neck Surg **3**:326-339, 1981.

220 Buchner A, Hansen LS, Merrell PW: Verruciform xanthoma of the oral mucosa. Report of five cases and review of the literature. Arch Dermatol **117**:563-565, 1981.

221 Chau MNY, Radden BG: Oral warty dyskeratoma. J Oral Pathol **13**:546-556, 1984.

222 Chen S-Y, Fantasia JE, Miller AS: Myxoid lipoma of oral soft tissue. A clinical and ultrastructural study. Oral Surg Oral Med Oral Pathol **57**:300-307, 1984.

223 Corio RL, Lewis DM: Intraoral rhabdomyomas. Oral Surg Oral Med Oral Pathol **48**:525-531, 1979.

224 Dunlap CL, Barker BF: Diagnostic problems in oral pathology. Semin Diagn Pathol **2**:16-30, 1985.

225 Eversole LR, Leider AS, Alexander G: Intraoral and labial keratoacanthoma. Oral Surg Oral Med Oral Pathol **54**:663-667, 1982.

226 Flaggert JJ III, Heldt LV, Keaton WM: Angiolipoma of the palate. Report of a case. Oral Surg Oral Med Oral Pathol **60**:333-336, 1986.

227 Gardner DG, Corio RL: Fetal rhabdomyoma of the tongue, with a discussion of the two histologic variants of this tumor. Oral Surg Oral Med Oral Pathol **56**:293-300, 1983.

228 Gardner DG, Corio RL: Multifocal adult rhabdomyoma. Oral Surg Oral Med Oral Pathol **56**:76-78, 1983.

229 Giansanti JS, Waldron CA: Peripheral giant cell granuloma. Review of 720 cases. J Oral Surg **27**:787-791, 1969.

230 Gorlin RJ, Sedano HO, Vickers RA, Cervenka J: Multiple mucosal neuromas, pheochromocytoma and medullary carcinoma of the thyroid. A syndrome. Cancer **22**:293-299, 1968.

231 Harrist TJ, Murphy GF, Mihm MC Jr: Oral warty dyskeratoma. Arch Dermatol **116**:929-931, 1980.

232 Janzer RC, Makek M: Intraoral malignant melanotic schwannoma. Ultrastructural evidence for melanogenesis by Schwann's cells. Arch Pathol Lab Med **107**:298-301, 1983.

233 Kameyama Y, Mizohata M, Takehana S, Murata H, Manabe H, Mukai Y: Ultrastructure of the congenital epulis. Virchows Arch [Pathol Anat] **401**:251-260, 1983.

234 Kaugars GE, Svirsky JA: Lung malignancies metastatic to the oral cavity. Oral Surg Oral Med Oral Pathol **51**:179-186, 1981.

235 Kay S, Elzay RP, Wilson MA: Ultrastructural observations on a gingival granular cell tumor (congenital epulis). Cancer **27**:674-680, 1971.

236 Kerr DA: Granuloma pyogenicum. Oral Surg Oral Med Oral Pathol **4**:158-176, 1951.

237 Kim RY, Perry SR, Levy DS: Metastatic carcinoma to the tongue. Cancer **43**:386-389, 1979.

238 Komori A, Takeda Y, Kakiichi T: Alveolar soft-part sarcoma of the tongue. Report of a case with electron microscopic study. Oral Surg Oral Med Oral Pathol **57**:532-539, 1984.

239 Lack EE, Perez-Atayde AR, McGill TJ, Vawter GF: Gingival granular cell tumor of the newborn (congenital "epulis"). Ultrastructural observations relating to histogenesis. Hum Pathol **13**:686-689, 1982.

240 Lack EE, Worsham GF, Callihan MD, Crawford BE, Vawter GF: Gingival granular cell tumors of the newborn (congenital "epulis"). A clinical and pathologic study of 21 patients. Am J Surg Pathol **5:**37-46, 1981.

241 Lifshitz MS, Flotte TJ, Greco MA: Congenital granular cell epulis. Immunohistochemical and ultrastructural observations. Cancer **53:**1845-1848, 1984.

242 Loeffler JR, Duray PH, Sasaki CT: Macroglossal lymphangioendotheliomatosis. Report of a case in a pregnant woman. Arch Otolaryngol **110:**600-603, 1984.

243 Lozada F, Silverman S Jr, Migliorati CA, Conant MA, Volberding PA: Oral manifestations of tumor and opportunistic infections in the acquired immunodeficiency syndrome (AIDS). Findings in 53 homosexual men with Kaposi's sarcoma. Oral Surg Oral Med Oral Pathol **56:**491-494, 1983.

244 MacDonald DG: Smooth muscle tumours of the mouth. Br J Oral Surg **6:**207-214, 1969.

245 MacVicar J, Dunn MF: Pregnancy tumour of the gums. J Obstet Gynaecol Br Commonw **76:**260-263, 1969.

246 Massarelli G, Tanda F, Salis B: Synovial sarcoma of the soft palate. Report of a case. Hum Pathol **9:**341-345, 1978.

247 Matthews JB, Mason GI: Oral granular cell myoblastoma. An immunohistochemical study. J Oral Pathol **11:**343-352, 1982.

248 Nagata M, Semba I, Ooya K, Urago A, Yonezawa S, Sakae K: Malignant endothelial neoplasm arising in the area of lymphangioma. Immunohistochemical and ultrastructural observation. J Oral Pathol **13:**560-572, 1984.

249 Natiella JR, Neiders ME, Greene GW: Oral leiomyoma. Report of six cases and a review of the literature. J Oral Pathol **11:**353-365, 1982.

250 Neville BW: The verruciform xanthoma. A review and report of eight new cases. Am J Dermatopathol **8:**247-253, 1986.

251 Neville BW, Weathers DR: Verruciform xanthoma. Oral Surg Oral Med Oral Pathol **49:**429-434, 1980.

252 Nowparast B, Howell FV, Rick GM: Verruciform xanthoma. A clinicopathologic review and report of fifty-four cases. Oral Surg Oral Med Oral Pathol **51:**619-625, 1981.

253 Oberman HA, Sullenger G: Neurogenous tumors of the head and neck. Cancer **20:**1992-2001, 1967.

254 Peters E, Altini M, Kola AH: Oral angiolymphoid hyperplasia with eosinophilia. Oral Surg Oral Med Oral Pathol **61:**73-79, 1986.

255 Piscioli F, Leonardi E, Scappini P, Cristofolini M: Primary angiosarcoma of the gingiva. Case report with immunohistochemical study. Am J Dermatopathol **8:**430-435, 1986.

256 Reyes JM, Vangore SK, Putong PB, Harwick R, Miller AS, Chen S-Y: Osteogenic sarcoma of the tongue. Oral Surg Oral Med Oral Pathol **51:**421-425, 1981.

257 Rohrer MD, Young SK: Congenital epulis (gingival granular cell tumor). Ultrastructural evidence of origin from pericytes. Oral Surg Oral Med Oral Pathol **53:**56-63, 1982.

258 Rusthoven JJ, Fine S, Thomas G: Adenocarcinoma of the rectum metastatic to the oral cavity. Two cases and a review of the literature. Cancer **54:**1110-1112, 1984.

259 Sadeghi EM, Sauk JJ Jr: Liposarcoma of the oral cavity. Clinical, tissue culture, and ultrastructure study of a case. J Oral Pathol **11:**263-275, 1982.

260 Saku T, Okabe H, Matsutani K, Sasaki M: Glomus tumor of the cheek. An immunohistochemical demonstration of actin and myosin. Oral Surg Oral Med Oral Pathol **60:**65-71, 1985.

261 Shmookler BM, Enzinger FM, Brannon RB: Orofacial synovial sarcoma. A clinicopathologic study of 11 new cases and review of the literature. Cancer **50:**269-276, 1982.

262 Slootweg P, de Wilde P, Vooijs P, Ramaekers F: Oral granular cell lesions. An immunohistochemical study with emphasis on intermediate-sized filaments proteins. Virchows Arch [Pathol Anat] **402:**35-45, 1983.

263 Wetzel W, Leipzig B, Grunow W, Kenna M, Kalderon A, Morgan B: Malignant granular cell tumor of the tongue. Arch Otolaryngol **108:**603-605, 1982.

264 Zarbo RJ, Lloyd RV, Beals TF, McClatchey KD: Congenital gingival granular cell tumor with smooth muscle cytodifferentiation. Oral Surg Oral Med Oral Pathol **56:**512-520, 1983.

265 Zohar Y, Ben-Tovim R, Gal R, Laurian N: Metastatic carcinoma of oral soft tissue. Head Neck Surg **7:**484-486, 1985.

6 Mandible and maxilla

Surgical pathology of the maxilla and mandible encompasses the spectrum of pathology, since both systemic and unique diseases have been documented in these locations. Conditions previously considered "dental" or removed from the consideration of the general surgical pathologist are being encountered with increasing frequency. The present discussion concentrates on commonly found and surgically related conditions of the jaws. A more detailed discussion of these conditions, as well as of others which are less common, may be found in specialized texts.[1,2]

INFLAMMATION

The majority of inflammatory conditions of the jaws have a dental origin. Dental caries eventually lead to inflammation of the pulpal or soft tissue portions of teeth that are unable to respond and heal adequately.[9,14,15] This results in inflammation of the cancellous bone and connective tissue surrounding the dental root apices that follows a predictable, if potentially variable, clinical and pathologic course. The histologic appearance of maxillary or mandibular inflammation in such circumstances is as variable as inflammation within any part of the body.

Dental granuloma or localized osteitis is ordinarily detected in a dental roentgenogram. Grossly, the lesion rarely measures over 1.5 cm in diameter. Microscopically, it consists of a rounded collection of chronic inflammatory cells rich in histiocytes and surrounded by dense fibrous tissue. Degeneration can occur in the center, leading to cavity formation and the development of a radicular or periapical cyst[11,12] (see p. 207).

Hyaline ring-like structures may be seen in areas of chronic periostitis. These rings enclose vessels, giant cells, other inflammatory cells, and bundles of collagen fibrils. This inconsequential microscopic oddity, variously referred to as pulse granuloma, lentil granuloma, oral vegetable granuloma, and giant cell hyaline angiopathy, has given rise to numerous theories about its nature, as can be deduced from the names[3,4,10,13] (Fig. 6-1). The two most popular hypotheses are a reaction to legume parenchymatous cells at various stages of digestion ("pulse" being the edible seed of legumes) and a degenerative change in vessel walls resulting from localized vasculitis.

Osteomyelitis of the jaws usually represents an additional consequence and extension of dental or periodontal infection. Acute, subacute, and chronic forms exist.[5,7,16] Hematogenous osteomyelitis has been encountered rarely.[17] Symptoms such as pain, fever, and soft tissue swelling or redness in later stages are usually present. Smooth, regular, and atrophic loss of the covering mucosa is a late finding, and the exposed bone appears dull and devitalized. Roentgenographic features of osteomyelitis are subtle, irregular, illdefined, and predominantly radiolucent lesions. A sequestrum is more often identified at the time of surgical exploration than during examination of x-ray films. Acute suppurative inflammation and resorptive scalloping of margins of nonvital bone within a large portion of maxilla or mandible are the main microscopic findings.

Staphylococcus aureus is the organism most commonly cultured. Recently, anaerobic bacteria have also been demonstrated to be important.[8] Tuberculosis, mucormycosis, aspergillosis, and candidiasis have all been causally identified in osteomyelitis of the jaws.[6]

SIMPLE BONE CYST

Simple bone cyst (traumatic or hemorrhagic extravasation cyst) presents as an intraosseous cavity not lined by epithelium and usually located in the mandible.[18,19,21] Such lesions may assume sizable proportions. Little is observed within the cavity at surgery, and it is this observation that often constitutes the basis for the final diagnosis. Surgical samples from the periphery, however, demonstrate a delicate fibrovascular connective tissue. Curettage and histopathologic examination of the material should be encouraged because aneurysmal bone cysts (especially those that are associated with benign fibro-osseous jaw lesions) and other conditions may present a similar surgical appearance but different histology and behavior. Surgical exploration and thorough curettage is the treatment of choice.[20] Recurrence has been observed but is distinctly uncommon.

Simple bone cyst usually occurs in young patients. Radiographically, it appears as a sharply outlined radiolucent

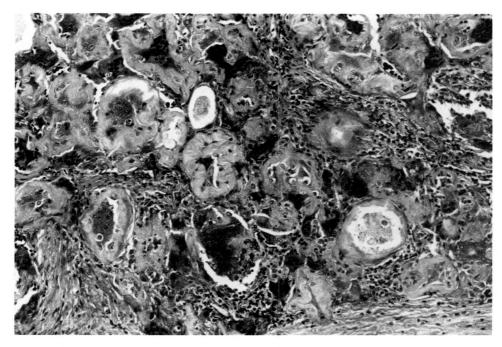

Fig. 6-1 So-called pulse granuloma. Hyaline ring-like structures are seen surrounded by chronic inflammatory infiltrate, some of them containing granular necrotic material in their centers.

mass (Fig. 6-2). There is a history of previous trauma in only one half of the patients, and the content of the cyst is hemorrhagic in only a small proportion of cases.[19] It may represent the counterpart of the lesion of long bones designated as solitary (unicameral) bone cyst. It should be

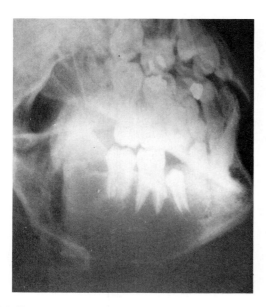

Fig. 6-2 Simple bone cyst of mandible in 11-year-old girl. Note thin shell of remaining mandible.

differentiated from other cystic lesions, including the "latent bone cavity," a symptomless open cavity situated below and behind the inferior dental canal near the angle of the mandible and often containing salivary gland tissue.[19]

CENTRAL GIANT CELL GRANULOMA AND OTHER GIANT CELL–CONTAINING LESIONS

Destructive lesions of the jaws that feature large numbers of benign, multinucleated giant cells histologically can be of several types, but the typical and most common example is only infrequently associated with aggressive behavior. Although giant cell tumor (osteoclastoma),[23,26,31,32] cherubism,[30] fibro-osseous lesions, bone lesion of hyperparathyroidism,[22] aneurysmal bone cyst, and other conditions feature benign, multinucleated giant cells, central giant cell granuloma is the most common entity in this group. Its pathogenesis is unknown. It has been suggested that it is the result of the organization of slow, minute, recurrent hemorrhages, hence the term *reparative giant cell granuloma*[29] used as an alternative. A history of trauma is often ascertained.

This condition affects children and young adults, predominantly females, and occurs almost twice as frequently in the mandible as in the maxilla, particularly in the anterior region.[29,32,34] It produces a cystic lesion of the bone which, microscopically, shows large numbers of giant cells, rather cellular vascular stroma, and often new bone formation (Figs. 6-3 and 6-4). The osteoclast-like giant cells have a patchy distribution usually associated with areas of hemorrhage. Ultrastructurally, the proliferating cells include fibroblasts, myofibroblasts, and histiocytes.[25]

The lesions of giant cell granuloma are treated by surgical removal and thorough curettage. Recurrence is treated similarly but only following reestablishment of the diagnosis.[24,32,34]

Hereditary and intraosseous fibrous swellings of the jaws (cherubism) is indistinguishable microscopically from the lesions of giant cell granuloma.[30] The bilateral presentation of mandibular and maxillary involvement in a young individual with an autosomal dominant mode of inheritance, the sometimes more delicate fibrovascular stroma without

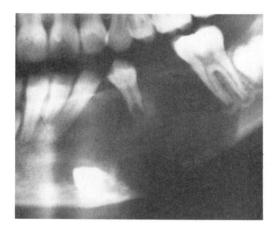

Fig. 6-3 Roentgenographic appearance of recurrent giant cell granuloma in 10-year-old girl. Inferior border of mandible has been eroded.

bone formation, and the differing behavior and response to treatment justify the nosologic separation between cherubism and giant cell granuloma.[33] The pathologist who relies only on the microscopic features in establishing the diagnosis of such conditions will eventually encounter a degree of clinical wrath. Surgical intervention in patients with cherubism should be carefully considered.[27]

Hyperparathyroidism, giant cell tumor, and other conditions containing areas resembling giant cell granuloma (especially at the periphery) may constitute a basis for histologic misinterpretation as well. Fortunately, these are encountered much less commonly and are usually associated with additional clinical or laboratory information that aids delineation.[28]

BENIGN FIBRO-OSSEOUS LESIONS

Numerous types of tumors and tumorlike conditions of the benign fibro-osseous type have been documented. The observation of different clinical behavior in patients having histologically similar lesions has added to the difficulty that pathologists experience when interpreting such diseases.[35-39]

Pathologists frequently receive samples of fibro-osseous jaw lesions without roentgenograms and adequate descriptions of the abnormality. Medical history, family history, dental history, roentgenographic appearance, operative appearance, skeletal survey, laboratory tests, course of disease, response to treatment and histologic appearance are all important diagnostic features. Pathologists or clinicians relying on one or few of these diagnostic features for interpretation and diagnosis will be less likely to contribute to the successful management of affected patients.

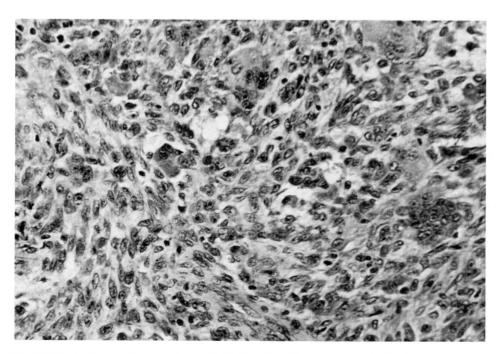

Fig. 6-4 Giant cell reparative granuloma with highly cellular fibrous tissue and collections of giant cells. Lesion occurred in maxilla of 10½-year-old girl.

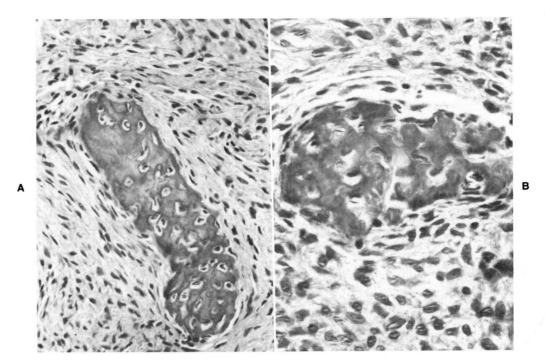

Fig. 6-5 Congenital mandibular fibrous dysplasia occurring in siblings. **A,** Female infant born in 1978. **B,** Male infant born in 1979. Consanguinity was denied.

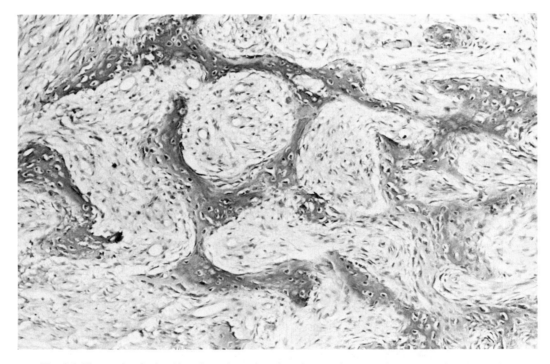

Fig. 6-6 Fibrous dysplasia of jaw. Irregular trabeculae of woven bone can be seen arising directly from fibrous stroma. Note absence of osteoblastic rimming. (Slide contributed by Dr. A. Schmaman, Johannesburg, South Africa.)

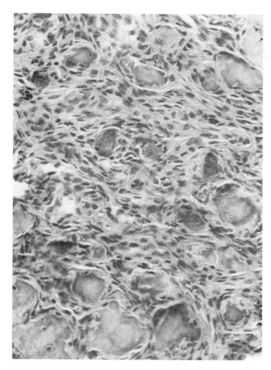

Fig. 6-7 Benign fibro-osseous lesion of cementifying fibroma type exhibiting numerous psammoma body—like spherules.

Fibrous dysplasia and related lesions

Fibrous dysplasia can be polyostotic or monostotic, the microscopic appearance of the two forms being essentially the same.[47,48] The polyostotic form may be accompanied by pigmented skin lesions, endocrine dysfunction presenting with precocious puberty in females, and other anomalies (Albright's syndrome). Fibrous dysplasia confined to jaw-bones is sometimes referred to as the *craniofacial form* of the disease. Congenital or hereditary fibrous dysplasia in siblings has been reported[40,46] and should not be confused with cherubism.

Clinically, painless swellings of the maxilla or mandible are observed that are characteristically unilateral. This feature is often dramatic. Young individuals of both sexes may be affected, the mean age at time of diagnosis in most series being from 25 to 35 years. The lesions tend to become static as skeletal maturity is reached.[44] The roentgenographic appearance varies from cystic or radiolucent to sclerotic or radiopaque, and the margins tend to be ill-defined.

The histologic appearance of fibrous dysplasia in its usual, most recognizable form is characterized by the presence of C-shaped or Chinese figurelike trabeculae of woven or immature bone within a proliferating fibroblastic stroma (Figs. 6-5 and 6-6). Osteoblastic rimming of these trabeculae is usually absent, but its presence focally does not rule out a diagnosis of fibrous dysplasia.

The two main morphologic variations in this theme are represented by lesions in which there is deposition of either lamellar bone with prominent osteoblastic rimming, or

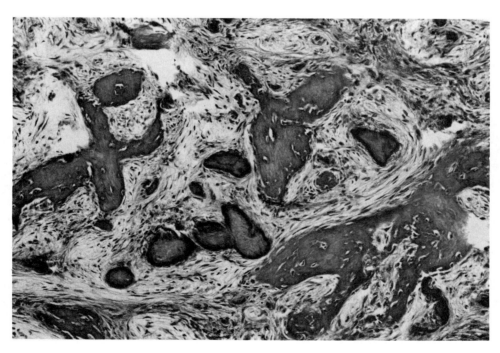

Fig. 6-8 Jaw lesion exhibiting predominant pattern of ossifying fibroma but also containing islands of cement. Mixture of these components suggests common histogenesis for this group of lesions.

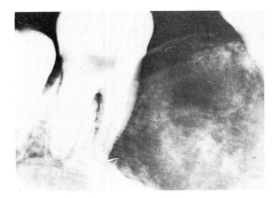

Fig. 6-9 Ossifying fibroma in 17-year-old girl. Note sharp border of lesion. (Courtesy Dr. C.A. Waldron, Atlanta, GA.)

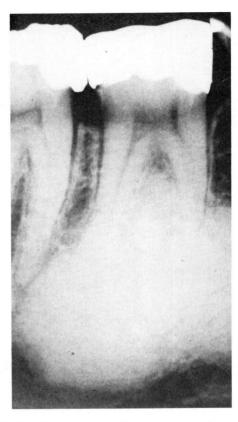

Fig. 6-10 Typical roentgenographic appearance of cementoblastoma. Dense, homogeneous mass is seen in continuity with tooth root. (Courtesy Dr. C.A. Waldron, Atlanta, GA.)

rounded psammoma-like masses resembling cement. The former have been designated as *ossifying fibroma* (fibrous osteoma), the latter as *cementifying fibroma,* and those lesions exhibiting both patterns as *cemento-ossifying fibroma*[41-43,45,49] (Figs. 6-7 to 6-9). It seems likely that all of these lesions have a periodontal ligament origin. These lesions show a marked predilection for females and for the molar-premolar region of the mandible. Some authors have stressed the importance of separating fibrous dysplasia from the "fibroma" group of lesions because the latter are well-demarcated lesions amenable to surgical enucleation or curettage.[41] Although these practical considerations justify a segregation for therapeutic and prognostic purposes, the pathogenetic relationship between these entities remains controversial.

Cementoma and related lesions

There are additional fibrous and ossifying, calcifying, or cementifying conditions of the jaws that may be linked to fibro-osseous lesions because of their histologic resemblance, although some of them may be of odontogenic nature.

Cementoma (periapical fibrous or cemental dysplasia) is a relatively common disorder, being detectable radiographically in 0.3% of the adult population. It is usually multiple and asymptomatic, it is limited to small regions surrounding apices of teeth, and ordinarily does not require treatment. An autosomal dominant form of this disorder has been described.[56]

Mandibular incisor regions of female adults usually are involved. Occasionally, a single tooth is affected, and this may become a surgical specimen. Tissue sections may convincingly mimic fibrous dysplasia. Trabeculae are less than entirely characteristic, although they are irregular, unassociated with osteoblastic rimming, and surrounded by a proliferative fibroblastic connective tissue.[50,55,58]

Benign osteoblastoma has been identified in the jaws, where it may assume an intimate relationship to a dental root surface—hence the alternate designation of *benign cementoblastoma* and *true cementoma*[54] (Fig. 6-10). Relatively few cases have been analyzed in the jaws, and studies

have suggested an innocuous clinical course.[51,54] Continued growth is not always observed, the lesion often stabilizing as a heavily calcified nodule in the jaw. Recurrence that necessitates additional surgical treatment has been observed, however, suggesting that surgical removal is the treatment of choice.

Microscopically, this lesion features irregular osteoid and bone formation (or cementum, the differences between these tissues being very subtle) within proliferative fibrovascular connective tissues.[57] Plump osteoblasts are seen rimming the newly formed trabeculae (Fig. 6-11). The potential for confusion between this feature and osteosarcoma exists. Delineation of "true cementoma" or "benign cementoblastoma" from benign osteoblastoma of other bones is not possible without identification of the relationship of the tumor to the dental root surface[51,54] (Fig. 6-12).

Other lesions of the jaw feature bone or cementum formation within proliferative fibrous connective tissue. Solitary *large* or *"gigantiform" cementomas, multiple cementomas* in black female patients, *osteomas* (especially those observed in patients with the osteomatosis-intestinal polyposis syndrome), and other lesions manifest a poorly understood, apparent relationship to each other. It should be noted here that inflammatory lesions of the jaws during their

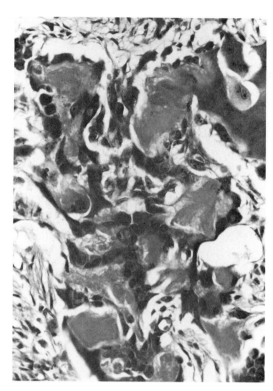

Fig. 6-11 Benign osteoblastoma or cementoblastoma of mandible. Irregular osteoid formation and large, atypical, and darkly staining osteoblasts. Isolated fields could be mistaken for osteosarcoma. (Courtesy Dr. W.G. Shafer, Indianapolis, IN., and Dr. C.A. Waldron, Atlanta, GA., and the American Academy of Oral Pathology.)

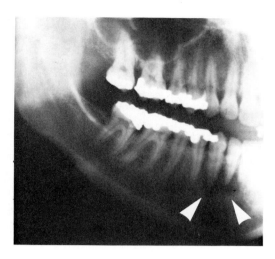

Fig. 6-12 Roentgenogram illustrating mandibular benign osteoblastoma or cementoblastoma without calcification that was associated with periapical regions of permanent premolars (arrows).

sclerotic or healing phases, as well as Paget's disease, constitute additional diagnostic problems.[52,53]

EPITHELIAL CYSTS

Epithelial-lined cysts of the maxilla or mandible are among the more commonly encountered oral diseases from both the clinician's and the pathologist's perspective.[109] Most cannot be identified specifically on the basis of their histologic appearance alone, with the exception of keratocysts and calcifying and keratinizing cysts. Therefore integration of radiographic, surgical, and microscopic findings is necessary to reach a specific diagnosis.[103,112]

A classification of cysts of the jaw acceptable to all has not yet been developed.[85,86,111] Odontogenic cysts arise from odontogenic epithelium and are observed within or, rarely, very close to the jaws. *Fissural* or *nonodontogenic* cysts are thought to arise from epithelial inclusions within soft or bony portions of the region. These epithelial formations lack the embryologic and tooth-forming heritage of odontogenic epithelium.

Odontogenic cysts
  Dentigerous cyst
  Eruption cyst
  Gingival cyst of newborn infants
  Lateral periodontal cysts
  Keratinizing and calcifying odontogenic cyst
  Radicular or periapical cyst
  Keratocysts
    Solitary or primordial
    Multiple (nevoid basal cell carcinoma syndrome)
Fissural and other nonodontogenic cysts
  Nasoalveolar cyst
  Nasopalatine cyst
  Fissural cysts of tongue and floor of the mouth
  Dermoid and epidermoid cysts
  Palatal cyst of newborn infants

Dentigerous cysts surround or are associated with unerupted teeth and usually are found in young adults. They are encountered in almost 1% of individuals having complete dental roentgenograms[72,87,96]; surgical removal is the treatment of choice. They arise following alteration of reduced enamel epithelium after development of enamel and are associated with the tooth crown, at least initially. Swelling and, rarely, pain are symptoms, but they occur late or with infection and inflammation.

While the dentigerous cyst ordinarily has an epithelial lining, inflammatory ulceration and tangential orientation may hinder its histologic identification. A stratified squamous epithelial lining without keratinization should be identified in order to make a diagnosis of dentigerous cyst.[72] Hyperplasia,[121] degeneration, inflammation, calcification,[87] metaplasia,[88] dysplasia,[80] and neoplasia[68,74,80,84] have been identified in epithelium of dentigerous cysts[96,97,114] (Fig. 6-13). Peripheral portions of dentigerous cyst walls consist of mature, collagenous tissue containing signs of chronic inflammation and prior hemorrhage, including lipofuscin pigment.[69]

Examples of cystlike, enlarged, pericoronal soft tissues and enlarged "follicles" may be encountered. While principally consisting of myxomatous fibrous tissue that is not inflamed, the epithelial lining of such tissues, when ob-

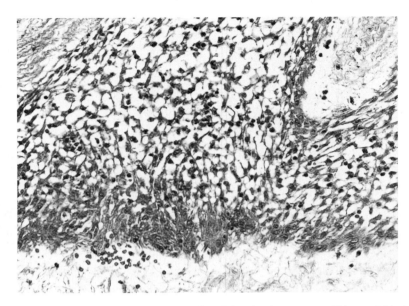

Fig. 6-13 Proliferative stratified squamous epithelium lining dentigerous cyst. This ameloblastomatous proliferation is probably hyperplasia rather than neoplasia. Compare with Fig. 6-30.

served, is probably degenerated dental organ epithelium and not stratified squamous epithelium. Frequently, dental organ epithelium remains attached to the enamel cuticle of the tooth.

Recurrence is not ordinarily considered a feature of dentigerous cysts. When it is observed, incomplete removal, keratocysts, other cystlike conditions of the jaws, and failure to recognize ameloblastoma in early or cystic examples should be considered.[120]

Eruption cyst is a subtype of dentigerous cyst that may be unilateral or bilateral, single or multiple. It presents as a gingival swelling above erupting primary or, rarely, permanent teeth. Surgical exposure of the affected tooth reveals a subacutely inflamed and hemorrhagic cyst wall lined by usually thin and nonkeratinizing stratified squamous epithelium.[88]

Gingival cysts of newborn infants are nodules or minute soft tissue cysts of the gingiva (Bohn's nodules); they are seen in most neonates and gradually disappear, usually in a matter of weeks.[87,96] Microscopically, they are stratified squamous epithelial inclusion cysts and may contain parakeratin.[73,83]

Lateral periodontal cysts probably originate from cyst formation of remnants of the dental lamina. They are remarkable by virtue of their anatomic location, usually apposing gingival or root surfaces of teeth in adults. Mandib-

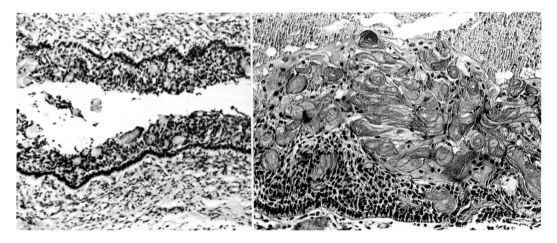

Fig. 6-14 Calcifying odontogenic cyst. Note pronounced basal layer with palisaded cells and large masses of partially keratinized "ghost" cells. (From Vickers RA, Gorlin RJ: Face, lips, teeth, mouth, jaws, salivary glands, and neck. In Anderson WAD, Kissane JM, eds: Pathology, ed. 7. St. Louis, 1977, The C.V. Mosby Co.)

ular premolar regions are the most frequent sites of occurrence. These cysts are lined by an extremely thin epithelium that may appear to be one or two layers thick.[117]

Keratinizing and calcifying odontogenic cyst is characterized by prominent basal palisading and large masses of keratinized "ghost" cells[59,62,63,82] (Fig. 6-14). Some of the cells may exhibit clear cell changes, and others may contain melanin pigment.[113] Histologically similar appearances have been observed in craniopharyngioma, some dermal tumors of sweat gland derivation, and—in very rare cases—some major salivary gland tumors.[88] The similarities between keratinizing and calcifying odontogenic cyst and craniopharyngioma are particularly striking, suggesting a related developmental pathogenesis.[65,94] Cases containing a malignant component have been reported, raising the possibility that at least some of the lesions included under this category are neoplasms rather than cysts.[64,79,93]

Radicular or periapical cysts are another sequela of dental inflammatory disease and represent the most frequently encountered cyst of the jaws.[102] They occur in all age groups but are more commonly diagnosed during the third and fourth decades. Those observed within the maxilla or the mandible following tooth extraction are called *residual cysts*. Roentgenographically, they present as a well-circumscribed radiolucency at the apex of the affected tooth (Fig. 6-15). Microscopically, they are lined by stratified

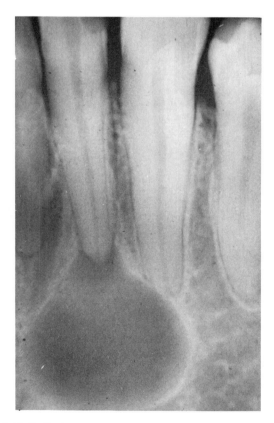

Fig. 6-15 Radicular periodontal cyst demonstrating continuity with pulp canal of nonvital tooth.

squamous epithelium, the thickness of which varies according to the degree of inflammation present. Ulceration is common, and epithelium may be difficult to identify. Metaplasia, calcification, and hyaline bodies occasionally may be identified in the epithelium. The inflammatory infiltrate in the wall may be acute, chronic, or mixed. Aggregates of cholesterol crystals, foamy macrophages, multinucleated giant cells, and plasma cells are common. The cyst usually is easily curetted from the surrounding bone, and recurrence is rare. At surgery, the cyst may be found attached to the apex of the extracted tooth.

Keratocysts constitute approximately 10% of cysts of the jaw and ordinarily can be diagnosed on the basis of their histologic features.[66,67,91,115,118] The importance of this recognition relates to the high rate of recurrence (60% in some studies) and the observation that approximately 10% of keratocysts are multiple and a component of the nevoid basal cell carcinoma syndrome (Gorlin's syndrome), together with cutaneous nevoid basal cell carcinomas and numerous skeletal abnormalities.[90,107] This syndrome is transmitted by an autosomal dominant gene having high penetrance and variable expressivity.[77,89]

Keratocysts have been observed most frequently in the third molar region of the mandible (Figs. 6-16 and 6-17). The mean age of the patients is 40 years. The cysts are more frequently multilocular and more commonly associated with swelling and pain than are dentigerous cysts.

Grossly, the cyst cavity contains a cheesy material consisting of keratinous debris which, when flushed away, reveals a white, subtly wrinkled surface. Microscopically, the epithelial lining is characterized by regimentation of the basal layer and a wavy, corrugated, or mildly verrucous surface of parakeratotic squamous epithelium.[99,104-106,114,123] Some authors have proposed to separate these from the cystic lesions exhibiting an orthokeratinized lining, on the basis of a lesser degree of aggressiveness associated with the latter.[122]

Several explanations for the recurrence of keratocysts have been proposed. Most surgeons note a certain friability and difficulty with curettement. Stoelinga et al.[118,119] also have identified epithelial remnants in human and experimental material that constitute an additional source of recurrent cyst formation. Budding of the epithelial lining with microcyst formation in the cyst wall seen histologically, multilocularity of the cysts, and enzymatic differences of epithelial and connective tissues may also be contributory factors.[78,101,105]

Nasoalveolar (Klestadt or nasolabial) cyst predominantly occurs in females. Bilateral examples are common. Originally thought to arise from epithelial rests at the embryologic junction of globular, lateral nasal, and maxillary processes, more recent theories of origin suggest development from the caudal end of the nasolacrimal rod or duct.[95,110] The nasoalveolar cyst is observed near the base of the nostril and is outside the alveolar process of the maxilla. It eventually obliterates the nasolabial fold and gently presses its way toward the nasal mucosa. Microscopically, various epithelial linings have been observed, including stratified squamous and respiratory types.

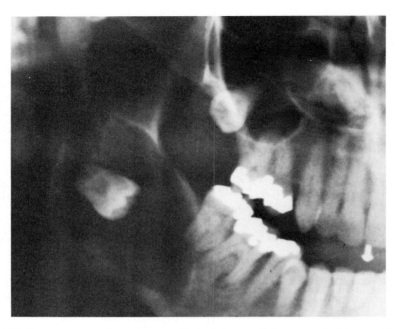

Fig. 6-16 Roentgenogram illustrating mandibular odontogenic keratocyst in 50-year-old man.

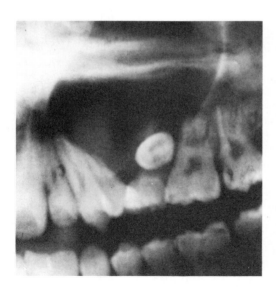

Fig. 6-17 Roentgenogram demonstrating portion of maxillary odontogenic keratocyst in 15-year-old youth with 2-week history of facial swelling.

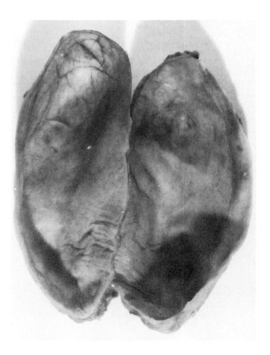

Fig. 6-18 Hemisectioned dermoid cyst of floor of mouth removed from 22-year-old male patient. It measured 6.5 cm in its greatest diameter.

Nasopalatine or *median anterior palatal cyst* may be intraosseous or within the soft tissues of the palatine papilla. It represents cyst formation of embryologic remnants of the incisive canal joining the oral and nasal cavities.[60] It is the most common fissural or nonodontogenic cyst and is lined by respiratory or oral epithelium or a combination of both.[70,76,108]

Fissural cysts of the tongue and floor of the mouth are infrequent.[61,81] "Globulomaxillary cysts" are probably not fissural cysts and justification for their inclusion in this category has been challenged.[75,100] The fissural and embryologic origin of "median mandibular cyst" is doubtful.[71,116]

Dermoid cysts have a squamous lining and cutaneous adnexae, whereas *epidermoid cysts* lack the latter component[92,98] (Fig. 6-18).

Palatal cysts in newborn infants (Epstein's pearls) appear at the junction of the hard and soft palate and are microscopically similar to gingival cysts.[83]

ODONTOGENIC TUMORS

Odontogenic tumors of the jaws arising from tooth-forming tissues are uncommon. There has been an interest in them, however, and classifications have been relatively numerous dating from that of Broca in 1867. In their classic study, Thoma and Goldman[131] classified odontogenic tumors according to their tissue of origin as epithelial, mesodermal, and mixed. Pindborg and Clausen,[128] in 1958, presented a classification that stressed the phenomenon of induction in addition to histogenesis. Subsequent authors have expanded on this slightly.[125-130] The subject is very complex because of the existence of numerous transitional forms,[124] most but not all of which are contemplated in the classification proposed by the World Health Organization.[129]

The following grouping presents odontogenic tumors in a simplified fashion. Moreover, it emphasizes clinical behavior in the traditional manner. It includes approximately 95% of the documented experience with these lesions. It is noteworthy that so many of these lesions are benign.

Benign tumors
    Adenomatoid odontogenic tumor
    Calcifying epithelial odontogenic tumor
    Squamous odontogenic tumor
    Clear cell odontogenic tumor
    Ameloblastic fibroma
    Odontoma
        Complex
        Compound
        Ameloblastic
    Cementoma
    Myxoma, myxofibroma, and odontogenic fibroma
Borderline tumors
    Ameloblastoma
Malignant tumors
    Ameloblastic carcinoma
    Ameloblastic fibrosarcoma

Benign tumors
Adenomatoid odontogenic tumor

Adenomatoid odontogenic tumor (adenoameloblastoma) is a benign lesion that probably arises from the preameloblast

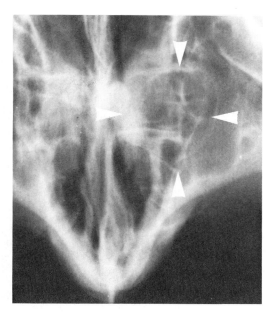

Fig. 6-19 Adenomatoid odontogenic tumor of maxilla in edentulous patient. Roentgenographically, a dentigerous cyst is suggested (arrows).

or inner enamel epithelium.[132-136,140] It appears to be more common in females, arises somewhat more often in the anterior region of the maxilla, and occurs most frequently in the second decade of life.[138] Frequently, it is associated with an unerupted canine tooth (Fig. 6-19) and may appear cystic roentgenographically. Although the tumor expands, it is not invasive and does not recur after conservative surgical therapy.[138]

Grossly, it is rounded and predominantly cystic, to the point that a diagnosis of odontogenic cyst may be suggested; however, focal solid areas may be present. The low-power microscopic appearance is also reminiscent of an odontogenic cyst. Examination of the thicker areas of the epithelial lining, however, reveals numerous ductal structures lined by cuboidal or tall columnar cells (Fig. 6-20). Homogeneous zones of hyaline material and calcified deposits may be scattered throughout the epithelial tissues.[132,134,139] Ultrastructurally there is clearcut evidence of glandular differentiation.[137]

Calcifying epithelial odontogenic tumor

Calcifying epithelial odontogenic tumor (Pindborg's tumor) occurs more commonly in the fourth and fifth decades.[141] There is no sex predilection. Several of the reported cases have arisen in the mandibular premolar-molar area in association with an embedded tooth,[149-151] and a few have been found peripherally located in a gingiva.[153] Roentgenographic features are variable (Fig. 6-21).

Microscopically, the tumor is composed of polyhedral epithelial cells with scanty stroma (Fig. 6-22). The closely packed cells frequently demonstrate nuclear pleomorphism. Intracellular degeneration results in numerous spheric spaces filled with eosinophilic homogeneous material that in time becomes calcified. This has been shown to be amyloid or

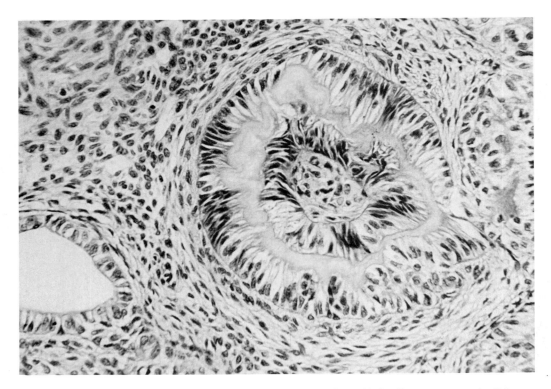

Fig. 6-20 Adenomatoid odontogenic tumor. Odontogenic epithelium with ductlike structures and cellular connective tissue stroma are demonstrated. (Slide contributed by Dr. J. Segura, San José, Costa Rica.)

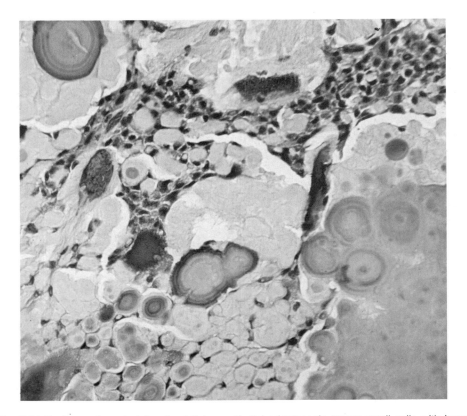

Fig. 6-21 Features characteristic of calcifying epithelial odontogenic tumor: small cells with hyperchromatic nuclei (upper right), large cells with faint eosinophilic cytoplasm and pyknotic nuclei pressed against cell membrane, and calcifying spherules developing within eosinophilic cytoplasm in various stages (exhibiting Liesegang's phenomenon) coalescing to form large calcific masses (lower right).

a similar substance.[143,147,148,152] Ultrastructurally, two cell populations exist.[146] High activity of alkaline phosphatase and ATPase has been found in the cytoplasmic membrane, similar to that of the stratum intermedium cells of the normal dental germ.[144] Hybrids of this neoplasm and adenomatoid odontogenic tumor have been described.[145]

Calcifying epithelial odontogenic tumor may be invasive and recur locally, but as a rule it is a less aggressive lesion than ameloblastoma.[151,154] A single instance of metastasis to a regional lymph node has been reported.[142]

Squamous odontogenic tumor

This recently described benign neoplasm occurs in a wide age range and has a predilection for the anterior maxilla and posterior mandible, tumors in the former location being somewhat more aggressive.[155,157,158] Radiographically, the lesion appears as a well-circumscribed semicircular radiolucency surrounded by a sclerotic border. Microscopically, it is composed of nests and islands of well-differentiated squamous epithelium lacking atypia or mitotic activity, located within a collagenous stroma of low to moderate cellularity.[155,156]

Clear cell odontogenic tumor

This rare epithelial lesion of the jaw of putative odontogenic origin may simulate a clear cell carcinoma of sali-vary gland type or of metastatic origin. The clear cells are arranged in nests surrounded by a mature collagenous stroma, are devoid of mucin, and contain glycogen.[159]

Ameloblastic fibroma

Ameloblastic fibroma often resembles a cyst roentgenographically (Fig. 6-23).In contrast to ameloblastoma, the tumor for which it is most commonly mistaken, ameloblastic fibroma usually occurs in a young age group, rarely being seen in individuals over 21 years of age.

Microscopically, this tumor is composed of strands and buds of epithelial cells in a cellular connective tissue stroma (Fig. 6-24). The presence of this mesenchymal component clearly differentiates this lesion from ameloblastoma. Hard tooth structures such as enamel or dentin are absent.[165] For the most part, the cells composing the epithelial strands are cuboid and two cell layers thick. Only occasionally a stellate reticulum is present. A granular variety of ameloblastic fibroma has been described.[161] The clinical behavior is benign.[160,163] In contrast to ameloblastoma, simple curettage of ameloblastic fibroma is usually adequate.[162-164]

Odontoma

Odontomas are defined as odontogenic tumors featuring production of calcified parts of teeth. They usually occur in the alveolar ridge of the mandible or maxilla, but a few

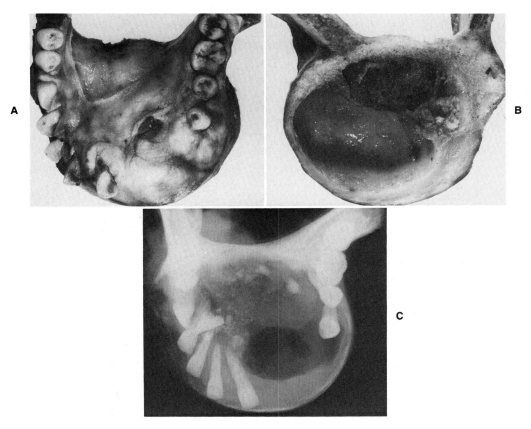

Fig. 6-22 Gross (**A** and **B**) and roentogenographic (**C**) appearance of calcifying epithelial odontogenic tumor removed from middle of mandible of 14-year-old New Guinean girl. (Courtesy Dr. R.A. Cooke, Queensland, Australia.)

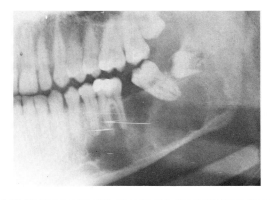

Fig. 6-23 Roentgenographic appearance of ameloblastic fibroma of mandible in 17-year-old youth. Defect is multilocular but suggests irregularity.

examples have been reported in the middle ear.[170] Three subtypes of odontoma are recognized.

Complex odontoma is a poorly differentiated lesion, with a variety of calcified patterns but not enough production of enamel, dentin, or cementum to reach a point where an actual tooth can be identified. It has been encountered most frequently in molar areas of the mandible in female patients. Although the tumors occasionally achieve considerable proportions, they are entirely benign. The lesions are frequently diagnosed after routine roentgenographic examinations (Fig. 6-25).

Compound odontoma presents a higher degree of differentiation than does complex odontoma, and the individual lesion characteristically consists of masses of small misshapen teeth. Some may have as few as three small teeth, whereas the exception has been reported containing 2000 denticles. These odontomas behave in an entirely benign fashion. They are more commonly encountered in anterior regions of the jaws and in the maxilla more often than in the mandible.

Ameloblastic odontoma (odonto-ameloblastoma) is characterized by the presence of a prominent epithelial component resembling ameloblastoma in addition to dental hard and soft tissues, such as enamel and dentin.[168,169,172] Occasionally, the lesion is predominantly cystic.[166,171] This tumor is currently regarded as a form of immature complex odontoma and different from both ameloblastoma and ameloblastic fibroma despite some morphologic resemblances.[167,173] This tumor is considered benign but, on occasion, it behaves more aggressively and recurs locally after conservative surgical removal.[168,169,171,172]

Cementoma

This lesion is discussed on p. 204.

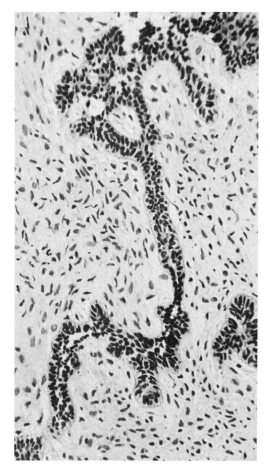

Fig. 6-24 Ameloblastic fibroma showing narrow strands of odontogenic epithelium within abundant uniform, immature, fibrous tissue. This type of tumor does not metastasize and only rarely recurs.

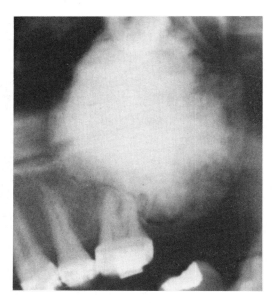

Fig. 6-25 Roentgenogram illustrating benign complex odontoma involving posterior maxilla of 16-year-old girl. Note molar superiorly and absence of one molar.

Myxoma, myxofibroma, and odontogenic fibroma

Myxoma of the jaws is generally regarded as of tooth germ origin and specifically derived from the dental papilla, hence its alternative designation as *odontogenic myxoma*.[174,177] Microscopically, it consists of loose stellate cells with long, branching cytoplasmic processes (Fig. 6-26). Occasionally, strands of odontogenic epithelium thought to represent rests of Malassez are noted.

Odontogenic fibroma differs microscopically from the myxoma by the presence of fibrous tissue and greater numbers of odontogenic epithelial rests.[175,178,179] Tumors in which the myxomatous and the fibrous components are equally represented are designated as *myxofibromas*.[180] Peripheral counterparts of these lesions occurring in the gingiva have been described.[176]

About 60% of these lesions occur during the second and third decades. The maxilla and mandible are equally affected. They often present as cystlike lesions on dental roentgenograms (Fig. 6-27) and are slow growing. Bony expression may be great (Fig. 6-28), however, producing obvious facial deformity, and recurrence following conservative removal has been observed.

Borderline tumors
Ameloblastoma

Ameloblastoma (adamantinoma) is the most common of the epithelial odontogenic tumors,[194] but it is still comparatively rare, comprising about 1% of tumors and cysts arising in the jaws. It may arise from the epithelial lining of a dentigerous cyst, from the remnants of the dental lamina

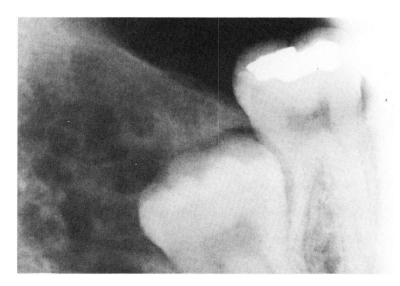

Fig. 6-26 Intraoral dental roentgenogram of odontogenic myxoma associated with unerupted mandibular third molar in 23-year-old woman.

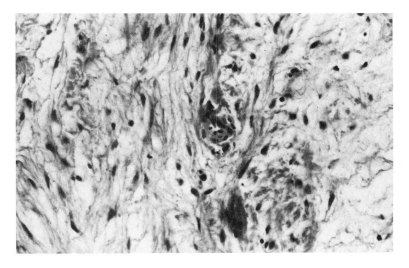

Fig. 6-27 Photomicrograph of same case shown in Fig. 6-26.

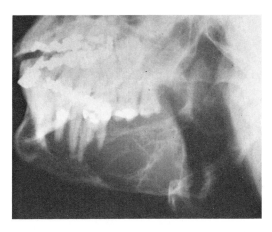

Fig. 6-28 Roentgenogram illustrating a large recurrent odontogenic myxoma of mandible in male adult.

and enamel organ, or from the basal layer of the oral mucosa[184,188,207,213,214] (see Chapter 5, Oral cavity).

Ameloblastoma appears most commonly in the third to fifth decades, but it has also been described in children.[183,208] No sex or racial preference is noted. Over 80% occur in the mandible, with 70% of these arising in the molar-ramus area. Clinical duration may range from a few weeks to 50 years[190,200,210] (Fig. 6-29).

Traditionally, ameloblastoma has been divided into solid and cystic types, but nearly all ameloblastomas demonstrate some cystic degeneration. Microscopically, many subtypes or patterns have been described: follicular, plexiform (Figs. 6-30 and 6-31), acanthomatous (Fig. 6-32), granular cell, and vascular.[181,182,189,204] However, two or more types may occur within the same tumor, and there is little evidence to suggest that one subtype is more aggressive than another.

The two predominant patterns are follicular and plexiform. In the follicular type, there is an attempt to mimic

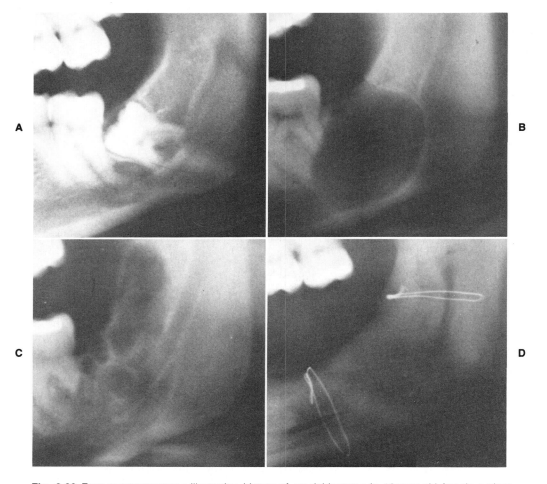

Fig. 6-29 Four roentgenograms illustrating history of ameloblastoma in 19-year-old female patient associated with impacted third molar tooth. **A** (April, 1971), Subtle, atypical radiolucency can be discerned below tooth. Tooth was surgically removed. No surgical specimen was obtained. **B** (September, 1974), Routine dental roentgenogram revealed residual or recurrent cystic lesion. Surgical curettage was performed and "early" ameloblastoma demonstrated. No further treatment was given. **C** (February, 1978), Multilocular radiolucency of more typical character. Tumor was resected. **D** (December, 1978), Current roentgenographic status. (Courtesy Dr. William Randall and Dr. Clark Borstad, Minneapolis, MN.)

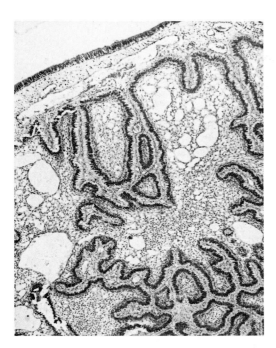

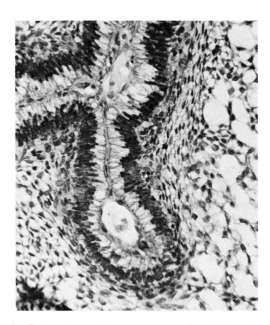

Fig. 6-30 Ameloblastoma of plexiform type. Similarity to odontogenic epithelium in normal enamel organ is well demonstrated. Early degeneration of stellate reticulum with microcyst formation is apparent. Respiratory eipthelium lining maxillary sinus can be seen at upper left.

Fig. 6-31 Same ameloblastoma shown in Fig. 6-30 under higher power, demonstrating polarized columnar cells resembling ameloblasts.

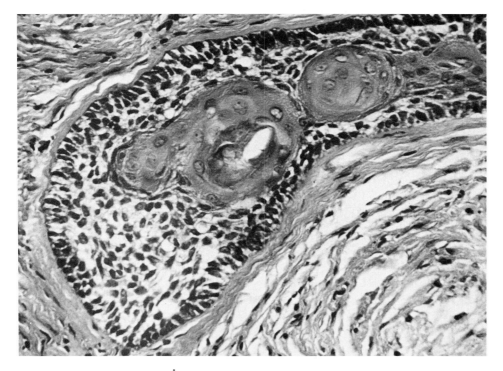

Fig. 6-32 Acanthomatous type of ameloblastoma. Squamous metaplasia within "stellate reticulum" must not be mistaken for squamous cell carcinoma.

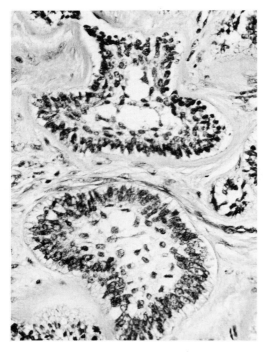

Fig. 6-33 Metastasizing ameloblastoma. One of the surgical excisions, which shows distinctive pattern of usual ameloblastoma with central areas suggesting stellate reticulum and tall peripheral palisaded cells. There is no microscopic evidence of malignancy.

the dental organ epithelium. The outermost cells resemble those of the inner dental epithelium of the developing tooth follicle—i.e., the ameloblastic layer. The cells are tall columnar, with polarization of the nuclei away from the basement membrane.[206] The central portion of the epithelial island is composed of a loose network of cells resembling stellate reticulum. Squamous metaplasia within the stellate reticulum gives rise to the acanthomatous type. The epithelial islands demonstrate little inductive influence upon the fibrous connective tissue stroma. Enamel and dentin are not formed by ameloblastoma. The plexiform pattern demonstrates irregular masses and inter-digitating cords of epithelial cells with a minimum of stroma.[188,197,206]

Immunohistochemically, the tumor cells exhibit strong reactivity for keratin and are surrounded by a continuous layer of laminin in a pattern similar to that seen in the developing tooth.[212]

Ultrastructurally, the tumor cells show clearcut evidence of epithelial differentiation in the form of bundles of tonofilaments and complex desmosomes, with some differences existing between the follicular and the plexiform types.[195,201,203] The granular variety shows the same type of lysosomal formations seen in granular cell tumor in other locations.[202,205,211]

Ameloblastoma has invasive properties and a tendency to recur. Distant metastases have been documented in rare instances, especially to the lungs[188,191,192,198,215] (Fig. 6-33). The term *malignant ameloblastoma* is reserved for those metastasizing tumors that retain the typical morphology of ameloblastoma.[209] In the majority of these cases, the distant metastases have been preceded by several local recurrences.[193]

A particularly vexing problem in this area is the differential diagnosis between ameloblastoma with cystic degeneration, ameloblastoma developing in odontogenic cyst, and

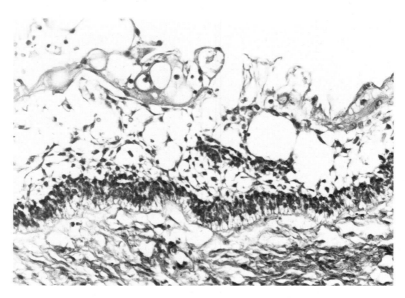

Fig. 6-34 Photomicrograph demonstrating epithelial lining of cystic lesion of mandible that is ameloblastoma. Microscopic tumor foci are likely already present in more than one half of such "cysts."

"ameloblastoid hyperplasia" in odontogenic cysts. Minimal criteria for the recognition of a true ameloblastoma in a cystic jaw lesion have been proposed and appear reliable[196,199,213] (Figs. 6-13 and 6-34). Controversy still exists, however, about the nature of the unilocular cystic lesions of jaw exhibiting a plexiform pattern of epithelial proliferation.[186] Fortunately, enucleation and careful follow-up are probably sufficient therapy for them.[185,187]

Malignant tumors
Ameloblastic carcinoma

Ameloblastic carcinoma is defined as a tumor having the microscopic features of ameloblastoma but also manifesting malignant cytologic features, such as marked nuclear atypia and numerous mitotic figures.[216] It is possible that at least some of the reported intraosseous carcinomas of the jaw represent ameloblastic carcinomas with a marked degree of squamous change[217] (Fig. 6-35).

Ameloblastic fibrosarcoma

Ameloblastic fibrosarcomas may present initially the histopathologic features of ameloblastic fibroma, but recurrences are characterized by increasing degrees of atypia, cellularity, diminution or absence of the epithelial component, and malignant behavior.[219] Ultrastructurally, most of the tumor cells have features of fibroblasts.[220]

Pain is a common symptom, a feature differing from other odontogenic tumors. Death follows extensive local recurrence and extension.[218,221] Metastases from this tumor have not been documented.

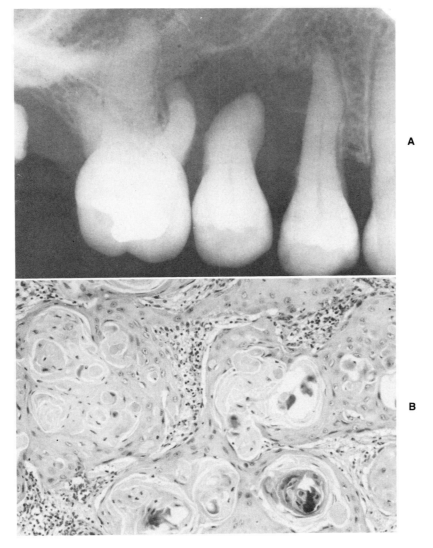

Fig. 6-35 Roentgenogram, **A,** and photomicrograph, **B,** of squamous cell carcinoma of maxilla in 70-year-old woman. Bony destruction was identified roentgenographically 9 months prior to time roentgenogram shown in **A** was taken and before clinical ulceration was evident, but proof of origin in bone was not possible. Note unusual calcification within pearls of neoplasm.

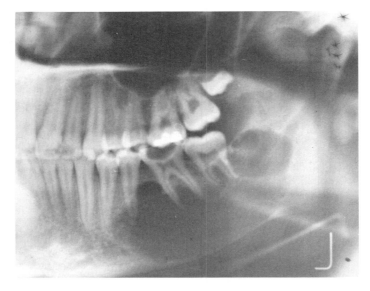

Fig. 6-36 Roentgenogram illustrating cyst-like appearance of aneurysmal bone cyst of mandible in 19-year-old man.

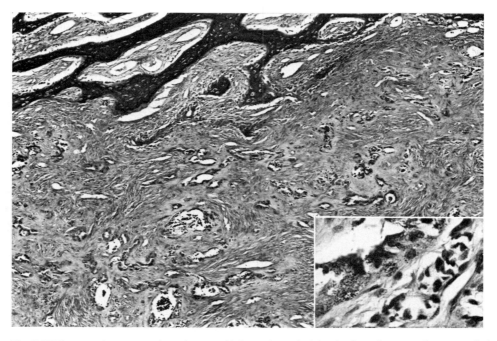

Fig. 6-37 Pigmented neuroectodermal tumor of infancy. Irregular islands of small tumor cells surrounded by cellular fibrous stroma are seen growing around bone trabeculae. **Inset** shows characteristic island of neuroblast-like cells adjacent to layer of larger cells containing melanin pigment.

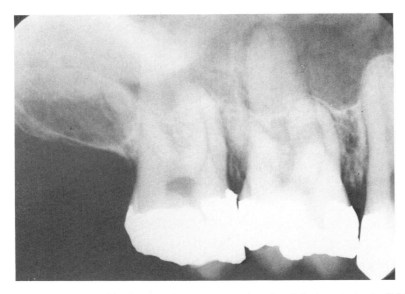

Fig. 6-38 Early roentgenographic changes of osteosarcoma in male adult who noted only slight change in position of tooth. Maxillary first molar periodontal space is wide. Also, slight irregularity of pattern of adjacent bone is appreciated.

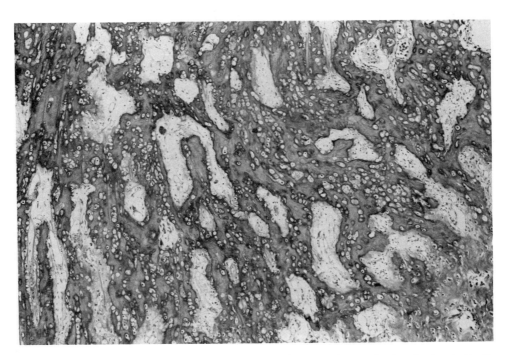

Fig. 6-39 Osteosarcoma of jaw. As is often case this location, tumor has predominantly chondroblastic appearance.

OTHER TUMORS AND TUMORLIKE CONDITIONS

Paget's disease of the mandible and maxilla can occur as a dominant clinical expression of a generalized process, or as the only localization in the monostotic form of the disease. The process may be complicated by the appearance of osteosarcoma or giant cell tumor. Actually, the possibility of Paget's disease should always be investigated when either of these two neoplasms is found in the jaw.

Eosinophilic granuloma (histiocytosis X) of bone has a marked predilection for the jaw—more often the mandible—where it causes a localized ragged zone of destruction.[239,251]

Aneurysmal bone cyst can produce massive expansion of the mandible (Fig. 6-36). Because of its high content of giant cells, the lesion can be confused microscopically with central giant cell granuloma.[226]

Benign tumors of the jaw include, among others, hemangioma of either cavernous or Masson's type,[248,266] benign peripheral nerve tumors,[241,256] non-ossifying fibroma[243] (not to be confused with the ossifying fibroma discussed on pp. 203-204), desmoplastic fibroma,[225,259,263] chondromyxoid fibroma,[236] chondroblastoma,[264] the already mentioned osteoblastoma, and so-called osteoma. The latter lesion occurs almost exclusively in the jaw and is present in more than 80% of patients with Gardner's syndrome.[246]

Salivary gland tumors may present as primary intraosseous masses; mucoepidermoid carcinoma is the most common type.[262]

Pigmented neuroectodermal tumor of infancy (melanotic progonoma; retinal anlage tumor) is a rare neoplasm of neuroectodermal derivation previously thought to arise from odontogenic epithelium[227] (Fig. 6-37). The maxilla is the most common location; however, it also occurs in the

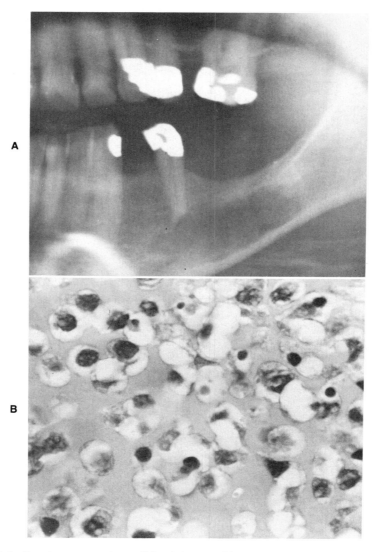

Fig. 6-40 A, Roentgenogram of mandible of 55-year-old woman who was found to have multiple myeloma following histologic identification from curetted mandibular tissue. **B,** Photomicrograph demonstrates numerous tumor cells. Amorphous interstitial material is amyloid.

mandible, skull, long bones, epididymis, mediastinum, and soft tissues of extremities.[247] Immunohistochemical and ultrastructural studies and the occasional demonstration of both neuronal differentiation and of vanilmandelic acid production have confirmed the neural nature of this neoplasm.[227] The behavior is generally benign, but some cases with aggressive local behavior and a few that have resulted in distant metastases have been documented.[238,247,257]

True giant cell tumors of the jawbone are exceptional[255]; most of them are seen in patients with Paget's disease. It should be remembered that the overwhelming majority of osteoclast-containing lesions of bone represent examples of entities other than giant cell tumor.

Osteosarcoma is the most common primary malignant tumor of the jaw. The mandible is affected slightly more often than the maxilla[244] (Fig. 6-38). Most cases arise *de novo*, but others represent complications of radiation therapy, Paget's disease, or fibrous dysplasia.[258] The majority are of the usual intramedullary type, but parosteal examples have been reported.[260] Microscopically, most have a conventional appearance, with many exhibiting a prominent chondroblastic component and some a telangiectatic quality that may lead to confusion with aneurysmal bone cyst[228] (Fig. 6-39). The prognosis for osteosarcoma of the jaw is, as a group, more favorable than for osteosarcoma of long bones. It is best for the tumors located in the mandibular symphysis and worst for those involving the maxillary antrum.[244]

Chondrosarcoma of the jaw shows a marked predilection for the maxilla.[230,267] It can be central or peripheral, and microscopically it may exhibit conventional, mesenchymal, or dedifferentiated features.[231]

Fibrosarcoma has a predilection for the mandible. It is slow-growing and locally aggressive.[235]

Ewing's sarcoma can present as a primary tumor of the jaw; most reported cases have been located in the maxilla.[224,229,261]

Other sarcomas of jaw include *leiomyosarcoma*,[249,254] *malignant schwannoma*,[247a] and *malignant fibrous histiocytoma*.[222,268] The latter is a very aggressive neoplasm.

Malignant lymphoma involving the jaws is nearly always of non-Hodgkin's type. In adults, most cases are of large cell type, whereas in children there is a predominance of undifferentiated types.[240] The high frequency of jaw involvement in Burkitt's lymphoma is well known.[240]

Hodgkin's disease with primary presentation in the jaw is a curiosity; less than a handful of cases have been reported, and the authenticity of some is in question,[233] particularly in the African cases.

Acute leukemia may involve the jaw and oral cavity in children, sometimes as the initial sign of the disease.[253,265]

Plasma cell myeloma can present in the jaw, either as part of a generalized process or as the prime manifestation of the disease[234,245] (Fig. 6-40).

Metastatic tumors to the jaw in adults most often originate from breast, lung, large bowel, prostate, kidney, thyroid, or testis[223,252] (Figs. 6-41 and 6-42).

The tooth-bearing area of the body and molar regions of the mandible are the most frequent sites for these metastases, possibly because of greater blood supply in these regions. In about one half of the cases, oral metastasis is the first sign of systemic disease. Swelling, pain, and anesthesia are the most common symptoms.[232,242,250]

In children, metastases to the jaw originate most frequently from adrenal neuroblastoma, embryonal rhabdomyosarcoma, and Wilms' tumor.[232,237]

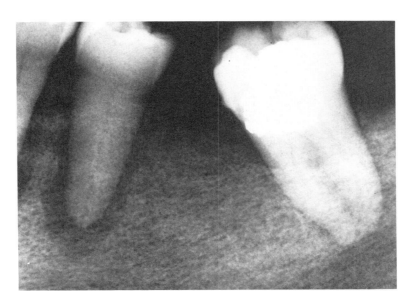

Fig. 6-41 Mandibular intraoral or periapical roentgenogram. Patient, 65-year-old man, had widespread bone metastases from adenocarcinoma of prostate.

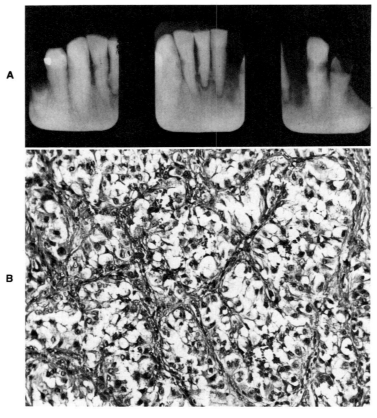

Fig. 6-42 Clinical roentgenographic **(A)** and histologic **(B)** appearance of metastatic adenocarcinoma of kidney. Similarity to inflammatory conditions of dental tissue in roentgenogram may be striking. (From Vickers RA, Gorlin RJ: Face, lips, teeth, mouth, jaws, salivary glands, and neck. In Anderson WAD, Kissane JM, eds: Pathology, ed. 7, St. Louis, 1977, The C.V. Mosby Co.)

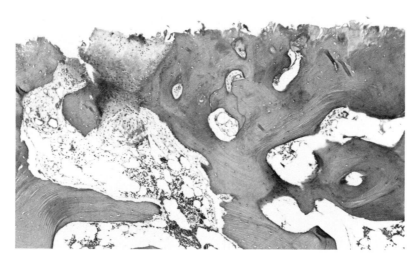

Fig. 6-43 Irregular articulating surface of mandibular condyle in osteoarthritis. Surface shows eburnation.

DISEASES OF THE TEMPOROMANDIBULAR JOINT

Hypoplasia of the mandibular condyle may be unilateral or bilateral, and it is characterized by facial asymmetry and abnormality of function. It often represents diminished or retarded development and may be associated with anomalies of the ear or temporal bone and with macrostomia. It may also be the result of acquired conditions, especially mandibular fracture or other traumas during the growth period.

Hyperplasia of the mandibular condyle usually manifests as a unilateral facial enlargement in adults as an isolated finding, but it may be associated with hemihypertrophy.[270] Grossly, the condyle appears larger than normal. Microscopic examination reveals a thick and irregular layer of hyaline or fibrohyaline cartilage covering the articular surface of the condyle. This disease is probably related to, if not identical with, *synovial chondromatosis* or *osteochondromatosis*.[269,271] When the cellularity of the cartilaginous nodules is marked, the possibility of overdiagnosing the case as chondrosarcoma exists.

Traumatic, inflammatory, and degenerative conditions may all result in the so-called *temporomandibular joint pain-dysfunction syndrome*. The features of this syndrome include limitation of jaw movement with discomfort or pain, tenderness of masticatory muscles, and, sometimes, clicking of the joint during mastication. The gross and microscopic anatomy of joint components (capsule, articulating portions of the mandibular condyle, and the meniscus) display markedly altered relationships in such instances. Less altered, individual components of the temporomandibular joint, such as a meniscus or condylar head, may be surgically removed and submitted for pathologic examination. While it is sometimes possible to demonstrate specific inflammatory or degenerative conditions of this joint such as rheumatoid arthritis, osteoarthritis (osteoarthrosis) (Fig. 6-43), or osteochondromatosis, in most cases the pathologic features are nonspecific.[272]

REFERENCES

1 Gorlin RJ, Goldman HM (eds): Thoma's oral pathology, ed. 6. St. Louis, 1970, The C.V. Mosby Co.
2 Pindborg JJ, Kramer IRH: Histologic typing of odontogenic tumours, jaw cysts, and allied lesions. In International Histological Classification of Tumours, no. 5, Geneva, 1971, World Health Organization.

INFLAMMATION

3 Barker BF, Dunlap CL: Hyaline rings of the oral cavity. The so-called "pulse" granuloma redefined. Semin Diagn Pathol **4:**237-242, 1987.
4 El-Labban NG, Kramer IRH: The nature of the hyaline rings in chronic periostitis and other conditions. An ultrastructural study. Oral Surg Oral Med Oral Pathol **51:**509-515, 1981.
5 Ellis DJ, Winslow JR, Indovina AA: Garre's osteomyelitis of the mandible. Report of a case. Oral Surg Oral Med Oral Pathol **44:**183-189, 1977.
6 Gorlin RJ, Goldman HM (eds): Thoma's oral pathology, ed. 6. St. Louis, 1970, The C.V. Mosby Co.
7 Jacobsson S, Heyden G: Chronic sclerosing osteomyelitis of the mandible. Histologic and histochemical findings. Oral Surg Oral Med Oral Pathol **43:**357-364, 1977.
8 Kannangara DW, Thadepalli H, McQuirter JL: Bacteriology and treatment of dental infections. Oral Surg Oral Med Oral Pathol **50:**103-109, 1980.
9 Massler M, Pawlak J: The affected and infected pulp. Oral Surg Oral Med Oral Pathol **43:**929-947, 1977.
10 McMillan MD, Kardos TB, Edwards JL, Thorburn DN, Adams DB, Palmer DK: Giant cell hyalin angiopathy or pulse granuloma. Oral Surg Oral Med Oral Pathol **52:**178-186, 1981.
11 Mortensen M, Winthee JE, Birn H: Periapical granulomas and cysts. An investigation of 1,600 cases. Scand J Dent Res **78:**241-250, 1970.
12 Moursh F: A roentgenographic study of dentigerous cysts. Oral Surg Oral Med Oral Pathol **18:**466-473, 1964.
13 Sapp JP, Jensvold J: The distribution and morphologic variation of hyaline deposits in odontogenic lesions. Oral Surg Oral Med Oral Pathol **55:**151-161, 1983.
14 Seltzer S, Rainey E, Gluskin AH: Correlation of scanning electron microscope and light microscope findings in uninflamed and pathologically involved human pulps. Oral Surg Oral Med Oral Pathol **43:**910-928, 1977.
15 Shaw JH: Causes and control of dental caries, N Engl J Med **317:**996-1002, 1987.
16 Titterington WP: Osteomyelitis and osteoradionecrosis of the jaws. J Oral Med **26:**7-16, 1971.
17 Waldvogel FA, Medoff G, Swartz MN: Osteomyelitis. Clinical features, therapeutic considerations and unusual aspects. Springfield, Ill., 1971, Charles C Thomas, Publisher.

SIMPLE BONE CYST

18 Gait C: Solitary bone cyst of the mandible. Report of a case. Br J Surg **13:**250-253, 1976.
19 Howe GL: "Haemorrhagic cysts" of the mandible. Br J Oral Surg **3:**55-76, 77-91, 1965.
20 Huebner GR, Turlington EG: So-called traumatic (hemorrhagic) bone cysts of the jaws. Oral Surg Oral Med Oral Pathol **31:**354-365, 1971.
21 Regezi JA, Courtney RM, Batsakis JG: The pathology of head and neck tumors. Part 12. Cysts of the jaws. Head Neck Surg **4:**48-57, 1981.

CENTRAL GIANT CELL GRANULOMA AND OTHER GIANT CELL–CONTAINING LESIONS

22 Black BK, Ackerman LV: Tumors of the parathyroid. A review of twenty-three cases. Cancer **3:**415-444, 1950.
23 Dahlin DC, Cupps RE, Johnson EW Jr: Giant-cell tumor. A study of 195 cases. Cancer **25:**1061-1070, 1970.
24 Dehner LP: Tumors of the mandible and maxilla in children. I. Clinicopathologic study of 46 histologically benign lesions. Cancer **31:**364-384, 1973.
25 El-Labban NG, Lee KW: Myofibroblasts in central giant cell granuloma of the jaws. An ultrastructural study. Histopathology **7:**907-918, 1983.
26 Goldenberg RR, Campbell CJ, Bonfiglio M: Giant cell tumor of bone. An analysis of two hundred and eighteen cases. J Bone Joint Surg [Br] **52:**619-664, 1970.
27 Hamner JE III, Ketcham AS: Cherubism. An analysis of treatment. Cancer **23:**1133-1143, 1969.
28 Huvos AG: Bone tumors. Diagnosis, treatment and prognosis. Philadelphia, 1980, W.B. Saunders Co.
29 Jaffe HL: Giant cell reparative granuloma, traumatic bone cyst, and fibrous (fibro-osseous) dysplasia of the jawbones. Oral Surg Oral Med Oral Pathol **6:**159-175, 1953.
30 Khosla VM, Korobkin M: Cherubism. Am J Dis Child **120:**458-461, 1970.
31 McGrath PJ: Giant-cell tumour of bone. An analysis of fifty-two cases. J Bone Joint Surg [Br] **54:**216-229, 1972.
32 Radcliffe A, Friedman I: Reparative giant-cell granuloma of the jaw. Br J Surg **45:**50-54, 1957.
33 Waldron CA: Intraosseous fibrous swelling of jaws. In Bergsma D (ed): Birth defects. Atlas and compendium. Baltimore, 1973, The Williams & Wilkins Co.
34 Waldron CA, Shafer WG: The central giant cell reparative granuloma of the jaws. An analysis of 38 cases. Am J Clin Pathol **45:**437-447, 1966.

BENIGN FIBRO-OSSEOUS LESIONS

35 Dehner LP: Tumors of the mandible and maxilla in children. I. Clinicopathologic study of 46 histologically benign lesions. Cancer **31:**364-384, 1973.
36 Eversole LR, Sabes WR, Rovin S: Fibrous dysplasia, a nosologic problem in the diagnosis of fibro-osseous lesions of the jaws. J Oral Pathol **1:**189-220, 1972.
37 Talib AN, Gaston GW: Biopsy technique for fibro-osseous and osteolytic lesions of the jaws. Oral Surg Oral Med Oral Pathol **44:**177-182, 1977.
38 Waldron CA: Intraosseous fibrous swelling of jaws. In Bergsma D (ed): Birth defects. Atlas and compendium. Baltimore, 1973, The Williams & Wilkins Co.
39 Waldron CA, Giansanti JS: Benign fibro-osseous lesions of the jaws. Oral Surg Oral Med Oral Pathol **35:**190-201, 340-350, 1973.

Fibrous dysplasia and related lesions

40 El Deeb M, Waite DE, Gorlin RJ: Congenital monostotic fibrous dysplasia. A new possibly autosomal recessive disorder. J Oral Surg 37:520-525, 1979.

41 Eversole LR, Leider AS, Nelson K: Ossifying fibroma. A clinicopathologic study of sixty-four cases. Oral Surg Oral Med Oral Pathol 60:505-511, 1985.

42 Eversole LR, Sabes WR, Rovin S: Fibrous dysplasia, a nosologic problem in the diagnosis of fibro-osseous lesions of the jaws. J Oral Pathol 1:189-220, 1972.

43 Hamner JE III, Scofield HH, Cornyn J: Benign fibrooseous jaw lesions of periodontal membrane origin. An analysis of 249 cases. Cancer 22:861-878, 1968.

44 Harris WH, Dudley HR, Barry RJ: The natural history of fibrous dysplasia. J Bone Joint Surg [Am] 44:207-233, 1962.

45 Phemister DB, Grimson KS: Fibrous osteoma of the jaws. Ann Surg 105:564-583, 1937.

46 Pierce AM, Wilson DF, Goss AN: Inherited craniofacial fibrous dysplasia. Oral Surg Oral Med Oral Pathol 60:403-409, 1985.

47 Reed RJ: Fibrous dysplasia of bone. Arch Pathol 75:480-495, 1963.

48 Schmaman A, Smith I, Ackerman LV: Benign fibro-osseous lesions of the mandible and maxilla. A review of 35 cases. Cancer 26:303-312, 1970.

49 Smith AG, Zavaleta A: Osteoma, ossifying fibroma, and fibrous dysplasia of facial and cranial bones. Arch Pathol 54:507-527, 1952.

Cementoma and related lesions

50 Chaudhry AP, Spink JH, Gorlin RJ: Periapical fibrous dysplasia (cementoma). J Oral Surg 22:218-226, 1964.

51 Corio RL, Crawford BE, Schaberg SJ: Benign cementoblastoma. Oral Surg Oral Med Oral Pathol 41:524-530, 1976.

52 Ellis DJ, Winslow JR, Indovina AA: Garre's osteomyelitis of the mandible. Report of a case. Oral Surg Oral Med Oral Pathol 44:183-189, 1977.

53 Jacobsson S, Heyden G: Chronic sclerosing osteomyelitis of the mandible. Histologic and histochemical findings. Oral Surg Oral Med Oral Pathol 43:357-364, 1977.

54 Larsson A, Forsberg O, Sjögren S: Benign cementoblastoma. Cementum analogue of benign osteoblastoma? J Oral Surg 36:299-303, 1978.

55 Pindborg JJ, Kramer IRH: Histologic typing of odontogenic tumours, jaw cysts, and allied lesions. In International Histological Classification of Tumours, no. 5, Geneva, 1971, World Health Organization.

56 Sedano HO, Kuba R, Gorlin RJ: Autosomal dominant cemental dysplasia. Oral Surg Oral Med Oral Pathol 54:642-646, 1982.

57 Steiner GC: Ultrastructure of osteoblastoma. Cancer 39:2127-2136, 1977.

58 Zegarelli EV, Ziskin DE: Cementomas. A report of 50 cases. Am J Orthod 29:285-292, 1943.

EPITHELIAL CYSTS

59 Abrams AM, Howell FV: The calcifying odontogenic cyst. Report of four cases. Oral Surg Oral Med Oral Pathol 25:594-606, 1968.

60 Abrams AM, Howell FV, Bullock WK: Nasopalatine cysts. Oral Surg Oral Med Oral Pathol 16:306-332, 1963.

61 Akinosi JO: Multiple sublingual dermoid cysts. Br J Oral Surg 12:235-239, 1974.

62 Altini M, Farman AG: The calcifying odontogenic cyst. Oral Surg Oral Med Oral Pathol 40:751-759, 1975.

63 Anneroth G, Nordenram A: Calcifying odontogenic cyst. Oral Surg Oral Med Oral Pathol 39:794-801, 1975.

64 Areen RG, McClatchey KD, Baker HL: Squamous cell carcinoma developing in an odontogenic keratocyst. Report of a case. Arch Otolaryngol 107:568-569, 1981.

65 Bernstein ML, Buchino JJ: The histologic similarity between craniopharyngioma and odontogenic lesions. A reappraisal. Oral Surg Oral Med Oral Pathol 56:502-511, 1983.

66 Brannon RB: The odontogenic keratocyst. Oral Surg Oral Med Oral Pathol 42:54-72, 1976.

67 Browne RM: The odontogenic keratocyst. Br Dent J 128:225-231, 1970; 131:249-259, 1971.

68 Browne RM, Gough NG: Malignant change in the epithelial lining of odontogenic cysts. Cancer 29:1199-1207, 1972.

69 Browne RM, Rippin JW: Autofluorescent granular cells in odontogenic cysts. Histopathology 8:937-945, 1984.

70 Buchner A, Mlinek A: Palatal opening of the nasopalatine duct. A developmental anomaly. Oral Surg Oral Med Oral Pathol 34:440-444, 1972.

71 Buchner A, Ramon Y: Median mandibular cyst. A rare lesion of debatable origin. Oral Surg Oral Med Oral Pathol 37:431-437, 1974.

72 Cabrini RL, Barras RE, Albano H: Cysts of the jaw. A statistical analysis. J Oral Surg 28:485-489, 1970.

73 Cataldo E, Berkman MD: Cysts of the oral mucosa in newborns. Am J Dis Child 116:44-48, 1968.

74 Chretien PB, Carpenter DF, White NS, Harrah JD, Lightbody PM: Squamous carcinoma arising in a dentigerous cyst. Presentation of a fatal case and review of four previously reported cases. Oral Surg Oral Med Oral Pathol 30:809-816, 1970.

75 Christ TF: The globulomaxillary cyst. An embryologic misconception. Oral Surg Oral Med Oral Pathol 30:515-526, 1970.

76 Courage GR, North AF, Hansen LS: Median palatine cysts. Review of the literature and report of a case. Oral Surg Oral Med Oral Pathol 37:745-753, 1974.

77 Donatsky O, Hjörting-Hansen E, Philipsen HP, Fejerskov O: Clinical, radiologic, and histopathologic aspects of 13 cases of nevoid basal cell carcinoma syndrome. Int J Oral Surg 5:19-28, 1976.

78 Donoff RB, Harper E, Guralnick C: Collagenolytic activity in keratocysts. J Oral Surg 30:879-884, 1972.

79 Ellis GL, Shmookler BM: Aggressive (malignant?) epithelial odontogenic ghost cell tumor. Oral Surg Oral Med Oral Pathol 61:471-478, 1986.

80 Eversole LR, Sabes WR, Rovin S: Aggressive growth and neoplastic potential of odontogenic cysts. With special reference to central epidermoid and muco-epidermoid carcinomas. Cancer 35:270-282, 1975.

81 Figi FA, Dix CR: Dermoid cyst of the floor of the mouth. Proc Staff Meet Mayo Clin 14:289-293, 1939.

82 Freedman PD, Lumerman H, Gee JK: Calcifying odontogenic cysts. A review and analysis of seventy cases. Oral Surg Oral Med Oral Pathol 40:93-106, 1975.

83 Fromm A: Epstein's pearls, Bohn's nodules and inclusion-cysts of the oral cavity. J Dent Child 34:275-287, 1967.

84 Gardner AF: A survey of odontogenic cysts and their relationship to squamous cell carcinoma. J Can Dent 41:161-167, 1975.

85 Gardner DG, Sapp JP, Wysocki GP: Odontogenic and "fissural" cysts of the jaws. Pathol Annu 13(Pt 1):177-200, 1978.

86 Gorlin RJ: Potentialities of oral epithelium manifest by mandibular dentigerous cysts. Oral Surg Oral Med Oral Pathol 10:271-284, 1957.

87 Gorlin RJ: Cysts of the jaws, oral floor, and neck. In Gorlin RJ, Goldman HM (eds): Thoma's oral pathology, ed. 6. St. Louis, 1970, The C.V. Mosby Co.

88 Gorlin RJ, Pindborg JJ, Clausen FP, Vickers RA: The calcifying odontogenic cyst. A possible analogue of the cutaneous calcifying epithelioma of Malherbe. An analysis of fifteen cases. Oral Surg Oral Med Oral Pathol 15:1235-1243, 1962.

89 Gorlin RJ, Pindborg JJ, Cohen MM Jr: Syndromes of the head and neck, ed 2. New York, 1976, McGraw-Hill Book Co.

90 Gorlin RJ, Vickers RA, Kelly E, Williamson JJ: The multiple basal cell nevi syndrome. Cancer 18:89-104, 1965.

91 Hodgkinson DJ, Woods JE, Dahlin DC, Tolman DE: Keratocysts of the jaw. Cancer 41:803-813, 1978.

92 Howell WE, Stein H, Tomaro AJ: Sublingual dermoid cyst in an infant. Report of a case. J Oral Surg 30:437-441, 1972.

93 Ikemura K, Horie A, Tashiro H, Nandate M: Simultaneous occurrence of a calcifying odontogenic cyst and its malignant transformation. Cancer 56:2861-2864, 1985.

94 Kalnins V: Calcification and amelogenesis in craniopharyngiomas. Oral Surg Oral Med Oral Pathol 31:366-379, 1971.

95 Karmody CS, Gallagher JC: Nasoalveolar cysts. Ann Otol Rhinol Laryngol 81:278-283, 1972.

96 Killey HC, Kay IW: An analysis of 471 benign cystic lesions of the jaws. Int Surg 46:540-545, 1966.

97 Killey HC, Kay IW: Benign cystic lesions of the jaws. Edinburgh, 1966, E.S. Livingstone Ltd., pp. 86-93.

98 Kinnman J, Suh KW: Dermoid cysts of the floor of the mouth. J Oral Surg 26:190-193, 1968.

99 Kramer IRH, Toller PA: The use of exfoliative cytology and protein estimations in preoperative diagnosis of odontogenic keratocysts. Int J Oral Surg 2:143-151, 1973.

100 Little JW, Jakobsen J: Origin of the globulomaxillary cyst. J Oral Surg 31:188-195, 1973.

101 Magnusson BC: Odontogenic keratocysts. A clinical and histological study with special reference to enzyme histochemistry. J Oral Pathol 7:8-18, 1978.

102 Mortensen M, Winther JE, Birn H: Periapical granulomas and cysts. An investigation of 1,600 cases. Scand J Dent Res 78:241-250, 1970.

103 Moursh F: A roentgenographic study of dentigerous cysts. Oral Surg Oral Med Oral Pathol 18:466-473, 1964.

104 Philipsen HP: Om keratocyster (kolesteatomer) i kaeberne. Tandlaegebladet **60**:963-980, 1956.

105 Philipsen HP, Fejerskov O, Donatsky O, Hjöting-Hansen E: Ultrastructure of epithelial lining of keratocysts in nevoid basal cell carcinoma syndrome. Int J Oral Surg **5**:71-81, 1976.

106 Pindborg JJ, Kramer IRH: Histologic typing of odontogenic tumours, jaw cysts, and allied lesions. In International Histological Classification of Tumours, no. 5, Geneva, 1971, World Health Organization.

107 Rayner CRW, Towers JF, Wilson JSP: What is Gorlin's syndrome? The diagnosis and management of the basal cell naevus syndrome, based on a study of thirty-seven patients. Br J Plast Surg **30**:62-67, 1977.

108 Redman RS: Nasopalatine duct cyst with pigmented lining suggestive of olfactory epithelium. Oral Surg Oral Med Oral Pathol **37**:421-428, 1974.

109 Regezi JA, Courtney RM, Batsakis JG: The pathology of head and neck tumors. Part 12. Cysts of the jaws. Head Neck Surg **4**:48-57, 1981.

110 Roed-Petersen B: Nasolabial cysts. A presentation of five patients with a review of the literature. Br J Oral Surg **7**:84-95, 1969.

111 Shear M: Cysts of the oral region. Bristol, 1976, John Wright & Sons, Ltd.

112 Sherman RS: Resume of the roentgen diagnosis of tumors of the jawbones. Oral Surg Oral Med Oral Pathol **4**:1427-1443, 1951.

113 Soames JV: A pigmented calcifying odontogenic cyst. Oral Surg Oral Med Oral Pathol **53**:395-400, 1982.

114 Sonesson A: Odontogenic cysts and cystic tumors of the jaws. Acta Radiol **81**[Suppl]:1-159, 1950.

115 Soskolne WA, Shear M: Observations on the pathogenesis of primordial cysts. Br Dent J **123**:321-326, 1967.

116 Soskolne WA, Shteyer A: Median mandibular cyst. Oral Surg Oral Med Oral Pathol **44**:84-88, 1977.

117 Standish SM, Shafter WG: The lateral periodontal cyst. J Periodontol **29**:27-33, 1958.

118 Stoelinga PJ, Peters JH: A note on the origin of keratocysts of the jaws. Int J Oral Surg **2**:37-44, 1973.

119 Stoelinga PJW, Cohen MM Jr, Morgan AF: The origin of keratocysts in the basal cell nevus syndrome. J Oral Surg **33**:659-663, 1975.

120 Vickers RA, Gorlin RJ: Ameloblastoma. Delineation of early histopathologic features of neoplasia. Cancer **26**:699-710, 1970.

121 Wright JM: Squamous odontogenic tumor-like proliferation in odontogenic cysts. Oral Surg Oral Med Oral Pathol **47**:354-358, 1979.

122 Wright JM: The odontogenic keratocyst. Orthokeratinized variant. Oral Surg Oral Med Oral Pathol **51**:609-618, 1981.

123 Wysocki GP, Sapp JP: Scanning and transmission electromicroscopy of odontogenic keratocysts. Oral Surg Oral Med Oral Pathol **40**:494-501, 1975.

ODONTOGENIC TUMORS

124 Anneroth G, Hansen LS: Variations in keratinizing odontogenic cysts and tumors. Oral Surg Oral Med Oral Pathol **54**:530-546, 1982.

125 Eversole LR, Tomich CE, Cherrick HM: Histogenesis of odontogenic tumors. Oral Surg Oral Med Oral Pathol **32**:569-581, 1971.

126 Gorlin RJ: Odontogenic tumors. In Gorlin RJ, Goldman HM (eds): Thoma's oral pathology, ed. 6. St. Louis, 1970, The C.V. Mosby Co.

127 Gorlin RJ, Chaudhry AP, Pindborg JJ: Odontogenic tumors. Classification, histopathology, and clinical behavior in man and domesticated animals. Cancer **14**:73-101, 1961.

128 Pindborg JJ, Clausen F: Classification of odontogenic tumors. Suggestion. Acta Odontol Scand **16**:293-301, 1958.

129 Pindborg JJ, Kramer IRH: Histologic typing of odontogenic tumours, jaw cysts, and allied lesions. In International Histological Classification of Tumours, no. 5, Geneva, 1971, World Health Organization.

130 Spouge JD: Odontogenic tumors. Oral Surg Oral Med Oral Pathol **24**:392-403, 1967.

131 Thoma KH, Goldman HM: Odontogenic tumors. Classification based on observations of epithelial, mesenchymal and mixed varieties. Am J Pathol **22**:433-471, 1946.

Benign tumors
Adenomatoid odontogenic tumor

132 Abrams AM, Melrose RJ, Howell FV: Adenoameloblastoma. Cancer **22**:175-185, 1968.

133 Bhaskar SN: Adenoameloblastoma. Its histogenesis and report of 15 new cases. J Oral Surg **22**:218-226, 1964.

134 Chambers KS: The adenoameloblastoma. Br J Oral Surg **10**:310-320, 1973.

135 Courtney RM, Kerr DA: The odontogenic adenomatoid tumor. Oral Surg Oral Med Oral Pathol **39**:424-435, 1975.

136 Giansanti JS, Someren A, Waldron CA: Odontogenic adenomatoid tumor (adenoameloblastoma). Survey of 111 cases. Oral Surg Oral Med Oral Pathol **30**:69-88, 1970.

137 Hatakeyama S, Suzuki A: Ultrastructural study of adenomatoid odontogenic tumor. J Oral Pathol **7**:395-410, 1978.

138 Philipsen HP, Birn H: The adenomatoid odontogenic tumour. Ameloblastic adenomatoid tumour or adenoameloblastoma. Acta Pathol Microbiol Scand **75**:375-398, 1969.

139 Pindborg JJ, Kramer IRH: Histologic typing of odontogenic tumours, jaw cysts, and allied lesions. In International Histological Classification of Tumours, no. 5, Geneva, 1971, World Health Organization.

140 Spouge JD: The adenoameloblastoma. Oral Surg Oral Med Oral Pathol **23**:470-482, 1967.

Calcifying epithelial odontogenic tumor

141 Ai-Ru L, Zhen L, Jian S: Calcifying epithelial odontogenic tumors. A clinicopathologic study of nine cases. J Oral Pathol **11**:399-406, 1982.

142 Basu MK, Matthews JB, Sear AJ, Browne RM: Calcifying epithelial odontogenic tumour. A case showing features of malignancy. J Oral Pathol **13**:310-319, 1984.

143 Chaudhry AP, Hanks CT, Leifer C, Gargiulo EA: Calcifying epithelial odontogenic tumor. A histochemical and ultrastructural study. Cancer **30**:1036-1045, 1972.

144 Chomette G, Auriol M, Guilbert F: Histoenzymological and ultrastructural study of a bifocal calcifying epithelial odontogenic tumor. Characteristics of epithelial cells and histogenesis of amyloid-like material. Virchows Arch [Pathol Anat] **403**:67-76, 1984.

145 Damm DD, White DK, Drummond JF, Poindexter JB, Henry BB: Combined epithelial odontogenic tumor. Adenomatoid odontogenic tumor and calcifying epithelial odontogenic tumor. Oral Surg Oral Med Oral Pathol **55**:487-496, 1982.

146 El-Labban NG, Lee KW, Kramer IRH: The duality of the cell population in a calcifying epithelial odontogenic tumor (CEOT). Histopathology **8**:679-691, 1984.

147 El-Labban NG, Lee KW, Kramer IRH, Harris M: The nature of the amyloid-like material in a calcifying epithelial odontogenic tumor. An ultrastructural study. J Oral Pathol **12**:366-374, 1983.

148 Franklin CD, Martin MV, Clark A, Smith CJ, Hindle MO: An investigation into the origin and nature of "amyloid" in a calcifying epithelial odontogenic tumour. J Oral Pathol **10**:417-429, 1981.

149 Pindborg JJ: A calcifying epithelial odontogenic tumor. Cancer **11**:838-843, 1958.

150 Pindborg JJ: The calcifying epithelial odontogenic tumor. Review of the literature and report of an extra-osseous case. Acta Odontol Scand **24**:419-430, 1966.

151 Pindborg JJ, Kramer IRH: Histologic typing of odontogenic tumours, jaw cysts, and allied lesions. In International Histological Classification of Tumours, no. 5, Geneva, 1971, World Health Organization.

152 Ranlov P, Pindborg JJ: The amyloid nature of the homogeneous substance in the calcifying epithelial odontogenic tumour. Acta Pathol Microbiol Scand **68**:169-174, 1966.

153 Takeda Y, Suzuki A, Sekiyama S: Peripheral calcifying epithelial odontogenic tumor. Oral Surg Oral Med Oral Pathol **56**:71-75, 1983.

154 Vap DR, Dahlin DC, Turlington EG: Pindborg tumor. The so-called calcifying epithelial odontogenic tumor. Cancer **25**:629-636, 1970.

Squamous odontogenic tumor

155 Goldblatt LI, Brannon RB, Ellis GL: Squamous odontogenic tumor. Report of five cases and review of the literature. Oral Surg Oral Med Oral Pathol **54**:187-196, 1982.

156 Leventon GS, Happonen R-P, Newland JR: Squamous odontogenic tumor. Report of two cases and review of the literature. Am J Surg Pathol **5**:671-677, 1981.

157 McClatchey KD: Tumors of the dental lamina. A selective review. Semin Diagn Pathol **4**:200-204, 1987.

158 Pullon PA, Shafer WG, Elzay RP, Kerr DA, Corio RL: Squamous odontogenic tumor. Report of six cases of a previously undescribed lesion. Oral Surg Oral Med Oral Pathol **40**:616-630, 1975.

Clear cell odontogenic tumor

159 Eversole LR, Belton CM, Hansen LS: Clear cell odontogenic tumor. Histochemical and ultrastructural features. J Oral Pathol **14**:603-614, 1985.

Ameloblastic fibroma

160 Chuong R, Kaban LB: Diagnosis and treatment of jaw tumors in children. J Oral Maxillofac Surg **43**:323-332, 1985.

161 Couch RD, Morris EE, Vellios F: Granular cell ameloblastic fibroma. Report of 2 cases in adults, with observations of its similarity to congenital epulis. Am J Clin Pathol 37:398-404, 1962.

162 Pindborg JJ, Kramer IRH: Histologic typing of odontogenic tumours, jaw cysts, and allied lesions. In International Histological Classification of Tumours, no. 5, Geneva, 1971, World Health Organization.

163 Shafer WG: Ameloblastic fibroma. J Oral Surg 13:317-321, 1955.

164 Trodahl JN: Ameloblastic fibroma. A survey of cases from the Armed Forces Institute of Pathology. Oral Surg Oral Med Oral Pathol 33:547-558, 1972.

165 van Wyk CW, van der Vyver PC: Ameloblastic fibroma with dentinoid formation/ immature dentinoma. A microscopic and ultrastructural study of the epithelial-connective tissue interface. J Oral Pathol 12:37-46, 1983.

Odontoma

166 Dunlap CL, Fritlen TJ: Cystic odontoma with concomitant adenoameloblastoma. Oral Surg Oral Med Oral Pathol 34:450-457, 1972.

167 Gardner DG: The mixed odontogenic tumors. Oral Surg Oral Med Oral Pathol 58:166-168, 1984.

168 Hamner JE, Pizer ME: Ameloblastic odontoma. Am J Dis Child 115:332-336, 1968.

169 Jacobsohn PH, Quinn JH: Ameloblastic odontomas. Report of three cases. Oral Surg Oral Med Oral Pathol 26:829-836, 1968.

170 McClatchey KD, Hakimi M, Batsakis JG: Retrotympanic odontoma. Am J Surg Pathol 5:401-404, 1981.

171 Olech E, Alvares O: Ameloblastic odontoma. Oral Surg Oral Med Oral Pathol 23:487-492, 1967.

172 Pindborg JJ, Kramer IRH: Histologic typing of odontogenic tumours, jaw cysts, and allied lesions. In International Histological Classification of Tumours, no. 5, Geneva, 1971, World Health Organization.

173 Slootweg PJ: An analysis of the interrelationship of the mixed odontogenic tumors—ameloblastic fibroma, ameloblastic fibro-odontoma, and the odontomas. Oral Surg Oral Med Oral Pathol 51:266-276, 1981.

Myxoma, myxofibroma, and odontogenic fibroma

174 Barros RE, Dominguez FV, Cabrini RL: Myxoma of the jaws. Oral Surg Oral Med Oral Pathol 27:225-236, 1969.

175 Dunlap CL, Barker BF: Central odontogenic fibroma of the WHO type. Oral Surg Oral Med Oral Pathol 57:390-394, 1984.

176 Gardner DG: The peripheral odontogenic fibroma. An attempt at clarification. Oral Surg Oral Med Oral Pathol 54:40-48, 1982.

177 Hasleton PS, Simpson W, Craig RD: Myxoma of the mandible. A fibroblastic tumor. Oral Surg Oral Med Oral Pathol 46:396-406, 1978.

178 Heimdal A, Isacsson G, Nilsson L: Recurrent odontogenic fibroma. Oral Surg Oral Med Oral Pathol 50:140-145, 1980.

179 Wesley RK, Wysocki GP, Mintz SM: The central odontogenic fibroma. Oral Surg Oral Med Oral Pathol 40:235-245, 1975.

180 Zimmerman DC, Dahlin DC: Myxomatous tumors of jaws. Oral Surg Oral Med Oral Pathol 11:1069-1080, 1958.

Borderline tumors
Ameloblastoma

181 Burkes EJ Jr, Wallace DA: Granular cell ameloblastoma. J Oral Surg 34:742-744, 1976.

182 Campbell JAH: Adamantinoma containing tissue resembling granular-cell myoblastoma. J Pathol Bacteriol 71:45-49, 1956.

183 Daramola JO, Ajaglae HA, Oluwasanmi JO: Ameloblastoma of the jaws in Nigerian children. A review of sixteen cases. Oral Surg Oral Med Oral Pathol 40:458-463, 1975.

184 Gardner DG: Peripheral ameloblastoma. A study of 21 cases, including 5 reported as basal cell carcinoma of the gingiva. Cancer 39:1625-1633, 1977.

185 Gardner DG: Plexiform unicystic ameloblastoma. A diagnostic problem in dentigerous cysts. Cancer 47:1358-1363, 1981.

186 Gardner DG, Corio RL: The relationship of plexiform unicystic ameloblastoma to conventional ameloblastoma. Oral Surg Oral Med Oral Pathol 56:54-60, 1983.

187 Gardner DG, Corio RL: Plexiform unicystic ameloblastoma. A variant of ameloblastoma with a low-recurrence rate after enucleation. Cancer 53:1730-1735, 1984.

188 Gorlin RJ: Odontogenic tumors. In Gorlin RJ, Goldman HM (eds): Thoma's oral pathology, ed. 6. St. Louis, 1970, The C.V. Mosby Co.

189 Hartman KS: Granular-cell ameloblastoma. Oral Surg Oral Med Oral Pathol 38:241-243, 1974.

190 Hoffman PJ, Baden E, Rankow RM, Potter GD: Fate of uncontrolled ameloblastoma. Oral Surg Oral Med Oral Pathol 26:419-426, 1968.

191 Hoke HF Jr, Harrelson AB: Granular cell ameloblastomas with metastases to cervical vertebrae. Cancer 20:991-999, 1967.

192 Ikemura K, Tashiro H, Fujino H, Ohbu D, Nakajima K: Ameloblastoma of the mandible with metastasis to the lungs and lymph nodes. Cancer 29:930-940, 1972.

193 Kunze E, Donath K, Luhr HG, Engelhardt W, De Vivie R: Biology of metastasizing ameloblastoma. Pathol Res Pract 180:526-535, 1985.

194 Larsson Å, Almerén H: Ameloblastoma of the jaws. Acta Pathol Microbiol Scand [A] 86:337-349, 1978.

195 Lee KW, El-Labban NG, Kramer RH: Ultrastructure of a simple ameloblastoma. J Pathol 108:173-176, 1972.

196 Leider AS, Eversole LR, Barkin ME: Cystic ameloblastoma. A clinicopathologic analysis. Oral Surg Oral Med Oral Pathol 60:624-630, 1985.

197 Lucas RB: Pathology of tumours of the oral tissues, ed. 2. Edinburgh and London, 1972, Churchill Livingstone.

198 Madiedo G, Choi H, Kleinman JG: Ameloblastoma of the maxilla with distant metastases and hypercalcemia. Am J Clin Pathol 75:585-591, 1981.

199 McMillan MD, Smillie AC: Ameloblastomas associated with dentigerous cysts. Oral Surg Oral Med Oral Pathol 51:689-696, 1981.

200 Mehlisch DR, Dahlin DC, Masson JK: Ameloblastoma. A clinicopathologic report. J Oral Surg 30:9-22, 1972.

201 Mincer HH, McGinnis JP: Ultrastructure of three histologic variants of the ameloblastoma. Cancer 30:1036-1045, 1972.

202 Mori M: Histochemical evaluation of enzymes in ameloblastic tumors. Acanthomatous and granular-cell ameloblastoma. J Oral Surg 28:825-831, 1970.

203 Nasu M, Ishikawa G: Ameloblastoma. Light and electron microscopic study. Virchows Arch [Pathol Anat] 399:163-175, 1983.

204 Nasu M, Takagi M, Yamamoto H: Ultrastructural and histochemical studies of granular-cell ameloblastoma. J Oral Pathol 13:448-456, 1984.

205 Navarrete AR, Smith M: Ultrastructure of granular cell ameloblastoma. Cancer 27:948-955, 1971.

206 Pindborg JJ, Kramer IRH: Histologic typing of odontogenic tumours, jaw cysts, and allied lesions. In International Histological Classification of Tumours, no. 5, Geneva, 1971, World Health Organization.

207 Richardson JF, Greer RO: Ameloblastoma of mucosal origin. Arch Otolaryngol 100:174-175, 1974.

208 Sehdev MK, Huvos AG, Strong EW, Gerold FP, Willis GW: Ameloblastoma of maxilla and mandible. Cancer 33:324-333, 1974.

209 Slootweg PJ, Müller H: Malignant ameloblastoma or ameloblastic carcinoma. Oral Surg Oral Med Oral Pathol 57:168-176, 1984.

210 Small IA, Waldron CA: Ameloblastomas of the jaws. Oral Surg Oral Med Oral Pathol 8:281-297, 1955.

211 Tandler B, Rossi EP: Granular cell ameloblastoma. Electron microscopic observations. J Oral Pathol 6:401-412, 1977.

212 Thesleff I, Ekblom P: Distribution of keratin and laminin in ameloblastoma. Comparison with developing tooth and epidermoid carcinoma. J Oral Pathol 13:85-96, 1984.

213 Vickers RA, Gorlin RJ: Ameloblastoma. Delineation of early histopathologic features of neoplasia. Cancer 26:699-710, 1970.

214 Wesley RK, Borninski ER, Mintz S: Peripheral ameloblastoma. Report of a case and review of the literature. J Oral Surg 35:670-672, 1977.

215 White RM, Patterson JW: Distant skin metastases in a long-term survivor of malignant ameloblastoma. J Cutan Pathol 13:383-389, 1986.

Malignant tumors
Ameloblastic carcinoma

216 McClatchey KD: Tumors of the dental lamina. A selective review. Semin Diagn Pathol 4:200-204, 1987.

217 Shear M: Primary intra-alveolar epidermoid carcinoma of the jaw. J Pathol 97:645-651, 1969.

Ameloblastic fibrosarcoma

218 Cina MT, Dahlin DC, Gores RJ: Ameloblastic sarcoma. Report of two cases. Oral Surg Oral Med Oral Pathol 15:696-700, 1962.

219 Chomette G, Auriol M, Guilbert F, Delcourt A: Ameloblastic fibrosarcoma of the jaws—report of three cases. Clinico-pathologic, histoenzymological and ultrastructural study. Pathol Res Pract 178:40-47, 1983.

220 Nasu M, Matsubara O, Yamamoto H: Ameloblastic fibrosarcoma. An ultrastructural study of the mesenchymal component. J Oral Pathol 13:178-187, 1984.

221 Pindborg JJ: Pathology of the dental hard tissues. Philadelphia, 1970, W.B. Saunders Co.

OTHER TUMORS AND TUMORLIKE CONDITIONS

222 Abdul-Karim FW, Ayala AG, Chawla SP, Jing B-S, Goepfert H: Malignant fibrous histiocytoma of jaws. A clinicopathologic study of 11 cases. Cancer **56**:1590-1596, 1985.

223 Al-Ani S: Metastatic tumors to the mouth. J Oral Surg **31**:120-122, 1973.

224 Arafat A, Ellis GL, Adrian JC: Ewing's sarcoma of the jaws. Oral Surg Oral Med Oral Pathol **55**:589-596, 1983.

225 Bertoni F, Present D, Marchetti C, Bacchini P, Stea G: Desmoplastic fibroma of the jaw. The experience of the Istituto Beretta. Oral Surg Oral Med Oral Pathol **61**:179-184, 1986.

226 Bhaskar SN, Bernier JL, Godby F: Aneurysmal bone cyst and other giant cell lesions of the jaws. Report of 104 cases. J Oral Surg **17**:30-41, 1959.

227 Borello ED, Gorlin RJ: Melanotic neuroectodermal tumor of infancy. A neoplasm of neural crest origin. Cancer **19**:196-206, 1966.

228 Chan CW, Kung TM, Ma L: Telangiectatic osteosarcoma of the mandible. Cancer **58**:2110-2115, 1986.

229 Chan RC, Sutow WW, Lindberg RD, Samuels ML, Murray JA: Management and results of localized Ewing's sarcoma. Cancer **43**:1001-1006, 1979.

230 Chaudhry AP, Rabinovitch MR, Mitchell DF, Vickers RA: Chondrogenic tumors of the jaws. Am J Surg **102**:403-411, 1961.

231 Christensen RE Jr: Mesenchymal chondrosarcoma of the jaws. Oral Surg Oral Med Oral Pathol **54**:197-206, 1982.

232 Clausen F, Poulsen H: Metastatic carcinoma to the jaws. Acta Pathol Microbiol Scand **57**:361-374, 1963.

233 Cohen MA, Bender S, Struthers PJ: Hodgkin's disease of the jaws. Review of the literature and report of a case. Oral Surg Oral Med Oral Pathol **57**:413-417, 1984.

234 Corwin J, Lindberg RD: Solitary plasmacytoma of bone vs. extramedullary plasmacytoma and their relationship to multiple myeloma. Cancer **43**:1007-1013, 1979.

235 Dahlin DC, Unni KK: Bone tumors. General aspects and data on 8,542 cases, ed. 4, Springfield, Ill., 1986, Charles C Thomas, Publisher.

236 Damm DD, White DK, Geissler RH, Drummond JF, Gonty AA: Chondromyxoid fibroma of the maxilla. Electron microscopic findings and review of the literature. Oral Surg Oral Med Oral Pathol **59**:176-183, 1985.

237 Dehner LP: Tumors of the mandible and maxilla in children. II. A study of 14 primary and secondary malignant tumors. Cancer **32**:112-120, 1973.

238 Dehner LP, Sibley RK, Sauk JJ Jr, Vickers RA, Nesbit ME, Leonard AS, Waite DE, Neeley JE, Ophoven J: Malignant melanotic neuroectodermal tumor of infancy. Cancer **43**:1389-1410, 1979.

239 Domboski ML: Eosinophilic granuloma of bone manifesting mandibular involvement. Oral Surg Oral Med Oral Pathol **50**:116-123, 1980.

240 Eisenbud L, Sciubba J, Mir R, Sachs SA: Oral presentations in non-Hodgkin's lymphoma. A review of thirty-one cases. Part II. Fourteen cases arising in bone. Oral Surg Oral Med Oral Pathol **57**:272-280, 1984.

241 Ellis GL, Abrams AM, Melrose RJ: Intraosseous benign neural sheath neoplasms of the jaws. Report of seven new cases and review of the literature. Oral Surg Oral Med Oral Pathol **44**:731-743, 1977.

242 Ellis GL, Jensen JL, Reingold IM, Barr RJ: Malignant neoplasms metastatic to gingivae. Oral Surg Oral Med Oral Pathol **44**:238-245, 1977.

243 Elzay RP, Mills S, Kay S: Fibrous defect (nonossifying fibroma) of the mandible. Oral Surg Oral Med Oral Pathol **58**:402-407, 1984.

244 Garrington GE, Scofield HH, Cornyn J, Hooker SP: Osteosarcoma of the jaws. Analysis of 56 cases. Cancer **20**:377-391, 1967.

245 Henderson D, Rowe NL: Myelomatosis affecting the jaws. Br J Oral Surg **6**:161-172, 1969.

246 Ida M, Nakamura T, Utsunomiya J: Osteomatous changes and tooth abnormalities found in the jaws of patients with adenomatosis coli. Oral Surg Oral Med Oral Pathol **52**:2-11, 1981.

247 Johnson RE, Scheithauer BW, Dahlin DC: Melanotic neuroectodermal tumor of infancy. A review of seven cases. Cancer **52**:661-666, 1983.

247a Kameyama Y, Maeda H, Nakane S, Maeda S, Takai Y, Fukaya M: Malignant schwannoma of the maxilla in a patient without neurofibromatosis. Histopathology **11**:1205-1210, 1987.

248 Komori A, Koike M, Kinjo T, Azuma T, Yoshinari M, Inaba H, Hizawa K: Central intravascular papillary endothelial hyperplasia of the mandible. Virchows Arch [Pathol Anat] **403**:453-459, 1984.

249 Kratochvil FJ III, MacGregor SD, Budnick SD, Hewan-Lowe K, Allsup HW: Leiomyosarcoma of the maxilla. Report of a case and review of the literature. Oral Surg Oral Med Oral Pathol **54**:647-655, 1982.

250 McDaniel RK, Luna MA, Stimson PG: Metastatic tumors in the jaws. Oral Surg Oral Med Oral Pathol **31**:380-386, 1971.

251 McGavran MH, Spady HA: Eosinophilic granuloma of bone. A study of twenty-eight cases. J Bone Joint Surg [Am] **42**:979-992, 1960.

252 Meyer I, Shklar G: Malignant tumors metastatic to mouth and jaws. Oral Surg Oral Med Oral Pathol **20**:350-362, 1965.

253 Michaud M, Baehner RL, Bixler D, Kafrawy AH: Oral manifestations of acute leukemia in children. J Am Dent Assoc **95**:1145-1150, 1977.

254 Miettinen M, Lehto V-P, Ekblom P, Tasanen A, Virtanen I: Leiomyosarcoma of the mandible. Diagnosis as aided by immunohistochemical demonstration of desmin and laminin. J Oral Pathol **13**:373-381, 1984.

255 Mintz GA, Abrams AM, Carlsen GD, Melrose RJ, Fister HW: Primary malignant giant cell tumor of the mandible. Report of a case and review of the literature. Oral Surg Oral Med Oral Pathol **51**:164-171, 1981.

256 Murphy J, Giunta JL: Atypical central neurilemmoma of the mandible. Oral Surg Oral Med Oral Pathol **59**:275-278, 1984.

257 Navas Palacios JJ: Malignant melanotic neuroectodermal tumor. Light and electron microscopic study. Cancer **46**:529-536, 1980.

258 Present D, Bertoni F, Enneking WF: Osteosarcoma of the mandible arising in fibrous dysplasia. A case report. Clin Orthop **204**:238-244, 1986.

259 Rabhan WN, Rosai J: Desmoplastic fibroma. Report of ten cases and review of the literature. J Bone Joint Surg [Am] **50**:487-502, 1968.

260 Roca AN, Smith JL Jr, Jing B-S: Osteosarcoma and parosteal osteogenic sarcoma of the maxilla and mandible. Study of 20 cases. Am J Clin Pathol **54**:625-636, 1970.

261 Shepherd J, Woodward CG, Turnbull L: Epstein-Barr virus and jaw tumors in North Nigeria. Cancer **59**:1150-1153, 1987.

262 Silvergrade LB, Alvares OF, Olech E: Central mucoepidermoid tumors of the jaws. Review of the literature and case report. Cancer **22**:650-653, 1968.

263 Slootweg PJ, Müller H: Central fibroma of the jaw, odontogenic or desmoplastic. A report of five cases with reference to differential diagnosis. Oral Surg Oral Med Oral Pathol **56**:61-70, 1983.

264 Spahr J, Elzay RP, Kay S, Frable WJ: Chondroblastoma of the temporomandibular joint arising from articular cartilage. A previously unreported presentation of an uncommon neoplasm. Oral Surg Oral Med Oral Pathol **54**:430-435, 1982.

265 Stafford R, Sonis S, Lockhart P, Sonis A: Oral pathoses as diagnostic indicators in leukemia. Oral Surg Oral Med Oral Pathol **50**:134-139, 1980.

266 Taylor BG, Etheredge SN: Hemangiomas of mandible and maxilla presenting as surgical emergencies. Am J Surg **108**:574-577, 1964.

267 Terezhalmy GT, Bottomley WK: Maxillary chondrogenic sarcoma. Management of a case. Oral Surg Oral Med Oral Pathol **44**:539-546, 1977.

268 Thompson SH, Shear M: Fibrous histiocytomas of the oral and maxillofacial regions. J Oral Pathol **13**:282-294, 1984.

DISEASES OF THE TEMPOROMANDIBULAR JOINT

269 Blankestijn J, Panders AK, Vermey A, Scherpbier AJJA: Synovial chondromatosis of the temporo-mandibular joint. Report of three cases and a review of the literature. Cancer **55**:479-485, 1985.

270 Gorlin RJ, Pindborg JJ, Cohen MM Jr: Syndromes of the head and neck, ed. 2. New York, 1976, McGraw-Hill Book Co.

271 Sanders B, McKelvy B: Osteochondromatous exostosis of the condyle. J Am Dent Assoc **95**:1151-1153, 1977.

272 Shapiro BL: Disorders of the temporomandibular joint. In Gorlin RJ, Goldman HM (eds): Thoma's oral pathology, ed. 6. St. Louis, 1970, The C.V. Mosby Co.

7 Respiratory tract

Nasal cavity, paranasal sinuses, and nasopharynx
Larynx and trachea
Lung and pleura

Nasal cavity, paranasal sinuses, and nasopharynx

INFLAMMATORY ("ALLERGIC") POLYP

Nasal polyps are not true neoplasms. Their formation is associated with infection, allergy, or mucoviscidosis.[1] Clinically, they appear as soft polypoid masses often filling the entire nasal cavity. Bilaterality is the rule, and there is a high tendency for recurrence following local excision.

Microscopically, the polyps are composed of a loose mucoid stroma and mucous glands and are covered by respiratory epithelium, which often exhibits foci of squamous metaplasia. They are infiltrated by lymphocytes, plasma cells, and eosinophils. Prominent thickening of the basement membrane is a common finding. The polyps presumably associated with allergy usually have a very marked eosinophilic leukocytic infiltrate. Occasionally, the stromal cells are large and pleomorphic, with bizarre hyperchromatic nuclei, and can simulate rhabdomyosarcoma or other malignancies[3,6] (Fig. 7-1). These changes are of a reactive nature, as indicated by follow-up studies.[2]

From 6% to 10% of patients with mucoviscidosis (cystic fibrosis) develop polyps in the nasal cavity and paranasal sinuses. Therefore children with nasal polyps should be investigated for this condition. Microscopically, the polyps differ from the ordinary variety by the presence of large cystic glands with inspissated secretion in their lumina,[5] lack of extensive infiltration by eosinophils, a preponderance of neutral mucin, and lack of submucosal hyalinization.[4]

OTHER NON-NEOPLASTIC LESIONS

Mucocele of the maxillary sinus may gradually expand the cavity, cause destruction of contiguous bones, and thus be mistaken for a malignant neoplasm.[10] It represents focal accumulation of inflammatory exudate and mucin that lifts the epithelial lining of the sinus and the periosteum away from the underlying bone; the term *pesudocyst* has been proposed as an alternative designation.[9]

Mucormycosis is the most important mycotic infection of the paranasal sinuses. It occurs most often in association with poorly controlled diabetes mellitus, especially with

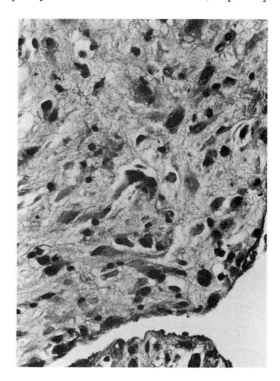

Fig. 7-1 Atypical stromal cells in nasal polyp. These cells have large hyperchromatic nuclei and irregular polygonal cytoplasm. These changes should not be misdiagnosed as sarcoma.

ketoacidosis. The infection may spread rapidly to involve orbit and brain. Characteristically, the organisms invade blood vessels and cause thrombosis, hemorrhage, and infarction.[13] Other paranasal mycotic infections include *Aspergillus* and *C. lunata*, both of which result in the formation of so-called allergic mucin, made up of pools of mucin-containing eosinophils, numerous Charcot-Leyden crystals, and fungal hyphae.[11,14]

Wegener's granulomatosis in its classic form is a rapidly progressive condition in which nasal involvement is accompanied by pulmonary and renal disease. Microscopically, a necrotizing vasculitis with secondary granulomatous reaction and epithelial ulceration is seen.[16] Multiple, deep biopsies may be necessary to find the diagnostic areas. Elastic tissue stains are helpful in identifying remnants of badly damaged vessels. Wegener's granulomatosis should be distinguished from tuberculosis and other specific infections, from so-called lethal midline granuloma (see p. 236), and from the recently described *eosinophilic angiocentric fibrosis*, a possible mucosal variant of granuloma faciale.[18]

Scleroma (rhinoscleroma) is an inflammatory disease of nose, pharynx, and larynx caused by an organism of the *Klebsiella* group. Microscopically, the predominant cells are foamy macrophages and plasma cells. Vasculitis, ulceration, and pseudoepitheliomatous hyperplasia may be present. The organisms can be identified with PAS or Hotchkiss-McManus stains, or by an immunocytochemical technique.[17] Scleroma should be distinguished from the upper respiratory tract lesions of sinus histiocytosis with massive lymphadenopathy.[8]

Granulomas of foreign body type can develop in nasal mucous membranes following local steroid injections.[20] They contain an amorphous foreign material in their center.

Myospherulosis is another iatrogenically induced granulomatous condition of the nose and paranasal sinuses.[12] It is a type of lipogranuloma that develops following hemostatic packing with petrolatum-based ointments and gauze and is microscopically analogous to a disease previously described in the subcutaneous tissues of East Africans.[15] Microscopically, its distinctive feature is the presence of large tissue spaces containing saclike structures with brown "spherules" resembling fungi. It turns out that these mysterious formations are simply erythrocytes that have been altered and clumped by the action of the petrolatum[19,19a] (Fig. 7-2).

Coup and Hopper[7] reported a case of *sarcoidosis* first presenting with nasal cavity lesions, and four cases of *cholesterol granulomas* of the paranasal sinuses.

TUMORS
Papilloma

Nasal and paranasal papillomas are benign neoplasms of the respiratory mucosa most commonly presenting in male adults with nasal stuffiness, nasal obstruction, or epistaxis (Fig. 7-3). Many adjectives have been attached to them, such as inverted, cylindric cell, transitional, squamous, and schneiderian.[22,29-31] Excluded from this group are the verrucal hyperkeratotic squamous papillomas arising from the

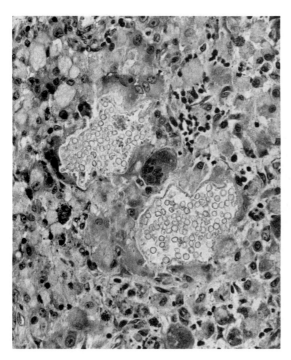

Fig. 7-2 Myospherulosis. Two large "bags" are present, surrounded by granulomatous reaction with multinucleated tumor cells. In their interior there are numerous "spherules," some of which appear collapsed. These spherules represent altered erythrocytes.

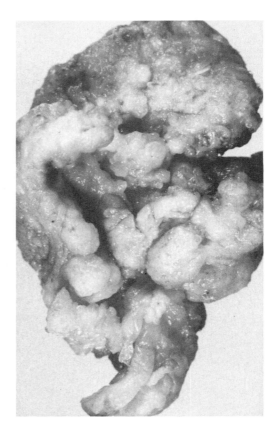

Fig. 7-3 Nasal papilloma, inverted type, in 57-year-old man.

stratified squamous epithelium lining the nasal vestibule, which are analogous to tumors occurring elsewhere in the skin. Nasal papillomas are not related to inflammatory polyps. The latter are bilateral in a high proportion of cases, but this was true only in six of 315 papillomas reviewed by Hyams.[24] Human papilloma virus types 6 and 11 have been demonstrated in a high proportion of cases by in situ hybridization techniques.[27] Microscopically, the papillomas are composed of proliferating columnar or squamous epithelial cells, with an admixture of mucin-containing cells.[28] Some tumors are partially or entirely composed of swollen, granular, eosinophilic cells with features of oncocytes.[21] Occasional mitoses are present in the basal layer. Atypia is mild to moderate, and there is an orderly maturation pattern. The tumor cells are able to synthesize secretory component and to take up IgA and IgM.[25]

The papillomas arising in the nasal septum are usually exophytic and mushroom shaped, with a thin central core of connective tissue (Fig. 7-4). Those located in the lateral wall (middle meatus or middle or inferior turbinate) are of the inverted type, with inward growth of the epithelium into the stroma. This last feature can be misinterpreted as invasion and the lesion incorrectly diagnosed as carcinoma.

They also have a complex and often misunderstood relationship with malignancy, which may manifest in three ways:

1 Development of obvious carcinoma months or years following the excision of a papilloma, with or without recurrences of the papilloma in the interim.[26] This event occurs in about 3% of all papillomas, and is associated with a 25% survival rate;

2 Presence of focal invasive carcinoma in an otherwise typical papilloma at the time of the first excision. This complication, seen in about 3% of the cases, is associated with an excellent prognosis.[23]

3 Occurrence of a tumor having a pattern of growth very similar to that of papilloma but with subtle cytologic features indicative of malignancy (see p. 232). The survival rate for this group is as poor as for carcinoma following papilloma, i.e., in the neighborhood of 25%.

Sinonasal carcinoma

Sinonasal carcinoma is an unusual tumor responsible for less than 1% of cancer deaths in the United States.[55] A marked left-sided preponderance has been noted for ethmoid tumors, suggestive of an exogenous pathogenesis.[54] An occupational group known to be at an increased risk is nickel refiners.[55] Of sixty-six carcinomas of the paranasal sinuses reviewed by Cheng and Wang,[39] fifty were in the maxillary sinus, eleven in the ethmoid sinus, four in the sphenoid sinus, and one in the frontal sinus. These tumors often are diagnosed late in their course, when extensive bone destruc-

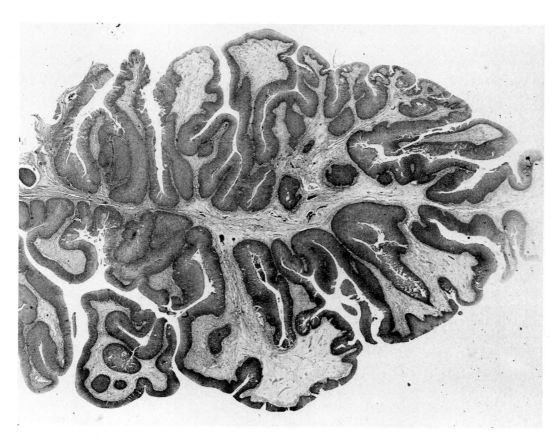

Fig. 7-4 Nasal papilloma of exophytic variety. Thick layer of mature squamous epithelium invaginates about central fibrovascular core.

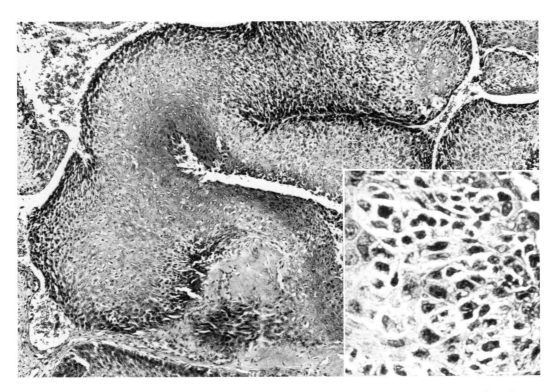

Fig. 7-5 Squamous cell carcinoma of nasal cavity. The well-differentiated nature of tumor and papillomatous pattern of growth often result in mistaken diagnosis of papilloma. **Inset,** High-power view, however, shows that tumor cells have atypical cytologic features.

tion is already present. Intranasal tumors may extend into the medial wall of the antrum, ethmoid sinuses, orbit, anterior skull bone, and upper lip. Tumors of the infrastructure of the maxillary sinus spread inferiorly into the alveolar process or gingivobuccal sulcus, anteriorly into the soft tissues of the cheek beneath the zygoma, or medially into the nasal cavity and hard palate. Those of the suprastructure may extend superiorly and medially into the orbit, ethmoid sinus, and cribriform plate; posterolaterally into the pterygoid space, sphenoid sinus, or base of the skull; anterolaterally into the zygoma; or posterolaterally into the infratemporal fossa.[35]

Microscopically, most sinonasal carcinomas are of *epidermoid (squamous cell)* type.[37,40,53] A closely related type is sometimes designated as *transitional* or *cylindric cell* carcinoma. The latter may contain foci of intracellular mucin. In most instances, the microscopic diagnosis is obvious because of the atypicality and stromal infiltration. There are, however, two varieties that can be erroneously diagnosed as benign: one is the type having a growth pattern quite similar to that of a papilloma (Fig. 7-5) (see p. 231). It often shows no obvious stromal invasion, and the differential diagnosis with papilloma has to be made on the basis of cellular abnormalities such as loss of polarity and atypical nuclear changes.[51] It should be remembered that mitoses and some degree of nuclear hyperchromasia also can be present in benign lesions. The second type is *verrucous*

carcinoma, of which we have seen several examples in the nasal cavity.

A rare type of epidermoid carcinoma exhibits *sarcoma-like* features similar to those seen more often in the oral cavity and pharynx.[52] An even more unusual occurrence is the formation of *yolk sac–like* features by the tumor.[49]

The recommended treatment for carcinoma of both nasal cavity and paranasal sinuses is a combination of surgery and radiation therapy.[33,38,48] The 5-year survival rates with this modality have been in the neighborhood of 60%.[48,58] No appreciable difference in the outcome has been noted between epidermoid and transitional cell carcinomas.[39] Prognostic factors are tumor stage and type of surgical procedure.[47] Tumor relapse occurs almost always within 2 years after the initial treatment.[46]

Adenocarcinomas without a specific salivary gland pattern usually arise on the middle turbinate or in the ethmoid sinus and from there extend laterally into the orbit and upward into the anterior cranial fossa. Microscopically, they show a wide range of differentiation[42] (Fig. 7-6). Some have an appearance strongly reminiscent of colorectal carcinoma, including the presence of goblet cells (colonic type).[34,56] Others resemble small intestinal mucosa (enteric type), with the formation of resorptive, goblet, Paneth, and argentaffin cells.[36,50,57]

An increased number of sinonasal adenocarcinomas has

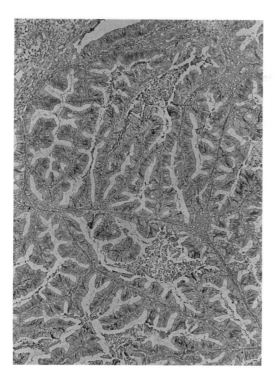

Fig. 7-6 Adenocarcinoma of nasal cavity with well-differentiated appearance.

been found in woodworkers of Europe, Australia, and North America.[32,44,45] These tumors are locally aggressive, with propensity for local recurrence, despite their well-differentiated nature.[50] Lymph node metastases are rare.

Undifferentiated carcinomas of the nasal cavity or paranasal sinuses are characterized microscopically by nests, trabeculae, and sheets of medium-sized cells having a high mitotic rate, extensive necrosis, and prominent vascular invasion. These neoplasms are extremely aggressive.[41,43]

Nasopharyngeal carcinoma

Carcinoma of the nasopharynx is a leading cause of death for large populations in southeast Asia. It is one of the most common malignant tumors in southern Chinese males, and it also occurs with increased frequency in northern Africa.[59] The age-incidence curve is bimodal, with a peak occurring between 15 and 25 years and another between 60 and 69 years.[66,73] In recent years, data have accumulated suggesting that genetic predisposition, environmental factors, and the Epstein-Barr virus play an important role in the pathogenesis of this tumor.[64,65,67,92] The consistent detection of IgG antibodies, which are directed against the early EBV antigen, and of IgA antibodies, which are directed against the capsid viral antigen, has been used to support a presumptive diagnosis of nasopharyngeal carcinoma[71,79,82]; however, the presence of 30% false positive results for the former test, and 9% to 18% for the latter indicate that the diagnosis of nasopharyngeal carcinoma cannot be based solely on serologic tests.

Grossly, the tumor may be very difficult to detect. Ran-

dom ("blind") biopsies from the nasopharyngeal area should be taken whenever the diagnosis is suspected, particularly from the fossa of Rosenmüller.

Microscopically, the crucial distinction to be made in nasopharyngeal carcinoma is between tumors that show clearcut evidence of keratinization and those that do not. The former, designated as *epidermoid* or *squamous cell carcinoma*, do not show the same association with EBV as the others and occur in an older age group.[88] The tumors in the second category, which represent the large majority, have been subdivided into *undifferentiated* and *nonkeratinizing*, with a spindle-cell subgroup.[61,77] A high proportion of these tumors is accompanied by a prominent inflammatory infiltrate rich in lymphocytes, a fact that is responsible for the designation of *lymphoepithelioma* that these neoplasms have traditionally received. The term is a misnomer, inasmuch as the lymphocytic population is not neoplastic. As a matter of fact, it may be accompanied by other inflammatory cells, such as plasma cells, eosinophils, and—on rare occasions—epithelioid and multinucleated giant cells; however, the term lymphoepithelioma, inaccurate as it may be, should perhaps be retained in view of the characteristic appearance of this neoplasm, which is not properly addressed by any of the alternative names that have been proposed.

Two patterns of growth may be seen, sometimes in combination. The first, inaccurately referred to as Regaud's type, consists of well-defined aggregates of epithelial cells surrounded by fibrous tissue and lymphoid cells (Fig. 7-7). In the second, designated just as incorrectly as the Schmincke type, the neoplastic epithelial cells grow in a diffuse fashion and are closely intermingled with inflammatory cells. It is the latter type that is apt to be confused with large cell malignant lymphoma (Fig. 7-8). Careful examination of the tumor cell nuclei should establish the diagnosis in most instances. The nuclei of nasopharyngeal carcinoma tend to be vesicular, with a smooth outline and a single, large, sharply etched eosinophilic nucleolus.[70] The nuclei of malignant lymphoma are usually more irregularly shaped, the chromatin is coarser, and the nucleoli are smaller and either basophilic or amphophilic.

Ultrastructurally, tonofilaments and complex desmosomes are present.[89] According to Lin et al.,[75] the tumor cells resemble those of transitional cell carcinoma and probably arise from the cells of the basal layers of pseudostratified and stratified epithelia. Immunohistochemically, there is reactivity for keratin (always), epithelial membrane antigen (usually), and CEA (occasionally).* Thus keratin is the most reliable marker for the identification of this neoplasm. Interestingly, a population of S-100 protein–positive dendritic cells may also be present[74]; this feature is allegedly associated with a better prognosis.[80] Rarely, amyloid is present in the tumor stroma.[84]

Nasopharyngeal carcinoma has a great propensity to metastasize to regional nodes; as a matter of fact, the appearance of unilateral cervical lymphadenopathy is the most common form of presentation. Microscopically, these nodal metastases may closely simulate a large cell lymphoma.[63]

---

*See references 62, 69, 76, 78, 81, and 94.

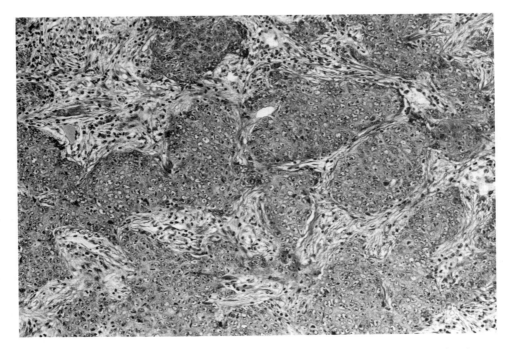

Fig. 7-7 Lymphoepithelioma of so-called Regaud's type. Tumor cells are arranged in well-defined nests separated by an inflamed stroma.

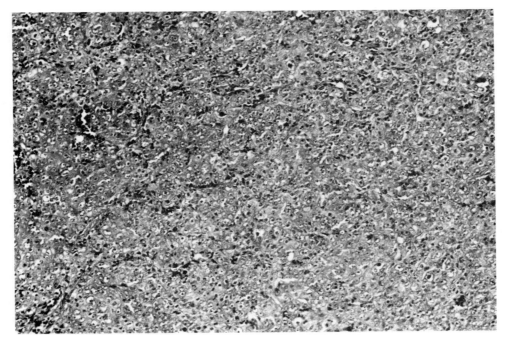

Fig. 7-8 Lymphoepithelioma of so-called Schmincke's type. Tumor cells grow in diffuse fashion that simulates malignant lymphoma.

The focal (predominantly sinusal) nature of the involvement and the large vesicular nuclei with a single prominent nucleolus seen in metastatic carcinoma are useful features in the differential dignosis. In some cases, the metastatic tumor is accompanied by a marked infiltration by eosinophils, which may result in a mistaken diagnosis of Hodgkin's disease.[68] In other cases the lymph node metastases are accompanied by an epithelioid cell reaction with varying degrees of caseation necrosis.[86] Metastases can also develop in distant sites, such as the skeletal system.[90]

The treatment of choice for nasopharyngeal carcinoma is radiation therapy, which cures over half of the patients.[83,85] Survival is significantly affected by patient age (better in young individuals) and the location of the regional metastases (better for homolateral rather than contralateral metastases, and for metastases that are limited to the upper neck as opposed to the lower cervical regions).[60] At a microscopic level, survival has been found to be worse for the keratinizing squamous cell carcinoma than for the others.[72,87] For the latter category, it has been claimed that the prognosis is worse for the tumors exhibiting marked anaplasia and/or pleomorphism[72] and for those lacking lymphocytic infiltration.[87]

Rare microscopic forms of nasopharyngeal carcinoma include *adenoid squamous cell carcinoma*[93] and *papillary adenocarcinoma*.[91] The latter tumor is gland-forming, papillary, mucin-producing, immunoreactive for keratin and CEA, and associated with an excellent prognosis.[91]

Salivary gland tumors

Tumors of minor salivary gland origin occur in the nasal cavity as well as in the sinuses. Of the latter, most are found in the maxillary sinus. Of thirty-seven cases reviewed by Rafla,[98] twenty-one were in the antrum, nine in the ethmoid, five in the nasal fossa, and two in the sphenoid. The large majority of the tumors of the paranasal sinuses are malignant; *adenoid cystic carcinoma* is the most common variety.[96] In the nasal cavity there is a relatively high proportion of benign tumors in the form of *benign mixed tumor*. Compagno and Wong[95] studied forty cases and found that the large majority arose from the mucosa of the bony or cartilaginous septum. Recurrence was rare. *Acinic cell carcinomas* have also been reported.[97]

Neurogenous and related tumors

Encephaloceles and *glial heterotopias* (commonly called *nasal gliomas*) are related malformational "tumors" usually affecting newborns and older infants.[103] They may present as subcutaneous masses at the base of the nose or as intranasal polyps. Microscopically, they are composed of mature glial tissue, with occasional multinucleated glial cells that may simulate neurons. Immunohistochemically, there is reactivity for both S-100 protein and GFAP.[111a] Exceptionally, a true neuronal component is also present.[119]

Associated bony defects are the rule with the encephaloceles, but they are unusual with the glial heterotopias, a feature to be evaluated at the time of removal.

Peripheral nerve tumors are extremely rare.[125,129] They presumably arise from the ophthalmic and maxillary branches of the trigeminal nerve and from branches of the autonomic nervous system. Robitaille at al.[127] reviewed the literature in 1975 and found twenty acceptable cases involving the paranasal sinuses: there were fifteen schwannomas, two neurofibromas, two plexiform neurofibromas, and one probable malignant schwannoma. The maxillary sinus was the most common location. Some extended to the nasal fossa or orbit. Two patients had Recklinghausen's disease.

Intracranial *meningiomas* may invade the sphenoid or frontal sinuses secondarily. They can also present as primary intranasal masses.[107,114,126]

Olfactory neuroblastoma (esthesioneuroblastoma) is a specific variant of neuroblastoma thought to arise from neuroepithelial elements in the olfactory membrane or neuroectodermal elements of the olfactory placode.[122,123] In the normal human fetus, this olfactory neuroepithelium extends from the roof of the nasal cavity to the midportion of the nasal septum and onto the superior turbinate in a continuous fashion. In the adult, many of these areas are replaced by respiratory epithelium.[120]

Olfactory neuroblastoma shows a wide range of age distribution (3 to 79 years), the median age being about 50 years.[118] Grossly, the tumor appears as a reddish gray, highly vascular polypoid mass of generally soft consistency located in the roof of the nasal fossa. Rare cases have been described as arising in the nasopharynx, maxillary sinus, and ethmoid sinus.[113,122] Microscopically, several patterns have been described.[104,115] These often merge with each other. The most easily recognizable and common appearance is that of a cellular tumor composed of uniform small cells with round nuclei, scanty cytoplasm, indistinct nuclear membrane, and a prominent fibrillary or reticular background, similar to that seen in other neurogenic tumors (such as ganglioneuroblastoma) (Fig. 7-9). Rosettes of the Homer Wright type may or may not be present, but differentiation into mature ganglion cells does not take place. Fibrovascular stroma may be abundant and separate the tumor cells in clusters. Exceptionally, melanin is found in the cytoplasm of the tumor cells.[102] The differential diagnosis of tumors with this appearance is with malignant lymphoma, plasmacytoma, and embryonal/alveolar rhabdomyosarcoma.

In other examples, the tumor cells are larger, have more abundant cytoplasm, and grow in solid nests, thus exhibiting an epithelial appearance. This type is often confused with undifferentiated carcinoma.[110]

Silva et al.[130] has made the interesting suggestion that these two patterns may correspond to two different tumor types, the former being true *neuroblastomas* and the latter representing *small cell neuroendocrine carcinomas*. The fact that in some of these tumors there is a component of adenocarcinoma or epidermoid carcinoma would seem to support their contention.[117] Taxy et al.[132] described a similar morphologic dichotomy, but they favored the existence of a spectrum of differentiation rather than the existence of two separate neoplasms, in view of the many shared ultrastructural and immunohistochemical features.

Catecholamines can be demonstrated by fluorescent techniques following formaldehyde vapor or glyoxylic acid treatment[106]; the enzyme dopamine β-hydroxylase and the

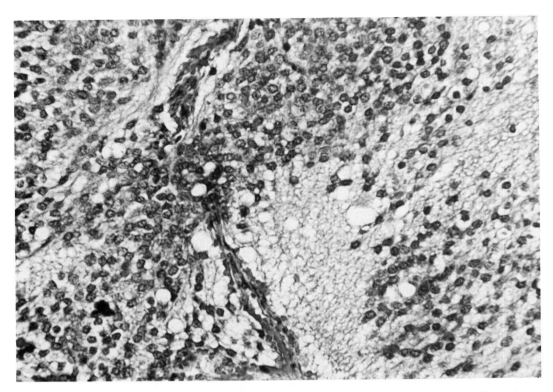

Fig. 7-9 Typical microscopic appearance of olfactory neuroblastoma. Compact nests of small round cells alternate with reticular areas formed by tangles of neurites emanating from tumor cells.

hormone ACTH have been detected by biochemical and immunocytochemical methods.[116] Other substances detected immunohistochemically in the tumor include neuron-specific enolase, chromogranin, neurofilaments, and keratin.[100,101a,132,134] In addition, S-100 protein has been found in isolated cells, often located at the edge of the tumor nests, and GFAP has been detected in scattered astrocyte-like cells.[101a,132]

Electron microscopy shows the consistent presence of neurofilaments, neurotubules, and dense-core neurosecretory cytoplasmic granules and may be of considerable help in difficult cases.[110,112,133] The behavior is mainly characterized by local invasiveness into the paranasal sinuses, nasopharynx, palate, orbit, base of skull, and brain.[105] Distant metastases occur in about one fifth of the cases; the most common sites are the cervical lymph nodes and lungs.[108] The 5-year survival rate is between 50% and 60%.[121] Late recurrence is common.[99,121] This tumor has been shown to be radiosensitive, and a combination of surgery and radiation therapy offers the best chances of cure.[101,109] No convincing relationship has been shown between microscopic pattern and behavior.[118,122]

Carcinoid tumor has been found in rare cases to present as an intranasal tumor. One such case, in a child, had oncocytic features and was associated with a bronchial carcinoid.[131]

Invasion of the nasal cavity by *pituitary adenomas* has been observed.[111]

Intranasal and nasopharyngeal *paragangliomas* have also been reported.[124,128]

Malignant melanoma

Primary malignant melanomas of the nasal cavity and paranasal sinuses usually present as solid polypoid growths.[135-138] They arise from melanocytes usually located in the epithelium and stroma of the respiratory mucosa.[139]

Holdcraft and Gallagher[137] collected thirty-nine cases, of which twenty-one were located in the nasal cavity, four in the antrum, two in the ethmoid, and one in both frontal and ethmoid sinuses. Of thirty-one patients in whom follow-up was available, twenty-six died as a result of metastatic disease (Fig. 7-10).

Lymphoid tumors and tumorlike conditions

Malignant lymphoma can present initially as a mass in the nasal cavity, sinus, or nasopharynx.[142,152,163,166] Most of these tumors are of large cell type.[150,156] Phenotypically, the majority are of T-cell type, at least in the Orient.[143]

Lethal midline granuloma is a clinical syndrome rather than a specific entity.[141,144,145,147,160,164] The term refers to the presence of a destructive lesion of the upper respiratory tract, including the nose, nasopharynx, palate, paranasal sinuses, and midface. It encompasses at least three different pathologic conditions. Some of these cases represent particularly aggressive examples of Wegener's granulomatosis. Others have the microscopic appearance of a conventional malig-

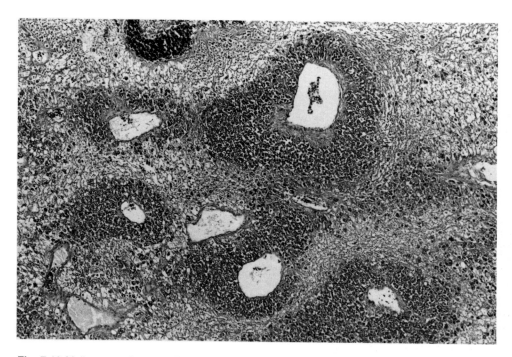

Fig. 7-10 Malignant melanoma of nasal cavity. Tumor grows in peritheliomatous appearance due to extensive necrosis associated with preservation of tumor cells around blood vessels. Diagnosis of malignant melanoma should always be considered in highly undifferentiated tumor in this location.

nant lymphoma, usually of large cell type.[155] Still others exhibit a polymorphic microscopic appearance unlike that of any conventional lymphoma; they have been designated as polymorphic reticulosis,[146] malignant histiocytosis,[140] and midline malignant reticulosis.[149] In this form, small lymphocytes alternate with large atypical cells. Erythrophagocytosis may be present,[159] sometimes in the form of so-called hemophagocytic syndrome.[161] According to Fechner and Lamppin,[149] it is the *polymorphism* that is crucial for its distinction from a conventional lymphoma. In some of these patients the disease remains localized; in an approximately equal number, dissemination occurs.[149,159] The suggestion has been advanced that this condition is microscopically identical and might be pathogenetically related to lymphomatoid granulomatosis of the lungs,[146] and the further proposal has been made that both of these conditions represent peripheral T-cell lymphomas with peculiar angiocentric properties.[143,144,153,158]

Plasma cell tumors arising in the nasal cavity or nasopharynx may present primarily in the nose as a soft bleeding mass.[151,154,157] Microscopic examination shows a monomorphic infiltration by immature plasma cells.[148,165] The majority of patients with apparently solitary plasma cell tumors of the upper air passages in whom there is adequate follow-up develop disseminated myeloma.[152] In some, this process takes 10 or more years to become manifest. Local control of the disease can usually be achieved with radiation therapy.[154]

Pseudolymphoma may present as a polypoid intranasal mass, but this is an extremely rare occurrence.[162]

Nasopharyngeal angiofibroma

Nasopharyngeal angiofibroma occurs almost exclusively in males between 10 and 25 years of age[171]; however, well-documented cases in older patients and in females are on record. The great predilection for young males strongly suggests that this neoplasm is androgen-dependent, a theory confirmed by the detection of specific testosterone and dihydrotestosterone-binding components in the tumor cytosol, but not estrogen or progesterone receptors.[172]

This neoplasm arises from a distinctive erectile-like fibrovascular stroma located in the posterior lateral wall of the roof of the nose, where the sphenoidal process of the palatine bone meets the horizontal ala of the vomer and the root of the pterygoid process of the sphenoid bone. Grossly, it presents as a polypoid mass that bleeds severely on manipulation and biopsy. It can grow to occlude the involved nares completely (Fig. 7-11). It may protrude below the free edge of the soft palate, extend into the antrum, and grow to the external orifice of the nares, posteriorly into the nasopharynx, or even into the orbit and cranial cavity.[170,171] Selective carotid arteriograms are helpful in determining the gross confines of the tumor (Fig. 7-12), although this goal can also be achieved now with noninvasive techniques such as CT scan and nuclear magnetic resonance.

Microscopically, the tumor is composed of an intricate mixture of blood vessels and fibrous stroma (Fig. 7-13). The latter varies from loose and edematous, with stellate fibroblasts and numerous mast cells, to a dense, acellular, and highly collagenized tissue. The vessels range from capillary size to venous size; the larger vessels are located at

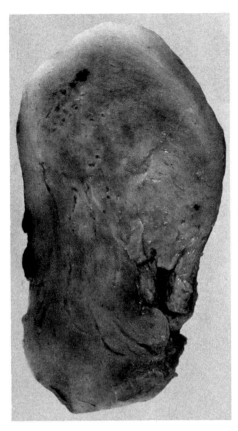

Fig. 7-11 Nasopharyngeal angiofibroma. Cut surface shows characteristic spongy appearance of erectile tissue and well-circumscribed outline. (Courtesy Dr. J. Costa, Lausanne, Switzerland.)

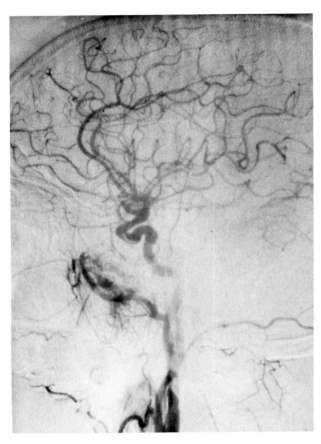

Fig. 7-12 Nasopharyngeal angiofibroma in 13-year-old boy well demonstrated by subtraction arteriography.

the base of the lesion, whereas the smaller capillary-like vessels with plump endothelial cells are particularly common at the "growing edge" of the tumor.[176] The large vessels may have an irregular or incomplete smooth muscle coat, but they lack elastic fibers. It is important to distinguish angiofibromas from capillary hemangiomas because of the different natural history of these lesions. In general, hemangiomas are accompanied by a lesser amount of fibrous tissue, and their vessels do not have the "erectile tissue" appearance so characteristic of nasopharyngeal angiofibroma. Location of the tumor is very important; a diagnosis of angiofibroma should be questioned in any tumor that is not located in the area described in the preceding paragraph.

Ultrastructurally, distinctive electron-dense granules composed of tightly bound RNA-protein complexes have been found in the nuclei of the proliferating cells.[177]

There is no doubt that some large angiofibromas regress after puberty, especially after incomplete surgical removal or radiation therapy. Spontaneous total regression, however, is very rare; in a patient with symptoms, treatment is indicated. There is controversy as to whether surgery or radiation is the treatment of choice.[168,174,178] Most of the post-therapy recurrences develop within the first year.[173] A few cases of sarcomatous transformation following radiation

therapy have been described.[167,175] Chemotherapy may be necessary for the more aggressive tumors.[169]

Other tumors and tumorlike conditions

Dermoid cysts are dorsal developmental defects located in the midline. They may be associated with bony defects and sinus tracts.[194]

Teratomas have been reported in the sinuses and nasopharynx of infants and children. The large majority are benign.[181, 194]

Vascular tumors are relatively common and include a large variety of types. *Capillary lobular hemangioma* is usually located in the nasal cavity, where it can reach a large size and be misdiagnosed as a nasopharyngeal angiofibroma[193] (Fig. 7-14). Twenty-three examples of a vascular neoplasm with features of *hemangiopericytoma* were described by Compagno and Hyams.[182] Most cases originated in a paranasal sinus and extended into the nasal cavity secondarily. The clinical diagnosis was often that of allergic polyp. Microscopically, the lesions appeared vascular and highly cellular, but with little atypia, necrosis, or mitotic activity (Fig. 7-15). Immunohistochemically, there is strong reactivity for vimentin and focal reactivity for actin.[183a] We view this tumor as a hybrid between heman-

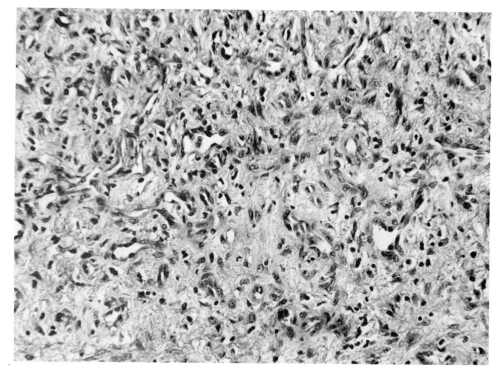

Fig. 7-13 Nasopharyngeal angiofibroma with typical prominent vessels and loose fibroblastic stroma.

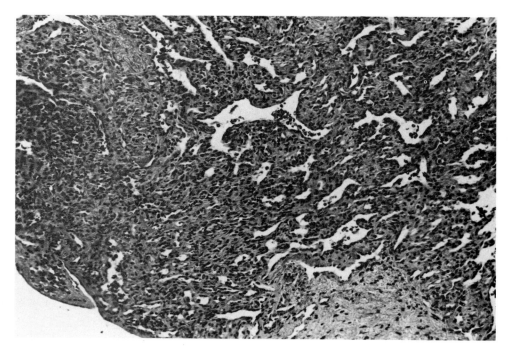

Fig. 7-14 Capillary lobular hemangioma arising from nasal septum. Branching central vessels are characteristic. This lesion should not be confused with nasopharyngeal angiofibroma.

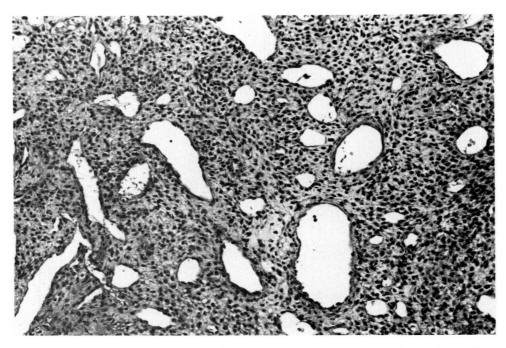

Fig. 7-15 Hemangiopericytoma-like tumor of nasal cavity. Appearance of this neoplasm is intermediate between that of hemangiopericytoma and glomus tumor.

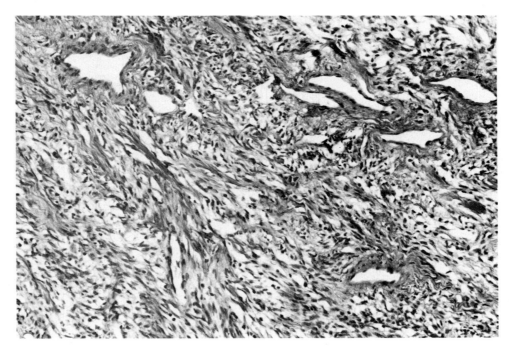

Fig. 7-16 Solitary fibrous tumor of nasopharynx. Appearance of this neoplasm is identical to that of so-called fibrous mesothelioma of pleura.

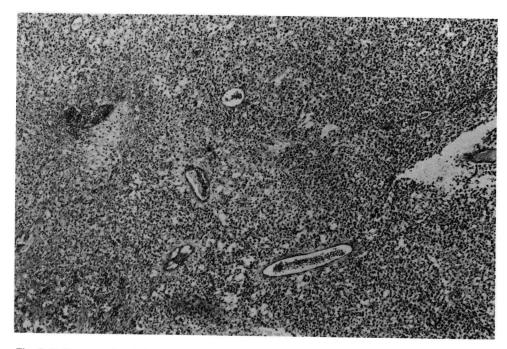

Fig. 7-17 Embryonal rhabdomyosarcoma of nasopharynx in child. This is small cell malignancy with areas of hypercellularity alternating with foci of edema and myxoid change.

giopericytoma and glomus tumor, perhaps closer to the latter. Recurrence is rare and metastases do not occur.

Other vascular tumors of the region include *hemangioma, lymphangioma, glomus tumor, Masson's hemangioma* (papillary endothelial neoplasia), *Kaposi's sarcoma,* and the exceptionally rare *angiosarcoma.*[180,184,193,201]

Solitary fibrous tumor of nasopharynx is a nasopharyngeal neoplasm morphologically analogous to solitary fibrous tumor of the pleura (so-called solitary fibrous mesothelioma), of which we have seen several examples[206] (Fig. 7-16).

Chordoma can present initially as an intranasal or nasopharyngeal mass.[179,203]

Embryonal rhabdomyosarcoma is one of the three most common types of nasopharyngeal malignancy in children, the other two being lymphoepithelioma and malignant lymphoma[183] (Fig. 7-17).

Teratoid carcinoma (teratocarcinosarcoma) is a unique sinonasal tract neoplasm that combines features of carcinosarcoma and teratoma. The patients are adults and the prognosis is poor, with 60% of the patients not surviving beyond 3 years.[195,204]

Soft tissue tumors of this region include, in addition to the entities already described, the following tumor types: osseous and fibro-osseous lesions,[185] cartilaginous tumors,[186,198] smooth muscle tumors,[187,196] skeletal muscle tumors,[188,192,197] fibrous tissue tumors,[189] myxomas,[190] adipose tissue tumors,[191] fibrous histiocytomas,[199,202] synovial sarcomas,[205] and extraskeletal Ewing's sarcomas.[200]

REFERENCES
INFLAMMATORY ("ALLERGIC") POLYP

1 Batsakis JG: The pathology of head and neck tumors. Nasal cavity and paranasal sinuses. Part 5. Head Neck Surg **2**:410-419, 1980.

2 Compagno J, Hyams VJ, Lepore ML: Nasal polyposis with stromal atypia. Review and follow-up study of 14 cases. Arch Pathol Lab Med **100**:224-226, 1976.

3 Kindblom L-G, Angervall L: Nasal polyps with atypical stroma cells. A pseudosarcomatous lesion. A light and electron-microscopic and immunohistochemical investigation with implications on the type and nature of the mesenchymal cells. Acta Pathol Microbiol Immunol Scand [A] **92**:65-72, 1984.

4 Oppenheimer EA, Rosenstein BJ: Differential pathology of nasal polyps in cystic fibrosis and atopy. Lab Invest **40**:445-449, 1979.

5 Schwachman H, Kulczycki LL, Mueller HL, Flake CG: Nasal polyposis in cystic fibrosis. Pediatrics **30**:389-401, 1962.

6 Smith CJ, Echevarria R, McLelland CA: Pseudosarcomatous changes in antrochoanal polyps. Arch Otolaryngol **99**:228-230, 1974.

OTHER NON-NEOPLASTIC LESIONS

7 Coup AJ, Hopper IP: Granulomatous lesions in nasal biopsies. Histopathology **4**:293-308, 1980.

8 Foucar E, Rosai J, Dorfman RF: Sinus histiocytosis with massive lymphadenopathy. Ear, nose and throat manifestations. Arch Otolaryngol **104**:687-693, 1978.

9 Gardner DG: Pseudocysts and retention cysts of the maxillary sinus. Oral Surg Oral Med Oral Pathol **58**:561-567, 1984.

10 Heffner DK: Problems in pediatric otorhinolaryngic pathology. I. Sinonasal and nasopharyngeal tumors and masses with myxoid features. Int J Pediatr Otorhinolaryngol **5**:77-91, 1983.

11 Katzenstein A-LA, Sale SR, Greenberger PA: Pathologic findings in allergic aspergillus sinusitis. A newly recognized form of sinusitis. Am J Surg Pathol **7**:439-443, 1983.

12 Kyriakos M: Myospherulosis of the paranasal sinuses, nose and middle ear. A possible iatrogenic disease. Am J Clin Pathol **67**:118-130, 1977.

13 Lehrer RI, Howard DH, Sypherd PS, Edwards JE, Segal GP, Winston DJ: Mucormycosis. Ann Intern Med **93**:93-108, 1980.

14 MacMillan RH III, Cooper PH, Body BA, Mills AS: Allergic fungal sinusitis due to *Curvularia lunata.* Hum Pathol **18**:960-964, 1987.

15 McClatchie S, Warambo MW, Bremner AD: Myospherulosis. A previously unreported disease? Am J Clin Pathol **51**:699-704, 1969.

16 McDonald TJ, DeRemee RA, Kern EB, Harrison EG Jr: Nasal manifestations of Wegener's granulomatosis. Layngoscope **84**:2101-2112, 1974.

17 Meyer PR, Shum TK, Becker TS, Taylor CR: Scleroma (rhinoscleroma). A histologic immunohistochemical study with bacteriologic correlates. Arch Pathol Lab Med **107**:377-383, 1983.

18 Roberts PF, McCann BG: Eosinophilic angiocentric fibrosis of the upper respiratory tract. A mucosal variant of granuloma faciale? A report of three cases. Histopathology **9**:1217-1225, 1985.

19 Rosai J: The nature of myospherulosis of the upper respiratory tract. Am J Clin Pathol **69**:475-481, 1978.

19a Travis WD, Li C-Y, Weiland LH: Immunostaining for hemoglobin in two cases of myospherulosis, Arch Pathol Lab Med **110**:763-765, 1986.

20 Wolff M: Granulomas in nasal mucoid membranes following local steroid injections. Am J Clin Pathol **62**:775-782, 1974.

TUMORS
Papilloma

21 Barnes L, Bedetti C: Oncocytic schneiderian papilloma. A reappraisal of cylindrical cell papilloma of the sinonasal tract. Hum Pathol **15**:344-351, 1984.

22 Christensen WN, Smith RRL: Schneiderian papillomas. A clinicopathologic study of 67 cases. Hum Pathol **17**:393-400, 1986.

23 Fechner RE, Alford DO: Inverted papilloma and squamous carcinoma. An unusual case. Arch Otolaryngol **88**:507-512, 1968.

24 Hyams VJ: Papillomas of the nasal cavity and paranasal sinuses. A clinicopathologic study of 315 cases. Ann Otol Rhinol Laryngol **80**:192-206, 1971.

25 Krisch I, Neuhold N, Krisch K: Demonstration of secretory component, IgA, and IgM by the peroxidase-antiperoxidase technique in inverted papillomas of the nasal cavities. Hum Pathol **15**:915-920, 1984.

26 Lasser A, Rothfeld RP, Shapiro RS: Epithelial papilloma and squamous cell carcinoma of the nasal cavity and paranasal sinuses. A clinicopathological study. Cancer **38**:2503-2510, 1976.

27 Luna M, Batsakis J, Weber R: In situ hybridization demonstrating human papilloma virus type 6/11 in schneiderian papillomas of the nasal cavity and paranasal sinuses (Abstract). Lab Invest **58**:58A, 1988.

28 Oberman HA: Papillomas of the nose and paranasal sinuses. Am J Clin Pathol **42**:245-258, 1964.

29 Ridolfi RL, Lieberman PH, Erlandson RA, Moore OS: Schneiderian papillomas. A clinicopathologic study of 30 cases. Am J Surg Pathol **1**:43-53, 1977.

30 Snyder RN, Perzin KH: Papillomatosis of nasal cavity and paranasal sinuses (inverted papilloma, squamous papilloma). A clinicopathologic study. Cancer **30**:668-690, 1972.

31 Vrabec DP: The inverted schneiderian papilloma. A clinical and pathological study. Laryngoscope **85**:186-220, 1975.

Sinonasal carcinoma

32 Acheson ED, Cowdall RH, Rang E: Adenocarcinoma of the nasal cavity and sinuses in England and Wales. Br J Industr Med **29**:21-30, 1972.

33 Ahmad K, Cordoba RB, Fayos JV: Squamous cell carcinoma of the maxillary sinus. Arch Otolaryngol **107**:48-51, 1981.

34 Barnes L: Intestinal-type adenocarcinoma of the nasal cavity and paranasal sinuses. Am J Surg Pathol **10**:192-202, 1986.

35 Barnes L, Johnson JT: Pathologic and clinical considerations in the evaluation of major head and neck specimens resected for cancer. Part 1. Pathol Annu **21**(Pt 1):173-250, 1986.

36 Batsakis JG, Mackay B, Ordoñez NG: Enteric-type adenocarcinoma of the nasal cavity. An electron microscopic and immunocytochemical study. Cancer **54**:855-860, 1984.

37 Batsakis JG, Rice DH, Solomon AR: The pathology of head and neck tumors. Squamous and mucous-gland carcinomas of the nasal cavity, paranasal sinuses, and larynx. Part 6. Head Neck Surg **2**:497-508, 1980.

38 Bush SE, Bagshaw MA: Carcinoma of the paranasal sinuses. Cancer **50**:154-158, 1982.

39 Cheng VST, Wang CC: Carcinomas of the paranasal sinuses. A study of sixty-six cases. Cancer **40**:3038-3041, 1977.

40 Frazell EL, Lewis JS: Cancer of the nasal cavity and accessory sinuses. Cancer **16**:1293-1301, 1963.

41 Frierson HF Jr, Mills SE, Fechner RE, Taxy JB, Levine PA: Sinonasal undifferentiated carcinoma. An aggressive neoplasm derived from schneiderian epithelium and distinct from olfactory neuroblastoma. Am J Surg Pathol **10**:771-779, 1986.

42 Heffner DK, Hyams VJ, Hauck KW, Lingeman C: Low-grade adenocarcinoma of the nasal cavity and paranasal sinuses. Cancer **50**:312-322, 1982.

43 Helliwell TR, Yeoh LH, Stell PM: Anaplastic carcinoma of the nose and paranasal sinuses. Light microscopy, immunohistochemistry and clinical correlation. Cancer **58**:2038-2045, 1986.

44 Ironside P, Matthews J: Adenocarcinoma of the nose and paranasal sinuses in woodworkers in the state of Victoria, Australia. Cancer **36**:1115-1121, 1975.

45 Klintenberg C, Olofsson J, Hellquist H, Sökjer H: Adenocarcinoma of the ethmoid sinuses. A review of 28 cases with special reference to wood dust exposure. Cancer **54**:482-488, 1984.

46 Kondo M, Inuyama Y, Ando Y, Tsutsui T, Yamashita S, Hashimoto T, Kunieda E, Uematsu M, Hashimoto S: Patterns of relapse of squamous cell carcinoma of the maxillary sinus. Cancer **53**:2206-2210, 1984.

47 Kondo M, Ogawa K, Inuyama Y, Yamashita S, Tominaga S, Shigematsu N, Nishiguchi I, Hashimoto S: Prognostic factors influencing relapse of squamous cell carcinoma of the maxillary sinus. Cancer **55**:190-196, 1985.

48 LeLiever WC, Bailey BJ, Griffiths C: Carcinoma of the nasal septum. Arch Otolaryngol **110**:748-751, 1984.

49 Manivel C, Wick MR, Dehner LP: Transitional (cylindric) cell carcinoma with endodermal sinus tumor-like features of the nasopharynx and paranasal sinuses. Clinicopathologic and immunohistochemical study of two cases. Arch Pathol Lab Med **110**:198-202, 1986.

50 Mills SE, Fechner RE, Cantrell RW: Aggressive sinonasal lesion resembling normal intestinal mucosa. Am J Surg Pathol **6**:803-809, 1982.

51 Osborn DA: Nature and behavior of transitional tumors in the upper respiratory tract. Cancer **25**:50-60, 1970.

52 Piscioli F, Aldovini D, Bondi A, Eusebi V: Squamous cell carcinoma with sarcoma-like stroma of the nose and paranasal sinuses. Report of two cases. Histopathology **8**:633-639, 1984.

53 Ringertz N: Pathology of malignant tumors arising in the nasal and paranasal cavities and maxilla. Acta Otolaryngol [Stockh] **27**(Suppl):1-405, 1938.

54 Robin PE, Shortridge RTJ: Lateralisation of tumours of the nasal cavity and paranasal sinuses and its relationship to aetiology. Lancet **1**:695-696, 1979.

55 Roush GC: Epidemiology of cancer of the nose and paranasal sinuses. Current concepts. Head Neck Surg **2**:3-11, 1979.

56 Sanchez-Casis G, Devine KD, Weiland LH: Nasal adenocarcinomas that closely simulate colonic carcinomas. Cancer **28**:714-720, 1971.

57 Schmid KO, Aubock L, Albegger K: Endocrine-amphicrine enteric carcinoma of the nasal mucosa. Virchows Arch [Pathol Anat] **383**:329-343, 1979.

58 St-Pierre S, Baker SR: Squamous cell carcinoma of the maxillary sinus. Analysis of 66 cases. Head Neck Surg **5**:508-513, 1983.

Nasopharyngeal carcinoma

59 Ablashi DV, Levine PH, Prasad U, Pearson GR: Fourth International Symposium on nasopharyngeal carcinoma. Application of field and laboratory studies to the control of NPC. Cancer Res **43**:2375-2378, 1983.

60 Baker SR, Wolfe RA: Prognostic factors of the nasopharyngeal malignancy. Cancer **49**:163-169, 1982.

61 Batsakis JG, Solomon AR, Rice DH: The pathology of head and neck tumors. Carcinoma of the nasopharynx. Part 11. Head Neck Surg **3**:511-524, 1981.

62 Bosq J, Gatter KC, Micheau C, Mason DY: Role of immunohistochemistry in diagnosis of nasopharyngeal tumours. J Clin Pathol **38**:845-848, 1985.

63 Carbone A, Micheau C: Pitfalls in microscopic diagnosis of undifferentiated carcinoma of nasopharyngeal type (lymphoepithelioma). Cancer **50**:1344-1351, 1982.

64 Chan SH, Day NE, Kunaratnam N, Chia KB, Simons MJ: HLA and nasopharyngeal carcinoma in Chinese. A further study. Int J Cancer **32**:171-176, 1983.

65 Dethe G, Ito Y (eds): Nasopharyngeal carcinoma. Etiology and control. (International Symposium on Nasopharyngeal Carcinoma. Etiology and control, Kyoto, Japan, April 4-6, 1977.) International Agency for Research on Cancer, Lyon, IARC Scientific Publications No. 20, 1978.

66 Easton JM, Levine PH, Hyams VJ: Nasopharyngeal carcinoma in the United States. A pathologic study of 177 U.S. and 30 foreign cases. Arch Otolaryngol **106**:88-91, 1980.

67 Editorial: Some progress with nasopharyngeal carcinoma. Lancet **1**:959-960, 1979.

68 Giffler RF, Gillespie JJ, Ayala AG, Newland JR: Lymphoepithelioma in cervical lymph nodes of children and young adults. Am J Surg Pathol **1**:293-302, 1977.

69 Gusterson BA, Mitchell DP, Warburton MJ, Carter RL: Epithelial markers in the diagnosis of nasopharyngeal carcinoma. An immunocytochemical study. J Clin Pathol **36**:628-631, 1983.

70 Heffner DK: Problems in pediatric otorhinolaryngic pathology. IV. Epithelial

and lymphoid tumors of the sinonasal tract and nasopharynx. Int J Pediatr Otorhinolaryngol **6**:219-237, 1983.

71 Henle G, Henle W: Epstein-Barr virus–specific IgA serum antibodies as an outstanding feature of nasopharyngeal carcinoma. Int J Cancer **17**:1-7, 1976.

72 Hsu H-C, Chen C-L, Hsu M-M, Lynn T-C, Tu S-M, Huang S-C: Pathology of nasopharyngeal carcinoma. Proposal of a new histologic classification correlated with prognosis. Cancer **59**:945-951, 1987.

73 Jenkin RDT, Anderson JR, Jereb B, Thompson JC, Pyesmany A, Wara WM, Hammond D: Nasopharyngeal carcinoma. A retrospective review of patients less than thirty years of age. A report from Children's Cancer Study Group. Cancer **47**:360-366, 1981.

74 Lauriola L, Michetti F, Sentinelli S, Cocchia D: Detection of S-100 labelled cells in nasopharyngeal carcinoma. J Clin Pathol **37**:1235-1238, 1984.

75 Lin H-S, Lin C-S, Yeh S, Tu S-M: Fine structure of nasopharyngeal carcinoma with special reference to the anaplastic type. Cancer **23**:390-405, 1969.

76 Madri JA, Barwick KW: An immunohistochemical study of nasopharyngeal neoplasms using keratin antibodies. Epithelial versus nonepithelial neoplasms. Am J Surg Pathol **6**:143-149, 1982.

77 Micheau C: What's new in histological classification and recognition of nasopharyngeal carcinoma (NPC). Pathol Res Pract **181**:249-253, 1986.

78 Miettinen M, Lehto V-P, Virtanen I: Nasopharyngeal lymphoepithelioma. Histological diagnosis as aided by immunohistochemical demonstration of keratin. Virchows Arch [Cell Pathol] **40**:163-169, 1982.

79 Naegele RF, Champion J, Murphy S, Henle G, Henle W: Nasopharyngeal carcinoma in American children. Epstein-Barr virus–specific antibody titers and prognosis. Int J Cancer **29**:209-212, 1982.

80 Nomori H, Watanabe S, Nakajima T, Shimosato Y, Kameya T: Histiocytes in nasopharyngeal carcinoma in relation to prognosis. Cancer **57**:100-105, 1986.

81 Oppedal BR, Bohler PJ, Marton PF, Brandtzaeg P: Carcinoma of the nasopharynx. Histopathological examination with supplementary immunohistochemistry. Histopathology **11**:1161-1169, 1987.

82 Pearson GR, Weiland LH, Neal HB III, Taylor W, Earle J, Mulroney SE, Goepfert H, Lanier A, Talvot ML, Pilch B, Goodman M, Huang A, Levine PH, Hyams V, Moran E, Henle G, Henle W: Application of Epstein-Barr virus (EBV) serology to the diagnosis of North American nasopharyngeal carcinoma. Cancer **51**:260-268, 1983.

83 Perez CA, Ackerman LV, Mill WB, Ogura JH, Powers WE: Cancer of the nasopharynx. Factors influencing prognosis. Cancer **24**:1-17, 1969.

84 Prathap K, Looi LM, Prasad U: Localized amyloidosis in nasopharyngeal carcinoma. Histopathology **8**:27-34, 1984.

85 Rahima M, Rakowsky E, Barzilay J, Sidi J: Carcinoma of the nasopharynx. An analysis of 91 cases and a comparison of differing treatment approaches. Cancer **58**:843-849, 1986.

86 Rennke H, Lennert K: Käsig-tuberkuloide Reaktion bei Lymphknoten-metastasen lymphoepithelialer Carcinome (Schmincke-Tumoren). Virchows Arch [Pathol Anat] **358**:241-247, 1973.

87 Shanmugaratnam K, Chan SH de-The G, Goh JEH, Khor TH, Simons MJ, Tye CY: Histopathology of nasopharyngeal carcinoma. Correlations with epidemiology, survival rates, and other biological characteristics. Cancer **44**:1029-1044, 1979.

88 Tamada A, Makimoto K, Yamabe H, Imai J, Hinuma Y, Oyagi A, Araki T: Titers of Epstein-Barr virus–related antibodies in nasopharyngeal carcinoma in Japan. Cancer **53**:430-440, 1984.

89 Taxy JB, Hidvegi DF, Battifora H: Nasopharyngeal carcinoma. Antikeratin immunohistochemistry and electron microscopy. Am J Clin Pathol **83**:320-325, 1985.

90 Tesh NB: Epidermoid carcinoma of the nasopharynx among Chinese. A study of 31 necropsies. J Pathol Bacteriol **73**:451-465, 1957.

91 Wenig B, Hyams V, Heffner D: Primary nasopharyngeal papillary adenocarcinoma (PNPA) (abstract). Lab Invest **58**:20A, 1988.

92 Yu MC, Ho JHC, Lai S-H, Henderson BE: Cantonese-style salted fish as a cause of nasopharyngeal carcinoma. Report of a case-control study in Hong Kong. Cancer Res **46**:956-961, 1986.

93 Zaatari GS, Santoianni RA: Adenoid squamous cell carcinoma of the nasopharynx and neck region. Arch Pathol Lab Med **110**:542-546, 1986.

94 Ziegels-Weissman J, Nadji M, Penneys NS, Morales AR: Prekeratin immunohistochemistry in the diagnosis of undifferentiated carcinoma of the nasopharyngeal type. Arch Pathol Lab Med **108**:588-589, 1984.

Salivary gland tumors

95 Compagno J, Wong RT: Intranasal mixed tumors (pleomorphic adenomas). A clinicopathologic study of 40 cases. Am J Clin Pathol **68**:213-218, 1977.

96 Goepfert H, Luna MA, Lindberg RD, White AK: Malignant salivary gland tumors of the paranasal sinuses and nasal cavity. Arch Otolaryngol **109**:662-668, 1983.

97 Perzin KH, Cantor JO, Johannessen JV: Acinic cell carcinoma arising in nasal cavity. Report of a case with ultrastructural observations. Cancer **47**:1818-1822, 1981.

98 Rafla S: Mucous gland tumors of paranasal sinuses. Cancer **24**:683-691, 1969.

Neurogenous and related tumors

99 Appelblatt NH, McClatchey KD: Olfactory neuroblastoma. A retrospective clinicopathologic study. Head Neck Surg **5**:108-113, 1982.

100 Axe S, Kuhajda FP: Esthesioneuroblastoma. Intermediate filaments, neuroendocrine, and tissue-specific antigens. Am J Clin Pathol **88**:139-145, 1987.

101 Bailey BJ, Barton S: Olfactory neuroblastoma. Management and prognosis. Arch Otolaryngol **101**:1-5, 1975.

101a Choi H-SH, Anderson PJ: Immunohistochemical diagnosis of olfactory neuroblastoma. J Neuropathol Exp Neurol **44**:18-31, 1985.

102 Curtis JL, Rubinstein LJ: Pigmented olfactory neuroblastoma. A new example of melanotic neuroepithelial neoplasm. Cancer **49**:2136-2143, 1982.

103 Fletcher CDM, Carpenter G, McKee PH: Nasal glioma. A rarity. Am J Dermatopathol **8**:341-346, 1986.

104 Gerard-Marchant R, Micheau C: Microscopical diagnosis of olfactory esthesioneuromas. General review and report of five cases. J Natl Cancer Inst **35**:75-82, 1965.

105 Harrison D: Surgical pathology of olfactory neuroblastoma. Head Neck Surg **7**:60-64, 1984.

106 Hirano T, Aida T, Moriyama M, Asano G, Suzuki I, Yuge K: Primary neuroblastoma of the nasal cavity and review of literature. Acta Pathol Jpn **35**:183-191, 1985.

107 Ho KL: Primary meningioma of the nasal cavity and paranasal sinuses. Cancer **46**:1442-1447, 1980.

108 Hutter RVP, Lewis JS, Foote FW Jr, Tollefsen HR: Esthesioneuroblastoma. Am J Surg **106**:748-753, 1963.

109 Kadish S, Goodman M, Wang CC: Olfactory neuroblastoma. A clinical analysis of 17 cases. Cancer **37**:1571-1576, 1976.

110 Kahn LB: Esthesioneuroblastoma. A light and electron microscopic study. Hum Pathol **5**:364-371, 1974.

111 Kay S, Lees JK, Stout AP: Pituitary chromophobe tumors of the nasal cavity. Cancer **3**:695-704, 1950.

111a Kindblom LG, Angervall L, Haglid K: An immunohistochemical analysis of S-100 protein and glial fibrillary acidic protein in nasal glioma. Acta Pathol Microbiol Immunol Scand [A] **92**:387-389, 1984.

112 Mackay B, Luna MA, Butler JJ: Adult neuroblastoma. Electron microscopic observations in nine cases. Cancer **37**:1334-1351, 1976.

113 Mashberg A, Thoma KH, Wasilewski EJ: Olfactory neuroblastoma (esthesioneuroepithelioma) of the maxillary sinus. Oral Surg Oral Med Oral Pathol **13**:908-912, 1960.

114 McGavran MH, Biller H, Ogura JH: Primary intranasal meningioma. Arch Otolaryngol **93**:95-97, 1971.

115 Mendeloff J: The olfactory neuroepithelial tumors. Cancer **10**:944-956, 1957.

116 Micheau C: A new histochemical and biochemical approach to olfactory esthesioneuroma. A nasal tumor of neural crest origin. Cancer **40**:314-318, 1977.

117 Miller DC, Goodman ML, Pilch BZ, Shi SR, Dickersin GR, Halpern H, Norris CM Jr: Mixed olfactory neuroblastoma and carcinoma. A report of two cases. Cancer **54**:2019-2028, 1984.

118 Mills SE, Frierson HF Jr: Olfactory neuroblastoma. A clinicopathologic study of 21 cases. Am J Surg Pathol **9**:317-327, 1985.

119 Mirra SS, Pearl SS, Hoffman JC, Campbell WG Jr: Nasal "glioma" with prominent neuronal component. Report of a case. Arch Pathol Lab Med **105**:540-541, 1981.

120 Nakashima T, Kimmelman CP, Snow JB Jr: Structure of human fetal and adult olfactory neuroepithelium. Arch Otolaryngol **110**:641-646, 1984.

121 Olsen KD, DeSanto LW: Olfactory neuroblastoma. Biologic and clinical behavior. Arch Otolaryngol **109**:797-802, 1983.

122 Oberman HA, Rice DH: Olfactory neuroblastomas. A clinicopathologic study. Cancer **38**:2494-2502, 1976.

123 Obert DJ, Devine KD, McDonald JR: Olfactory neuroblastomas. Cancer **13**:205-215, 1960.

124 Parisier SC, Sinclair GM: Glomus tumor of the nasal cavity. Laryngoscope **78**:2013-2024, 1968.

125 Perzin KH, Panyu H, Wechter S: Nonepithelial tumors of the nasal cavity, paranasal sinuses, and nasopharynx. A clinicopathologic study. XII. Schwann

cell tumors (neurilemoma, neurofibroma, malignant schwannoma). Cancer **50:**2193-2202, 1982.

126 Perzin KH, Pushparaj N: Nonepithelial tumors of the nasal cavity, paranasal sinuses, and nasopharynx. A clinicopathologic study. XIII. Meningiomas. Cancer **54:**1860-1869, 1984.

127 Robitaille Y, Seemayer TA, Deiry AE: Peripheral nerve tumors involving paranasal sinuses. A case report and review of the literature. Cancer **35:**1254-1258, 1975.

128 Schuller DE, Lucas JG: Nasopharyngeal paraganglioma. Report of a case and review of literature. Arch Otolaryngol **108:**667-670, 1982.

129 Shugar JMA, Som PM, Biller HF, Som ML, Krespi YP: Peripheral nerve sheath tumors of the paranasal sinuses. Head Neck Surg **4:**72-76, 1981.

130 Silva EG, Butler JJ, Mackay B, Goepfert H: Neuroblastomas and neuroendocrine carcinomas of the nasal cavity. A proposed new classification. Cancer **50:**2388-2405, 1982.

131 Siwersson U, Kindblom L-G: Oncocytic carcinoid of the nasal cavity and carcinoid of the lung in a child. Pathol Res Pract **178:**562-569, 1984.

132 Taxy JB, Bharani NK, Mills SE, Frierson HF Jr, Gould VE: The spectrum of olfactory neural tumors. A light-microscopic immunohistochemical and ultrastructural analysis. Am J Surg Pathol **10:**687-695, 1986.

133 Taxy JB, Hidvegi DF: Olfactory neuroblastoma. An ultrastructural study. Cancer **39:**131-138, 1977.

134 Trojanowski JQ, Lee V, Pillsbury N, Lee S: Neuronal origin of human esthesioneuroblastoma demonstrated with anti-neurofilament monoclonal antibodies. N Engl J Med **307:**159-161, 1982.

Malignant melanoma

135 Berthelsen A, Andersen AP, Jensen S, Hansen HS: Melanomas of the mucosa in the oral cavity and the upper respiratory passages. Cancer **54:**907-912, 1984.

136 Chaudhry AP, Hampel A, Gorlin RJ: Primary malignant melanoma of the oral cavity. Cancer **11:**923-928, 1958.

137 Holdcraft J, Gallagher JC: Malignant melanomas of the nasal and paranasal sinus mucosa. Ann Otol Rhinol Laryngol **78:**5-20, 1969.

138 Hormia M, Vuori EJ: Mucosal melanomas of the head and neck. J Laryngol **831:**349-359, 1969.

139 Uehara T, Matsubara O, Kasuga T: Melanocytes in the nasal cavity and paranasal sinus. Incidence and distribution in Japan. Acta Pathol Jpn **37:**1105-1114, 1987.

Lymphoid tumors and tumorlike conditions

140 Aozasa K: Biopsy findings in malignant histiocytosis presenting as lethal midline granuloma. J Clin Pathol **35:**599-605, 1982.

141 Batsakis JG, Luna MA: Midfacial necrotizing lesions, Semin Diagn Pathol **4:**90-116, 1987.

142 Birt BD: Reticulum cell sarcoma of the nose and paranasal sinuses. J Laryngol Otol **84:**615-630, 1970.

143 Chan JKC, Ng CS, Lau WH, Lo STH: Most nasal/nasopharyngeal lymphomas are peripheral T-cell neoplasms. Am J Surg Pathol **11:**418-429, 1987.

144 Costa J, Delacretaz F: The midline granuloma syndrome. Pathol Annu **21** (Pt 1):159-171, 1986.

145 Crissman JD, Weiss MA, Gluckman J: Midline granuloma syndrome. A clinicopathologic study of 13 patients. Am J Surg Pathol **6:**335-346, 1982.

146 DeRemee RA, Weiland LH, McDonald TJ: Polymorphic reticulosis, lymphomatoid granulomatosis. Two diseases or one? Mayo Clin Proc **53:**634-640, 1978.

147 Eichel BS, Harrison EG Jr, Devine KD, Brown HA: Primary lymphoma of the nose including relationship to lethal midline granuloma. Am J Surg **112:**597-605, 1966.

148 Ewing MR, Foote FW Jr: Plasma-cell tumors of the mouth and upper air passages. Cancer **5:**499-513, 1952.

149 Fechner RE, Lamppin DW: Midline malignant reticulosis. A clinicopathologic entity. Arch Otolaryngol **95:**467-476, 1972.

150 Frierson HF Jr, Mills SE, Innes DJ Jr: Non-Hodgkin's lymphomas of the sinonasal region. Histologic subtypes and their clinicopathologic features. Am J Clin Pathol **81:**721-727, 1984.

151 Fu Y-S, Perzin KH: Nonepithelial tumors of the nasal cavity, paranasal sinuses and nasopharynx. A clinicopathologic study. IX. Plasmacytomas. Cancer **42:**2399-2406, 1978.

152 Fu Y-S, Perzin KH: Nonepithelial tumors of the nasal cavity, paranasal sinuses and nasopharynx. A clinicopathologic study. X. Malignant lymphomas. Cancer **43:**611-621, 1979.

153 Ishii Y, Yamanaka N, Ogawa K, Yoshida Y, Takami T, Matsuura A, Isago H, Kataura A, Kikuchi K: Nasal T-cell lymphoma as a type of so-called "lethal midline granuloma." Cancer **50:**2336-2344, 1982.

154 Kapadia SB, Desai U, Cheng VS: Extramedullary plasmacytoma of the head and neck. A clinicopathologic study of 20 cases. Medicine (Baltimore) **61:**317-328, 1982.

155 Kassel SH, Echevarria RA, Guzzo FP: Midline malignant reticulosis (so-called lethal midline granuloma). Cancer **23:**920-935, 1969.

156 Kluin PM, Slootweg PJ, Schuurman HJ, Go DMDS, Rademakers LHPM, Van der Putte SCJ, Van Unnik JAM: Primary B-cell malignant lymphoma of the maxilla with a sarcomatous pattern and multilobated nuclei. Cancer **54:**1598-1605, 1984.

157 Kotner LM, Wang CC: Plasmacytoma of the upper air and food passages. Cancer **30:**414-418, 1972.

158 Lippman SM, Grogan TM, Spier CM, Kopmann CF Jr, Gall EP, Shimm DS, Durie BGM: Lethal midline granuloma with a novel T-cell phenotype as found in peripheral T-cell lymphoma. Cancer **59:**936-939, 1987.

159 Michaels L, Gregory MM: Pathology of "non-healing (midline) granuloma." J Clin Pathol **30:**317-327, 1977.

160 Nelson JF, Finkelstein MW, Acevedo A, Gonzales GM: Midline "nonhealing" granuloma. Oral Surg Oral Med Oral Pathol **58:**554-560, 1984.

161 Ng C-S, Chan JKC, Cheng PNM, Szeto S-C: Nasal T-cell lymphoma associated with hemophagocytic syndrome. Cancer **58:**67-71, 1986.

162 Rimarenko S, Schwartz IS: Polypoid nasal pseudolymphoma. Am J Clin Pathol **83:**507-509, 1985.

163 Robbins KT, Fuller LM, Vlasak M, Osborne B, Jing BS, Velasquez WS, Sullivan JA: Primary lymphomas of the nasal cavity and paranasal sinuses. Cancer **56:**814-819, 1985.

164 Tsokos M, Fauci AS, Costa J: Idiopathic midline destructive disease (IMDD). A subgroup of patients with the "mid-line granuloma" syndrome. Am J Clin Pathol **77:**162-168, 1982.

165 Webb HE, Harrison EG, Masson JK, ReMine WH: Solitary extramedullary myeloma (plasmacytoma) of the upper part of the respiratory tract and oropharynx. Cancer **15:**1142-1155, 1962.

166 Wilder WH, Harner SG, Banks PM: Lymphoma of the nose and paranasal sinuses. Arch Otolaryngol **109:**310-312, 1983.

Nasopharyngeal angiofibroma

167 Chen KTK, Bauer FW: Sarcomatous transformation of nasopharyngeal angiofibroma. Cancer **49:**369-371, 1982.

168 Cummings BJ: Relative risk factors in the treatment of juvenile nasopharyngeal angiofibroma. Head Neck Surg **3:**21-26, 1980.

169 Goepfert H, Cangir A, Lee Y-Y: Chemotherapy for aggressive juvenile nasopharyngeal angiofibroma. Arch Otolaryngol **111:**285-289, 1985.

170 Harma RA: Nasopharyngeal angiofibroma. Acta Otolaryngol [Stockh] **146** (Suppl):1-74, 1958.

171 Hicks JL, Nelson JF: Juvenile nasopharyngeal angiofibroma. Oral Surg Oral Med Oral Pathol **35:**807-817, 1973.

172 Lee DA, Rao BR, Meyer JS, Prioleau PG, Bauer WC: Hormonal receptor determination in juvenile nasopharyngeal angiofibromas. Cancer **46:**547-551, 1980.

173 McGavran MH, Sessions DG, Dorfman RD, Davis DO, Ogura JH: Nasopharyngeal angiofibroma. Arch Otolaryngol **90:**94-104, 1969.

174 Neel HB III, Whicker JH, Devine KD, Weiland LH: Juvenile angiofibroma. Review of 120 cases. Am J Surg **126:**547-556, 1973.

175 Spagnolo DV, Papadimitriou JM, Archer M: Postirradiation malignant fibrous histiocytoma arising in juvenile nasopharyngeal angiofibroma and producing alpha-1-antitrypsin. Histopathology **8:**339-352, 1984.

176 Sternberg SS: Pathology of juvenile nasopharyngeal angiofibroma. A lesion of adolescent males. Cancer **7:**15-28, 1954.

177 Topilko A, Zakrzewski A, Pichard E, Viron A: Ultrastructural cytochemistry of intranuclear dense granules in nasopharyngeal angiofibroma. Ultrastruct Pathol **6:**221-228, 1984.

178 Waldman SR, Levine HL, Astor F, Wood BG, Weinstein M, Tucker HM: Surgical experience with nasopharyngeal angiofibroma. Arch Otolaryngol **107:**677-682, 1981.

Other tumors and tumorlike conditions

179 Batsakis JG, Solomon AR, Rice DH: The pathology of head and neck tumors. Neoplasms of cartilage, bone, and the notochord. Part 7. Head Neck Surg **3:**43-57, 1980.

180 Beneck D, Abati AD, Greco MA: Lymphangioma presenting as a nasal polyp in an infant. Arch Pathol Lab Med **109:**773-775, 1985.

181 Boies LR Jr, Harris D: Nasopharyngeal dermoid of the newborn. Laryngoscope **75:**763-767, 1965.

182 Compagno J, Hyams VJ: Hemangiopericytoma-like intranasal tumors. A clinicopathologic study of 23 cases. Am J Clin Pathol **66:**672-683, 1976.

183 Deutsch M, Mercado R Jr, Parsons JA: Cancer of the nasopharynx in children. Cancer **41:**1128-1133, 1978.

183a Eichhorn JH, Bhan AK, Dickersin GR, Pilch BZ, Goodman ML: Intranasal hemangiopericytoma. An ultrastructural, immunocytologic study (abstract). Lab Invest **58:**26A, 1988.

184 Fu Y-S, Perzin KH: Nonepithelial tumors of the nasal cavity, paranasal sinuses and nasopharynx. A clinicopathologic study. I. General features and vascular tumors. Cancer **33:**1275-1288, 1974.

185 Fu Y-S, Perzin KH: Nonepithelial tumors of the nasal cavity, paranasal sinuses and nasopharynx. A clinicopathologic study. II. Osseous and fibro-osseous lesions, including osteoma, fibrous dysplasia, ossifying fibroma, osteoblastoma, giant cell tumor, and osteosarcoma. Cancer **33:**1289-1305, 1974.

186 Fu Y-S, Perzin KH: Nonepithelial tumors of the nasal cavity, paranasal sinuses and nasopharynx. A clinicopathologic study. III. Cartilaginous tumors (chondroma, chondrosarcoma). Cancer **34:**453-463, 1974.

187 Fu Y-S, Perzin KH: Nonepithelial tumors of the nasal cavity, paranasal sinuses and nasopharynx. A clinicopathologic study. IV. Smooth muscle tumors (leiomyoma, leiomyosarcoma). Cancer **35:**1300-1308, 1975.

188 Fu Y-S, Perzin KH: Nonepithelial tumors of the nasal cavity, paranasal sinuses and nasopharynx. A clinicopathologic study. V. Skeletal muscle tumors (rhabdomyoma and rhabdomyosarcoma). Cancer **37:**364-376, 1976.

189 Fu Y-S, Perzin KH: Nonepithelial tumors of the nasal cavity, paranasal sinuses and nasopharynx. A clinicopathologic study. VI. Fibrous tissue tumors (fibroma, fibromatosis, fibrosarcoma). Cancer **37:**2912-2928, 1976.

190 Fu Y-S, Perzin KH: Nonepithelial tumors of the nasal cavity, paranasal sinuses and nasopharynx. A clinicopathologic study. VII. Myxomas. Cancer **39:**195-203, 1977.

191 Fu Y-S, Perzin KH: Nonepithelial tumors of the nasal cavity, paranasal sinuses and nasopharynx. A clinicopathologic study. VIII. Adipose tissue tumors (lipoma and liposarcoma). Cancer **40:**1314-1317, 1977.

192 Gale N, Rott T, Kambič: Nasopharyngeal rhabdomyoma. Report of case (light and electron microscopic studies) and review of the literature. Pathol Res Pract **178:**454-460, 1984.

193 Heffner DK: Problems in pediatric otorhinolaryngic pathology. II. Vascular tumors and lesions of the sinonasal tract and nasopharynx. Int J Pediatr Otorhinolaryngol **5:**125-138, 1983.

194 Heffner DK: Problems in pediatric otorhinolaryngic pathology. III. Teratoid and neural tumors of the nose, sinonasal tract, and nasopharynx. Int J Pediatr Otorhinolaryngol **6:**1-21, 1983.

195 Heffner DK, Hyams VJ: Teratocarcinosarcoma (malignant teratoma?) of the nasal cavity and paranasal sinuses. A clinicopathologic study of 20 cases. Cancer **53:**2140-2154, 1984.

196 Kawabe Y, Kondo T, Hosoda S: Two cases of leiomyosarcoma of the maxillary sinuses. Arch Otolaryngol **90:**492-495, 1969.

197 Manon JK, Soule EH: Embryonal rhabdomyosarcoma of the head and neck. Report on eighty-eight cases. Am J Surg **110:**585-591, 1965.

198 McCoy JM, McConnel FMS: Chondrosarcoma of the nasal septum. Arch Otolaryngol **107:**125-127, 1981.

199 Perzin KH, Fu Y-S: Non-epithelial tumors of the nasal cavity, paranasal sinuses and nasopharynx. A clinicopathologic study. XI. Fibrous histiocytomas. Cancer **45:**2616-2626, 1980.

200 Pontius KI, Sebek BA: Extraskeletal Ewing's sarcoma arising in the nasal fossa. Light- and electron-microscopic observations. Am J Clin Pathol **75:**410-415, 1981.

201 Potter AJ Jr, Khatib G, Peppard SB: Intranasal glomus tumor. Arch Otolaryngol **110:**755-756, 1984.

202 Rice DH, Batsakis JG, Headington JT, Boles R: Fibrous histiocytomas of the nose and paranasal sinuses. Arch Otolaryngol **100:**398-401, 1974.

203 Richter HJ, Batsakis JG, Boles R: Chordomas. Nasopharyngeal presentation and atypical long survival. Ann Otol Rhinol Laryngol **84:**327-332, 1975.

204 Shanmugaratnam K, Kunaratnam N, Chia KB, Chiang GSC, Finniah R: Teratoid carcinosarcoma of the paranasal sinuses. Pathology **15:**413-419, 1983.

205 Shmookler BM, Enzinger FM, Brannon RB: Orofacial synovial sarcoma. Cancer **50:**269-276, 1982.

206 Witkin GB, Rosai J: Solitary fibrous tumor of nasopharynx. The upper respiratory tract counterpart of so-called solitary fibrous mesothelioma. (In preparation.)

Larynx and trachea

Larynx
CYSTS AND LARYNGOCELE

The two most common types of *cysts* of the larynx have been divided by DeSanto et al.[1] according to their mechanism of formation into *saccular* (24%) and *ductal* (75%). The former arise from cystic distention of the laryngeal saccule. They are large and deep and are often found inside the ventricle. Saccular cysts differ from laryngoceles only in that they contain mucus, whereas the latter contain air. Ductal cysts, which are the result of dilatation of mucous glands, are small and superficial and are usually located in the true cord or epiglottis. Both types can be lined by either squamous or respiratory epithelium or a combination of both.

A third type of laryngeal cyst, which perhaps represents a subtype of the ductal cyst, is referred to as *oncocytic cyst* because of the fact that it is lined partially or completely by oncocytes.[5] Papillary infoldings are usually present, but the condition is regarded as a metaplastic and hyperplastic change rather than a true neoplasia.[2] In rare cases, the entire larynx is involved in a diffuse fashion by this process.[6] Oncocytic cysts have a tendency to recur.[2]

A fourth type of laryngeal cyst has been described as *tonsillar cyst*.[4] It has squamous-lined crypt-like structures and abundant follicular lymphoid tissue in the wall.

The term *laryngocele* refers to an air-containing saccular dilatation of the appendix of the laryngeal ventricle, communicating with the lumen of the ventricle by a narrow stalk.[3] The internal variety presents with hoarseness, dyspnea, or reflex cough, whereas the external type appears as a soft mass in the lateral aspect of the neck. Combined forms occur.

INFLAMMATION

Chronic *nonspecific laryngitis* can be the result of infection, overuse of the voice, exposure to chemical or physical agents, or irritation by tobacco and alcohol. Microscopically, a lymphocytic infiltrate is seen beneath the mucosa with an inconstant admixture of plasma cells and histiocytes accompanied by some hyperplasia of the overlying epithelium.

Acute epiglottitis (acute supraglottitis) is a relatively rare but potentially lethal disease, because of respiratory tract obstruction caused by massive edema.[11] It is usually a disease of children but also occurs in adults.[15] As a matter of fact, it has been suggested that George Washington died of it.[18] It is a bacterial infection, and *Haemophilus influenzae* type B is the most common organism involved. Grossly, the epiglottis appears red and edematous; microscopically, there is an intense acute inflammatory infiltrate associated with edema that extends to the adjacent soft tissues.

Tuberculosis of the larynx begins with edema of the posterior interarytenoid space, from which it spreads to epiglottis, aryepiglottic fold, and vocal cords.[7] It can simulate carcinoma on laryngoscopic examination.[20] Roentgenographic examination of the chest often shows active advanced tuberculosis although not as frequently as in the past.[16] Laryngeal biopsy shows typical granulomas, with or without caseation necrosis. Demonstration of acid-fast bacilli is necessary to document the diagnosis.

Histoplasmosis and *blastomycosis* are the two most common types of mycotic laryngitis in this country. In histoplasmosis, the early lesions are frequently located in the vocal cords and epiglottis[10] (Fig. 7-18). A granulomatous lesion involving *only* the anterior portions of the larynx (especially the epiglottis) or having associated oral lesions is more likely to be histoplasmosis than tuberculosis. *Aspergillus* may also involve the larynx and induce pseudoepitheliomatous changes in the overlying epithelium.[17]

Crohn's disease can be accompanied by ulcerative and granulomatous lesions in the larynx, particularly the epiglottis.[9,13]

Laryngeal *granulomas* due to endotracheal trauma caused by intubation can occur bilaterally on the vocal process of the arytenoid cartilage and be mistaken for a neoplasm.[8] Injection of *Teflon* into paralyzed vocal cords, used as a means of augmentation in cases of recurrent nerve paralysis, may lead to the formation of an exuberant *foreign body granuloma*. A case of laryngeal *malakoplakia* has been described.[14] *Radiation therapy* may result in granulation tissue-type reactions with bizarre mesenchymal cells that can simulate malignancy.[19] *Arthritis* of the cricoarytenoid joint is commonly associated with generalized arthritis of a rheumatoid nature.[12]

LARYNGEAL NODULE

Laryngeal nodules represent a peculiar non-inflammatory reaction to injury causing hoarseness and appear in people who misuse their voices. They occur chiefly on the anterior

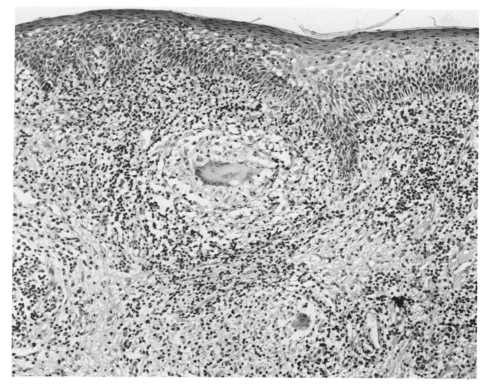

Fig. 7-18 Histoplasmosis of larynx. Well-developed granulomas are present in the stroma.

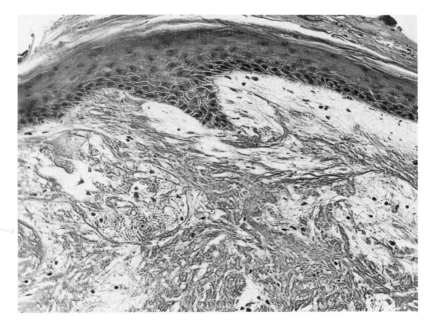

Fig. 7-19 Laryngeal nodule. Note amorphous eosinophilic material beneath intact epithelium.

third of the vocal cords and have been variously called singers' nodules, amyloid tumors, polyps, and varices.

Microscopically, these nodules have varying patterns, depending on their stage of evolution.[21] In the early stages, they show edema and proliferation of young fibroblasts. Later, dilated blood vessels and hyalinization of the stroma appear. Cases with a prominent vascular component are frequently mistaken for hemangioma. The hyaline stage is the one previously designated "amyloid tumor" (Fig. 7-19). This is a misnomer, because the material is hyalinized collagen rather than amyloid.

A lesion sometimes erroneously equated with laryngeal nodule but actually having a different presentation, histology, and behavior is known to otorhinolaryngologists as *posterior commissure ulcer* or contact (granulomatous) ulcer. As the first name implies, the lesion is almost always found at the level of the posterior commissure, in the area of the vocal process of the arytenoid cartilage, at a site where the amount of subepithelial stroma is scantier. Microscopically, it has the appearance of exuberant granulation tissue; it is often confused with a pyogenic granuloma but lacks the characteristic lobular pattern of the latter.[22] It stubbornly recurs following local excision, but eventually it subsides. Conservative management is to be recommended.

OTHER NON-NEOPLASTIC LESIONS

Amyloidosis may involve the tracheobronchial tree as a localized phenomenon.[23,24]

Eosinophilic angiocentric fibrosis is a term recently proposed for a peculiar inflammatory lesion of the upper respiratory tract thought to represent a mucosal variant of granuloma faciale; one of the reported cases involved the subglottis.[25] The differential diagnosis includes Wegener's granulomatosis and specific infections.

TUMORS AND TUMORLIKE CONDITIONS
Papillomatosis

Juvenile laryngeal papillomas present in children or adolescents with multiple papillary tumors on the true cords, from which they may spread to the false cords, epiglottis, and subglottic area, and, in rare cases, even to the trachea and bronchi.[31] When extensive, papillomatosis may cause extreme respiratory difficulty and even death (Fig. 7-20).

The viral etiology of juvenile laryngeal papillomatosis has been proved by ultrastructural examination,[30] by immunohistochemical demonstration of human papillomavirus antigens,[27] and by DNA hybridization techniques.[38] Viral DNA has also been found in uninvolved sites in patients with active disease and also in patients in remission.[38] The types of HPV that have been specifically associated with laryngeal papillomas are HPV-11 and HPV-6.[26]

The microscopic appearance is that of a papillary or acanthotic growth of well-differentiated squamous cells with an orderly maturation pattern[32] (Fig. 7-21). Mitotic activity is common, and some degree of koilocytosis and nuclear atypia are the rule.[33] When the process involves the respiratory mucosa, the maturation pattern, which is constant in the squamous epithelium, is not so apparent (Fig. 7-22). This may lead to an overdiagnosis of carcinoma in situ.

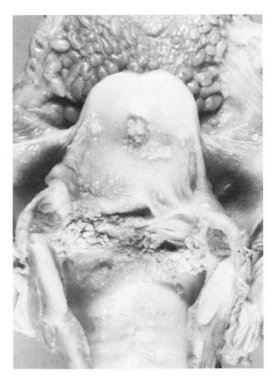

Fig. 7-20 Extensive papillomatosis in 18-year-old boy. Patient had had almost fifty resections of this process, beginning at 7 years of age, and finally died of suffocation.

Mild chronic inflammation and hyperemia are usually present beneath the epithelium.[32]

These tumors tend to recur over a long period of time. Exceptionally, they may extend into the tracheostomy stoma and soft tissues of the larynx, or wrap around the carotid artery, while maintaining its well-differentiated nature. Such a process has been designated *invasive papillomatosis.*[28] Treatment has included hormones, drugs, vaccines, cautery, cryosurgery, and interferon, with mixed but generally limited results.[36] In very extensive disease, laryngectomy may become necessary.[35]

Rarely, an obviously malignant squamous cell carcinoma develops in association with laryngeal papillomatosis. In practically all the reported cases of this complication, irradiation therapy had been administered previously for the papillomas; however, a few cases have been documented in which malignancy developed in the absence of radiation therapy. The carcinoma is usually located in the larynx, but in cases with extensive papillomatosis of the tracheobronchial tree, it may also arise in the trachea or bronchi.[26,34,37]

Adult laryngeal papillomas have a male predominance, are most commonly solitary, show a greater degree of inflammatory reaction, do not tend to spread, and recur less frequently than the juvenile form. Immunohistochemical staining for human papillomavirus is usually negative in them,[27] but hybridization techniques still reveal viral DNA.[38]

Verruca vulgaris is another HPV-related lesion that may occur in the larynx and be confused with epidermoid or verrucous carcinoma.[29]

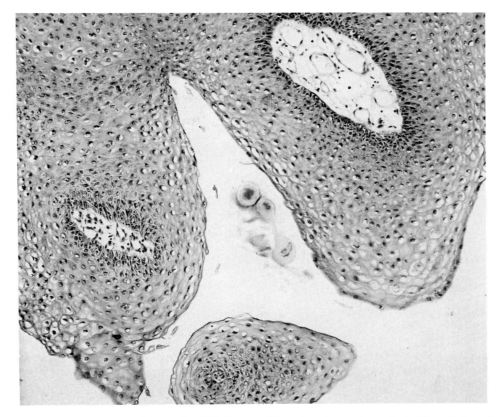

Fig. 7-21 Papillomatosis of larynx in child. Note papillary character and excellent differentiation of epithelium.

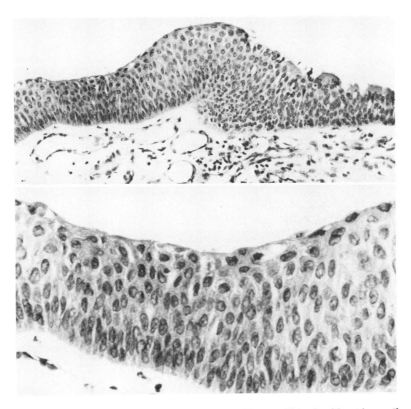

Fig. 7-22 Papillomatosis involving respiratory epithelium of larynx. This should not be confused with carcinoma in situ.

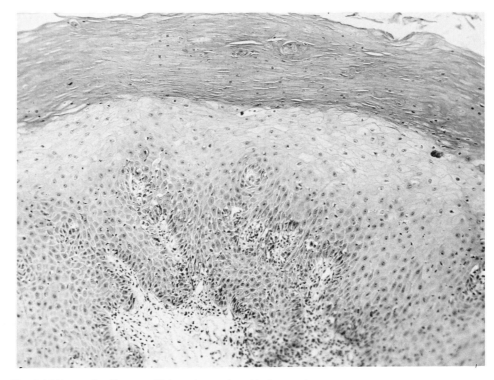

Fig. 7-23 Keratosis of larynx with hyperkeratotic epithelium and acanthosis. Basal membrane is intact.

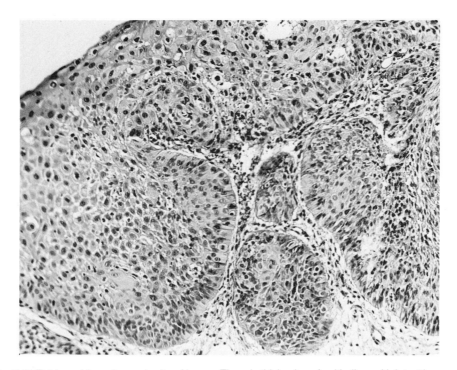

Fig. 7-24 Epidermoid carcinoma in situ of larynx. There is thickening of epithelium with intact basement membrane and complete disorganization of all layers.

Keratosis

Keratosis of the larynx involves the true cords and interarytenoid area. This lesion often occurs in smokers, in singers, and in those who use their voices excessively.[42] Laryngoscopic examination shows thickening of the vocal cord. Biopsy reveals hyperkeratotic epithelium, often with a granular layer, with downgrowth of the underlying squamous cells (Fig. 7-23).

Cellular atypia or dysplasia, when present, is graded as mild, moderate, or severe.[40]

The chances for patients with keratosis to develop carcinoma are related to the degree of atypia but on the whole are rather small. In a series of eighty-four patients with laryngeal keratosis followed between 5 and 15 years, only three developed carcinoma, and only one of these patients died as a result.[44] Other series have resulted in similar figures.[39,43] We believe, therefore, that conservative therapy is indicated, even for the lesions with severe atypia, if proper periodic examinations are carried out. The usual treatment is in the form of stripping.[41]

Carcinoma in situ

Epidermoid carcinoma in situ of the larynx is now recognized as a definite entity. In most cases, it is seen at the peripheral margin of an invasive cancer; it has been estimated that 75% of invasive squamous cell carcinomas have an associated in situ component.[46] In other instances, it may represent the only lesion present. These patients present with hoarseness and may show slight reddening of the true cord. Traditionally, the microscopic criteria for diagnosis have been the same as for its more common counterpart in the uterine cervix; i.e., the presence of atypical changes throughout the epithelium without evidence of surface maturation[45] (Fig. 7-24); however, some authors accept the diagnosis of laryngeal carcinoma in situ in the presence of surface maturation in the form of keratinization if nuclear atypia is prominent enough.[48] Aneuploid patterns have been found by microspectrophotometry in both types of lesion.[47]

It is likely that most cases of untreated carcinoma in situ will eventually develop into invasive carcinoma, but the interval may be very long. It is not unusual for patients to have documented carcinoma in situ for 5 years or more without an invasive component developing during this period.[50]

Carcinoma in situ of the larynx can be treated by biopsy, local excision, laryngeal fissure, stripping, or radiation therapy.[49,50] It is very important to rule out the presence of invasion before embarking on definitive treatment.

Invasive carcinoma
General features

Carcinoma of the larynx accounts for 2.2% of all cancers in men and 0.4% in women. Most patients are in their fifth

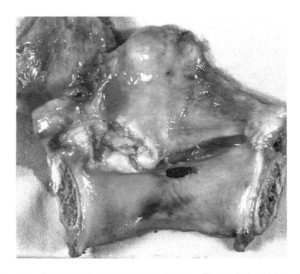

Fig. 7-25 Transglottic laryngeal carcinoma. Tumor is involving true cords, crossing ventricle of Morgagni and extending into supraglottic region. (Courtesy Dr. J. Costa, Lausanne, Switzerland.)

Table 7-1 "T" classification for carcinoma of the larynx

	Supraglottic	Glottic	Subglottic
Tis	Carcinoma in situ	Carcinoma in situ	Carcinoma in situ
T1	Tumor confined to site of origin with normal mobility	Tumor confined to vocal cord(s) with normal mobility	Tumor confined to the subglottic region
T2	Tumor involves adjacent supraglottic site or glottis without fixation	Supraglottic and/or subglottic extension of tumor with normal or impaired cord mobility	Tumor extension to vocal cords with normal or impaired cord mobility
T3	Tumor limited to larynx with fixation and/or extension to involve postcricoid area, medial wall of pyriform sinus or preepiglottic space	Tumor confined to larynx with cord fixation	Tumor confined to larynx with cord fixation
T4	Massive tumor extending beyond the larynx to involve oropharynx, soft tissues of neck, or destruction of thyroid cartilage	Massive tumor with thyroid cartilage destruction and/or extension beyond the confines of the larynx	Massive tumor with cartilage destruction and/or extension beyond the confines of the larynx

Beahrs OH, Myers MH (eds): *Manual for staging of cancer*, American Joint Committee on Cancer, ed. 2. Philadelphia, 1983, J.B. Lippincott Co., pp. 38-39.

decade of life or beyond, but cases occurring in much younger patients are on record.[54,55] About 96% of the patients are males. Smoking is the main risk factor, this risk being enhanced by heavy alcohol consumption.[52,53] Interestingly, a difference in the incidence of the various topographic sites

within the larynx has been found depending on geographic location.[51] Hoarseness is a common early symptom for glottic tumors but not for those located elsewhere.

The "T" classification for cancer of the larynx is shown in Table 7-1.

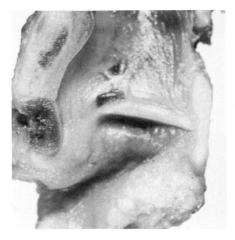

Fig. 7-26 Sagittal section of gross specimen of larynx showing small carcinoma of true cord.

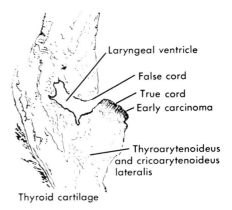

Fig. 7-27 Schematic representation and anatomy of lesion shown in Fig. 7-26.

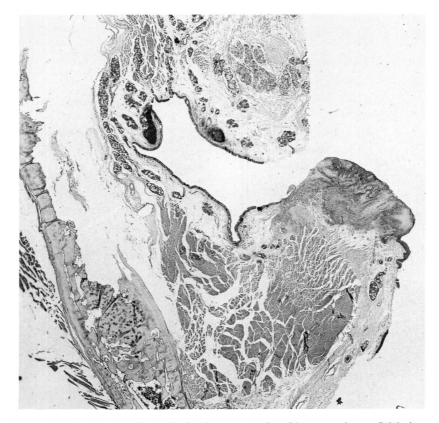

Fig. 7-28 Lesion illustrated in Fig. 7-26 showing topography of larynx and superficial character of carcinoma. Lesion could have been cured as well by good radiation therapy as by laryngectomy.

Types, spread, and therapy

Spread of laryngeal carcinoma can be accurately predicted from the site of origin and knowledge of the anatomic barriers produced by the different laryngeal compartments.[57] Accordingly, these tumors are divided, depending on their location, into four major types[58] (Figs. 7-25 to 7-28). This classification is largely based on laryngoscopic evaluation, but it seems likely that new radiographic modalities such as CT scan will result in greater accuracy.[56] The four types are:

1 *Glottic* (60% to 65% of all cases). These tumors arise from the true vocal cords, the anterior third of the glottis being the most common location. They tend to remain localized for long periods because of the surrounding cartilaginous wall and the paucity of lymphatic vessels. In time, they may spread across the anterior commissure to the opposite cord, posteriorly to involve the arytenoids, superiorly to involve the supraglottic portion, inferiorly to extend into the subglottic, and anteriorly to penetrate the thyroid cartilage with subsequent growth into the soft tissues of the anterior neck. In one series, ipsilateral lymph node metastases were not found in any of forty-one T1 lesions and in only 7.3% of T2 tumors[75];

therefore, prophylactic lymph node dissection is not indicated.

Early cases can be treated by irradiation therapy with excellent results[60,68,71,77] (Fig. 7-29). If irradiation fails, surgery will still save most of the patients.[64,67] Actually, small, superficially invasive ("microinvasive") epidermoid carcinomas of the true cord can be cured by endoscopic removal alone with results essentially identical to those obtained in carcinoma in situ.[59a,81] T2 glottic cancers are best treated by hemilaryngectomy.[59,76]

2 *Supraglottic* (30% to 35% of all cases). These tumors involve the false cord, the ventricle (including those arising in a laryngocele[65]), and/or the laryngeal or lingual surface of the epiglottis.[66] One third of the supraglottic cancers arise from the latter structure. These tumors have a marked tendency to spread toward the pre-epiglottic space, but the oropharynx is protected by the thick hyoepiglottic ligament.[73,79] They may erupt at the laryngeal surface of the epiglottis, leading to confusion with primary tumors of this area. Only 1% of supraglottic carcinomas invade the glottis. Invasion of cartilage is also rare and is largely restricted to those

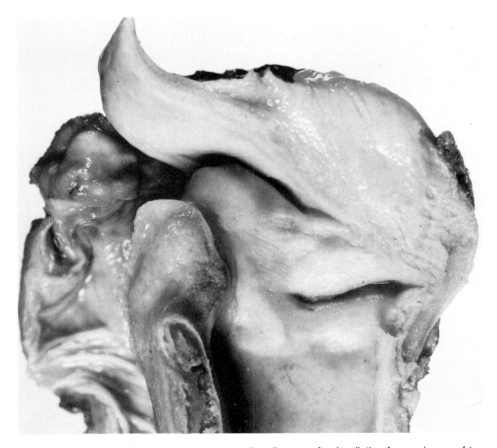

Fig. 7-29 Hemisection of larynx at autopsy more than 5 years after irradiation for carcinoma of true cord. Note perfectly normal true and false cords. Patient died of cardiovascular disease.

cases in which the cartilage had undergone bony metaplasia.[62]

The incidence of lymph node metastases averages 40%. About 20% to 35% of patients with clinically negative nodes will harbor occult metastases on microscopic examination.[57] Supraglottic tumors can be treated by irradiation or laryngectomy.[60,70]

3 *Transglottic* (less than 5% of all cases). This term is applied to cancers that cross the laryngeal ventricle.[74] They have the highest incidence of lymph node involvement (52%). Of sixteen transglottic cancers examined by McGavran et al.,[72] five (31%) had clinically undetected node metastases. This figure indicates that elective lymph node dissection should be performed for tumors in this location, in addition to a total laryngectomy.[78]

4 *Infraglottic* (subglottic) (less than 5% of all cases). Under this category are included cancers involving the true cord with a subglottic extension of more than 1 cm (Fig. 7-30) as well as tumors entirely confined to the subglottic area. The latter are very unusual[80] (Fig. 7-31). Lateral spread to the cricoid cartilage is the rule. Also common is destruction by tumor of the weak interthyrocricoid membrane, with invasion of the prelaryngeal wall and thyroid gland.[69,73] Because of the frequent extension to the trachea, this structure should be resected as distally as possible. Metastases to cervical nodes occur in 15% to 20% of the cases, and metastases to paratracheal nodes in about 50%.[57,72] Therefore radical node dissection with clearance of paratracheal nodes is indicated.

Tumors situated on the pyriform sinus or postcricoid areas are considered of pharyngeal origin.

The most common sites of metastases from laryngeal carcinoma, regardless of site of the primary tumor, are the regional lymph nodes, followed by the lungs. Thyroid gland and jugular vein involvement is usually the result of direct extension; the latter is seen only in the presence of extensive nodal involvement and is accompanied by a high probability of systemic dissemination.[61] Cervical node metastases can be accurately diagnosed with the technique of fine needle aspiration.[63]

Pathologic features

Grossly, most laryngeal carcinomas usually measure from 1 to 4 cm in diameter. They are usually described as a protruding pink to gray mass that is often ulcerated. Vocal cord lesions tend to have a keratotic appearance.

Microscopically, over 90% of laryngeal carcinomas are of epidermoid (squamous cell) type. They are graded into well, moderately, and poorly differentiated.[82] Most glottic carcinomas are well to moderately differentiated, whereas a high percentage of those located in other regions of the larynx (particularly in the subglottis) are moderately to poorly differentiated. In general, the smaller the tumor, the better differentiated its appearance. Those neoplasms in which the stromal invasion is limited to the most superficial layers are designated as superficially invasive, microinvasive, or "early." The latter term should be avoided, since it may be inaccurate, and also because it is used by clinicians

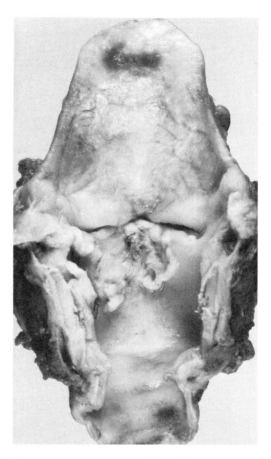

Fig. 7-30 Laryngeal carcinoma involving both true cords and extending into subglottic area for distance of 1.7 cm. This type is classified as infraglottic (subglottic) carcinoma.

with a somewhat different meaning, i.e., to indicate whether the mobility of the cord is normal or impaired.

The diagnosis of post-radiation persistence of carcinoma is often a difficult one to make. If dysplastic or atypical cells are present but limited to the mucosa, it is better to err on the conservative side because of the great difficulty in distinguishing tumor recurrence from post-irradiation atypia.[83]

Other microscopic types

Verrucous carcinoma is a rare variant of epidermoid carcinoma with a distinctly polypoid appearance and an extremely well-differentiated microscopic appearance[91] (Fig. 7-32). Like its counterpart in the oral cavity and other locations, it may show extensive local invasion but practically never metastasizes.[93] Human papillomavirus sequences have been demonstrated both in the tumor and in adjacent normal tissues.[84] Verrucous carcinoma should be distinguished from the verrucous form of keratosis (verrucous hyperplasia). The differential diagnosis is based on the presence or absence of invasion and can therefore be impossible to make on a small biopsy.[88]

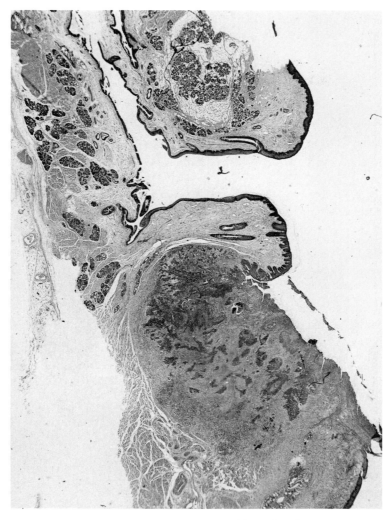

Fig. 7-31 True infraglottic epidermoid carcinoma in 42-year-old man. Hemilaryngectomy was performed. All margins were free. This was third infraglottic carcinoma out of 600 consecutive laryngectomies.

Small cell (oat cell, neuroendocrine) carcinoma has a light microscopic appearance identical to that of its pulmonary counterpart.[98] Similarly, it contains dense core secretory granules on ultrastructural examination and may exhibit immunoreactivity for neural markers.[86] As in other sites, it may be pure or associated with other patterns.[97,99] Cervical, nodal, and distal metastases are very common, and the prognosis is dismal.[97]

Basaloid-squamous carcinoma is a term recently proposed for a highly malignant laryngeal tumor characterized by areas of typical in situ and/or invasive epidermoid carcinoma associated with nests of small crowded cells. These cells have hyperchromatic nuclei, scant cytoplasm, small cystic spaces, necrosis, prominent hyalinization, and peripheral palisading.[101] This tumor, which also occurs in the tongue, pharynx, and esophagus, should not be confused with adenoid cystic carcinoma or mucoepidermoid carcinoma. Its behavior is extremely aggressive.[101]

Adenocarcinoma of nonsalivary gland type is a very rare neoplasm; most of the reported cases have been in the supraglottic or infraglottic regions[87,90] (Fig. 7-33).

Epidermoid carcinoma with sarcoma-like stroma (spindle epidermoid carcinoma; pseudosarcoma; carcinosarcoma) is a peculiar neoplasm with a high predilection for the upper aerodigestive tracts.[85,92] Tumors of this type located in the larynx, as elsewhere, often have a polypoid configuration[100] (Fig. 7-34) and may simulate a laryngeal polyp. Most are located in the supraglottic region. Microscopically, they have an element of epidermoid carcinoma (often inconspicuous and frequently in situ) and a pleomorphic sarcoma-like component, which makes up the bulk of the lesion. The sarcomatoid component may be as bland as to simulate granulation tissue or have a bizarre appearance reminiscent of malignant fibrous histiocytoma, malignant giant cell tumor of soft parts, or osteosarcoma[96] (Fig. 7-35).

Lymph node metastases may be composed of the carci-

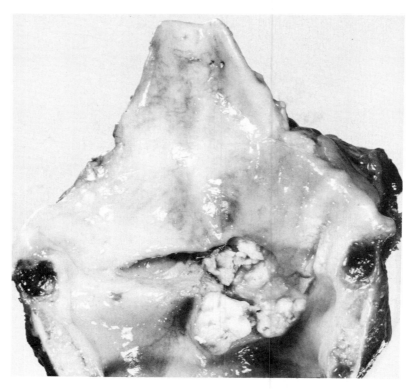

Fig. 7-32 Verrucous carcinoma of larynx with obliteration of right vocal cord and extension into subglottis. (From Kraus FT, Perez-Mesa C: Verrucous carcinoma. Clinical and pathologic study of 105 cases involving oral cavity, larynx, and genitalia. Cancer **19:**26-28, 1966.)

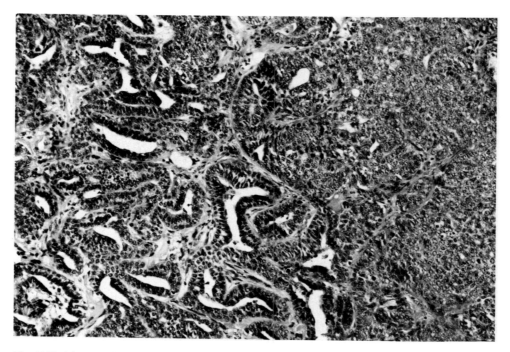

Fig. 7-33 Adenocarcinoma of larynx with solid areas. Appearance of this tumor does not correspond to any well-known minor salivary gland neoplasm.

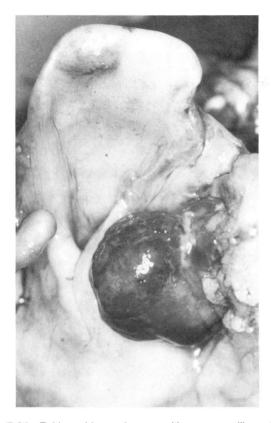

Fig. 7-34 Epidermoid carcinoma with sarcoma-like stroma ("pseudosarcoma") involving pharyngeal wall. Note typical polypoid configuration. (From Cornes JS, Lewis MS: Polypoid carcinomas of the pharynx with sarcomatous or pseudosarcomatous stroma. Br J Surg **53:**340-344, 1966.)

nomatous component alone, both patterns as in the primary tumor, or—in rare cases—the sarcoma-like elements exclusively. Whether the sarcoma-like stroma is of mesenchymal derivation or a carcinoma in disguise has been a matter of controversy since the time the entity was described.[95] Current evidence strongly favors the latter interpretation. Immunohistochemical markers of epithelial differentiation such as keratin are detected in at least some of the spindle cells in most cases, even in those with a monophasic appearance.[89,103] Reactivity for alpha-1-antitrypsin and alpha-1-chymotrypsin can also be detected; this should not be construed as evidence of histiocytic differentiation.[89]

Surgical excision is the treatment of choice.[100] The prognosis is better for the polypoid tumors than for deeply invasive neoplasms.[94,102]

Prognosis

The prognosis of laryngeal carcinoma is related to clinical stage, tumor location, and—to a lesser degree—microscopic grading.[104,105] The approximate 5-year survival rates for the different types are as follows, allowing for the usual differences from series to series:

Glottic: 80%
    I: 90%; II: 85%; III: 60%; IV: <5%
Supraglottic: 65%
    I: 85%; II: 75%; III: 45%; IV: <5%
Transglottic: 50%
Subglottic: 40%

Salivary gland–type tumors

The most common form of salivary gland–type tumor of the larynx is *adenoid cystic carcinoma*[109] (Fig. 7-36). Al-

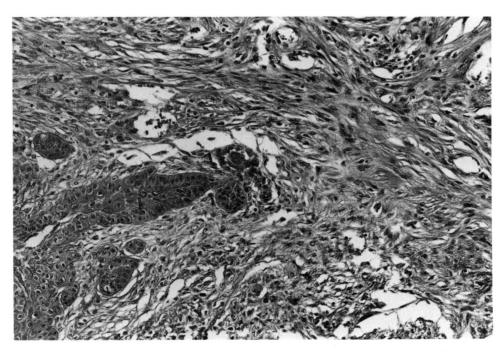

Fig. 7-35 Epidermoid carcinoma with sarcoma-like stroma. Islands of squamous cell carcinoma are surrounded by bulky tumor component with spindle sarcomatous appearance.

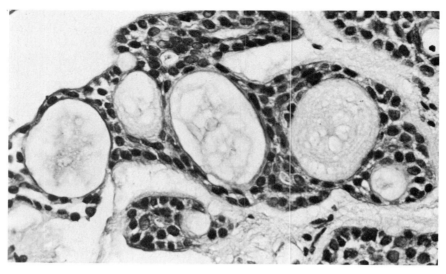

Fig. 7-36 Adenoid cystic carcinoma arising from mucous glands of larynx. Extensive lymph node and pulmonary metastases were present at time of this biopsy.

most all of them are located in areas other than the true vocal cords. They grow slowly but eventually prove fatal in most instances.[108]

Other neoplasms in this category include mucoepidermoid carcinoma,[111,112] acinic cell carcinoma,[106,110] and benign mixed tumor (pleomorphic adenoma).[107]

Carcinoid tumor and paraganglioma

In addition to small cell carcinoma, the larynx can be the site of two other tumors with endocrine differentiation, i.e., carcinoid tumor and paraganglioma.

Carcinoid tumor looks in all respects like its more common bronchial counterpart, including the presence of argyrophilia and dense-core neurosecretory granules.[114,120] Some of the tumors are predominantly composed of oncocytic cells ("oncocytic carcinoid tumors").[119] As in the lung, an *atypical* variety exists characterized by pleomorphism, mitotic activity, necrosis, and aggressive behavior.[115,116,120]

Paraganglioma is usually located in the supraglottic region, from where it often extends to the ipsilateral aryepiglottic fold.[113] Metastases have been documented in about a fifth of the reported cases.[117] Calcitonin and VIP have been detected in some of the cases, in addition to the usual endocrine markers.[118]

Other tumors

Hemangioma of larynx characteristically presents in infants as a sessile, poorly circumscribed mass in the subglottic area, immediately beneath the true vocal cord. Symptoms of upper respiratory tract obstruction may be severe. One half of the patients have associated hemangiomas in the skin, an important diagnostic sign. Biopsy can precipitate massive bleeding. The treatment of choice is radiation therapy, sometimes preceded by tracheotomy.[137]

Angiosarcoma can present as a polypoid mass in the epiglottis (Fig. 7-37).

Granular cell tumor may involve the true cord or other sites in the larynx.[129] Most are located posteriorly.[128] They are small and yellow and are covered by epithelium. The clinical diagnosis is usually that of laryngeal papilloma or nodule. Their microscopic appearance is typical, but they can be mistaken microscopically for epidermoid carcinoma because of the pseudoepitheliomatous hyperplasia that often accompanies this lesion.[125]

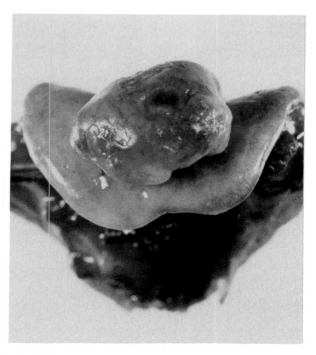

Fig. 7-37 Well-differentiated angiosarcoma of epiglottis. Tumor has distinctly polypoid appearance and is partially ulcerated. (Courtesy Dr. J. Costa, Lausanne, Switzerland.)

Fibromatosis of the larynx in a neonate may result in severe laryngeal obstruction.[135]

Rhabdomyoma has a predilection for the head and neck area, including the larynx. Cross striations are often found in the tumor cells in addition to peculiar crystal-like intracytoplasmic particles.[123]

Rhabdomyosarcoma also occurs; it is restricted to infancy and childhood and is almost always of the embryonal variety.[122]

Cartilaginous tumors of the larynx often arise from the cricoid cartilage and appear posteriorly in the subglottic region (Fig. 7-38). Goethals et al.[133] classified four of their twenty-two cases as benign and all of the others as chondrosarcomas by applying the same microscopic criteria used for the skeletal tumors; however, none of the tumors metastasized, and only six recurred locally. Although subsequently there have been reported cases with pulmonary metastases, these findings indicate that surgery should be as conservative as possible for cartilaginous neoplasms occurring in this location.

Osteosarcomas also occur[131]; they should be distinguished from chondrosarcomas with osseous metaplasia.

Liposarcoma of the well-differentiated type can present as a pedunculated laryngeal mass.[121]

Malignant fibrous histiocytomas of the larynx also have been described,[132] but one wonders how many of them actually represent carcinomas with sarcoma-like stroma, in which the epithelial component (which may be very inconspicuous) has either been overlooked or else has been destroyed by tumor ulceration.

Malignant melanoma can be primary in the larynx, but the possibility of metastasis should always be ruled out before entertaining such a diagnosis.[126]

Lymphoid lesions can also involve the larynx, although the event is rare. Reported cases include non-Hodgkin's lymphoma, mycosis fungoides, and plasmacytoma.[127,136] Although the latter lesion may appear localized, dissemination is likely to occur.[130] Acute leukemia can present initially with laryngeal obstruction.[134,138] We have also seen a case of a pseudolymphoma presenting as a polypoid intralaryngeal mass.

Metastatic tumors to the larynx can arise from a variety of sites; skin (melanoma), kidney, breast, and lung are the most common primary sites.[124]

Trachea
NON-NEOPLASTIC LESIONS

Tracheopatia osteoplastica presents as multiple submucosal nodules composed of mature bone and cartilage.[139] Its etiology is unknown.

Amyloidosis of the tracheobronchial tree is characterized by the formation of solitary or multiple nodules, usually asymptomatic.

Papilloma and *papillomatosis* of the trachea are morphologically similar to the lesions seen in the larynx (Fig. 7-39). Those cases seen in conjunction with laryngeal lesions usually begin in infancy and have a very low incidence of malignant transformation. Those limited to the trachea and bronchi usually begin in adulthood and have a greater tendency for malignant change. As in the larynx, some of these well-differentiated papillomatous tumors exhibit invasive tendencies.[140]

TUMORS

Epidermoid (squamous cell) carcinoma is the most common primary malignant tumor of the trachea[146,155] (Fig. 7-40). The majority arise in the lower third of the trachea. The clinical course is rapid and the prognosis is poor. The treatment is surgical, usually consisting of circumferential resection of the involved segment with end-to-end anastomosis.[152]

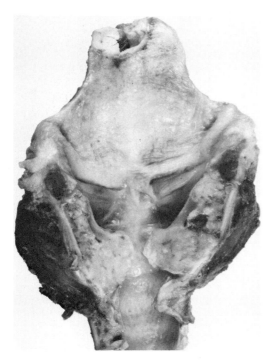

Fig. 7-38 Chondrosarcoma of larynx. Large white mass with foci of calcification replaces most of cricoid cartilage.

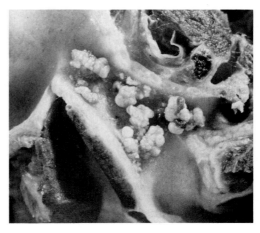

Fig. 7-39 Extensive papillomatosis of trachea and bronchi.

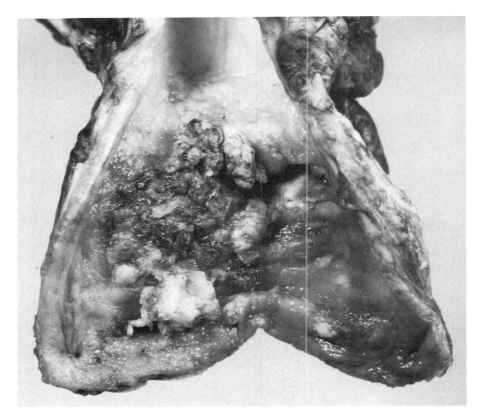

Fig. 7-40 Squamous cell carcinoma of trachea, excised following course of radiation therapy (6,000 R). Patient is alive and without evidence of disease 4 years later.

Adenoid cystic carcinoma is the second most common type. Its appearance is similar to that of the homonymous tumor in the major salivary glands. Most cases are located in the upper third of the trachea.[144] The clinical course is very slow, but the long-term prognosis is poor.

Small cell (oat cell, neuroendocrine) carcinoma has an appearance and a behavior similar to that of the bronchial tumor of the same type, an extension from which should always be considered in the differential diagnosis.[145]

Adenocarcinoma (mucin-producing) has also been observed in the lower third of the organ.[144]

Carcinoid tumor may arise in the trachea and be cured by segmental resection with primary reconstruction.[142]

Benign mixed tumors (pleomorphic adenomas) and other salivary gland–type tumors occur, but not nearly as often as adenoid cystic carcinoma.[145,149]

Other primary tumors of the trachea, all exceptionally rare, include glomus tumor,[143] hemangiopericytoma,[141] granular cell tumor,[151] "fibromyxoma,"[153] neurilemoma,[150] paraganglioma,[148] benign clear cell tumor ("sugar tumor"),[147] fibrosarcoma,[152] benign and malignant fibrous histiocytoma,[154] plasmacytoma and malignant lymphoma. Hodgkin's disease can present initially as a tracheal mass as a result of invasion from adjacent nodes.

Secondary tumors are much more common than primary neoplasms. Most of them arise in the bronchi, esophagus, or larynx and involve the trachea by direct extension.

REFERENCES
Larynx
CYSTS AND LARYNGOCELE

1 DeSanto LW, Devine KD, Weiland LH: Cysts of the larynx. Classification. Laryngoscope **80**:145-176, 1970.
2 Gallagher JC, Puzon BQ: Oncocytic lesions of the larynx. Ann Otol Rhinol Laryngol **78**:307-318, 1969.
3 Giovaniello J, Grieco RV, Bartone NF: Laryngocele. Am J Roentgenol Radium Ther Nucl Med **108**:825-829, 1970.
4 Newman BH, Taxy JB, Laker HI: Laryngeal cysts in adults. A clinicopathologic study of 20 cases. Am J Clin Pathol **81**:715-720, 1984.
5 Oliveira CA, Roth JA, Adams GL: Oncocytic lesions of the larynx. Laryngoscope **87**:1718-1725, 1977.
6 Yamase HT, Putman HC: Oncocytic papillary cystadenomatosis of the larynx. A clinicopathologic entity. Cancer **44**:2306-2311, 1979.

INFLAMMATION

7 Bailey CM, Windle-Taylor PC: Tuberculous laryngitis. A series of 37 patients. Laryngoscope **91**:93-100, 1981.
8 Barton RT: Observation on the pathogenesis of laryngeal granuloma due to endotracheal anesthesia. N Engl J Med **248**:1097-1099, 1953.
9 Basu MK, Asquith P, Thompson RA, Coake WT: Oral manifestations of Crohn's disease. Gut **16**:249-254, 1975.
10 Bennett DE: Histoplasmosis of the oral cavity and larynx. A clinicopathologic study. Arch Intern Med **120**:417-427, 1967.
11 Berenberg W, Kevy S: Acute epiglottitis in childhood. A serious emergency, readily recognized at the bedside. N Engl J Med **258**:870-874, 1958.
12 Bienestock H, Ehrlich GE, Freyberg RH: Rheumatoid arthritis of the cricoarytenoid joint. A clinicopathologic study. Arthritis Rheum **6**:48-63, 1963.
13 Croft CB, Wilkinson AR: Ulceration of the mouth, pharynx, and larynx in Crohn's disease of the intestine. Br J Surg **59**:249-252, 1972.
14 Gabrielides CG, Karkavelas G, Triarides C, Kouloulas A: Malakoplakia of the larynx. Pathol Res Pract **172**:53-57, 1981.

15 Hawkins DB, Miller AH, Sachs GB, Benz RT: Acute epiglottitis in adults. Laryngoscope **83**:1211-1220, 1973.

16 Hunter AM, Millar JW, Wightman AJA, Horne NW: The changing pattern of laryngeal tuberculosis. J Laryngol Otol **95**:393-398, 1981.

17 Kheir SM, Flint A, Moss JA: Primary aspergillosis of the larynx simulating carcinoma. Hum Pathol **14**:184-186, 1983.

18 Scheidemandel HH: Did George Washington die of quinsy? Arch Otolaryngol **102**:519-521, 1976.

19 Weidner N, Askin FB, Berthrong M, Hopkins MB, Kute TE, McGuirt FW: Bizarre (pseudomalignant) granulation-tissue reactions following ionizing-radiation exposure. A microscopic, immunohistochemical, and flow-cytometric study. Cancer **59**:1509-1514, 1987.

20 Yarnal JR, Golish JA, van der Kuyp F: Laryngeal tuberculosis presenting as carcinoma. Arch Otolaryngol **107**:503-505, 1981.

LARYNGEAL NODULE

21 Ash JE, Schwartz L: The laryngeal (vocal cord) nodule. Trans Am Acad Ophthalmol Otolaryngol **48**:323-332, 1944.

22 Fechner RE, Cooper PH, Mills SE: Pyogenic granuloma of the larynx and trachea. A causal and pathologic misnomer for granulation tissue. Arch Otolaryngol **107**:30-32, 1981.

OTHER NON-NEOPLASTIC LESIONS

23 Hui AN, Koss MN, Hochholzer L, Wehunt WD: Amyloidosis presenting in the lower respiratory tract. Clinicopathologic, radiologic, immunohistochemical, and histochemical studies on 48 cases. Arch Pathol Lab Med **110**:212-218, 1986.

24 Kamberg S, Loitman BS, Holtz S: Amyloidosis of the tracheobronchial tree. N Engl J Med **266**:587-591, 1962.

25 Roberts PF, McCann BG: Eosinophilic angiocentric fibrosis of the upper respiratory tract. A mucosal variant of granuloma faciale? A report of three cases. Histopathology **9**:1217-1225, 1985.

TUMORS AND TUMORLIKE CONDITIONS
Papillomatosis

26 Byrne JC, Tsao M-S, Fraser RS, Howley PM: Human papilloma virus-11 DNA in a patient with chronic laryngotracheobronchial papillomatosis and metastatic squamous-cell carcinoma of the lung. N Engl J Med **317**:873-878, 1987.

27 Costa J, Howley PM, Bowling MC, Howard R, Bauer WC: Presence of human papilloma viral antigens in juvenile multiple laryngeal papilloma. Am J Clin Pathol **75**:194-197, 1981.

28 Fechner RE, Goepfert H, Alford BR: Invasive laryngeal papillomatosis. Arch Otolaryngol **99**:147-151, 1974.

29 Fechner RE, Mills SE: Verruca vulgaris of the larynx. A distinctive lesion of probable viral origin confused with verrucous carcinoma. Am J Surg Pathol **6**:357-362, 1982.

30 Incze JS, Lui PS, Strong MS, Vaughan CW, Clements MP: The morphology of human papillomas of the upper respiratory tract. Cancer **39**:1634-1646, 1977.

31 Moore RL, Lattes R: Papillomatosis of the larynx and bronchi. Cancer **12**:117-126, 1959.

32 Nikolaidis ET, Trost DC, Buchholz CL, Wilkinson EJ: The relationship of histologic and clinical factors in laryngeal papillomatosis. Arch Pathol Lab Med **109**:24-29, 1985.

33 Quick CA, Foucar E, Dehner LP: Frequency and significance of epithelial atypia in laryngeal papillomatosis. Laryngoscope **89**:550-560, 1979.

34 Rabbett WF: Juvenile laryngeal papillomatosis. Relation of irradiation to malignant degeneration in this disease. Ann Otol Rhinol Laryngol **74**:1149-1163, 1965.

35 Robbins KT, Howard D: Multiple laryngeal papillomatosis requiring laryngectomy. Arch Otolaryngol **109**:765-769, 1983.

36 Robbins KT, Woodson GE: Current concepts in the management of laryngeal papillomatosis. Head Neck Surg **6**:861-866, 1984.

37 Runckler D, Kessler S: Bronchogenic squamous carcinoma in nonirradiated juvenile laryngotracheal papillomatosis. Am J Surg Pathol **4**:293-296, 1980.

38 Steinberg BM, Topp WC, Schneider PS, Abramson AL: Laryngeal papillomavirus infection during clinical remission. N Engl J Med **308**:1261-1264, 1983.

Keratosis

39 Crissman JD: Laryngeal keratosis and subsequent carcinoma. Head Neck Surg **1**:386-391, 1979.

40 Crissman JD: Laryngeal keratosis preceding laryngeal carcinoma. A report of four cases. Arch Otolaryngol **108**:445-448, 1982.

41 Gillis TM, Incze J, Strong MS, Vaughan CW, Simpson GT: Natural history and

management of keratosis, atypia, carcinoma in situ and microinvasive cancer of the larynx. Am J Surg **146**:512-516, 1983.

42 Goodman ML: Keratosis (leukoplakia) of the larynx. Otolaryngol Clin North Am **17**:179-183, 1984.

43 Hellquist H, Lundgren J, Olofsson J: Hyperplasia, dysplasia and carcinoma in situ of the vocal cords. A follow-up study. Clin Otolaryngol **7**:11-27, 1982.

44 McGavran MH, Bauer WC, Ogura JH: Isolated laryngeal keratosis. Its relation to carcinoma of the larynx based on a clinicopathologic study of 87 consecutive cases with long-term follow-up. Laryngoscope **70**:932-951, 1960.

Carcinoma in situ

45 Altman F, Ginsberg I, Stout AP: Intraepithelial carcinoma (cancer in situ) of the larynx. Arch Otolaryngol **56**:121-133, 1952.

46 Bauer WC, McGavran MH: Carcinoma-in-situ and evaluation of epithelial changes in laryngo-pharyngeal biopsies. JAMA **221**:72-75, 1972.

47 Crissman JD, Fu YS: Intraepithelial neoplasia of the larynx. A clinicopathologic study of six cases with DNA analysis. Arch Otolaryngol Head Neck Surg **112**:522-528, 1986.

48 Crissman JD, Grepp DR, Goodman ML, Hellquist H, Johns ME: Preinvasive lesions of the upper aerodigestive tract. Histologic definitions and clinical implications. Pathol Annu **22**(Pt 1):311-352, 1987.

49 Elman AJ, Goodman M, Wang CC, Pilch B, Busse J: In situ carcinoma of the vocal cords. Cancer **43**:2422-2428, 1979.

50 Hintz BL, Kagan AR, Nussbaum H, Rao AR, Chan PY, Miles J: A 'watchful waiting' policy for in situ carcinoma of the vocal cords. Arch Otolaryngol **107**:746-751, 1981.

Invasive carcinoma
General features

51 Barnes L, Johnson JT: Pathologic and clinical considerations in the evaluation of major head and neck specimens resected for cancer. Pathol Annu **21**(Pt 1):173-250, 1986.

52 DeStefani E, Correa P, Oreggia F, Leiva J, Rivero S, Fernandez G, Deneo-Pellegrini H, Zavala D, Fontham E: Risk factors for laryngeal cancer. Cancer **60**:3087-3091, 1987.

53 Elwood JM, Pearson JCG, Skippen DH, Jackson SM: Alcohol, smoking, social and occupational factors in the aetiology of cancer of the oral cavity, pharynx, and larynx. Int J Cancer **34**:603-612, 1984.

54 Lee S-S, Ro JY, Luna MA, Batsakis JG: Squamous cell carcinoma of the larynx in young adults. Semin Diagn Pathol **4**:150-152, 1987.

55 Mendez P Jr, Maves MD, Panje WR: Squamous cell carcinoma of the head and neck in patients under 40 years of age. Arch Otolaryngol **111**:762-764, 1985.

Types, spread, and therapy

56 Archer CR, Yeager VL, Herbold DR: Improved diagnostic accuracy in laryngeal cancer using a new classification based on computed tomography. Cancer **53**:44-57, 1984.

57 Barnes L, Johnson JT: Pathologic and clinical considerations in the evaluation of major head and neck specimens resected for cancer. Pathol Annu **21**(Pt 1):173-250, 1986.

58 Bauer WC, Edwards DL, McGavran MH: A critical analysis of laryngectomy in the treatment of epidermoid carcinoma of the larynx. Cancer **15**:263-270, 1962.

59 Biller HF, Ogura JH, Pratt LL: Hemilaryngectomy for T2 glottic cancers. Arch Otolaryngol **93**:238-243, 1971.

59a Crissman, JD, Zarbo RJ: Carcinoma in-situ and microinvasive carcinoma of the laryngeal glottis. Lab Invest **58**:20A, 1988 (Abstract).

60 DeSanto LW: The options in early laryngeal carcinoma. N Engl J Med **306**:910-912, 1982.

61 Djalilian M, Weiland LH, Devine KD, Beahrs OH: Significance of jugular vein invasion by metastatic carcinoma in radical neck dissection. Am J Surg **126**:566-569, 1973.

62 Dyess CL, Carter D, Kirchner JA, Baron RE: A morphometric comparison of the changes in the laryngeal skeleton associated with invasion by tumor and by external-beam radiation. Cancer **59**:1117-1122, 1987.

63 Feldman PS, Kaplan MJ, Johns ME, Cantrell RW: Fine-needle aspiration in squamous cell carcinoma of the head and neck. Arch Otolaryngol **109**:735-742, 1983.

64 Fisher AJ, Caldarelli DD, Chacko DC, Holinger LD: Glottic cancer. Surgical salvage for radiation failure. Arch Otolaryngol Head Neck Surg **112**:519-521, 1986.

65 Gerard-Marchant R, Micheau C, Cachin Y: Epithélioma laryngé et laryngocèle—une forme anatomo-clinique particulière. Compte-rendu de 7 observations. Ann Otolaryngol **86**:437-442, 1969.

66 Johns ME, Farrior E, Boyd JC, Cantrell RW: Staging of supraglottic cancer. Arch Otolaryngol 108:700-702, 1982.

67 Jose B, Calhoun DL, Mohammed A: Recurrences after irradiation in early vocal cord cancer with literature review. J Surg Oncol 27:224-227, 1984.

68 Kaplan MJ, Johns ME, Clark DA, Cantrell RW: Glottic carcinoma. The roles of surgery and irradiation. Cancer 53:2641-2648, 1984.

69 Lam KH: Extralaryngeal spread of cancer of the larynx. A study with whole-organ sections. Head Neck Surg 5:410-424, 1983.

70 Maceri DP, Lampe HB, Makielski KH, Passamani PP, Krause CJ: Conservation laryngeal surgery. A critical analysis. Arch Otolaryngol 111:361-365, 1985.

71 Marks RD Jr, Fitz-Hugh GS, Constable WC: Fourteen years' experience with cobalt-60 radiation therapy in the treatment of early cancer of the true vocal cords. Cancer 28:571-576, 1971.

72 McGavran MH, Bauer WC, Ogura JH: The incidence of cervical lymph node metastases from epidermoid carcinoma of the larynx and their relationship to certain characteristics of the primary tumor. A study based on the clinical and pathological findings for 96 patients treated by primary en bloc laryngectomy and radical neck dissection. Cancer 14:55-65, 1961.

73 Michaeu C, Luboinski B, Sancho H, Cachin Y: Modes of invasion of cancer of the larynx. A statistical, histological, and radioclinical analysis of 120 cases. Cancer 38:346-360, 1976.

74 Mittal B, Marks JE, Ogura JH: Transglottic carcinoma. Cancer 53:151-161, 1984.

75 Ogura JH, Biller HF: Neck dissection for carcinoma of the larynx and hypopharynx. Proceedings of the Sixth National Cancer Conference. Philadelphia, 1970, J.B. Lippincott Co., pp. 671-675.

76 Ogura JH, Sessions DG, Spector GJ: Analysis of surgical therapy for epidermoid carcinoma of the laryngeal glottis. Laryngoscope 85:1522-1530, 1975.

77 Perez CA, Holtz S, Ogura JH, Dedo HH, Powers WE: Radiation therapy of early carcinoma of the true vocal cords. Cancer 21:764-771, 1968.

78 Robbins KT, Michaels L: Feasibility of subtotal laryngectomy based on whole-organ examination. Arch Otolaryngol 111:356-360, 1985.

79 Russ JE, Sullivan C, Gallager HS, Jesse RH: Conservation surgery of the larynx. A reappraisal based on whole organ study. Am J Surg 138:588-596, 1979.

80 Sessions DG, Ogura JH, Fried MP: Carcinoma of the subglottic area. Laryngoscope 85:1417-1423, 1975.

81 Stutsman AC, McGavran MH: Ultraconservative management of superficially invasive epidermoid carcinoma of the true vocal cord. Ann Otol Rhinol Laryngol 80:507-512, 1971.

Pathologic features

82 Chung CK, Stryker JA, Abt AB, Cunningham DE, Strauss M, Connor GH: Histologic grading in the clinical evaluation of laryngeal carcinoma. Arch Otolaryngol 106:623-624, 1980.

83 Crissman JD, Ghepp DR, Goodman ML, Hellquist H, Johns ME: Preinvasive lesions of the upper aerodigestive tract. Histologic definitions and clinical implications (a symposium). Pathol Annu 22(Pt 1):311-352, 1987.

Other microscopic types

84 Abramson AL, Brandsma J, Steinberg B, Winkler B: Verrucous carcinoma of the larynx. Possible human papillomavirus etiology. Arch Otolaryngol 111:709-715, 1985.

85 Appelman HD, Oberman HA: Squamous cell carcinoma of the larynx with sarcoma-like stroma. A clinicopathologic assessment of spindle cell carcinoma and "pseudosarcoma." Am J Clin Pathol 44:135-145, 1965.

86 Benisch BM, Tawfik B, Breitenbach EE: Primary oat cell carcinoma of the larynx. An ultrastructural study. Cancer 36:145-148, 1975.

87 Cady B, Rippey JH, Frazell EL: Non-epidermoid cancer of the larynx. Ann Surg 167:116-120, 1968.

88 Crissman JD, Ghepp DR, Goodman ML, Hellquist H, Johns ME: Preinvasive lesions of the upper aerodigestive tract. Histologic definitions and clinical implications (a symposium). Pathol Annu 22(Pt 1):311-352, 1987.

89 Ellis GL, Langloss JM, Heffner DK, Hyams VJ: Spindle-cell carcinoma of the aerodigestive tract. An immunohistochemical analysis of 21 cases. Am J Surg Pathol 11:335-342, 1987.

90 Ferlito A. Histological classification of larynx and hypopharynx cancers and their clinical implications. Acta Otolaryngol (Suppl.) 342:1-88, 1976.

91 Ferlito A, Recher G: Ackerman's tumor (verrucous carcinoma) of the larynx. A clinicopathologic study of 77 cases. Cancer 46:1617-1630, 1980.

92 Goellner JR, Devine KD, Weiland LH: Pseudosarcoma of the larynx. Am J Clin Pathol 59:312-326, 1973.

93 Kraus FT, Perez-Mesa C: Verrucous carcinoma. Clinical and pathologic study of 105 cases involving oral cavity, larynx, and genitalia. Cancer 19:26-28, 1966.

94 Lambert PR, Ward PH, Berci G: Pseudosarcoma of the larynx. A comprehensive analysis. Arch Otolaryngol 106:700-708, 1980.

95 Lane N: Pseudosarcoma (polypoid sarcoma like masses) associated with squamous cell carcinoma of the mouth, fauces and larynx. Report of ten cases. Cancer 10:19-41, 1957.

96 Lasser KH, Naeim F, Higgins J, Cove H, Waisman J: "Pseudosarcoma" of the larynx. Am J Surg Pathol 3:397-404, 1979.

97 Mills SE, Cooper PH, Garland TA, Johns ME: Small cell undifferentiated carcinoma of the larynx. Report of two patients and review of 13 additional cases. Cancer 51:116-120, 1983.

98 Olofsson J, van Nostrand AWP: Anaplastic small cell carcinoma of larynx. Ann Otol Rhinol Laryngol 81:284-287, 1972.

99 Paladugu RR, Nathwani BN, Goodstein J, Dardi LE, Memoli VE, Gould VE: Carcinoma of the larynx with mucosubstance production and neuroendocrine differentiation. An ultrastructural and immunohistochemical study. Cancer 49:343-349, 1982.

100 Randall G, Alonso WA, Ogura JH: Spindle cell carcinoma (pseudosarcoma) of the larynx. Arch Otolaryngol 101:63-66, 1975.

101 Wain SL, Kier R, Vollmer RT, Bossen EH: Basaloid-squamous carcinoma of the tongue, hypopharynx, and larynx. Report of 10 cases. Hum Pathol 17:1158-1166, 1986.

102 Weidner N: Sarcomatoid carcinoma of the upper aerodigestive tract. Semin Diagn Pathol 4:157-168, 1987.

103 Zarbo RJ, Crissman JD, Venkat H, Weiss MA: Spindle-cell carcinoma of the upper aerodigestive tract mucosa. An immunohistologic and ultrastructural study of 18 biphasic tumors and comparison with seven monophasic spindle-cell tumors. Am J Surg Pathol 10:741-753, 1986.

Prognosis

104 Barnes L, Johnson JT: Pathologic and clinical considerations in the evaluation of major head and neck specimens resected for cancer. Pathol Annu 21(Pt 1):173-250, 1986.

105 Pera E, Moreno A, Galindo L: Prognostic factors in laryngeal carcinoma. A multifactorial study of 416 cases. Cancer 58:928-934, 1986.

Salivary gland–type tumors

106 Crissman JD, Rosenblatt A: Acinous cell carcinoma of the larynx. Arch Pathol Lab Med 102:233-236, 1978.

107 MacMillan RH III, Fechner RE: Pleomorphic adenoma of the larynx. Arch Pathol Lab Med 110:245-247, 1986.

108 Olofsson J, van Nostrand AWP: Adenoid cystic carcinoma of the larynx. A report of four cases and a review of the literature. Cancer 40:1307-1313, 1977.

109 Spiro RH, Hajdu SI, Lewis JS, Strong EW: Mucus gland tumors of the larynx and laryngopharynx. Ann Otol 85:498-503, 1976.

110 Squires JE, Mills SE, Cooper PH, Innes DJ Jr, McLean WC: Acinic cell carcinoma. Its occurrence in the laryngotracheal junction after thyroid radiation. Arch Pathol Lab Med 105:266-268, 1981.

111 Tomita T, Lotuaco L, Talbott L, Watanabe I: Mucoepidermoid carcinoma of the subglottis. An ultrastructural study. Arch Pathol Lab Med 101:145-148, 1977.

112 Whicker JH, Weiland LH, Neel HB III, Devine KD: Adenocarcinoma of the larynx. Ann Otol Rhinol Laryngol 83:487-490, 1974.

Carcinoid tumor and paraganglioma

113 Gallivan MVE, Chun B, Rowden G, Lack EE: Laryngeal paraganglioma. Case report with ultrastructural analysis and literature review. Am J Surg Pathol 3:85-92, 1979.

114 Goldman NC, Hood CI, Singleton GT: Carcinoid of the larynx. Arch Otolaryngol 90:64-67, 1969.

115 Mills SE, Johns ME: Atypical carcinoid tumor of the larynx. A light microscopic and ultrastructural study. Arch Otolaryngol 110:58-62, 1984.

116 Nonomura A, Shintani T, Kono N, Kamimura R, Ohta G: Primary carcinoid tumor of the larynx and review of the literature. Acta Pathol Jpn 33:1041-1049, 1983.

117 Ohsawa M, Kurita Y, Horie A, Kurita K: Malignant chemodectoma (paraganglioma) of the larynx. A case report with electron microscopy and biochemical assay. Acta Pathol Jpn 33:1279-1288, 1983.

118 Sneige N, Mackay B, Ordonez NG, Batsakis JG: Laryngeal paraganglioma. Report of two tumors with immunohistochemical and ultrastructural analysis. Arch Otolaryngol 109:113-117, 1983.

119 Stanley RJ, DeSanto LW, Weiland LH: Oncocytic and oncocytoid carcinoid tumors (well-differentiated neuroendocrine carcinomas) of the larynx. Arch Otolaryngol Head Neck Surg 112:529-535, 1986.

120 Tamai S, Iri H, Maruyama T, Kasahara M, Akatsuka S, Sakurai S, Murakami Y: Laryngeal carcinoid tumor. Light and electron microscopic studies. Cancer 48:2256-2259, 1981.

Other tumors

121 Allsbrook WC Jr, Harmon JD, Chongchitnant N, Erwin S: Liposarcoma of the larynx. Arch Pathol Lab Med **109:**294-296, 1985.

122 Batsakis JG, Fox JE: Rhabdomyosarcoma of the larynx. Arch Otolaryngol **91:**136-140, 1970.

123 Batsakis JG, Fox JE: Supporting tissue neoplasms of the larynx. Surg Gynecol Obstet **131:**989-997, 1970.

124 Batsakis JG, Luna MA, Byers RM: Metastases to the larynx. Head Neck Surg **7:**458-460, 1984.

125 Booth JB, Osborn DA: Granular cell myoblastoma of the larynx. Acta Otolaryngol (Stockh) **70:**279-293, 1970.

126 Cady B, Rippey JH, Frazell EL: Non-epidermoid cancer of the larynx. Ann Surg **167:**6-120, 1968.

127 Chen KTK: Localized laryngeal lymphoma. J Surg Oncol **26:**208-209, 1984.

128 Coates HL, Devine KD, McDonald TJ, Weiland LH: Granular cell tumors of the larynx. Ann Otol **85:**504-507, 1976.

129 Compagno J, Hyams VJ, Ste-Marie P: Benign granular cell tumors of the larynx. A review of 36 cases with clinicopathologic data. Ann Otol **84:**308-314, 1975.

130 Costen JB: Plasmacytoma. A case with original lesion of the epiglottis and metastasis to the tibia. Laryngoscope **61:**266-270, 1951.

131 Dahm LJ, Schaefer SD, Carder HM, Vellios F: Osteosarcoma of the soft tissue of the larynx. Report of a case with light and electron microscopic studies. Cancer **42:**2343-2351, 1978.

132 Ferlito A: Histiocytic tumors of the larynx. A clinicopathological study with review of the literature. Cancer **42:**611-622, 1978.

133 Goethals PL, Dahlin DC, Devine KD: Cartilaginous tumors of the larynx. Surg Gynecol Obstet **117:**77-82, 1963.

134 Jones RV: Laryngeal involvement in acute leukemia. J Laryngol **82:**123-128, 1968.

135 Rosenberg HS, Vogler C, Close LG, Warshaw HE: Laryngeal fibromatosis in the neonate. Arch Otolaryngol **107:**513-517, 1981.

136 Swerdlow JB, Merl SA, Davey FR, Gacek RR, Gottlieb AJ: Non-Hodgkin's lymphoma limited to the larynx. Cancer **53:**2546-2549, 1984.

137 Tefft M: The radiotherapeutic management of subglottic hemangioma in children. Radiology **85:**207-214, 1966.

138 Ti M, Villafuerte R, Chase PH, Dosik H: Acute leukemia presenting as laryngeal obstruction. Cancer **34:**427-430, 1974.

Trachea
NON-NEOPLASTIC LESIONS

139 Ashley DJ: Bony metaplasia in trachea and bronchi. J Pathol **102:**186-188, 1970.

140 Fechner RE, Fitz-Hugh GS: Invasive tracheal papillomatosis. Am J Surg Pathol **4:**79-86, 1980.

TUMORS

141 Ballard RW, Yarington CT Jr: Hemangiopericytoma of the tracheal wall. Arch Otolaryngol **107:**558-560, 1981.

142 Briselli M, Mark GJ, Grillo HC: Tracheal carcinoids. Cancer **42:**2870-2879, 1978.

143 Fabich DR, Hafez G-R: Glomangioma of the trachea. Cancer **45:**2337-2341, 1980.

144 Hajdu SI, Huvos AG, Goodner JT, Foote FW Jr, Beattie EJ Jr: Carcinoma of the trachea. Clinicopathologic study of 41 cases. Cancer **25:**1448-1456, 1970.

145 Heard BE, Dewar A, Firmin RK, Lennox SC: One very rare and one new tracheal tumour found by electron microscopy. Glomus tumour and acinic cell tumour resembling carcinoid tumours by light microscopy. Thorax **37:**97-103, 1982.

146 Houston HE, Payne WS, Harrison EG Jr, and Olsen AM: Primary cancers of the trachea. Arch Surg **99:**132-140, 1969.

147 Küng M, Landa JF, Lubin J: Benign clear cell tumor ("sugar tumor") of the trachea. Cancer **54:**517-519, 1984.

148 Liew S-H, Leong A S-Y, Tang HMK: Tracheal paraganglioma. A case report with review of the literature. Cancer **47:**1387-1393, 1981.

149 Ma CK, Fine G, Lewis J, Lee MW: Benign mixed tumor of the trachea. Cancer **44:**2260-2266, 1979.

150 Ma CK, Raju U, Fine G, Lewis JW Jr: Primary tracheal neurilemoma. Report of a case with ultrastructural examination. Arch Pathol Lab Med **105:**187-189, 1981.

151 Muthuswamy PP, Alrenga DP, Marks P, Barker WL: Granular cell myoblastoma. Rare localization in the trachea. Report of a case and review of the literature. Am J Med **80:**714-718, 1986.

152 Olmedo G, Rosenberg M, Fonseca R: Primary tumors of the trachea. Clinicopathologic features and surgical results. Chest **81:**701-706, 1982.

153 Pollak ER, Naunheim KS, Little AG: Fibromyxoma of the trachea. A review of benign tracheal tumors. Arch Pathol Lab Med **109:**926-929, 1985.

154 Sandstrom RE, Proppe KH, Trelstad RL: Fibrous histiocytoma of the trachea. Am J Clin Pathol **70:**429-433, 1978.

155 Weber AL, Grillo HC: Tracheal tumors. Radiol Clin North Am **16:**227-246, 1978.

Lung and pleura

Pleura
NORMAL ANATOMY

Both pleural layers have a lining of mesothelial cells endowed with a continuous basement membrane and resting on a layer of well-vascularized connective tissue. All of these elements are mesodermally derived. The normal mesothelial cell is flat or low cuboidal. Ultrastructurally, it features apical tight junctions, desmosomes, surface microvilli, and bundles of cytoplasmic tonofilaments. Immunohistochemically, it shows reactivity for both low- and high-molecular weight keratins.[1,2,3]

The normal subserosal cells have the ultrastructural features of fibroblasts and express the intermediate filament vimentin but not keratin; however, when these "multipotential subserosal cells" proliferate in reactive conditions, they co-express keratin and vimentin, and develop surface differentiation.[1]

PLEURITIS AND OTHER NON-NEOPLASTIC LESIONS

Inflammatory diseases of the lung may spread to the pleura. The pulmonary lesion may completely resolve but leaves a pleural symphysis (fusion between the two layers) secondary to prominent pleural fibrosis, which can be several centimeters thick. The underlying lung parenchyma may be perfectly normal, but its expansion is prevented by the surrounding rigid and contracted thickened pleura. If this thickened pleura is peeled off, pulmonary function will improve markedly. It is likely that the process designated "shrinking pleuritis with atelectasis," "folded lung syndrome," or "round atelectasis" represents a variation on this theme.[6,9]

Marked inflammatory pleural thickening may also occur as the result of organization of a hematoma formed following a penetrating wound of the thorax, a condition well-known to military surgeons. The best time to perform a decortication of this lesion is 3 to 5 weeks after the injury.[11] Microscopically, the material obtained represents an organized hematoma made up of fibrous tissue. Elastic fibers are absent, an indication that the underlying pleura is not part of the process.

Tuberculosis has been seen to involve the pleura in a variety of ways: as a complication of a subpleural infection, by direct extension from reinfection disease, as a complication of pneumothorax in the pre-chemotherapy era, and as a result of hematogeneous spread.[5]

Rheumatoid disease occasionally involves the lung and pleura (see p. 295). In the latter site, it induces a diffuse inflammatory reaction with effusion.[10] The microscopic appearance of the pleural biopsy is often nonspecific. In some instances, however, the presence of palisaded spindle histiocytes underlying a layer of fibrin and arranged perpendicularly to the pleural surface should make the pathologist suspect a rheumatoid etiology.[4,8] Cytologically, the pleural fluid shows epithelioid cells, giant cells, and cholesterol crystals, but there is a remarkable paucity of mesothelial cells.[7]

Endometriosis of the pleura and diaphragm has been reported. Most of the cases have occurred in the right side and have been associated with widespread intra-abdominal endometriosis.[12]

Amyloidosis can involve the pleura; the diagnosis is possible with needle biopsy.[7a]

ASBESTOSIS AND THE PLEURA

Asbestos is a family of fibrous hydrated silicates that are divided into two groups: the serpentines and the amphiboles.[16] Those of commercial importance are chrysolite in the first group and crocidolite and amosite in the second.[18,19] These minerals are a component of a large variety of manufactured products, particularly in the construction industry. Proof of the widespread use of this material is the finding of asbestos bodies in lung smears (particularly in the lower lobes) in approximately 40% of persons autopsied in the United States.[13,14] Inhalation of these fibers from the ambient air can result in various pathologic processes, which are dependent upon the type of mineral, the dimensions and concentration of the fibers, and the duration of the exposure. The pleural manifestations of asbestos exposure are pleural plaques and mesothelioma.

Pleural plaques are made up of hyalinized fibrous tissue. They are usually but not always associated with asbestos exposure.[20,22] The occurrence of these plaques correlates well with the duration and intensity of exposure. They are characteristically located on the parietal side, mainly in the intercostal spaces on the anterior and posterolateral aspects of the chest wall, and on the dome of the diaphragm at sites where the visceral and parietal pleuras approximate during respiratory excursions.[26] Over time, they become calcified and therefore detectable on chest x-rays. Amosite and crocidolite are responsible for most cases.[28]

The relationship between asbestos and *mesothelioma,* first identified by Wagner et al.[27] in South Africa, has now been documented all over the world.[17,21,25] The prevalence

of mesothelioma in people with prolonged heavy exposure to asbestos is 2% to 3% and has reached up to 10% in some series. The latency period is usually 20 years or longer. It should be pointed out that one third of mesothelioma cases are not associated with a history of asbestos exposure.[24] Crocidolite and amosite are the fiber types found in most cases of mesothelioma.[15]

Asbestos bodies are more commonly found in the lung than within the mesothelioma. Microscopic examination is a very insensitive and nonspecific method for the detection and identification of asbestos bodies. Extraction methods to increase their yield and biophysical techniques (such as electron microprobe analysis) are necessary to properly study their true incidence and composition.[13,23]

TUMORS
Mesothelioma

Benign "epithelial" mesothelioma is relatively common in the peritoneal cavity (see Chapter 26) but very rare in the pleura. Grossly, it presents as a soft friable mass, mottled pink, gray, and yellow. Microscopically, papillary processes lined by one or several layers of cuboidal mesothelial cells are seen. The distinction with malignant epithelial mesothelioma is made on the basis of the lack of significant atypia and the well-circumscribed, solitary nature of the lesion.

Malignant mesothelioma is usually seen in adults and typically presents with chest pain and pleural effusion. It often involves the lower half of a hemithorax but may spread to the entire pleural space, both pleura, interlobular septa, pericardium, chest wall, diaphragm, or even the peritoneum.[32] Extension into the subpleural portions of the lung is also common, but presence of nodular masses within the lung parenchyma favors a primary lung cancer with prominent pleural spread. Distant metastases in mesothelioma generally occur late in the course of the disease, if at all.[55] Presence of prominent hilar and supraclavicular lymphadenopathy at the time of initial presentation also favors carcinoma more than mesothelioma; however, we have seen pleural mesotheliomas that have presented initially with lymph node involvement in the cervical or axillary region.[60]

Grossly, multiple gray or white ill-defined nodules are seen in a diffusely thickened pleura. Pleural effusion is almost always present. Microscopically, the neoplastic formations may form papillae or pseudoacini or grow as solid nests (Fig. 7-41). The cytoplasm is abundant and acidophilic. Early cases must be distinguished from reactive mesothelial hyperplasia, as seen in association with lung inflammatory disease or sometimes with no apparent cause.[39] Features in favor of malignancy include infiltration of deep tissues, obvious cytologic atypia, prominent cell groupings, and necrosis.[54] In case of doubt, a conservative approach is indicated; if the lesion is a mesothelioma, usually this will become obvious in a few months.[54]

Obviously malignant mesotheliomas need to be distinguished from metastatic carcinoma, particularly pulmonary adenocarcinoma. This may be a very difficult or even impossible task in a biopsy specimen. In general, the cells of mesothelioma are more uniform and regular than those of

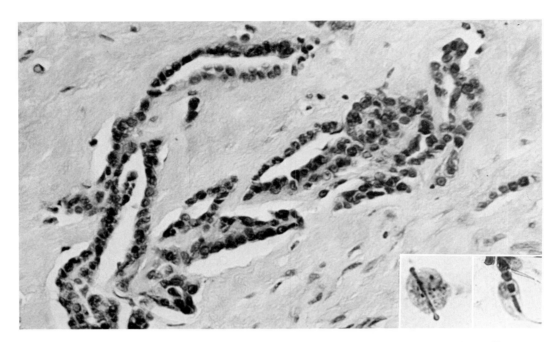

Fig. 7-41 Malignant diffuse mesothelioma of epithelial type. Gland-like spaces grow in dense fibrous stroma. **Insets,** Asbestos bodies found in patient's sputum.

adenocarcinoma. Histochemical stains can be of some help. Mesotheliomas usually produce large amounts of hyaluronic acid, which can be demonstrated both intracellularly and extracellularly with the Alcian blue or colloidal iron stains.[43,47] This material is nearly always mucicarmine negative, and the Alcian blue can be removed almost entirely by pretreatment with hyaluronidase. The presence of obvious droplets of mucicarmine-positive or PAS-positive material in the cytoplasm of the tumor cells strongly favors a diagnosis of adenocarcinoma over that of mesothelioma. Electron-microscopic examination can also aid in this differential diagnosis, the microvilli of mesothelioma cells being longer and more slender than those of adenocarcinoma.[33,36,61,66] A greater discriminatory capacity is provided by immunocytochemical techniques. The cells of mesothelioma are always positive for keratin; often positive for vimentin, epithelial membrane antigen, and S-100 protein; and nearly always negative for CEA, Leu-M1, and secretory component.[31,42,46,56,57] The cells of pulmonary adenocarcinoma are also positive for keratin, but in addition show consistently strong reactivity for EMA, CEA, Leu-M1, and secretory component.[35,41,59,65] A variety of monoclonal antibodies raised against adenocarcinoma cell lines has been recently described; this promises to offer a greater degree of specificity in the distinction between these two tumor types.[50,62] Differences have also been described regarding lectin-binding patterns, but they do not seem to have a sharp discriminatory ability.[43a]

Some mesotheliomas are predominantly or entirely composed of spindle cells. These *spindle cell* or *sarcomatoid* tumors tend to be more nodular and less plaque-like than those composed of cuboidal mesothelial cells and are often

accompanied by hemorrhage, necrosis, and cystic change.[58] Pleural effusion is present in most but not all of the cases. Microscopically, the tumor is highly cellular, formed by interwoven bundles of spindle cells. Nuclear atypia is present, and mitotic figures are common (Fig. 7-42). In rare cases, foci of osseous and cartilaginous metaplasia are encountered.[37,67] Cases in which spindle tumor cells co-exist with plumper epithelial-like cells may show a resemblance to synovial sarcoma.[53] Spindle cell (sarcomatoid) mesotheliomas show consistent immunohistochemical positivity for keratin.[54a]

Some spindle cell or mixed mesotheliomas are accompanied by a very abundant deposition of fibrous tissue and are referred to as *desmoplastic mesotheliomas*.[34] The main differential diagnosis of this form of malignant pleural mesothelioma is with the more cellular types of solitary fibrous tumors of pleura, some of which may be malignant themselves. Immunohistochemical positivity for keratin is the best evidence in favor of the former. Ultrastructurally, rudimentary evidence of epithelial differentiation may be demonstrated.[44]

Desmoplastic mesotheliomas also need to be distinguished from areas of dense inflammatory fibrosis. A claim was made to the effect that immunohistochemical positivity for keratin in the spindle cells established a diagnosis of mesothelioma, but this turned out not to be the case; the reactive mesothelial cells entrapped in the fibrous plaques are just as positive, as one would have predicted.[38] Thus, the differential diagnosis is largely based on the appearance of the proliferating cells in the routinely stained sections. Features favoring malignancy are nuclear atypia, necrosis, presence of well-developed fascicular, storiform, or other

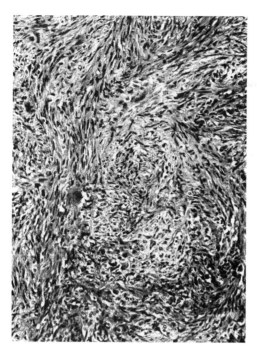

Fig. 7-42 Sarcomatoid malignant mesothelioma. Tumor cells have spindle-cell appearance and fascicular arrangement that simulate soft tissue sarcoma. Some of these cells showed immunocytochemical positivity for keratin.

complex tissue patterns, and infiltration of adjacent tissues.[54] As in the case of the proliferation of the more typical cuboidal mesothelial cells, a conservative approach is strongly recommended in dubious cases.

Malignant mesotheliomas with squamous differentiation (pleural squamous cell carcinomas) have been described in patients with a history of chronic empyema or therapeutic pneumothorax,[40] but some of these might have been lung carcinomas with extensive pleural extension.

The prognosis of pleural mesothelioma is uniformly poor.[48,51,52,63] Fifteen of the sixteen patients reported by Ratzer et al.[58] died from the tumor within 11 to 58 months following the onset of symptoms. Spindle cell (sarcomatoid) tumors have been associated with shorter survival than the conventional type.[29,49] Systemic chemotherapy, sometimes combined with resection of the bulk of the tumor and/or radiation therapy, has resulted in some prolonged remissions.[30,45,64]

Solitary fibrous tumor of pleura

Solitary fibrous tumor of pleura (so-called solitary fibrous mesothelioma) is always well circumscribed and sometimes even encapsulated. It is usually asymptomatic, although on occasion patients present with pain, cough, dyspnea, and/or prominent pulmonary osteoarthropathy that rapidly regresses when the tumor is removed.[68,75] It is not associated with asbestosis. Grossly, the lesion is firm, lobulated, gray-white to yellow-white, with frequent whorling and fasciculation. The mean diameter is 6 cm. The appearance is reminiscent of uterine leiomyoma (Fig. 7-43). Cystic de-

generation is very unusual, but we have seen examples presenting as a mural nodule within a large pleural-lined cyst. It may be found attached to the visceral pleura (80%), parietal pleura, within an interlobar fissure, or sometimes within the lung parenchyma without a pleural connection.[79a] We have seen lesions with an identical microscopic appearance in the mediastinum (see Chapter 8) and nasopharynx (see Chapter 7).

Microscopically, there is a tangled network of fibroblast-like cells, accompanied by deposition of abundant reticulin and collagen fibers. The degree of cellularity varies a great deal from case to case. Hemangiopericytoma-like areas are frequent. The most cellular types may be misdiagnosed as fibrosarcoma or malignant schwannoma (Fig. 7-44). If proper attention is paid to the lack of nuclear aberrations and the rarity or absence of mitoses, confusion is unlikely to occur. In some instances, clusters of cuboidal cells forming papillae, tubules, or solid nests are found at the periphery of predominantly fibrous tumors. It is not clear if they are a constituent of the neoplasm, or merely entrapped mesothelium or pulmonary epithelium, but the latter seems more likely.[71,76]

This neoplasm has been regarded for many years as a form of mesothelioma, largely on the basis of the pattern of growth that the tumor cells exhibit in tissue culture[79]; however, on ultrastructural examination these cells show fibroblast-like rather than mesothelial-like features, and by immunohistochemistry they are reactive for vimentin and sometimes desmin rather than keratin.* The most likely interpretation of this tumor, therefore, is that it arises from noncommitted mesenchymal cells present in the areolar tissue subjacent to the mesothelial lining.[73] This has led to the proposal of alternative terms such as submesothelioma or submesothelial fibroma.

Almost 90% of these neoplasms are cured by surgical excision. In a thorough review of the literature, Briselli et al.[68] found that 12% had caused death because of extensive intrathoracic growth. Indicators of good prognosis were presence of a pedicle, good circumscription, and absence of nuclear pleomorphism or mitotic activity.

Other primary tumors

Vascular tumors of either the epithelioid (histiocytoid) hemangioendothelioma or angiosarcoma types may grow diffusely in the pleura in a fashion simulating mesothelioma.[81,82]

In rare cases, *thymomas* can present as primary pleural lesions (see Chapter 8).

Malignant lymphoma of the pleural cavity has been reported, developing from a long-standing pyothorax.[80]

Metastatic tumors

About 75% of metastatic tumors in the pleura are of a carcinomatous nature. As a matter of fact, metastatic carcinoma is the most common malignant tumor in the pleura. It is second only to congestive heart failure as the cause of pleural effusions in patients over 50 years of age. Dyspnea, cough, and chest pain are the most common presenting

*See references 69, 70, 72, 74, 76a, 77, and 78.

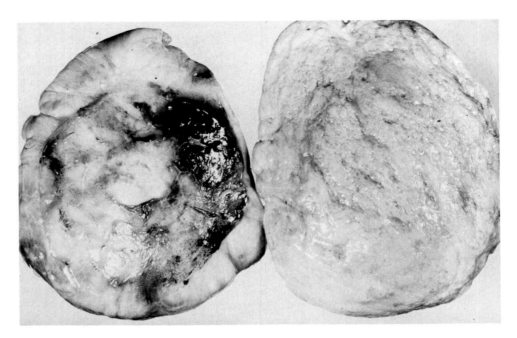

Fig. 7-43 Large, asymptomatic, benign solitary fibrous tumor of pleura.

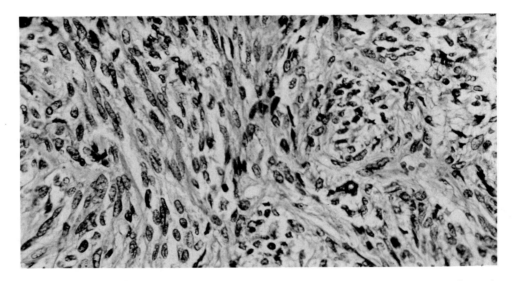

Fig. 7-44 Highly cellular solitary fibrous tumor of pleura. Changes shown may cause incorrect diagnosis of sarcoma.

symptoms. Most malignant pleural effusions are greater than 500 ml. The fluid is most often serous to serosanguinous, but it may be frankly hemorrhagic.

In one series,[83] the most common sites for the primary lesion were lung (33%), breast (20.9%), and stomach (7.3%). Ninety-two per cent of the lung, breast, and ovarian malignant effusions were ipsilateral to the primary lesion. A malignant pleural effusion was the first evidence of the existence of cancer in 46% of the patients.

Biopsy and cytology

Needle biopsy of the parietal pleura is very useful for the differential diagnosis between inflammatory disease and malignancy.[99,101] Aaron et al.[84] combined pleural biopsy with biopsy of the lung parenchyma and hilar lymph nodes in the study of eighty-nine patients with diffuse pulmonary disease and/or hilar adenopathy and persistent pleural effusion. A definite diagnosis was reached in sixty-two cases. If tuberculosis is suspected, part of the pleural biopsy should be cultured. Levine et al.[95] found that culture of a single specimen from pleural biopsy was positive with greater frequency than multiple cultures of pleural fluid.

Whenever the possibility of malignancy is considered in the presence of pleural effusion, a cytologic examination of the pleural fluid should always be performed, regardless of its gross appearance.

Traditionally, long-standing pleural effusions have been regarded as probably malignant if bloody and probably tuberculous if serous. Actually, there is very little relation between the appearance of the fluid and the nature of the disease.[86,91] The differential cell count of the effusion is of no great help either, since 93% of the effusions caused by tuberculosis and 67% of those caused by cancer are predominantly lymphocytic[97]; however, the presence of numerous mesothelial cells essentially excludes tuberculosis.

There is probably no area in diagnostic cytology that is more difficult to interpret than that of effusions in serous cavities.[93,98] This is mainly because proliferating reactive mesothelial cells can acquire features dangerously similar to those of cells of mesothelioma and even metastatic carcinoma. The cells of mesotheliomas can occur singly or in clusters with scalloped borders. The cytoplasm is dense and often has small, regular, centrally located vacuoles.[85] Nuclei are atypical, the nucleo-cytoplasmic ratio is greatly altered, and multinucleated forms may be present. Cytologic preparations can be stained for PAS, mucicarmine, various enzymes, keratin or CEA, and also examined ultrastructurally.[88,90,92,96] In the huge series by Johnston,[94] a cytopathologic diagnosis conclusive for cancer was obtained in the first specimen of fluid in 90.5% of the cases; there were no false-positive diagnoses.

The presence of a high content of hyaluronic acid in a pleural effusion favors the diagnosis of mesothelioma.[87,100] Chromosomal analysis has also been used in conjunction with cytologic analysis in order to improve the diagnostic yield.[89]

Lung
NORMAL ANATOMY

The two main components of the lung parenchyma are the bronchi and bronchioles (airways) and the alveoli. The alveoli are lined by type I pneumocytes and type II (granular) pneumocytes; the latter produce surfactant and are the main proliferating component following alveolar injury. The alveolar walls contain capillaries whose basement membrane fuses with that of the alveolar epithelium to consitute a single alveolar capillary membrane.

The main cell types of the bronchial-bronchiolar epithelium are basal cells, Kultschitsky's cells, ciliated cells, serous cells, Clara cells, and goblet cells. Goblet and ciliated cells decrease in number as one approaches the terminal bronchioles, whereas the number of Clara cells increases proportionally. The vasculature of the lung derives from the pulmonary vessels and bronchial vessels, the latter belonging to the systemic circulation. Pulmonary arteries have both an internal and external elastic membrane, whereas pulmonary veins have a single elastic layer.

Structures sometimes seen in alveolar luminae, which are of no diagnostic significance by themselves, are fresh red blood cells (usually the result of surgical trauma), scattered alveolar macrophages, corpora amylacea (common in elderly people), and blue bodies (composed primarily of calcium carbonate). The interstitium of the lung in adult city dwellers invariably contains variable amounts of anthracotic pigment (carbon); scattered birefringent silica crystals may also be found, a feature which by itself is not diagnostic of silicosis (see p. 290).

It is not rare to find scattered megakarycocytes in the alveolar walls; the large, hyperchromatic, and distorted nuclei of these cells should not be misinterpreted as evidence of malignancy or viral infection.[101a]

NON-NEOPLASTIC LESIONS
Biopsy

It is imperative for the pathologist to know the clinical history and radiographic findings of the case before attempting to interpret a lung biopsy, especially in nonneoplastic lesions. Basic facts such as localized versus diffuse pattern of the process, presence and degree of functional impairment, and occupational or travel history are extremely important in this regard.

The type of lung biopsy obtained is also of importance. Transbronchial biopsies are useful for infections, sarcoidosis, and neoplasms but not for the usual interstitial pneumonia.[105] For the latter, open lung biopsy represents the ideal material.[102] The lingula or right middle lobe tips should be avoided because of their tendency to show more fibrosis than elsewhere.[104] Areas of extreme scarring and honeycombing are likely to show only end-stage disease and therefore are not very informative. Ideally, samples from two or three different areas should be obtained.[103]

Cystic diseases

Congenital cystic disease is a generic term for any cystic process of the lung thought to be already present at birth. The condition is often overdiagnosed. It can be simulated by a variety of acquired processes, such as a healed abscess. The absence of coal pigment in the cystic area has been used as a sign that the lesion is congenital but is not pathognomonic. Morphologic types of congenital cystic disease include pulmonary sequestration (see p. 270), congenital lobar emphysema, bronchogenic cyst, the nebulous "congenital bronchiectasis," and cystic adenomatoid transformation.[113,115]

Congenital lobar emphysema (congenital lobar hyperinflation) presents in young children. It only affects one of the upper lobes or the right middle lobe of the lung. Theories for its occurrence include mucosal folds, mucous plugs, and deficiencies in the bronchial cartilages. The pathologic change consists of massive overdistension of the alveolar spaces, not accompanied by tissue destruction. It is therefore not truly a cystic or an emphysematous process. Severe compression of the other pulmonary lobes may result from this lesion.

Cystic adenomatoid transformation is characterized by the presence of variously sized intercommunicating cysts

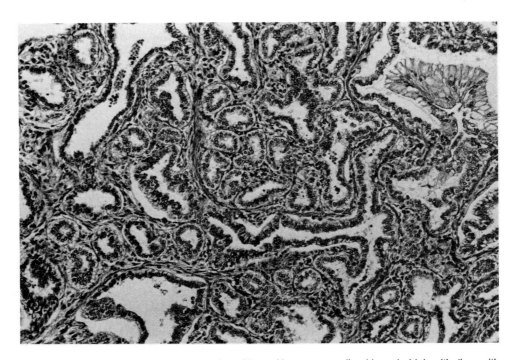

Fig. 7-45 Cystic adenomatoid transformation of lung. Air spaces are lined by cuboidal epithelium with an adenomatoid appearance.

lined by an "adenomatoid" cuboidal-to-ciliated pseudostratified columnar epithelium[107,114] (Fig. 7-45). It may be seen in association with bronchial atresia. It usually presents with respiratory distress in neonates, but it has also been found in older children and in adults.[108] Three morphologic varieties have been described depending on the size and number of the cysts.[114] Solitary lesions usually involve a lower lobe. Some of the patients have associated pulmonary or extrapulmonary anomalies. Lobectomy is the treatment of choice.[110]

Most *acquired cystic diseases* of the lung result from emphysema or honeycombing. The latter represents the end stage of interstitial pneumonia or other inflammatory diseases and is discussed on p. 281.

Emphysema is defined as an increase beyond the normal in the size of airspaces distal to the terminal bronchiole associated with destruction of their walls.[112] Emphysematous *bullae* are large cystic spaces covered by a thin, stretched pleura. Symptoms may result from hemorrhage, infection, compression of adjacent lung, or pneumothorax. Large bullae can be treated by simple excision of the walls with closure of bronchiolar fistulas and obliteration of the pleural space.[106,111] *Blebs* are formed by the rupture of an alveolus directly beneath the pleura and the escape of air into the areolar layer of the pleura, which results in interstitial emphysema. A bleb may rupture into the free pleural space, causing pneumothorax.

Mesenchymal cystic hamartoma is the name recently given by Mark[109] to a multifocal and bilateral lung lesion characterized by the formation of small (up to 1 cm) cysts

lined by normal or metaplastic respiratory epithelium resting on a cellular "cambium layer" of mesenchymal cells.

Bronchopulmonary sequestration

Bronchopulmonary sequestration is characterized by partial or complete separation of a portion of a lobe of the lung, with no connection to the bronchial tree.

In the *extralobar* variety, the tissue is enveloped by its own pleural covering and exists as a nodule apart from the lung, at any level from the thoracic inlet to the diaphragm, or even within the abdominal cavity. About 90% of the cases occur in the left side. Other congenital malformations, especially diaphragmatic hernias, occur in approximately 20% of the patients.[119] An association with polyhydramnios and edema has been observed.[122] The arterial supply is usually by one or several small arteries from the aorta or one of its branches. The venous drainage is into the azygos system.

The *intralobar* variety, which is much more likely to be symptomatic, is characteristically located within the lower lobe, especially in the posterior basal segment.[116,123] About 60% of the cases occur on the left side. The segment is supplied by a *large* artery arising from the aorta or one of its branches; this artery arises above the diaphragm in 75% of the patients and below the diaphragm in the remainder. Failure of the surgeon to appreciate this fact may result in death from hemorrhage. Despite its origin, the artery is always of the elastic pulmonary type. Shunts between the anomalous arteries and intrapulmonary vessels have been demonstrated.[117]

Intralobular sequestrations have been divided into types

I, II, and III, depending on whether the overlap between the pulmonary and the anomalous systemic arteries is extensive, slight, or absent, respectively.[121] Venous blood flows into the pulmonary venous system. Grossly, the sequestered portion may present as a single cyst, as a multicystic area, or as a solid mass. Microscopically, there is usually chronic inflammation and fibrosis. Obliterative changes of blood vessels are prominent. The pathogenesis of this condition is controversial. Persistence of the systemic arterial supply[118] and defects in the pulmonary arterial development[120] have been postulated. Other authors favor an acquired origin related to repeated episodes of chronic pneumonia, citing in favor of this interpretation the almost complete absence of this disease in neonates or infants, the infrequency of associated anomalies, and the almost universal presence of chronic inflammation and fibrosis.[121]

Bronchiectasis

Bronchiectasis refers to the dilatation of bronchial lumina, usually associated with destruction of some elements of the bronchial wall and inflammatory changes in the surrounding lung parenchyma. It is a disease usually contracted in youth; 69% of the cases studied in a large series[132] first manifested during the first two decades of life. A history of antecedent pulmonary infection can often be elicited: in a group of children with bronchiectasis reported by Field in 1949,[126] there was a history of pneumonia in 35% and of pertussis in 30%. Bronchial obstruction by a neoplasm, a foreign body, an inflammatory process in the bronchial wall, a greatly enlarged lymph node, or the inspissated mucous secretions of cystic fibrosis (mucoviscidosis) may lead to bronchiectasis; most cases of cystic fibrosis are complicated by sinusitis and bronchiectasis.[124,131] Two other disorders associated with chronic sinonasal infection and frequent formation of bronchiectasis are *Kartagener's* or *immobile cilia syndrome,* associated with complete situs inversus and infertility, and *Young's syndrome,* associated with infertility caused by azoospermia but lacking ultrastructural ciliary abnormalities.[127,133]

The most common pathogenetic sequence for the formation of bronchiectasis seems to be bronchial obstruction, pneumonitis, atelectasis, and bronchial dilatation.[126,130]

In atelectasis, intrapleural pressure becomes more negative and is then transmitted through the solid nonexpansible pulmonary tissue to the elastic and expansible bronchial walls.

Bronchiectasis involves the left lung more often than the right, possibly because of a difficulty in draining caused by the physiologic constriction imposed on the left bronchus by the pulmonary artery. The lower lobes are the more frequent sites of the disease. However, bronchiectasis of the left lower lobe is almost always accompanied by involvement of the lingular division of the left upper lobe and bronchiectasis of the right lower lobe by involvement of the right middle lobe and pectoral branch of the right upper lobe. It is important to realize that the process is usually focal and that the extent of the disease is entirely dependent on the primary insult. Once bronchiectasis has become established in an area of the lung, it tends to remain confined to that area *unless* there is additional pulmonary infection and atelectasis. For instance, of 114 patients reported by Perry and King,[132] only six developed a spread of the disease, and all of them had intercurrent pneumonia.

Grossly, the pleura is frequently thickened and the lung

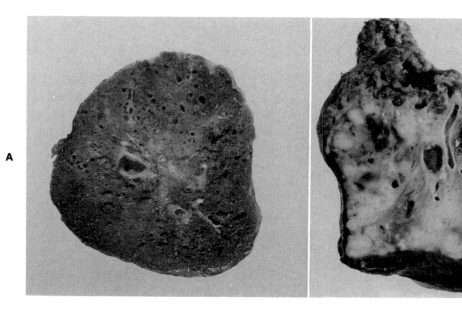

A   **B**

Fig. 7-46 A, Extralobar type of pulmonary sequestration. Lung has spongy appearance and is covered by normal pleura. **B,** Intralobar type of pulmonary sequestration. As is often the case with this variety, there are extensive secondary inflammatory changes. (Courtesy Dr. J. Costa, Lausanne, Switzerland.)

is heavier than normal. Bronchiectasis is broadly classified into saccular, cystic, and cylindric types, according to the shape of the bronchial dilatation (Figs. 7-46 and 7-47). The region of involvement is usually in the secondary bronchi; it can be segmental or diffuse. The bronchial walls are irregularly thickened. The bronchial cartilage may undergo

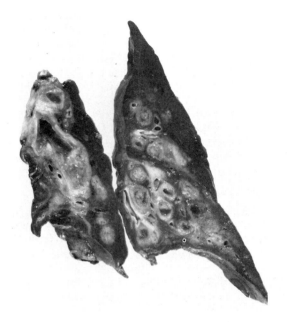

Fig. 7-47 Bronchiectasis in patient with cystic fibrosis. Lesions are cylindric and accompanied by marked fibrotic and inflammatory changes in surrounding parenchyma. (Courtesy Dr. J. Costa, Lausanne, Switzerland.)

ossification and ulcerate into the lumen. The intervening lung parenchyma shows variable degrees of inflammation and fibrosis; peribronchial abscesses may be seen. Infrequently, pleural perforation and empyema occur.

Microscopically, chronic inflammation of the bronchial wall is a constant finding. Lymphocytes predominate, and germinal centers can be encountered, particularly in younger patients (Fig. 7-48). Areas of ulceration are common, but the persistent epithelium is usually ciliated and otherwise normal; squamous metaplasia can occur, but is unusual. With advanced changes, granulation tissue develops in the lamina propria, the cartilage is fragmented or destroyed, and the muscle is erased or undergoes focal hyperplastic changes. The mucous glands persist longer than other structures. The bronchial arteries often become greatly enlarged, tortuous, and thick-walled.[129] Anastomoses between them and branches of the pulmonary artery develop along the bronchi of the fourth order. The changes in the lung parenchyma vary from none to advanced organizing pneumonia. Multiple small solid foci of proliferating spindle cells may be seen microscopically in association with saccular bronchiectasis.[125] These formations, traditionally known as *tumourlets*, represent nodular hyperplasia of Kultschitsky's type neuroendocrine cells and are histogenetically related to carcinoid tumors (see p. 312).

Various immunologic abnormalities have been reported in patients with bronchiectasis, and several types of immune-mediated diseases have been shown to be associated with this disease.[128]

Complications of bronchiectasis such as bronchopleural fistula with empyema, brain abscess, and amyloidosis are no longer frequent. At present, conservative medical treatment for the cases with an infectious etiology is sufficient

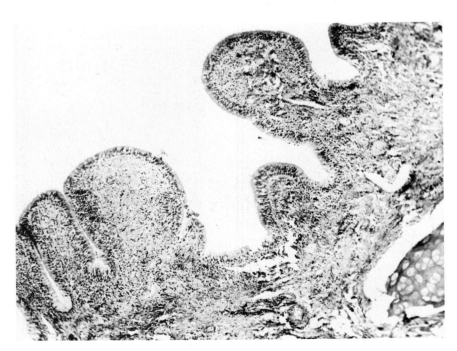

Fig. 7-48 Bronchiectasis, in which epithelium is still present, showing diffuse chronic inflammation, absence of muscle layer, and fragmented bronchial cartilage.

to control the disease in most instances. Surgical resection is indicated in patients with predominantly unilateral disease and in those with hemorrhage and/or repeated pulmonary infections.

Abscess

In the pre-antibiotic era, solitary lung abscesses often followed tonsillectomies and other ENT operations. Presently, most lung abscesses follow the aspiration of foreign material or represent secondary infections of lung carcinomas (Fig. 7-49). Embolism from distant sources does not cause unilocular abscesses but can cause multiple bilateral abscesses.

The most common locations of lung abscesses are the right lower lobe, the right upper lobe (particularly the subapical segment), and the left lower lobe, in that order of frequency[134,135] (Fig. 7-50). The apical segment of the lower lobes is particularly vulnerable in patients who must assume a supine position. Anaerobic organisms are the agents most commonly responsible.[135]

Chronic abscesses have thick fibrotic walls and are surrounded by areas of organizing pneumonia. The bronchi communicating with them show prominent bronchiectasis. Lung abscesses and other long-standing pulmonary cavities

may be complicated by the growth of fungi, particularly *Mucor* and *Aspergillus* (Fig. 7-51). For small unilocular abscesses, partial resection of the lobe may be curative.[136] However, in most cases lobectomy is preferable because complications such as bronchopleural fistula and empyema are much less frequent.

Complications of untreated lung abscesses include spread of the process to other portions of the lung, massive hemorrhage, bronchopleural fistula with empyema, and brain abscess.

Granulomatous inflammation

A large number of granulomatous processes involve the lung; some of them radiographically and grossly simulate a neoplastic process. Often, microscopic examination is insufficient to establish a specific diagnosis; therefore, it is important to submit a sample for bacteriologic and mycologic examination and to perform stains for mycobacteria and fungi in the sections in every case.[137,138]

Tuberculosis

The material received in the pathology laboratory in cases of pulmonary tuberculosis may be a biopsy obtained with the fiberoptic bronchoscope,[143] material procured via fine

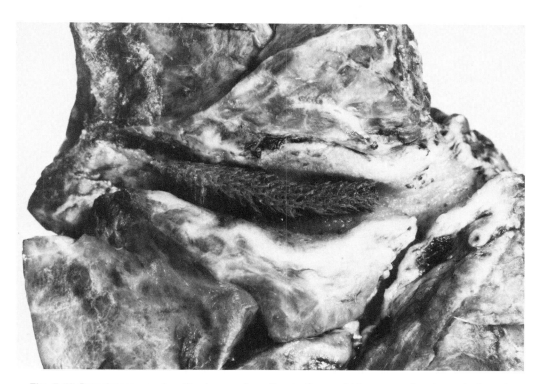

Fig. 7-49 Bronchopneumonia with abscess formation in 2-year-old boy secondary to aspiration of foreign body (Timothy grass inflorescence). (From Kissane JM: Pathology of infancy and childhood, ed. 2. St. Louis, 1975, The C.V. Mosby Co.) First recorded case of this condition seems to be that recorded in book entitled *Some account of Lord Boringdon's accident on July 21st, 1817, and its consequences* as follows: "In 1662, Armand de Boutree, son of the Compte de Nogent, was seized with a violent fever, accompanied by a great difficulty in breathing, a dry cough, afterwards spotting of blood, sleeplessness, and great pain in the right side. A tumor at length appeared on that side, and a surgeon extracted from it an ear of barley almost entire which was quite green and had undergone no change."

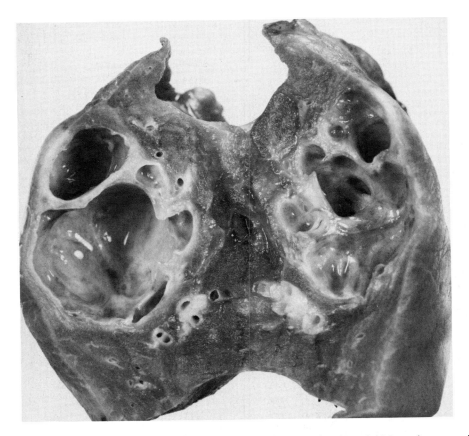

Fig. 7-50 Chronic abscess of right lower lobe of lung in child following 2-week history of pneumonia. Abscess is well delimited with smooth walls.

needle aspiration,[141] an open-lung biopsy,[146] or a surgical specimen. Despite the use of modern drugs, there is still an appreciable number of patients who, because of inadequate response to drug therapy, become candidates for surgery. Most of the surgical procedures done at the present time for tuberculosis are resectional—wedge excision, subsegmental resection, lobectomy, and pneumonectomy. Strieder et al.[149] summarized the indications for pulmonary resection as follows:

  1 Open cavity (with or without positive sputum) after a suitable period (4 to 6 months) on a satisfactory drug regimen
  2 Residual caseous or fibrocaseous disease, with or without positive sputum
  3 Irreversible destructive lesion, such as bronchostenosis or bronchiectasis
  4 Recurrent or persistent hemorrhage, usually arising in a cavity or bronchiectasis
  5 Thoracoplasty failure
  6 Unexpandable lobe or lung, with associated chronic encapsulated tuberculous empyema
  7 Suspected neoplasm

In most reported series of surgically treated tuberculous patients, 80% to 85% have inactive disease 2 to 5 years after surgery. Most complications of surgery, such as bronchopleural fistula, occur in patients with positive sputum preoperatively.[145]

Grossly, most of the tissue resected consists of inflamed, fibrotic, and otherwise nonfunctioning lung parenchyma. Bronchial involvement may lead to stricture formation, with distal bronchiectasis, atelectasis, and superimposed infection [147] (Figs. 7-52 and 7-53). The bronchiectatic changes are more often accompanied by extensive active tuberculosis in the lower than in the upper lobe because of differences in drainage. Peribronchial tuberculous lymph nodes may infect the bronchial mucous glands by direct extension or penetrate the bronchial wall and erode into the lumen, especially when these nodes are calcified.

Tuberculous cavities removed in patients following prolonged antimicrobial therapy may show healing by the process of approximation of the walls, granulation tissue, fibrosis, and the formation of a stellate scar.[151] In other patients, the lesion stabilizes as a chronic open cavity. Potential danger exists when this healing occurs with inspissation of caseous material, because of the long-term persistence of viable organisms in this material.[139] The most complete form of healing, relatively rare, results in a thin fibrous wall with a smooth surface that has no lining except for a short squamous segment at the point at which the bronchus enters the cavity (Fig. 7-54).[140,152] Examination of these healed cavities for acid-fast organisms is invariably negative.[150]

Tuberculomas are usually seen in adults and are an expression of tuberculous reinfection rather than a primary Ghon focus. In the series by Steele,[148] tuberculomas made

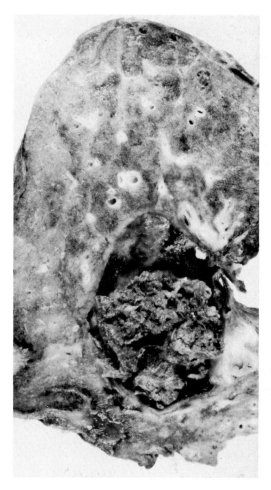

Fig. 7-51 Chronic pulmonary abscess complicated by growth of "fungous ball."

up 25% of the solitary lung granulomas and 14% of all solitary pulmonary nodules. In only 14% of the cases of tuberculoma, there was a previous history of tuberculosis. Grossly, they present as round discrete firm nodules; they are usually solitary and located immediately beneath a white or slightly yellowish pleura. On section the lesions may show concentric laminations, central calcification, or cavitation (Figs. 7-55 and 7-56).[142] Microscopically, there are often persistent areas of caseation, in which acid-fast bacilli may be found. A thick fibrous wall surrounds the caseous center, with a variable number of Langhans' giant cells, epithelioid histiocytes, and lymphocytes in between. There is also prominent subpleural fibrous thickening. Communication of the tuberculoma with a bronchus and small active tubercles may be found in the immediate vicinity of the main lesion.

Tuberculomas are treated surgically because of the difficulty of ruling out malignancy and the fact that they represent the nidus for potential spread of infection.

It should be remarked that there is not a single microscopic feature that is pathognomonic of tuberculosis in any of its forms. The identification of the organism, therefore, is essential for diagnosis. This is usually done by staining the sections with the Ziehl-Neelsen technique, but fluorescent and immunoperoxidase techniques are also available.[144]

Atypical mycobacteriosis

An increasing number of granulomatous infections of the lung is caused by "atypical" or "unclassified" acid-fast mycobacteria.[156] Many of these cases are seen in the immune-compromised host.[153] These infections cannot be distinguished from tuberculosis on the basis of their microscopic appearance, and therefore culture of the organism is required; however, the diagnosis can be suspected from the appearance of the organisms in acid-fast preparations, since

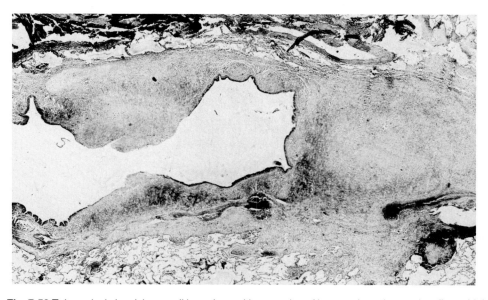

Fig. 7-52 Tuberculosis involving small bronchus, with narrowing of lumen, ulceration, and peribronchial involvement.

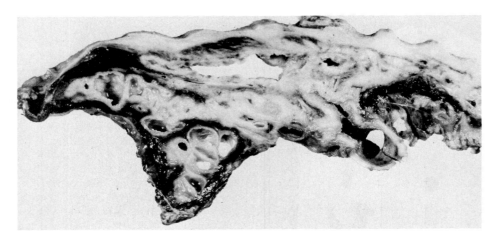

Fig. 7-53 Extensive tuberculosis involving entire left lung with prominent bronchiectasis, cavitation, and thickened pleura. It is obvious that compression therapy cannot cure such lesions.

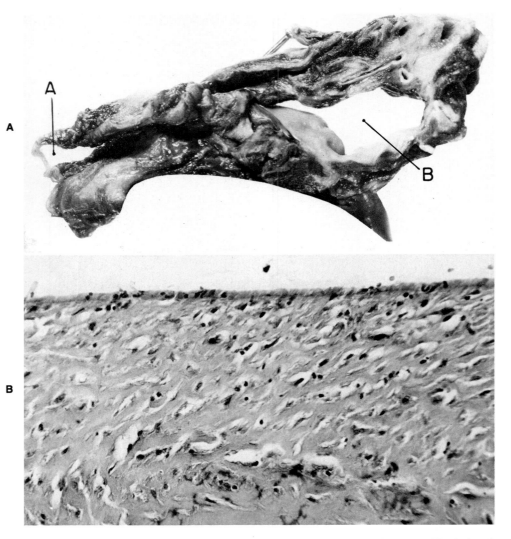

Fig. 7-54 A, Two apparently healed cavities, *A* and *B,* of right middle lobe. **B,** Lining of healed cavity shown in **A.** There is no epithelium and no evidence of activity of process. (**A,** From Auerbach O, Small MJ: The syndrome of persistent cavitation and noninfectious sputum during chemotherapy and its relation to the open healing of cavities; **B,** slide contributed by Dr. O. Auerbach, East Orange, NJ.)

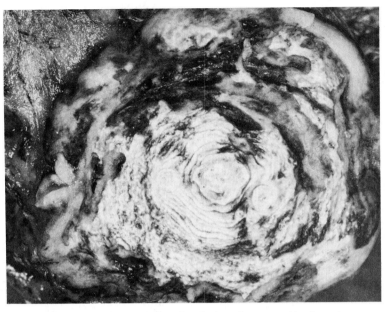

Fig. 7-55 Large granuloma that elevated pleural surface and presented laminated appearance. These laminated lesions often are caused by histoplasmosis.

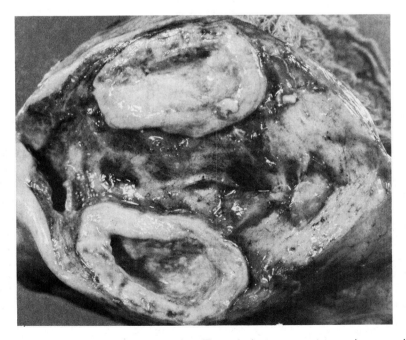

Fig. 7-56 Tuberculoma with central cavitation. These lesions may rupture and cause widespread dissemination.

they tend to be longer (about 20 μm), thicker, more coarsely beaded, and much more bent than tubercle bacilli.[155] The surgical approach follows the same general rules as for tuberculosis.[154]

Sarcoidosis

Sarcoidosis can present in the thoracic cavity in a variety of ways: moderate to marked perihilar node involvement without pulmonary disease, diffuse pulmonary disease without roentgenographic evidence of node involvement, a combination of lymph node enlargement and diffuse pulmonary disease, pulmonary interstitial fibrosis, and localized bronchostenosis with distal bronchiectasis and atelectasis. The great majority of the cases fall into the first and third categories. Microscopically, the hallmark of the disease is a noncaseating granuloma mainly composed of epithelioid cells but also containing Langhans' giant cells and lymphocytes (Fig. 7-57). The latter are predominantly of helper T-cell type, many of which show features of activation.[159] However, there are many variations in this theme.

Hyalinization of the granuloma and diffuse interstitial fibrosis may render the diagnosis difficult. Small foci of necrosis having a bright eosinophilic ("fibrinoid") appearance may be found in the center of some granulomas. Intracellular and extracellular inclusions of several kinds may be seen, but none is specific (see Chapter 21). Most of the granulomas in sarcoidosis are located in the interstitium and seem to be distributed along lymphatic pathways. They are often seen surrounding bronchioles (but not larger bronchi); because of this, transbronchial lung biopsy is positive in more than 80% of the cases.[160] Pleural involvement is less common, in the neighborhood of 10%.[164] The granulomas also can be present around blood vessels and even within the walls of branches of the pulmonary artery and may result in pulmonary hypertension.[163]

Necrotizing sarcoid granulomatosis is the name proposed by Liebow[162] for a pulmonary disease characterized by extensive vascular granulomas that infiltrate, destroy, and occlude pulmonary arteries and veins and are accompanied by widespread necrosis of lung tissue. It is not clear whether this condition is a variant of sarcoidosis or a type of sarcoid-like granulomatous vasculitis, although the former interpretation is favored.[157,158] Most of the patients are female adults and often are asymptomatic. The lesions may be bilateral or unilateral, diffuse or localized. Response to steroid and immunosuppressive drugs is good, and excision of the localized lesion is usually curative.[161]

Wegener's granulomatosis

Wegener's granulomatosis is the better known member of the group of diseases designated as *pulmonary angiitis and granulomatosis*. It is becoming apparent that the latter term comprises a number of totally unrelated entities, and it is doubtful whether it should be retained.[166,168]

Classic Wegener's granulomatosis is characterized by the triad of necrotizing angiitis, aseptic necrosis (both involving the upper respiratory tract and lungs) and focal glomerulitis. If left untreated, it runs an accelerated clinical course[169]; however, it has proved quite responsive to cytotoxic drugs (particularly cyclophosphamide). The main

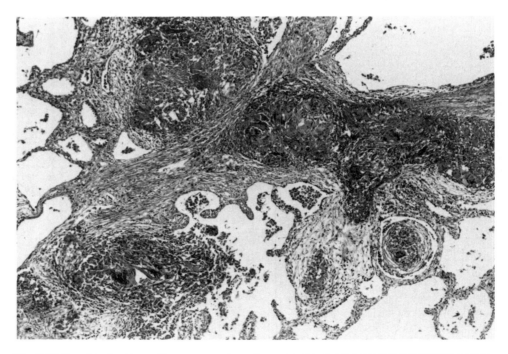

Fig. 7-57 Sarcoidosis of lung. Numerous noncaseating granulomas are present in interstitium, accompanied by fibrosis and nonspecific chronic inflammatory infiltrate, which partially obliterates air spaces.

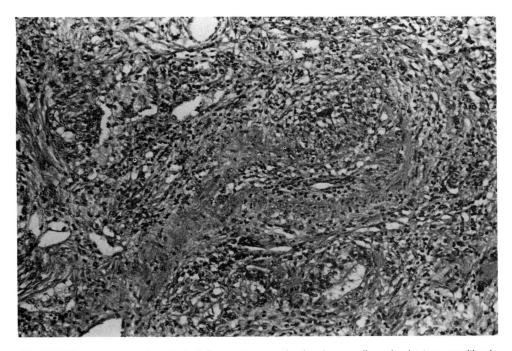

Fig. 7-58 Wegener's granulomatosis. Inflammatory reaction involves medium-sized artery, resulting in nearly complete obliteration of lumen.

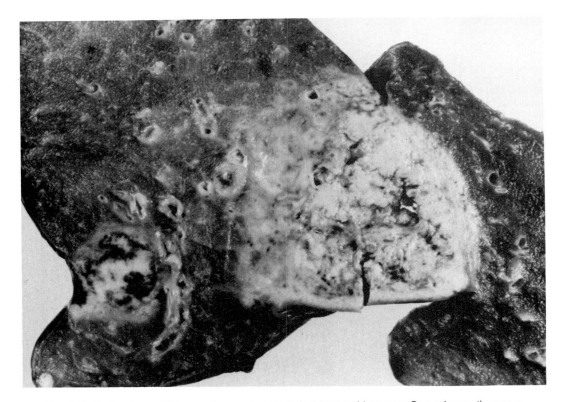

Fig. 7-59 Limited form of Wegener's granulomatosis in 69-year-old woman. Several necrotic granulomatous foci are evident. Largest has infarct-like shape, a feature of diagnostic significance.

morphologic changes in the lungs are liquefactive and/or coagulative necrosis, a large number of eosinophils, scanty benign-appearing lymphocytes and plasma cells, multinucleated giant cells that generally do not form well-defined granulomas as in tuberculosis or sarcoidosis, and a destructive, leukocytolytic angiitis involving arteries and veins[167,173] (Fig. 7-58). A *fulminant type* with a predominance of exudative changes and a *fibrous scar type* with abundant deposition of collagen also exist.[173] In rare cases, the disease is accompanied by diffuse pulmonary hemorrhage.[171]

Limited Wegener's granulomatosis, as described by Carrington and Liebow,[165] is confined to the lungs and has a more protracted clinical course. Specifically, there is no glomerulitis. Steroids and cytotoxic drugs are highly effective. Grossly, there are multiple, bilateral nodules, some round and other infarctlike, frequently located in the lower lobes (Fig. 7-59). Microscopically, the disease is indistinguishable from the classic variety. As in the latter, lymphocytes and plasma cells are scanty, a fact that led Saldana et al.[170] to suggest the alternative term *lymphocyte-depleted angiitis and granulomatosis* for both the classic and the limited forms of Wegener's granulomatosis. Angiitis is a requisite for the diagnosis. However, it should be recognized that vessels located within ordinary infectious (tuberculous or mycotic) granulomas can exhibit secondary inflammatory changes. Therefore, the presence of angiitis away from the areas of necrosis and massive inflammation should be searched for to document the diagnosis. The diagnosis of Wegener's granulomatosis should be made with great cau-

tion, if at all, in granulomas that appear solitary by roentgenographic examination.[172]

Bronchocentric granulomatosis and allergic granulomatosis

Bronchocentric granulomatosis has been defined by Liebow[181] as a pulmonary granulomatous disease in which all or nearly all the granulomas are centered in bronchi and bronchioles, leading to their destruction. Most of his original nine patients were adults, and some were remarkably asymptomatic despite the extensive nature of the process. The lesions are usually solitary and appear on chest roentgenograms as areas of consolidation or atelectasis rather than discrete nodules. The involved bronchi contain an extremely viscous material, which is composed microscopically of a mixture of mucus, neutrophils, and eosinophils, sometimes agglutinated into a dense mass that is surrounded by foreign body giant cells (Fig. 7-60). This condition is always limited to the lungs, in contrast to the pulmonary granulomatous angiitides, which frequently are accompanied by extrapulmonary manifestations.[182] The prognosis is generally favorable.

Cases of bronchocentric granulomatosis occurring in asthmatics tend to contain numerous eosinophils and are usually the result of *allergic bronchopulmonary aspergillosis*[173a]; most of those seen in non-asthmatics show a predominance of neutrophils and the sensitizing agent is usually not identified.[178]

Mucus or *mucoid impaction* is a process in which proximal bronchi become filled with thick inspissated mucus. This

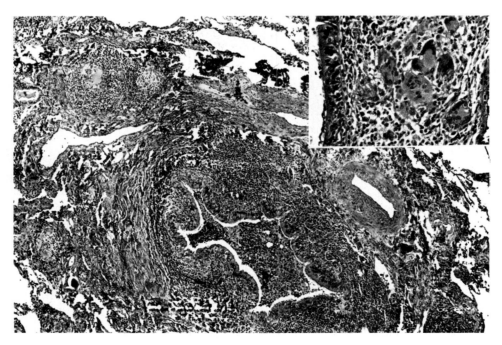

Fig. 7-60 Bronchocentric granulomatosis. Granulomatous infiltrate is seen centered on medium-sized bronchus. **Inset** shows collection of multinucleated giant cells in wall of bronchus.

change, when extensive, may cast a staghorn shadow on the x-ray films.[175] The disease can also involve smaller bronchi and bronchioles. It overlaps microscopically with allergic bronchopulmonary aspergillosis and bronchocentric granulomatosis, but it lacks granulomatous inflammation.[176,183]

Allergic granulomatosis (Churg-Strauss syndrome) presents a clinical picture of systemic vasculitis resembling polyarteritis nodosa but is typically associated with a history of asthma, peripheral eosinophilia (up to 80%), and a high incidence of pulmonary involvement.[174,179]

Microscopically, both the pulmonary and the extrapulmonary lesions are characterized by a prominent eosinophilic infiltrate, foci of necrosis (some associated with eosinophils and some unrelated to them), a granulomatous reaction around some of these necrotic foci, and eosinophilic vasculitis.[177] The disease is very rare, and some authors even doubt that it represents a distinct entity.[180]

Other granulomatous inflammations

Other granulomatous diseases of the lung that may be encountered in biopsies or surgical specimens are those caused by *histoplasmosis*,[189] *blastomycosis, sporotrichosis*,[188] *cryptococcosis*[186,190] *coccidioidomycosis*,[194] *mucormycosis*,[184] *actinomycosis*,[192] and *aspergillosis*.[193] The latter disease may present as a secondary colonization of a lung abscess or some other cavitary process, in the form of allergic bronchopulmonary aspergillosis (see p. 280) or as invasive or necrotizing pulmonary aspergillosis; the latter usually occurs in the immunocompromised host.[185,193] Granulomas may also be seen in eosinophilic pneumonia (see p. 286), bronchial chondromalacia, as a result of exposure to talc in drug abusers through inhalation,[191] from industrial exposure to metal dust,[187] and as an expression of hypersensitivity in the group of disorders known as extrinsic allergic alveolitis (see p. 290).

Interstitial pneumonia

Interstitial pneumonia (interstitial lung disease) is the generic name given to a pattern of pulmonary reaction in which the infiltrate has a predominantly interalveolar or interstitial distribution.[202]

Some cases are the result of viral, mycoplasmal, or chemical pneumonia, whereas others represent the residue of a diffuse granulomatous process. An increasing number of cases are seen following chemotherapy,[223,228] particularly with alkylating agents (such as busulfan,[230] cyclophosphamide[219] and bleomycin[220]). A drug recently added to the list of causative agents is amiodarone, used for the treatment of refractory arrhythmias.[203,222] Some instances of interstitial pneumonia show a pattern of familial incidence suggestive of genetic predisposition,[198] and others are associated with neurofibromatosis[234] or pulmonary veno-occlusive disease (see p. 291). Still others are associated with immune-mediated diseases, such as systemic lupus erythematosus, rheumatoid arthritis, scleroderma, Sjögren's syndrome, chronic active hepatitis, Raynaud's phenomenon, ulcerative colitis, and thyroid disease. In a study of 130 cases of idiopathic interstitial fibrosis, rheumatoid arthritis was found

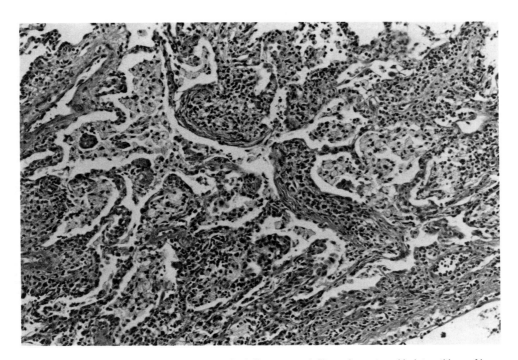

Fig. 7-61 Early phase of interstitial pneumonia. Inflammatory infiltrate is centered in interstitium of lung accompanied by little fibrosis and some outpouring of inflammatory cells in alveolar spaces.

in 18%, transient polyarthritis in 12%, and Sjögren's syndrome in 3%.[233] Approximately 30% of patients with idiopathic interstitial fibrosis have circulating antinuclear antibodies. Immunofluorescent studies in the lung tissue have demonstrated deposition of immunoglobulins and C3,[233] and the presence of circulating immune complexes has been documented in most cases.[204] All these facts suggest that most cases of idiopathic interstitial fibrosis represent a form of immune-complex lung disease.[226]

If the course of the disease is rapid, with death occurring within a matter of weeks or months, the terms *acute interstitial pneumonia* or *Hamman-Rich syndrome* are used.[212] Most of the cases, however, have an insidious onset and a chronic evolution, many of the patients dying of respiratory failure after an average of 4 to 5 years.

In the early stages, the disease is characterized by necrosis, hyaline membrane formation, fibrin deposition, outpouring of inflammatory cells, and hyperplasia of alveolar cells (Fig. 7-61). This combination of changes has been referred to as *diffuse alveolar damage (DAD)*. Mallory body–like structures may be found in the cytoplasm of the alveolar cells,[227] and "blue bodies" may be seen within the alveolar lumina.[215] Foamy macrophages are said to be more common in the cases associated with amiodarone toxicity.[222] Damage to the terminal bronchioles may also be present in the form of bronchiolitis, but this is not a prominent feature (see p. 285). Atypia of the bronchiolar and alveolar epi-

thelium plus squamous metaplasia of the former are particularly pronounced in the cases caused by chemotherapy.[219,230]

Ultrastructural studies suggest that the fibrosis results largely from migration of activated mesenchymal cells through defects in the epithelial lining and its basement membrane, from the interstitial into the intraluminal compartment.[196,200] Other mechanisms that may contribute to the changes are permanent apposition of alveolar walls and incorporation of intra-alveolar exudates.[211]

In the late stages, there is irregular fibrosis, smooth-muscle proliferation, and microcystic formation. *Honeycombing* is a gross descriptive term applied to a localized or diffuse area of coarsening of the lung parenchyma with increased porosity, distinguishable from emphysema by virtue of the fibrosis present and representing the end result of interstitial pneumonia or other inflammatory parenchymal disorders, such as histiocytosis X (Figs. 7-62 and 7-63). It should be regarded neither as an entity nor as indicative of a specific lung disease.

The term *bronchiolar emphysema* has been used inappropriately for this condition in the past. There is no evidence that honeycombing is ever of congenital origin. The superior portions of the upper and lower lobes are the most common sites of involvement. Atypical foci of acinar and squamous proliferation are often seen in late stages of honeycombing. Meyer and Liebow[221] consider this a precancerous change, in view of its frequent association with ma-

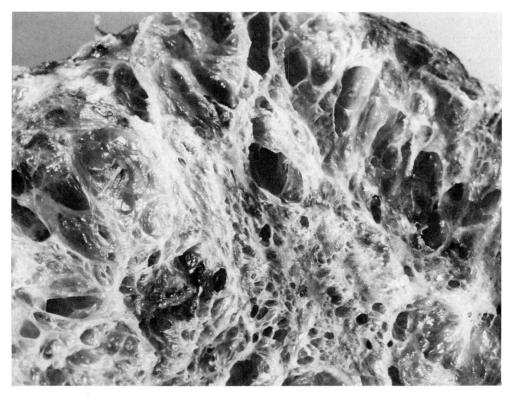

Fig. 7-62 Extensive honeycombing of right upper lobe in 63-year-old woman who had associated adenocarcinoma. Regional lymph nodes were negative.

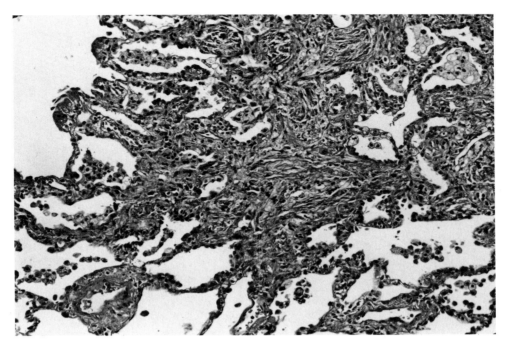

Fig. 7-63 Later phase of interstitial pneumonia. There is extensive deposition of collagen in interstitium, leading to progressive obliteration of air spaces.

lignant tumors, particularly adenocarcinomas. Several cases of carcinoma arising in lungs with diffuse interstitial fibrosis have been reported.[207,214]

Liebow[216] proposed to divide interstitial pneumonia into four more or less distinct varieties on the basis of their morphologic features. According to this scheme, the process previously described constitutes the usual or classic type of interstitial pneumonia (UIP). *Desquamative interstitial pneumonia* (DIP) is characterized by a filling of the alveolar spaces by large mononuclear cells, associated with relatively minor interstitial changes[208,218] (Fig. 7-64). In cases examined electron microscopically, the desquamated cells have features of macrophages rather than of granular pneumocytes, although hyperplasia of the latter is present in the alveolar wall. Necrosis, hyaline membranes, and fibrin are absent. Roentgenographically, a ground-glass type of opacification is seen bilaterally in the periphery of the lung bases. Most cases are seen in adults, but pediatric cases also have been reported.[229] Good response to steroids was noted by Liebow et al[218] in their original series of eighteen patients.

Lymphoid or *lymphocytic interstitial pneumonia* is characterized by a lymphocytic infiltrate, often admixed with histiocytes and plasma cells, occupying the lung interstitium.[209,217] Serum immunoglobulin abnormalities may be present. A third of the cases have been associated with Sjögren's syndrome.[197] The roentgenographic appearance is that of consolidation and perivascular infiltrative densities.[210] Response to steroids is poor.

The differential diagnosis includes *follicular bronchitis and bronchiolitis,* a nonspecific inflammatory reaction in which reactive germinal centers are seen adjacent to airways in the absence of chronic obstructive pulmonary disease.[235] It also includes well-differentiated lymphocytic lymphoma (see p. 322), a difficult problem further complicated by the occasional instances of lymphoma developing in cases of long-standing lymphoid interstitial pneumonia.[195]

Giant cell interstitial pneumonia is the rarest form of interstitial pneumonia. As the name indicates, it contains multinucleated giant cells mixed with the other inflammatory components.

Scadding and Hinson[224,225] use the pathogenetically more satisfactory term *diffuse* or *cryptogenic fibrosing alveolitis* to designate this group of conditions. They consider Liebow's UIP and DIP, which they call the "mural type" and the "desquamative type" of diffuse fibrosing alveolitis, respectively, as the opposite ends of a continuous spectrum rather than as two separate entities.[205] Specifically, the proposal is that DIP represents the cellular phase of fibrosing alveolitis.[201,231] Regardless of which viewpoint is correct, it seems clear that it is worthwhile to separate the two conditions in view of their different course and response to therapy. In the series of Carrington et al.,[199] the mortality in DIP was 27.5% and mean survival 12.2 years, in contrast with 66% and 5.6 years in UIP.

Without treatment, 21.9% of the patients with DIP but none with UIP improved. With corticosteroid therapy, 61.5% with DIP and only 11.5% with UIP improved, whereas 27% and 69.2% worsened, respectively. Other series have shown a closer correlation with patient's age, duration of symptoms, functional and radiographic findings, and initial response to steroid therapy than with differences in microscopic appearance.[232]

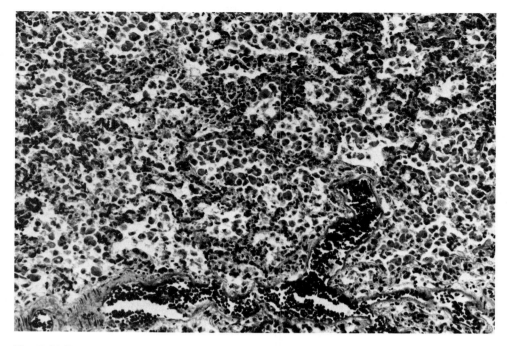

Fig. 7-64 Desquamative interstitial pneumonia. Numerous macrophages are seen within alveolar spaces, accompanied by little interstitial inflammation.

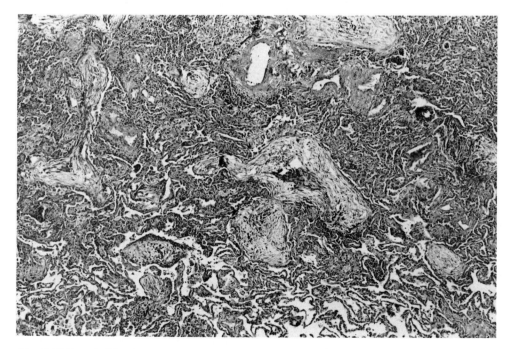

Fig. 7-65 Broncholitis obliterans organizing pneumonia. Cellular mesenchymal proliferation is seen expanding lumen of several bronchioles accompanied by some interstitial changes in surrounding parenchyma.

Bronchiolitis obliterans organizing pneumonia is a term recently proposed for a pulmonary lesion that has been traditionally included among the interstitial pneumonias.[206,213] Clinically, it has a more acute onset, often associated with fever. Radiographically, it has a more patchy distribution. Microscopically, bronchiolitis obliterans refers to the presence of granulation tissue plugs within the lumen of small airways, sometimes associated with descrition of the walls and extending into the alveolar ducts (Fig. 7-65). The interstitium is spared. The prognosis is much better than for the usual interstitial pneumonia.[206,213]

Organizing pneumonia

Pneumonia is not usually considered a surgical problem. However, if the disease—instead of resolving—organizes, shadows occurring in the lung may be mistaken for tumor (Fig. 7-66). The patients present with cough, hemoptysis, and weight loss, further suggesting the existence of a malignant process.[236]

Grossly, the involved area is sharply outlined and very firm, but the pattern of the lung persists. The process extends to the pleura, which is invariably thickened. Microscopically, there is an exudate in various degrees of organization, sometimes accompanied by necrotizing changes in the bronchi. Bacteriologic study has not been rewarding. The variant of this process known as bronchiolitis obliterans organizing pneumonia has been discussed in the preceding section.

Lipoid pneumonia

Lipoid pneumonia is often a complication of debilitating disease found as an incidental postmortem finding. However, the local expression of this process may be confused with a malignant neoplasm and consequently may become a surgical problem.

Lipoid pneumonia can be divided into two types: exogenous and endogenous. In the *exogenous* type, now seen only rarely, lipoid material from nasal sprays or other sources reaches the lung through the tracheobronchial tree. The *endogenous* type is associated with bronchial obstruction by carcinoma or some other process; the fat accumulated is of endogenous origin.

Grossly, the lesion is well circumscribed and firm[237] (Fig. 7-67). In the exogenous type, the lymphatic vessels over the surface of the lung are often prominent, suggesting lymphatic permeation by carcinoma, and fat droplets may be seen flowing from the fresh cut surface.[238] Microscopically, both forms exhibit sudanophilic lipoid material, inflammatory cells, proliferating alveolar cells, and young fibroblasts occupying large spaces (Fig. 7-68). There may also be reactive endarteritis. The marked hyperplasia of alveolar

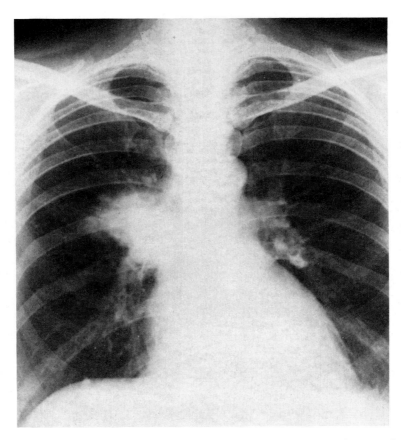

Fig. 7-66 Hilar mass that was considered roentgenographically to be carcinoma but proved pathologically to be organizing pneumonia.

cells and histiocytes may cause confusion in cytology or frozen section interpretation.

Eosinophilic pneumonia

Liebow and Carrington[240] group under the term *eosinophilic pneumonia* all pulmonary infiltrations associated with eosinophilia, as well as infiltrations of the lung by eosinophils with or without peripheral eosinophilia (Fig. 7-69). Histiocytosis X (eosinophilic granuloma) is excluded. The acute form of eosinophilic pneumonia, characterized by fleeting pulmonary infiltrates accompanied by eosinophilia and lasting no more than a month, is commonly referred to as *Löffler's syndrome*. Most cases of eosinophilic pneumonia are of a chronic nature, although the onset can be quite sudden. This is a disease of women, usually between the ages of 20 and 50 years.

Clinically, it is characterized by fever, weight loss, dyspnea, frequent peripheral eosinophilia, and pulmonary infiltrates. The radiographic appearance is very characteristic because of the distinctly peripheral distribution of the infiltrate. The most notable microscopic change is alveolar and interstitial infiltration by eosinophils, but there are also plasma cells and histiocytes. Charcot-Leyden crystals may be found. Occasional features include mild angiitis, granulomatosis with giant cell formation, some fibrosis with organization, mucous plugging, and bronchiolitis with necrosis. It has been described in association with rheumatoid arthritis, polyarteritis nodosa, malignant lymphoma, breast carcinoma, nephrotic syndrome, scleroderma, ulcerative colitis, and hypersensitivity to nitrofurantoin, a drug used in the treatment of urinary tract infection.[239,241]

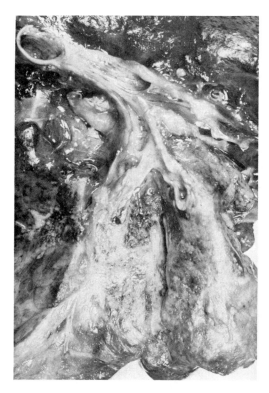

Fig. 7-67 Exogenous lipoid pneumonia producing firm, indurated area that, grossly, was considered to be carcinoma.

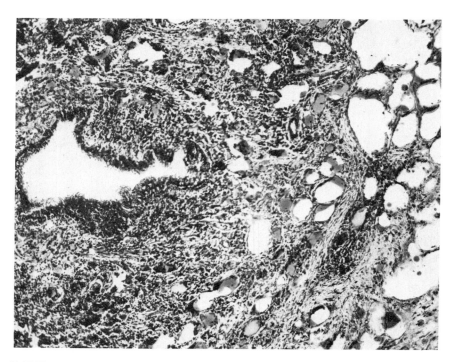

Fig. 7-68 Exogenous lipoid pneumonia demonstrating fibrosis and empty spaces that contained sudanophilic material.

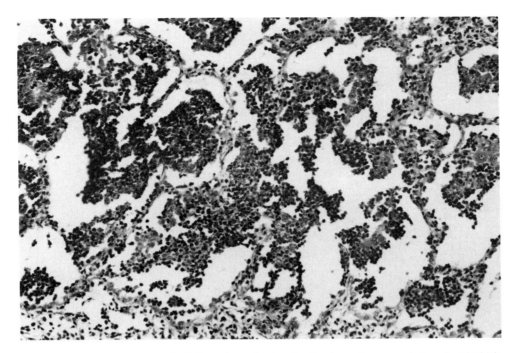

Fig. 7-69 Eosinophilic pneumonia. Infiltrate is predominantly alveolar and composed almost exclusively of mature eosinophils.

Helminths, drugs, *Filaria*, *Dirofilaria*, and especially *Aspergillus* have been identified as the etiologic agents in some of the cases.[242] When chronic eosinophilic pneumonia develops in a patient with longstanding asthma, it is usually on the basis of allergic aspergillosis.[243] If the changes of eosinophilic pneumonia are accompanied by necrotizing vasculitis, there is a good probability of extrapulmonary involvement. In *dirofilariasis*, the presentation may also be in the form of single or multiple subpleural infarcts with a central thrombosed artery containing the parasite.[243a]

Other pneumonias

Pneumocystis carinii pneumonia is a nonbacterial opportunistic infection. Most cases are seen in individuals who are chronically debilitated and immunosuppressed, such as patients receiving therapy for neoplastic disease or patients with AIDS.[248,260,264] The diagnosis depends on the microscopic identification of the organism, since at present there are no reliable microbiologic or serologic tests available.[253] Furthermore, Weber et al.[266] have found that the microscopic features supposed to be characteristic of this infection—i.e., a foamy or honeycombed intra-alveolar exudate accompanied by a lymphoplasmacytic interstitial infiltrate—may be absent (Fig. 7-70). Conversely, they described changes not usually regarded as typical of *Pneumocystis carinii* infection, such as epithelioid granulomas, focal multinucleated giant cells, marked interstitial fibrosis, and severe infiltration by alveolar macrophages.

The organism can be identified in sputum or pulmonary secretions, transbronchial and percutaneous biopsy, and open biopsy performed through a small thoracotomy incision.[261] The specimen should be cultured (to rule out the possibility of other infectious processes), imprints should be taken, and the rest of the tissue should be either fixed in formalin and processed routinely or subjected to frozen section examination.[259] If *Pneumocystis carinii* is present, the imprints will almost invariably be positive. The most reliable stain for detecting the organism is Gomori's methenamine silver (GMS). Its disadvantage has been the fact that in its original description it takes 3 hours to perform; recently, technical modifications that cut down the time to less than 20 minutes have been described.[254] Immunoperoxidase techniques using monoclonal antibodies have also been described.[252a]

The cyst forms of the organism appear with this stain as round structures, up to 5 μm in diameter, containing single or paired discrete "intracystic bodies" measuring 1 to 2 μm.[263,265] Some of the cysts are crumpled and others are collapsed, with a crescentic shape.

Cytomegalovirus pneumonia is usually seen in immunocompromised patients, such as those with AIDS, lymphoid malignancies, transplant recipients, and those receiving cytotoxic drugs. Radiographically, it may present in the form of small (2 to 4 cm) peripherally located nodules, as an acute miliary pattern, or as a diffuse interstitial process. Coalescence and consolidation may occur. Microscopically, a predominantly mononuclear inflammatory infiltrate is seen in conjunction with edema and hyperplasia of the alveolar epithelium. In the diffuse pattern, these changes are associated with spheric areas of hemorrhagic necrosis. Viral inclusion bodies can be detected in most but not all of the cases (Fig. 7-71). These are found both in the nucleus and

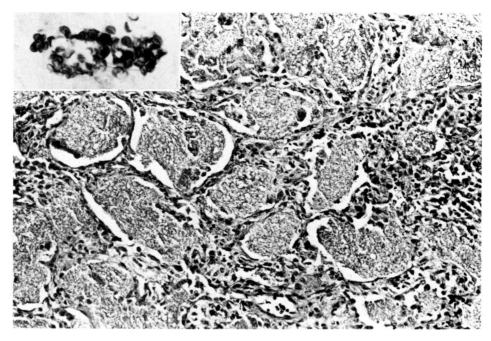

Fig. 7-70 *Pneumocystis carinii* pneumonia. Frothy exudate fills alveolar spaces and is accompanied by mild degree of interstitial inflammation. **Inset** shows organisms stained with Grocott technique.

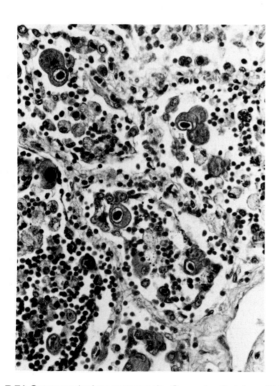

Fig. 7-71 Cytomegalovirus pneumonia. Several cells lying within alveolar spaces contain typical intranuclear inclusions.

in the cytoplasm. The latter are stained with both PAS and GMS, a fact that may lead to a mistaken diagnosis of *Pneumocystis carinii* pneumonia.[250]

Herpes simplex pneumonia may result in an interstitial process with mononuclear inflammation and alveolar cell hyperplasia, or in a necrotizing bronchopneumonia.[251] Intranuclear viral inclusions can be found at the edge of the necrotic areas, but they are less numerous than in cytomegalovirus pneumonia.

Adenovirus pneumonia has a more characteristic microscopic appearance, by virtue of the combination of smudged nuclei, bricklike intranuclear inclusions in epithelial cells, and bronchiolitis obliterans.[244,245,262]

Legionnaires' disease became an instant media sensation in 1976, when it occurred in a small epidemic form among persons attending a convention in a hotel in downtown Philadelphia.[247] It turns out that this is anything but a new disease; apparently, sporadic cases have been seen by the thousands over the previous decades.[246] Occasionally, an open or transbronchial lung biopsy is performed in these patients. Microscopically, the process is characterized by intra-alveolar accumulation of neutrophils, macrophages, and fibrin.[268] In this respect, it does not differ much from lobar pneumococcal pneumonia. However, many cases also show a leukocytoclastic neutrophilic inflammatory infiltrate, small vessel vasculitis, and necrosis.[269] The Dieterle silver impregnation stain has proved to be the most reliable for identifying the responsible organism, a short Gram-negative bacillus. Involvement of the hilar lymph nodes occurs in

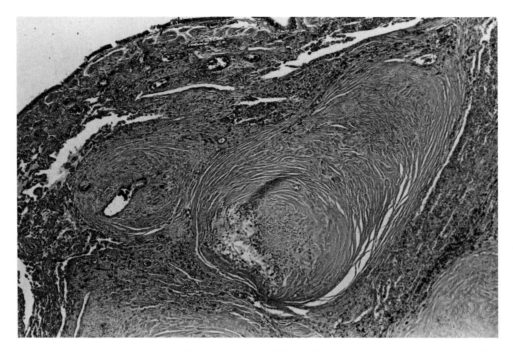

Fig. 7-72 Silicotic nodule in lung. Nodule has dense fibrohyaline appearance and is surrounded by moderated nonspecific chronic inflammation. Silica particles were identified on examination with polarized light.

nearly half of the autopsied cases, and in about one quarter of the cases there is hematogenous spread to other organs.[267]

Nocardiosis is another opportunistic lung infection, whose frequency appears to be increasing.[256] Approximately one half of the patients have been treated with organ transplantation, immunosuppression, steroids, or chemotherapy.[249,257] The diagnosis may require an open lung biopsy. Microscopically, the picture is that of a focal bronchopneumonia, with formation of microabscesses and ill-defined granulomas. Gram stain shows slender, slightly beaded, branching filamentous bacilli.

Mycoplasma pneumoniae pneumonia. formerly known as *atypical pneumonia,* is dominated by bronchiolitis and shifting pulmonary infiltrates. Parenchymal disease takes the form of both interstitial and intra-alveolar involvement; it presents as a pneumonia or bronchopneumonia and may be accompanied by regional lymph node involvement.[255] Microscopically, there is a nonspecific neutrophilic infiltrate in the bronchiolar lumina, bronchiolar metaplasia, lymphoplasmacytic infiltrate in the bronchial wall, and hyperplasia of granular pneumocytes.[258]

Malakoplakia of the lung is very rare; its microscopic appearance is the same as in other locations.[252]

Lung in AIDS

Pulmonary disease occurs frequently during the course of AIDS and often necessitates bronchoalveolar lavage, transbronchial biopsy, or open lung biopsy for appropriate management.[270,271] The open lung biopsy gives the highest

diagnostic yield, but the combination of lavage and transbronchial biopsy comes very close to these figures.[274,276] The abnormalities that can be seen in this background include cytomegalovirus pneumonia, *Pneumocystis* pneumonia, atypical mycobacteriosis and tuberculosis, candidiasis, toxoplasmosis, cryptococcosis, histoplasmosis, blastomycosis, and Kaposi's sarcoma, often in combination.[275,277a] Sometimes the morphologic changes are nonspecific, the features being those of usual, desquamative, or lymphocytic interstitial pneumonia.[272,273,277]

Lung in bone marrow transplantation

Most nonleukemic deaths following bone marrow transplantation are caused by graft-versus-host disease and interstitial pneumonia. The incidence of the latter ranges from 20% to 50%, with a fatality rate of 50% to 70%. The most common type is infectious, with cytomegalovirus as the most frequently encountered pathogen.[278] The other, labeled idiopathic, probably results from pulmonary toxicity of chemotherapy and irradiation, although the possibility has been suggested that some cases represent the pulmonary manifestation of graft-versus-host disease.[279]

Anthracosis and silicosis

Anthracosis refers to the presence of carbon particles in the lung and it is not a pathologic condition *per se.* The particles are concentrated around bronchovascular bundles, in interlobular septa, and beneath the pleura i.e., along the lymphatic vessel network. Carbon is relatively inert and even if present in large amounts, it elicits little or no fibrosis.

Silicosis results from the deposition in the lung of particles of silica (quartz, silicon dioxide). The lesions are characterized by micronodular scars along the lymphatic network, particularly around bronchovascular bundles. Early lesions appear as cellular nodules composed of fibroblasts and histiocytes containing abundant silica particles; older nodules are less cellular and hyalinized (Fig. 7-72). They may fuse to produce large masses, undergo necrosis, and cavitate. The edges of the nodule have a characteristic stellate shape. The arteries often show intimal and medial thickening.

The silica particles are best demonstrated under polarized light. They appear as birefringent spicules with pointed ends, 5 μm or less in length. They may be found intracellularly or extracellularly. It should be emphasized that the mere presence of silica particles in a lung specimen does not establish the diagnosis of silicosis. Such a diagnosis should be reserved for those cases showing silica in association with the characteristic fibrous scars.[280]

Asbestosis

The chemical and environmental features of asbestos fibers and the pleural manifestations of the disease are discussed on p. 265. In the lung parenchyma, asbestosis manifests in the early stages by interstitial pneumonia with predominantly "mural" or desquamative features. Hyperplastic alveolar cells may contain intracytoplasmic Mallory's hyaline, a finding that is not specific for this disorder.[281] In later stages, the interstitial fibrosis becomes more diffuse and results in honeycomb lung. The involvement is more prominent in the basal segments. The morphologic features are not specific, and the diagnosis of asbestosis therefore requires the identification of asbestos bodies in the lesions, either by conventional microscopy, electron microscopy, or incineration. The typical asbestos body is a long, thin, symmetric beaded structure with bulbous ends. It is usually straight but it may be bent or branched. Its core is translucent, and its coat brown because of the iron content.

Extrinsic allergic alveolitis

Extrinsic allergic alveolitis (hypersensitivity alveolitis) is the generic term given to an inflammatory process centered in the alveoli and representing a tissue reaction to an inhaled allergen.[282a,283,284] Patients suffering from this condition have both cellular and humoral immune processes directed against the organic particulate. In a typical case, fever and dyspnea develop a few hours after inhalation of the material. With repeated exposures, a chronic lung disease develops.

Microscopically, there is interstitial and intra-alveolar alveolitis with a predominance of lymphocytes, granulomas, intra-alveolar "buds" made up of fibroblasts and other mesenchymal cells, and fibrosis.[283]

Some of the diseases included in this category are farmer's lung, maple-bark stripper's lung, pigeon-breeder's lung, budgerigar-fancier's lung, and mushroom-picker's lung. Thermophylic actinomycetes from air conditioners or humidifiers can produce acute pulmonary infiltrates or a chronic granulomatous process.[282]

Silo-filler's disease should be clearly separated from the aforementioned group, since it is a form of chemical pneumonitis secondary to nitrogen dioxide inhalation and is not characterized by the presence of granulomas.

Histiocytosis X

Histiocytosis X (eosinophilic granuloma) of the lung is most commonly seen in the third and fourth decades of life.[287] It can be circumscribed or diffuse.[289] It predominates

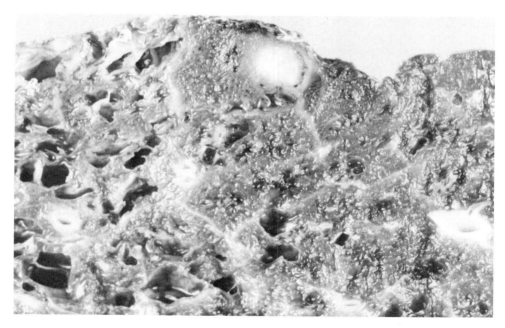

Fig. 7-73 Eosinophilic granuloma of lung. Small solid subpleural nodule is associated with extensive honeycombing of adjacent parenchyma.

in the upper lobes and can produce nodular as well as cavitary lesions. Honeycombing of the lung is a characteristic feature in the late stage of the disease (Fig. 7-73). In approximately 20% of the patients, there is associated extrapulmonary involvement, usually in bones or the pituitary region. Spontaneous pneumothorax is a common complication. Microscopically, there is a compact interstitial infiltrate, often subpleural, composed of Langerhans' cells, numerous eosinophils, and reactive mesothelial cells (Fig. 7-74). Langerhans' cells are the most important element for the diagnosis; they have an abundant acidophilic cytoplasm and a vesicular nucleus, with typical grooves and indentations (however, similar grooves also can be seen in reactive mesothelial cells). Hemosiderin deposition and foci of necrosis are common.[291] Vasculitis may be present. In the healing stage, the disease may be no longer diagnosable microscopically. In these instances, immunohistochemical staining for S-100 protein, HLA-DR, and OKT6 can be very helpful.[288,293,294] These stains can also be applied to cells from bronchoalveolar lavage fluid.[286]

The typical microscopic appearance of eosinophilic granuloma can be obscured by a superimposed infection, such as *Pneumocystis carinii* pneumonia; in these cases, electron microscopic search for Langerhans' granules may be necessary to document the diagnosis.[290] Another source of confusion is *"reactive eosinophilic pleuritis,"* an apparently nonspecific reaction to pleural injury that may closely simulate eosinophilic granuloma because of the mixture of eosinophils and mesothelial cells (which can look very similar to the Langerhans' cells) (Fig. 7-75); in contrast to true eosinophilic granuloma, this lesion lacks interstitial lung disease by roentgenographic examination and Langerhans' granules by electron microscopic examination.[285] In most patients with eosinophilic granuloma of the lung, the disease resolves or stabilizes, with few or no residual foci. A few patients develop progressive pulmonary disease that is ultimately fatal.[289]

Four cases of co-existent pulmonary histiocytosis X and carcinoma have been reported, but it is not clear whether the two processes are pathogenetically related.[292]

Vascular diseases

Open lung biopsies are sometimes performed in patients with congenital heart disease and pulmonary hypertension in order to decide whether the state of the pulmonary vessels would allow corrective surgery.[295,299] Sections should be examined after hematoxylin-eosin and elastic tissue stains. The status of the arteries, veins, lymphatics, and lung parenchyma should be evaluated. Wagenvoort[301] considers pulmonary vascular disease reversible when the arterial lesions are restricted to medial hypertrophy, intimal thickening on the basis of longitudinal smooth muscle, post-thrombotic intimal fibrosis, or cellular intimal proliferation. Concentric-laminar intimal fibrosis of moderate or severe degree probably does not regress. Fibrinoid necrosis and/or plexiform lesions are regarded as contraindications to surgery unless the nature of the defect is such that one lung is spared.

Pulmonary veno-occlusive disease predominantly affects children and adolescents, especially females.[296,300] Pulmonary hypertension is present because of the widespread

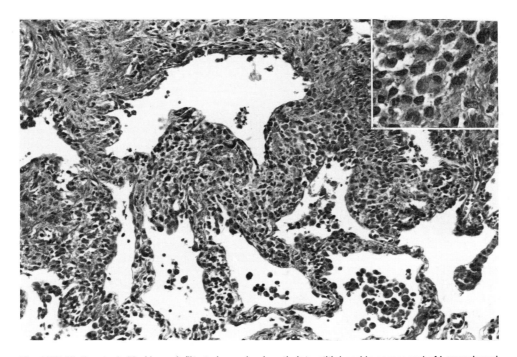

Fig. 7-74 Histiocytosis X of lung. Infiltrate is predominantly interstitial and is composed of Langerhans' cells, lymphocytes, and eosinophils. Characteristic features of Langerhans' cells are better seen in **inset**.

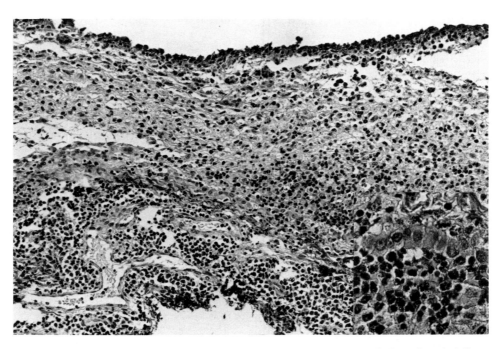

Fig. 7-75 Reactive eosinophilic pleuritis. Beneath hyperplastic pleural mesothelium, there is infiltrate composed of lymphocytes, eosinophils, and histiocytes. This reactive lesion can be confused with histiocytosis X. Inset shows cluster of histiocytes covered by row of reactive mesothelial cells.

occlusion of many large and medium-sized branches of the pulmonary veins, accompanied by recanalization and pseudoangiomatous changes.[302] Arterial thickening, as well as prominent hemosiderosis, also are present.[298] The etiology of the disease is unknown; an influenza-like illness has been found to precede many cases of this condition, and an immune-complex pathogenesis has been suggested.[297]

Other non-neoplastic diseases

Arteriovenous fistulas (aneurysms) are roentgenographically discernible, frequently multiple, and occur often in the right lower and middle lobes (Figs. 7-76 and 7-77). These probably congenital lesions are made up of large vascular channels with arteriovenous communications.[319] Microscopically, the vessels are abnormal, often showing deficiencies and excesses of muscle, which make it impossible to distinguish artery from vein. Because of the shunt, there are bruit, cyanosis, polycythemia, and low oxygen content of arterial blood. Excision is curative.

Broncholithiasis can be seen as a complication of food aspiration, bronchiectasis, or granulomatous diseases (particularly tuberculosis and histoplasmosis).[304,315] The term *broncholith* has been used for any calcification that impinges upon and distorts a bronchus. Others prefer to restrict the term to a calcified tissue fragment that is found floating within the bronchial lumen.

Infarcts are usually identified as such on roentgenographic examination. However, occasionally they simulate a malignant tumor and are resected surgically (Fig. 7-78).

Alveolar proteinosis is perihilar in distribution, roentgenographically resembling the picture of pulmonary edema. It is being increasingly recognized as an important cause of diffuse pulmonary disease in immunocompromised patients.[306] Consequently, it may be regarded as a type of response to alveolar injury rather than as a specific entity. Its occasional coexistence with other conditions, such as nocardiosis, histoplasmosis, cryptococcosis, aspergillosis, tuberculosis, cytomegalovirus infection, and a wide range of hematologic malignancies support this contention.[305,323,327]

Microscopically, the hallmark of the process is the accumulation of an amorphous eosinophilic (but sometimes basophilic) PAS-positive material of predominantly phospholipid nature in the alveolar lumina, associated with some proliferation and desquamation of granular pneumocytes, small lymphoid accumulations in the interstitium, and some degree of fibrosis[324] (Fig. 7-79). The disease seems to be the result of either increased secretion of lamellar bodies by granular pneumocytes or abnormal uptake and handling of lamellar bodies by alveolar macrophages.[325] It is usually treated by whole-lung lavage.[310]

Idiopathic hemosiderosis classically presents in young adults with hemoptysis and refractory anemia.[326] Roentgenograms of the lung often show a granular perihilar infiltrate. Microscopically, large accumulations of hemosiderin-laden macrophages in the alveolar lumina are accompanied by proliferation of alveolar lining cells. Necrosis, vasculitis, granulomas, and lymphoid follicles do not occur, and there are no deposits of IgG on the alveolar basement mem-

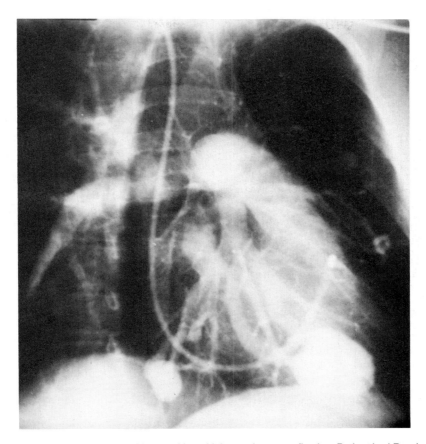

Fig. 7-76 Angiogram of 28-year-old man with multiple arteriovenous fistulas. Patient had Rendu-Osler-Weber syndrome. After left lower lobectomy, oxygen saturation went from 86% to 95%.

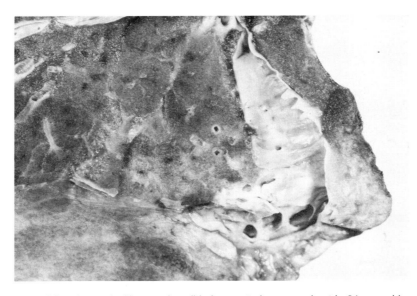

Fig. 7-77 Dilated vessel with smooth wall in large arteriovenous shunt in 24-year-old woman.

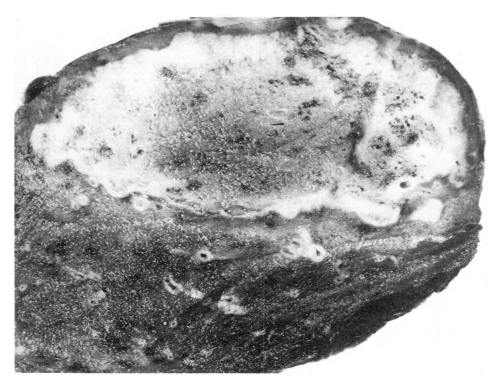

Fig. 7-78 Well-delimited infected infarct in 51-year-old man that was thought possibly to be primary carcinoma.

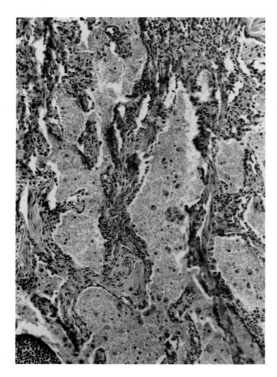

Fig. 7-79 Pulmonary alveolar proteinosis. Alveolar spaces are filled by granular amorphous material with only occasional admixture of histiocytes and other cells. Mild chronic inflammatory infiltrate is present in interstitium.

branes.[309] The latter finding is important in the differential diagnosis with Goodpasture's syndrome, which it may simulate in the routine sections.[303,308] In *Goodpasture's syndrome* there is an associated glomerulonephritis, circulating antiglomerular basement membrane antibodies, and linear deposits of IgG along glomerular and alveolar basement membranes. The differential diagnosis of hemorrhagic lung disorders also includes those diseases known to cause secondary pulmonary alveolar bleeding and hemosiderosis, such as mitral stenosis, periarteritis nodosa, lupus erythematosus, and other forms of systemic vasculitis.[311,317,320]

Hematoma of the lung can present as a distinct round mass that radiographically resembles a neoplasm; it usually develops as a result of blunt trauma to the thorax.[313]

Amyloidosis of the lung can be divided into four categories on the basis of distribution: vascular (never a serious clinical problem), nodular bronchial, nodular parenchymal, and diffuse alveolar septal.[307,318,328] Roentgenographically, lesions in the second and third categories can simulate tuberculosis or a metastatic neoplasm. Lesions of the fourth type lead to a severe impairment of lung function, a diffuse infiltrate upon roentgenographic examination, and a poor prognosis.[318]

Hyalinizing granuloma, a lesion described by Engleman et al.,[312] is usually multiple and bilateral. Microscopically, the central portion undergoes hyalinization and elicits a foreign body response, thus simulating nodular amyloidosis. However, special stains for amyloid are negative. No infectious agents have been identified, and the pathogenesis remains unknown. Four of the cases reported by Engleman et al.[312] were complicated by sclerosing mediastinitis and one by retroperitoneal fibrosis. In another series, more than half of the patients had autoimmune phenomena or previous exposures to mycobacterial or fungal antigens.[330] This suggests that hyalinizing granuloma represents a peculiar immune reaction.

Endometriosis of the lung may present with recurrent catamenial hemoptysis, or as asymptomatic nodules discovered on routine chest x-rays.[316] Most of the reported cases have been located on the right side (see p. 265).

Pulmonary alveolar microlithiasis is a rare disease characterized by the presence of microliths or calcospherites within the alveoli of an otherwise normal lung. The process is diffuse and bilateral, and the clinical course is extremely long. The chest x-ray appearance is virtually diagnostic.[322]

Rheumatoid lung disease can present in a wide variety of patterns: diffuse interstitial fibrosis, bronchiolitis obliterans, coarse scarring, marked arterial sclerosis, necrotizing vasculitis, interstitial lymphocytic infiltration with germinal center formation, nodular fibrosis associated with pneumoconiosis (Caplan's syndrome), juxtabronchiolar microgranulomas, rheumatoid nodules, and pleuritis.[314,321,329] The latter is discussed on p. 265.

CARCINOMA
General features

Carcinoma of the lung has become increasingly frequent during the past 50 years. This is due not only to increased recognition through better radiographic, bronchoscopic, and cytologic techniques but also to an actual rise in incidence. This increase is seen both in male and female patients and is true for all the major microscopic types.

Much has been written about the cause for this increase. Many factors thought in the past to be of pathogenetic importance—such as tuberculosis, tarring of roads, the 1918 influenza epidemic, anthracosis, and anthracosilicosis—are now considered to be totally unrelated to cancer or to account for only a minimal fraction of cases. Exposure to asbestos; polycyclic aromatic hydrocarbons; arsenic, nickel and chromium compounds; BCME; CMME; vinyl chloride; uranium; and other occupational agents undoubtedly accounts for some of the cases.* However, the significance of these factors pales by comparison with the role played by cigarette smoking, both in males and in females.[344] The fact that smokers living in urban areas and/or exposed to asbestos are at a higher risk for lung carcinoma than others suggests the potentiating effect of air pollution and asbestos upon the carcinogenic effect of tobacco, a possibility that is supported by some experimental models.[338] Interestingly, there is a nearly total absence in animals of spontaneous lung tumors that are histologically similar to the smoking-related human lung cancers.[340]

The relationship of cigarette smoking with malignant and premalignant alterations of the tracheobronchial tree has also been thoroughly documented by the meticulous histologic observations of Auerbach et al.[332]; at autopsy they found an almost linear correlation between the severity of the changes and the degree of cigarette consumption.

Another factor thought to be related to the development of carcinoma is pulmonary fibrosis, through a preceding stage of atypical proliferation of the terminal bronchiolar epithelium. Malignant tumors arising at the site of scars resulting from bullets or other foreign bodies have been well-documented, but these constitute an infinitesimal fraction of lung cancers. In most of the peripheral lung tumors diagnosed as "scar carcinomas," the scar is probably the result rather than the cause of the cancer (see p. 297). A somewhat related problem is that posed by the diffuse fibrosis seen in interstitial lung disease with honeycombing; of 153 resected lung tumors studied by Meyer and Liebow,[347] 22% were associated with—and presumably preceded by—honeycombing and atypical epithelial proliferation. Most of these tumors were in the upper lobe, and one third of them were adenocarcinomas.

A few cases of lung carcinomas have arisen as a malignant transformation of papillomatosis of the respiratory tract.[335]

Lung carcinoma is more common in males than females, but the difference is becoming smaller because of a proportionally higher increase in women. The current male:female ratio is 4:1. More than 90% of the patients are over 40 years old at the time of the diagnosis. Lung carcinoma is multiple in about 5% of the cases and is associated with independent cancer of the head and neck region in about 20% of the cases.[346]

Most lung cancers are of considerable size when first detected, and about 60% are incurable as a result of extensive local spread and/or distant metastases. Symptoms and signs develop relatively late in the course of the disease, are usually related to partial or complete bronchial obstruction, and may lead to confusion with a primary inflammatory process. Peripherally located lesions are clinically silent until they reach a sufficient size to ulcerate into a bronchus or to involve the pleural space. Carcinomas located in the superior pulmonary sulcus result in a clinical picture peculiar to their location, known as *Pancoast's syndrome*.[350] This is characterized by pain in the distribution of the ulnar nerve and is often accompanied by Horner's syndrome secondary to involvement of the sympathetic chain.

Sometimes lung carcinoma presents as a solitary circumscribed mass ("coin lesion") on the chest x-ray of an asymptomatic individual. About 35% to 50% of pulmonary coin lesions in adults represent lung carcinoma.[337,352] The percentage is higher for patients older than 60 years and for noncalcified lesions. The incidence of malignancy in coin lesions exhibiting obvious calcification is less than 1%.[337]

Lung neoplasms are sometimes associated with extrapulmonary manifestations not related to the presence of metastatic disease. Although exceptions occur, there is a fairly good correlation between some morphologic parameters and the systemic effect produced.[354] These are summarized in Table 7-2. These manifestations are caused by the secretion by the tumor of biologically active compounds. Additional substances that have been detected in some cases of lung carcinoma include amylase, calcitonin, CEA, AFP, beta-1-pregnancy-specific glycoprotein, and epidermal growth factor receptors. A preponderance of small cell car-

---

*See references 331, 341, 343, 345, 349, 351, and 353.

Table 7-2 Systemic effects of lung cancer and their relationship with tumor type

Systemic effect and hormone responsible	Tumor type
Cushing syndrome (ACTH)	Small cell carcinoma Bronchial carcinoid
Carcinoid syndrome	Bronchial carcinoid Small cell carcinoma
Hyponatremia (ADH)	Small cell carcinoma
Hyperparathyroidism (parathormone)	Squamous cell carcinoma
Gynecomastia (HCG)	All tumor types
Clubbing of fingers and hypertrophic pulmonary osteoarthopathy	Unrelated to tumor type; mainly dependent on proximity to pleural surface
Mental syndromes (i.e., toxic confusional psychosis)	Small cell carcinoma
Cortical cerebellar degeneration	All tumor types
Encephalomyelitis	Small cell carcinoma
Sensory neuropathy	Small cell carcinoma
Myopathic-myasthenic syndrome	Small cell carcinoma

cinomas exists in this group; however, the correlation between the presence of a tumor marker and the microscopic type is generally poor.*

Pathologic features

Several microscopic classifications of lung carcinoma exist. The one we use has been slightly modified from the classifications of Kreyberg[364] and the World Health Organization[367,367a] and includes the following categories:

1 Squamous cell (epidermoid) carcinoma
  a Well differentiated
  b Moderately differentiated
  c Poorly differentiated
2 Adenocarcinoma
  a Not otherwise specified (NOS)
  b Bronchioloalveolar
3 Adenosquamous carcinoma
4 Small cell carcinoma
  a Oat cell carcinoma
  b Intermediate
5 Undifferentiated large cell carcinoma
6 Giant cell carcinoma

Several independent studies have shown the applicability and reproducibility of this classification and the fact that there is a very close correlation in tumor type between the biopsy specimen, the surgical specimen, and the lymph node metastases.[363] The greater degree of interobserver variability is found in the identification of undifferentiated large cell carcinomas *vis a vis* poorly differentiated adenocarcinomas and poorly differentiated squamous cell carci-

---

*See references 333, 334, 336, 339, 342, 348, and 355.

noma.[358,362] Fortunately, these morphologic distinctions have very few practical implications. Greater specificity will be obtained if ultrastructural examination is carried out in every tumor, but one fails to appreciate the practical value of such a costly effort.[356]

Part of the difficulty in sharply separating lung carcinomas into the previously described categories stems from the fact that many of them will show a combination of patterns.[357] In a study of 100 consecutive cases of lung carcinoma in which either the entire tumor or ten blocks were examined, only 34% were composed of a single histologic type.[365] Early hopes that immunocytochemical determinations would provide a sharper separation into distinct types have not materialized; on the contrary, there is evidence for considerable overlap of antigenic profile between different histologic types.[359,360] At a practical level, one should also realize that the method used to classify the tumors will greatly influence the end results. Thus adenosquamous carcinoma will make a much higher proportion of cases in series studied by electron microscopy than in those based exclusively on routine light microscopy.[361,366]

Squamous cell (epidermoid) carcinoma

Over 80% of squamous cell carcinomas occur in males. Most cases are centered in segmental bronchi (Fig. 7-80) and therefore present as hilar or perihilar masses in chest roentgenograms. However, they can also be found peripherally and even subpleurally. As a group, they are larger than the other types at the time of the diagnosis.[368] Signs of bronchial obstruction, such as obstructive pneumonitis or atelectasis, are found in approximately one half of the patients. The tumors have a special tendency to undergo central necrosis with cavitation. Thus of forty-four tumors with roentgenographically demonstrable cavitation examined by Strang and Simpson,[374] thirty-six were of squamous cell type. On the other hand, calcification is extremely unusual. Rarely, squamous cell carcinoma presents as an intrabronchial polypoid mass with only minor extrabronchial spread.[371]

Microscopically, the diagnosis of malignancy is based on cell atypia and invasiveness, and the diagnosis of squamous cell type on the detection of keratin and/or intercellular bridges (Fig. 7-81). Keratin formation may be seen in isolated cells or, more commonly, in the form of "keratin pearls." Isolated necrotic cells should not be confused with keratinized cells. Whorl formation and definite stratification of tumor cells have been used by some as presumptive evidence of squamous differentiation in the absence of the above features, but according to the WHO classification these tumors should be placed in an undifferentiated large cell category.

Electron microscopic examination shows abundant tonofilaments and complex desmosomes (Fig. 7-82).[370] Immunohistochemically, there is reactivity for high-molecular–weight keratin and for involucrin.[372,373] The latter is a precursor of the cross-linked envelope protein or marginal band present in human stratum corneum. The bronchial mucosa adjacent to the tumor usually shows squamous metaplasia and sometimes carcinoma in situ, occasionally extending several centimeters from the main mass.[369]

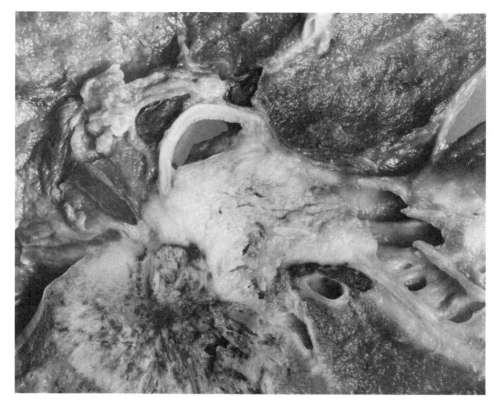

Fig. 7-80 Bronchial carcinoma arising in major bronchus. Tumor replaces portion of bronchial wall and extends into surrounding parenchyma. Organizing pneumonia can be seen peripherally.

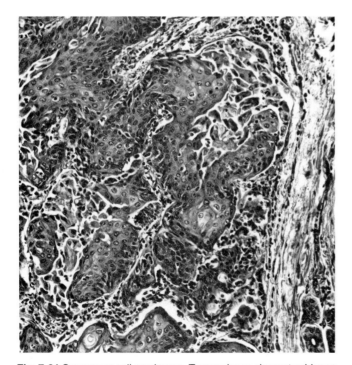

Fig. 7-81 Squamous cell carcinoma. Tumor shows clearcut evidence of keratin formation.

Adenocarcinoma

Adenocarcinomas comprise approximately half of all lung cancers in females, whereas the proportion in males is lower.[379,397] In absolute numbers, however, they are more common in males than in females. There is epidemiologic evidence suggesting that adenocarcinoma is becoming progressively more prevalent as compared to other microscopic types of lung cancer,[386b,396] to the extent that in some recent series it has become the most common form.[381,395] Grossly, adenocarcinomas usually present as poorly circumscribed gray-yellowish lesions. If they secrete mucin, they have a mucoid, glairy appearance. Cavitation is very unusual. About 65% of the cases are located peripherally and 77% involve the visceral pleura at the time of excision (Fig. 7-83) Occasionally, a small peripheral adenocarcinoma spreads massively into the pleural space and coats both pleural layers so as to closely simulate the appearance of diffuse mesothelioma[384] (Fig. 7-84). Even rarer is the presentation of adenocarcinoma as a large endobronchial polypoid mass.[388]

A high percentage of adenocarcinomas arise in association with a peripheral scar or honeycombing and may show foci of atypical acinar proliferation in the neighboring air spaces.[376,391] In a series of eighty-two "scar cancers" reviewed by Auerbach et al.,[375] 72% were adenocarcinomas and 18% were squamous cell carcinomas, the rest being large cell undifferentiated carcinomas. There were no small

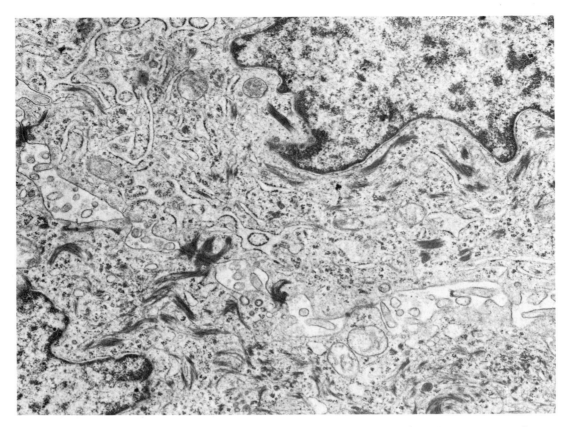

Fig. 7-82 Squamous cell carcinoma of lung. Neoplastic cells with numerous tonofilaments, some of them attached to desmosomes. This is characteristics of squamous differentiation. ($\times$ 16,850.)

cell carcinomas. Some controversy has arisen as to whether the scar precedes the appearance of the carcinoma or whether the fibrosis represents a desmoplastic host reaction to the tumor. Immunophenotyping of the collagen present in the scar suggests that the latter mechanism is the most prevalent.[378,380,389,390]

Microscopically adenocarcinomas exhibit a wide range of differentiation, one extreme blending with bronchiolo-alveolar carcinoma and the other with undifferentiated large cell carcinoma. The two morphologic signs of glandular differentiation, often found together, are formation of tubules or papillae and secretion of mucin (Fig. 7-85). In this context, it should be remembered that lining of tumor cells along alveolar walls, a pattern of growth that many primary or metastatic tumor types may exhibit, can simulate gland formation. A few cases exhibit prominent eosinophilic intracytoplasmic globules.[393a] By electron microscopy, neoplastic counterparts of all the major cells lining the bronchial tree may be found; this includes goblet cells, mucous cells, nonciliated bronchiolar cells, and Clara cells.[382,385,387] Immunohistochemically, there is reactivity for low-molecular-weight keratins, epithelial membrane antigens, CEA, and secretory components.[377,386a,392,393] Sometimes there is coexpression of keratin and vimentin.[394] S-100 protein-positive Langerhans' cells are frequent in the stroma.[383] In about half of the cases there is positivity for surfactant apoprotein, a feature of utility in the differential diagnosis with other types

of primary lung carcinoma and—most important—with metastatic adenocarcinoma.[391a] Lung adenocarcinomas also show consistent expression of Lewis X and Y blood group antigens, a feature that may be of some differential diagnostic value.[386]

Blood vessel invasion was identified by Bennett et al.[379] in 86% of the 100 adenocarcinomas they examined. In the same series, metastases to peribronchial or hilar lymph nodes were found in one half of the patients. The resectability rate was 71%, about twice the overall rates for bronchogenic carcinoma.

Undifferentiated large cell carcinoma

Undifferentiated large cell carcinomas are pleomorphic epithelial tumors without definite evidence of either squamous or glandular differentiation.[405] The tumor cells are large, at least in comparison with those of small cell carcinoma (Fig. 7-86). These tumors probably do not represent a specific entity but are rather poorly differentiated variants of squamous cell carcinoma, adenocarcinoma, and perhaps even small cell carcinoma.[406] Electron microscopic studies have supported this interpretation by demonstrating intracellular and extracellular lumina (as evidence of glandular differentiation) or well-formed desmosomes with numerous tonofilaments (as evidence of squamous cell carcinoma).[398,401,403] The location of these tumors (as seen radiographically) and the combination of ultrastructural and im-

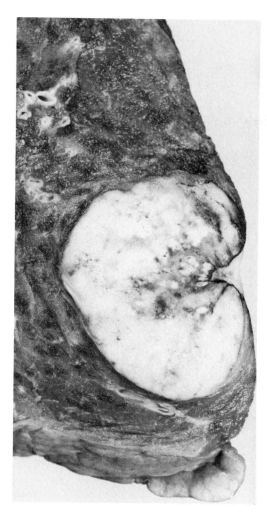

Fig. 7-83 Large peripheral carcinoma with marked pleural retraction. Latter finding is seen much more commonly in primary rather than in metastatic tumors.

munohistochemical features suggests a closer relation to adenocarcinoma than to the other tumor types.[400,402] Some large cell carcinomas are associated with marked peripheral eosinophilia or leukocytosis.[399,404]

Giant cell carcinoma

Giant cell carcinoma is a distinctive and lethal form of lung cancer.[408,409] Bizarre multinucleated giant cells alternate with mononuclear forms in a solid fashion that simulates sarcoma (Fig. 7-87). A heavy neutrophilic infiltration can be seen between and inside the tumor cells and may be accompanied by leukocytosis. Most tumors are peripheral in location and quite extensive at the time of diagnosis. In some cases, foci of glandular differentiation and/or mucin production have been identified; because of this, some authors regard this tumor as a poorly differentiated variant of adenocarcinoma.[407] Others include it with the large cell undifferentiated carcinomas. Because of their distinctive light-microscopic appearance, electron-microscopic features, and behavior, we and others prefer to identify giant cell carcinoma as a specific tumor type.

Clear cell carcinoma

Clear cell carcinoma is defined as a type of lung carcinoma predominantly or exclusively composed of clear cells.[411] This lesion probably does not represent a specific microscopic type of lung cancer.[409,410] Focal or extensive areas of clear cell changes can be seen both in squamous cell carcinoma and adenocarcinoma. These clear cells usually contain abundant glycogen and may also contain mucin. The possibility of metastatic renal cell carcinoma should always be considered in the presence of a lung tumor with a prominent clear cell component.

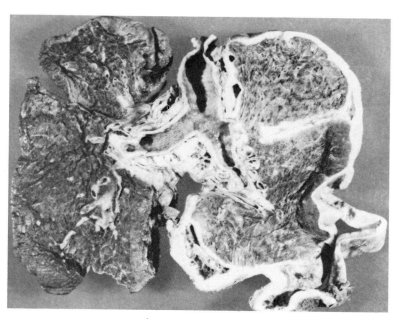

Fig. 7-84 Peripheral adenocarcinoma of lung spreading diffusely to pleural surfaces and closely simulating gross appearance of malignant mesothelioma. Note metastases in perihilar and intertracheobronchial nodes.

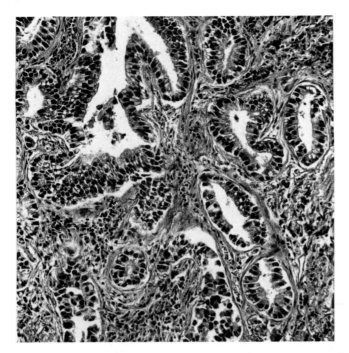

Fig. 7-85 Adenocarcinoma. Tumor is well-differentiated, with most of glands having tubular configuration. Glands were positive for mucin stains.

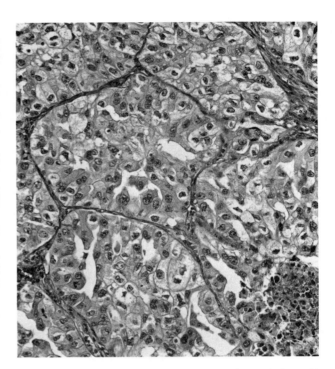

Fig. 7-86 Undifferentiated large cell carcinoma. Tumor is formed by large cells growing in solid nests without evidence of glandular or squamous differentiation.

Bronchioloalveolar carcinoma

Bronchioloalveolar carcinoma can present in a variety of forms that bear an important relationship to its prognosis: a single peripheral nodule, multiple nodules, and a diffuse, pneumonic-like infiltrate[416,419] (Fig. 7-88, *A* and *B*). The latter two forms may involve several lobes or even be bilateral. Grossly, the mass may have a mucoid surface. Often the surgeon is not aware that the lesion is a neoplasm. Microscopically, this tumor is formed by well-differentiated mucin-containing columnar cells that line respiratory spaces without invading the stroma (Fig. 7-89). Intranuclear inclusion bodies can be present[420] (Fig. 7-90). The tumor nodules have a topographic association with bronchioles rather than bronchi. Continuity between tumor cells lining alveoli and the epithelium of respiratory bronchioles or alveolar ducts can be demonstrated.[423] Inflammatory cells, fat-filled macrophages, and areas of interstitial fibrosis frequently are associated with the tumor. Psammoma bodies are present in 13% of the cases.[413]

The differential diagnosis includes primary adenocarcinoma of the conventional type and metastatic adenocarcinoma. Bennett and Sasser[413] compared thirty cases of bronchioalveolar carcinomas with 100 cases of ordinary lung adenocarcinoma and found frequent overlapping patterns. The main differences encountered were a higher incidence of multiplicity and a slightly better survival rate in the patients with bronchioalveolar carcinoma. Furthermore, multiple foci of bronchioalveolar carcinoma can be found in association with conventional adenocarcinoma.[424a] The pat-

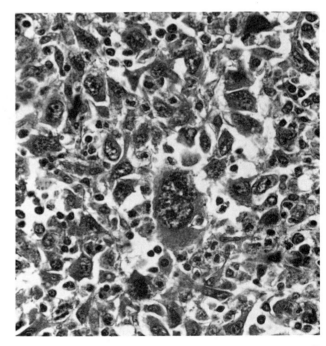

Fig. 7-87 Giant cell carcinoma. Bizarre tumor cells with huge hyperchromatic nuclei are seen growing in solid fashion. Scattered neutrophils are present in stroma and also in cytoplasm of some tumor cells.

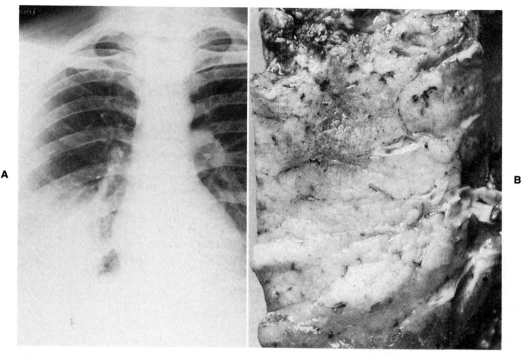

Fig. 7-88 Bronchioalveolar carcinoma. **A,** Typical roentgenogram. Note poorly defined shadow in right lower lung field. **B,** Typical gross appearance: mucoid surface, appearance somewhat like organizing pneumonia, and poorly defined borders.

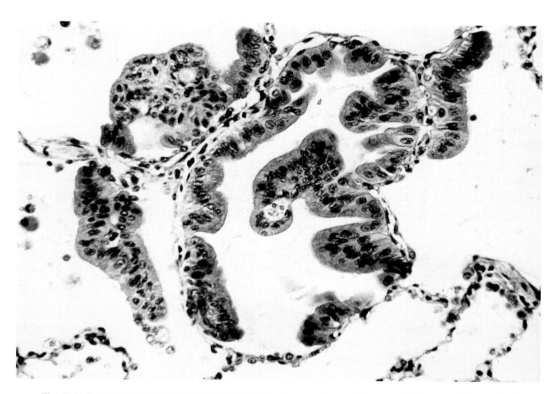

Fig. 7-89 Typical well-differentiated bronchioloalveolar carcinoma. Tumor cells line wall of terminal air spaces.

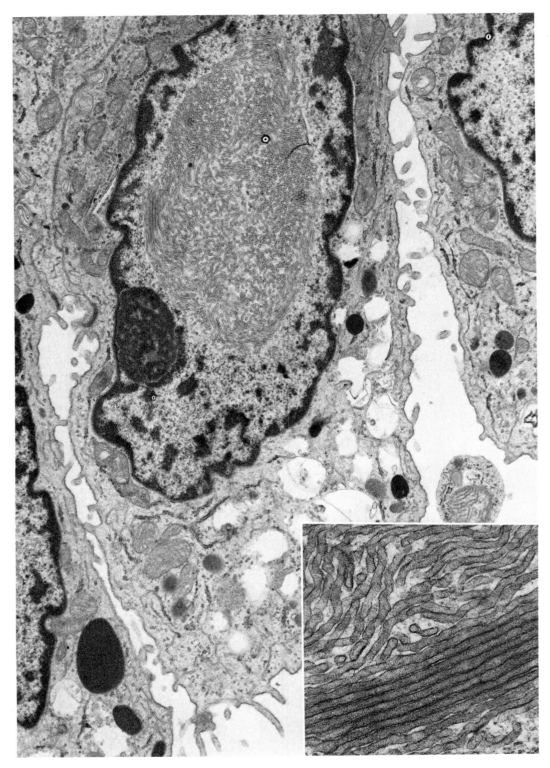

Fig. 7-90 Electron micrograph of bronchioloalveolar carcinoma showing an intranuclear inclusion formed by serpiginous and parallel tubular arrays, better appreciated in high-power **inset.** Short microvilli protrude from surface. Scattered dense bodies may be seen in cytoplasm. Significance of intranuclear inclusion is uncertain. (×11,200; **inset,** ×41,000.)

tern of bronchioloalveolar carcinoma can be closely simulated by metastatic well-differentiated adenocarcinomas, particularly from the pancreas.[430]

Sputum or bronchial washing cytology is almost invariably negative in cases that present as single peripheral nodules but is often positive (up to 88% of the cases) for the multinodular and pneumonic-like forms.[436,437] Percutaneous fine needle aspiration has been successfully used for the detection of this tumor.[432]

The histogenesis of this neoplasm has been debated for many years.[417] Electron-microscopic studies[422] have given support to the theory that in most instances the tumor arises from terminal bronchiolar epithelium[412,422] and that it may contain cells with the ultrastructural and biochemical features of Clara cells, a property it shares with conventional adenocarcinoma and other carcinoma types.[415,421,429,431] Granular pneumocytes are sometimes found admixed in the lesion; it is not clear whether they are part of the tumor or whether they represent a reactive component. However, it would appear from the available evidence that the majority of bronchioloalveolar carcinomas are primarily of bronchiolar epithelial (including Clara cell) origin, with secondary spread to, and admixture with, alveolar epithelium.[425] Alpha-1-antitrypsin has been proposed as a useful marker for Clara cell differentiation.[437a]

It has become increasingly evident that the tumor having the features previously described constitutes only one form (albeit the most frequent) of bronchioloalveolar carcinoma: this form has been designated as type I and could be properly regarded as a *bronchiolar carcinoma*.

According to this view, type II bronchioalveolar carcinoma is largely or entirely comprised of type II (granular) pneumocytes and could therefore be regarded as a neoplasm of this specific type of alveolar cell. It differs from type I by virtue of mucin-negativity, the cuboidal shape of the tumor cells, the ultrastructural evidence of lamellar inclusion bodies, and immunohistochemcial positivity for surfactant apoprotein.[414,426,433,435] The latter substance may be found both in the cytoplasm and in the nucleus, in which it manifests in the form of PAS-positive intranuclear inclusions.[434] S-100 protein-positive cells are numerous in the stroma.[427] The type II tumor is more likely to be solitary and has a much better prognosis than type I neoplasm.[424] The existence of a benign counterpart of this lesion has been recently postulated, and the term *papillary adenoma* has been proposed for it.[418,428] Another benign tumor allegedly composed of type II pneumocytes is so-called sclerosing hemangioma (see p. 319).

Adenosquamous carcinoma

The term adenosquamous carcinoma is used for lung tumors in which unquestionable evidence of squamous and glandular differentiation is found in the same neoplasm in a roughly equivalent amount[438] (Fig. 7-91). Squamous cell carcinomas having occasional mucin-producing cells or adenocarcinomas with minute foci of squamous differentiation are named according to their predominant component. Thus defined, adenosquamous carcinomas comprise less than 10% of lung cancers. Most of the cases are located peripherally and often are associated with a scar, suggesting a

closer relationship with adenocarcinoma than with squamous cell carcinoma.

Small cell carcinoma

Small cell carcinoma comprises 10% to 20% of all lung cancers. Over 80% of the patients are males, and 85% or more are smokers.[451] It is typically a lesion of the central portions of the lung, but occasionally it is found in a peripheral location.[446a] Bronchoscopic biopsy is often positive, even if no gross abnormalities are seen. Small cell carcinoma should be viewed as a distinctive tumor type rather than as an undifferentiated form of lung cancer. The pattern of growth is generally solid, but there may be streams and ribbons, rosettes and pseudorosettes, tubules and ductules.[439] From a cytologic standpoint, this neoplasm has been traditionally divided into three types. The most common (42% of cases) is referred to as *lymphocyte-like* or *oat cell type* and is characterized by small round or oval cells resembling lymphocytes (Fig. 7-92). The nuclei are extremely hyperchromatic, and the cytoplasm is so scanty as to be unrecognizable in routine preparations. A very common artifact, particularly prominent in small biopsy specimens, is elongation of the nuclei, with deformation, clumping, and diffusion of the chromatin. If present throughout the specimen, it may render the diagnosis impossible. Chromatin diffusion secondary to necrosis may spread to the wall of the blood vessels, which appear strongly hematoxyphilic.[439] These foci, sometimes referred to as Azzopardi's effect, are positive for the Feulgen reaction.

Another morphologic variant of this tumor (29% of the cases) is known as *fusiform*. As the name indicates, most if not all of the tumor cells have an elongated shape. The good nuclear preservation and the larger cell size distinguishes this type from the artifactual elongation previously described. The third morphologic variant, referred to as *polygonal cell type* (29%), is composed of medium-sized cells with relatively abundant cytoplasm. It is often confused with other types of lung cancer, but its overall architecture, electron-microscopic appearance, and clinical behavior indicate that it belongs in the small cell carcinoma category.

In the revised WHO classification,[464] three categories of small cell carcinomas are accepted: oat cell carcinoma, intermediate cell type (which combines the fusiform and polygonal cell types of the former classification), and combined type. The latter represents an admixture of small cell–large cell carcinoma and large cell carcinoma.[456] In rare cases small cell carcinomas that are otherwise typical may contain scattered giant tumor cells; this change is seen more commonly following chemotherapy, but it can also be encountered in the initial specimen.[440]

The key factor in determining whether a lung tumor belongs in the small cell category or not, either in a pure or a combined form, is not the detection of neuroendocrine differentiation discussed in the following paragraph or the nuclear size but rather the chromatin and nucleolar patterns. The chromatin should be finely dispersed, without prominent clumps; more importantly, nucleoli should be inconspicuous, if detectable at all.

Cytoplasmic argyrophilia may be found in some of the cases.[460] Ultrastructurally, a few dense-core neurosecretory-type granules are found in at least some of the cells in most cases[441,445] (Fig. 7-93). Immunohistochemically, there is variable positivity for neural markers, such as neurofilaments,[452,462] Leu 7,[454] and neuron-specific enolase[442,458]; the latter marker has also been found to be elevated in the serum of many of these patients, rendering it useful for the monitoring of the disease.[446,449] Despite earlier claims, the tumor cells also exhibit positivity for keratin,[462] often simultaneously with the neural markers.

This combination of morphologic, ultrastructural, and immunohistochemical features, plus the well-known association of small cell carcinoma with a wide variety of endocrine syndromes—including the carcinoid syndrome[457,463]—suggests that the cells of this neoplasm are differentiating in the direction of neuroendocrine (Kultschitsky's-type) cells. A further argument favoring this interpretation is the existence of cases with a microscopic appearance that is intermediate between small cell carcinoma and bronchial carcinoid, known as atypical carcinoid tumors (see p. 317).[453] However, these considerations do not necessarily indicate that small cell carcinoma arises from bronchial Kultschitsky's cells, as some have claimed.[461] It is more likely that it originates in primitive cells of the basal bronchial epithelium, which in the process of neoplastic change under-

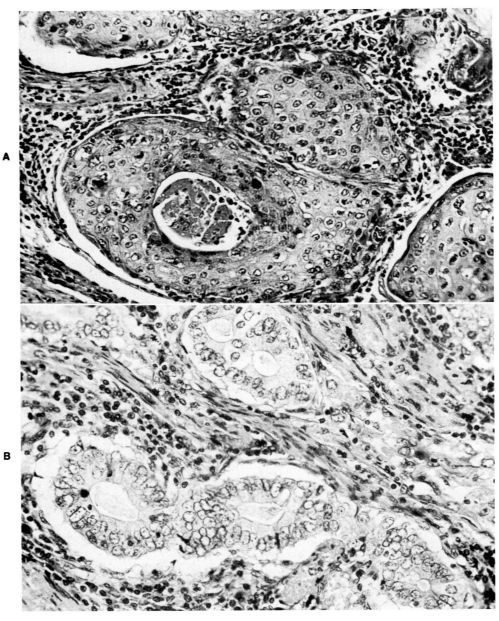

Fig. 7-91 A, Carcinoma of lung showing squamous differentiation. **B,** Same tumor shown in **A** demonstrating adenocarcinoma in adjacent zone.

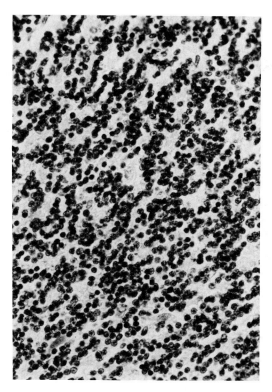

Fig. 7-92 Small cell carcinoma of round cell (lymphocyte-like) type.

goes partial differentiation toward so-called neuroendocrine cells.[443,459,465] Such an occurrence would explain why small cell carcinoma is so closely related epidemiologically to the other types of lung carcinoma, why some tumors with the small cell carcinoma pattern lack neurosecretory granules by electron microscopy and contain instead desmosomes and tonofilaments,[444,447] and why—as previously indicated—one may see in the same tumor a mixture of small cell carcinoma and squamous cell carcinoma, adenocarcinoma, or undifferentiated large cell carcinoma.

A somewhat related problem stems from the fact that occasionally one finds ultrastructural and/or immunohistochemical features of endocrine differentiation in lung carcinomas lacking the morphologic features of small cell carcinoma.[448,450,455] One should name these tumors according to their overall appearance (adenocarcinoma, undifferentiated large cell carcinoma, etc.), and simply add ". . . . with endocrine differentiation" to the diagnostic term. There is no evidence that the presence of this type of differentiation changes in any way the behavior or prognosis of these neoplasms.

A recent finding of great interest is the detection of a deletion in chromosome 3 (p14-p23) in the cell of small cell carcinoma.[454a]

Carcinoma in situ

It has been shown that squamous cell carcinomas of the lung have a long preclinical stage in which the lesion progresses from dysplasia to carcinoma in situ, microinvasive

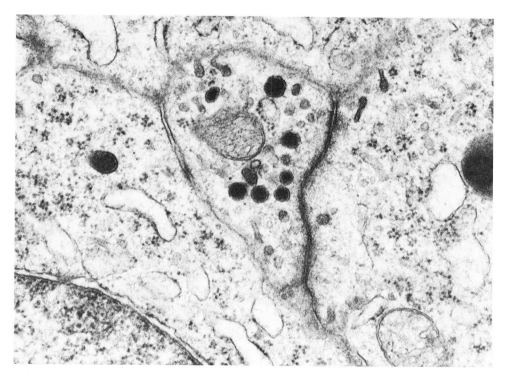

Fig. 7-93 Small cell carcinoma of lung. A few of uniform, round, dense-core, membrane-bound granules are present. These granules are difficult to find and are usually present at periphery of cells. (× 41,200).

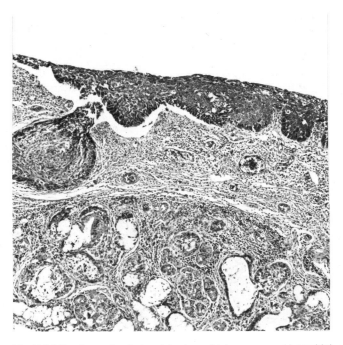

Fig. 7-94 Carcinoma in situ involving bronchial mucosa and bronchial gland. Artifactual detachment from stroma is similar to that often seen in carcinoma in situ of uterine cervix.

carcinoma, and frank invasive cancer.[467,468,471] Detailed morphologic studies of these very early cases have shown that the site of origin is a segmental bronchus in most instances and that most cases are unifocal in origin[466,471] (Fig. 7-94). One would think that identification of tumors at this early stage should lead to an increase in the cure rate. Woolner et al.[472] collected twenty-eight such cases seen at the Mayo Clinic in a 23-year period. The prognosis in their series was good: only three patients died of the cancer; in two of the three there was evidence of multicentricity. More recent studies from this group and from other authors have not substantiated these early optimistic figures, quoting a high death rate as a result of recurrence or development of a second tumor.[470,473]

Unfortunately, mass roentgenogram screening programs have not been successful in the detection of early carcinoma.[469] Cytologic screening programs have also been tried. Melamed et al.[471] screened 4,000 asymptomatic cigarette-smokers over the age of 45 in New York City and found lung cancer in nine men with normal chest roentgenograms. Seven had in situ or incipient invasive epidermoid carcinomas.

In another project, conducted by the Mayo Clinic, a high-risk population was screened by means of periodic sputum cytology examinations and chest x-rays; 54% of incidence cancers in the group that were being rescreened every 4 months were detected at an early, potentially curable stage. Sputum cytology proved highly effective for the early detection of epidermoid carcinoma, but not for adenocarcinomas or undifferentiated large cell carcinomas; there were very few small cell carcinomas.[474]

Biopsy

The advent of fiberoptic bronchoscopy has dramatically expanded the potential of the bronchoscopic biopsy. The instrument is easily inserted, is better accepted by patients, enables exploration of both segmental and subsegmental bronchi, and can be performed at the bedside in acutely ill patients.[484] Biopsy with the rigid bronchoscope provided positive specimens in only one third of operable patients with lung carcinomas,[480] but the fiberoptic bronchoscope has increased these figures substantially, particularly for peripherally located lesions.[475,478,483,486] However, it has made things more difficult for the pathologist because of the smaller size of the sample obtained, in comparison with the use of the rigid bronchoscope.[476]

Careful correlation between the bronchoscopic appearance, site of the biopsy, and microscopic evaluation is important. A fragment with the microscopic features of carcinoma in situ may be representative of the entire lesion if taken from the center of an area of slight thickening or irregularity of the mucosa but may represent just the peripheral component of an invasive lesion if taken at the edge of a polypoid or ulcerating mass. The presence of squamous metaplasia in a bronchial biopsy should be regarded as a non-specific change that may be present by itself or accompanied by inflammation, dysplasia, in situ or invasive carcinoma, or even carcinoid tumor (Fig. 7-95). Sometimes, the main bronchial specimen is unremarkable but clumps of cells with diagnostic features of carcinoma are present separately from it (Fig. 7-96).

One of the most serious problems in small bronchial biopsies is the identification of small crushed blue nuclei as belonging to a small cell carcinoma, as opposed to a lymphoma or even a reactive lymphocytic population. Careful handling of the material will reduce the problem, but will not eliminate it entirely. In some cases, this artifactual distortion is of such magnitude that a differential diagnosis simply becomes impossible, even in the presence of a large number of these cells, much to the bewilderment and irritation of the bronchoscopist.

Biopsy of various lymph node groups has been advocated in the preoperation evaluation of patients with suspected lung carcinomas, in order to avoid thoracotomy in inoperable patients.[482] The nodes most commonly sampled are cervical (especially scalene) and mediastinal. The latter can be obtained through limited incisions in the second intercostal space[481] or—with increasing frequency—by mediastinoscopy.[477,485] By biopsying both cervical and mediastinal lymph nodes simultaneously, Paulson[481] obtained positive results in 45% of his 182 patients; in 60% of these positive cases, the mediastinum appeared normal on chest x-ray examination.

If bronchoscopic biopsy (with or without lymph node biopsy) fails to establish the diagnosis of carcinoma, but the clinical suspicion is high, an exploratory thoracotomy should be performed without delay. At the present time, this procedure carries practically no operative mortality. Early exploratory thoracotomy will increase the number of tumors suitable for resection.

Thoracotomy with lung biopsy is also indicated in patients with bilateral disseminated disease in which bronchoscopic

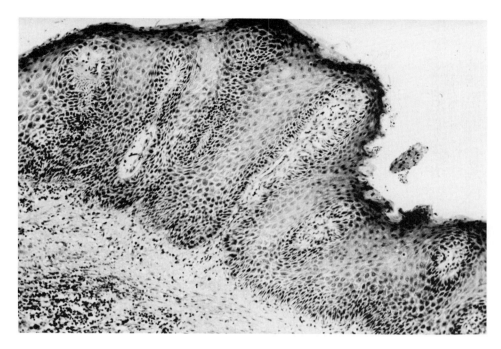

Fig. 7-95 Prominent squamous metaplasia of bronchus.

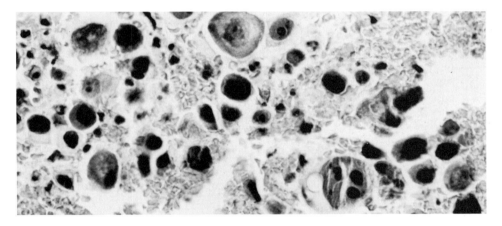

Fig. 7-96 Clump of malignant cells seen in bronchoscopic biopsy specimen. Note variation in cell size and atypical nuclei.

biopsies and other procedures have failed to establish a diagnosis. By this method not only can the pathologic diagnosis be made, but bacterial studies and chemical analyses can also be carried out. The site of the incision is planned according to the distribution of the lesions.[479]

Cytology

Pulmonary cytology has reached a high level of accuracy since Wandall's classic monograph.[488,490,491,493,507] By examination of the sputum and/or bronchial brushings, it is now possible to make a diagnosis in 80% to 90% of patients with cancer.[491,497] Most authors agree that bronchial washing does not add significant information to that obtained from

the brushings and that the preparations are of inferior quality.[487,495,502,503] A single sputum specimen will be positive in 40% to 60% of the patients with lung cancer, but this rate rises to 80% or more when five sputum specimens are examined.[489]

In most instances, the tumor cells are easily recognized (Figs. 7-97, 7-98 and 7-99). False positive diagnoses have been made in patients with infarct, bronchiectasis, fungous disease, viral pneumonia, irradiation changes, and lipoid pneumonia (Fig. 7-100). Usually, the cells that are misinterpreted as cancer are either macrophages or altered alveolar lining cells.

The diagnosis of exfoliative material from sputum spec-

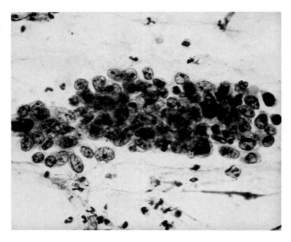

Fig. 7-97 Clump of malignant cells from patient with small cell carcinoma. Piling up of cells and their grouping in strands are characteristic of this tumor type.

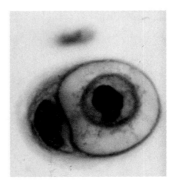

Fig. 7-98 Apparent "cannibalism" of one tumor cell by another. In actuality, one cell overrides other. This is more frequently seen in epidermoid carcinoma but may be found in other tumor types as well.

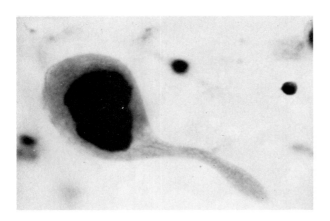

Fig. 7-99 Tadpole-shaped cell in patient with epidermoid cell carcinoma. Large "ink spot" type of nucleus is common in this tumor type.

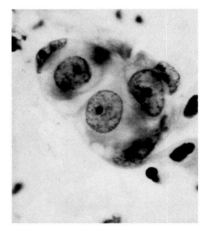

Fig. 7-100 Clump of reactive macrophages mistaken for malignant tumor. Resection of lobe demonstrated only lipoid pneumonia.

imens should be made on a conservative basis. Our reports read as follows:

1 "Unsatisfactory (saliva only)" when no macrophages are present in the smear
2 "Negative" when no abnormal cells are observed in a technically satisfactory smear
3 "Benign atypia" when epithelial bronchial cells with hyperplastic and metaplastic changes secondary to inflammation are identified
4 "Suspicious but not diagnostic" (this report is an indication for repeat examination)
5 "Positive for cancer cells"

It should be remembered that malignant cells present in sputum may also originate in any portion of the upper aerodigestive tract.[497a] If a patient with a negative chest x-ray is found to have a positive sputum cytology, a thorough inspection of the bronchial tree with the fiberoptic scope should be carried out together with a complete ENT examination.[508a]

An increasingly popular cytologic specimen is that provided by fine needle aspiration. The technique is associated with minimal morbidity, and the diagnostic yield is very high, especially for peripherally located lesions.[501,505,508]

Yet another source of cytologic material is pleural fluid. The incidence of false negatives is higher in this specimen type than in others, particularly for small cell carcinoma.[500,504]

In addition to making a diagnosis of carcinoma, the pathologist examining cytologic specimens from any of these sites should attempt to establish the specific cell type involved. The overall agreement rate between cytology and histology ranges from 70% to 90%.[498,506] It is particularly high for well-differentiated squamous cell carcinoma, well-differentiated adenocarcinoma, and small cell carcinoma.[492,494,496,499] Most difficulties are encountered in the differential diagnosis between poorly differentiated squamous cell carcinoma and large cell undifferentiated carcinoma.

Frozen section

Frozen section is an important procedure in debatable lesions of the lung and has its greatest value in peripherally located lesions. In patients with resectable lung carcinoma, bronchoscopic and cytologic examination will be positive in about 80% of the cases. This means that a number of patients with cancer will undergo surgery without a definite preoperative diagnosis. For peripheral lesions, it is better to excise them entirely with a margin of normal lung. This excision may imply lobectomy. Frozen section is then done. Frequently, the lesion proves to be a benign process such as tuberculoma, hamartoma, or organizing pneumonia. If it is cancer, the thoracic surgeon decides the extent of resection.

It is much more important that the pathologist make a definite diagnosis in lesions of the lung than in lesions of the breast, for a second thoracotomy carries with it considerable morbidity and additional risk. One must not be misled into making a diagnosis of carcinoma in highly cellular inflammatory lesions such as organizing pneumonia, lipoid pneumonia, or inflammatory pseudotumor. Conversely, some of the poorly differentiated neoplasms of the lung may have a considerable inflammatory infiltrate and be incorrectly diagnosed as non-neoplastic.

Spread and metastases

Lung cancer spreads by direct extension proximally and distally along the bronchus of origin and may reach the trachea at the level of the carina. It also grows into the lung parenchyma, from where it may reach the mediastinum or pleura. The latter event may result in seeding in both pleural layers and extension into the chest wall and diaphragm. Invasion of blood vessels is also common; sometimes, this may lead to extensive tumor emboli and cor pulmonale, a phenomenon seen more commonly with adenocarcinoma.[511]

Lymph node metastases occur first in the hilar region, then in the mediastinal and lower cervical groups, and less commonly in axillary and subdiaphragmatic sites.

Distant metastases are more common in liver, other areas of lung, adrenal, bone and bone marrow, kidney, and central nervous system.[514,515] Less common sites include the gastrointestinal tract, pancreas, thyroid, spleen, pituitary gland, skin, and skeletal muscle.[513,516] Brain metastases seem to be more common in adenocarcinoma.[509] The occurrence of metastases to the lung raises the differential diagnosis with a second primary lung cancer, an event detected by LeGal and Bauer[512] in 6.4% of sixty-three patients who had survived at least 30 months following excision of a lung cancer. Presence of distant metastases at the time of initial diagnosis is particularly high in small cell carcinoma. In one series, 84% of the patients had "extensive" or extrathoracic disease at the time of diagnosis, 14% had metastases to the central nervous system, and 47% had bone marrow metastases.[510]

Treatment

The standard therapy for operable non-small cell carcinoma of the lung is complete surgical excision through thoracotomy. The excision can be in the form of pneumonectomy, lobectomy, or (very rarely) segmental resection, depending on the location and type of the tumor.[518]

The first successful lung resection for epidermoid carcinoma was performed by Dr. Evarts A. Graham at Barnes Hospital in 1933. The patient, a physician, died 30 years later of an unrelated disease (Fig. 7-101). Ironically, he survived Dr. Graham, who died as a result of lung carcinoma.

Of every 100 patients with lung cancer, about 60% will be explored, and about 60% of these (or 35% of the total) will be resectable.[518]

Radiation therapy can effectively control the local growth of lung cancer and sometimes results in long-term survival,[528] but, like surgery, it fails to cure most patients, mainly because as many as 50% of them have distant metastases when diagnosed or shortly following the initial diagnosis.[525,527] It also fails to decrease the incidence of recurrence in the cases showing microscopic evidence of involvement of the bronchial margin.[522] It can reduce local recurrences after resection of squamous cell carcinoma, but it does not increase survival rates.[523] The role of radiation therapy seems to be greater, whether given alone or as a preoperative measure, for tumors of the superior pulmonary sulcus[517,520,521,524] and as an adjunctive measure in the treatment of small cell carcinoma.[519,526]

Multidrug chemotherapy is currently the treatment of choice for small cell carcinoma, although some workers believe that a selected group is still best treated with surgery alone.[529] There is no question that the initial tumor response to chemotherapy and its short-term results are distinctly better than for the other types of lung carcinoma; yet, long-term cures are rarely achieved.

Prognosis

The long-term prognosis of lung carcinoma remains disappointingly poor, no substantial improvement having been made in recent years in long-term survival rates. In a series of 1008 cases of lung carcinoma treated at a single institution from 1948 to 1955, the 5-year survival rate was 21.3% for the resected cases and 8% for the entire group.[532] Similar figures have been obtained from various other groups during the last 30 years.[541,558]

The prognosis of lung carcinomas has been related to a large number of factors:

1 *Age.* Patients who are younger than 40 years of age have a very poor prognosis, probably because most have advanced disease at presentation.[560]

2 *Sex.* Women have been found to have a worse survival rate than men; this has been partially attributed to the fact that they have a higher incidence of advanced lesions and of tumors with an adenocarcinoma pattern.[547,548]

3 *Location.* It is claimed that tumors of the superior pulmonary sulcus have a better prognosis than the others, the reported 5-year survival rates oscillating between 20% and 34%.[530,538,550,559] For squamous cell

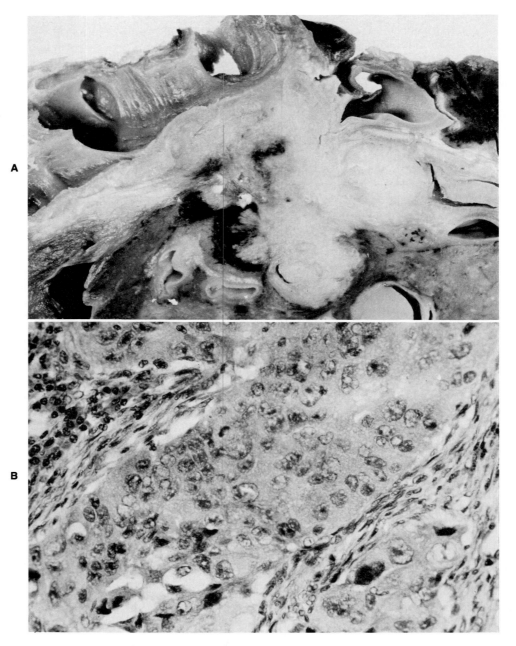

Fig. 7-101 A, Epidermoid carcinoma of lung resected by Dr. Evarts A. Graham in 1933. Note extension into surrounding lung and involvement of two regional lymph nodes. Patient died in 1962 without evidence of cancer. **B,** Poorly differentiated squamous carcinoma shown in **A.**

carcinomas, those located at the periphery are said to do better than those located centrally.[567a]

4 *Stage.* A direct relationship is evident between clinical stage and survival rates (Table 7-3).[540] Actually, TNM stage is regarded by most as the single most important prognostic parameter in lung carcinoma.[542]

5 *Tumor size.* Large tumors have a worse prognosis than smaller neoplasms of the same histologic type.[552] For the peripheral neoplasms, this relationship no longer

holds once the tumor reaches a diameter of 6 cm.[568]

6 *Cell type* and *degree of differentiation.* Squamous cell carcinoma is the most curable form of lung cancer.[533,566] In series of long-term survivors of lung carcinomas, about half of the cases are squamous cell carcinomas.[546] The 5-year survival rate in patients undergoing resection for cure is about 40% for well-differentiated tumors, 20% for moderately differentiated tumors, and 7% for the poorly differentiated

Table 7-3 Definitions for staging lung carcinoma (American Joint Committee on Cancer Staging, 1973)

Description
T0: No evidence of primary tumor
TX: Tumor proved by the presence of malignant cells in bronchopulmonary secretions but not visualised roentgenographically or bronchoscopically, or any tumor that cannot be assessed
TIS: Carcinoma in situ
T1: A tumor that is 3 cm or less in greatest diameter, surrounded by lung or visceral pleura, and without evidence of invasion proximal to a lobar bronchus at bronchoscopy
T2: A tumor more than 3 cm in greatest diameter, or a tumor of any size that either invades the visceral pleura or has associated atelectasis or obstructive pneumonitis extending to the hilar region. At bronchoscopy, the proximal extent of demonstrable tumor must be within a lobar bronchus or at least 2 cm distal to the carina. Any associated atelectasis or obstructive pneumonitis must involve less than an entire lung, and there must be no pleural effusion
T3: A tumor of any size with direct extension into an adjacent structure such as the parietal pleura or chest wall, the diaphragm, or the mediastinum and its contents, or a tumor demonstrable bronchoscopically to involve a main bronchus less than 2 cm distal to the carina; or any tumor associated with atelectasis or obstructive pneumonitis of any entire lung or pleural effusion
N0: No demonstrable metastasis to regional lymph nodes
N1: Metastasis to lymph nodes in the peribronchial or the ipsilateral hilar region, or both, including direct extension
N2: Metastasis to lymph nodes in the mediastinum
M0: No (known) distant metastasis
M1: Distant metastasis such as in scalene cervical or contralateral hilar lymph nodes, brain, bones, liver, or contralateral lung

Summary of staging

Stage I (operable)	T1	N0	M0
	T1	N1	M0
	T2	N0	M0
Stage II (operable)	T2	N1	M0
Stage III (inoperable)	T3 any N or M		
	N2 any T or M		
	M1 any T or N		

From Spiro SG, Goldstraw P: The staging of lung cancer. Thorax **39**:401–407, 1984.

tumors. For adenocarcinomas, the corresponding figure is about 25%, apparently not influenced by the degree of differentiation.

As a group, the prognosis of bronchioloalveolar carcinoma is not substantially different from that of ordinary adenocarcinoma.[531] However, the localized form of the former (usually of type II histology) is curable in a high proportion of cases.[534,553,555] Undifferentiated large cell carcinomas give a figure close to 15%. In one recent series, undifferentiated large cell histology and presence of tumor giant cells in any histologic type were significantly associated with a

worse outcome.[552] Giant cell carcinoma is practically never curable.[545]

Small cell carcinoma has been traditionally associated with a dismal prognosis, the 5-year survival rate being less than 2% in most early series.[544] A substantial short-term improvement has come as a result of chemotherapy, but the long-term outlook remains bleak. Much has been written about the relationship between the small cell carcinoma subtypes and prognosis.[537,543,557] Although some controversy persists, the consensus is that no appreciable prognostic differences exist between lymphocyte-like (oat cell) carcinoma and the intermediate type, but that pure small cell carcinoma is associated with a longer survival period than small cell/large cell carcinoma.[543,563,569]

7 *Blood vessel invasion.* This feature has ominous prognostic connotations.[536] When associated with lymph node metastases, the adverse effect upon survival is additive.[565]

8 *Chest wall invasion.* Surprisingly, tumors associated with obvious invasion of the chest wall have been found to have a prognosis not significantly different than those lacking this feature, when all other staging parameters are the same; the operative mortality, however, is substantially higher.[561]

9 *Presence of a scar.* It has been claimed that peripheral adenocarcinomas or undifferentiated large cell carcinomas associated with a well-defined fibrotic area (scar) have a worse prognosis than tumors lacking this feature.[564]

10 *Lymph node involvement.* This parameter, which is a component of the staging system, is one of the most important prognostic determinators. This applies not only to the presence of nodal metastasis but also to the anatomic level of these deposits.[552,556] It should be pointed out, however, that a 5-year disease-free survival is possible in patients with involvement of mediastinal nodes.[554]

11 *Inflammatory reaction.* The presence of a prominent lymphoplasmacytic reaction around the tumor is a favorable prognostic sign.[552] Also, it has been claimed that tumors associated with regional lymph nodes showing lymphocyte or germinal center predominance have a better prognosis than those in which the nodes have lymphocyte depletion or appear unstimulated.[549]

12 *DNA ploidy.* Preliminary information is at hand to suggest that determination of tumor DNA ploidy by flow cytometry can contribute significantly to the prognostic assessment of lung carcinoma, provided that material is obtained by multiple site sampling.[533a,567]

13 *Oncogene expression.* It has been reported that the expression of *ras* oncogene is enhanced in non-small cell carcinoma, and amplification of at least three *mic* genes has been shown in small cell carcinoma lines.[535,551,562] Whether analysis of these protooncogenes will provide insight into the pathogenesis of lung cancer and aid in predicting its behavior remains to be determined. Preliminary claims have been made that increased expression of N-myc in small cell cancer predicts poor prognosis.[539]

OTHER PRIMARY TUMORS
Hamartoma

Hamartoma (chondroid hamartoma; chondroid adenoma; chondroma) is a relatively rare benign tumor that generally occurs in adults. It is usually solitary but can be multiple.[574] Its most common location is the lung parenchyma just beneath the pleura, and it presents in most instances as an asymptomatic clearcut shadow in a chest x-ray. It is usually small, although occasionally it may occupy the entire lobe. Grossly, it is sharply delineated and lobulated. The cut surface is characterized by glistening nodules of cartilage separated by ill-defined clefts. A less common presentation is as a polypoid mass inside a large bronchus[572]; this type may result in symptoms caused by bronchial obstruction.[576]

This lesion has been designated as a hamartoma because it conforms to the definition of this term by Albrecht[570]: "Hamartomata are tumor-like malformations in which occur only abnormal mixing of the normal components of the organ. The abnormalities may take the form of a change in quantity, arrangement, or degree, or may comprise all three."*

Microscopically, the peripheral hamartoma is made up of normal cartilage arranged in islands, fat, smooth muscle,

---

*From Albrecht E: Ueber Hamartome. Verh Dtsch Pathol Ges 7:153-157, 1904.

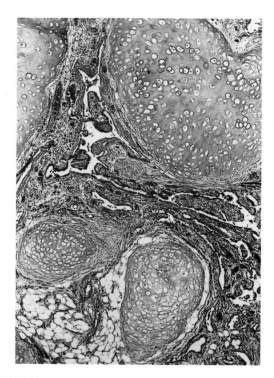

Fig. 7-102 Hamartoma of lung. Lesion is composed of sharply defined islands of mature cartilage separated by islands of adipose tissue and bronchial epithelium growing in cleft-like fashion.

and clefts lined by ciliated or nonciliated respiratory epithelium (Fig. 7-102). The cartilage often shows calcification and, rarely, ossification. Anthracotic pigment is absent. The endobronchial lesions have fewer epithelial clefts, a decreased proportion of cartilage, and an increase in the amount of the adipose tissue component.[576]

There is clinical, morphologic, and ultrastructural evidence to suggest that this lesion is acquired and that it represents a primary overgrowth of mesenchymal tissues of the bronchial wall, with secondary entrapment of bronchial epithelium in the more peripheral lesions.[571,575] This lesion is easily diagnosed on gross inspection and frozen section and is treated by local resection only. Carney[573] has identified a familial syndrome characterized by pulmonary chondromas, gastric epithelioid leiomyosarcomas, and functioning extra-adrenal paragangliomas.

Carcinoid tumor and related endocrine neoplasms

Carcinoid tumor is the most common form of the tumor formerly known as bronchial adenoma, a term to be discarded.[578,581] It comprises less than 5% of primary pulmonary neoplasms. For the purposes of discussion, it is advisable to divide pulmonary carcinoid tumor into three major categories, acknowledging the existence of intermediate forms, and the fact that all of them differentiate in the direction of Kultschitsky's type neuroendocrine cells as normally seen in the bronchial mucosa.[577,579,580,582] These categories are central, peripheral, and atypical carcinoid tumors.

Central carcinoid tumor

Central carcinoid tumor is the most common type. It usually presents as a slow-growing, solitary polypoid mass within a major bronchus; because of its location and high vascularity, hemoptysis and pulmonary infection caused by blockage of distal bronchi are common.[592] Most cases occur in adults, but they have also been observed in children. As a matter of fact, they constitute the most common primary neoplasm in the latter age group.[599] The sex incidence is almost equal. Most cases are endocrinologically silent at the clinical level. However, cases with typical carcinoid syndrome and elevated 5-HIAA in the urine have been documented. In some instances, the tumor has been found to secrete 5-hydroxytryptophan instead of serotonin.[609] Cases have been reported to be associated with Cushing's syndrome caused by ACTH production[595,596] with endocrine tumors of other sites[597] and with multiple endocrine adenomatosis.[618] It is likely that, in addition, these tumors secrete as yet unidentified peptide hormones analogous to those of their gastrointestinal counterparts.[589]

Grossly, central carcinoids are predominantly intrabronchial but also infiltrate the bronchial wall, may extend to the surrounding parenchyma, and even reach the pleura or the myocardium (Fig. 7-103, A and B). Some examples show a predominant extrabronchial component. They are covered by bronchial mucosa, which is only rarely ulcerated. The cut surface is grayish yellow, sometimes divided by fibrous septa, and very well vascularized. Islands of bronchial cartilage totally surrounded by tumor may be evident.

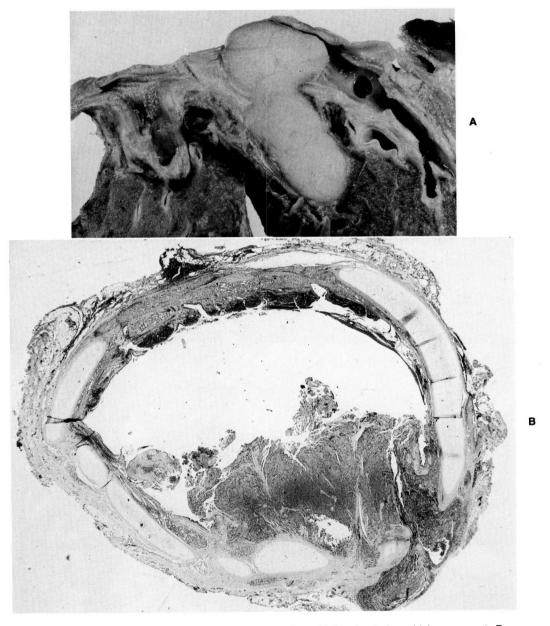

Fig. 7-103 A, Bronchial carcinoid with prominent intrabronchial and extrabronchial component. **B,** Typical growth pattern of bronchial carcinoid. Most of tumor is endobronchial and polypoid, but a portion is infiltrating wall and invading peribronchial soft tissues.

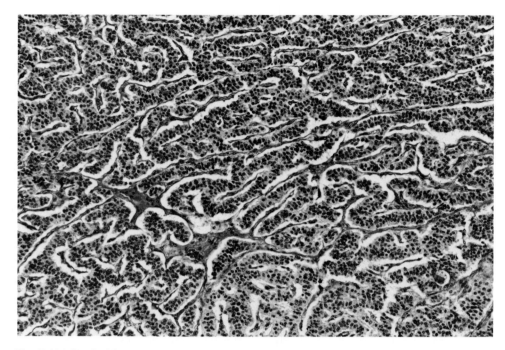

Fig. 7-104 Carcinoid tumor of central (classic) type. There is prominent trabecular arrangement of tumor cells, which are supported by delicate fibrovascular stroma.

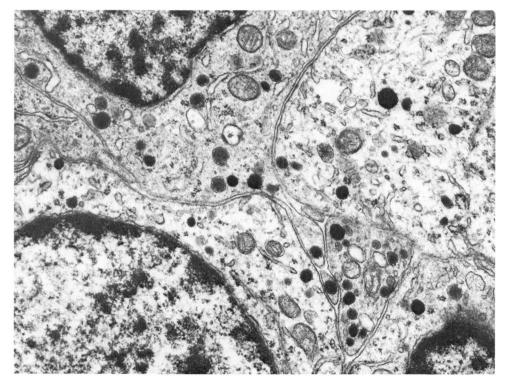

Fig. 7-105 Carcinoid tumor of lung in a woman with multiple endocrine adenomatosis. Moderate numbers of fairly uniform electron-dense neurosecretory granules are present. ($\times$25,270.)

Microscopically, the tumor is made up of small and uniform cells having central nuclei with scanty or no mitotic activity and a moderate amount of finely granular cytoplasm (Fig. 7-104). It may grow in the form of compact nests, ribbons, and festoons, in a diffuse solid fashion and—rarely—in a pseudopapillary or true papillary configuration.[604] Small glands with a rosette-like appearance are only rarely present. Vascularity is pronounced. The stroma can be heavily hyalinized and may exhibit focal calcification or ossification. Some of the bone present may represent osseous metaplasia by entrapped bronchial cartilage.

Mucin stains are usually negative, but focal positivity may be found in the glandular lumina.[608]

Argentaffin cells are rare in formalin-fixed, parafin-embedded sections of bronchial carcinoid, whereas argyrophilic cells (as demonstrated by the Grimelius or Sevier-Munger techniques) are the rule.

The histochemical features of bronchial carcinoid thus resemble those of carcinoid tumors arising from other foregut derivatives, such as stomach and duodenum, and differ from the more common carcinoid tumors of the appendix and distal small bowel.[587,617] By electron microscopy, the cells contain dense-core secretory granules, sometimes aligned along the cell membrane[584] (Fig. 7-105). Some variability in the appearance of these granules exists from case to case, suggesting the involvement of at least two different endocrine cell types.[593] Occasionally, abundant cytoplasmic fibrillary inclusions are found.[585]

Immunohistochemically, there is variable reactivity for keratin, serotonin, neuron-specific enolase, chomogranin, synaptophysin, opioid peptides, Leu 7, and neurofilaments.[591,602,603,612,620] In addition, many peptide hormones have been detected in individual tumors, sometimes in combination. They include the following: somatostatin, bombesin, gastrin-releasing peptide, gastrin, substance P, pancreatic polypeptide, VIP, ACTH, and calcitonin* (Fig. 7-106).

Metastases to regional lymph nodes occur in about 5% of the cases; rare instances of distant metastases have also been documented. Interestingly, those located in bone are characteristically of the osteoblastic type.[613]

The tumors are easily identifiable with the bronchoscope in the large majority of cases.[615] Bronchoscopic biopsy is usually positive, although severe hemorrhage may result because of the marked vascularity of the tumors. The microscopic diagnosis is generally easy, although small samples with crushing artifact can be confused with small cell carcinoma.[600,605] The diagnosis can also be made on cytologic examination, but the well-differentiated nature of the tumor cells and the fact that the tumor is usually covered

---

*See references 590, 594, 606, 610, 614, and 619.

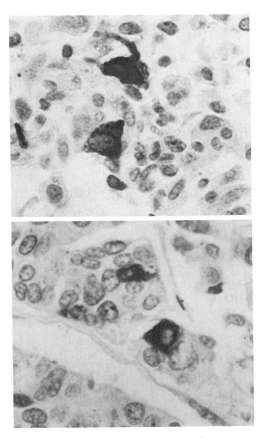

Fig. 7-106 Ectopic ACTH production in bronchial carcinoid shown by immunoperoxidase technique.

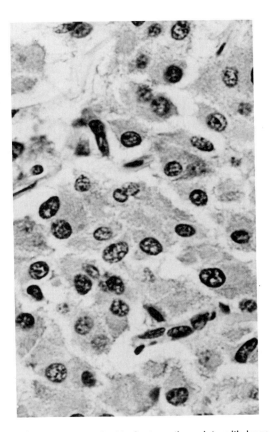

Fig. 7-107 Bronchial carcinoid of oncocytic variety with large cells, eosinophilic cytoplasm, small nucleus, and no mitotic figures.

by normal or metaplastic mucosa conspire to render most specimens nondiagnostic.[598]

The treatment is surgical. Removal through the bronchoscope is not adequate, because of the infiltrative nature of the tumor.[615] Depending on the location of the tumor along the bronchial tree and the status of the distal lung, operation may be a segmental bronchial resection, a lobectomy (the usual procedure), or a pneumonectomy.[583,615,616] The overall prognosis is excellent. In one series, the overall 10-year cumulative survival was 70%; for resected cases only, it was 82%, whereas of eleven patients treated by bronchoscopic methods, only one was alive.[615] It has been suggested that carcinoid tumors exhibiting immunoreactivity for CEA are associated with a more aggressive behavior manifested by a greater propensity for nodal metastases.[586]

Oncocytic carcinoid is a variant of central carcinoid tumor in which the tumor cells have an abundant, granular acidophilic cytoplasm[588,601] (Fig. 7-107). At the ultrastructural level, the cytoplasm contains numerous mitochondria and also dense-core secretory granules.[607,611] The differential diagnosis is with oncocytoma (see p. 326), and the behavior seems to be similar to that of central carcinoid tumor of the usual type.

Peripheral carcinoid tumor

As the name indicates, this type of carcinoid tumor arises in the peripheral lung, often immediately beneath the pleura. It tends to be multiple and presents grossly as non-encapsulated gray to tan nodules.[624] Microscopically, they are composed of spindle cells that may closely simulate the appearance of smooth muscle cells; it is not unusual for this lesion to be misdiagnosed as leiomyoma[621,624] (Fig. 7-108). The arrangement of the cells is disorderly; there is a certain degree of pleomorphism and occasional mitoses.[627] The stroma can be prominent, sometimes of such a degree and amount as to produce restrictive and obstructive lung disease when multiple tumors are present.[626]

Amyloid and melanin may be found, and calcitonin reactivity may be demonstrated immunohistochemically[625]; these features establish a close histogenetic link between peripheral lung carcinoid, thymic carcinoid, and thyroid medullary carcinoma. Most other immunohistochemical reactions are similar to those of central carcinoid tumor.[629]

The behavior of peripheral carcinoid tumor is excellent; regional node metastases are very rare, and most cases are cured by limited surgery.[627] Lobectomy is preferable to wedge resection because of the possibility of multicentricity; enucleation should not be attempted.

Tumourlet is the term given to nodular proliferation of small spindle cells seen in relation to bronchioles, often in association with bronchiectasis. These cells have been found to have the same ultrastructural and immunohistochemical features of those of peripheral carcinoid tumor.[622,630] Therefore they could be regarded as either nodular proliferations of endocrine cells or minute carcinoid tumors; indeed, sometimes one sees them in association with a typical peripheral carcinoid.[628] They almost always represent an incidental microscopic finding, and their behavior is generally benign, although isolated instances of metastatic behavior have been reported.[623]

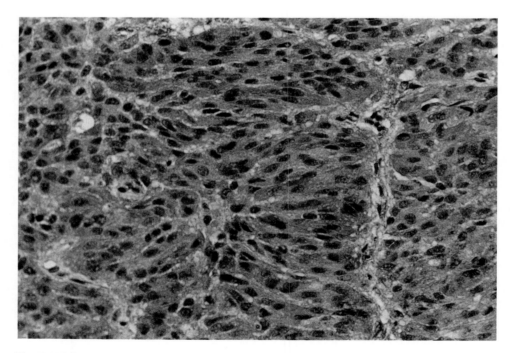

Fig. 7-108 Peripheral carcinoid tumor. Tumor cells have spindle shape and vaguely fascicular arrangement that can induce confusion with mesenchymal and neural neoplasms.

Atypical carcinoid tumor

Some lung tumors exhibit the overall architectural, ultrastructural, and immunohistochemical features of carcinoid tumor but also exhibit atypical features in the form of increased mitotic activity, nuclear hyperchromasia, and foci of necrosis[631,634] (Fig. 7-109). Exceptionally, stromal amyloid is present.[630a] It has been suggested that these atypical (intermediate, grade IV) carcinoids represent a link between the typical carcinoid tumor and small cell carcinoma.[635] Whether such a histogenetic link exists or not—and there is strong evidence against it[632,633]—there is no question that, for prognostic and therapeutic purposes, typical carcinoid tumors of either the central or peripheral types should be sharply separated from the atypical variety.[636] We view this tumor as a form of lung carcinoma exhibiting a greater or lesser degree of neuroendocrine differentiation. Along similar lines, some authors prefer to designate it as a well-differentiated neuroendocrine carcinoma (small cell carcinoma being the poorly differentiated counterpart).[633a]

In one series, the incidence of lymph node metastases for atypical carcinoid was almost 70%, as opposed to an incidence of about 5% for the typical carcinoid.[631] Therefore the treatment should be more aggressive and not different from that for ordinary lung carcinoma of non–small cell type.[637]

Paraganglioma

Primary paragangliomas occur rarely in the lung, presenting as solitary (usually peripheral) masses. Their histologic appearance is identical to that of paragangliomas in other sites, including carotid body tumors,[639,641] and their behavior is usually benign. The differential diagnosis with carcinoid tumor may be difficult or impossible, even after applying electron-microscopic and immunohistochemical techniques. Presence of ribbons, festoons, rosettes, and positivity for mucin, keratin, and CEA favor carcinoid, while the presence of a population of S-100 protein-positive sustentacular cells at the periphery of the nests favors paraganglioma.

Occasionally, a patient with a paraganglioma of the carotid body will present with a miliary pulmonary infiltrate made up of innumerable paraganglioma nodules intimately connected with blood vessels.[642] These have been interpreted as pulmonary metastases from such tumor, but the possibility of multicentric growth for at least some of these cases also needs to be considered.

An altogether different condition is mentioned here only because it was originally interpreted as *multiple pulmonary chemodectomas*. It is occasionally seen as an incidental finding in surgically excised lung, the lesions presenting as 1 to 3 mm tan yellow nodules having an intimate connection with blood vessels. Ultrastructural studies have shown a total lack of neurosecretory granules or other features suggestive of a neuroendocrine derivation. The cells have instead an appearance similar to that of arachnoidal cells and the cells of meningioma.[638,640] Immunohistochemically, they are negative for keratin and positive for vimentin and CEA, a pattern again similar to that of meningothelial cells.[638b] However, some authors have also found positivity

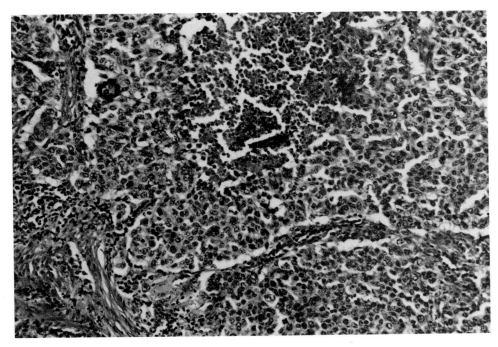

Fig. 7-109 So-called atypical carcinoid tumor. Presence of marked pleomorphism, mitotic activity, and necrosis distinguish this tumor from usual carcinoid. Hematoxyphilic staining of vessel wall is seen at center.

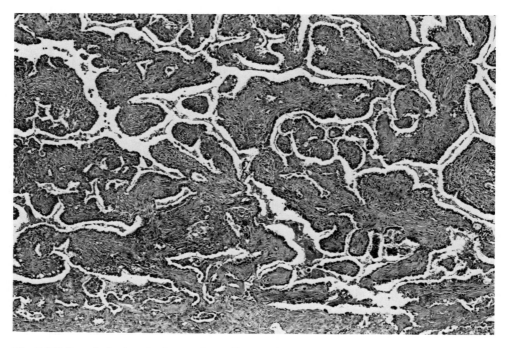

Fig. 7-110 So-called sclerosing hemangioma. Tumor has papillary configuration, papillae having stout fibrous cores and lining of single layer of cuboidal cells.

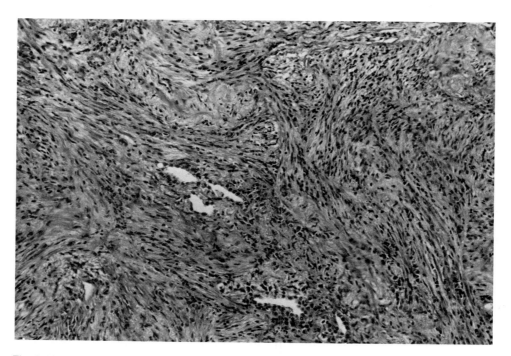

Fig. 7-111 Inflammatory pseudotumor of lung. Fascicles of proliferating mesenchymal cells separated by collagen fibers and chronic inflammatory cells are present. A few residual air spaces can still be appreciated.

for muscle-specific actin, suggesting an origin from smooth muscle cells or myofibroblasts.[638a]

So-called sclerosing hemangioma

This distinctive lesion occurs mostly in adult females, being generally detected as an asymptomatic small solitary nodule on chest x-ray. On serial films, the lesion is found to be stable or, at the most, very slow-growing. Grossly, it is well-circumscribed but not encapsulated, solid, tan or yellow, sometimes with hemorrhagic areas. Microscopically, there is a compact growth of polygonal cells with relatively abundant eosinophilic cytoplasm, arranged in a solid as well as a papillary or sclerotic pattern; this growth may be continuous with that of identifiable bronchiolar epithelium[651] (Fig. 7-110). Aggregates of xanthoma cells may be present. The histogenesis of this lesion has been highly controversial since its description as an entity. The polygonal cells thought to represent the neoplastic elements have been variously interpreted as endothelial, histiocytic, mesothelial, and epithelial.[645,647-650,653] Immunohistochemically, the positivity that has been obtained in them for EMA, keratin, and surfactant apoprotein strongly suggests a derivation from epithelial cells, specifically type II (granular) pneumocytes, with or without an accompanying mesenchymal component.[646,652] Accordingly, the proposal has been made to designate this lesion as *papillary* or *sclerosing pneumocytoma*.[643,644,646] This entity is generally benign and curable by limited excision, but a case with metastasis in a hilar node has been reported.[654]

Fibroxanthoma and related lesions

There is a group of pulmonary lesions presenting as more or less circumscribed nodules, having as a common feature the presence of large numbers of inflammatory cells (Figs. 7-111 and 7-112). Wide variations on this basic theme occur from case to case or even within the same case and are responsible for the many names and histogenetic interpretations that this group of lesions has received. These variations include vascular proliferation, fibrosis, hyalinization, myxoid change, fat accumulation with formation of xanthoma cells, hemosiderin deposition, proliferation of alveolar cells, and presence of inflammatory cells, such as lymphocytes and plasma cells.[656,662]

We believe that many of the lesions diagnosed as inflammatory pseudotumor, plasma cell granuloma, and histiocytoma are closely related processes.[660] Some cases diagnosed as sclerosing hemangioma and hyalinizing granuloma probably fall into this category as well. As with fibroxanthomas elsewhere, their inflammatory versus neoplastic nature is in doubt.[658] Many cases, however, seem to have a clearly reactive appearance.[661] We have seen these lesions confused with hemangiopericytoma, carcinoid tumor, plasmacytoma, amyloid tumor, and metastatic carcinoma.

Most cases of this entity occur in adults, but a good number of those rich in plasma cells are seen in children. Actually, they constitute the most common isolated primary lesion of the lung in patients below 16 years of age. The majority present as asymptomatic small peripheral nodules, yellow and firm, covered by an intact pleura. In rare instances there is extension to pleura or mediastinum. Other cases present as polypoid endobronchial masses and may lead to distal inflammatory changes.[655,659] Their behavior is benign and excision is usually curative. Radiation therapy is an acceptable therapeutic option for selected cases.[657] We have seen a single instance of malignant transformation in a long-standing lesion, and two similar cases have been reported.[660]

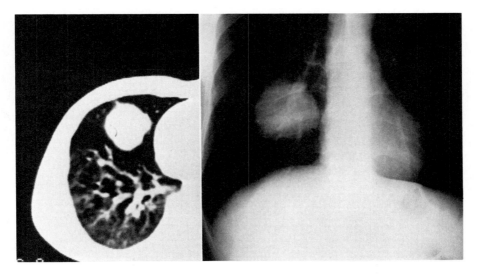

Fig. 7-112 CT scan and plain radiographic appearance of inflammatory pseudotumor of lung. Lesion has sharply outlined nodular quality that closely simulates a neoplastic process. (Courtesy Dr. J. Costa, Lausanne, Switzerland.)

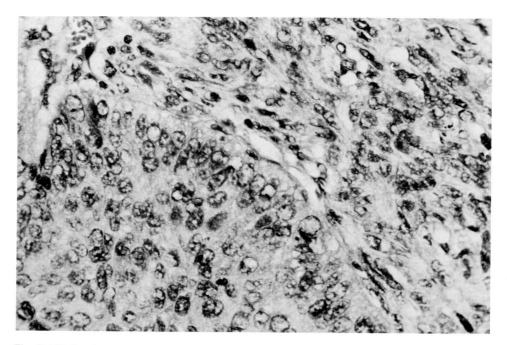

Fig. 7-113 Carcinosarcoma showing rather sharp demarcation between squamous carcinoma and sarcoma.

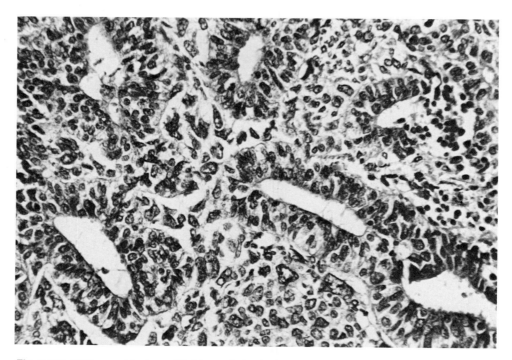

Fig. 7-114 Pulmonary blastoma. Well-formed glands are surrounded by very cellular stroma of "embryonal" appearance.

Carcinosarcoma and blastoma

Carcinosarcoma of the lung is a rare neoplasm that usually presents in adults as a centrally located, often intrabronchial, polypoid mass.[665] Microscopically, there is an intermingling of carcinomatous and sarcoma-like elements (Fig. 7-113). The carcinomatous component is usually of squamous cell type. The sarcoma-like component is usually spindle-shaped, with an appearance reminiscent of fibrosarcoma or malignant fibrous histiocytoma, and occasionally of chondrosarcoma, osteosarcoma, or rhabdomyosarcoma.[667b] Osteoclast-like giant cells can also be present.[671] The sarcoma-like component is probably of epithelial nature, this neoplasm representing the pulmonary analogue of carcinoma with sarcoma-like stroma of the upper aerodigestive tract.[663,667b] Bronchoscopic biopsy may show one or both elements. Despite earlier claims, the prognosis of this tumor has been found to be poor, comparable to that of bronchial carcinoma of the conventional type.[666,677] In one series, distant metastases were found in nine of twenty-four cases.[677]

Pulmonary blastoma, also known as embryoma, may present in adults or children, even neonates.[664,667,678] It is usually peripherally located. Microscopically, it is characterized by the presence of well-differentiated glands in a cellular stroma composed of undifferentiated spindle cells[668] (Fig. 7-114). The overall appearance resembles fetal lung and is also reminiscent of Wilms' tumor.[674] The stromal component may show differentiation toward skeletal muscle, cartilage, or bone.[667a] Intestinal differentiation has been found in some cases.[673] A few examples of the tumor have occurred in patients with pre-existent or concurrent cystic lung disease.[679] Metastases supervened in five of twelve cases reviewed by Stackhouse et al.[677]

The prognosis of carcinosarcoma and blastoma is similar, despite early claims to the contrary.[666] The occasional presence of transitional forms between these two tumors and their very similar ultrastructural appearance suggests that they are histogenetically closely related and that in a given case the distinction may not be possible or even warranted.[676]

A lung tumor with a glandular component similar to that of blastoma but lacking the sarcomatous elements has been described as *pulmonary endodermal tumor* or *adenocarcinoma of fetal type*[669,675]; in some cases, the tumor cells have been found to have endocrine features.[670,672]

Vascular tumors

Vascular tumors of the lung are extremely rare. Bonafide *hemangioma* should not be equated with so-called sclerosing hemangioma, a lesion that is of a nonvascular nature (see p. 319). *Capillary hemangiomatosis* presents with symptoms and signs of pulmonary hypertension.[696] *Hemangiopericytoma* and *glomus tumor* of the lung probably exist,[680,691] but most cases diagnosed as such probably represent misdiagnoses. A particularly notorious trap is to misdiagnose as hemangiopericytoma a solitary lung metastasis from an endometrial stromal sarcoma of the uterus.

Kaposi's sarcoma primary in the lung is usually a manifestation of AIDS[692,693] but can also occur in immunocompetent individuals.[681,693] The distribution of the disease typically follows lymphatic channels.[693]

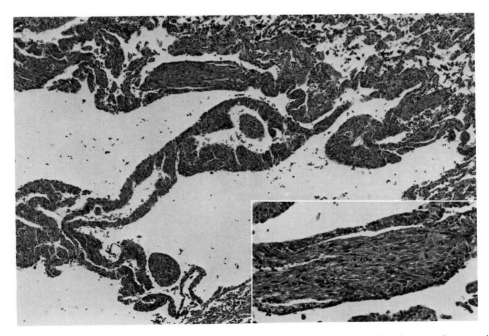

Fig. 7-115 Lymphangiomyomatosis of lung. Proliferating smooth muscle cells related to vessels expand pulmonary interstitium. Smooth muscle nature of these elements is better appreciated in **inset.**

Angiosarcoma can present as diffuse pulmonary infiltrates as an expression of a primary malignancy, but the more likely possibility of metastases should always be ruled out.[699]

Lymphangiomyomatosis may diffusely involve both lungs.[684] It occurs *exclusively* in women. Some patients are affected by tuberous sclerosis and renal angiomyolipomas.[689,694] It often leads to respiratory insufficiency, spontaneous pneumothorax, and chylous pleural effusion. The microscopic features are the same as those of the similarly named lesion of soft tissues (Fig. 7-115) (see Chapter 25). Progesterone receptors have been identified in the tumor cells, and objective response to progestational agents or oophorectomy has been documented.[682,688,690]

Intravascular bronchioloalveolar tumor (IV-BAT) is a neoplastic process of the lung that typically appears as multiple nodules. Many of the patients are young adults, and over 80% are females.[685] Microscopically, a thin rim of plump acidophilic cells that may resemble epithelium, histiocytes, cartilage, or decidua are seen surrounding an eosinophilic mass of hyalinized stroma, which is sometimes calcified (Fig. 7-116). These polypoid formations fill alveoli and occasionally bronchioles. The lumen of both arteries and veins may be filled with tumor, even at a distance from the main mass. Although originally interpreted as a variant of bronchioloalveolar carcinoma, ultrastructural and immunohistochemical studies have shown that the tumor is composed of endothelial cells and that it represents the pulmonary form of epithelioid (histiocytoid) hemangioendothelioma.[683,686,698]

The tumor grows in a very slow but progressive fashion, with a tendency to remain restricted to the thoracic cavity.[695] Some patients die as a result of pulmonary insufficiency.[685] Most of these tumors are primary in the lung, but others with an identical appearance have been interpreted as representing lung metastases from epithelioid hemangioendotheliomas located elsewhere, particularly the liver.[687,697] The alternative possibility of these being multicentric tumors has also been considered.

Lymphoid tumors and tumorlike conditions

The lung can be involved by a variety of lymphoproliferative processes, either secondarily or as the only manifestation of the disease. For purposes of discussion, these can be divided into six broad categories: large cell lymphoma of conventional type, the small lymphocytic pulmonary infiltrates, plasmacytoma, Hodgkin's disease, the leukemias, and lymphomatoid granulomatosis.[704]

Large cell lymphoma of conventional type presents as a large mass, occupying most of a lobe and often accompanied by foci of necrosis (Fig. 7-117). Occasionally, the pattern of growth is predominantly intrabronchial.[725] Microscopically, a monomorphic infiltrate of large lymphoid cells is present. Most cases belong to the large noncleaved or B-immunoblastic sarcoma categories.[712]

Small lymphocytic proliferations resulting in pulmonary nodules are often difficult to interpret. Most of the patients are elderly and asymptomatic, the lesion presenting as a solitary nodule or infiltrate on a chest x-ray. Grossly, they appear as a relatively well-defined but encapsulated mass,

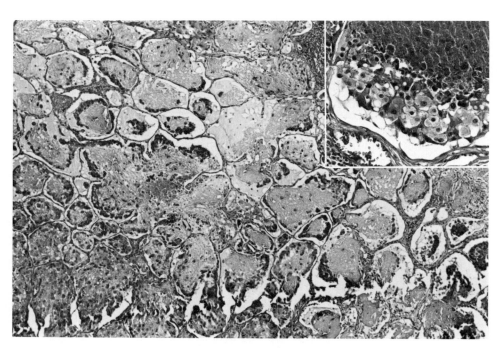

Fig. 7-116 Intravascular bronchioloalveolar tumor. Lesion grows in well-defined nests containing plump tumor cells and abundant amorphous eosinophilic material. Epithelioid features of tumor cells can be appreciated in **inset.**

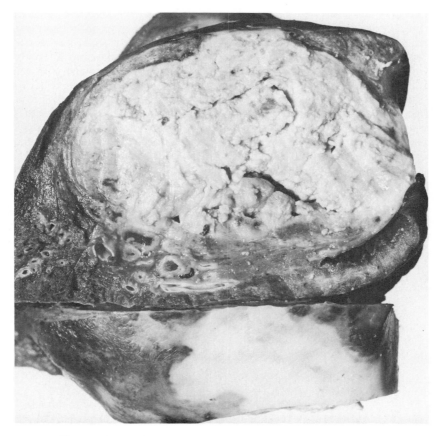

Fig. 7-117 Huge large cell lymphoma of lung in 45-year-old woman.

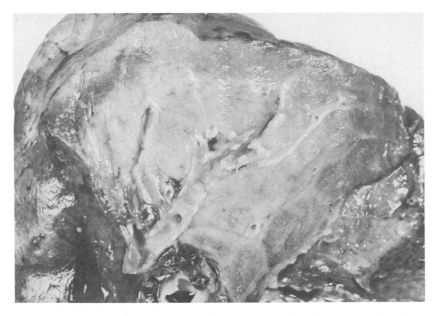

Fig. 7-118 Homogeneous localized area of small lymphocytic proliferation occurring in left upper lobe in 74-year-old woman. Regional lymph nodes were hyperplastic. Pneumonectomy was done by Dr. Evarts A. Graham. Patient died 5 years later without evidence of cancer.

which on cut surface show a homogeneous gray appearance (Fig. 7-118). Some of these lesions are of reactive nature and have been traditionally referred to as *pseudolymphomas*.[713,727] Microscopic features favoring a benign diagnosis are absence of hilar lymph node involvement, numerous germinal centers, and presence of other inflammatory cells.[727] In rare cases, this reactive lymphoid hyperplasia acquires the features of Castleman's disease.[718]

Other lesions are neoplastic in nature and represent either well-differentiated lymphocytic lymphomas (with or without plasmacytoid differentiation) or small cleaved lymphocytic lymphomas.[712,715] Features in favor of malignancy are the generally monomorphic nature of the infiltrate; the presence of plasmacytoid features (as opposed to mature plasma cells); the invasion of bronchial cartilage, wall of large vessels, or visceral pleura; and a lymphangitic pattern of infiltration.[711,712,731] Amyloid may be present in the stroma, another feature favoring malignancy.[713]

In recent years, there has been a reassessment of the well-differentiated lymphocytic lesions of the lung on the basis of immunohistochemical evaluations, the consensus being that the majority of these lesions are monoclonal in nature and therefore malignant, even when exhibiting morphologic features suggestive of benignancy[709,711,715,722,733] The main problem is that it is very difficult to predict on the basis of the morphologic and even the immunohistochemical features the evolution of these lesions.[705,711] By and large, they run a very indolent clinical course and have an excellent outcome,[731] which is upset in a minority of cases by the emergence of a high-grade lymphoma.[711,714]

Plasmacytoma should be used as a diagnostic term only for neoplastic lesions composed almost entirely of mature

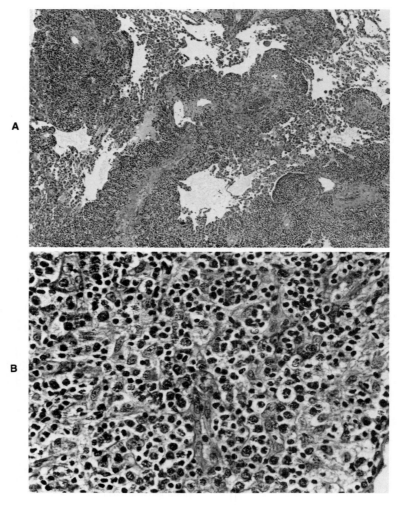

Fig. 7-119 Lymphomatoid granulomatosis of lung. **A,** Extensive lymphoid infiltrate is seen invading lung, with tendency to surround and infiltrate blood vessels. **B,** On higher magnification, infiltrate is seen to be composed of polymorphic population of lymphoid cells among which large cells with prominent nuclei and mitotic activity can be appreciated.

and immature plasma cells. Tumors with a prominent lymphoid component should be classified with the malignant lymphomas. Plasmacytomas of lung may be intraparenchymal or endobronchial, may be associated with nodal or bone involvement, and usually exhibit production of an M-protein,[700,730,735] which may appear in the tissue in the form of nodular deposits.[719]

Hodgkin's disease involving the lung parenchyma is usually associated with nodal involvement, direct extension from mediastinal nodes being frequent in the nodular sclerosis form. However, rare cases of primary pulmonary Hodgkin's disease have been well documented. They occur most frequently in women and older individuals and usually appear as nodular lesions on chest x-ray.[729,736] Endobronchial involvement can also occur, either in the form of a plaque-like infiltrate or as a polypoid mass.[708]

Leukemic involvement of the lung is found at autopsy in 30% to 40% of the chronic lymphocytic forms, in about 15% to 20% of the chronic myelogenous types, and in over 60% of the adult acute forms, but most of them are not manifested clinically.[720,732] Occasionally, however, significant pulmonary impairment results from the infiltrate of chronic lymphocytic leukemia acquiring a selective bronchiolocentric distribution.[720] In rare cases, acute granulocytic leukemia will present with widespread pulmonary nodules (granulocytic sarcoma).[701]

Lymphomatoid granulomatosis, originally included in the "pulmonary angiitis and granulomatosis" group[716,717] is now placed among the lymphoproliferative disorders. It usually presents in middle age with well-defined bilateral rounded mass densities, which roentgenographically may resemble the appearance of metastases.[721] Cases have been reported in immunosuppressed renal transplant recipients[707] and in association with Sjögren's syndrome.

The key microscopic picture is the presence of a polymorphic infiltrate rich in plasma cells, immunoblasts, and atypical large lymphoid cells, with a tendency to involve the walls of pulmonary vessels and to collect in the subendothelial spaces (Fig. 7-119). The multinucleated giant cells and necrotizing changes of Wegener's granulomatosis are lacking in this condition.

Extrapulmonary involvement occurs in over 80% of the cases.[726] The most common sites are the skin (particularly in the form of vasculitis in the lower extremities), central nervous system, and kidneys. Other sites include liver, spleen, adrenals, heart, and gastrointestinal tract.[723] The histologic appearance is quite similar in all of these sites. Exceptionally, the microscopic changes of lymphomatoid granulomatosis are seen in an extrapulmonary site in the absence of pulmonary involvement.[702,728] Furthermore, it has been postulated that midline malignant reticulosis represents the upper-respiratory-tract equivalent of lymphomatoid granulomatosis.

In recent years it has become evident that both the morphologic features of lymphomatoid granulomatosis and its clinical course are more in keeping with a malignant than a reactive process[726] and that it is common for large cell lymphomas of lung to exhibit vascular infiltration.[703] Accordingly, lymphomatoid granulomatosis is currently viewed as a primary lymphoproliferative disease that either

is or has a great tendency to become malignant lymphoma. Response to steroids is poor, but multidrug chemotherapy induces complete remission in about half of the cases.[706] The larger the number of atypical lymphoid cells, the worse the prognosis. In the series of 152 cases reported by Katzenstein et al.,[710] 63.5% died as a result of the disease, the median survival being 14 months. Most of the deaths were caused by extensive destruction of the pulmonary parenchyma, sepsis being a common complication. At autopsy, an infiltrate similar to that seen in the lungs was often found in the kidneys, liver, brain, and spleen. Eighteen patients (12%) developed a monomorphic large cell lymphoid infiltrate with the features of malignant lymphoma of the large cell type. Many of these lymphomas fulfill the morphologic criteria for immunoblastic sarcoma. Some cases are generalized, whereas others are found restricted to the central nervous system.[724]

A problem of nosology and terminology arises with the occasional pulmonary processes that show angiitis associated with a prominent but benign-appearing lymphocytic infiltrate. These lesions are not Wegener's granulomatosis of either the classic or limited type, but it is not clear whether they represent a variant of lymphoid interstitial pneumonia with angiitis, a cytologically bland form of lymphomatoid granulomatosis, or a distinct entity. Saldana et al.[726] and others[734] favor the third interpretation and propose the term *benign lymphocytic angiitis and granulomatosis* for them.

Salivary gland–type tumors

Several types of epithelial tumors with patterns analogous to those of salivary gland neoplasm occur in the lung, probably arising from submucous bronchial glands. Most of them are located within the main bronchi; in the past, the tendency was to group them under the term bronchial adenoma, an unfortunate practice because the term also included bronchial carcinoid tumor, a totally unrelated entity.

The most common type of bronchial salivary gland tumor-type neoplasm is *adenoid cystic carcinoma*[745] (Fig. 7-120). It arises in the major bronchi and often involves the trachea.[738] Metastases to regional lymph nodes and lung parenchyma are frequent (Fig. 7-121). If this tumor is diagnosed by bronchoscopic biopsy, pneumonectomy is indicated. Irradiation therapy may induce marked regression, but it is not curative. The total duration of the disease is long, but the ultimate prognosis is very poor.[745]

Mucoepidermoid carcinomas of the lung can be divided into low-grade and high-grade varieties, like their salivary gland counterparts. Only the low-grade type can be confidently identified as being of mucous gland origin, and perhaps it is the only one in this location that deserves to be regarded as of salivary gland type and to be designated mucoepidermoid carcinoma. Several of these cases have occurred in children.[743] It has a low malignant potential, characterized mainly by local invasion[744,748,751b]; some of these cases behave in an unexpectedly aggressive fashion.[737] Most cases of high-grade mucoepidermoid carcinoma are probably equivalent to the adenosquamous carcinoma and arise in all likelihood from the surface bronchial epithelium. Not surprisingly, they carry a very poor prognosis.[751]

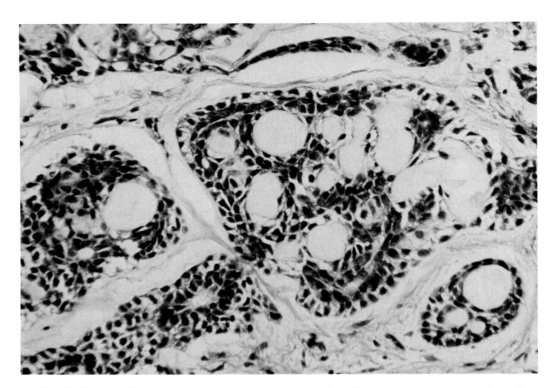

Fig. 7-120 Adenoid cystic carcinoma arising in major bronchus. Microscopic appearance is identical to homologous salivary gland neoplasm.

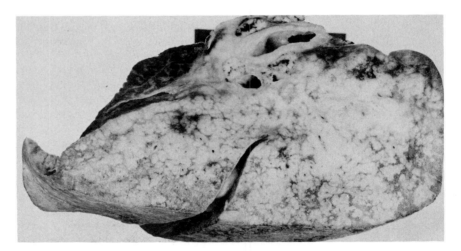

Fig. 7-121 Extensive involvement of lung, bronchi, and regional lymph nodes by adenoid cystic carcinoma.

Two cases of lung carcinoma with adenosquamous features, suggestion of myoepithelial cell differentiation (such as positivity for S-100 protein), and amyloid-like stroma made up of basement membrane material have been recently reported.[751a]

Other tumors in this category include *mucous gland adenoma*,[740,742,750] *benign mixed tumor* (pleomorphic adenoma),[747] *acinic cell tumor*,[741] *cystadenoma*, and pure *on-*

cocytoma.[739,749] The latter, which can be malignant, should be distinguished from oncocytic carcinoid tumor, a task that may require ultrastructural or immunohistochemical evaluation.[746]

Benign clear cell tumor

Benign clear cell tumor ("sugar tumor") presents grossly as a round or ovoid mass of small size, usually located in the peripheral lung.[756] It occurs in adults and children.[754] Microscopically, it is made up of large cells with clear cytoplasm crowded with glycogen granules. Fat is absent. Mitoses are not seen. By electron microscopy, most of the glycogen is usually membrane-bound in lysosome-like organelles, in a pattern reminiscent of glycogenosis II.[753,755] Its histogenesis is unknown: pericytes, smooth muscle cells, neuroendocrine cells, Clara cells, and epithelial serous cells have been implicated.[752] The differential diagnosis includes primary carcinoma with clear cell pattern and metastatic carcinoma, particularly from the kidney.[756]

Muscle tumors

Smooth muscle tumors of lung are rare. Primary solitary leiomyomas exist,[764,766,767] but some peripheral cases so diagnosed are actually spindle carcinoid tumors.

Occasionally, a middle-aged asymptomatic or minimally symptomatic female will present with innumerable small pulmonary nodules made up of well-differentiated smooth muscle, sometimes enclosing epithelial-lined clefts.[763] Concomitant uterine smooth muscle tumors are invariably present. A controversy exists as to whether the pulmonary nodules represent metastases from an extremely well-differentiated uterine leiomyosarcoma (so-called benign metastasizing leiomyoma)[765,769] or multicentric benign leiomyomatous growths.[759,763] We favor the latter interpretation, at least for the cases that we have personally examined. Support for this interpretation is provided by the fact that regression of these lesions during pregnancy or following oophorectomy has been observed.[758,760]

Leiomyosarcoma primary in the lung has been described,[761,768] but in the presence of a malignant smooth muscle tumor in the lung—even if solitary—the chances are overwhelming that the lesion is metastatic.

Rhabdomyosarcoma can present as a pleomorphic type in the lungs of adults,[757] or as an expression of the embryonal variety in the lungs of children; interestingly, the latter tends to occur against a background of cystic adenomatoid transformation.[762]

Miscellaneous primary tumors

Squamous papillomas of the large bronchi can occur alone or, more commonly, in association with tracheal and laryngeal involvement;[780,781] cases of this condition presenting in adulthood have a tendency for malignant transformation.[788,789]

Granular cell tumor can present as a polypoid intrabronchial mass and produce signs of bronchial obstruction.[776] Multicentric lesions have been described.[793]

Other rare benign lung tumors include intrapulmonary *thymoma*,[791] *neurilemoma*,[786,787] *neurofibroma*, *ganglioneuroblastoma*,[773] and bronchial *lipoma*[774] (Fig. 7-122). The latter is probably of malformative nature and related to hamartoma[792] (see p. 312). *Solitary fibrous tumor of pleura* can be entirely intrapulmonary and should therefore be considered in the differential diagnosis of spindle cell tumors of this organ (see p. 267). It is possible that the tumors reported as primary *meningiomas* of lung[772,777] arise from related stromal cells.

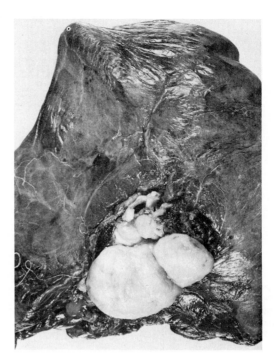

Fig. 7-122 Large, bright yellow lipoma involving bronchus.

Primary sarcomas of lung other than those already mentioned are rare. *Fibrosarcoma*,[770,782] *malignant fibrous histiocytoma*,[778,779,780a] *chondrosarcoma*,[775,790] *osteosarcoma*,[785] and *malignant schwannoma*[786] have been described in the lung. However, in the presence of any of these tumors, all efforts should be made to rule out the possibility of a primary tumor elsewhere and/or of a primary lung carcinoma with a sarcoma-like appearance. A similar warning applies to the diagnosis of *malignant melanoma*.[771,784] Although convincing examples of primary melanomas of the lung exist, the large majority represent metastatic deposits from known or occult primaries. Finally, several cases interpreted as primary pulmonary *choriocarcinoma* have been described.[783]

METASTATIC TUMORS

The lung is a very common site of metastatic disease. Most metastases are multiple, sharply outlined, and rapidly growing; this is particularly true for metastases from breast or stomach. Other metastases (particularly from stomach, breast, pancreas, and prostate) present as widespread neoplastic involvement of the pulmonary lymphatics (so-called lymphangitic carcinomatosis), which may result in severe dyspnea and pulmonary hypertension.

In other instances, the metastases present as isolated nodules and may simulate the appearance of primary tumors (Fig. 7-123). Sometimes, intraparenchymal or nodal metastases may penetrate the wall of a major bronchus and appear as polypoid intrabronchial masses, closely simulating a primary neoplasm.[806] We have seen this occur in testicular tumors, carcinoma of the kidney, and carcinoma of the rectum (Fig. 7-124).

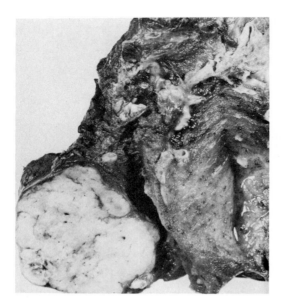

Fig. 7-123 Well-defined chondrosarcoma metastatic to lung in patient who had had this type of tumor in tibia several years before.

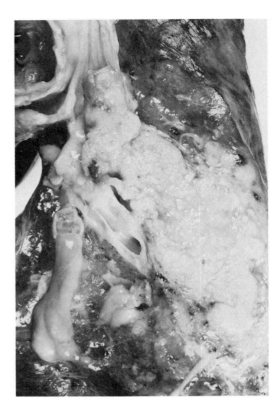

Fig. 7-124 Metastatic carcinoma of rectum forming polypoid mass in bronchus—a rare occurrence.

The differential diagnosis between primary and metastatic lung carcinoma can be difficult and sometimes is impossible. Multiplicity of lesions and extensive lymphatic permeation favor a metastasis. The presence of atypical or in situ changes in the bronchial mucosa adjacent to an epidermoid carcinoma and of honeycombing and atypical hyperplasia of bronchiolar epithelium in the parenchyma surrounding an adenocarcinoma favor a primary tumor. It should be remembered that many metastatic cancers to the lung line the alveolar walls in a fashion simulating bronchioloalveolar carcinomas. In one series, this was true for 25% of metastases from the kidney, 15% from the pancreas, 6% from the large bowel, and 6% from the breast.[804]

It has been claimed that the presence of microvilli having core rootlets and glycocalyceal bodies on ultrastructural examination of the cells of an adenocarcinoma favors a metastasis from the gastrointestinal tract, but the number of exceptions is such as to severely limit the value of this determination.[797]

When the pulmonary metastatic foci are few and sharply circumscribed, they are amenable to surgical excision.[807] Generally, the neoplasms most favorable for resection are well-differentiated sarcomas, and the least favorable are melanomas.[798-800,802] These resectable tumors do not usually cause any pulmonary symptoms and are discovered on roentgenograms of the chest taken at properly spaced intervals. The most important prognostic sign is the interval between the primary operation and the appearance of a metastasis. This was found to be directly proportional to survival time thereafter in the series of Edlich et al.[796] when the group was considered as a whole. Bad prognostic signs are multiplicity of metastases as seen in tomograms and presence of lymph node involvement.[801,805]

In recent years, a particularly aggressive approach has been taken towards lung metastases in children, particularly those from osteosarcoma or Wilms' tumor; the excision may be followed by radiation therapy or chemotherapy, depending on the nature of the tumor.[794] Five-year-survival rates of 25% to 40% have been obtained.[795,803]

REFERENCES
Pleura
NORMAL ANATOMY

1 Bolen JW, Hammar SP, McNutt MA: Reactive and neoplastic serosal tissue. A light-microscopic, ultrastructural, and immunocytochemical study. Am J Surg Pathol **10**:34-47, 1986.

2 Whitaker D, Papadimitriou JM, Walters MNI: The mesothelium. Techniques for investigating the origin, nature, and behaviour of mesothelial cells. J Pathol **132**:263-271, 1980.

3 Whitaker D, Papadimitriou JM, Walters MNI: The mesothelium. A histochemical study of resting mesothelial cells. J Pathol **132**:273-284, 1980.

PLEURITIS AND OTHER NON-NEOPLASTIC LESIONS

4 Aru A, Engel U, Francis D: Characteristic and specific histological findings in rheumatoid pleurisy. Acta Pathol Microbiol Immunol Scand [A] **94**:57-62, 1986.

5 Auerbach O: Pleural, peritoneal and pericardial tuberculosis. A review of 209 cases uncomplicated by treatment of secondary infection. Am Rev Tuberc **61**:845-861, 1950.

6 Dernevik L, Gatzinsky P, Hultman E, Selin K, William-Olsson G, Zettergren L: Shrinking pleuritis with atelectasis. Thorax **37**:252-258, 1982.

7 Engel U, Aru A, Francis D: Rheumatoid pleurisy. Specificity of cytological findings. Acta Pathol Microbiol Immunol Scand [A] **94**:53-56, 1986.

7a Knapp MJ, Roggli VL, Kim J, Moore JO, Shelburne JD: Pleural amyloidosis. Arch Pathol Lab Med **112**:57-60, 1988.

8 Martel W, Abell RM, Mikkelsen WM, Whitehouse WM: Pulmonary and pleural lesions in rheumatoid disease. Radiology **90**:641-653, 1968.

9 Menzies R, Fraser R: Round atelectasis. Pathologic and pathogenetic features. Am J Surg Pathol **11**:674-681, 1987.

10 Petty TL, Wilkins M: The five manifestations of rheumatoid lung. Dis Chest **49:**75-82, 1966.

11 Samson PC, Burford TH: Total pulmonary decortication. J Thorac Surg **16:**127-145, 1947.

12 Yeh TJ: Endometriosis within the thorax. Metaplasia, implantation, or metastasis? J Thorac Cardiovasc Surg **53:**201-205, 1967.

ASBESTOSIS AND THE PLEURA

13 Bhagavan BS, Koss LG: Secular trends in prevalence and concentration of pulmonary asbestos bodies—1940 to 1972. Arch Pathol Lab Med **100:**539-541, 1976.

14 Cauna D, Totten RS, Gross P: Asbestos bodies in human lungs at autopsy. JAMA **192:**371-373, 1965.

15 Churg A: Malignant mesothelioma in British Columbia in 1982. Cancer **55:**672-674, 1985.

16 Churg AM, Warnock ML: Asbestos and other ferruginous bodies. Their formation and clinical significance. Am J Pathol **102:**447-456, 1981.

17 Craighead JE: Current pathogenetic concepts of diffuse malignant mesothelioma. Hum Pathol **18:**544-557, 1987.

18 Craighead JE, Mossman BT: The pathogenesis of asbestos-associated diseases. N Engl J Med **306:**1446-1455, 1982.

19 Gaensler EA, Addington WW: Asbestos or ferruginous bodies. N Engl J Med **280:**288-292, 1969.

20 Hourihane DO'B, Lessof L, Richardson PC: Hyaline and calcified pleural plaques as an index of exposure to asbestos. A study of radiological and pathological features of 100 cases with a consideration of epidemiology. Br Med J **1:**1069-1074, 1966.

21 Kannerstein M, Churg J, McCaughey WTE: Asbestos and mesothelioma. A review. Pathol Annu **13**(Pt 1):81-129, 1978.

22 Kannerstein M, Churg J, McCaughey WTE, Selikoff IJ: Pathogenic effects of asbestos. Arch Pathol Lab Med **101:**623-628, 1977.

23 Langer AM, Rubin IB, Selikoff LJ: Chemical characterization of asbestos body cores by electron microprobe analysis. J Histochem Cytochem **20:**723-734, 1972.

24 Peterson JT Jr, Greenberg SD, Buffler PA: Non-asbestos-related malignant mesothelioma. A review. Cancer **54:**951-960, 1984.

25 Roggli VL, Kolbeck J, Sanfilippo F, Shelburne JD: Pathology of human mesothelioma. Etiologic and diagnostic considerations. Pathol Annu **22:**(Pt 2)91-131, 1987.

26 Rous V, Studeny J: Aetiology of pleural plaques. Thorax **25:**270-284, 1970.

27 Wagner JC, Sleggs CA, Marchand P: Diffuse pleural mesothelioma and asbestos exposure in the North Western Cape Province. Br J Intern Med **17:**260-271, 1960.

28 Warnock ML, Prescott BT, Kuwahara TJ: Numbers and types of asbestos fibers in subjects with pleural plaques. Am J Pathol **109:**37-46, 1982.

TUMORS
Mesothelioma

29 Adams VI, Unni KK, Muhm JR, Jett JR, Ilstrup DM, Bernatz PE: Diffuse malignant mesothelioma of pleura. Diagnosis and survival in 92 cases. Cancer **58:**1540-1551, 1986.

30 Aisner J, Wiernik PH: Chemotherapy in the treatment of malignant mesothelioma. Semin Oncol **8:**335-343, 1981.

31 Battifora H, Kopinski MI: Distinction of mesothelioma from adenocarcinoma. An immunohistochemical approach. Cancer **55:**1679-1685, 1985.

32 Brenner J, Sordillo PP, Magill GB, Golbey RB: Malignant mesothelioma of the pleura. Review of 123 patients. Cancer **49:**2431-2435, 1982.

33 Burns TR, Greenberg SD, Mace ML, Johnson EH: Ultrastructural diagnosis of epithelial malignant mesothelioma. Cancer **56:**2036-2040, 1985.

34 Cantin R, Al-Jabi M, McCaughey WTE: Desmoplastic diffuse mesothelioma. Am J Surg Pathol **6:**215-222, 1982.

35 Corson JM, Pinkus GS: Mesothelioma. Profile of keratin proteins and carcinoembryonic antigen. Am immunoperoxidase study of 20 cases and comparison with pulmonary adenocarcinomas. Am J Pathol **108:**80-87, 1982.

36 Dardick I, Jabi M, McCaughey WTE, Deodhare S, van Nostrand AWP, Srigley JR: Diffuse epithelial mesothelioma. A review of the ultrastructural spectrum. Ultrastruct Pathol **11:**503-533, 1987.

37 Donna A, Betta PG: Differentiation towards cartilage and bone in a primary tumour of pleura. Further evidence in support of the concept of mesodermoma. Histopathology **10:**101-108, 1986.

38 Epstein JI, Budin RE: Keratin and epithelial membrane antigen immunoreactivity in nonneoplastic fibrous pleural lesions. Implications for the diagnosis of desmoplastic mesothelioma. Hum Pathol **17:**514-519, 1986.

39 Hansen RM, Caya JG, Clowry LJ Jr, Anderson T: Benign mesothelial proliferation with effusion. Clinicopathologic entity that may mimic malignancy. Am J Med **77:**887-892, 1984.

40 Hillerdal G, Berg J: Malignant mesothelioma secondary to chronic inflammation and old scars. Two new cases and review of the literature. Cancer **55:**1968-1972, 1985.

41 Holden J, Churg A: Immunohistochemical staining for keratin and carcinoembryonic antigen in the diagnosis of malignant mesothelioma. Am J Surg Pathol **8:**277-279, 1984.

42 Jasani B, Edwards RE, Thomas ND, Gibbs AR: The use of vimentin antibodies in the diagnosis of malignant mesothelioma. Virchows Arch [Pathol Anat] **406:**441-448, 1985.

43 Kannerstein M, Churg J, Magner D: Histochemistry in the diagnosis of malignant mesothelioma. Ann Clin Lab Sci **3:**207-211, 1973.

43a Kawai T, Greenberg SD, Truong LD, Mattioli CA, Klima M, Titus JL: Differences in lectin binding of malignant pleural mesothelioma and adenocarcinoma of the lung. Am J Pathol **130:**401-410, 1988.

44 Klima M, Bossart MI: Sarcomatous type of malignant mesothelioma. Ultrastruct Pathol **4:**349-358, 1983.

45 Klima M, Spjut HJ, Seybold WD: Diffuse malignant mesothelioma. Am J Clin Pathol **65:**583-600, 1976.

46 Kondi-Paphitis A, Addis BJ: Secretory component in pulmonary adenocarcinoma and mesothelioma. Histopathology **10:**1279-1287, 1986.

47 Kwee WS, Veldhuizen RW, Golding RP, Mullink H, Stam J, Donner R, Boon ME: Histologic distinction between malignant mesothelioma, benign pleural lesion and carcinoma metastasis. Evaluation of the application of morphometry combined with histochemistry and immunostaining. Virchows Arch [Pathol Anat] **397:**287-299, 1982.

48 Law MR, Gregor A, Hodson ME, Bloom HJG, Turner-Warwick M: Malignant mesothelioma of the pleura. A study of 52 treated and 64 untreated patients. Thorax **39:**255-259, 1984.

49 Law MR, Hodson ME, Heard B: Malignant mesothelioma of the pleura. Relation between histological type and clinical behaviour. Thorax **37:**810-815, 1982.

50 Lee I, Radosevich JA, Chejfec G, Ma Y, Warren WH, Rosen ST, Gould VE: Malignant mesotheliomas. Improved differential diagnosis from lung adenocarcinomas using monoclonal antibodies 44-3A6 and 624A12, Am J Pathol **123:**497-507, 1986.

51 Legha SS, Muggia FM: Pleural mesothelioma. Clinical features and therapeutic implications. Ann Intern Med **87:**613-621, 1977.

52 Lerner HJ, Schoenfeld DA, Martin A, Falkson G, Borden E: Malignant mesothelioma. The Eastern Cooperative Oncology Group (ECOG) experience. Cancer **52:**1981-1985, 1983.

53 Lewis RJ, Sisler GE, Mackenzie JW: Diffuse, mixed malignant pleural mesothelioma. Ann Thorac Surg **31:**53-60, 1981.

54 McCaughey WTE, Al-Jabi M: Differentiation of serosal hyperplasia and neoplasia in biopsies. Pathol Annu **21**(Pt 1):271-293, 1986.

54a Montag AG, Pinkus GS, Corson JM: Keratin protein immunoreactivity of sarcomatoid and mixed types of diffuse malignant mesothelioma. An immunoperoxidase study of 30 cases. Hum Pathol **19:**336-342, 1988.

55 Nauta RJ, Osteen RT, Antman KH, Koster JK: Clinical staging and the tendency of malignant pleural mesotheliomas to remain localized. Ann Thorac Surg **34:**66-70, 1982.

56 Otis CN, Carter D, Cole S, Battifora H: Immunohistochemical evaluation of pleural mesothelioma and pulmonary adenocarcinoma. A bi-institutional study of 47 cases. Am J Surg Pathol **11:**445-456, 1987.

57 Rasmussen OO, Larsen KE: S-100 protein in malignant mesotheliomas. Acta Pathol Microbiol Immunol Scand [A] **93:**199-201, 1985.

58 Ratzer ER, Pool JL, Melamed MR: Pleural mesotheliomas. Clinical experiences with thirty-seven patients. Am J Roentgenol Radium Ther Nucl Med **99:**863-880, 1967.

59 Sheibani K, Battifora H, Burke JS: Antigenic phenotype of malignant mesotheliomas and pulmonary adenocarcinomas. An immunohistologic analysis demonstrating the value of Leu M1 antigen. Am J Pathol **123:**212-219, 1986.

60 Sussman J, Rosai J: Lymphadenopathy as the initial manifestation of malignant mesothelioma (abstract). Lab Invest **58:**90A, 1988.

61 Suzuki Y, Churg J, Kannerstein M: Ultrastructure of human malignant diffuse mesothelioma. Am J Pathol **85:**241-252, 1976.

62 Szpak CA, Johnston WW, Roggli V, Kolbeck J, Lottich C, Vollmer R, Thor A, Schlom J: The diagnostic distinction between malignant mesothelioma of the pleura and adenocarcinoma of the lung as defined by monoclonal antibody (B72.3). Am J Pathol **122:**252-260, 1986.

63 Vogelzang NJ, Schultz SM, Iannucci AM, Kennedy BJ: Malignant mesothelioma. The University of Minnesota experience. Cancer **53:**377-383, 1984.

64 Wanebo HJ, Martini N, Melamed MR, Hilaris B, Beattie EJ Jr: Pleural mesothelioma. Cancer 38:2481-2488, 1976.

65 Wang NS, Huang SN, Gold P: Absence of carcinoembryonic antigen–like material in mesothelioma. An immunohistochemical differentiation from other lung cancers. Cancer 44:937-943, 1979.

66 Warhol MJ, Corson JM: An ultrastructural comparison of mesotheliomas with adenocarcinomas of the lung and breast. Hum Pathol 16:50-55, 1985.

67 Yousem SA, Hochholzer L: Malignant mesotheliomas with osseous and cartilaginous differentiation. Arch Pathol Lab Med 111:62-66, 1987.

Solitary fibrous tumor of pleura

68 Briselli M, Mark EJ, Dickersin GR: Solitary fibrous tumors of the pleura. Eight new cases and review of 360 cases in the literature. Cancer 47:2678-2689, 1981.

69 Dalton WT, Zolliker AS, McCaughey WTE, Jacques J, Kannerstein M: Localized primary tumors of the pleura. An analysis of 40 cases. Cancer 44:1465-1475, 1979.

70 Dervan PA, Tobin B, O'Connor M: Solitary (localized) fibrous mesothelioma. Evidence against mesothelial cell origin. Histopathology 10:867-875, 1986.

71 Foster EA, Ackerman LV: Localized mesotheliomas of the pleura. The pathologic evaluation of 18 cases. Am J Clin Pathol 34:349-364, 1960.

72 Hernandez FJ, Fernandez BB: Localized fibrous tumors of pleura. A light and electron microscopic study. Cancer 34:1667-1674, 1974.

73 Janssen JP, Wagenaar SJSC, van den Bosch JMM, Vanderschueren RGJRA, Planteydt HT: Benign localized mesothelioma of the pleura. Histopathology 9:309-313, 1985.

74 Kawai T, Zakumaru K, Mikata A, Kageyama K, Torikata C: Solitary (localized) pleural mesothelioma. A light- and electron-microscopic study. Am J Surg Pathol 2:365-375, 1978.

75 McPeak CJ, Papaiannou AN: Nonpancreatic tumors associated with hypoglycemia. Arch Surg 93:1019-1024, 1966.

76 Ratzer ER, Pool JL, Melamed MR: Pleural mesotheliomas. Clinical experiences with thirty-seven patients. Am J Roentgenol Radium Ther Nucl Med 99:863-880, 1967.

76a Rayburn JL, Godwin TA: Fibrous tumor of the pleura. An immunohistochemical study (abstract). Lab Invest 58:76A, 1988.

77 Said JW, Nash G, Banks-Schlegel S, Sassoon AF, Shintaku IP: Localized fibrous mesothelioma. An immunohistochemical and electron microscopic study. Hum Pathol 15:440-443, 1984.

78 Scharifker D, Kaneko M: Localized fibrous ''mesothelioma'' of pleura (submesothelial fibroma). A clinicopathologic study of 18 cases. Cancer 43:627-635, 1979.

79 Stout AP, Murray MR: Localized pleural mesothelioma. Investigation of its characteristics and histogenesis by the method of tissue culture. Arch Pathol 34:50-64, 1951.

79a Yousem SA, Flynn SD: Intrapulmonary localized fibrous tumor. Intraparenchymal so-called localized fibrous mesothelioma. Am J Clin Pathol 89:365-369, 1988.

Other primary tumors

80 Iuchi K, Ichimiya A, Akashi A, Mizuta T, Lee Y-E, Tada H, Mori T, Sawamura K, Lee Y-S, Furuse K, Yamamoto S, Aozasa K: Non-Hodgkin's lymphoma of the pleural cavity developing from long-standing pyothorax. Cancer 60:1771-1775, 1987.

81 McCaughey WTE, Dardick I, Barr JR: Angiosarcoma of serous membranes. Arch Pathol Lab Med 107:304-307, 1983.

82 Yousem SA, Hochholzer L: Unusual thoracic manifestations of epithelioid hemangioendothelioma. Arch Pathol Lab Med 111:459-463, 1987.

Metastatic tumors

83 Chernow B, Sahn SA: Carcinomatous involvement of the pleura. An analysis of 96 patients. Am J Med 63:695-702, 1977.

Biopsy and cytology

84 Aaron BL, Bellinger SB, Shepard BM, Doohen DJ: Open lung biopsy. A strong stand. Chest 59:18-22, 1971.

85 Boon ME, Veldhuizen RW, Ruinaard C, Snieders MW, Kwee WS: Qualitative distinctive differences between the vacuoles of mesothelioma cells and of cells from metastatic carcinoma exfoliated in pleural fluid. Acta Cytol [Baltimore] 28:443-449, 1984.

86 Broghamer WL Jr, Richardson ME, Faurest SE: Malignancy-associated serosanguinous pleural effusions. Acta Cytol [Baltimore] 28:46-50, 1984.

87 Chiu B, Churg A, Tengblad A, Pearce R, McCaughey WTE: Analysis of hyaluronic acid in the diagnosis of malignant mesothelioma. Cancer 54:2195-2199, 1984.

88 Cibas ES, Corson JM, Pinkus GS: The distinction of adenocarcinoma from malignant mesothelioma in cell blocks of effusions. The role of routine mucin histochemistry and immunohistochemical assessment of carcinoembryonic antigen, keratin proteins, epithelial membrane antigen, and milk fat globule–derived antigen. Hum Pathol 18:67-74, 1987.

89 Dewald G, Dines DE, Weiland LH, Gordon H: Usefulness of chromosome examination in the diagnosis of malignant pleural effusions. N Engl J Med 295:1494-1500, 1976.

90 Ehya H: The cytologic diagnosis of mesothelioma. Semin Diagn Pathol 3:196-203, 1986.

91 Ferguson TB, Burford TH: The role of surgery in the management of unilateral pleural effusion. Ann Intern Med 50:981-998, 1959.

92 Herbert A, Gallagher PJ: Interpretation of pleural biopsy specimens and aspirates with the immunoperoxidase technique. Thorax 37:822-827, 1982.

93 Jarvi OH, Kunnas RJ, Laitio MT, Tyrkko JES: The accuracy and significance of cytologic cancer diagnosis of pleural effusions. Acta Cytol [Baltimore] 16:152-158, 1972.

94 Johnston WW: The malignant pleural effusion. A review of cytopathologic diagnoses of 584 specimens from 472 consecutive patients. Cancer 56:905-909, 1985.

95 Levine H, Metzger W, Lacera D, Kay L: Diagnosis of tuberculous pleurisy by culture of pleural biopsy specimen. Arch Intern Med 126:269-271, 1970.

96 Li C-Y, Lazcano-Villareal O, Pierre RV, Yam LT: Immunocytochemical identification of cells in serous effusions. Technical considerations. Am J Clin Pathol 88:696-706, 1987.

97 Light RW, Erozan YS, Ball WC: Cells in pleural fluid. Their value in differential diagnosis. Arch Intern Med 132:854-860, 1973.

98 Lopez Cardozo P: A critical evaluation of 3000 cytologic analyses of pleural fluid, ascitic fluid and pericardial fluid. Acta Cytol [Baltimore] 10:455-460, 1966.

99 Rao V, Jones PO, Greenberg SD, Bahar D, Daysog AO Jr, Schweppe HI Jr, Jenkins DE: Needle biopsy of parietal pleura in 124 cases. Arch Intern Med 115:34-51, 1965.

100 Roboz J, Greaves J, Silides D, Chahinian AP, Holland JF: Hyaluronic acid content of effusions as a diagnostic aid for malignant mesothelioma. Cancer Res 45:1850-1854, 1985.

101 Von Hoff DD, LiVolsi V: Diagnostic reliability of needle biopsy of the parietal pleura. A review of 272 biopsies. Am J Clin Pathol 64:200-203, 1975.

Lung
NORMAL ANATOMY

101a Colby TV, Yousem SA: Pulmonary histology for the surgical pathologist. Am J Surg Pathol 12:223-239, 1988.

NON-NEOPLASTIC LESIONS
Biopsy

102 Burt ME, Flye W, Webber BL, Wesley RA: Prospective evaluation of aspiration needle, cutting needle, transbronchial, and open lung biopsy in patients with pulmonary infiltrates. Ann Thorac Surg 32:146-153, 1981.

103 Churg A: Pathologist and pulmonologist. Ever the two shall meet? Hum Pathol 17:763-764, 1986.

104 Newman SI, Michel RP, Wang NS: Lingular lung biopsy. Is it representative? Am Rev Respir Dis 132:1084-1086, 1985.

105 Wall CP, Gaensler EA, Carrington CB, Wall CP, Gaensler EA, Carrington CB, Hayes JA: Comparison of transbronchial and open biopsies in diffuse infiltrative lung disease. Am Rev Respir Dis 123:280-285, 1981.

Cystic diseases

106 Allbritten FF Jr, Templeton JY: Treatment of giant cysts of the lung. J Thorac Surg 20:749-760, 1950.

107 Alt B, Shikes RH, Stanford RE, Silverberg SG: Ultrastructure of congenital cystic adenomatoid malformation of the lung. Ultrastruct Pathol 3:217-228, 1982.

108 Avitabile AM, Greco MA, Hulnick DH, Feiner HD: Congenital cystic adenomatoid malformation of the lung in adults. Am J Surg Pathol 8:193-202, 1984.

109 Mark EJ: Mesenchymal cystic hamartoma of the lung. N Engl J Med 315:1255-1259, 1986.

110 Nishibayashi SW, Andrassy RJ, Woolley MM: Congenital cystic adenomatoid malformation. A 30-year experience. J Pediatr Surg 16:704-706, 1981.

111 Potgieter PD, Benatar SR, Hewitson RP, Ferguson AD: Surgical treatment of bullous lung disease. Thorax 36:885-890, 1981.

112 Pride NB: Definitions of emphysema, chronic bronchitis, asthma, and airflow obstruction. 25 years on from the Ciba symposium. Thorax 39:81-85, 1984.

113 Stocker JT, Drake RM, Madewell JE: Cystic and congenital lung disease in the newborn. Perspect Pediatr Pathol **4**:93-154, 1978.

114 Stocker JT, Madewell JE, Drake RM: Congenital cystic adenomatoid malformation of the lung. Classification and morphologic spectrum. Hum Pathol **8**:155-171, 1977.

115 Wesley JR, Heidelberger KP, DiPietro MA, Cho KJ, Coran AG: Diagnosis and management of congenital cystic disease of the lung in children. J Pediatr Surg **3**:202-207, 1986.

Bronchopulmonary sequestration

116 Bruwer A, Clagett OT, McDonald JR: Intralobar bronchopulmonary sequestration. Med Clin North Am **38**:1081-1090, 1954.

117 Johnston DG: Inflammatory and vascular lesions of bronchopulmonary sequestration. Am J Clin Pathol **26**:636-644, 1956.

118 Pryce DM, Sellors TH, Blair LG: Intralobar sequestration of lung associated with an abnormal pulmonary artery. Br J Surg **35**:18-29, 1947.

119 Savic B, Birtel FJ, Tholen W, Funke HD, Knoche R: Lung sequestration. Report of seven cases and review of 540 published cases. Thorax **34**:96-101, 1979.

120 Smith RA: Some controversial aspects of intralobar sequestration of the lung. Surg Gynecol Obstet **114**:57-68, 1962.

121 Stocker JT: Sequestrations of the lung. Semin Diagn Pathol **3**:106-121, 1986.

122 Stocker JT, Kagan-Hallet K: Extralobar pulmonary sequestration. Analysis of 15 cases. Am J Clin Pathol **72**:917-926, 1979.

123 Telander RL, Lennox C, Sieber W: Sequestration of the lung in children. Mayo Clin Proc **51**:578-584, 1976.

Bronchiectasis

124 Bolman RM III, Wolfe WG: Bronchiectasis and bronchopulmonary sequestration. Surg Clin North Am **60**:867-881, 1980.

125 Cunningham GJ, Nassau E, Walter JB: The frequency of tumour-like formations in bronchiectatic lungs. Thorax **13**:64-68, 1958.

126 Field CE: Bronchiectasis in childhood. Pediatrics **4**:21-45, 1949; **4**:231-248, 1949; **4**:355-372, 1949.

127 Handelsman DJ, Conway AJ, Boylan LM, Turtle JR: Young's syndrome. Obstructive azoospermia and chronic sinopulmonary infections. N Engl J Med **310**:3-9, 1984.

128 Hilton AM, Hasleton PS, Bradlow A, Leahy BC, Cooper KM, Moore M: Cutaneous vasculitis and immune complexes in severe bronchiectasis. Thorax **39**:185-191, 1984.

129 Liebow AA, Hales MR, Lindskog GE: Enlargement of the bronchial arteries and their anastomoses with the pulmonary arteries in bronchiectasis. Am J Pathol **25**:211-232, 1949.

130 Mallory TB: The pathogenesis of bronchiectasis, bronchial infection and atelectasis. N Engl J Med **237**:795-798, 1947.

131 Oppenheimer EH, Esterly JR: Pathology of cystic fibrosis. Review of the literature and comparison with 146 autopsied cases. Perspect Pediatr Pathol **2**:241-278, 1975.

132 Perry KMA, King DS: Bronchiectasis. Study of prognosis based on follow-up of 400 patients. Am Rev Tuberc **41**:531-548, 1940.

133 Smallman LA, Gregory J: Ultrastructural abnormalities of cilia in the human respiratory tract. Hum Pathol **17**:848-855, 1986.

Abscess

134 Bosher LH Jr: A review of surgically treated lung abscess. J Thorac Surg **21**:370-376, 1951.

135 Hagan JL, Hardy JD: Lung abscess revisited. A survey of 184 cases. Ann Surg **197**:755-762, 1983.

136 Myers RT, Bradshaw HH: Conservative resection of chronic lung abscess. Ann Surg **131**:985-993, 1950.

Granulomatous inflammation

137 Ulbright TM, Katzenstein AL: Solitary necrotizing granulomas of the lung. Differentiating features and etiology. Am J Surg Pathol **4**:13-28, 1980.

138 Zimmerman LE: Demonstration of *Histoplasma* and *Coccidioides* in so-called tuberculomas of lung. Arch Intern Med **94**:690-699, 1954.

Tuberculosis

139 Auerbach O, Hobby GL, Small MJ, Lenert TF, Comer JV: The clinicopathologic significance of the demonstration of viable tubercle bacilli in resected lesions. J Thorac Surg **29**:109-132, 1955.

140 Auerbach O, Small MJ: The syndrome of persistent cavitation and noninfectious sputum during chemotherapy and its relation to the open healing of cavities. Am Rev Tuberc **75**:242-258, 1957.

141 Bailey TM, Akhtar M, Ali MA: Fine needle aspiration biopsy in the diagnosis of tuberculosis. Acta Cytol [Baltimore] **29**:732-736, 1985.

142 Black H, Ackerman LV: The clinical and pathologic aspects of tuberculoma of the lung. An analysis of 18 cases. Surg Clin North Am **30**:1279-1297, 1950.

143 Danek SJ, Bower JS: Diagnosis of pulmonary tuberculosis by flexible fiberoptic bronchoscopy. Am Rev Respir Dis **119**:677-679, 1979.

144 Humphrey DM, Weiner MH: Mycobacterial antigen detection by immunohistochemistry in pulmonary tuberculosis. Hum Pathol **18**:701-708, 1987.

145 Malave G, Foster ED, Wilson JA, Munro DD: Bronchopleural fistula. Present-day study of an old problem. A review of 52 cases. Ann Thorac Surg **11**:1-10, 1971.

146 Marchevsky A, Damsker B, Gribetz A, Tepper S, Geller SA: The spectrum of pathology of nontuberculous mycobacterial infections in open-lung biopsy specimens. Am J Clin Pathol **78**:695-700, 1982.

147 Parker EF, Brailsford LE, Gregg DB: Tuberculous bronchiectasis. Am Rev Respir Dis **98**:240-249, 1968.

148 Steele JD: The solitary pulmonary nodule. Springfield, Ill., 1964, Charles C Thomas, Publisher.

149 Strieder JW, Laforet EG, Lynch JP: The surgery of pulmonary tuberculosis. N Engl J Med **276**:960-965, 1967.

150 Sutinen S: Evaluation of activity in tuberculous cavities of the lung. A histopathologic and bacteriologic study of resected specimens with clinical and roentgenographic correlations. Scand J Respir Dis **67**(Suppl):5-78, 1968.

151 Sweany HC, Seiler HH: The pathology and bacteriology of resected lesions in pulmonary tuberculosis. Dis Chest **29**:119-152, 1956.

152 Thompson JR: "Open healing" of tuberculous cavities. Am Rev Tuberc **72**:601-612, 1955.

Atypical mycobacteriosis

153 Chester AC, Winn WC Jr: Unusual and newly recognized patterns of nontuberculous mycobacterial infection with emphasis on the immunocompromised host. Pathol Annu **21**(Pt 1):251-270, 1986.

154 Hattler BG Jr, Young WG Jr, Sealy WC, Gentry WH, Cox CB: Surgical management of pulmonary tuberculosis due to atypical mycobacteria. J Thorac Cardiovasc Surg **59**:366-371, 1970.

155 Snijder J: Histopathology of pulmonary lesions caused by atypical mycobacteria. J Pathol Bacteriol **90**:65-73, 1965.

156 Wolinsky E: Nontuberculous mycobacteria and associated diseases. Am Rev Respir Dis **119**:107-159, 1979.

Sarcoidosis

157 Churg A: Pulmonary angiitis and granulomatosis revisited. Hum Pathol **14**:868-883, 1983.

158 Churg A, Carrington CB, Gupta R: Necrotizing sarcoid granulomatosis. Chest **76**:406-413, 1979.

159 Hancock WW, Kobzik L, Colby AJ, O'Hara CJ, Cooper AG, Godleski JJ: Detection of lymphokines and lymphokine receptors in pulmonary sarcoidosis. Am J Pathol **123**:1-8, 1986.

160 Koerner SK, Sakowitz AJ, Appelman RI, Becker NH, Schoenbaum SW: Transbronchial lung biopsy for the diagnosis of sarcoidosis. N Engl J Med **293**:268-270, 1975.

161 Koss MN, Hochholzer L, Feigin DS, Garancis JC, Ward PA: Necrotizing sarcoid-like granulomatosis. Clinical, pathologic, and immunopathologic findings. Hum Pathol **11**:510-519, 1980.

162 Liebow AA: Pulmonary angiitis and granulomatosis. Am Rev Respir Dis **108**:1-18, 1973.

163 Rosen Y, Moon S, Huang C-T, Gourin A, Lyons HA: Granulomatous pulmonary angiitis in sarcoidosis. Arch Pathol Lab Med **101**:170-174, 1977.

164 Wilen SB, Rabinowitz JG, Ulreich S, Lyons HA: Pleural involvement in sarcoidosis. Am J Med **57**:200-209, 1974.

Wegener's granulomatosis

165 Carrington CB, Liebow AA: Limited forms of angiitis and granulomatosis of Wegener's type. Am J Med **41**:497-527, 1966.

166 Churg A: Pulmonary angiitis and granulomatosis revisited. Hum Pathol **14**:868-883, 1983.

167 Fienberg R: The protracted superficial phenomenon in pathergic (Wegener's) granulomatosis. Hum Pathol **12**:458-467, 1981.

168 Leavitt RY, Fauci AS: Pulmonary vasculitis. Am Rev Respir Dis **134**:149-166, 1986.

169 Nielsen K, Christiansen I, Jensen E: Wegener's granulomatosis. A survey and three cases. Acta Med Scand **181**:577-582, 1967.

170 Saldana MJ, Patchefsky AS, Israel HI, Atkinson GW: Pulmonary angiitis and granulomatosis. The relationship between histological features, organ involvement, and response to treatment. Hum Pathol **8**:391-409, 1977.

171 Travis WD, Carpenter HA, Lie JT: Diffuse pulmonary hemorrhage. An uncommon manifestation of Wegener's granulomatosis. Am J Surg Pathol **11**:702-708, 1987.

172 Ulbright TM, Katzenstein AL: Solitary necrotizing granulomas of the lung. Differentiating features and etiology. Am J Surg Pathol **4**:13-28, 1980.

173 Yoshikawa Y, Watanabe T: Pulmonary lesions in Wegener's granulomatosis. A clinicopathologic study of 22 autopsy cases. Hum Pathol **17**:401-410, 1986.

Bronchocentric granulomatosis and allergic granulomatosis

173a Bosken CH, Myers JL, Greenberger PA, Katzenstein A-LA: Pathologic features of allergic bronchopulmonary aspergillosis. Am J Surg Pathol **12**:216-222, 1988.

174 Churg A: Pulmonary angiitis and granulomatosis revisited. Hum Pathol **14**:868-883, 1983.

175 Jelihovsky T: The structure of bronchial plugs in mucoid impaction, bronchocentric granulomatosis and asthma. Histopathology **7**:153-167, 1983.

176 Katzenstein AL, Liebow AA, Friedman PJ: Bronchocentric granulomatosis, mucoid impaction, and hypersensitivity reaction to fungi. Am Rev Respir Dis **111**:497-537, 1975.

177 Koss MN, Antonovych T, Hochholzer L: Allergic granulomatosis (Churg-Strauss syndrome). Pulmonary and renal morphologic findings. Am J Surg Pathol **5**:21-28, 1981.

178 Koss MN, Robinson RG, Hochholzer L: Bronchocentric granulomatosis. Hum Pathol **12**:632-638, 1987.

179 Lanham JG, Elkon KB, Pusey CD, Hughes GR: Systemic vasculitis with asthma and eosinophilia. A clinical approach to the Churg-Strauss syndrome. Medicine [Baltimore] **63**:65-81, 1984.

180 Leavitt RY, Fauci AS: Pulmonary vasculitis. Am Rev Respir Dis **134**:149-166, 1986.

181 Liebow AA: Pulmonary angiitis and granulomatosis (The J. Burns Amberson Lecture). Am Rev Respir Dis **108**:1-18, 1973.

182 Saldana MJ: Bronchocentric granulomatosis. Clinicopathologic observations in 17 patients (abstract). Lab Invest **40**:281-282, 1979.

183 Urschel HC Jr, Paulsen DL, Shaw RR: Mucoid impaction of the bronchi. Ann Thorac Surg **2**:1-16, 1966.

Other granulomatous inflammations

184 Bigby TD, Serota ML, Tierney LM Jr, Matthay MA: Clinical spectrum of pulmonary mucormycosis. Chest **89**:435-439, 1986.

185 Binder RE, Faling LJ, Pugatch RD, Mahasaen C, Snider GL: Chronic necrotizing pulmonary aspergillosis. A discrete clinical entity. Medicine [Baltimore] **61**:109-124, 1982.

186 Campbell GD: Primary pulmonary cryptococcosis. Am Rev Respir Dis **94**:236-243, 1966.

187 Chen WJ, Monnat RJ Jr, Chen M, Mottet NK: Aluminum induced pulmonary granulomatosis. Hum Pathol **9**:705-711, 1978.

188 England DM, Hochholzer L: Primary pulmonary sporotrichosis. Report of eight cases with clinicopathologic review. Am J Surg Pathol **9**:193-204, 1985.

189 Goodwin RA Jr, Des Prez RM: Histoplasmosis. Am Rev Respir Dis **117**:929-956, 1978.

190 Hammerman KJ, Powell KE, Christianson CS, Huggin PM, Larsh HW, Vivas JR, Tosh FE: Pulmonary cryptococcosis. Clinical forms and treatment. Am Rev Respir Dis **108**:1116-1123, 1973.

191 Hopkins GB, Taylor DG: Pulmonary talc granulomatosis. A complication of drug abuse. Am Rev Respir Dis **101**:101-104, 1970.

192 Oddò D, Gonzalez S: Actinomycosis and nocardiosis. A morphologic study of 17 cases. Pathol Res Pract **181**:320-326, 1986.

193 Rafferty P, Biggs BA, Crompton GK, Grant IWB: What happens to patients with pulmonary aspergilloma? Analysis of 23 cases. Thorax **38**:579-583, 1983.

194 Zimmerman LE: Demonstration of *Histoplasma* and *Coccidioides* in so-called tuberculomas of lung. Arch Intern Med **94**:690-699, 1954.

Interstitial pneumonia

195 Banerjee D, Ahmad D: Malignant lymphoma complicating lymphocytic interstitial pneumonia. A monoclonal B-cell neoplasm arising in a polyclonal lymphoproliferative disorder. Hum Pathol **13**:780-782, 1982.

196 Basset F, Ferrans VJ, Soler P, Takemura T, Fukuda Y, Crystal RG: Intraluminal fibrosis in interstitial lung disorders. Am J Pathol **122**:443-461, 1986.

197 Bloch KJ, Buchanan WW, Wohl MJ, Bunim JJ: Sjogren's syndrome. A clinical, pathological, and serological study of sixty-two cases. Medicine (Baltimore) **44**:187-231, 1965.

198 Bonanni PP, Frymoyer JW, Jacox RF: A family study of idiopathic pulmonary fibrosis. Am J Med **39**:411-421, 1965.

199 Carrington CB, Gaensler EA, Coutu RE, Fitzgerald MX, Gupta RG: Natural history and treated course of usual and desquamative interstitial pneumonia. N Engl J Med **298**:801-809, 1978.

200 Coalson JJ: The ultrastructure of human fibrosing alveolitis. Virchows Arch [Pathol Anat] **395**:181-199, 1982.

201 Crystal RG: Alveolitis. The key to the interstitial lung disorders. Thorax **37**:1-10, 1982.

202 Crystal RG, Bitterman PB, Rennard SI, Hance AJ, Keogh BA: Interstitial lung diseases of unknown cause. Disorders characterized by chronic inflammation of the lower respiratory tract. N Engl J Med **310**:154-166; 235-244, 1984.

203 Darmanata JI, van Zandwijk N, Düren DR, van Royen EA, Mooi WJ, Plomp TA, Jansen HM, Durrer D: Amiodarone pneumonitis. Three further cases with a review of published reports. Thorax **19**:57-64, 1984.

204 Dreisin RB, Schwartz MI, Theofilopoulos AN, Stanford RE: Circulating immune complexes in the idiopathic interstitial pneumonias. N Engl J Med **298**:353-357, 1978.

205 Editorial: Interstitial pneumonia (fibrosing alveolitis). Lancet **2**:191-192, 1978.

206 Epler GR, Colby TV, McLoud TC, Carrington CB, Gaensler EA: Bronchiolitis obliterans organizing pneumonia. N Engl J Med **312**:152-158, 1985.

207 Fraire AE, Greenberg SD: Carcinoma and diffuse interstitial fibrosis of lung. Cancer **31**:1078-1086, 1973.

208 Gaensler EA, Goff AM, Prowse CM: Desquamative interstitial pneumonia. N Engl J Med **274**:113-128, 1966.

209 Greenberg SD, Haley MD, Jenkins DE, Fischer SP: Lymphoplasmacytic pneumonia with accompanying dysproteinemia. Arch Pathol **96**:73-80, 1973.

210 Heitzman ER, Markarian B, DeLise CT: Lymphoproliferative disorders of the thorax. Semin Roentgenol **10**:73-81, 1975.

211 Katzenstein A-LA: Pathogenesis of "fibrosis" in interstitial pneumonia. An electron microscopic study. Hum Pathol **16**:1015-1024, 1985.

212 Katzenstein A-LA, Myers JL, Mazur MT: Acute interstitial pneumonia. A clinicopathologic, ultrastructural, and cell kinetic study. Am J Surg Pathol **10**: 256-267, 1986.

213 Katzenstein A-LA, Myers JL, Prophet WD, Corley LS III, Shin MS: Bronchiolitis obliterans and usual interstitial pneumonia. A comparative clinicopathologic study. Am J Surg Pathol **10**:373-381, 1986.

214 Kitamura H, Kitamura H, Tsugu S: Combined epidermoid and adenocarcinoma in diffuse interstitial pulmonary fibrosis. Hum Pathol **13**:580-583, 1982.

215 Koss MN, Johnson FB, Hochholzer L: Pulmonary blue bodies. Hum Pathol **12**:258-266, 1981.

216 Liebow AA: New concepts and entities in pulmonary disease. In Liebow AA, Smith DE (eds): The lung (Monograph of the International Academy of Pathology). Baltimore, 1968, The Williams & Wilkins Co., pp. 332-365.

217 Liebow AA, Carrington CB: Diffuse pulmonary lymphoreticular infiltrations associated with dysproteinemia. Med Clin North Am **57**:809-843, 1973.

218 Liebow AA, Steer A, Billingsley JG: Desquamative interstitial pneumonia. Am J Med **39**:369-404, 1965.

219 Littler WA, Kay JM, Hasleton PS, Heath D: Busulfan lung. Thorax **24**:639-655, 1969.

220 Luna MA, Bedrossian CWM, Lichtiger B, Salem PA: Interstitial pneumonitis associated with bleomycin therapy. Am J Clin Pathol **58**:501-510, 1972.

221 Meyer EC, Liebow AA: Relationship of interstitial pneumonia honeycombing and atypical epithelial proliferation to cancer of the lung. Cancer **18**:322-351, 1965.

222 Myers JL, Kennedy JI, Plumb VJ: Amiodarone lung. Pathologic findings in clinically toxic patients. Hum Pathol **18**:349-354, 1987.

223 Rosenow EC III: The spectrum of drug-induced pulmonary disease. Ann Intern Med **77**:977-991, 1972.

224 Scadding JG: Diffuse pulmonary alveolar fibrosis. Thorax **29**:271-281, 1974.

225 Scadding JG, Hinson KFW: Diffuse fibrosing alveolitis (diffuse interstitial fibrosis of the lungs). Correlation of histology at biopsy with prognosis. Thorax **22**:291-304, 1967.

226 Schatz M, Patterson R, Fink J: Immunologic lung disease. N Engl J Med **300**:1310-1320, 1979.

227 Shimizu S, Kobayashi H, Watanabe H, Ohnishi Y: Mallory body–like structures in the lung. Acta Pathol Jpn **36**:105-112, 1986.

228 Sostman HD, Mattay RA, Putman CE: Cytotoxic drug-induced lung disease. Am J Med **62**:608-615, 1977.

229 Stillwell PC, Norris DG, O'Connell EJ, Rosenow EC, Weiland LH, Harrison EG Jr: Desquamative interstitial pneumonia in children. Chest **77**:165-171, 1980.

230 Topilow AA, Rothenberg SP, Cottrell TS: Interstitial pneumonia after prolonged treatment with cyclophosphamide. Am Rev Respir Dis **108**:114-117, 1973.

231 Tubbs RR, Benjamin SP, Reich NE, McCormack LJ, Van Ordstrand HS: Desquamative interstitial pneumonitis. Cellular phase of fibrosing alveolitis. Chest **72**:159-165, 1977.

232 Tukiainen P, Taskinen E, Holsti P, Korhola O, Valle M: Prognosis of cryptogenic fibrosing alveolitis. Thorax **38**:349-355, 1983.

233 Turner-Warwick M: Phillip Ellman lecture. Immunological aspects of systemic diseases of the lungs. Proc R Soc Med **67**:541-547, 1974.

234 Webb WR, Goodman PC: Fibrosing alveolitis in patients with neurofibromatosis. Radiology **122**:289-293, 1977.

235 Yousem SA, Colby TV, Carrington CB: Follicular bronchitis/bronchiolitis. Hum Pathol **16**:700-706, 1985.

Organizing pneumonia

236 Ackerman LV, Elliott GV, Alanis M: Localized organizing pnemonia. Its resemblance to carcinoma. Review of its clinical, roentgenographic and pathologic features. Am J Roentgenol **71**:988-996, 1954.

Lipoid pneumonia

237 Berg R Jr, Burford TH: Pulmonary paraffinoma (lipoid pneumonia). J Thorac Surg **20**:418-428, 1950.

238 Wagner JC, Adler DI, Fuller DN: Foreign body granulomata of the lungs due to liquid paraffin. Thorax **10**:157-170, 1955.

Eosinophilic pneumonia

239 Grantham JG, Meadows JA III, Gleich GJ: Chronic eosinophilic pneumonia. Evidence for eosinophil degranulation and release of major basic protein. Am J Med **80**:89-94, 1986.

240 Liebow AA, Carrington CB: The eosinophilic pneumonias. Medicine (Baltimore) **48**:251-285, 1969.

241 Magee F, Wright JL, Chan N, Currie W, Karr G, Hogg J, Thurlbeck WM: Two unusual pathological reactions to nitrofurantoin. Case reports. Histopathology **10**:701-706, 1986.

242 Neafie RC, Piggott J: Human pulmonary dirofilariasis. Arch Pathol **92**:342-349, 1971.

243 Warnock ML, Fennessy J, Rippon J: Chronic eosinophilic pneumonia. A manifestation of allergic aspergillosis. Am J Clin Pathol **62**:73-81, 1974.

243a White V, Luna M, Green L, Ayala A: Pulmonary dirofilariasis (abstract). Lab Invest **58**:96A, 1988.

Other pneumonias

244 Aherne W, Bird T, Court SDM, Gardner PS, McQuillin J: Pathologic changes in virus infections of the lower respiratory tract in children. J Clin Pathol **23**:7-18, 1970.

245 Becroft DMO: Histopathology of fatal adenovirus infection of the respiratory tract in young children. J Clin Pathol **20**:561-569, 1967.

246 Blackmon JA, Chandler FW, Cherry WB, England AC III, Feeley JC, Hicklin MD, McKinney RM, Wilkinson HW: Legionellosis. Am J Pathol **103**:429-465, 1981.

247 Blackmon JA, Hicklin MD, Chandler FW: Legionnaires' disease. Pathological and historical aspects of a 'new' disease. Arch Pathol Lab Med **102**:337-343, 1978.

248 Burke B, Good RA: *Pneumocystis carinii* infection. Medicine **52**:23-51, 1973.

249 Frazier AR, Rosenow EC III, Roberts GD: Nocardiosis. A review of 25 cases occurring during 24 months. Mayo Clin Proc **50**:657-663, 1975.

250 Gorelkin L, Chandler FW, Ewing EP Jr: Staining qualities of cytomegalovirus inclusions in the lungs of patients with the acquired immunodeficiency syndrome. A potential source of diagnostic misinterpretation. Hum Pathol **17**:926-929, 1986.

251 Graham BS, Snell JD Jr: Herpes simplex virus infection of the adult lower respiratory tract. Medicine **62**:384-393, 1983.

252 Hodder RV, St. George-Hyslop P, Chalvardjian A, Bear RA, Thomas P: Pulmonary malakoplakia. Thorax **39**:70-71, 1984.

252a Kovacs JA, Ng VL, Masur H, Leoung G, Hadley WK, Evans G, Lane HC, Ognibene FP, Shelhamer J, Parrillo JE, Gill VJ: Diagnosis of pneumocystis carinii pneumonia. Improved detection in sputum with use of monoclonal antibodies. N Engl J Med **318**:589-593, 1988.

253 Macfarlane JT: *Pneumocystis carinii* pneumonia. Thorax **40**:561-570, 1985.

254 Mahan CT, Sale GE: Rapid methenamine silver stain for pneumocystis and fungi. Arch Pathol Lab Med **102**:351-352, 1978.

255 Murray HW, Masur H, Senterfit LB, Roberts RB: The protean manifestations of Mycoplasma pneumoniae infection in adults. Am J Med **58**:229-242, 1975.

256 Oddó D, Gonzalez S: Actinomycosis and nocardiosis. A morphologic study of 17 cases. Pathol Res Pract **181**:320-326, 1986.

257 Palmer DL, Harvey RL, Wheeler JK: Diagnostic and therapeutic considerations in *Nocardia asteroides* infection. Medicine [Baltimore] **53**:391-401, 1974.

258 Rollins S, Colby T, Clayton F: Open lung biopsy in Mycoplasma pneumoniae pneumonia. Arch Pathol Lab Med **110**:34-41, 1986.

259 Rosen PP: Frozen section management of a lung biopsy for suspected *Pneumocystis* pneumonia. Am J Surg Pathol **1**:79-82, 1977.

260 Rosen PP, Armstrong DA, Ramos C: *Pneumocystis carinii* pneumonia. A clinicopathologic study of 20 patients with neoplastic diseases. Am J Med **53**:428-436, 1972.

261 Rosen PP, Martini N, Armstrong DA: *Pneumocystis carinii* pneumonia. Diagnosis by lung biopsy. Am J Med **56**:794-802, 1975.

262 Schaefer HE: Inflammatory disease of the human lung of definite or presumed viral origin. Cytologic and histologic topics. Curr Topics Pathol **73**:153-206, 1983.

263 Schwartz DA, Munger RG, Katz SM: Plastic embedding evaluation of *Pneumocystis carinii* pneumonia in AIDS. Simultaneous demonstration of cyst and sporozoite forms. Am J Surg Pathol **11**:304-309, 1987.

264 Walzer PD, Perl P, Krogstad DJ, Rawson PG, Schultz MG: *Pneumocystis carinii* pneumonia in the United States. Ann Intern Med **80**:83-93, 1974.

265 Watts JC, Chandler FW: *Pneumocystis carinii* pneumonitis. The nature and diagnostic significance of the methenamine silver-positive "intracystic bodies." Am J Surg Pathol **9**:744-751, 1985.

266 Weber WR, Askin FB, Dehner LP: Lung biopsy in *Pneumocystis carinii* pneumonia. A histopathologic study of typical and atypical features. Am J Clin Pathol **67**:11-19, 1977.

267 Weisenburger DD, Helms CM, Renner ED: Sporadic Legionnaires' disease. A pathologic study of 23 fatal cases. Arch Pathol Lab Med **105**:130-137, 1981.

268 Winn WC Jr, Glavin FL, Perl DP, Keller JL, Andres TL, Brown TM, Coffin CM, Sensecqua JE, Roman LN, Craighead JE: The pathology of Legionnaires' disease. Fourteen fatal cases from the 1977 outbreak in Vermont. Arch Pathol Lab Med **102**:344-350, 1978.

269 Winn WC Jr, Myerowitz RL: The pathology of the Legionella pneumonias. A review of 74 cases and the literature. Hum Pathol **12**:401-442, 1981.

Lung in AIDS

270 Blumenfeld W, Wagar E, Hadley WK: Use of the transbronchial biopsy for diagnosis of opportunistic pulmonary infections in acquired immunodeficiency syndrome (AIDS). Am J Clin Pathol **81**:1-5, 1984.

271 Gal AA, Klatt EC, Koss MN, Strigle SM, Boylen CT: The effectiveness of bronchoscopy in the diagnosis of *Pneumocystis carinii* and cytomegalovirus pulmonary infections in acquired immunodeficiency syndrome. Arch Pathol Lab Med **111**:238-241, 1987.

272 Joshi VV, Oleske JM, Minnefor AB, Saad S, Klein KM, Singh R, Zabala M, Dadzie C, Simpser M, Rapkin RH: Pathologic pulmonary findings in children with the acquired immunodeficiency syndrome. A study of ten cases. Hum Pathol **16**:241-246, 1985.

273 Marchevsky A, Rosen MJ, Chrystal G, Kleinerman J: Pulmonary complications of the acquired immunodeficiency syndrome. A clinicopathologic study of 70 cases. Hum Pathol **16**:659-670, 1985.

274 McKenna RJ Jr, Campbell A, McMurtrey MJ, Mountain CF: Diagnosis for interstitial lung disease in patients with acquired immunodeficiency syndrome (AIDS). A prospective comparison of bronchial washing, alveolar lavage, transbronchial lung biopsy, and open-lung biopsy. Ann Thorac Surg **41**:318-321, 1986.

275 Nash G, Fligiel S: Pathologic features of the lung in the acquired immune deficiency syndrome (AIDS). An autopsy study of seventeen homosexual males. Am J Clin Pathol **81**:6-12, 1984.

276 Orenstein M, Webber CA, Cash M, Heurich AE: Value of bronchoalveolar lavage in the diagnosis of pulmonary infection in acquired immune deficiency syndrome. Thorax **41**:345-349, 1986.

277 Ramaswamy G, Jagadha V, Tchertkoff V: Diffuse alveolar damage and interstitial fibrosis in acquired immunodeficiency syndrome patients without concurrent pulmonary infection. Arch Pathol Lab Med **109**:408-412, 1985.

277a Travis WD, Lack EE, Ognibene FP, Suffredini AF, Shelhamer J: Pathology of the lung in the acquired immune deficiency syndrome (AIDS) (abstract). Am J Clin Pathol **89**:431-432, 1988.

Lung in bone marrow transplantation

278 Sloane JP, Depledge MH, Powles RL, Morgenstern GR, Trickey BS, Dady PJ: Histopathology of the lung after bone marrow transplantation. J Clin Pathol **36**:546-554, 1983.

279 Urbanski SJ, Kossakowska AE, Curtis J, Chan CK, Hutcheon MA, Hyland RH, Messner H, Minden M, Sculier JP: Idiopathic small airways pathology in patients with graft-versus-host disease following allogeneic bone marrow transplantation. Am J Surg Pathol **11**:965-971, 1987.

Anthracosis and silicosis

280 Naeye RL: The anthracotic pneumoconioses. Curr Top Pathol 55:37-68, 1971.

Asbestosis

281 Kuhn C III, Kuo TT: Cytoplasmic hyalin in asbestosis. Arch Pathol 95:190-194, 1973.

Extrinsic allergic alveolitis

282 Fink JN, Banaszak EF, Baroriak JJ, Hensley GT, Kurup VP, Scanlon GT, Schleuter DP, Sosman AJ, Thiede WH, Unger GF: Interstitial lung disease due to contamination of forced air systems. Ann Intern Med 85:406-413, 1976.

282a Hammar S: Hypersensitivity pneumonitis. Pathol Annu 23(Pt 1):195-215, 1988.

283 Kawanami O, Basset F, Barrios R, Lacronique JG, Ferrans VJ, Crystal RG: Hypersensitivity pneumonitis in man. Light- and electron-microscopic studies of 18 lung biopsies. Am J Pathol 110:275-289, 1983.

284 Nicholson DP: Extrinsic allergic pneumonias. Am J Med 53:131-136, 1972.

Histiocytosis X

285 Askin FB, McCann BG, Kuhn C: Reactive eosinophilic pleuritis. A lesion to be distinguished from pulmonary eosinophilic granuloma. Arch Pathol Lab Med 101:187-191, 1977.

286 Chollet S, Soler P, Dournovo P, Richard MS, Ferrans VJ, Basset F: Diagnosis of pulmonary histiocytosis X by immunodetection of Langerhans' cells in bronchoalveolar lavage fluid. Am J Pathol 115:225-232, 1984.

287 Colby TV, Lombard C: Histiocytosis X in the lung. Hum Pathol 14:847-856, 1983.

288 Flint A, Lloyd RV, Colby TV, Wilson BW: Pulmonary histiocytosis X. Immunoperoxidase staining for HLA-DR antigen and S 100 protein. Arch Pathol Lab Med 110:930-933, 1986.

289 Friedman PJ, Liebow AA, Sokoloff J: Eosinophilic granuloma of lung. Clinical aspects of primary pulmonary histiocytosis in the adult. Medicine 60:385-396, 1981.

290 Gold J, L'Heureux P, Dehner LP: Ultrastructure in the differential diagnosis of pulmonary histiocytosis and pneumocystosis. Arch Pathol Lab Med 101:243-247, 1977.

291 Lewis JG: Eosinophilic granuloma and its variants with special reference to lung involvement. Q J Med 33:337-359, 1964.

292 Lombard CM, Medeiros LJ, Colby TV: Pulmonary histiocytosis X and carcinoma. Arch Pathol Lab Med 111:339-341, 1987.

293 Soler P, Chollet S, Jacque C, Fukuda Y, Ferrans VJ, Basset F: Immunocytochemical characterization of pulmonary histiocytosis X cells in lung biopsies. Am J Pathol 118:439-451, 1985.

294 Webber D, Tron V, Askin F, Churg A: S-100 staining in the diagnosis of eosinophilic granuloma of lung. Am J Clin Pathol 84:447-453, 1985.

Vascular diseases

295 Bjornsson J, Edwards WD: Primary pulmonary hypertension. A histopathologic study of 80 cases. Mayo Clin Proc 60:16-25, 1985.

296 Carrington CB, Liebow AA: Pulmonary veno-occlusive disease. Hum Pathol 1:322-324, 1970.

297 Corrin B, Spencer H, Turner-Warwich M, Beales SJ, Hamblin JJ: Pulmonary veno-occlusion. An immune complex disease? Virchows Arch [Pathol Anat] 364:81-91, 1974.

298 Hasleton PS, Ironside JW, Whittaker JS, Kelly W, Ward C, Thompson GS: Pulmonary veno-occlusive disease. A report of four cases. Histopathology 10:933-944, 1986.

299 Hughes JD, Rubin LJ: Primary pulmonary hypertension. An analysis of 28 cases and a review of the literature. Medicine 65:56-72, 1986.

300 Thadani U, Burrow C, Whitaker W, Heath D: Pulmonary veno-occlusive disease. Q J Med 44:133-159, 1975.

301 Wagenvoort CA: Open lung biopsies in congenital heart disease for evaluation of pulmonary vascular disease. Predictive value with regard to corrective operability. Histopathology 9:417-436, 1985.

302 Wagenvoort CA, Wagenvoort N: The pathology of pulmonary veno-occlusive disease. Virchows Arch [Pathol Anat] 364:69-79, 1974.

Other non-neoplastic diseases

303 Abboud RT, Chase WH, Ballon HS: Goodpasture's syndrome. Diagnosis by transbronchial lung biopsy. Ann Intern Med 89:635-638, 1978.

304 Arrigoni MG, Bernatz PE, Donoghue FE: Broncholithiasis. J Thorac Cardiovasc Surg 62:231-237, 1971.

305 Carnovale R, Zornoza J, Goldman AM, Luna M: Pulmonary alveolar proteinosis.

Its association with hematologic malignancy and lymphoma. Radiology 122:303-306, 1977.

306 Colon AR, Lawrence RD, Mills SD, O'Connell EJ: Childhood pulmonary alveolar proteinosis (PAP). Report of a case and review of the literature. Am J Dis Child 121:481-485, 1971.

307 Da Costa P, Corrin B: Amyloidosis localized to the lower respiratory tract. Probable immunoamyloid nature of the tracheobronchial and nodular pulmonary forms. Histopathology 9:703-710, 1985.

308 Donald KJ, Edwards RL, McEvoy JDS: Alveolar capillary basement membrane lesions in Goodpasture's syndrome and idiopathic pulmonary hemosiderosis. Am J Med 59:642-649, 1975.

309 Donlan CJ Jr, Srodes CH, Duffy FD: Idiopathic pulmonary hemosiderosis. Electron microscopic, immunofluorescent, and iron kinetic studies. Chest 68:577-580, 1975.

310 Du Bois RM, McAllister WAC, Branthwaite MA: Alveolar proteinosis. Diagnosis and treatment over a 10-year period. Thorax 38:360-363, 1983.

311 Eagen JW, Memoli VA, Roberts JL: Pulmonary hemorrhage in systemic lupus erythematosus. Medicine (Baltimore) 57:545-560, 1978.

312 Engleman P, Liebow AA, Gmelich J, Friedman PJ: Pulmonary hyalinizing granuloma. Am Rev Respir Dis 115:997-1008, 1977.

313 Errion GD, Hauk VN, Kettering DL: Pulmonary hematoma due to blunt non-penetrating thoracic trauma. Am Rev Respir Dis 88:384-392, 1963.

314 Geddes DM, Corrin B, Brewerton DA, Davies RJ, Turner-Warwick M: Progressive airway obliteration in adults and its association with rheumatoid disease. Q J Med 46:427-444, 1977.

315 Groves LK, Effler DB: Broncholithiasis. A review of twenty-seven cases. Am Rev Tuberc 73:19-30, 1956.

316 Hibbard LT, Schumann WR, Goldstein GE: Thoracic endometriosis. A review and report of two cases. Am J Obstet Gynecol 140:227-232, 1981.

317 Leatherman JW, Davies SF, Hoidal JR: Alveolar hemorrhage syndromes. Diffuse microvascular lung hemorrhage in immune and idiopathic disorders. Medicine 63:343-360, 1984.

318 Lee S-C, Johnson HA: Multiple nodular pulmonary amyloidosis. A case report and comparison with diffuse alveolar-septal pulmonary amyloidosis. Thorax 30:178-185, 1975.

319 Lingskog GE, Liebow AA, Kausel H, Janzen A: Pulmonary arteriovenous aneurysm. Ann Surg 132:591-606, 1950.

320 Mark EJ, Ramirez JF: Pulmonary capillaritis and hemorrhage in patients with systemic vasculitis. Arch Pathol Lab Med 109:413-418, 1985.

321 Petty IL, Wilkins M: The five manifestations of rheumatoid lung. Dis Chest 49:75-82, 1966.

322 Prakash UBS, Barham SS, Rosenow EC III, Brown ML, Payne WS: Pulmonary alveolar microlithiasis. A review including ultrastructural and pulmonary function studies. Mayo Clin Proc 58:290-300, 1983.

323 Ranchod M, Bissell M: Pulmonary alveolar proteinosis and cytomegalovirus infection. Arch Pathol Lab Med 103:139-142, 1979.

324 Rosen SH, Castleman B, Liebow AA: Pulmonary alveolar proteinosis. N Engl J Med 258:1123-1142, 1958.

325 Schober R, Bensch KG, Kosek JC, Northway WH: On the origin of the membranous intraalveolar material in pulmonary alveolar proteinosis. Exp Mol Pathol 21:246-258, 1974.

326 Soergel KH, Sommers SC: Idiopathic pulmonary hemosiderosis and related syndromes. Am J Med 32:499-511, 1962.

327 Steer A: Focal pulmonary alveolar proteinosis in pulmonary tuberculosis. Arch Pathol 87:347-352, 1969.

328 Thompson PJ, Citron KM: Amyloid and the lower respiratory tract. Thorax 38:84-87, 1983.

329 Walker WC, Wright V: Pulmonary lesions and rheumatoid arthritis. Medicine (Baltimore) 47:501-520, 1968.

330 Yousem SA, Hochholzer L: Pulmonary hyalinizing granuloma. Am J Clin Pathol 87:1-6, 1987.

CARCINOMA
General features

331 Auerbach O, Garfinkel L, Parks VR, Conston AS, Galdi VA, Joubert L: Histologic type of lung cancer and asbestos exposure. Cancer 54:3017-3021, 1984.

332 Auerbach O, Gere JB, Forman JB, Petrick TG, Smolin HJ, Muehsam GE, Kassouny DY, Stout AP: Changes in the bronchial epithelium in relation to smoking and cancer of the lung. N Engl J Med 256:97-104, 1957.

333 Fukayama M, Hayashi Y, Koike M, Hajikano H, Endo S, Okumura H: Human chorionic gonadotropin in lung and lung tumors. Immunohistochemical study on unbalanced distribution of subunits. Lab Invest 55:433-443, 1986.

334 Harach HR, Skinner M, Gibbs AR: Biological markers in human lung carcinoma. An immunopathological study of six antigens. Thorax **38**:937-941, 1983.

335 Helmuth RA, Strate RW: Squamous carcinoma of the lung in a nonirradiated, nonsmoking patient with juvenile laryngotracheal papillomatosis. Am J Surg Pathol **11**:643-650, 1987.

336 Hirata Y , Matsukura S, Imura H, Yakura T, Ihjima S, Nagase C, Itoh M: Two cases of multiple hormone-producing small cell carcinoma of the lung. Coexistence of tumor ADH, ACTH, and β-MSH. Cancer **38**:2575-2582, 1976.

337 Hood RT Jr, Good CA, Clagett OT, McDonald JR: Solitary circumscribed lesions of the lung. JAMA **152**:1185-1191, 1953.

338 Humphrey EW, Ewing SL, Wrigley JV, Northrup WF III, Kersten TE, Mayer JE, Varco RL: The production of malignant tumors of the lung and pleura in dogs from intratracheal asbestos instillation and cigarette smoking. Cancer **47**:1994-1999, 1981.

339 Hwang DL, Tay Y-C, Lin SS, Lev-Ran A: Expression of epidermal growth factor receptors in human lung tumors. Cancer **58**:2260-2263, 1986.

340 Ilgren EB, Griner L, Benirschke K, Pang LSC: A comparative study of pulmonary tumors from the San Diego Zoological Gardens and the tumor reference collection, Imperial Cancer Research Fund, London. Pathol Annu **17**(Pt 2):331-351, 1982.

341 Kannerstein M, Churg J: Pathology of carcinoma of the lung associated with asbestos exposure. Cancer **30**:14-21, 1972.

342 Krauss S, Macy S, Ichiki AT: A study of immunoreactive calcitonin (CT), adrenocorticotropic hormone (ACTH) and carcinoembryonic antigen (CEA) in lung cancer and other malignancies. Cancer **47**:2485-2492, 1981.

343 Kvale G, Bjelke E, Heuch I: Occupational exposure and lung cancer risk. Int J Cancer **37**:185-193, 1986.

344 Loeb LA, Ernster VL, Warner KE, Abbotts J, Laszio J: Smoking and lung cancer. An overview. Cancer Res **44**:5940-5958, 1984.

345 Machle W, Gregorius F: Cancer of the respiratory system in United States chromate-producing industry. Public Health Rep **63**:1114-1127, 1948.

346 Marks PH, Schechter FG: Multiple primary carcinomas of the head, neck, and lung. Ann Thorac Surg **33**:324-332, 1982.

347 Meyer EC, Liebow AA: Relationship of interstitial pneumonia honeycombing and atypical epithelial proliferation to cancer of the lung. Cancer **18**:322-351, 1965.

348 Miyake M, Ito M, Mitsuoka A, Taki T, Wada H, Hitomi S, Kino T, Matsui Y: Alpha-fetoprotein and human chorionic gonadotropin–producing lung cancer. Cancer **59**:227-232, 1987.

349 Pastorino U, Berrino F, Gervasio A, Pesenti V, Riboli E, Crosignani P: Proportion of lung cancers due to occupational exposure. Int J Cancer **33**:231-237, 1984.

350 Paulson DL: Carcinomas in the superior pulmonary sulcus. J Thorac Cardiovasc Surg **70**:1095-1104, 1975.

351 Sikl H: The present status of knowledge about the Jachymov disease (cancer of the lungs in the miners of the radium mines). Acta Un Int Cancer **6**:1366-1375, 1950.

352 Toomes H, Delphendahl A, Manke H-G, Vogt-Moykopf I: The coin lesion of the lung. A review of 955 resected coin lesions. Cancer **51**:534-537, 1983.

353 Warnock ML, Kuwahara TJ, Wolery G: The relation of asbestos burden to asbestosis and lung cancer. Pathol Annu **18**(Pt 2):109-145, 1983.

354 Yesner R: Spectrum of lung cancer and ectopic hormones. Pathol Annu **13**(Pt 1):207-240, 1978.

355 Yokoyama M, Natsuizaka T, Ishii Y, Ohshima S, Kasagi A, Tateno S: Amylase-producing lung cancer. Ultrastructural and biochemical studies. Cancer **40**:766-772, 1977.

Pathologic features

356 Auerbach O, Frasca JM, Parks VR, Carter HW: A comparison of World Health Organization (WHO) classification of lung tumors by light and electron microscopy. Cancer **50**:2079-2088, 1982.

357 Dunnill MS, Gatter KC: Cellular heterogeneity in lung cancer. Histopathology **10**:461-475, 1986.

358 Feinstein AR, Gelfman NA, Yesner R, Auerbach O, Hackel DB, Pratt PC: Observer variability in the histopathologic diagnosis of lung cancer. Am Rev Respir Dis **101**:671-684, 1970.

359 Gatter KC, Dunnill MS, Heryet A, Mason DY: Human lung tumours. Does intermediate filament co-expression correlate with other morphological or immunocytochemical features? Histopathology **11**:705-714, 1987.

360 Gatter KC, Dunnill MS, Pulford KAF, Heryet A, Mason DY: Human lung tumours. A correlation of antigenic profile with histological type. Histopathology **9**:805-823, 1985.

361 Hammar SP, Bolen JW, Bockus D, Remington F, Friedman S: Ultrastructural and immunohistochemical features of common lung tumors. An overview. Ultrastruct Pathol **9**:283-318, 1985.

362 Haratake J, Horie A, Tokudome S, Era S, Fujii H, Kawachi J, Miyamoto Y, Suko S, Tokunaga M, Tsuji K, Ikeda M, Kuratsune M: Inter- and intra-pathologist variability in histologic diagnoses of lung cancer. Acta Pathol Jpn **37**:1053-1060, 1987.

363 Hinson KFW, Miller AB, Tall R: An assessment of the World Health Organization classification of the histologic typing of lung tumors applied to biopsy and resected material. Cancer **35**:399-405, 1975.

364 Kreyberg L: Main histological types of primary epithelial lung tumours. Br J Cancer **15**:206-210, 1961.

365 Roggli VL, Vollmer RT, Greenberg SD, McGavran MH, Spjut HJ, Yesner R: Lung cancer heterogeneity. A blinded and randomized study of 100 consecutive cases. Hum Pathol **16**:569-579, 1985.

366 Saba SR, Espinoza CG, Richman AV, Azar HA: Carcinomas of the lung. An ultrastructural and immunocytochemical study. Am J Clin Pathol **80**:6-13, 1983.

367 World Health Organization: The World Health Organization histological typing of lung tumors. Am J Clin Pathol **77**:123-136, 1982.

367a Yesner R: Histopathology of lung cancer. Semin Ultrasound **9**:4-26, 1988.

Squamous cell (epidermoid) carcinoma

368 Bateson EM: The solitary circumscribed bronchogenic carcinoma. A radiological study of 100 cases. Br J Radiol **37**:598-607, 1964.

369 Black H. Ackerman LV: The importance of epidermoid carcinoma in situ in the histogenesis of carcinoma of the lung. Ann Surg **136**:44-55, 1952.

370 Dingemans KP, Mooi WJ: Ultrastructure of squamous cell carcinoma of the lung. Pathol Annu **19**(Pt 1):249-273, 1984.

371 Dulmet-Brender E, Jaubert F, Huchon G: Exophytic endobronchial epidermoid carcinoma. Cancer **57**:1358-1364, 1986.

372 Nelson WG, Sun T-T: The 50- and 58-kdalton keratin classes as molecular markers for stratified squamous epithelia. Cell culture studies. J Cell Biol **97**:244-251, 1983.

373 Said JW, Nash G, Sassoon AF, Shintaku IP, Banks-Schlegel S: Involucrin in lung tumors. A specific marker for squamous differentiation. Lab Invest **49**:563-568, 1983.

374 Strang C, Simpson JA: Carcinomatous abscess of the lung. Thorax **8**:11-28, 1953.

Adenocarcinoma

375 Auerbach O, Garfinkel L, Parks VR: Scar cancer of the lung. Increase over a 21 year period. Cancer **43**:636-642, 1979.

376 Bakris GL, Mulopulos GP, Korchik R, Ezdinli EZ, Ro J, Yoon B-H: Pulmonary scar carcinoma. A clinicopathologic analysis. Cancer **52**:493-497, 1983.

377 Banks-Schlegel SP, McDowell EM, Wilson TS, Trump BF, Harris CC: Keratin proteins in human lung carcinomas. Combined use of morphology, keratin immunocytochemistry, and keratin immunoprecipitation. Am J Pathol **114**:273-286, 1984.

378 Barsky SH, Huang SJ, Bhuta S: The extracellular matrix of pulmonary scar carcinomas is suggestive of a desmoplastic origin. Am J Pathol **124**:412-419, 1986.

379 Bennett DE, Sasser WF, Ferguson T: Adenocarcinoma of the lung in men. A clinicopathologic study of 100 cases. Cancer **23**:431-439, 1969.

380 Cagle PT, Cohle SD, Greenberg SD: Natural history of pulmonary scar cancers. Clinical and pathologic implications. Cancer **56**:2031-2035, 1985.

381 Cox JD, Yesner RA: Adenocarcinoma of the lung. Recent results from the Veterans Administration Lung Group. Am Rev Respir Dis **120**:1025-1029, 1979.

382 Eimoto T, Teshima K, Shirakusa T, Kikuchi M: Ultrastructure of well-differentiated adenocarcinomas of the lung with special reference to bronchioloalveolar carcinoma. Ultrastruct Pathol **8**:177-190, 1985.

383 Furukawa T, Watanabe S, Kodama T, Sato Y, Shimosato Y, Suemasu K: T-zone histiocytes in adenocarcinoma of the lung in relation to postoperative prognosis. Cancer **56**:2651-2656, 1985.

384 Harwood TR, Gracey DR, Yokoo H: Pseudomesotheliomatous carcinoma of the lung. A variant of peripheral lung cancer. Am J Clin Pathol **65**:159-167, 1976.

385 Horie A, Kotoo Y, Ohta M, Kurita Y: Relation of fine structure to prognosis for papillary adenocarcinoma of the lung. Hum Pathol **15**:870-879, 1984.

386 Jordon D, Jagirdar J: Lewis X and Y blood group expression in malignant mesothelioma and adenocarcinoma (abstract). Lab Invest **58**:44A, 1988.

386a Kawai T, Torikata C, Suzuki M: Immunohistochemical study of pulmonary adenocarcinoma. Am J Clin Pathol **89**:455-462, 1988.

386b Khiyami A, Tomashefski JF Jr, Kleinerman J: Patterns of primary lung carcinoma from 1956-1987 (abstract). Am J Clin Pathol **89**:431, 1988.

387 Kimula Y: A histochemical and ultrastructural study of adenocarcinoma of the lung. Am J Surg Pathol 2:253-264, 1978.

388 Kodama T, Shimosato Y, Koide T, Watanabe S, Yoneyama T: Endobronchial polypoid adenocarcinoma of the lung. Histological and ultrastructural studies of five cases. Am J Surg Pathol 8:845-854, 1984.

389 Kung ITM, Lui IOL, Loke SL, Khin MA, Mok CK, Lam WK, So SY: Pulmonary scar cancer. A pathologic reappraisal. Am J Surg Pathol 9:391-400, 1985.

390 Madri JA, Carter D: Scar cancers of the lung. Origin and significance. Hum Pathol 15:625-631, 1984.

391 Meyer EC, Liebow AA: Relationship of interstitial pneumonia honeycombing and atypical epithelial proliferation to cancer of the lung. Cancer 18:322-351, 1965.

391a Mizutani Y, Nakajima T, Morinaga S, Gotoh M, Shimosato Y, Akino T, Suzuki A: Immunohistochemical localization of pulmonary surfactant apoproteins in various lung tumors. Special reference to nonmucus producing lung adenocarcinomas. Cancer 61:532-537, 1988.

392 Ramaekers F, Puts J, Moesker O, Kant A, Jap P, Vooijs P: Demonstration of keratin in human adenocarcinomas. Am J Pathol 111:213-223, 1983.

393 Said JW, Nash G, Tepper G, Banks-Schlegel S: Keratin proteins and carcinoembryonic antigen in lung carcinoma. An immunoperoxidase study of fifty-four cases, with ultrastructural correlations. Hum Pathol 14:70-76, 1983.

393a Scroggs MW, Roggli VL, Fraire AE, Sanfilippo F: Eosinophilic intracytoplasmic globules in pulmonary adenocarcinomas. A histologic histochemical and immunohistochemical study of six cases (abstract). Lab Invest 58:82A, 1988.

394 Upton MP, Hirohashi S, Tome Y, Miyazawa N, Suemasu K, Shimosato Y: Expression of vimentin in surgically resected adenocarcinomas and large cell carcinomas of lung. Am J Surg Pathol 10:560-567, 1986.

395 Valaitis J, Warren S, Gamble D: Increasing incidence of adenocarcinoma of the lung. Cancer 47:1042-1046, 1981.

396 Vincent RG, Pickren JW, Lane WW, Bross I, Takita H, Houten L, Gutierrez AC, Rzepka T: The changing histopathology of lung cancer. A review of 1682 cases. Cancer 39:1647-1655, 1977.

397 Vincent TN, Satterfield JV, Ackerman LV: Carcinoma of the lung in women. Cancer 18:559-570, 1965.

Undifferentiated large cell carcinoma

398 Albain KS, True LD, Golomb HM, Hoffman PC, Little AG: Large cell carcinoma of the lung. Ultrastructural differentiation and clinicopathologic correlations. Cancer 56:1618-1623, 1985.

399 Ascensao JL, Oken MM, Ewing SL, Goldberg RJ, Kaplan ME: Leukocytosis and large cell lung cancer. A frequent association. Cancer 60:903-905, 1987.

400 Byrd RB, Miller WE, Carr DT, Payne WS, Woolner LB: The roentgenographic appearance of large cell carcinoma of the bronchus. Mayo Clin Proc 43:333-336, 1968.

401 Churg A: The fine structure of large cell undifferentiated carcinoma of the lung. Evidence for its relation to squamous cell carcinomas and adenocarcinomas. Hum Pathol 9:143-156, 1978.

402 Hammar S: Adenocarcinoma and large cell undifferentiated carcinoma of the lung. Ultrastruct Pathol 11:263-291, 1987.

403 Horie A, Ohta M: Ultrastructural features of large cell carcinoma of the lung with reference to the prognosis of patients. Hum Pathol 12:423-432, 1981.

404 Kodama T, Takada K, Kameya T, Shimosato Y, Tsuchiya R, Okabe T: Large cell carcinoma of the lung associated with marked eosinophilia. A case report. Cancer 54:2313-2317, 1984.

405 Shimosato Y, Sobin L, Spencer H, et al. (eds): Histological typing of lung tumours. Geneva, World Health Organization, 1981.

406 Yesner R: Large cell carcinoma of the lung. Semin Diagn Pathol 2:255-269, 1985.

Giant cell carcinoma

407 Herman DL, Bullock WK, Waken JK: Giant cell adenocarcinoma of the lung. Cancer 19:1337-1346, 1966.

408 Nash AD, Stout AP: Giant cell carcinoma of the lung. Cancer 11:369-376, 1958.

409 Wang N-S, Seemayer TA, Ahmed MN, Knaack J: Giant cell carcinoma of the lung. A light and electron microscopic study. Hum Pathol 7:3-16, 1976.

Clear cell carcinoma

409 Edwards C, Carlile A: Clear cell carcinoma of the lung. J Clin Pathol 38:880-885, 1985.

410 Katzenstein A-LA, Prioleau PG, Askin FB: The histologic spectrum and significance of clear-cell change in lung carcinoma. Cancer 45:943-947, 1980.

411 Morgan AD, Mackenzie DH: Clear-cell carcinoma of the lung. J Pathol Bacteriol 87:25-27, 1964.

Bronchioloalveolar carcinoma

412 Bedrossian CWM, Weilbaecher DG, Bentinck DC, Greenberg SD: Ultrastructure of human bronchioloalveolar cell carcinoma. Cancer 36:1399-1413, 1975.

413 Bennett DE, Sasser WF: Bronchiolar carcinoma. A valid clinicopathologic entity? A study of 30 cases. Cancer 24:876-887, 1969.

414 Bonikos DS, Hendrickson M, Bensch KG: Pulmonary alveolar cell carcinoma. Fine structural and in vitro study of a case and critical review of this entity. Am J Surg Pathol 1:93-108, 1977.

415 Dermer GB: Origin of bronchioloalveolar carcinoma and peripheral bronchial adenocarcinoma. Cancer 49:881-887, 1982.

416 Donaldson JC, Kaminsky DB, Elliott RC: Bronchiolar carcinoma. Report of 11 cases and review of the literature. Cancer 41:250-258, 1978.

417 Edwards CW: Alveolar carcinoma. A review. Thorax 39:166-174, 1984.

418 Fantone JC, Geisinger KR, Appelman HD: Papillary adenoma of the lung with lamellar and electron dense granules. An ultrastructural study. Cancer 50:2839-2844, 1982.

419 Greco RJ, Steiner RM, Goldman S, Cotler H, Patchefsky A, Cohn HE: Bronchoalveolar cell carcinoma of the lung. Ann Thorac Surg 41:652-656, 1986.

420 Greenberg SD, Smith MN, Spjut HJ: Bronchiolo-alveolar carcinoma. Cell of origin. Am J Clin Pathol 63:153-167, 1975.

421 Jacques J, Currie W: Bronchiolo-alveolar carcinoma. Clara cell tumor? Cancer 40:2171-2180, 1977.

422 Kuhn C III: Fine structure of bronchioloalveolar cell carcinoma. Cancer 30:1107-1118, 1972.

423 Laipply TC, Sherrick JC, Cape WE: Bronchiolar (alveolar cell) tumors. Arch Pathol 59:35-50, 1955.

424 Manning JT Jr, Spjut HJ, Tschen JA: Bronchioloalveolar carcinoma. The significance of two histopathologic types. Cancer 54:525-534, 1984.

424a Miller RR, Nelems B, Evans KG, Muller NL, Ostrow DN: Glandular neoplasia of the lung. A proposed analogy to colonic tumors. Cancer 61:1009-1014, 1988.

425 Montes M, Binette JP, Chaudhry AP, Adler RH, Guarino R: Clara cell adenocarcinoma. Light and electron microscope studies. Am J Surg Pathol 1:245-253, 1977.

426 Morningstar WA, Hassan MO: Bronchiolo-alveolar carcinoma with nodal metastases. Am J Surg Pathol 3:273-278, 1979.

427 Nakajima T, Kodama T, Tsumuraya M, Shimosato Y, Kameya T: S-100 protein-positive Langerhans cells in various human lung cancers, especially in peripheral adenocarcinomas. Virchows Arch [Pathol Anat] 407:177-189, 1985.

428 Noguchi M, Kodama T, Shimosato Y, Koide T, Naruke T, Singh G, Katyal SL: Papillary adenoma of type 2 pneumocytes. Am J Surg Pathol 10:134-139, 1986.

429 Ogata T, Endo K: Clara cell granules of peripheral lung cancers. Cancer 54:1635-1644, 1984.

430 Rosenblatt MB, Lisa JR, Collier F: Primary and metastatic bronchioloalveolar carcinoma. Dis Chest 52:147-152, 1967.

431 Sidhu GS, Forrester EM: Glycogen-rich Clara cell-type bronchioloalveolar carcinoma. Light and electron microscopic study. Cancer 40:2209-2215, 1977.

432 Silverman JF, Finley JL, Park HK, Strausbauch P, Unverferth M, Carney M: Fine needle aspiration cytology of bronchioloalveolar-cell carcinoma of the lung. Acta Cytol 29:887-896, 1985.

433 Singh G, Katyal SL, Torikata C: Carcinoma of type II pneumocytes. Immunodiagnosis of a subtype of "bronchioloalveolar carcinomas." Am J Pathol 102:195-208, 1981.

434 Singh G, Katyal SL, Torikata C: Carcinoma of type II pneumocytes. PAS staining as a screening test for nuclear inclusions of surfactant specific apoprotein. Cancer 50:946-948, 1982.

435 Singh G, Scheithauer BW, Katyal SL: The pathobiologic features of carcinomas of type II pneumocytes. An immunocytologic study. Cancer 57:994-999, 1986.

436 Spriggs AI, Cole M, Dunnill MS: Alveolar-cell carcinoma. A problem in sputum cytodiagnosis. J Clin Pathol 35:1370-1379, 1982.

437 Tao LC, Delarue NC, Sanders D, Weisbrod G: Bronchiolo-alveolar carcinoma. A correlative clinical and cytologic study. Cancer 42:2759-2767, 1978.

437a Tomashefski JF Jr, Buzatu T, Petrelli M, Kleinerman J: αI-Antitrypsin is a marker for Clara cell carcinomas of the lung (abstract). Lab Invest 58:94A, 1988.

Adenosquamous carcinoma

438 Fitzgibbons PL, Kern WH: Adenosquamous carcinoma of the lung. A clinical and pathologic study of seven cases. Hum Pathol 16:463-466, 1985.

Small cell carcinoma

439 Azzopardi JG: Oat cell carcinoma of the bronchus. J Pathol Bacteriol 78:513-519, 1959.

440 Begin P, Sahai S, Wang N-S: Giant cell formation in small cell carcinoma of the lung. Cancer **52:**1875-1879, 1983.

441 Bensch KG, Corrin B, Pariente R, Spencer H: Oat-cell carcinoma of the lung. Its origin and relationship to bronchial carcinoid. Cancer **22:**1163-1172, 1968.

442 Bergh J, Esscher T, Steinholtz L, Nilsson K, Påhlman S: Immunocytochemical demonstration of neuron-specific enolase (NSE) in human lung cancers. Am J Clin Pathol **84:**1-7, 1985.

443 Carter D: Small-cell carcinoma of the lung. Am J Surg Pathol **7:**787-795, 1983.

444 Churg A, Johnston WH, Stulbarg M: Small cell and squamous–small cell anaplastic carcinomas of the lung. Am J Surg Pathol **4:**255-263, 1980.

445 Elema JD, Keuning HM: The ultrastructure of small cell lung carcinoma in bronchial biopsy specimens. Hum Pathol **16:**1133-1140, 1985.

446 Esscher T, Steinholtz L, Bergh J, Nou E, Nilsson K, Påhlman S: Neurone specific enolase. A useful diagnostic serum marker for small cell carcinoma of the lung. Thorax **40:**85-90, 1985.

446a Gephardt GN, Grady KJ, Ahmad M, Tubbs RR, Mehta AC, Shepard KV: Peripheral small cell undifferentiated carcinoma of the lung. Clinicopathologic features of 17 cases. Cancer **61:**1002-1008, 1988.

447 Hage E, Hansen M, Hirsch FR: Electron microscopic sub-classification of small cell carcinoma of the lung. Acta Pathol Jpn **33:**671-681, 1983.

448 Hammond ME, Sause WT: Large cell neuroendocrine tumors of the lung. Clinical significance and histopathologic definition. Cancer **56:**1624-1629, 1985.

449 Johnson DH, Marangos PJ, Forbes JT, Hainsworth JD, Van Welch R, Hande KR, Greco FA: Potential utility of serum neuron–specific enolase levels in small cell carcinoma of the lung. Cancer Res **44:**5409-5414, 1984.

450 Kameya T, Shimosato Y, Kodama T, Tsumuraya M, Koide T, Yamaguchi K, Abe K: Peptide hormone production by adenocarcinomas of the lung. Its morphologic basis and histogenetic considerations. Virchows Arch [Pathol Anat] **400:**245-257, 1983.

451 Kato Y, Ferguson TB, Bennett DE, Burford TH: Oat cell carcinoma of the lung. A review of 138 cases. Cancer **23:**517-524, 1969.

452 Lehto VP, Stenman S, Miettinen M, Dahl D, Virtanen I: Expression of a neural type of intermediate filament as a distinguishing feature between oat cell carcinoma and other lung cancers. Am J Pathol **110:**113-118, 1983.

453 Mark EJ, Ramirez JF: Peripheral small-cell carcinoma of the lung resembling carcinoid tumor. A clinical and pathologic study of 14 cases. Arch Pathol Lab Med **109:**263-269, 1985.

454 Michels S, Swanson PE, Robb JA, Wick MR: Leu-7 in small cell neoplasms. An immunohistochemical study with ultrastructural correlations. Cancer **60:**2958-2964, 1987.

454a Naylor SL, Johnson BE, Minna JD, Sakaguchi AY: Loss of heterozygosity of chromosome 3p markers in small-cell lung cancer. Nature **329:**451-454, 1987.

455 Neal MH, Kosinski R, Cohen P, Orenstein JM: Atypical endocrine tumors of the lung. A histologic, ultrastructural, and clinical study of 19 cases. Hum Pathol **17:**1264-1277, 1986.

456 Radice PA, Matthews MJ, Ihde DC, Gazdar AF, Carney DN, Bunn PA, Cohen MH, Fossieck BE, Makuch RW, Minna JD: The clinical behavior of "mixed" small cell/large cell bronchogenic carcinoma compared to "pure" small cell subtypes. Cancer **50:**2894-2902, 1982.

457 Salyer D, Eggleston JC: Oat cell carcinoma of the bronchus and the carcinoid syndrome. Arch Pathol **99:**513-515, 1975.

458 Sheppard MN, Corrin B, Bennett MH, Marangos PJ, Bloom SR, Polak JM: Immunocytochemical localization of neuron specific enolase in small cell carcinomas and carcinoid tumours of the lung. Histopathology **8:**171-181, 1984.

459 Sidhu GS: The endodermal origin of digestive and respiratory tract APUD cells. Histopathologic evidence and a review of the literature. Am J Pathol **96:**5-20, 1979.

460 Tateishi R, Horai T, Hattori S: Demonstration of argyrophil granules in small cell carcinoma of the lung. Virchows Arch [Pathol Anat] **377:**203-210, 1978.

461 Tischler AS: Small cell carcinoma of the lung. Cellular origin and relationship to other neoplasms. Semin Oncol **5:**244-252, 1978.

462 van Muijen G NP, Ruiter DJ, van Leeuwen C, Prins FA, Rietsema K, Warnaar SO: Cytokeratin and neurofilament in lung carcinomas. Am J Pathol **116:**363-369, 1984.

463 Williams ED, Azzopardi JG: Tumors of lung and carcinoid syndrome. Thorax **15:**30-36, 1960.

464 World Health Organization: The World Health Organization histological typing of lung tumours. Am J Clin Pathol **77:**123-136, 1982.

465 Yesner R: Small cell tumors of the lung. Am J Surg Pathol **7:**775-785, 1983.

Carcinoma in situ

466 Carter D: Pathology of early squamous cell carcinoma of the lung. Pathol Annu **13**(Pt 1):131-147, 1978.

467 Carter D: Squamous cell carcinoma of the lung. An update. Semin Diagn Pathol **2:**226-234, 1985.

468 Carter D, Marsh BR, Baker R, Erozan YS, Frost JK: Relationships of morphology to clinical presentation in ten cases of early squamous cell carcinoma of the lung. Cancer **37:**1389-1396, 1976.

469 Cohen MH: Lung cancer. A status report (editorial). J Natl Cancer Inst **55:**505-511, 1975.

470 Mason MK, Jordan JW: Outcome of carcinoma in situ and early invasive carcinoma of the bronchus. Thorax **37:**453-456, 1982.

471 Melamed MR, Zaman MB, Flehinger BJ, Martini N: Radiologically occult in situ and incipient invasive epidermoid lung cancer. Detection by sputum cytology in a survey of asymptomatic cigarette smokers. Am J Surg Pathol **1:**5-16, 1977.

472 Woolner LB, David E, Fontana RS, Andersen HA, Bernatz PE: In situ and early invasive bronchogenic carcinoma. Report of 28 cases with postoperative survival data. J Thorac Cardiovasc Surg **60:**275-290, 1970.

473 Woolner LB, Fontana RS, Cortese DA, Sanderson DR, Bernatz PE, Payne WS, Pairolero PC, Piehler JM, Taylor WF: Roentgenographically occult lung cancer. Pathologic findings and frequency of multicentricity during a 10-year period. Mayo Clin Proc **59:**453-466, 1984.

474 Woolner LB, Fontana RS, Sanderson DR, Miller WE, Muhm JR, Taylor WF, Uhlenhopp MA: Mayo lung project. Evaluation of lung cancer screening through December 1979. Mayo Clin Proc **56:**544-555, 1981.

Biopsy

475 Bibbo M, Fennessy JJ, Lu C-T, Strauss FH, Variakojis D, Wied GL: Bronchial brushing technique for the cytological diagnosis of peripheral lung lesions. A review of 693 cases. Acta Cytol [Baltimore] **17:**245-251, 1973.

476 Chuang MT, Marchevsky A, Teirstein AS, Kirschner P, Kleinerman J: Diagnosis of lung cancer by fibreoptic bronchoscopy. Problems in the histological classification of non-small cell carcinomas. Thorax **39:**175-178, 1984.

477 Coughlin M, Deslauriers J, Beaulieu M, Fournier B, Piraux M, Rouleau J, Tardif A: Role of mediastinoscopy in pretreatment staging of patients with primary lung cancer. Ann Thorac Surg **40:**556-560, 1985.

478 Fennessy JJ, Fry WA, Manalo-Estrella P, Hidvegi DVSF: The bronchial brushing technique for obtaining cytologic specimens from peripheral lung lesions. Acta Cytol [Baltimore] **14:**25-30, 1970.

479 Grant LJ, Trivedi SA: Open lung biopsy for diffuse pulmonary lesions. Br Med J **1:**17-21, 1960.

480 Koss LG, Melamed MR, Goodner JT: Pulmonary cytology. A brief survey of diagnostic results from July 1st, 1952 until December 31st, 1960. Acta Cytol [Baltimore] **8:**104-113, 1964.

481 Paulson DL: A philosophy of treatment for bronchogenic carcinoma. Ann Thorac Surg **5:**289-299, 1968.

482 Pearson FG, Nelems JM, Henderson RD, Delarue NC: The role of mediastinoscopy in the selection of treatment for bronchial carcinoma with involvement of superior mediastinal lymph nodes. J Thorac Cardiovasc Surg **64:**382-390, 1972.

483 Pearson FG, Thompson DW, Delarue NC: Experience with the cytologic detection, localization, and treatment of radiographically undemonstrable bronchial carcinoma. J Thorac Cardiovasc Surg **54:**371-382, 1967.

484 Sackner MA: Bronchofiberscopy. Am Rev Respir Dis **111:**62-88, 1975.

485 Unruh H, Chu-Jeng R: Mediastinal assessment for staging and treatment of carcinoma of the lung. Ann Thorac Surg **41:**224-229, 1986.

486 Zavala DC: Diagnostic fiberoptic bronchoscopy. Techniques and results of biopsy in 600 patients. Chest **68:**12-19, 1975.

Cytology

487 Chopra SK, Genovesi MG, Simmons DH, Gothe B: Fiberoptic bronchoscopy in the diagnosis of lung cancer. Comparison of pre- and post-bronchoscopy sputa washings, brushings and biopsies. Acta Cytol [Baltimore] **21:**524-527, 1977.

488 Erozan YS: Cytopathologic diagnosis of pulmonary neoplasms in sputum and bronchoscopic specimens. Semin Diagn Pathol **3:**188-195, 1986.

489 Fontana RS, Carr DT, Woolner LB, Miller FK: An evaluation of methods of inducing sputum production in patients with suspected cancer of the lung. Proc Staff Meet Mayo Clin **37:**113-121, 1962.

490 Greenberg SD: Recent advances in pulmonary cytopathology. Hum Pathol **14:**901-912, 1983.

491 Hess FG, Jr, McDowell EM, Trump BF: Pulmonary cytology. Current status of cytologic typing of respiratory tract tumors. Am J Pathol **103:**323-333, 1981.

492 Johnston WW, Bossen EH: Ten years of respiratory cytopathology at Duke University Medical Center. II. The cytopathologic diagnosis of lung cancer during the years 1970 to 1974, with a comparison between cytopathology and

histopathology in the typing of lung cancer. Acta Cytol [Baltimore] **25:**499-505, 1981.

493 Johnston WW, Frable WJ: The cytopathology of the respiratory tract. A review. Am J Pathol **84:**372-414, 1976.

494 Kanhouwa SB, Matthews MJ: Reliability of cytologic typing of lung cancer. Acta Cytol [Baltimore] **20:**229-232, 1976.

495 Kvale PA, Frederick RB, Kini S: Diagnostic accuracy in lung cancer. Comparison of techniques used in association with flexible fiberoptic bronchoscopy. Chest **69:**752-757, 1976.

496 Lange E, Hoeg K: Cytologic typing of lung cancer. Acta Cytol [Baltimore] **16:**327-330, 1972.

497 Ng ABP, Horak GC: Factors significant in the diagnostic accuracy of lung cytology in bronchial washing and sputum samples. I. Bronchial washings. Acta Cytol [Baltimore] **27:**391-396, 1983.

497a Pearson FG, Thompson DW, Delarue NC: Experience with the cytologic detection, localization, and treatment of radiographically undemonstrable bronchial carcinoma. J Thorac Cardiovasc Surg **54:**371-382, 1967.

498 Pilotti S, Rilke F, Gribaudi G, Spinelli P: Cytologic diagnosis of pulmonary carcinoma on bronchoscopic brushing material. Acta Cytol [Baltimore] **26:**655-660, 1982.

499 Roger V, Nasiell M, Linden M, Enstad I: Cytologic differential diagnosis of bronchioloalveolar carcinoma and bronchogenic adenocarcinoma. Acta Cytol [Baltimore] **20:**303-307, 1976.

500 Salhadin A, Nasiell M, Nasiell K, Silfverswärd C, Hjerpe A, Wadas AM, Enstad I: The unique cytologic picture of oat cell carcinoma in effusions. Acta Cytol [Baltimore] **20:**298-302, 1976.

501 Sinner WN: Pulmonary neoplasms diagnosed with transthoracic needle biopsy. Cancer **43:**1533-1540, 1979.

502 Skitarelie K, Von Haam E: Bronchial brushings and washings. A diagnostically rewarding procedure? Acta Cytol [Baltimore] **18:**321-324, 1974.

503 Solomon DA, Solliday NH, Gracey DR: Cytology in fiberoptic bronchoscopy. Comparison of bronchial brushing, washing and post bronchoscopy sputum. Chest **65:**616-619, 1974.

504 Spriggs AI, Boddington MM: Oat-cell bronchial carcinoma. Identification of cells in pleural fluid. Acta Cytol [Baltimore] **20:**525-529, 1976.

505 Todd TRJ, Weisbrod G, Tao LC, Sanders DE, Delarue NC, Chamberlain DW, Ilves R, Pearson FG, Cass W, Cooper JD: Aspiration needle biopsy of thoracic lesions. Ann Thorac Surg **32:**154-161, 1981.

506 Truong LD, Underwood RD, Greenberg SD, McLarty JW: Diagnosis and typing of lung carcinomas by cytopathologic methods. A review of 108 cases. Acta Cytol **23:**379-384, 1985.

507 Wandall HH: A study on neoplastic cells in sputum as a contribution to the diagnosis of primary lung cancer. Acta Chir Scand **91**[Suppl 93]:1-143, 1944.

508 Zaman MB, Hajdu SI, Melamed MR, Watson RC: Transthoracic aspiration cytology of pulmonary lesions. Semin Diagn Pathol **3:**176-187, 1986.

508a Zavala DC: Diagnostic fiberoptic bronchoscopy. Techniques and results of biopsy in 600 patients. Chest **68:**12-19, 1975.

Spread and metastases

509 Cox JD, Yesner RA: Adenocarcinoma of the lung. Recent results from the Veterans Administration Lung Group. Am Rev Respir Dis **120:**1025-1029, 1979.

510 Eagan RT, Maurer LH, Forcier RJ, Tulloh M: Small cell carcinoma of the lung. Staging, paraneoplastic syndromes, treatment, and survival. Cancer **33:**527-532, 1974.

511 Gonzalez-Vitale JC, Garcia-Bunuel R: Pulmonary tumor emboli and cor pulmonale in primary carcinoma of the lung. Cancer **38:**2105-2110, 1976.

512 LeGal Y, Bauer WG: Second primary bronchogenic carcinoma. J Thorac Cardiovasc Surg **41:**114-124, 1961.

513 McNeill PM, Wagman LD, Neifeld JP: Small bowel metastases from primary carcinoma of the lung. Cancer **59:**1486-1489, 1987.

514 Onuigbo WIB: Patterns in metastasis in lung cancer. A review. Cancer Res **21:**1077-1085, 1961.

515 Rosen ST, Aisner J, Makuch RW, Matthews MJ, Ihde DC, Whitacre M, Glatstein EJ, Wiernik PH, Lichter AS, Bunn PA Jr: Carcinomatous leptomeningitis in small cell lung cancer. A clinicopathologic review of the National Cancer Institute experience. Medicine **61:**45-53, 1982.

516 Sridhar KS, Rao RK, Kunhardt B: Skeletal muscle metastases from lung cancer. Cancer **59:**1530-1534, 1987.

Treatment

517 Ahmad K, Fayos JV, Kirsh MM: Apical lung carcinoma. Cancer **54:**913-917, 1984.

518 Burford TH, Ferguson TB, Spjut HJ: Results in the treatment of bronchogenic carcinoma. J Thorac Surg **36:**316-328, 1958.

519 Choi NC, Carey RW, Kaufman SD, Grillo HC, Younger J, Wilkins EW Jr: Small cell carcinoma of the lung. A progress report of 15 years' experience. Cancer **59:**6-14, 1987.

520 Devine JW, Mendenhall WM, Million RR, Carmichael MJ: Carcinoma of the superior pulmonary sulcus treated with surgery and/or radiation therapy. Cancer **57:**941-943, 1986.

521 Komaki R, Roh J, Cox JD, Lopes da Conceicao A: Superior sulcus tumors. Results of irradiation of 36 patients. Cancer **48:**1563-1568, 1981.

522 Law MR, Henk JM, Lennox SC, Hodson ME: Value of radiotherapy for tumour on the bronchial stump after resection for bronchial carcinoma. Thorax **37:**496-499, 1982.

523 Lung Cancer Study Group: Effects of postoperative mediastinal radiation on completely resected stage II and stage III epidermoid cancer of the lung. N Engl J Med **315:**1377-1381, 1986.

524 Paulson DL: Carcinomas in the superior pulmonary sulcus. J Thorac Cardiovasc Surg **70:**1095-1104, 1975.

525 Perez CA: Radiation therapy in the management of carcinoma of the lung. Cancer **39:**901-916, 1977.

526 Perry MC, Eaton WL, Propert KJ, Ware JH, Zimmer B, Chahinian AP, Skarin A, Carey RW, Kreisman H, Faulkner C, Comis R, Green MR: Chemotherapy with or without radiation therapy in limited small-cell carcinoma of the lung. N Engl J Med **316:**912-918, 1987.

527 Petrovich Z, Stanley K, Cox JD, Paig C: Radiotherapy in the management of locally advanced lung cancer of all cell types. Final report of randomized trial. Cancer **48:**1335-1340, 1981.

528 Sherman DM, Weichselbaum R, Hellman S: The characteristics of long-term survivors of lung cancer treated with radiation. Cancer **47:**2575-2580, 1981.

529 Sørensen HR, Lund C, Alstrup P: Survival in small cell lung carcinoma after surgery. Thorax **41:**479-482, 1986.

Prognosis

530 Ahmad K, Fayos JV, Kirsh MM: Apical lung carcinoma. Cancer **54:**913-917, 1984.

531 Bennett DE, Sasser WF: Bronchiolar carcinoma. A valid clinicopathologic entity? A study of 30 cases. Cancer **24:**876-887, 1969.

532 Burford TH, Ferguson TB, Spjut HJ: Results in the treatment of bronchogenic carcinoma. J Thorac Surg **36:**316-328, 1958.

533 Carter D: Squamous cell carcinoma of the lung. An update. Semin Diagn Pathol **2:**226-234, 1985.

533a Cibas E, Melamed M, Zaman M, Kimmel M: Prognostic significance of tumor DNA content, tumor size, and TNM classification for patients with stage I adenocarcinoma of the lung (abstract). Lab Invest **58:**18A, 1988.

534 Clayton F: Bronchioloalveolar carcinomas. Cell types, patterns of growth, and prognostic correlates. Cancer **57:**1555-1564, 1986.

535 Cline MJ, Battifora H: Abnormalities of protooncogenes in non-small cell lung cancer. Correlations with tumor type and clinical characteristics. Cancer **60:**2669-2674, 1987.

536 Collier FC, Blakemore WS, Kyle RH, Enterline HT, Kirby CK, Johnson J: Carcinoma of the lung. Factors which influence five-year-survival with special reference to blood vessel invasion. Ann Surg **146:**417-423, 1957.

537 Davis S, Stanley KE, Yesner R, Kuang DT, Morris JF: Small-cell carcinoma of the lung. Survival according to histologic subtype. A veterans administration lung group study. Cancer **47:**1863-1866, 1981.

538 Devine JW, Mendenhall WM, Million RR, Carmichael MJ: Carcinoma of the superior pulmonary sulcus treated with surgery and/or radiation therapy. Cancer **57:**941-943, 1986.

539 Funa K, Steinholtz L, Nou E, Bergh J: Increased expression of N-myc in human small cell lung cancer biopsies predicts lack of response to chemotherapy and poor prognosis. Am J Clin Pathol **88:**216-220, 1987.

540 Gail MH, Eagan RT, Feld R, Ginsberg R, Goodell B, Hill L, Holmes EC, Lukeman JM, Mountain CF, Oldham RK, Pearson FG, Wright PW, Lake WH Jr, The Lung Cancer Study Group: Prognostic factors in patients with resected stage I non-small cell lung cancer. A report from the Lung Cancer Study Group. Cancer **54:**1802-1813, 1984.

541 Gibbon JH Jr, Albritten FF Jr, Templeton JY III, Nealon TF Jr: Cancer of the lung. An analysis of 532 consecutive cases. Ann Surg **138:**489-501, 1953.

542 Greenberg SD, Fraire AE, Kinner BM, Johnson EH: Tumor cell type versus staging in the prognosis of carcinoma of the lung. Pathol Annu **22**(Pt 2):387-405, 1987.

543 Hirsch FR, Østerlind K, Hansen HH: The prognostic significance of histopath-

ologic subtyping in small cell carcinoma of the lung according to the classification of the World Health Organization. A study of 375 consecutive patients. Cancer **52:**2144-2150, 1983.

544 Kato Y, Ferguson TB, Bennett DE, Burford TH: Oat cell carcinoma of the lung. A review of 138 cases. Cancer **23:**517-524, 1969.

545 Kemeny M, Block LR, Braun DW Jr, Martini N: Results of surgical treatment of carcinoma of the lung by stage and cell type. Surg Gynecol Obstet **147:**865-871, 1978.

546 Kern WH, Tucker BL: The pathology of lung cancer in ten-year survivors (abstract). Am J Clin Pathol **86:**397, 1986.

547 Kirsh MM, Rotman H, Argenta L, Bove E, Cimmino V, Tashian J, Ferguson P, Sloan H: Carcinoma of the lung. Results of treatment over ten years. Ann Thorac Surg **21:**371-377, 1976.

548 Kirsh MM, Tashian J, Sloan H: Carcinoma of the lung in women. Ann Thorac Surg **34:**34-39, 1982.

549 Kitaichi M, Asamoto H, Izumi T, Furuta M: Histological classification of regional lymph nodes in relation to postoperative survival in primary lung cancer. Hum Pathol **12:**1000-1005, 1981.

550 Komaki R, Roh J, Cox JD, Lopes da Conceicao A: Superior sulcus tumors. Results of irradiation of 36 patients. Cancer **48:**1563-1568, 1981.

551 Lee I, Gould VE, Radosevich JA, Thor A, Ma Y, Schlom J, Rosen ST: Immunohistochemical evaluation of ras oncogene expression in pulmonary and pleural neoplasms. Virchows Arch [B] **53:**146-152, 1987.

552 Lipford EH III, Eggleston JC, Lillemoe KD, Sears DL, Moore GW, Baker RR: Prognostic factors in surgically resected limited-stage, non small cell carcinoma of the lung. Am J Surg Pathol **8:**357-365, 1984.

553 Manning JT Jr, Spjut HJ, Tschen JA: Bronchioloalveolar carcinoma. The significance of two histopathologic types. Cancer **54:**525-534, 1984.

554 Martini N, Flehinger BJ, Zaman MB, Beattie EJ Jr: Results of resection in non-oat cell carcinoma of the lung with mediastinal lymph node metastases. Ann Surg **198:**386-397, 1983.

555 Miller WT, Husted J, Freiman D, Atkinson B, Pietra GG: Bronchioloalveolar carcinoma. Two clinical entities with one pathologic diagnosis. AJR **130:**905-912, 1978.

556 Naruke T, Suemasu K, Ishikawa S: Lymph node mapping and curability at various levels of metastasis in resected lung cancer. J Thorac Cardiovasc Surg **76:**832-839, 1978.

557 Nixon DW, Murphy GF, Sewell CW, Kutner M, Lynn MJ: Relationship between survival and histologic type in small cell anaplastic carcinoma of the lung. Cancer **44:**1045-1049, 1979.

558 Nõu E: The natural five-year course in bronchial carcinoma. Epidemiologic results. Cancer **53:**2211-2216, 1984.

559 Paulson DL: Carcinomas in the superior pulmonary sulcus. J Thorac Cardiovasc Surg **70:**1095-1104, 1975.

560 Pemberton JH, Nagorney DM, Gilmore JC, Taylor WF, Bernatz PE: Bronchogenic carcinoma in patients younger than 40 years. Ann Thorac Surg **36:**509-515, 1983.

561 Piehler JM, Pairolero PC, Weiland LH, Offord KP, Payne WS, Bernatz PE: Bronchogenic carcinoma with chest wall invasion. Factors affecting survival following en bloc resection. Ann Thorac Surg **34:**684-691, 1982.

562 Rodenhuis S, van de Wetering ML, Mooi WJ, Evers SG, van Zandwijk N, Bos JL: Mutational activation of the K-ras oncogene. A possible pathogenetic factor in adenocarcinoma of the lung. N Engl J Med **319:**929-935, 1987.

563 Sehested M, Hirsch FR, Østerlind K, Olsen JE: Morphologic variations of small cell lung cancer. A histopathologic study of pretreatment and posttreatment specimens in 104 patients. Cancer **57:**804-807, 1986.

564 Shimosato Y, Hashimoto T, Kodama T, Kameya T, Suzuki A, Nishiwaki Y, Yoneyama T: Prognostic implications of fibrotic focus (scar) in small peripheral lung cancers. Am J Surg Pathol **4:**365-373, 1980.

565 Spjut HJ, Roper CL, Butcher HR Jr: Pulmonary cancer and its prognosis. A study of the relationship of certain factors to survival of patients treated by pulmonary resection. Cancer **14:**1251-1258, 1961.

566 Temeck BK, Flehinger BJ, Martini N: A retrospective analysis of 10-year survivors from carcinoma of the lung. Cancer **53:**1405-1408, 1984.

567 Tirindelli-Danesi D, Teodori L, Mauro F, Modini C, Botti C, Cicconetti F, Stipa S: Prognostic significance of flow cytometry in lung cancer. A 5-year study. Cancer **60:**844-851, 1987.

567a Tomashefski FJ Jr, Rosenthal E, Conners AF Jr: Peripheral versus central squamous cell carcinoma of the lung. A comparison of clinical features, histopathology and survival (abstract). Lab Invest **58:**94A, 1988.

568 Treasure T, Belcher JR: Prognosis of peripheral lung tumours related to size of the primary. Thorax **36:**5-8, 1981.

569 Vollmer RT, Birch R, Ogden L, Crissman JD: Subclassification of small cell cancer of the lung. The Southeastern Cancer Study Group experience. Hum Pathol **16:**247-252, 1985.

OTHER PRIMARY TUMORS
Hamartoma

570 Albrecht E: Ueber Hamartome. Verh Dtsch Pathol Ges **7:**153-157, 1904.

571 Bateson EM: So-called hamartoma of the lung. A true neoplasm of fibrous connective tissue of the bronchi. Cancer **31:**1458-1467, 1973.

572 Butler C, Kleinerman J: Pulmonary hamartoma. Arch Pathol **88:**584-592, 1969.

573 Carney JA: The triad of gastric epithelioid leiomyosarcoma, functioning extra-adrenal paraganglioma, and pulmonary chondroma. Cancer **43:**374-382, 1979.

574 King TE Jr, Christopher KL, Schwarz MI: Multiple pulmonary chondromatous hamartomas. Hum Pathol **13:**496-497, 1982.

575 Perez-Atayde AR, Seiler MW: Pulmonary hamartoma. An ultrastructural study. Cancer **53:**485-492, 1984.

576 Tomashefski JF Jr: Benign endobronchial mesenchymal tumors. Their relationship to parenchymal pulmonary hamartomas. Am J Surg Pathol **6:**531-540, 1982.

Carcinoid tumor and related endocrine neoplasms

577 Bonikos DS, Bensch KG: Endocrine cells of bronchial and bronchiolar epithelium. Am J Med **63:**765-771, 1977.

578 Corrin B: Lung endocrine tumours. Invest Cell Pathol **3:**195-206, 1980.

579 Gmelich JT, Bensch KG, Liebow AA: Cells of Kultschitsky type in bronchioles and their relation to the origin of peripheral carcinoid tumor. Lab Invest **17:**88-98, 1967.

580 Gould VE, Linnoila RI: Pulmonary neuroepithelial bodies, neuroendocrine cells, and pulmonary tumors. Hum Pathol **13:**1064-1066, 1982.

581 Markel SF, Abell MR, Haight C, French AJ: Neoplasms of bronchus commonly designated as adenomas. Cancer **17:**590-608, 1964.

582 Tateishi R: Distribution of argyrophil cells in adult human lungs. Arch Pathol **96:**198-202, 1973.

Central carcinoid tumor

583 Attar S, Miller JE, Hankins J, Thompson BW, Suter CM, Kleger PJ, McLaughlin JS: Bronchial adenoma. A review of 51 patients. Ann Thorac Surg **40:**126-132, 1985.

584 Bensch KG, Gordon GB, Miller LR: Electron microscopic and biochemical studies on the bronchial carcinoid tumor. Cancer **18:**592-602, 1965.

585 Berger G, Berger F, Bejui F, Bouvier R, Rochet M, Feroldi J: Bronchial carcinoid with fibrillary inclusions related to cytokeratins. An immunohistochemical and ultrastructural study with subsequent investigation of 12 foregut APUDomas. Histopathology **8:**245-257, 1984.

586 Bishopric GA Jr, Ordóñez NG: Carcinoembryonic antigen in primary carcinoid tumors of the lung. Cancer **58:**1316-1320, 1986.

587 Black WC III: Enterochromaffin cell types and corresponding carcinoid tumors. Lab Invest **19:**473-486, 1968.

588 Black WC III: Pulmonary oncocytoma. Cancer **23:**1347-1357, 1969.

589 Bonikos DS, Bensch KG: Endocrine cells of bronchial and bronchiolar epithelium. Am J Med **63:**765-771, 1977.

590 Bostwick DG, Bensch KG: Gastrin releasing peptide in human neuroendocrine tumours. J Pathol **147:**237-244, 1985.

591 Bostwick DG, Null WE, Holmes D, Weber E, Barchas JD, Bensch KG: Expression of opioid peptides in tumors. N Engl J Med **317:**1439-1443, 1987.

592 Brandt B III, Heintz SE, Rose EF, Ehrenhaft JL: Bronchial carcinoid tumors. Ann Thorac Surg **38:**63-65, 1984.

593 Capella C, Gabrielli M, Polak JM, Buffa R, Solcia E, Bordi C: Ultrastructural and histological study of 11 bronchial carcinoids. Evidence for different types. Virchows Arch [Pathol Anat] **381:**313-329, 1979.

594 Christen B, Trojanowski JQ, Pietra GG: Immunohistochemical demonstration of phosphorylated and nonphosphorylated forms of human neurofilament subunits in human pulmonary carcinoids. Hum Pathol **18:**997-1001, 1987.

595 Cohen RB, Toll GD, Castleman B: Bronchial adenomas in Cushing's syndrome. Their relation to thymomas and oat cell carcinomas associated with hyperadrenocorticism. Cancer **13:**812-817, 1960.

596 DeStephano DB, Lloyd RV, Schteingart DE: Cushing's syndrome produced by a bronchial carcinoid tumor. Hum Pathol **15:**890-892, 1984.

597 Eusebi V, Pileri S, Usellini L, Grassigli A, Capella C: Primary endocrine carcinoma of the parotid salivary gland associated with a lung carcinoid. A possible new association. J Clin Pathol **35:**611-616, 1982.

598 Gephardt GN, Belovich DM: Cytology of pulmonary carcinoid tumors. Acta Cytol [Baltimore] **26:**434-438, 1982.

599 Hartman GE, Shochat SJ: Primary pulmonary neoplasms of childhood. A review. Ann Thorac Surg **36:**108-119, 1983.

600 Hurt R, Bates M: Carcinoid tumours of the bronchus. A 33 year experience. Thorax **39:**617-623, 1984.

601 Kuwahara T, Maruyama K, Mochizuki S, Seki Y, Sawada K: Oncocytic carcinoid of the lung. An ultrastructural observation. Acta Pathol Jpn **34:**355-359, 1984.

602 Lehto V-P, Miettinen M, Dahl D, Virtanen I: Bronchial carcinoid cells contain neural-type intermediate filaments. Cancer **54:**624-628, 1984.

603 Lehto V-P, Miettinen M, Virtanen I: A dual expression of cytokeratin and neurofilaments in bronchial carcinoid cells. Int J Cancer **35:**421-425, 1985.

604 Mark EJ, Quay SC, Dickersin GR: Papillary carcinoid tumor of the lung. Cancer **48:**316-324, 1981.

605 Markel SF, Abell MR, Haight C, Franch AJ: Neoplasms of bronchus commonly designated as adenomas. Cancer **17:**590-608, 1964.

606 Said JW, Vimadalal S, Nash G, Shintaku IP, Heusser RC, Sassoon AF, Lloyd RV: Immunoreactive neuron-specific enolase, bombesin, and chromogranin as markers for neuroendocrine lung tumors. Hum Pathol **16:**236-240, 1985.

607 Sajjad SM, Mackay B, Lukeman JM: Oncocytic carcinoid tumor of the lung. Ultrastruct Pathol **1:**171-176, 1980.

608 Salyer DC, Salyer WR, Eggleston JC: Bronchial carcinoid tumors. Cancer **36:**1522-1537, 1975.

609 Sandler M, Scheuer PJ, Watt PJ: 5-Hydroxytryptophan-secreting bronchial carcinoid tumour. Lancet **2:**1067-1069, 1961.

610 Sano T, Saito H, Yamasaki R, Hamaguchi K, Ooiwa K, Shimoda T, Hosoi E, Saito S, Hizawa K: Immunoreactive somatostatin and calcitonin in pulmonary neuroendocrine tumor. Cancer **57:**64-68, 1986.

611 Sklar JL, Churg A, Bensch KG: Oncocytic carcinoid tumor of the lung. Am J Surg Pathol **4:**287-292, 1980.

612 Springall DR, Lackie P, Levene MM, Marangos PJ, Polak JM: Immunostaining of neuron-specific enolase is a valuable aid to the cytological diagnosis of neuroendocrine tumours of the lung. J Pathol **143:**259-265, 1984.

613 Thomas BM: Three unusual carcinoid tumours, with particular reference to osteoblastic bone metastases. Clin Radiol **19:**221-225, 1968.

614 Warren WH, Memoli VA, Gould VE: Immunohistochemical and ultrastructural analysis of bronchopulmonary neuroendocrine neoplasms. I. Carcinoids. Ultrastruct Pathol **6:**15-27, 1984.

615 Wilkins EW Jr, Darling RC, Soutter L, Sniffen RC: A continuing clinical survey of adenomas of the trachea and bronchus in a general hospital. J Thorac Cardiovasc Surg **46:**279-291, 1963.

616 Wilkins EW Jr, Grillo HC, Moncure AC, Scannell JG: Changing times in surgical management of bronchopulmonary carcinoid tumor. Ann Thorac Surg **38:**339-344, 1984.

617 Williams ED: The classification of carcinoid tumours. Lancet **1:**238-239, 1963.

618 Williams ED, Celestin LR: The association of bronchial carcinoid and pluriglandular adenomatosis. Thorax **17:**120-127, 1962.

619 Wilson TS, McDowell EM, Marangos PJ, Trump BF: Histochemical studies of dense-core granulated tumors of the lung. Neuron-specific enolase as a marker for granulated cells. Arch Pathol Lab Med **109:**613-620, 1985.

620 Yang K, Ulich T, Taylor I, Cheng L, Lewin KJ: Pulmonary carcinoids. Immunohistochemical demonstration of brain-gut peptides. Cancer **52:**819-823, 1983.

Peripheral carcinoid tumor

621 Bonikos DS, Bensch KG, Jamplis RW: Peripheral pulmonary carcinoid tumors. Cancer **37:**1977-1998, 1976.

622 Churg A, Warnock ML: Pulmonary tumorlet. A form of peripheral carcinoid. Cancer **37:**1469-1477, 1976.

623 D'Agati VD, Perzin KH: Carcinoid tumorlets of the lung with metastasis to a peribronchial lymph node. Report of a case and review of the literature. Cancer **55:**2472-2476, 1985.

624 Felton WL II, Liebow AA, Lindskog GE: Peripheral and multiple bronchial adenomas. Cancer **6:**555-567, 1953.

625 Grazer R, Cohen SM, Jacobs JB, Lucas P: Melanin-containing peripheral carcinoid of the lung. Am J Surg Pathol **6:**73-78, 1982.

626 Miller MA, Mark GJ, Kanarek D: Multiple peripheral pulmonary carcinoids and tumorlets of carcinoid type, with restrictive and obstructive lung disease. Am J Med **65:**373-378, 1978.

627 Ranchod M, Levine GD: Spindle-cell carcinoid tumors of the lung. A clinicopathologic study of 35 cases. Am J Surg Pathol **4:**315-331, 1980.

628 Salyer DC, Salyer WR, Eggleston JC: Bronchial carcinoid tumors. Cancer **36:**1522-1537, 1975.

629 Tamai S, Kameya T, Yamaguchi K, Yanai N, Abe K, Yanaihara N, Yamazaki H, Kageyama K: Peripheral lung carcinoid tumor producing predominantly gastrin-releasing peptide (GRP). Cancer **52:**273-281, 1983.

630 Torikata C, Mukai M, Kawakita H, Kageyama K: Neurofilaments of Kulchitsky cells in human lung. Acta Pathol Jpn **36:**93-104, 1986.

Atypical carcinoid tumor

630a Al-Kaisi N, Abdul-Karim FW, Mendelsohn G, Jacobs G: Bronchial carcinoid tumor with amyloid stroma. Arch Pathol Lab Med **112:**211-214, 1988.

631 Arrigoni MG, Woolner LB, Bernatz PE: Atypical carcinoid tumors of the lung. J Thorac Cardiovasc Surg **64:**413-421, 1972.

632 Fisher ER, Palekar A, Paulson JD: Comparative histopathologic, histochemical, electron microscopic and tisse culture studies of bronchial carcinoids and oat cell carcinomas of lung. Am J Clin Pathol **69:**165-172, 1978.

633 Godwin JD II, Brown CC: Comparative epidemiology of carcinoid and oat-cell tumors of the lung. Cancer **40:**1671-1673, 1977.

633a Memoli VA, Warren WH, Gould VE, Ball ED: MOAB SCCL 175 distinguishes small cell carcinoma (SCC) from well-differentiated neuroendocrine carcinoma (WDNC) of lung (abstract). Lab Invest **58:**63A, 1988.

634 Mills SE, Cooper PH, Walker AN, Kron IL: Atypical carcinoid tumor of the lung. A clinicopathologic study of 17 cases. Am J Surg Pathol **6:**643-654, 1982.

635 Paladugu RR, Benfield JR, Pak HY, Ross RK, Teplitz RL: Bronchopulmonary Kulchitsky cell carcinomas. A new classification scheme for typical and atypical carcinoids. Cancer **55:**1303-1311, 1985.

636 Warren WH, Memoli VA, Gould VE: Immunohistochemical and ultrastructural analysis of bronchopulmonary neuroendocrine neoplasms. II. Well-differentiated neuroendocrine carcinomas. Ultrastruct Pathol **7:**185-199, 1984.

637 Wilkins EW Jr, Grillo HC, Moncure AC, Scannell JG: Changing times in surgical management of bronchopulmonary carcinoid tumor. Ann Thorac Surg **38:**339-344, 1984.

Paraganglioma

638 Churg AM, Warnock ML: So-called "minute pulmonary chemodectoma." A tumor not related to paragangliomas. Cancer **37:**1759-1769, 1976.

638a Cole SR, Pedersen CA, Kryzmowski GA, Knibbs DR, Cartun RW: Histogenesis of so-called minute pulmonary chemodectomas. A study of 18 tumors by immunocytochemistry (abstract). Lab Invest **58:**19A, 1988.

638b Gaffey MJ, Mills SE, Askin FB: Minute pulmonary meningothelial-like nodules. A clinicopathologic study of so-called minute pulmonary chemodectoma. Am J Surg Pathol **12:**167-175, 1988.

639 Heppleston AG: A carotid-body–like tumour in the lung. J Pathol Bacteriol **75:**461-464, 1958.

640 Kuhn C III, Askin FB: The fine structure of so-called minute pulmonary chemodectomas. Hum Pathol **6:**681-691, 1975.

641 Singh G, Lee RE, Brooks DH: Primary pulmonary paraganglioma. Report of a case and review of the literature. Cancer **40:**2286-2289, 1977.

642 Tu H, Bottomley RH: Malignant chemodectoma presenting as a miliary pulmonary infiltrate. Cancer **33:**244-249, 1974.

So-called sclerosing hemangioma

643 Chan K-W, Gibbs AR, Lo WS, Newman GR: Benign sclerosing pneumocytoma of lung (sclerosing haemangioma). Thorax **37:**404-412, 1982.

644 Eggleston JC: The intravascular bronchioloalveolar tumor and the sclerosing hemangioma of the lung. Misnomers of pulmonary neoplasia. Semin Diagn Pathol **2:**270-280, 1985.

645 Haas JE, Yunis EJ, Totten RS: Ultrastructure of a sclerosing hemangioma of the lung. Cancer **30:**512-518, 1972.

646 Haimoto H, Tsutsumi Y, Nagura H, Nakashima N, Watanabe K: Immunohistochemical study of so-called sclerosing haemangioma of the lung. Virchows Arch [Pathol Anat] **407:**419-430, 1985.

647 Hill GS, Eggleston JC: Electron microscopic study of so-called "pulmonary sclerosing hemangioma." Report of a case suggesting epithelial origin. Cancer **30:**1092-1106, 1972.

648 Katzenstein A-LA, Gmelich JT, Carrington CB: Sclerosing hemangioma of the lung. A clinicopathologic study of 51 cases. Am J Surg Pathol **4:**343-356, 1980.

649 Katzenstein A-LA, Weise DL, Fulling K, Battifora H: So-called sclerosing hemangioma of the lung. Evidence for mesothelial origin. Am J Surg Pathol **7:**3-14, 1983.

650 Kay S, Still WJS, Borochovitz D: Sclerosing hemangioma of the lung. An endothelial or epithelial neoplasm? Hum Pathol **8:**468-474, 1977.

651 Liebow AA, Hubbel DS: Sclerosing hemangioma (histiocytoma, xanthoma) of lung. Cancer **9:**53-75, 1956.

652 Nagata N, Dairaku M, Ishida T, Sueishi K, Tanaka K: Sclerosing hemangioma of the lung. Immunohistochemical characterization of its origin as related to surfactant apoprotein. Cancer **55**:116-123, 1985.

653 Navas Palacios JJ, Escribano PM, Toledo J, Garzon A, Larrú E, Palomera J: Sclerosing hemangioma of the lung. An ultrastructural study. Cancer **44**:949-955, 1979.

654 Spencer H, Nambu S: Sclerosing haemangiomas of the lung. Histopathology **10**:477-487, 1986.

Fibroxanthoma and related lesions

655 Buell R, Wang N-S, Seemayer TA, Ahmed MN: Endobronchial plasma cell granuloma (xanthomatous pseudotumor). A light and electron microscopic study. Hum Pathol **7**:411-426, 1976.

656 Chen HP, Lee SS, Berardi RS: Inflammatory pseudotumor of the lung. Ultra-structural and light microscopic study of a myxomatous variant. Cancer **54**:861-865, 1984.

657 Imperato JP, Folkman J, Sagerman RH, Cassady JR: Treatment of plasma cell granuloma of the lung with radiation therapy. A report of two cases and a review of the literature. Cancer **57**:2127-2129, 1986.

658 Katzenstein A-LA, Mauer JJ: Benign histiocytic tumor of lung. A light- and electron-microscopic study. Am J Surg Pathol **3**:61-68, 1979.

659 Lund C, Sørensen IM, Axelsen F, Larsen K: Pulmonary histiocytomas. Eur J Respir Dis **64**:141-149, 1983.

660 Spencer H: The pulmonary plasma cell/histiocytoma complex. Histopathology **8**:903-916, 1984.

661 Titus JL, Harrison EG, Clagett OT, Anderson MW, Knaff LJ: Xanthomatous and inflammatory pseudotumors of the lung. Cancer **15**:522-538, 1962.

662 Wentworth P, Lynch MJ, Fallis JC, Turner JAP, Lowden JA, Conen PE: Xan-thomatous peudotumor of lung. A case report with electron microscope and lipid studies. Cancer **22**:345-355, 1968.

Carcinosarcoma and blastoma

663 Addis BJ, Corrin B: Pulmonary blastoma, carcinosarcoma and spindle-cell car-cinoma. An immunohistochemical study of keratin intermediate filaments. J Pathol **147**:291-301, 1985.

664 Ashworth TG: Pulmonary blastoma. A true congenital neoplasm. Histopathology **7**:585-594, 1983.

665 Bergmann M, Ackerman LV, Kemler RL: Carcinosarcoma of the lung. Review of the literature and report of two cases treated by pneumonectomy. Cancer **4**:919-929, 1951.

666 Davis MP, Eagan RT, Weiland LH, Pairolero PC: Carcinosarcoma of the lung. Mayo Clinic experience and response to chemotherapy. Mayo Clin Proc **59**:598-603, 1984.

667 Francis D, Jacobsen M: Pulmonary blastoma. Curr Top Pathol **73**:265-294, 1983.

667a Heckman CJ, Truong LD, Cagle PT, Font RL: Pulmonary blastoma with rhab-domyosarcomatous differentiation. An electron microscopic and immunohisto-chemical study. Am J Surg Pathol **12**:35-40, 1988.

667b Humphrey PA, Scroggs MW, Roggli VL, Shelburne JD: Pulmonary carcinomas with a sarcomatoid element. An immunocytochemical and ultrastructural anal-ysis. Hum Pathol **19**:155-165, 1988.

668 Jacobsen M, Francis D: Pulmonary blastoma. A clinico-pathological study of 11 cases. Acta Pathol Microbiol Scand [A] **88**:151-160, 1980.

669 Kodama T, Shimosato Y, Watanabe S, Koide T, Naruke T, Shimase J: Six cases of well-differentiated adenocarcinoma simulating fetal lung tubules in pseudo-glandular stage. Comparison with pulmonary blastoma. Am J Surg Pathol **8**:735-744, 1984.

670 Kradin RL, Young RH, Dickersin GR, Kirkham SE, Mark EJ: Pulmonary blas-toma with argyrophil cells and lacking sarcomatous features (pulmonary endo-dermal tumor resembling fetal lung). Am J Surg Pathol **6**:165-172, 1982.

671 Love GL, Daroca PJ Jr: Bronchogenic sarcomatoid squamous cell carcinoma with osteoclast-like giant cells. Hum Pathol **14**:1004-1006, 1983.

672 Manning JT Jr, Ordóñez NG, Rosenberg HS, Walker WE: Pulmonary endo-dermal tumor resembling fetal lung. Report of a case with immunohistochemical studies. Arch Pathol Lab Med **109**:48-50, 1985.

673 Marcus PB, Dieb TM, Martin JH: Pulmonary blastoma. An ultrastructural study emphasizing intestinal differentiation in lung tumors. Cancer **49**:1829-1833, 1982.

674 Minken SL, Craver WL, Adams JT: Pulmonary blastoma. Arch Pathol **86**:442-446, 1968.

675 Müller-Hermelink HK, Kaiserling E: Pulmonary adenocarcinoma of fetal type. Alternating differentiation argues in favour of a common endodermal stem cell. Virchows Arch [Pathol Anat] **409**:195-210, 1986.

676 Roth JA, Elguezabal A: Pulmonary blastoma evolving into carcinosarcoma. A case study. Am J Surg Pathol **2**:407-413, 1978.

677 Stackhouse EM, Harrison EG Jr, Ellis FH: Primary mixed malignancies of lung, carcinosarcoma and blastoma. J Thorac Cardiovasc Surg **57**:385-399, 1969.

678 Valderrama E, Saluja G, Shende A, Langkowsky P, Berkman J: Pulmonary blastoma. Report of two cases in children. Am J Surg Pathol **2**:415-422, 1978.

679 Weinblatt ME, Siegel SE, Isaacs H: Pulmonary blastoma associated with cystic lung disease. Cancer **49**:669-671, 1982.

Vascular tumors

680 Alt B, Huffer WE, Belchis DA: A vascular lesion with smooth muscle differ-entiation presenting as a coin lesion in the lung. Glomus tumor versus heman-giopericytoma. Am J Clin Pathol **80**:765-771, 1983.

681 Antman KH, Nadler L, Mark EJ, Montella DL, Kirkpatrick P, Halpern J: Primary Kaposi's sarcoma of the lung in an immunocompetent 32-year-old heterosexual white man. Cancer **54**:1696-1698, 1984.

682 Banner AS, Carrington CB, Emory WB, Kittle F, Leonard G, Ringus J, Taylor P, Addington WW: Efficacy of oophorectomy in lymphangioleiomyomatosis and benign metastasizing leiomyoma. N Engl J Med **305**:204-209, 1981.

683 Bhagavan BS, Dorfman HD, Murthy MSN, Eggleston JC: Intravascular bron-chiolo-alveolar tumor (IVBAT). A low-grade sclerosing epithelioid angiosar-coma of lung. Am J Surg Pathol **6**:41-52, 1982.

684 Corring B, Liebow AA, Friedman PJ: Pulmonary lymphangiomyomatosis. Am J Pathol **79**:348-382, 1975.

685 Dail DH, Liebow AA, Gmelich JT, Friedman PJ, Miyai K, Myer W, Patterson SD, Hammar SP: Intravascular, bronchiolar, and alveolar tumor of the lung (IVBAT). An analysis of twenty cases of a peculiar sclerosing endothelial tumor. Cancer **51**:452-464, 1983.

686 Eggleston JC: The intravascular bronchioloalveolar tumor and the sclerosing hemangioma of the lung. Misnomers of pulmonary neoplasia. Semin Diagn Pathol **2**:270-280, 1985.

687 Gledhill A, Kay JM: Hepatic metastases in a case of intravascular bronchio-loalveolar tumour. J Clin Pathol **37**:279-282, 1984.

688 Graham ML II, Spelsberg TC, Dines DE, Payne WS, Bjornsson J, Lie JT: Pulmonary lymphangiomyomatosis. With particular reference to steroid-receptor assay studies and pathologic correlation. Mayo Clin Proc **59**:3-11, 1984.

689 Lack EE, Dolan MF, Finisio J, Grover G, Singh M, Triche TJ: Pulmonary and extrapulmonary lymphangioleiomyomatosis. Report of a case with bilateral renal angiomyolipomas, multifocal lymphangioleiomyomatosis, and a glial polyp of the endocervix. Am J Surg Pathol **10**:650-657, 1986.

690 McCarty KS Jr, Mossler JA, McLelland R, Sieker HO: Pulmonary lymphan-giomyomatosis responsive to progesterone. N Engl J Med **303**:1461-1465, 1980.

691 Meade JB, Whitwell F, Bickford BJ, Waddington KB: Primary haemangio-pericytoma of lung. Thorax **29**:1-15, 1974.

692 Nash G, Fligiel S: Kaposi's sarcoma presenting as pulmonary disease in the acquired immunodeficiency syndrome. Diagnosis by lung biopsy. Hum Pathol **15**:999-1001, 1984.

693 Purdy LJ, Colby TV, Yousem SA, Battifora H: Pulmonary Kaposi's sarcoma. Premortem histologic diagnosis. Am J Surg Pathol **10**:301-311, 1986.

694 Sobonya RE, Quan SF, Fleishman JS: Pulmonary lymphangioleiomyomatosis. Quantitative analysis of lesions producing airflow limitation. Hum Pathol **16**:1122-1128, 1985.

695 Taguchi T, Tsuji K, Matsuo K, Takebayashi S, Kawahara K, Hadama T: Intra-vascular bronchioloalveolar tumor. Report of an autopsy case and review of literature. Acta Pathol Jpn **35**:631-642, 1985.

696 Tron V, Magee F, Wright JL, Colby T, Churg A: Pulmonary capillary heman-giomatosis. Hum Pathol **17**:1144-1150, 1986.

697 Verbeken E, Beyls J, Moerman P, Knockaert D, Goddeeris P, Lauweryns JM: Lung metastasis of malignant epithelioid hemangioendothelioma mimicking a primary intravascular bronchioalveolar tumor. A histologic, ultrastructural, and immunohistochemical study. Cancer **55**:1741-1746, 1985.

698 Weldon-Linne CM, Victor TA, Christ ML, Fry WA: Angiogenic nature of the 'intravascular bronchioloalveolar tumor' of the lung. An electron microscopic study. Arch Pathol Lab Med **105**:174-179, 1981.

699 Yousem SA: Angiosarcoma presenting in the lung. Arch Pathol Lab Med **110**:112-115, 1986.

Lymphoid tumors and tumorlike conditions

700 Amin R: Extramedullary plasmacytoma of the lung. Cancer **56**:152-156, 1985.

701 Callahan M, Wall S, Askin F, Delaney D, Koller C, Orringer EP: Granulocytic sarcoma presenting as pulmonary nodules and lymphadenopathy. Cancer **60**:1902-1904, 1987.

702 Chen KTK: Abdominal form of lymphomatoid granulomatosis. Hum Pathol **8:**99-108, 1977.

703 Colby TV, Carrington CB: Pulmonary lymphomas simulating lymphomatoid granulomatosis. Am J Surg Pathol **6:**19-32, 1982.

704 Colby TV, Yousem SA: Pulmonary lymphoid neoplasms. Semin Diagn Pathol **2:**183-196, 1985.

705 Evans HL: Extranodal small lymphocytic proliferation. A clinicopathologic and immunocytochemical study. Cancer **49:**84-96, 1982.

706 Fauci AS, Haynes BF, Costa J, Katz P, Wolff SM: Lymphomatoid granulomatosis. Prospective clinical and therapeutic experience over 10 years. N Engl J Med **306:**68-74, 1982.

707 Hammar S, Mennemeyer R: Lymphomatoid granulomatosis in a renal transplant recipient. Hum Pathol **7:**111-116, 1976.

708 Harper PG, Fisher C, McLennan K, Souhami RL: Presentation of Hodgkin's disease as an endobronchial lesion. Cancer **53:**147-150, 1984.

709 Herbert A, Wright DH, Isaacson PG, Smith JL: Primary malignant lymphoma of the lung. Histopathologic and immunologic evaluation of nine cases. Hum Pathol **15:**415-422, 1984.

710 Katzenstein A-LA, Carrington CB, Liebow AA: Lymphomatoid granulomatosis. A clinicopathologic study of 152 cases. Cancer **43:**360-373, 1979.

711 Kennedy JL, Nathwani BN, Burke JS, Hill LR, Rappaport H: Pulmonary lymphomas and other pulmonary lymphoid lesions. A clinicopathologic and immunologic study of 64 patients. Cancer **56:**539-552, 1985.

712 Koss MN, Hochholzer L, Nichols PW, Wehunt WD, Lazarus AA: Primary non-Hodgkin's lymphoma and pseudolymphoma of lung. A study of 161 patients. Hum Pathol **14:**1024-1038, 1983.

713 Kradin RL, Mark EJ: Benign lymphoid disorders of the lung, with a theory regarding their development. Hum Pathol **14:**857-867, 1983.

714 Kradin RL, Young RH, Kradin LA, Mark EJ: Immunoblastic lymphoma arising in chronic lymphoid hyperplasia of the pulmonary interstitium. Cancer **50:**1339-1343, 1982.

715 L'Hoste RJ Jr, Filippa DA, Lieberman PH, Bretsky S: Primary pulmonary lymphomas. A clinicopathologic analysis of 36 cases. Cancer **54:**1397-1406, 1984.

716 Liebow AA: Pulmonary angiitis and granulomatosis (The J. Burns Amberson Lecture). Am Rev Respir Dis **108:**1-18, 1973.

717 Liebow AA, Carrington CRB, Friedman PJ: Lymphomatoid granulomatosis. Hum Pathol **3:**457-558, 1972.

718 Mohamedani AA, Bennett MK: Angiofollicular lymphoid hyperplasia in a pulmonary fissure. Thorax **40:**686-687, 1985.

719 Morinaga S, Watanabe H, Gemma A, Mukai K, Nakajima T, Shimosato Y, Goya T, Shinoda T: Plasmacytoma of the lung associated with nodular deposits of immunoglobulin. Am J Surg Pathol **11:**989-995, 1987.

720 Palosaari DE, Colby TV: Bronchiolocentric chronic lymphocytic leukemia. Cancer **58:**1695-1698, 1986.

721 Patton WF, Lynch JP III: Lymphomatoid granulomatosis. Clinicopathologic study of four cases and literature review. Medicine **61:**1-11, 1982.

722 Peterson H, Snider HL, Yam LT, Bowlds CF, Arnn EH, Li CY: Primary pulmonary lymphoma. A clinical and immunohistochemical study of six cases. Cancer **56:**805-813, 1985.

723 Rattinger MD, Dunn TL, Christian CD Jr, Donnell RM, Collins RD, O'Leary JP, Flexner JM: Gastrointestinal involvement in lymphomatoid granulomatosis. Report of a case and review of the literature. Cancer **51:**694-700, 1983.

724 Reddick RL, Fauci AS, Valsamis MP, Mann RB: Immunoblastic sarcoma of the central nervous system in a patient with lymphomatoid granulomatosis. Cancer **42:**652-659, 1978.

725 Rose RM, Grigas D, Strattemeir E, Harris NL, Linggood RM: Endobronchial involvement with non-Hodgkin's lymphoma. A clinical-radiologic analysis. Cancer **57:**1750-1755, 1986.

726 Saldana MJ, Patchefsky AS, Israel HI, Atkinson GW: Pulmonary angiitis and granulomatosis. The relationship between histological features, organ involvement, and response to treatment. Hum Pathol **8:**391-409, 1977.

727 Saltzstein SL: Pulmonary malignant lymphomas and pseudolymphomas. Classification, therapy, and prognosis. Cancer **16:**928-955, 1963.

728 Singh G, Hellstrom HR: Lymphomatoid granulomatosis. Report of a case without pulmonary lesions and with ischemic colitis, probably a sequel to granulomatosis. Hum Pathol **9:**364-366, 1978.

729 Strum SB, Weiss A, McDermed JE, Rosen VJ: Intrathoracic Hodgkin's disease. A case presentation with multiple pulmonary nodules in the absence of mediastinal or hilar node disease. Cancer **56:**1953-1956, 1985.

730 Tenholder MF, Scialla SJ, Weisbaum G: Endobronchial metastatic plasmacytoma. Cancer **49:**1465-1468, 1982.

731 Turner RR, Colby TV, Doggett RS: Well-differentiated lymphocytic lymphoma.

A study of 47 patients with primary manifestation in the lung. Cancer **54:**2088-2096, 1984.

732 Wardman AG, Cooke NJ: Pulmonary infiltrates in adult acute leukaemia. Empirical treatment or lung biopsy? Thorax **39:**647-650, 1984.

733 Weiss LM, Yousem SA, Warnke RA: Non-Hodgkin's lymphomas of the lung. A study of 19 cases emphasizing the utility of frozen section immunologic studies in differential diagnosis. Am J Surg Pathol **9:**480-490, 1985.

734 Weiss MA, Rolfes DB, Alvira MA, Cohen LJ: Benign lymphocytic angiitis and granulomatosis. A case report with evidence of an autoimmune etiology. Am J Clin Pathol **81:**110-116, 1984.

735 Wile A, Olinger G, Peter JB, Dornfeld L: Solitary intraparenchymal pulmonary plasmacytoma associated with production of an M-protein. Report of a case. Cancer **37:**2338-2342, 1976.

736 Yousem SA, Weiss LM, Colby TV: Primary pulmonary Hodgkin's disease. A clinicopathologic study of 15 cases. Cancer **57:**1217-1224, 1986.

Salivary gland–type tumors

737 Barsky SH, Martin SE, Matthews M, Gazdar A, Costa JC: "Low grade" mucoepidermoid carcinoma of the bronchus with "high grade" biological behavior. Cancer **51:**1505-1509, 1983.

738 Conlan AA, Payne WS, Wollner LB, Sanderson DR: Adenoid cystic carcinoma (cylindroma) and mucoepidermoid carcinoma of the bronchus. J Thorac Cardiovasc Surg **76:**369-377, 1978.

739 Fechner RE, Bentinck BR: Ultrastructure of bronchial oncocytoma. Cancer **31:**1451-1457, 1973.

740 Heard BE, Corrin B, Dewar A: Pathology of seven mucous cell adenomas of the bronchial glands with particular reference to ultrastructure. Histopathology **9:**687-701, 1985.

741 Katz DR, Bubis JJ: Acinic cell tumor of the bronchus. Cancer **38:**830-832, 1976.

742 Kroe DJ, Pitcock JA: Benign mucous gland adenoma of the bronchus. Arch Pathol **84:**539-542, 1967.

743 Lack EE, Harris GBC, Eraklis AJ, Vawter GF: Primary bronchial tumors in childhood. A clinicopathologic study of six cases. Cancer **51:**492-497, 1983.

744 Leonardi HK, Jung-Legg Y, Legg A, Neptune WB: Tracheobronchial mucoepidermoid carcinoma. J Thorac Cardiovasc Surg **76:**431-438, 1978.

745 Markel SF, Abell MR, Haight C, French AJ: Neoplasms of bronchus commonly designated as adenomas. Cancer **17:**590-608, 1964.

746 Nielsen AL: Malignant bronchial oncocytoma. Case report and review of the literature. Hum Pathol **16:**852-854, 1985.

747 Payne WS, Schier J, Woolner LB: Mixed tumors of the bronchus (salivary gland type). J Thorac Cardiovasc Surg **49:**663-668, 1965.

748 Reichle FA, Rosemond GP: Mucoepidermoid tumors of the bronchus. J Thorac Cardiovasc Surg **51:**443-448, 1966.

749 Santos-Briz A, Terrón J, Sastre R, Romero L, Valle A: Oncocytoma of the lung. Cancer **40:**1330-1336, 1977.

750 Spencer H: Bronchial gland tumours. Virchows Arch [Pathol Anat] **383:**101-115, 1979.

751 Turnbull AD, Huvos AG, Goodner JT, Foote FW Jr: Mucoepidermoid tumors of bronchial glands. Cancer **28:**539-544, 1971.

751a Yousem SA: Pulmonary carcinomas with amyloid-like stroma. Am J Clin Pathol (in press).

751b Yousem SA, Hochholzer L: Mucoepidermoid tumors of the lung. Cancer **60:**1346-1352, 1987.

Benign clear cell tumor

752 Andrion A, Mazzucco G, Gugliotta P, Monga G: Benign clear cell ('sugar') tumor of the lung. A light microscopic, histochemical, and ultrastructural study with a review of the literature. Cancer **56:**2657-2663, 1985.

753 Becker NH, Soifer L: Benign clear cell tumor ("sugar tumor") of the lung. Cancer **27:**712-719, 1971.

754 Fukuda T, Machinami R, Joshita T, Nagashima K: Benign clear cell tumor of the lung in an 8-year-old girl. Arch Pathol Lab Med **110:**664-666, 1986.

755 Hoch WS, Patchefsky AS, Takeda M, Gordon G: Benign clear cell tumor of the lung. An ultrastructural study. Cancer **33:**1328-1336, 1974.

756 Liebow AA, Castleman B: Benign clear cell ("sugar") tumors of the lung. Yale J Biol Med **43:**213-222, 1971.

Muscle tumors

757 Avagnina A, Elsner B, DeMarco L, Bracco AN, Nazar J, Pavlovsky H: Pulmonary rhabdomyosarcoma with isolated small bowel metastasis. A report of a case with immunohistochemical and ultrastructural studies. Cancer **53:**1948-1951, 1984.

758 Banner AS, Carrington CB, Emory WB, Kittle F, Leonard G, Ringus J, Taylor P, Addington WW: Efficacy of oophorectomy in lymphangioleiomyomatosis and benign metastasizing leiomyoma. N Engl J Med **305:**204-209, 1981.

759 Burkhardt A, Otto HF, Kaukel E: Multiple pulmonary (hamartomatous?) leiomyomas. Light and electron microscopic study. Virchows Arch [Pathol Anat] **394:**133-141, 1981.

760 Horstmann JP, Pietra GG, Harman JA, Cole NG Jr, Grinspan S: Spontaneous regression of pulmonary leiomyomas during pregnancy. Cancer **39:**314-321, 1977.

761 Jimenez JF, Uthman EO, Townsend JW, Gloster ES, Seibert JJ: Primary bronchopulmonary leiomyosarcoma in childhood. Arch Pathol Lab Med **110:**348-351, 1986.

762 Krous HF, Sexauer CL: Embryonal rhabdomyosarcoma arising within a congenital bronchogenic cyst in a child. J Pediatr Surg **16:**506-508, 1981.

763 Silverman JF, Kay S: Multiple pulmonary leiomyomatous hamartomas. Report of a case with ultrastructure examination. Cancer **38:**1199-1204, 1976.

764 Taylor TL, Miller DR: Leiomyoma of the bronchus. J Thorac Cardiovasc Surg **57:**284-288, 1969.

765 Tench WD, Dail D, Gmelich JT, Matani N: Benign metastasizing leiomyomas. A review of 21 cases (abstract). Lab Invest **38:**367, 1978.

766 Vera-Román JM, Sobonya RE, Gomez-Garcia JL, Sanz-Bondia JR, Paris-Romeu F: Leiomyoma of the lung. Literature review and case report. Cancer **52:**936-941, 1983.

767 White SH, Ibrahim NBN, Forrester-Wood CP, Jeyasingham K: Leiomyomas of the lower respiratory tract. Thorax **40:**306-311, 1985.

768 Wick MR, Scheithauer BW, Piehler JM, Pairolero PC: Primary pulmonary leiomyosarcomas. A light and electron microscopic study. Arch Pathol Lab Med **106:**510-514, 1982.

769 Wolff M, Silva F, Kaye F: Pulmonary metastases (with admixed epithelial elements) from smooth muscle neoplasms. Report of nine cases, including three males. Am J Surg Pathol **3:**325-342, 1979.

Miscellaneous primary tumors

770 Black H: Fibrosarcoma of the bronchus. J Thorac Surg **19:**123-134, 1950.

771 Carstens PHB, Kuhns JG, Ghazi C: Primary malignant melanomas of the lung and adrenal. Hum Pathol **15:**910-914, 1984.

772 Chumas JC, Lorelle CA: Pulmonary meningioma. A light- and electron-microscopic study. Am J Surg Pathol **6:**795-801, 1982.

773 Cooney TP: Primary pulmonary ganglioneuroblastoma in an adult. Maturation, involution and the immune response. Histopathology **5:**451-463, 1981.

774 Crutcher RR, Waltuck TL, Ghosh AK: Bronchial lipoma. J Thorac Cardiovasc Surg **55:**422-425, 1968.

775 Daniels AC, Conner GH, Straus FH: Primary chondrosarcoma of the tracheobronchial tree. Report of a unique case and brief review. Arch Pathol **84:**615-624, 1967.

776 Gallivan GJ, Dolan CT, Stam RE, Eggerston BS Jr, Tovey JD: Granular cell myoblastoma of the bronchus. J Thorac Cardiovasc Surg **52:**875-881, 1966.

777 Kemnitz P, Spormann H, Heinrich P: Meningioma of lung. First report with light and electron microscopic findings. Ultrastruct Pathol **3:**359-365, 1982.

778 Kern WH, Hughes RK, Meyer BW, Harley DP: Malignant fibrous histiocytoma of the lung. Cancer **44:**1793-1801, 1979.

779 Lee JT, Shelburne JD, Linder J: Primary malignant fibrous histiocytoma of the lung. A clinicopathologic and ultrastructural study of five cases. Cancer **53:**1124-1130, 1984.

780 Maxwell RJ, Gibbons JR, O'Hara MD: Solitary squamous papilloma of the bronchus. Thorax **40:**68-71, 1985.

780a McDonnell T, Kyriakos M, Roper C, Mazoujian G: Malignant fibrous histiocytoma of the lung. Cancer **61:**137-145, 1988.

781 Moore RL, Lattes R: Papillomatosis of larynx and bronchi. Cancer **12:**117-126, 1959.

782 Nascimento AG, Unni KK, Bernatz PE: Sarcomas of the lung. Mayo Clin Proc **57:**355-359, 1982.

783 Pushchak MJ, Farhi DC: Primary choriocarcinoma of the lung. Arch Pathol Lab Med **111:**477-479, 1987.

784 Reid JD, Mehta VT: Melanoma of the lower respiratory tract. Cancer **19:**627-631, 1966.

785 Reingold LM, Amromin GD: Extraosseous osteosarcoma of the lung. Cancer **28:**491-498, 1971.

786 Roviaro G, Montorsi M, Varoli F, Binda R, Cecchetto A: Primary pulmonary tumours of neurogenic origin. Thorax **38:**942-945, 1983.

787 Silverman JF, Leffers BR, Kay S: Primary pulmonary neurilemoma. Report of a case with ultrastructural examination. Arch Pathol Lab Med **100:**644-648, 1976.

788 Smith PS, McClure J: A papillary endobronchial tumor with a transitional cell pattern. Arch Pathol Lab Med **106:**503-506, 1982.

789 Spencer H, Dail DH, Arneaud J: Non-invasive bronchial epithelial papillary tumors. Cancer **45:**1486-1497, 1980.

790 Sun C-CJ, Kroll M, Miller JE: Primary chondrosarcoma of the lung. Cancer **50:**1864-1866, 1982.

791 Thorburn JD, Stephens HB, Grimes OF: Benign thymoma in the hilus of the lung. J Thorac Surg **24:**540-543, 1952.

792 Tomashefski JR Jr: Benign endobronchial mesenchymal tumors. Their relationship to parenchymal pulmonary hamartomas. Am J Surg Pathol **6:**531-540, 1982.

793 Young CD, Gay RM: Multiple endobronchial granular cell myoblastomas discovered at bronchoscopy. Hum Pathol **15:**193-194, 1984.

METASTATIC TUMORS

794 Baldeyrou P, Lemoine G, Zucker JM, Schweisguth O: Pulmonary metastases in children. The place of surgery. A study of 134 patients. J Pediatr Surg **19:**121-125, 1984.

795 Beattie EJ Jr: Surgical treatment of pulmonary metastases. Cancer **54:**2729-2731, 1984.

796 Edlich RF, Shea MA, Foker JE, Grondin C, Castaneda AR, Varco RL: A review of 26 years' experience with pulmonary resection for metastatic cancer. Dis Chest **49:**587-594, 1966.

797 Engstrand DA, England DM, Oberley TD: Limitations of the usefulness of microvillous ultrastructure in distinguishing between carcinoma primary in and metastatic to the lung. Ultrastruct Pathol **11:**53-58, 1987.

798 Feldman PS, Kyriakos M: Pulmonary resection for metastatic sarcoma. J Thorac Cardiovasc Surg **64:**784-799, 1972.

799 Flye MW, Woltering G, Rosenberg SA: Aggressive pulmonary resection for metastatic osteogenic and soft tissue sarcomas. Ann Thorac Surg **37:**123-127, 1984.

800 Habein HC Jr, Clagett OT, McDonald JR: Pulmonary resection for metastatic tumors. Arch Surg **78:**716-723, 1959.

801 Katzenstein AL, Purvis R Jr, Gmelich J, Askin F: Pulmonary resection for metastatic renal adenocarcinoma. Pathologic findings and therapeutic value. Cancer **41:**712-723, 1978.

802 Mountain CF, McMurtrey MJ, Hermes KE: Surgery for pulmonary metastasis. A 20-year experience. Ann Thorac Surg **38:**323-330, 1984.

803 Putnam JB Jr, Roth JA, Wesley MN, Johnston MR, Rosenberg SA: Survival following aggressive resection of pulmonary metastases from osteogenic sarcoma. Analysis of prognostic factors. Ann Thorac Surg **36:**516-523, 1983.

804 Rosenblatt MB, Lisa JR, Collier F: Primary and metastatic bronchioloalveolar carcinoma. Dis Chest **52:**147-152, 1967.

805 Roth JA, Putnam JB Jr, Wesley MN, Rosenberg SA: Differing determinants of prognosis following resection of pulmonary metastases from osteogenic and soft tissue sarcoma patients. Cancer **55:**1361-1366, 1985.

806 Shepherd MP: Endobronchial metastatic disease. Thorax **37:**362-365, 1982.

807 Shepherd MP: Thoracic metastases. Thorax **37:**366-370, 1982.

8 Mediastinum

GENERALITIES

The mediastinum is the portion of the thoracic cavity located between the pleural cavities, extending anteroposteriorly from the sternum to the spine and sagittally from the thoracic inlet to the diaphragm. The large number of organs and structures it contains make it a veritable Pandora's box. Congenital cysts, benign tumors, and primary and malignant neoplasms occur in it.

An arbitrary division of the mediastinum into *superior, anterior, middle,* and *posterior* compartments has proved useful, since most cysts and neoplasms have a predilection for one compartment over the others. The most common mediastinal lesions are noted in Fig. 8-1 according to their frequency and most common site of occurrence.[1,5,7,10]

About half of the patients with mediastinal cysts and tumors are asymptomatic, the lesions being discovered incidentally on chest x-ray films. When symptoms develop, they usually result from compression and/or invasion of adjacent structures, and include chest pain, cough, and dys-

pnea. Development of the superior vena cava syndrome is usually indicative of malignancy, the two most common causes being metastatic lung carcinoma and malignant lymphoma[6,8]; however, it can also occur with benign conditions, such as fibrosing mediastinitis.[2] Pulmonary stenosis can also occur with mediastinal tumors as a result of compression of the pulmonary artery or the right ventricular outflow tract.[3]

The location of lesions in the mediastinum, together with their configuration, may give a hint about the specific diagnosis, but many lesions (both benign and malignant) give similar roentgenographic shadows, even with newer modalities such as CT scan.[4] Exploration is therefore mandatory in most instances. Preoperative irradiation should be avoided whenever possible because the changes resulting from it may render the pathologic interpretation difficult or even impossible. Core needle and fine needle aspiration of mediastinal masses has been used successfully, particularly in lesions of the anterosuperior compartment.[9]

INFLAMMATORY DISEASES

Acute mediastinitis is usually the result of traumatic perforation of the esophagus,[19] or descent of infection from within the neck through the "danger space" anterior to the prevertebral fascia[11,19]; in both cases, it involves predominantly the posterior portion of the mediastinum. Abscess formation usually takes place and generally requires surgical drainage.

Chronic mediastinitis can produce compression of the vena cava and simulate a malignant process. The typical location is the anterior mediastinum, in front of the tracheal bifurcation. Microscopically, one may find granulomas, fibrosis, or a combination of both.[22] In some of these cases, a mycotic (usually histoplasmosis) or tuberculous etiology has been documented.[12,14,21,23] Goodwin et al.[14] studied thirty-eight cases of mediastinal granuloma or fibrosis and found, either by histology or cultures, that they were caused by *Histoplasma* in twenty-six cases and by *Mycobacteria* in twelve. Those caused by *Histoplasma* often were characterized by the formation of a thick fibrous capsule; in those caused by *Mycobacteria* the capsule was quite thin. Cases of *Nocardia* mediastinitis resulting in superior vena cava syndrome have also been reported.[20]

In many instances of chronic mediastinitis, a specific etiology cannot be demonstrated.[13,15] Some of these cases represent examples of *fibrosing mediastinitis* (idiopathic mediastinal fibrosis), a member of the group of idiopathic fibrosing (sclerosing) inflammatory conditions, which also includes retroperitoneal fibrosis, sclerosing cholangitis, Riedel's struma, and inflammatory pseudotumor of the orbit. Indeed, fibrosing mediastinitis can be seen in association with one or more of these conditions, particularly retroperitoneal fibrosis.[16,18] This disease should be suspected when

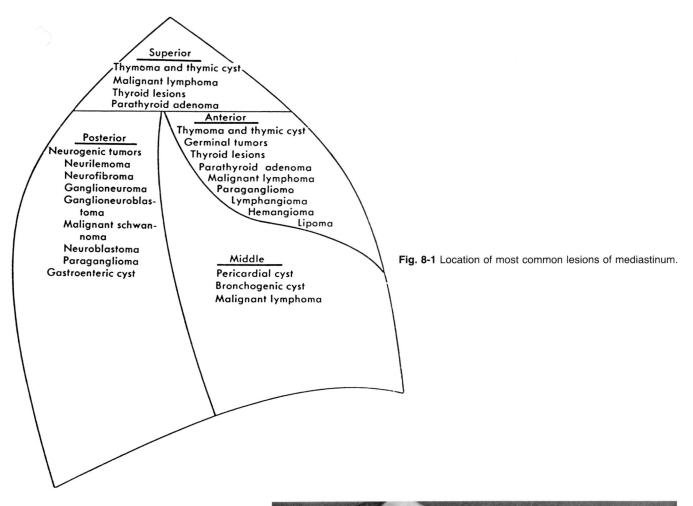

Superior
Thymoma and thymic cyst
Malignant lymphoma
Thyroid lesions
Parathyroid adenoma

Anterior
Thymoma and thymic cyst
Germinal tumors
Thyroid lesions
Parathyroid adenoma
Malignant lymphoma
Paraganglioma
Lymphangioma
Hemangioma
Lipoma

Posterior
Neurogenic tumors
Neurilemoma
Neurofibroma
Ganglioneuroma
Ganglioneuroblas-
toma
Malignant schwan-
noma
Neuroblastoma
Paraganglioma
Gastroenteric cyst

Middle
Pericardial cyst
Bronchogenic cyst
Malignant lymphoma

Fig. 8-1 Location of most common lesions of mediastinum.

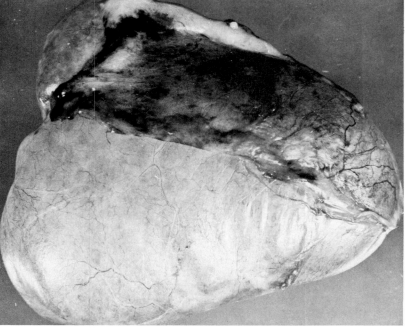

Fig. 8-2 Unilocular thin-walled pericardial cyst.

the fibrous reaction is particularly cellular, when the inflammatory infiltrate is rich in plasma cells and eosinophils, and particularly in the presence of phlebitis. At the same time, one should always keep in mind that some neoplastic disorders—particularly Hodgkin's disease—may contain extensive areas in which only fibrosis and chronic inflammation are seen. The treatment of fibrosing mediastinitis includes steroid therapy and surgical excision.[17]

CYSTS (OTHER THAN THYMIC)
Pericardial (coelomic) cysts

The pericardial sac is formed by the fusion of multiple disconnected lacunae. Failure of one of the lacunar cavities to merge with the others results in the development of a pericardial (coelomic) cyst. Such cysts are usually located at the right cardiophrenic angle.[24] They are soft and unilocular, usually loosely adherent to the pericardium and attached to the diaphragm; sometimes they communicate with the pericardial cavity (Fig. 8-2). Less commonly, they are seen in a suprapericardial position. At times, multiple cysts may be present. They contain clear fluid unless infected. The blood supply comes from the pericardium. The inner surface of the cyst wall is covered by a thin layer of mesothelium.

Foregut cysts

In the embryonic stage, fusion of the lateral walls that form the tracheoesophageal septum begins caudally. If a small bud or diverticulum of the foregut is pinched off during this process, it will be carried into the mediastinum by the downward growth of the lungs. This structure contains the endoderm and mesoderm that were destined to become part of the trachea, bronchi, esophagus, stomach, or intestine.[25]

Bronchial cysts occur along the tracheobronchial tree, their most common location being posterior to the carina. Rarely, they are located just above the diaphragm.[29,30] They can be missed on plain films but are easily detectable on barium-swallow studies.[28] These cysts contain clear or gelatinous fluid, are usually unilocular, thin-walled, and spherical, and have an average diameter of 3 to 4 cm[31] (Fig. 8-3). Microscopically, they usually are lined by ciliated columnar epithelium, but focal or extensive squamous metaplasia and/or extreme attenuation of the mucosa can occur (Fig. 8-4). The wall may contain hyaline cartilage, smooth muscle, bronchial glands, and nerve trunks.

Esophageal cysts probably arise from a persistence, in the wall of the foregut, of vacuoles that form during the solid tube stage of development. Most of them are found embedded in the wall of the lower half of the organ. The lining may be squamous, ciliated, columnar, or a mixture. Distinction from bronchial cyst may be difficult or even impossible, especially because the latter can be found entirely within the wall of the esophagus. The best evidence that a cyst in this location is of esophageal type is the presence of a definite double layer of smooth muscle in the wall.

Gastric and *enteric cysts* usually are located in the posterior mediastinum in a paravertebral location, attached to the wall of the esophagus or even embedded within the muscle layer of this organ. Nearly all cases are associated

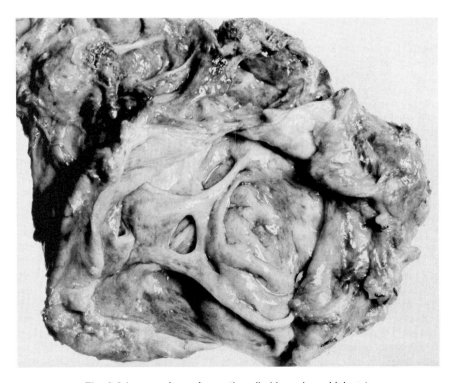

Fig. 8-3 Inner surface of smooth-walled large bronchial cyst.

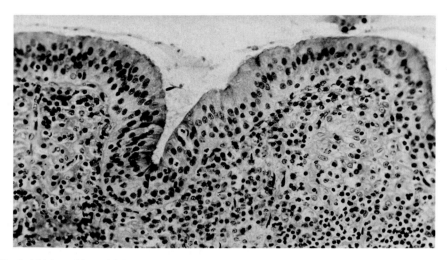

Fig. 8-4 Lining of bronchial cyst shown in Fig. 8-3. Surface epithelium is ciliated and columnar.

with vertebral malformations. The gastric variety is made up of the same coats as the stomach, whereas the enteric type simulates the wall of normal intestine. Combined forms occur and are designated as *gastroenteric cysts.* Nerve fibers and ganglia are often present in them.[25]

• • •

This group of congenital cysts only exceptionally communicates with the tracheobronchial tree or the esophagus. They are not neoplasms, and malignant change takes place within them only exceptionally.[27] Symptoms from these cysts depend on their size and location; they are related to pressure phenomena and consist of cough, dysphagia, recurrent pulmonary infection, dyspnea, pain, and rarely hemoptysis. Most bronchial, esophageal, and enteric cysts are asymptomatic and are found incidentally in a routine chest roentgenogram. In contrast, gastric and gastroenteric cysts are often symptomatic and even life-threatening because of the occurrence of gastric secretion and the resulting hemorrhage, peptic ulcer, or perforation.[26]

Other cysts

Cases of mediastinal cysts arising from the *thoracic duct* have been reported.[33] Some of these perhaps represent examples of cystic lymphangiomas.

Pancreatic pseudocysts may have a primarily mediastinal presentation.[32]

THYROID AND PARATHYROID LESIONS

Thyroid tumors and tumorlike conditions of several types can present as superior mediastinal masses. The most common pathologic change in mediastinal thyroid glands is nodular hyperplasia, which can reach huge proportions and cause compression symptoms.[35] Thyroid nodular hyperplasia in the mediastinum tends to occur in the form of seemingly independent nodules, a fact which may lead the unwary to regard the lesion as malignant. Actually, malignant change in mediastinal thyroid is too unusual to justify ex-

cision on this basis; the main rationale for surgery is the relief of compression symptoms.[34] Nearly all of these lesions can be removed through a collar suprasternal incision.

From a pathogenetic standpoint, the nodular hyperplasia in most instances probably does not arise from ectopic thyroid tissue but rather from cervical thyroid that has been pulled down either into the anterior prevascular compartment or the retrotracheal compartment (so-called posterior descending goiter) by the nodular enlargement. Support for this interpretation comes from the fact that these masses retain their cervical blood supply through a narrow pedicle. Radioactive iodine scanning yields a positive result in over half of the cases.

Parathyroid tumors and tumor-like conditions can also occur in the mediastinum, a not surprising event in view of the embryologic origin of the parathyroid glands and their intimate relationship with the thymus. About 7% of parathyroid adenomas are found in the superior mediastinum, and most of them can be excised through a collar suprasternal incision. Because of their location, these adenomas can grow to much larger size than their equivalents in the neck. Mediastinal parathyroid carcinomas have also been reported, some of them being nonfunctioning.[36]

THYMUS
Normal anatomy

The thymus is a lobulated organ covered by a capsule and divided into cortical and medullary portions, the cortex being further subdivided into a subcapsular (outer) and a deep region. The two major cell types are endodermally derived epithelial cells and bone marrow–derived lymphocytes. The epithelial cells have been divided into several subtypes on the basis of their location, appearance, and some preliminary immunohistochemical data: cortical (dendritic), subcapsular, medullary, and Hassall's corpuscle–related.[43,47,48,49] These epithelial cells are keratin-positive and express HLA-DR antigens. They are thought to be responsible for the differentiation of T lymphocytes, a process perhaps modulated through the secretion of thymic hormones.[37,44]

The thymic lymphocytes (traditionally known as thymocytes) have a T-cell phenotype; a whole range of differentiation exists among them, the better defined stages being those of subcapsular thymocyte, cortical thymocyte, medullary thymocyte, and mature (peripheral type) T lymphocyte.[41,42,48]

Other cells normally present in the thymus include interdigitating reticulum cells, Langerhans' cells,[38] mast cells, eosinophils (particularly in neonates),[40] and the usual stromal cells.

The thymus undergoes marked involution in chronic wasting diseases, regardless of their etiology.[39,40] These changes can be marked and should not be misinterpreted as evidence of a primary thymic disorder.

The thymus undergoes atrophy after puberty, although it never disappears completely.[45,46] Islands of thymic tissue are consistently found on microscopic examination of the prepericardial fat. The islands predominantly composed of lymphocytes may be confused with lymph nodes; those mainly made up of epithelial cells show trabecular or rosette-like formations and may be misinterpreted as carcinomatous or neuroendocrine.

Cysts

Thymic cysts can occur in the neck or the mediastinum.[50,53,54] The former can be seen anywhere along a line extending from the angle of the mandible to the manubrium sterni.[55] The only distinguishing feature at the microscopic level is the presence of thymic tissue in the wall. The epithelial lining may be squamous or columnar (Fig. 8-5). Degenerative and inflammatory changes are common, with formation of cholesterol granulomas. Sometimes the lining epithelium participates in this reactive proliferation and acquires the features of *pseudoepitheliomatous hyperplasia;* we have seen several instances of this phenomenon that had been originally misinterpreted as examples of malignant transformation. It is possible, however, that true epidermoid carcinomas may exceptionally arise from these cysts.[52]

Some thymic cysts are of developmental origin and originate from a remnant of the third branchial pouch–derived thymopharyngeal duct. Others are probably acquired and of either a degenerative or reactive nature, arising from cystic dilatation of Hassall's corpuscles. The so-called *Dubois' abscesses* described in the thymuses of neonates with congenital syphilis belong to the latter category. A large proportion of "nonspecific cysts" of the anterosuperior portion of the mediastinum are probably of thymic origin. Care should always be exercised in excluding the possibility of thymoma with cystic degeneration, a not uncommon occurrence.[51] It should also be remembered that Hodgkin's disease and, less frequently, non-Hodgkin's lymphoma and seminoma can be accompanied by prominent secondary cystic changes of the thymic parenchyma.

Primary immunodeficiencies

The morphologic abnormalities of the thymus in the various primary immunodeficiency diseases are poorly defined.

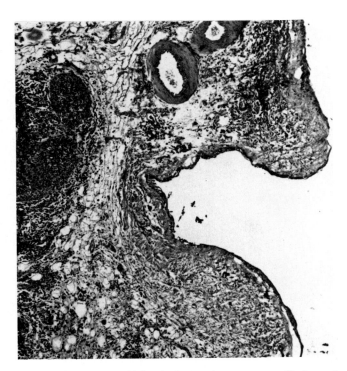

Fig. 8-5 Thymic cyst. Lining is flattened squamous epithelium of nondescript type. Nature of cyst is made evident by presence of thymic lobules in wall (left upper corner).

Autopsy studies are hampered by the fact that atrophic changes caused by superimposed infections and wasting complicate the microscopic picture. Thymic biopsies have been performed in some of these patients, and attempts at morphologic classification and correlations with the immunologic status have begun. The most important task is to distinguish atrophic secondary changes from primary "dysplastic" abnormalities.[56] In simple atrophy, there is prominent lymphocytic depletion, but the lobular architecture is preserved and Hassall's corpuscles can be identified. In the better-defined form of dysplasia, cortico-medullary differentiation is absent, the epithelial cells have an oval to spindle shape, there is formation of primitive tubules and rosettes without central lumina, and lymphocytes are generally lacking. Variants of dysplasia showing cortico-medullary differentiation or features similar to those of severe atrophy have been described, the whole issue being rather confusing at this point.[56]

Other non-neoplastic diseases

Ectopic thymus with an entirely normal microscopic appearance can present as a mass in the neck or pleural cavity.[68]

Ectopic tissues sometimes found in a normally located thymus include *parathyroid gland* (not surprising in view of their common embryogenesis) and *sebaceous glands*.[75]

Thymic involution is a constant feature of chronic, debilitating diseases.[69] These changes are of a secondary nature and should not be misinterpreted as evidence of a primary immune defect. In AIDS patients, thymic involution is particularly pronounced and is accompanied by effacement of

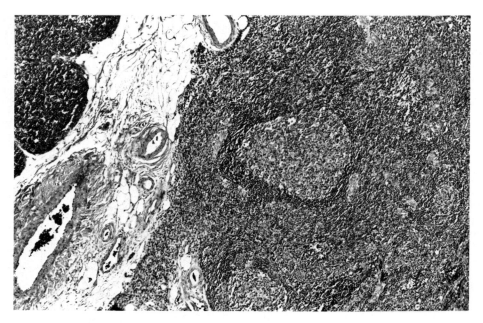

Fig. 8-6 Lymphoid hyperplasia of thymus in patient with myasthenia gravis. Large germinal centers are present through lymphoid tissue.

the cortico-medullary junction, marked lymphocytic depletion, variable degrees of plasma cell infiltration and fibrosis, and lack or paucity of Hassall's corpuscles.[64,72]

True thymic hyperplasia is defined as thymic enlargement beyond the upper limits of normal for the age (as determined by the classic Hammar's table) but accompanied by a microscopically normal gland. It has been most often described in infants or children,[58,66] but it has also been found in adults, sometimes following successful chemotherapy for malignant disease.[61]

Thymic follicular hyperplasia (often called simply thymic hyperplasia, a misleading term) is defined as the presence of lymphoid follicles in the thymus independent of the size of the gland. Actually, the weight of most of the thymuses with lymphoid hyperplasia is within normal limits.[74] These follicles are of secondary type, with germinal center formation (Fig. 8-6). Accordingly, they are largely composed of B lymphocytes, most of which contain immunoglobulins of the IgM and IgD classes.[67] According to some authors, this is accompanied by a disorderly arrangement and hypertrophy of medullary epithelial cells.[59,70]

Follicular hyperplasia is seen in about 65% of the patients with myasthenia gravis (see p. 358). It is also commonly present in patients with hyperthyroidism, Addison's disease, lupus erythematosus, and other immune-mediated diseases.[71] A few germinal centers also may be found in the apparently normal thymus, especially during infancy and childhood; therefore only their presence in a substantial number in adult patients can be viewed as a distinctly abnormal finding.

Histiocytosis X can present as a thymic mass in children,

either alone or together with involvement of other sites. The microscopic appearance is characteristic, and the overall prognosis is excellent.[73] One case has been seen in association with myasthenia gravis.[60] Granulomas containing numerous eosinophils and simulating histiocytosis X can develop in the thymic capsule as a result of diagnostic pneumomediastinum, a procedure that has been largely abandoned[62]; they are probably equivalent to the reactive eosinophilic pleuritis seen in patients with pneumothorax.[57]

Other diseases that can occasionally involve the thymus are *allergic angitis and granulomatosis* (Churg-Strauss disease)[63] and *Castleman's disease* (giant lymph node hyperplasia).[65]

Thymoma
General features

Thymoma is a term that should be restricted to neoplasms of thymic epithelial cells, independently of the presence or number of lymphocytes.[85,87,88] Seminoma, carcinoid, Hodgkin's disease, and non-Hodgkin's disease can involve the thymus; thus they can be viewed as thymic tumors but should not be regarded as variants of thymoma.

Nearly all thymomas present in adult life. Thymomas in children are exceptional; most of the cases so diagnosed actually represent lymphoblastic lymphomas of the thymus.[78] However, some well-documented cases exist, most of them occurring near the age of puberty, with an appearance and behavior equivalent to that of their adult counterpart, including an occasional association with myasthenia gravis.[76,79] Some younger children are found to have highly malignant thymic neoplasms with unusual morphologic fea-

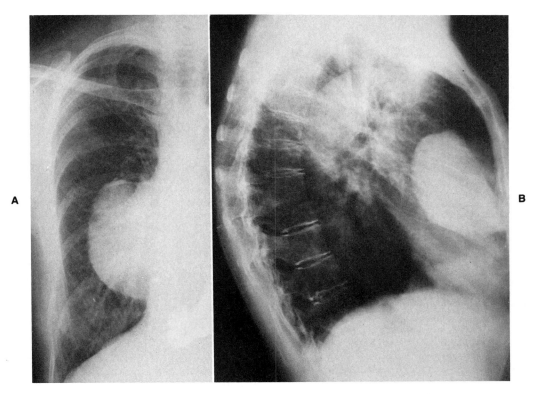

Fig. 8-7 Lobulated large benign thymoma located in anterior portion of mediastinum.

tures, the nature of which has not yet been thoroughly elucidated.[78] Familial incidence of thymoma has been recorded
only exceptionally.[90]

The usual location of thymoma is the anterosuperior mediastinum; however, it can also occur in other mediastinal
compartments (although a posterior location is very rare),
in the neck,[86,91] within the thyroid, in the pulmonary hilum,
lung parenchyma,[81,84] or in the pleura itself, coating it in a
mesothelioma-like fashion.[82]

Roentgenographically, thymoma usually results in a lobulated shadow that may be calcified (Fig. 8-7). Internal
mammary artery arteriography and thymic venography have
been used to further delineate the mass,[80] but these invasive
procedures have now been largely abandoned after the advent of CT scan and nuclear magnetic resonance techniques.[83] Fine needle aspiration has been used with success,
the diagnosis of thymoma based on the finding of a dual
population of epithelial cells and lymphocytes.[77,89]

Pathologic features

Grossly, the typical thymoma is largely or entirely solid,
yellowish gray, and separated in lobules by connective tissue
septa[100,106,110] (Fig. 8-8). In approximately 80% of the cases,
the tumor is well encapsulated and can be removed with
ease. In the remainder, infiltration of surrounding structures
is noted at surgery. Most clinically evident tumors are large,
but widespread performance of coronary by-pass surgery
recently has led to discovery of a large number of small

asymptomatic thymomas. Cystic degeneration is common,
particularly among larger tumors. Sometimes the entire tumor undergoes cystic change, many sections being needed
to identify residual diagnostic areas (Fig. 8-9).

Microscopically, nearly all thymomas are composed of a
mixture of neoplastic epithelial cells and non-neoplastic
lymphocytes, the proportion among them varying widely
from case to case and in different lobules of the same tumor
(Fig. 8-10). The epithelial cells may have a round-oval
("plump") or a spindle shape (Figs. 8-11 and 8-12). The
nuclei are vesicular and of smooth contour; the nucleolus
may be conspicuous, but unduly large eosinophilic nucleoli
should be of concern (see p. 362). The lymphocytes may
appear mature (inactive) or show varying degrees of "activation" manifested by a larger nuclear size, open chromatin
pattern, visible nucleolus, an identifiable cytoplasmic rim,
and mitotic activity; however, they should not appear convoluted or cleaved. Thymomas with a sizable component of
epithelial cells often show one or more features suggestive of
organoid differentiation. These include perivascular spaces
containing lymphocytes, proteinaceous fluid, red blood
cells, foamy macrophages, or fibrous tissue; rosettes without
central lumina; gland-like formations within the tumor or,
more often, in the tumor capsule; true glandular structures
(an exceptional event); and whorls suggestive of abortive
Hassall's corpuscle formation[105,106,109] (Fig. 8-13). Well-
formed Hassall's corpuscles are occasionally found within
thymomas, but their presence in large numbers is usually

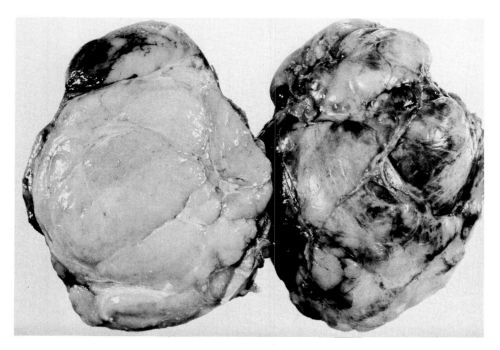

Fig. 8-8 Large lobulated thymoma showing encapsulation, no necrosis, and connective tissue trabeculae.

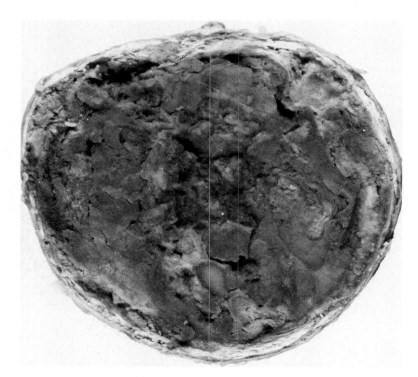

Fig. 8-9 Thymoma with extensive cystic degeneration. Only one of many microscopic sections showed residual neoplasm. Confusion with thymic cyst is likely in this case.

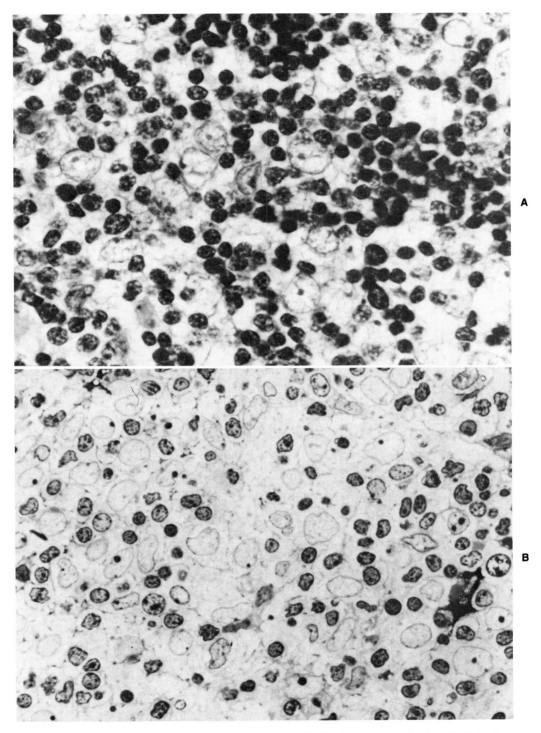

Fig. 8-10 Typical microscopic appearance of thymoma. Distinction between neoplastic epithelial cells and accompanying lymphocytes is evident both in paraffin-embedded, hematoxylin-eosin section, **A,** and in epoxy-embedded, toluidine blue–stained material, **B.**

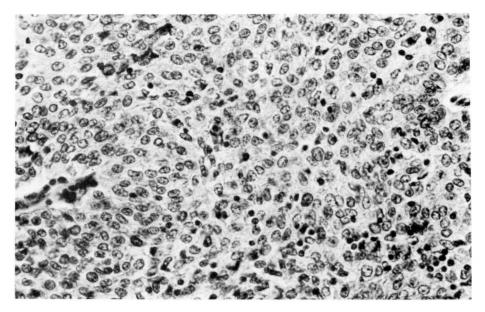

Fig. 8-11 Thymoma in patient with myasthenia gravis. Note plump appearance of epithelial cells.

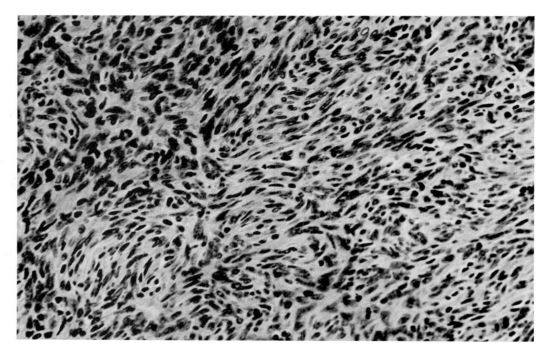

Fig. 8-12 Light microscopic appearance of thymoma composed of spindle cells. Large masses of spindle tumor cells alternate with occasional lymphocytes.

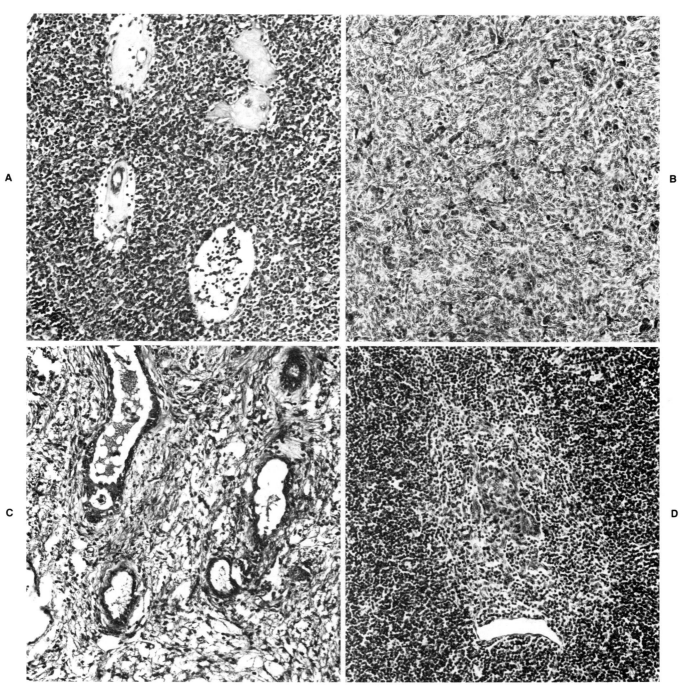

Fig. 8-13 Various architectural features of thymoma. **A,** Perivascular spaces. Some of the spaces contain lymphocytes, whereas others are hyalinized. **B,** Rosette-like formations in thymoma. These structures are formed by cytoplasm and cytoplasmic prolongations of tumor cells and lack a central lumen. **C,** Gland-like formations in thymoma. Lining of these structures is made up of neoplastic epithelial cells. **D,** Abortive Hassall's corpuscle in center of area of medullary differentiation.

an indication of pre-existing structures surrounded by a tumor and is actually more common in other neoplasms (such as malignant lymphoma) than in thymoma. Presence of rosettes with well-defined lumina should suggest a diagnosis of thymic carcinoid rather than thymoma. In thymomas with great lymphocyte predominance, it is common to find round, lighter foci of medullary differentiation, an important clue to the diagnosis. Other helpful diagnostic features of this variant of thymoma are the thick, often calcified fibrous capsule, the lobular arrangement induced by these fibrous bands, the sharp interphase between tumor lobules and fibrous tracts, and the angular shape of some of the lobules. Vascularization may be prominent and may result in a mistaken diagnosis of hemangiopericytoma. Microcystic and pseudopapillary formations may be focally prominent.

By electron microscopy, the neoplastic epithelial cells exhibit branching tonofilaments, complex desmosomes, elongated cell processes, and basal lamina[101,102,115] (Fig. 8-14). These characteristics are very useful in the differential diagnosis of thymoma from other anterior mediastinal tumors, such as thymic carcinoid, malignant lymphoma, seminoma, and fibrous mesothelioma[102] (Fig. 8-15; Table 8-1).

Immunohistochemically, the epithelial cells of thymoma exhibit reactivity for keratin[92,103,114] (Color plate 2, *B*). They have also been found to react for A_2B_5 (an antibody that recognizes neuroendocrine cells),[103] anti-p19 (an antibody against the internal protein of HTLV),[103] Leu-7,[93] and CEA.[112] One group has also claimed to detect reactivity for

the thymic hormones thymulin and thymosin $\alpha 1$, a finding that if confirmed would represent a most specific marker for this neoplasm.[113]

The lymphocytes of thymoma are of T-cell derivation (except for those located in follicles of patients with myasthenia gravis). Most of these T lymphocytes do not have the enzymatic and immunohistochemical phenotype of mature (peripheral) T-cells, but rather of immature thymocytes.[98,107,117] They are also positive for Ki67, a monoclonal antibody that reacts with cells in the proliferative phase of the cell cycle.[94] A remarkable correlation has been found between the morphologic features of the tumor and the phenotype of the lymphocyte. In lymphocyte-rich areas, the lymphocytes have the features of cortical (very immature) thymocytes; in areas of medullary differentiation they acquire features of medullary (less immature) thymocytes; and in predominantly epithelial tumors there is a preponderance of T lymphocytes of peripheral (mature) type[95,98,111] (Figs. 8-16 and 8-17). It should be pointed out that since both the lymphocytes of thymoma and those of lymphoblastic lymphoma usually exhibit an immature T phenotype, cell marker studies cannot be used to separate these two disorders. Instead, it has been shown that the lymphocytes of thymoma do not show evidence of rearrangement of the T-cell receptor gene.[96a] This finding not only provides another criterion for distinguishing the two entities but also offers further evidence for the non-neoplastic nature of the lymphocytes of thymoma.

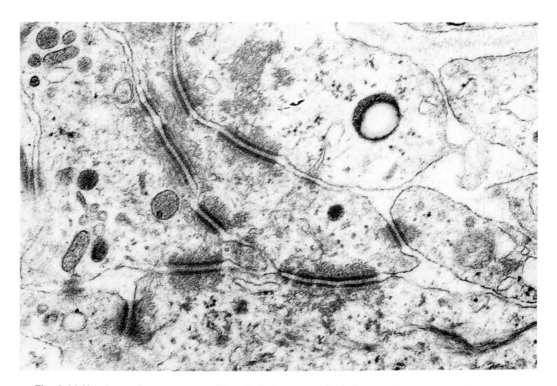

Fig. 8-14 Numerous desmosomes and tonofibrils in tumor cells indicate epithelial origin of thymoma composed of spindle cells. (Uranyl acetate–lead citrate; ×54,500; from Levine G.D., Bensch KG: Epithelial nature of spindle cell thymoma. An ultrastructural study. Cancer **30**:500-511, 1972.)

Table 8-1 Differential features of tumors of the anterior mediastinum*

Features	Thymoma*	Large cell lymphoma	Lymphoblastic lymphoma	Thymic Hodgkin's disease	Thymic seminoma	Thymic carcinoid
Patterns (low-power observation)	Sharply defined, angular lobules Fibrous bands and capsule Mottling and trabeculation (caused by epithelial-lymphocyte admixture)	Diffuse growth Variable fibrosis with occasional compartmentalizing sclerotic pattern Residual cystic thymus	Diffuse growth or pseudonodular pattern (both in lymph nodes and in thymus)	Extensive fibrosis with rounded lobules of tumor Prominent cysts seen at low power	Subdivided by fine fibrous trabeculae into variable-sized compartments	Ribbons, festoons, punctate calcified necrosis producing discrete and rounded masses of tumor
Nuclei	Often fine chromatin contrasting with well-defined nuclear membrane Usually inconspicuous nucleoli; great variation, including spindle shape Epithelial mitoses usually rare	Vesicular with prominent nucleoli Marked folding of nuclei ("cloverleaf") Variable chromatin pattern Mitotic figures variable (usually readily found)	Even chromatin ("dusky" at low power) Scant inconspicuous nucleoli Numerous mitotic figures	Cytologic features—those of nodular sclerosing Hodgkin's disease complicated by admixture with thymic epithelium and cysts	Coarse chromatin, marked prominence of nucleoli, variable numbers of mitotic figures	Rounded nuclei with sharp stippling of chromatin Variable number of mitotic figures (note spindle cell variant)
Cytoplasm	Great variation from scant to squamoid to squamous Intracytoplasmic cysts (emperipolesis) Gland-like spaces	Variable, occasionally abundant and rich in RNA (methyl green–pyronine positive)	Scant	Lacunar cells often prominent	Marked retraction of cytoplasm; often glycogen rich	Polyhedral cells with finely granular eosinophilic cytoplasm True gland formation
Associated features	Germinal centers in surrounding thymus (in cases of myasthenia gravis) Incorporation of non-neoplastic thymus (13%)	Residual lymphocytes often form tight perivascular cuffs Necrosis frequent Markedly invasive	Residual Hassall's corpuscles		Germinal centers, epithelioid and giant cells	
Electron microscopy	Well-formed desmosomes Bundles of tonofilaments	Nuclear blebs Absence of epithelial features	Nuclear blebs Fine chromatin Absence of epithelial features	Absence of epithelial characteristics in Reed-Sternberg cells	Even chromatin Prominent nucleoli Glycogen-rich Scant desmosomes Only rare tonofilaments	Dense-core granules Desmosomes inconspicuous or poorly formed Tonofilaments only rarely prominent

Slightly modified from Levine GD, Rosai J: Thymic hyperplasia and neoplasia. A review of current concepts. Hum Pathol 9:495-515, 1978.
*Nuclear and cytoplasmic features refer only to epithelium.

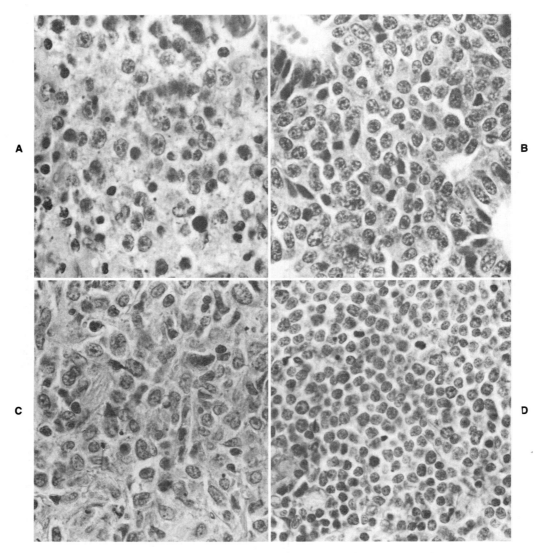

Fig. 8-15 Cytologic comparison of four types of malignant mediastinal tumor of thymic region. **A,** Seminoma. **B,** Thymic carcinoid. **C,** Large cell lymphoma. **D,** Lymphoblastic lymphoma.

In addition to epithelial cells and lymphocytes, thymomas often contain an important population of S-100 protein-positive cells, presumably non-neoplastic and of interdigitating reticulum cell nature.[97,99]

Many classifications of thymoma have been proposed over the years. We have found the division of thymomas into epithelial, lymphoepithelial, lymphocytic, spindle cell, rosette-forming, and other types to be conceptually incorrect and also difficult to use in practice because of the many transitions and admixtures that exist in this neoplasm.[96,109] Recently, proposals for newer classifications have been made based on the phenotypes of the epithelial cells as determined by a battery of monoclonal antibodies.[103,104,114] We view these proposals as premature, not only because the immunotypes of the normal thymic epithelial cells are still poorly defined but also because thymomas are likely to show heterogeneity for these markers.[116]

We prefer to diagnose our cases simply as thymomas and to list the features that may be of importance for the purposes of clinicopathologic correlation and prognosis, according to the following scheme[108]:

1 Shape of epithelial cells: round-oval ("plump"), spindle, or a mixture of the two
2 Number of lymphocytes: few, moderate, or many
3 Ancillary features: perivascular spaces, rosettes, gland-like spaces, Hassall's corpuscles, etc.
4 Staging/grading (see also p. 365)
   a Benign (encapsulated)
   b Malignant, type I (invasive); specify degree and type of invasion
   c Malignant, type II (thymic carcinoma); specify type

Myasthenia gravis

A definite relationship exists between thymic abnormalities and myasthenia gravis, although the precise nature of this association is still unclear.[130,135] In patients with my-

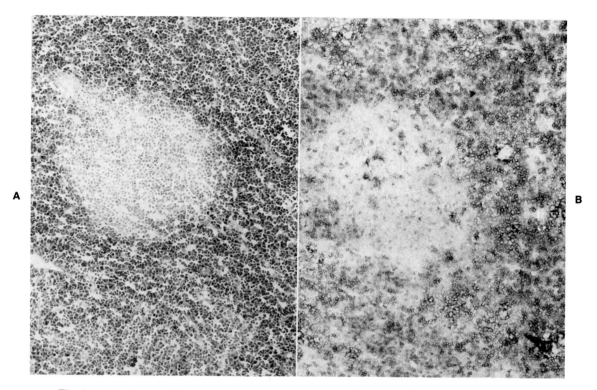

Fig. 8-16 Lymphocyte-rich thymoma with area of medullary differentiation in center. Lymphocytes in outer portion, morphologically resembling normal thymic cortex, stain for markers of cortical thymocytes, such as TdT **(A)** and OKT6 **(B).**

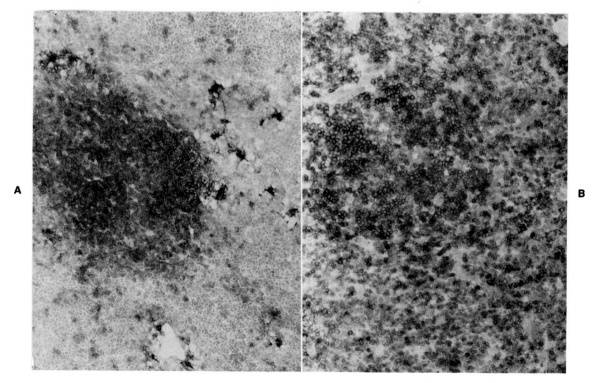

Fig. 8-17 Same cells as Fig. 8-16. Lymphocytes within central area of medullary differentiation stain for markers of medullary thymocytes, such as A1G3 **(A)** and OKT3 **(B).** (From Mokhtar N, Hsu S-M, Ladd RP, Haynes BF, Jaffe ES: Thymoma. Lymphoid and epithelial components mirror the phenotype of normal thymus. Hum Pathol **15:**378-384, 1984.)

asthenia gravis, the thymus will show follicular hyperplasia (see p. 350) as the only abnormality in about 65% of the cases, a thymoma (with or without follicular hyperplasia in the non-neoplastic portion) in 10%, and no gross or microscopic abnormalities in 25%.[145] Viewed from another angle, this relationship is shown by the fact that about 30% to 45% of patients with thymoma develop myasthenia.[129,143] The tumor may be diagnosed during the investigation of a myasthenic patient, or the myasthenia may develop months or years after the tumor has been excised[119,134]; a patient with myasthenia is more likely to have a thymoma if the person is a male and/or develops symptoms after the age of 50.[131] The incidence of malignancy in these tumors seems to be similar than among those unassociated with myasthenic symptoms.[120,132,140] Thymomas associated with myasthenia gravis almost always have epithelial cells of "plump" shape (although the reverse is not necessarily true) (see Fig. 8-11). The relative proportion of epithelial cells and lymphocytes does not correlate with the presence of myasthenia. No consistent ultrastructural or immunohistochemical differences have been found between myasthenic and non-myasthenic thymomas.[146] Actually, the best and simplest way to predict the presence of myasthenia in a patient with thymoma is to find lymphoid follicles in the adjacent thymic tissue or, exceptionally, even in the thymoma itself.[118]

In the not too distant past, the presence of myasthenia in a patient with thymoma had a profound influence on survival. Thus in a large series reported by Wilkins et al.,[145] the 10-year cumulative survival rate for patients with thymoma without myasthenia gravis was 67% and in those with thymoma with myasthenia gravis it was 32%. Most of the deaths in the latter group resulted from myasthenic crisis. As a result of marked improvements in the medical treatment of myasthenia, this is no longer the case.[124] As a matter of fact, the presence or absence of myasthenia in recent series of patients with thymomas shows that this association is no longer of prognostic significance.

The pathogenesis of myasthenia gravis has been found to be related to a defect in the acetylcholine receptor molecule in the subsynaptic membrane of the neuromuscular junction, probably as a result of circulating antibodies directed against this molecule.[122,123,127,141] Patients with thymomas and myasthenia have other autoantibodies to striated muscle antigens that also react with the thymoma cells.[126] Furthermore, a material similar to the acetylcholine receptor seems to be present in the thymus.[127b,138] Finally, the normal thymus contains striated muscle cells ("myoid cells") and other cells containing myoglobin, desmin, and other muscle antigens.[121,128] These findings suggest that the autosensitization may be initiated in the thymus.[142] The immune-mediated nature of myasthenia is also manifested by the fact that 12% of these patients have other autoimmune diseases, such as Graves' disease and rheumatoid arthritis.[133] Another most peculiar association is between myasthenia and generalized hair follicle hamartoma of the skin.[144]

Myasthenia gravis should be distinguished from the Lambert-Eaton syndrome, a clinically somewhat similar condition that is frequently associated with pulmonary small cell carcinoma and also immune-related.[127a]

The treatment of myasthenia includes a thymectomy. This indication also applies to cases that began in childhood[147] and probably also those with only ocular symptoms.[139] In the absence of a sizable tumor, the operation can usually be carried out through a transcervical route. Symptomatic improvement is more likely if the thymus is the site of follicular hyperplasia than if it is normal or involved by thymoma.[137] The long-term results of the operation are somewhat related to the duration and severity of the myasthenic symptoms but not to the age of the patient; however, substantial differences in this regard exist among the various published series.[125,130,131,137] Persistence of symptoms has been attributed to residual thymic tissue with lymphoid hyperplasia.[136]

Other associated diseases

In addition to myasthenia gravis, thymoma has been found to be associated with a large number of systemic disorders, nearly all of which are immune-mediated. These include hypogammaglobulinemia (12% of the cases), erythroid hypoplasia (5%),[149] and, more rarely, white blood cell aplasia,[147a] myositis, myocarditis, dermatomyositis, lupus erythematosus, rheumatoid arthritis, scleroderma, Sjögren's disease, multiple myeloma, subacute motor neuronopathy,[155] inappropriate antidiuretic hormone secretion,[151] bullous dermatoses, hyperglobulinemic purpura, mucocutaneous candidiasis,[150,152] peripheral T-cell lymphocytosis,[148] and T-cell chronic lymphocytic leukemia.[156] In addition, it has been claimed that patients with thymoma have an increased incidence of malignant tumors, including lymphoma.[153,154] Most of the thymomas associated with hypogammaglobulinemia or erythroid hyperplasia are composed of spindle-shaped epithelial cells, in sharp contrast to those linked with myasthenia gravis.

Ectopic hamartomatous variant

This is a distinct type of thymic lesion that occurs in the lower neck of young patients and seems to share features of hamartoma and benign neoplasia.[157] Most of the mass is made up of epithelial cells that are so spindle shaped that they easily cause a misdiagnosis of the lesion as of mesenchymal or peripheral nerve nature. The other component is represented by solid squamous nests and epithelial-lined cysts. The behavior is perfectly benign. We have not seen examples of this entity within the mediastinum.

Malignant thymoma

About 70% to 80% of all thymomas with the microscopic features previously described are totally encapsulated and classified as benign. The remainder represent the group of malignant lymphoma. These have been further divided into two categories, allowing for the existence of transitional forms.

Type I malignant thymoma, which is by far the most common, is composed of tumors with all the clinical, morphologic, and cytologic attributes of thymoma as already described (including their association with a variety of systemic disorders) but which exhibit aggressiveness in the form of local invasion, pleural or pericardial implants, or distant metastases[158] (Figs. 8-18 and 8-19). The latter event

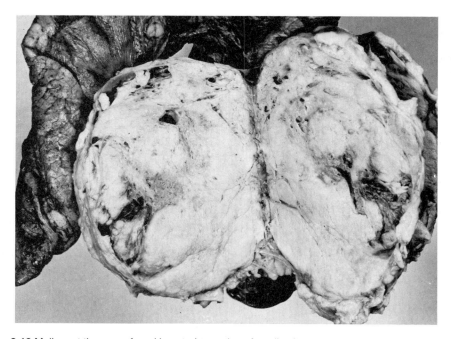

Fig. 8-18 Malignant thymoma found in anterior portion of mediastinum at autopsy. There was invasion of surrounding structures but no distant metastases.

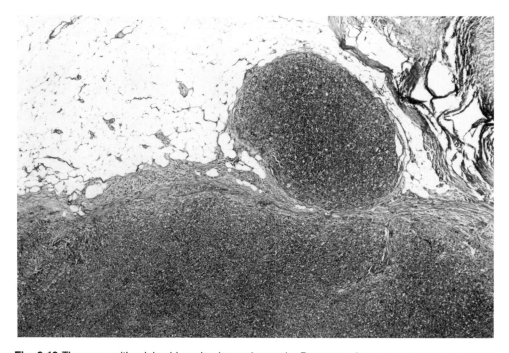

Fig. 8-19 Thymoma with minimal invasion beyond capsule. Presence of tumor nests growing in mediastinal fat outside capsule is a sign of invasiveness and indication for postoperative radiation therapy.

is exceptional but has been fully documented; the most common sites of involvement are mediastinal and cervical lymph nodes, lungs, liver, and bone (particularly spine).[159,163] We have seen a case in which a supraclavicular node metastasis was the first manifestation of the disease. The locally invasive features may be obvious to the surgeon at the time of the thoracotomy or may become apparent only on pathologic examination. These tumors, which some authors prefer to designate as *invasive thymomas*, cannot be confidently distinguished from the benign encapsulated types on cytologic or architectural grounds. As a group they tend to be predominantly epithelial; most of these epithelial cells are of round-oval ("plump") shape; their nuclei are perhaps larger and their nucleoli more prominent than in benign thymoma[163,165a] (Fig. 8-20). However, numerous exceptions occur,[171] and therefore the diagnosis of malignancy should be largely based on the documentation of invasion.[161] Thus sampling becomes of great importance. Complete capsular breaks, tumor islands in the mediastinal fat, or presence of large nerves surrounded by tumor are evidence of invasiveness and therefore of clinical malignancy. The suggestion has recently been made that the expression of *ras* p21 protein is increased in malignant thymomas.[164a]

Type II malignant thymoma is identified as such on cytoarchitectural grounds, although it also exhibits as a rule clearcut invasive features. Some authors prefer to designate this tumor type as *thymic carcinoma*.[172] As a group, these lesions lack the organoid features of benign or type I ma-

lignant thymomas (such as perivascular spaces) and are never associated with myasthenia gravis or other systemic manifestations. Although very rare, they display a wide variety of morphologic patterns, which are listed below. The first two comprise over 90% of the cases.[162]

Squamous cell carcinoma. This is a form of malignant thymoma rich in atypical epithelial cells, many of which undergo keratinization[167] (Fig. 8-21). The appearance is indistinguishable from that of squamous cell carcinoma in other sites; however, the lobular pattern of growth is generally maintained and the tumor lobules are, if anything, even more widely separated from each other by fibrous bands than in the benign tumors. Before making a diagnosis of primary squamous cell carcinoma of the thymus, the alternative possibility of metastatic carcinoma (particularly from the lung) should always be considered.

Lymphoepithelioma-like carcinoma. As the name implies, this tumor has a microscopic appearance that is essentially identical to that of so-called lymphoepithelioma of the tonsil and nasopharynx. Large, deeply acidophilic nucleoli that are sharply outlined and perfectly round are the hallmark of the tumor cells of this neoplasm (Fig. 8-22). Keratinization and intercellular bridges are absent; however, the tumor cells are consistently immunoreactive for keratin. The lymphocytes of this tumor have the phenotype of mature peripheral T-cells rather than the immature thymocytic phenotype seen in ordinary lymphoma.[166] The finding of the Epstein-Barr virus (EBV) genome in one case of this entity suggests that the similarity with nasopharyngeal carcinoma may be more than morphologic.[164]

Sarcomatoid carcinoma (carcinosarcoma). This cytologically malignant tumor simulates a mesenchymal neoplasm by virtue of its diffuse pattern of growth and the prominent spindling of tumor cells. The diagnosis is made by finding, somewhere in the tumor, foci of epithelial appearance.[168] The sarcoma-like areas may include foci of cartilaginous and skeletal muscle differentiation (Fig. 8-23). We have seen one such case that superimposed itself upon a long-standing benign thymoma (Fig. 8-24). Skeletal muscle differentiation has also been described in benign thymomas.[160,165] The differential diagnosis includes germ cell tumors and malignant schwannoma ("triton tumor").

Clear cell carcinoma. In this rare variant, the presence of large amounts of glycogen-rich, clear cytoplasm in the tumor cells results in a striking resemblance with renal cell carcinoma.[168,169,173]

Basaloid carcinoma. This tumor is formed by well-defined epithelial islands with prominent peripheral palisading. It may present as a mural nodule in what otherwise looks like a squamous-lined thymic cyst.[168]

Mucoepidermoid carcinoma. Areas of squamous and mucin-producing glandular differentiation alternate in this neoplasm. Some of the mucin may become extracellular and elicit an inflammatory reaction.[168,170]

Small cell carcinoma and small cell–squamous cell carcinoma. These are discussed on p. 365.

• • •

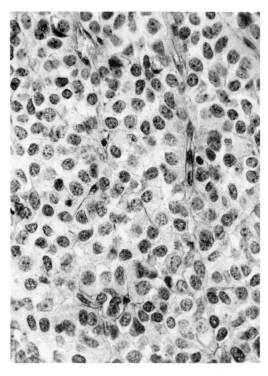

Fig. 8-20 Malignant thymoma. Tumor appears well differentiated, yet tumor implants and blood vessel invasion were present.

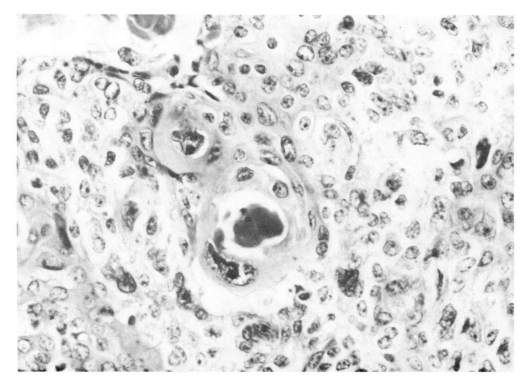

Fig. 8-21 Squamous cell carcinoma of thymus. Keratinizing pearls composed of highly atypical cells are present.

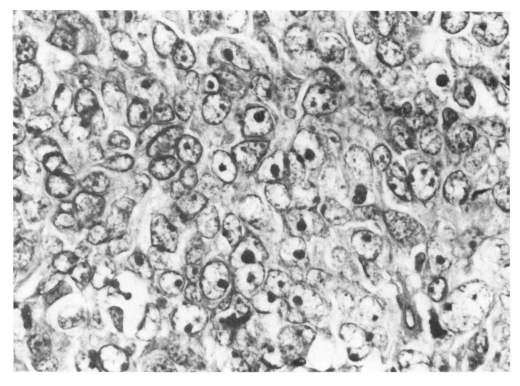

Fig. 8-22 Malignant thymoma with lymphoepithelioma-like pattern. Note extremely prominent nucleoli and large vesicular nuclei.

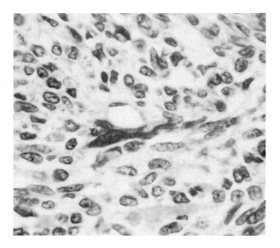

Fig. 8-23 Sarcomatoid carcinoma of thymus. Focal rhabdomyosarcomatous differentiation is demonstrated by presence of myoglobin with immunoperoxidase technique. Cross striations were demonstrated by light and electron microscopy.

These morphologic varieties have in common a clearcut epithelial look, a fact of importance in the differential diagnosis. If an obviously malignant mediastinal tumor lacks such an appearance, the chances are high that it does not represent a thymoma.

As a group, type II malignant thymomas are very aggressive neoplasms. Local invasion is the rule and distant metastases are common.[172] This does not seem to apply to the few reported mucoepidermoid and basaloid carcinomas, the outlook of which has been rather favorable.

Treatment and prognosis

The primary treatment of thymoma is surgical excision. For the entirely encapsulated thymomas that have been removed *in toto*, no additional therapy is necessary; however, if there is any question about the possibility of having left some tumor behind, postoperative radiation therapy should be considered.

For the type I malignant thymomas associated with gross invasion or implants, excision should be supplemented with radiation therapy.[178] There is not enough information in the literature to know for certain whether post-operative radiation therapy is also needed in those thymomas that exhibit

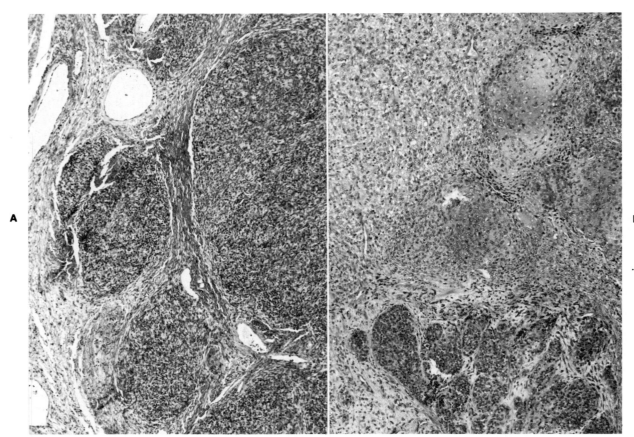

Fig. 8-24 Sarcomatoid thymoma with areas of cartilaginous differentiation arising on pre-existing benign thymoma. **A** represents the benign component and **B** the highly malignant neoplasm.

only minimal invasion, but our bias has been to recommend it. When distant metastases are present, chemotherapy has been added; combination regimes containing cis-platinum have shown the best results.[174]

Type II malignant thymomas of squamous or lympho-epithelioma-like type are treated with surgery plus radiation therapy, with chemotherapy added in cases of massive local disease or distant spread.

The prognosis of benign (encapsulated) thymoma following surgical excision is excellent, regardless of the shape of the epithelial cells and the relative number of lymphocytes. Recurrence will supervene in only about 2% of the cases, either as a solitary mediastinal mass or pleural implants.[175] As already indicated, presence or absence of myasthenic symptoms has lost much of its prognostic significance.[176,179]

The prognosis of type I malignant thymomas greatly depends on the completeness of the original excision.[176,179] In most series, it has also been found to correlate with the degree of invasiveness, a fact that has been used to propose various staging systems for this tumor.[177,179] According to this scheme, the prognosis of minimally invasive (stage I) thymomas is not significantly different from that of encapsulated tumors, but it drops markedly for the tumors showing gross invasion or implants and even more for the few cases associated with distant metastases.[177]

The prognosis of type II malignant thymomas is poor.[176,180] In the series of Wick et al.,[180] sixteen of their twenty patients died of tumor, all of them within 5 years of the initial diagnosis.

Carcinoid tumor and oat cell carcinoma

Carcinoid tumor of the thymus is a distinct clinicopathologic entity that for many years has been confused with true thymoma. It is composed of thymic neuroendocrine cells, and its morphologic appearance and natural history are similar to those of carcinoid tumors elsewhere, particularly those of foregut derivation. It is a malignant tumor that often invades locally and metastasizes distantly, sometimes after a long interval; in one series, the incidence of distant metastases was 73%.[194] Well-circumscribed tumors, however, are often cured by local excision.[188] Thymic carcinoid usually lacks endocrine manifestations, and we have yet to see a case accompanied by the carcinoid syndrome; however, it is associated in one third of the cases with Cushing's syndrome and other distant manifestations[190,194]; we believe that all of the reported cases of thymomas associated with Cushing's syndrome are, in reality, examples of thymic carcinoids.[191]

Thymic carcinoid can be associated with carcinoid tumor of other sites, such as bronchus or ileum. It can also occur as a component of multiple endocrine adenomatosis (MEA) type I or IIa[189,190] or *formes frustes* of these syndromes.[193] In these patients and in those with Cushing's syndrome, the tumor runs a more aggressive clinical course.[189]

Grossly, thymic carcinoid is solid, usually well-circumscribed but not encapsulated, and lacks the distinct lobulations of thymoma.

Microscopically, the typical thymic carcinoid tumor ex-

hibits ribbon and festoon formation, rosette-like glands with central lumina, "balls" of cells with central necrosis and calcification, marked vascularization, and frequent lymphatic and blood vessel invasion (Fig. 8-25). Lymphocytes, perivascular spaces, and other features of thymoma are absent. The tumor cells have a more granular cytoplasm than those of thymoma, the nuclear chromatin is slightly coarser, and mitotic activity is frequent. In this regard, it should be noted that if one were to apply to thymic carcinoids the criteria currently used for the homonymous bronchial lesion, most of them would fall into the category of *atypical* carcinoid tumor. This probably explains the fact that as a group, thymic carcinoid is a more aggressive neoplasm than bronchial carcinoid, in which the atypical form represents a small minority.

Special techniques are very useful for confirmation of a diagnosis of thymic carcinoid. Some of the tumor cells are argyrophilic, although not argentaffin. Electron microscopy shows short interdigitating cell processes, focal basal lamina, scanty junctional processes, and practically no complex desmosomes or tonofilaments. The cytoplasm contains dense-core granules and sometimes perinuclear whorls of microfilaments[182,190,196] (Fig. 8-26). Immunohistochemically, there is reactivity for keratin, neuron-specific enolase, chromogranin, and other general endocrine markers. In addition, the tumors associated with Cushing's syndrome show positivity for ACTH. Other substances detected in this tumor include serotonin, somatostatin, cholecystokinin, neurotensin, and met-enkephalin.[181,183,187,196]

Morphologic variants of thymic carcinoid tumor include lesions with a spindle-cell pattern[186] and with melanin.[184,185] There are also tumors containing amyloid and calcitonin, and therefore closely related to medullary thyroid carcinoma.[190] Finally, there is a thymic neoplasm with morphologic features identical to those of pulmonary *small cell (oat cell) carcinoma.*[190,195] The decision of whether to place this tumor in the family of neuroendocrine carcinomas alongside carcinoid tumor or to regard it as an undifferentiated type of thymic carcinoma presents the same conceptual difficulties as it does in the lung. A further analogy between the two sites is represented by the thymic tumors formed by an admixture of *small cell and squamous cell carcinoma.*[192]

At a practical level, it is important to emphasize that the diagnosis of primary small cell carcinoma of the thymus can only be entertained once the more likely possibility of a mediastinal metastasis from a pulmonary small cell carcinoma has been ruled out.

Thymolipoma and other stromal tumors

Thymolipoma is an encapsulated benign thymic lesion that can attain a huge size and can simulate radiographically cardiomegaly or pulmonary sequestration. The large majority of the cases are asymptomatic, but isolated instances of association with myasthenia gravis, aplastic anemia, and Graves' disease are on record.[198] Grossly, the lesion has the appearance of a lipoma except for the focal presence of whitish solid areas. Microscopically, there is an admixture in various proportions of mature adipose tissue and unremarkable thymic tissue. The amount of the latter is well in

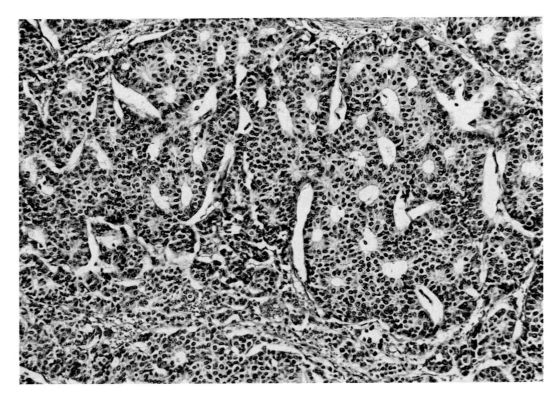

Fig. 8-25 Carcinoid tumor of thymus. Tumor cells of uniform appearance and predominantly solid pattern of growth form regularly distributed rosettes.

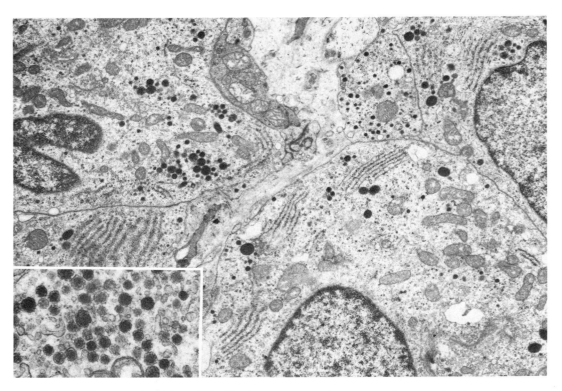

Fig. 8-26 Thymic carcinoid characterized by dense-core secretory granules that separate this neoplasm from other thymic tumors. These cells also have prominent rough endoplasmic reticulum, Golgi apparatus, and scattered mitochondria. **Inset,** Note uniform, membrane-bound, dense-core granules with peripheral halo. (×7,450; **inset** ×25,270.)

excess of that normally expected for the patient's age.

We have seen two examples of **thymic liposarcoma**, which could perhaps be interpreted as the malignant counterpart of thymolipoma.[197] A case of **osteosarcoma**, presumably arising in an ectopic hamartomatous thymus, has been described.[199]

GERM CELL TUMORS

Germ cell tumors account for approximately 20% of the mediastinal tumors and cysts. Their histogenesis, like that of extragonadal germ cell tumors in general, remains obscure, although origin from misplaced germ cells is presently favored.[203] This theory has received strong support from the anatomic demonstration of a widespread pathway of germ cell migration during embryogenesis. Germ cell neoplasms are often seen in close anatomic relation with the thymus and may actually be found totally within this organ; however, they have no histogenetic relationship with true thymoma and should not be labeled as such. The possibility of any mediastinal germ cell tumor representing a metastasis from a testicular or ovarian primary lesion should always be investigated, although in the presence of a single upper mediastinal tumor with negative retroperitoneal lymphangiogram the chances of this being the case are remote.[221,224]

Some cases of mediastinal germ cell tumors have occurred in association with Klinefelter's syndrome; it has been estimated that the incidence of this syndrome among patients with mediastinal germ cell neoplasms is thirty to forty times

that seen in the general population.[212,219] Another interesting association is that between mediastinal germ cell tumors and hematologic malignancies.[204,214]

A definite relationship exists between the patient's sex and the incidence of the various mediastinal germ cell tumors. Seminoma (germinoma), for all practical purposes, affects only males; we have yet to see a convincing case in a female. Embryonal carcinoma, endodermal sinus tumor, teratocarcinoma, and choriocarcinoma show a great male predilection, but unquestionable cases in females have been reported.[206,223] Mature cystic teratoma affects both sexes equally.

Seminoma (germinoma) of the mediastinum arises almost always within the thymus but—as already stated—should be regarded as a germ cell tumor rather than a true thymoma (Fig. 8-27). The microscopic appearance is identical to that of its testicular counterpart (Fig. 8-28). Some of the tumors show a degree of atypicality and mitotic activity that places them in the category of *anaplastic seminoma,* but it is not clear whether this carries any prognostic significance. The differential diagnosis includes thymoma and large cell lymphoma. Presence of fibrous septa infiltrated by lymphocytes and plasma cells, epithelioid granulomas, numerous germinal centers, large amounts of cytoplasmic glycogen, and presence of an irregular, skein-like nucleolus favor a diagnosis of seminoma. The diagnosis may be obscured by the presence of a very prominent granulomatous reaction, reactive follicular hyperplasia, epithelial-lined cystic formations of thymic origin, and fibrosis.[200]

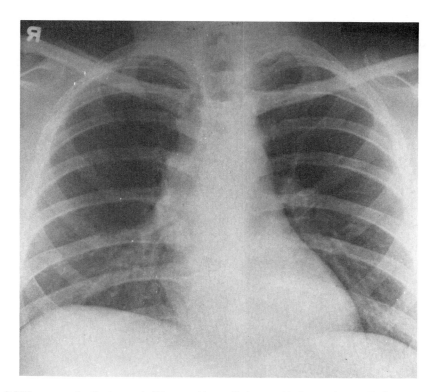

Fig. 8-27 Large mediastinal mass in 24-year-old man that proved to be seminoma. Patient was treated by irradiation and has survived over 10 years.

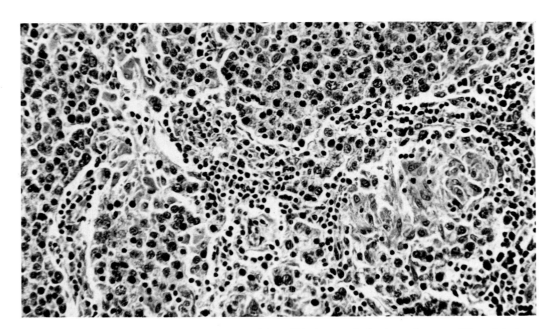

Fig. 8-28 Primary seminoma of mediastinum arising within thymus. Collections of large undifferentiated cells are separated by fibrous strands containing numerous lymphocytes and epithelioid cell granulomas.

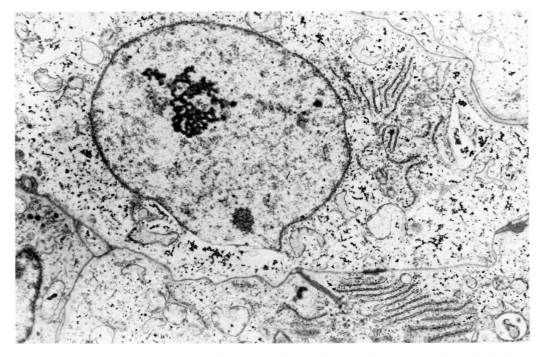

Fig. 8-29 Ultrastructural appearance of tumor cells in seminoma of thymus. (Uranyl acetate–lead citrate; ×8,800; from Levine GD: Primary thymic seminoma. A neoplasm ultrastructurally similar to testicular seminoma and distinct from epithelial thymoma. Cancer **31:**729-741, 1973.)

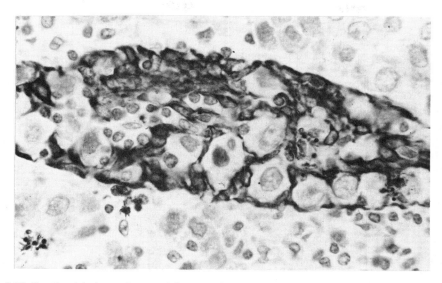

Fig. 8-30 Keratin stain in seminoma of thymus, showing island of keratin-positive thymic epithelium surrounded and invaded by keratin-negative seminoma cells.

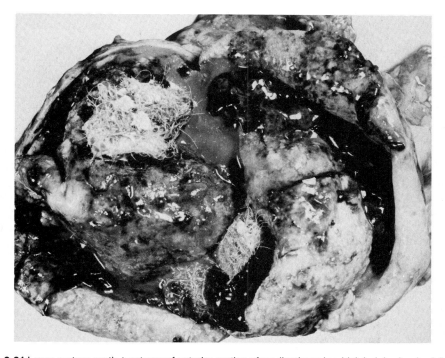

Fig. 8-31 Large mature cystic teratoma of anterior portion of mediastinum in which hair is clearly visible.

Electron microscopic and immunohistochemical evaluation can be very useful to confirm the diagnosis[216] (Fig. 8-29). Seminomas are immunoreactive for placental alkaline phosphatase and often for Leu 7, but they are negative for leukocyte antigen and usually negative for keratin. One should be careful not to misinterpret entrapped thymic epithelial cells as neoplastic elements (Fig. 8-30). The primary treatment is with radiation therapy, and the prognosis is good.[201,215,225] In the series of Shantz et al.,[225] one patient died following resection, but the sixteen with adequate follow-up were alive and well. In the series of Bush et al.[201] the 10-year actuarial survival was 69%.

Mature cystic teratoma is the most common type of mediastinal germ cell neoplasm. It usually becomes clinically apparent in early adult life. It may grow to a large size and has a distinct, sharply delineated wall that often becomes calcified. The cut surface is predominantly cystic (Fig. 8-31). Adherence to surrounding structures is common. If the sebaceous material within it escapes, a prominent xanthogranulomatous inflammatory reaction follows. Perforation into the tracheobronchial tree may occur, and the patient coughs up sebaceous oily material and hair.

The microscopic appearance resembles that of the more common mature cystic teratoma of ovary. The cysts are lined by stratified squamous epithelium and contain sebaceous glands and hair follicles (Fig. 8-32). Other common components are neural tissue, gastrointestinal tract, cartilage, and respiratory structures. Pancreatic tissue is also quite frequent[224,228]; it may be accompanied by islet cell elements and result in hypoglycemia. It has been suggested that the dense adhesions often found in this tumor may be the result of pancreatic enzyme secretion.[227]

Immature teratoma is defined, as in other sites, as a germ cell tumor similar to mature teratoma but also containing immature epithelial, mesenchymal, or neural elements without a component of embryonal carcinoma; the number of cases reported is too small to know what to expect in terms of behavior.[202] This condition should be distinguished both from teratocarcinoma and from malignant transformation of mature cystic teratoma, the latter being a very rare event.

Embryonal carcinoma is an invasive, highly necrotic neoplasm. Its microscopic appearance is, by definition, poorly differentiated. Immunohistochemically, there is often reactivity for placental alkaline phosphatase and Leu 7. It is very important for the pathologist to consider the possibility of germ cell tumor in the presence of a poorly differentiated malignant neoplasm of the mediastinum, especially if the patient is a young male, instead of automatically relegating it to the category of "undifferentiated malignant tumor"; otherwise he might be denying the patient the opportunity of remission or even cure with current chemotherapeutic regimes.[205,207,222]

Endodermal sinus tumor (yolk sac tumor) also occurs[229,230] (Fig. 8-33). The prognosis is very poor,[211] although the few tumors in this category that are found to be encapsulated have a better outlook.[220]

Teratocarcinoma, defined as the combination of embryonal carcinoma and mature teratoma and usually also containing elements of immature teratoma, comprises about 5% of all mediastinal germ cell tumors. It grows rapidly and

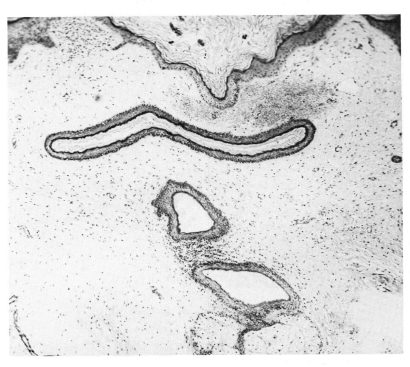

Fig. 8-32 Usual lining of mature cystic teratoma showing stratified squamous epithelium and abundant sebaceous glands.

infiltrates widely. Grossly, areas of hemorrhage and necrosis are present (Fig. 8-34). Microscopically, areas of embryonal carcinoma alternate with mature foci, with an abundance of foci of intermediate differentiation (Fig. 8-35). In some cases, a sarcomatous component of adult type is present, such as angiosarcoma or rhabdomyosarcoma.[218,231] As a rule, this component is not responsive to the chemotherapeutic regime given for germ cell tumors.

Primary *choriocarcinomas* of the mediastinum occur, for the most part, in the third decade of life.[208,226,232] They are often associated with gynecomastia and invariably accompanied by elevated serum levels of hCG. The prognosis is extremely poor. Before accepting a diagnosis of primary mediastinal choriocarcinoma, the possibility of a metastasis from an occult testicular tumor should always be investigated. That choriocarcinoma can occur as a primary lesion in the mediastinum has been demonstrated rather convincingly by serially sectioning both testes and finding no abnormalities in them.[213,217] It should be emphasized, however, that it is in choriocarcinoma, more than any other germ cell

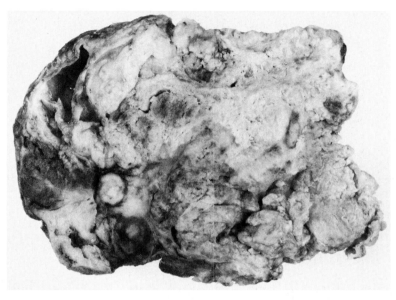

Fig. 8-33 Yolk sac tumor of mediastinum. As is often the case with this tumor, there are extensive areas of necrosis and hemorrhage. (Courtesy Dr. W. Robert Weber, Gainesville, FL.)

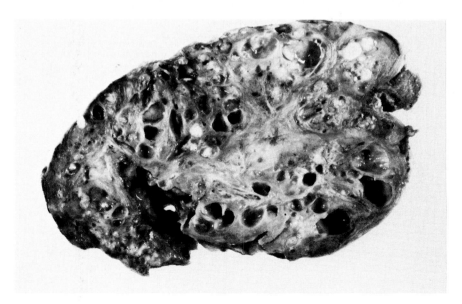

Fig. 8-34 Teratocarcinoma of mediastinum. Tumor has markedly variegated appearance with areas of cystic change, solid portions, necrosis, and hemorrhage. (Courtesy Dr. J. Costa, Lausanne, Switzerland.)

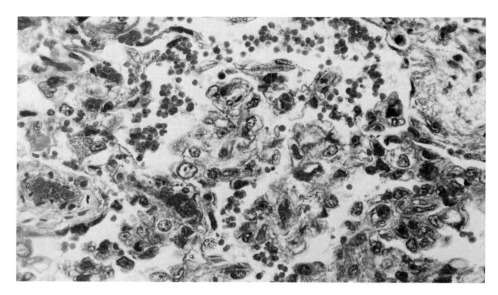

Fig. 8-35 Teratocarcinoma of mediastinum. This area has embryonal carcinoma pattern. Other foci of tumor were well differentiated.

tumor, that the possibility of an occult testicular primary lesion exists because of the tendency for this tumor type to be quite small and even burnt out at the time that the metastases develop. The case of testicular choriocarcinoma measuring only 2 mm in diameter reported by Greenwood et al.[208] is very illustrative in this regard. The distinction, however, is mainly of academic interest inasmuch as the treatment (systemic chemotherapy) and the prognosis are similar whether or not an occult testicular tumor can be identified.

Malignant nonseminomatous germ cell tumors are accompanied by serum elevation of hCG and/or AFP in about 90% of the patients, but these markers are usually negative in pure seminoma.[210]

As in other extragonadal locations and in the gonads, admixtures of various types of germ cell tumors are common. These tumors are collectively referred to as *mixed germ cell tumors*, but it is important to describe accurately the components present. One such combination is between seminomatous and nonseminomatous elements.[209]

MALIGNANT LYMPHOMA

Malignant lymphoma can present as an anterior, superior, or middle mediastinal mass, in this order of frequency.[235] It represents the most common primary neoplasm of the middle portion of the mediastinum. It may appear in this area as a manifestation of a disseminated process, or it may present as a primary mediastinal disease.[234,235] The diagnosis can be suspected on clinicoradiographic grounds, and sometimes it can be confirmed with fine needle aspiration biopsy or a small tissue biopsy obtained through a suprasternal collar incision.[233] However, in most instances a formal thoracotomy will be needed to establish a precise diagnosis.

The large majority of malignant lymphomas presenting as primary mediastinal neoplasms fall into three categories. The general features of these lymphomas are discussed in Chapter 21; only those pertaining specifically to their mediastinal location will be mentioned here.

Hodgkin's disease

Mediastinal Hodgkin's disease can involve primarily the thymus or the lymph nodes or both sites.[240] Most patients are young adults, and there is a predilection for females. The disease may present with local pressure symptoms (dyspnea, cough, chest pain) or be found incidentally in a chest x-ray examination. One case of thymic Hodgkin's disease has been seen in association with myasthenia gravis[244] and another with red cell hypoplasia.[245] Primary Hodgkin's disease of the mediastinum is nearly always of nodular sclerosis type. When affecting the nodes, its gross and microscopic appearance is similar to that seen elsewhere. When involving the thymus, it is usually sharply outlined and sometimes surrounded by a thick capsule not too dissimilar from that of a thymoma. The nodules may be multiple (a very rare event in true thymoma), and residual thymic tissue may be identified. The consistency is hard, and the cut surface is vaguely or distinctly nodular (Fig. 8-36). It is not uncommon to find within the mass variously sized cysts containing clear or grumous fluid. Occasionally, the entire lesion has a gross appearance indistinguishable from that of a benign thymic cyst.[246] This is the result of a peculiar reaction of the thymic epithelium, which is also seen in other disorders but which is undoubtedly more common in Hodgkin's disease. The low-power appearance may resemble that of true thymoma by virtue of the presence of cellular nodules encircled by fibrous bands. In thymoma, however, the interphase between the fibrous strands and the neoplastic nodules is usually sharper, and the shape of the nodules tends to be

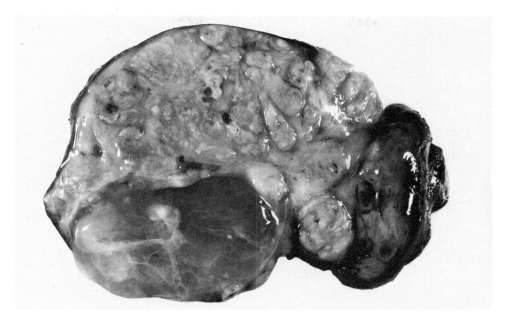

Fig. 8-36 Hodgkin's disease of nodular sclerosis type involving thymus. Area of cystic degeneration is present. (Courtesy Dr. J. Costa, Lausanne, Switzerland.)

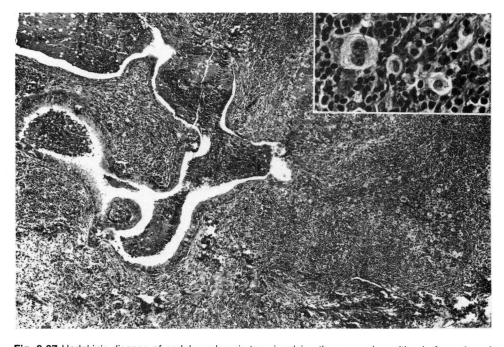

Fig. 8-37 Hodgkin's disease of nodular sclerosis type involving thymus and resulting in formation of thymic cysts lined by ciliated epithelium. **Inset** shows lacunar Reed-Sternberg cells.

angular rather than round.[243] The infiltrate tends to be polymorphic, with lymphocytes, plasma cells, eosinophils, histiocytes, and the elements that provide the diagnosis, i.e., Reed-Sternberg cells, their mononuclear variants, and lacunar cells. These are often seen in intimate association with epithelial-lined cysts, Hassall's corpuscles, and isolated thymic epithelial cells (Fig. 8-37). This feature has led in the past to a misinterpretation of the lesion as a granulomatous thymoma.[238,239,242] Immunohistochemical stains for Leu M1 and keratin will sharply delineate the lymphoid neoplastic and epithelial reactive components, respectively. Another confusing pattern results from the arrangement of these cells in compact and rather monomorphic clusters, often surrounding foci of necrosis. These foci may simulate non-Hodgkin's lymphoma, germ cell tumor, and carcinoma. Conversely, some foci—especially at the periphery—may show only a nonspecific chronic inflammatory infiltrate and fibrosis and be misdiagnosed as sclerosing mediastinitis. In some instances, the disease is accompanied by the formation of lymphoid follicles with prominent germinal centers, so that a mistaken diagnosis of Castleman's disease may result. In cases of this sort, if there is a strong radiographic suspicion of malignancy, a new biopsy should be requested from a more centrally located area. An important differential diagnostic point about the fibrosis is that in addition to wide bands, it also manifests itself as a fine network that entraps small groups of cells or even individual cells, this resulting in a blurring of the boundaries of the nodules. This is not a feature of thymoma, although it can also be seen in large cell lymphoma. The prognosis of mediastinal Hodgkin's disease is similar whether the neoplasm involves the thymus, the mediastinal lymph nodes, or both.[240] It seldom spreads subdiaphragmatically in the absence of supraclavicular lymph node involvement. Therefore routine staging laparotomy is not indicated.

The primary treatment is in the form of radiation therapy, although it may be appropriate to precede this by surgical excision if the lesion found at operation is of well-circumscribed nature.[237,247] Sometimes, administration of radiation therapy is followed by the appearance of a large epithelial-lined thymic cyst, which may simulate radiographically tumor relapse.[236,241]

Lymphoblastic lymphoma

Lymphoblastic (convoluted cell) lymphoma has a particular predilection for the thymic region. It is usually of T-cell type, but a certain degree of phenotypic heterogeneity occurs.[249] Its typical presentation is in the form of acute respiratory distress in an adolescent, sometimes requiring emergency radiation therapy.[251] Grossly, it is generally solid, soft, and nonencapsulated. Some preservation of the thymic shape can be appreciated in early cases. Microscopically, the infiltrate involves the thymic parenchyma and can be confused with a lymphocyte-rich thymoma. However, the lymphocytes are atypical (with a blastic appearance, very fine chromatin pattern, frequent nuclear convolutions, and numerous mitotic figures), there is usually extension into the perithymic fat, and blood vessel invasion is frequent. Residual thymic lobules and Hassall's corpuscles that have been expanded and infiltrated by the lymphoma cells should

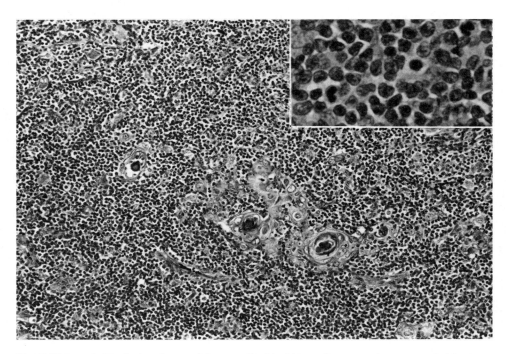

Fig. 8-38 Lymphoblastic lymphoma of thymus. Residual Hassall's corpuscles surrounded by tumor may induce mistaken diagnosis of thymoma. **Inset** shows fine nuclear convolutions in tumor cells.

not be interpreted as evidence of thymoma (Fig. 8-38). It also should be remembered that true thymomas in children are exceptional. Fibrosis and formation of epithelial-lined cysts can be seen in thymic lymphoblastic lymphoma, but both phenomena are distinctly less common than in Hodgkin's disease. Occasionally, there is a scattering of eosin-

ophils, and we have seen a case accompanied by focal granulomatous reaction. Necrosis can be very extensive, whether spontaneous or radiation-induced, to the extent that the entire biopsy may show only necrotic lymphoma tissue. Under these circumstances, if the clinicoradiographic features are compatible, the possibility of lymphoblastic lym-

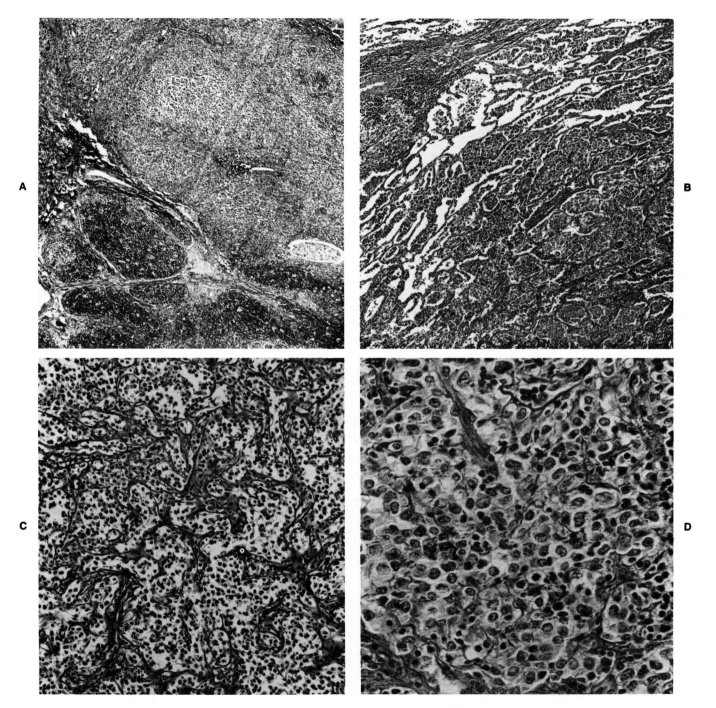

Fig. 8-39 Malignant lymphoma of large cell type with sclerosis. **A,** Diffuse involvement of thymus. Residual thymic parenchyma is seen at the tumor edge. **B,** Extension of tumor in lung parenchyma. **C,** Compartmentalization of tumor induced by fibrous strands, highlighted by PAS stain. **D,** High-power view of tumor, showing large size and irregularities of nuclei and clear appearance of cytoplasm, which may lead to confusion with seminoma or thymoma.

phoma should be suspected and a new biopsy should be requested.

The differential diagnosis of lymphoblastic lymphoma also includes the rare case of **granulocytic sarcoma** (chloroma, myeloblastoma), presenting initially as a mediastinal mass.[248,250]

Large cell lymphoma

Mediastinal large cell lymphoma can present as a mass in the thymus with or without lymph node involvement. Most patients are young adult females, and presentation with superior vena cava syndrome is frequent.[255,257,258] The tumor has grossly invasive features; extension into pericardium, pleura, lung, sternum, and chest wall is common.[253,257] The consistency is generally firm; foci of necrosis are often seen. Microscopically, a sometimes striking feature is the presence of wide bands of fibrosis, which results in compartmentalization of the tumor cells and a microscopic appearance that simulates an epithelial, germ cell, or endocrine neoplasm.[257] Other reasons why this tumor is so often incorrectly diagnosed are the following: perivascular collections of lymphocytes, which may be misinterpreted as the perivascular spaces of thymoma; artifactual clearing of the cytoplasm induced by formalin fixation (not present in B5 or Zenker's fixed material); and entrapment of thymic epithelium.[256] The latter feature can also create problems when the tumor is examined ultrastructurally or when immunostained for keratin.[257] Parenthetically, another immunohistochemical pitfall is represented by lysozyme and other histiocytic markers, in the sense that the sometimes abundant reactive histiocytic population may lead to a mistaken diagnosis of true histiocytic lymphoma.

A diagnosis of large cell lymphoma should be favored in the presence of tumor cells with large, vesicular, irregularly shaped nuclei (indented, kidney-shaped, polylobated); entrapment of intrathymic and perithymic fat; invasion of blood vessel wall, pleura, or lung; and the fact that the fibrosis is manifested not only in the form of wide hyaline bands but also as a fine network that entraps individual cells (Fig. 8-39). Immunohistochemical reactivity for leukocyte common antigen is the rule. Of the tumors studied with cell markers, the majority have been found to be of B-cell nature,[252,254,257,260] but T-cell malignancies are also represented.[259] Its peculiar morphologic attributes suggest that it may represent a neoplasm of a specific subset of lymphoid cells. It should be kept in mind that in young females with a clinically and microscopically malignant mediastinal tumor in which the differential diagnosis is between malignant thymoma, seminoma (germinoma), and large cell malignant lymphoma, the correct diagnosis will be the latter entity in the large majority of the cases.

Large cell malignant lymphoma of mediastinum is usually restricted to the intrathoracic region at the time of initial presentation. A good response to radiation therapy and chemotherapy is the rule, but in many instances the tumor recurs massively within the chest and spreads to other sites, including peripheral lymph nodes. We have been impressed by the high frequency with which the kidneys have been found to be involved in recurrent disease.[257]

NEUROGENIC TUMORS

Neurogenic tumors make up a high proportion of the posterior mediastinal neoplasms, but they can also occur in other compartments.[261,264] The two major categories are tumors of the sympathetic nervous system and tumors of the peripheral nerve sheath. A definite relationship between age and the relative incidence of these tumors exists.[263] In a series of 160 cases,[262] the majority of the tumors occurring in patients under the age of 10 years belonged to the sympathetic nervous system category, and all of those in patients under 1 year of age were neuroblastomas or ganglioneuroblastomas. Most ganglioneuromas, paragangliomas, and tumors of nerve sheath origin were seen after the age of 20 years.

Roentgenographically, most tumors of the sympathetic nervous system have an elongated tapered appearance, whereas benign tumors of nerve sheath origin are round and well-circumscribed.[262]

Tumors of sympathetic nervous system

The general features of these tumors are discussed in Chapter 16. The main difference between the mediastinal and retroperitoneal (particularly adrenal) tumors is the greater degree of differentiation seen in the former. Thus **neuroblastoma** is rather unusual in this location, appearing as an infiltrative mass with areas of necrosis and calcification, usually high in the posterior mediastinum and seen almost exclusively in children. Most of the mediastinal tumors of this group in children are examples of **ganglioneuroblastoma**, a tumor with an intermediate degree of differentiation and which is probably homologous to differentiating neuroblastoma and immature ganglioneuroma[265] (Fig. 8-40) (see Chapter 16). Grossly it tends to be better circumscribed than the neuroblastoma and is sometimes surrounded by a well-formed capsule.

Ganglioneuroma occurs in older children and in adults and is the most common of the three tumors.[267] Grossly, it forms a smooth, well-encapsulated mass, usually in the posterior portion of the mediastinum. The consistency is soft, and the cut surface is yellowish gray; it may contain cystic areas and fatty degeneration, but fresh necrosis is generally absent (Fig. 8-41). Microscopically, an admixture of mature ganglion cells and spindle cells, which could be viewed either as Schwann's cells or satellite cells, is present (Figs. 8-42 and 8-43). The ganglion cells may have several nuclei and are often arranged in clusters. Focal collections of lymphocytes are often present; they should not be confused with the immature cells of ganglioneuroblastoma.[268] These tumors can be multiple and can occur in different locations, with various degrees of differentiation.[270]

The survival rate in patients with tumors of the sympathetic nervous system is directly related to the degree of differentiation of the tumor. Since thoracic neoplasms tend to be better differentiated than their retroperitoneal (particularly adrenal) counterparts, this probably explains why as a group they are associated with a better prognosis.[266,269] Adequate excision effects cure in all patients with ganglioneuromas. The prognosis in patients with ganglioneuroblastomas that contain both elements is somewhat unpre-

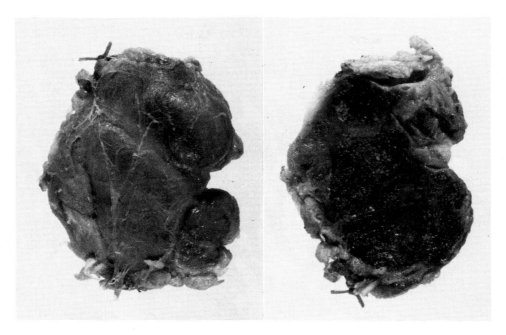

Fig. 8-40 Ganglioneuroblastoma of posterior mediastinum. Tumor contains areas of hemorrhage and calcification. (Courtesy Dr. J. Costa, Lausanne, Switzerland.)

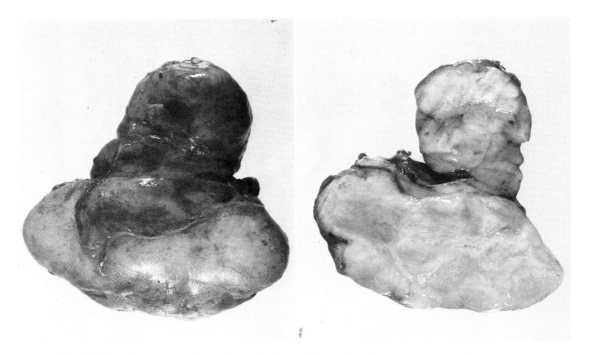

Fig. 8-41 Ganglioneuroma of posterior mediastinum. Tumor shows homogeneous whorling appearance and lacks areas of necrosis or hemorrhage. (Courtesy Dr. J. Costa, Lausanne, Switzerland.)

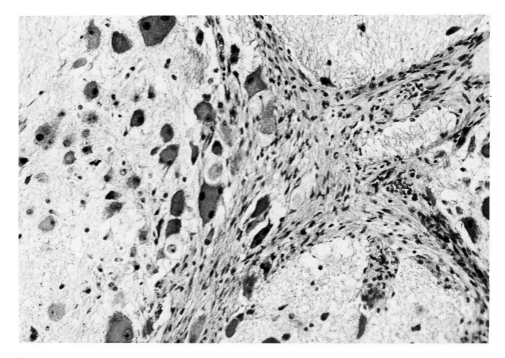

Fig. 8-42 Mediastinal ganglioneuroma with collections of ganglion cells, schwannian sheath proliferation, and cobwebby material. (From Ackerman, LV, Taylor FH: Neurogenous tumors within the thorax. A clinical pathologic evaluation of forty-eight cases. Cancer **4:**669-691, 1951.)

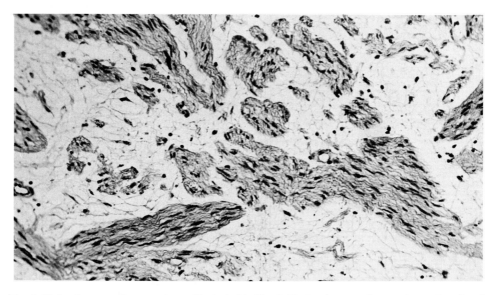

Fig. 8-43 Another area in same tumor illustrated in Fig. 8-42 showing prominent schwannian sheath proliferation. (From Ackerman LV, Taylor FH: Neurogenous tumors within the thorax. A clinical pathologic evaluation of forty-eight cases. Cancer **4:**669-691, 1951.)

dictable, but cure is achieved in most instances.[265] The prognosis in neuroblastoma is the least favorable for the entire group.

Tumors of peripheral nerves

The three major tumors in this category are neurilemoma, neurofibroma, and malignant schwannoma[272,273] (Fig. 8-44). The general features of these tumors are discussed in Chapter 25. It is interesting to note that whereas neurofibroma in most other locations is a nonencapsulated tumor, in the mediastinum it is often surrounded by a complete fibrous capsule, perhaps owing to the large size that it can reach at this site. Therefore presence of encapsulation cannot be used as a distinguishing feature between the two types of benign peripheral nerve tumor.

Another feature common to these neoplasms, perhaps again the result of their sometimes unduly large size, is the high frequency of regressive change within them, such as fatty degeneration, hemorrhage, and cystic formation (Fig. 8-45). Some can become completely cystic, and their recognition may be difficult. Neurilemomas exhibiting prominent cystic and other regressive changes have been designated *ancient neurilemomas,* under the assumption that they have been present for a very long time. Indeed, most benign peripheral nerve sheath tumors are asymptomatic and are discovered incidentally on chest x-ray examinations.

Some neurilemomas can be very cellular and can be confused with sarcoma (Fig. 8-46). A point to remember is that despite their marked cellularity, they have practically no mitotic activity. The prognosis for both neurilemoma and neurofibroma is excellent, excision being curative in nearly every instance.

Malignant schwannoma of mediastinum may arise *de novo* or, more commonly, in the setting of Recklinghausen's disease.[271] In the initial stages of the malignant transformation of a neurofibroma the change may be barely perceptible microscopically, the only suggestion being some slight increase in cellularity. With outspoken malignant change, the tumor cells become bizarre, and it may then be impossible to recognize the malignant tumor as originating from a pre-existing neurofibroma (Figs. 8-47 and 8-48). In these instances, the presence of Recklinghausen's disease, previous biopsy, or the presence of other neurofibromas may suggest the diagnosis.

Some mediastinal malignant schwannomas have areas of glandular differentiation or rhabdomyoblastic features (so-called "triton tumor"). The prognosis is extremely poor.

TUMORS OF PARAGANGLIA

Most mediastinal paragangliomas occur in association with the aorticopulmonary chemoreceptor bodies and therefore occur in the anterosuperior mediastinum close to the

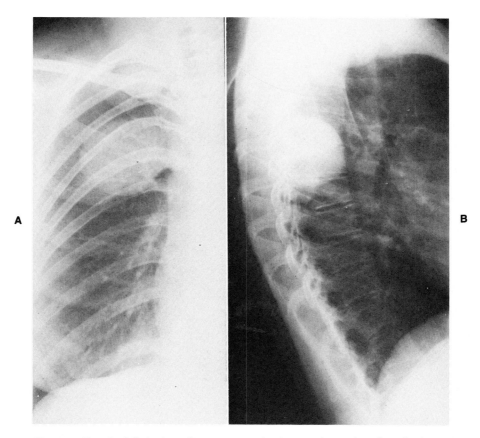

Fig. 8-44 Sharply delimited neurilemoma occurring in posterior portion of mediastinum.

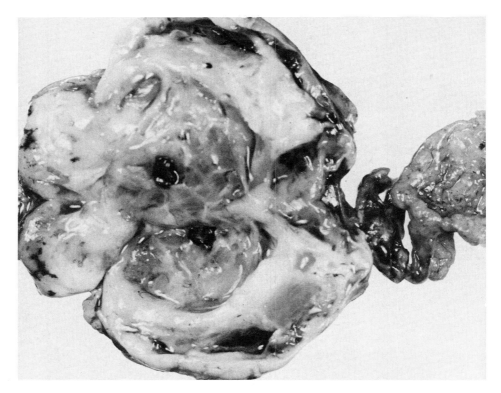

Fig. 8-45 Gross appearance of neurilemoma. The tumor is encapsulated and shows extensive cystic degeneration (same case as Fig. 8-44).

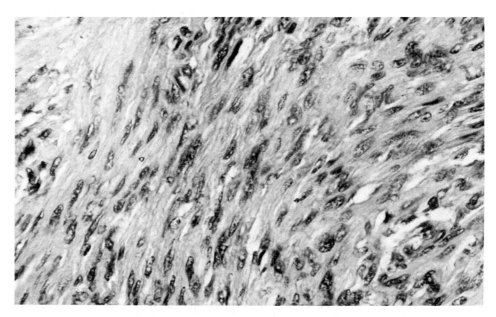

Fig. 8-46 Highly cellular neurilemoma that was benign but incorrectly diagnosed as malignant because of cellularity. (From Ackerman LV, Taylor FH: Neurogenous tumors within the thorax. A clinical pathologic evaluation of forty-eight cases. Cancer **4:**669-691, 1951.)

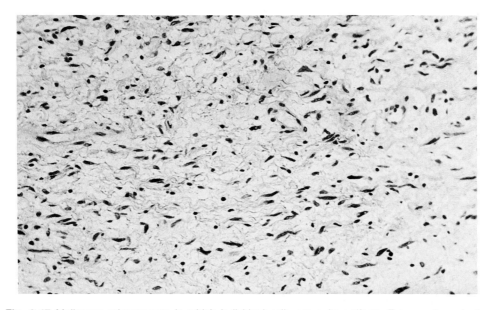

Fig. 8-47 Malignant schwannoma in which individual cells are quite uniform. From such a single microscopic field, it would be difficult, if not impossible, to tell that the tumor was malignant. (From Ackerman LV, Taylor FH: Neurogenous tumors within the thorax. A clinical pathologic evaluation of forty-eight cases. Cancer **4:**669-691, 1951.)

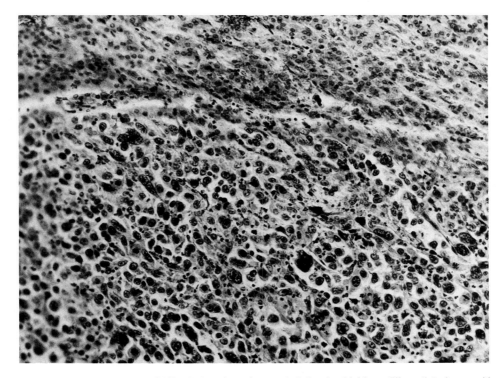

Fig. 8-48 Same tumor shown in Fig. 8-47 at later time period showing highly undifferentiated area with numerous tumor giant cells.

base of the heart.[276] Others arise from mediastinal aortico-sympathetic paraganglia and occur posteriorly, along the costovertebral sulcus. Their morphologic appearance is identical to paragangliomas in other locations, such as the carotid body (see Chapter 16).

The large majority of these tumors are nonfunctioning. Some, however (particularly when related to the sympathetic system), can result in hypertension and are sometimes referred to as extra-adrenal pheochromocytomas.[274] However, it is now agreed to reserve the designation of pheochromocytomas for paragangliomas located in the adrenal medulla, whether they are functioning or not.

Traditionally, mediastinal paragangliomas have been regarded as generally benign in nature. However, a critical long-term follow-up study of thirty-five reported cases revealed that the tumor had behaved in an aggressive fashion in sixteen (46%), resulting in important morbidity and sometimes in death.[275]

MESENCHYMAL TUMORS

Lipoma is one of the most common benign mesenchymal neoplasms of the mediastinum. It is often very large and located just above the diaphragm. Occasionally, it extends into both pleural cavities, making complete removal difficult.[282,285] Presence of thymic tissue should be sought in mediastinal lipomas to rule out a diagnosis of thymolipoma (see p. 365). The other differential diagnoses are with *lipomatosis*, a diffuse accumulation of mature adipose tissue that may occur in association with obesity, Cushing's disease, or steroid therapy,[283] and with *lipoblastomatosis* of infancy.[280]

Lymphangioma is another common mediastinal neoplasm (Fig. 8-49). Most cases are seen in the anterosuperior mediastinum of children, often in continuity with a cervical component.[278] *Lymphangioma* and *lymphangiomyomatosis* occur exclusively in females, the distinction among the two depending on their circumscribed versus infiltrative pattern of growth, respectively (see Chapter 25).

Hemangioma in adults is usually of the cavernous variety. Microscopically, it is composed of dilated vessels lined by attenuated endothelium, separated by fine septa. Foci of thrombosis, calcification, and cholesterol granulomas may be present. Excision is usually curative.[288] In children, the hemangiomas may have a very cellular appearance (benign hemangioendotheliomas).[277] *Hemangiopericytomas* probably occur, but most anterosuperior mediastinal tumors with a hemangiopericytoma-like pattern are well-vascularized thymomas. Other vascular mediastinal tumors include histiocytoid (epithelioid) hemangioendothelioma and angiosarcoma.[281] Some of the latter arise on the background of a malignant germ cell tumor.[284]

Solitary fibrous tumor of the mediastinum is the mediastinal equivalent of solitary fibrous tumor of the pleura (so-called solitary fibrous mesothelioma). It is possible that

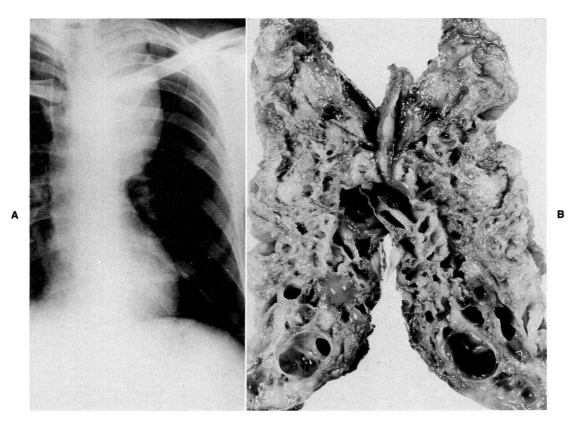

Fig. 8-49 A, Lymphangioma of anterior portion of mediastinum. **B,** Lymphangioma demonstrating large, cystic, smooth-walled spaces.

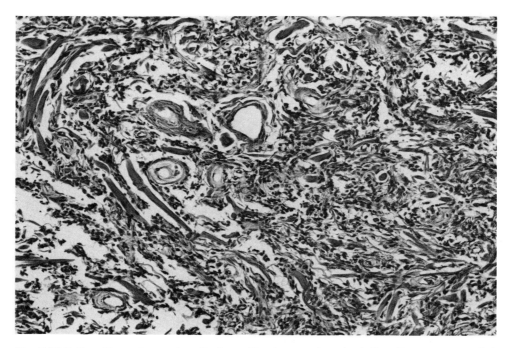

Fig. 8-50 Solitary fibrous tumor of mediastinum. Bland mesenchymal spindle cells are accompanied by deposition of prominent bands of collagen fibers. Thick-walled blood vessels are irregularly scattered throughout tumor.

some of these tumors grow into the mediastinum from the medial pleura, but we think that most originate from the mediastinal (including thymic) stroma. Their microscopic appearance and behavior seem to be similar to those of their pleural counterparts[290] (Fig. 8-50).

Liposarcoma predominates among the malignant mesenchymal neoplasms.[286] Sometimes it is seen in conjunction with liposarcoma of thigh or retroperitoneum as an example of multicentric disease. Some mediastinal liposarcomas containing thymic tissue can be viewed as the malignant counterpart of thymolipomas (i.e., as thymoliposarcomas) (see p. 367).

Synovial sarcoma can present as a primary mediastinal neoplasm, its morphologic appearance being the same as that of the most common type occurring in the extremities.[289]

Other malignant mesenchymal tumors that have been observed in the mediastinum include *leiomyosarcoma,*[287] *malignant mesenchymoma,* and *malignant fibrous histiocytoma.*[279,285]

OTHER PRIMARY TUMORS AND TUMORLIKE CONDITIONS

Castleman's disease (giant lymph node hyperplasia) has a special predilection for the mediastinum. In the past, it was often confused with thymoma because the hyalinized germinal centers that constitute the hallmark of the most common form of this disease were misinterpreted as Hassall's corpuscles[292] (Fig. 8-51). It usually involves mediastinal nodes, but exceptionally it may be located within the thymus.[291] This disorder is more thoroughly discussed in Chapter 21.

Extramedullary hematopoiesis may present as large solitary mediastinal masses, usually located along the paravertebral column. The primary disease in most patients is hereditary spherocytosis or thalassemia.[293]

Meningioma has been reported in the posterior mediastinum in association with the sympathetic chain, presumably arising from the stellate ganglion.[294]

METASTATIC TUMORS

Some tumors metastatic to the mediastinum can mimic clinically and radiographically a primary tumor. Small cell carcinoma of the lung is the most notorious example, often appearing as a huge mediastinal mass in the presence of a small, radiographically undetectable bronchial lesion. Other types of lung carcinoma may produce a similar picture, either by direct extension or nodal metastases.

Direct mediastinal extension can also occur with tumors of the esophagus, pleura, chest wall, vertebra, or trachea. Other tumors that we have seen metastasizing to the mediastinum and confused with primary neoplasms—sometimes even at the microscopic level—are carcinomas of the breast, thyroid, larynx, kidney, and prostate; testicular germ cell tumors; and malignant melanoma.[295,296] Since most of these tumors are located, at least initially, in mediastinal lymph nodes, they are usually centered in the middle mediastinum (where most lymph nodes are situated), and they may exhibit a residual nodal component at their periphery.

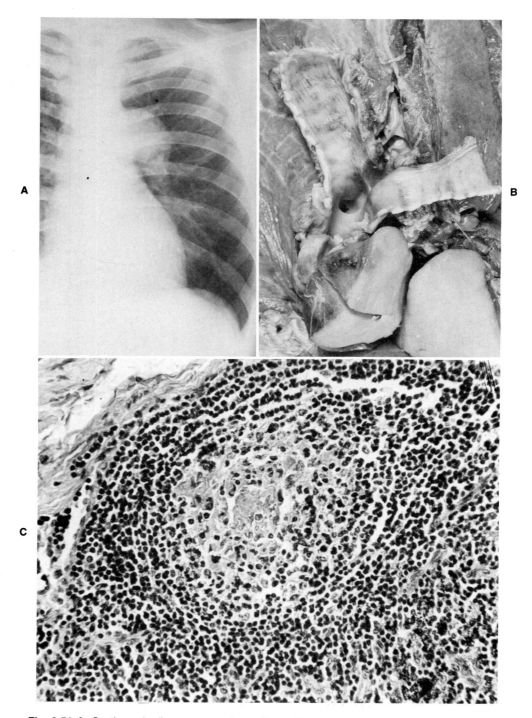

Fig. 8-51 A, Castleman's disease presenting radiographically as a hilar mass. **B,** At operation, firm mass intimately associated with bronchus was thought to represent neoplasm. **C,** Microscopically, mass proved to be example of giant lymph node hyperplasia.

REFERENCES

GENERALITIES

1 Hodge J, Aponte G, McLaughlin E: Primary mediastinal tumors. J Thorac Surg **37:**730-744, 1959.
2 Mahajan V, Strimlan V, Van Ordstrand HS, Loop FD: Benign superior vena cava syndrome. Chest **68:**32-35, 1975.
3 Marshall ME, Trump DL: Acquired extrinsic pulmonic stenosis caused by mediastinal tumors. Cancer **49:**1496-1499, 1982.
4 Marvasti MA, Mitchell GE, Burke WA, Meyer JA: Misleading density of mediastinal cysts on computerized tomography. Ann Thorac Surg **31:**167-170, 1981.
5 Oldham HN Jr, Sabiston DC Jr: Primary tumors and cysts of the mediastinum. Monogr Surg Sci **4:**243-279, 1967.
6 Parish JM, Marschke PF Jr, Dines DE, Lee RE: Etiologic considerations in superior vena cava syndrome. Mayo Clin Proc **56:**407-413, 1981.
7 Ringertz N, Lidholm SO: Mediastinal tumors and cysts. J Thorac Surg **31:**458-487, 1956.
8 Schechter MM: The superior vena cava syndrome. Am J Med Sci **227:**46-56, 1954.
9 Sterrett G, Whitaker D, Glancy J: Fine-needle aspiration of lung, mediastinum, and chest wall. A clinicopathologic exercise. Pathol Annu **17**(Pt 2):197-228, 1982.
10 Wychulis AR, Payne WS, Clagett OT, Woolner LB: Surgical treatment of mediastinal tumors. A 40 year experience. J Thorac Cardiovasc Surg **62:**379-392, 1971.

INFLAMMATORY DISEASES

11 Cogan MIC: Necrotizing mediastinitis secondary to descending cervical cellulitis. Oral Surg Oral Med Oral Pathol **36:**307-320, 1973.
12 Dines DE, Payne WS, Bernatz PE, Pairolero PC: Mediastinal granuloma and fibrosing mediastinitis. Chest **75:**320-324, 1979.
13 Ferguson TB, Burford TH: Mediastinal granuloma. A 15-year experience. Ann Thorac Surg **1:**125-141, 1965.
14 Goodwin RA, Nickell JA, Des Prez RM: Mediastinal fibrosis complicating healed primary histoplasmosis and tuberculosis. Medicine [Baltimore] **51:**227-246, 1972.
15 Light AM: Idiopathic fibrosis of mediastinum. A discussion of three cases and review of the literature. J Clin Pathol **31:**78-88, 1978.
16 Magee JF, Wright JL, Dodek A, Tutassaura H: Mediastinal and retroperitoneal fibrosis with fibrotic pulmonary nodules. A case report. Histopathology **9:**995-999, 1985.
17 Mitchell IM, Saunders HR, Maher O, Lennox SC, Walker DR: Surgical treatment of idiopathic mediastinal fibrosis. Report of five cases. Thorax **41:**210-214, 1986.
18 Mitchinson MJ: The pathology of idiopathic retroperitoneal fibrosis. J Clin Pathol **23:**681-689, 1970.
19 Payne WS, Larson RH: Acute mediastinitis. Surg Clin North Am **49:**999-1009, 1969.
20 Rankin RS, Wescott JL: Superior vena cava syndrome caused by *Nocardia* mediastinitis. Am Rev Respir Dis **108:**361-363, 1973.
21 Salyer JM, Harrison HN, Winn DF Jr, Taylor RR: Chronic fibrous mediastinitis and superior vena caval obstruction due to histoplasmosis. Dis Chest **35:**364-377, 1959.
22 Schowengerdt CG, Suyemoto R, Main FB: Granulomatous and fibrous mediastinitis. A review and analysis of 180 cases. J Thorac Cardiovasc Surg **57:**365-379, 1969.
23 Strimlan CV, Dines DE, Payne WS: Mediastinal granuloma. Mayo Clin Proc **50:**702-705, 1975.

CYSTS (OTHER THAN THYMIC)
Pericardial (coelomic) cysts

24 Lillie WI, McDonald JR, Clagett OT: Pericardial celomic cysts and pericardial diverticula. A concept of etiology and report of cases. J Thorac Surg **20:**494-504, 1950.

Foregut cysts

25 Abell MR: Mediastinal cysts. Arch Pathol **61:**360-379, 1956.
26 Chitale AR: Gastric cyst of the mediastinum. A distinct clinicopathological entity. J Pediatr **75:**104-110, 1969.
27 Chuang MT, Barba FA, Kaneko M, Teirstein AS: Adenocarcinoma arising in an intrathoracic duplication cyst of foregut origin. A case report with review of the literature. Cancer **47:**1887-1890, 1981.

28 Eraklis AJ, Griscom NT, McGovern JB: Bronchogenic cysts of the mediastinum in infancy. N Engl J Med **281:**1150-1155, 1969.
29 Laipply TC: Cysts and cystic tumors of the mediastinum. Arch Pathol **39:**153-161, 1945.
30 Maier HC: Bronchiogenic cysts of the mediastinum. Ann Surg **127:**476-502, 1948.
31 Salyer DC, Salyer WR, Eggleston JC: Benign developmental cysts of the mediastinum. Arch Pathol **101:**136-139, 1977.

Other cysts

32 Johnston RH Jr, Owensby LC, Vargas GM, Garcia-Rinaldi R: Pancreatic pseudocyst of the mediastinum. Ann Thorac Surg **41:**210-212, 1986.
33 Sambrook Gowar FJ: Mediastinal thoracic duct cyst. Thorax **33:**800-802, 1978.

THYROID AND PARATHYROID LESIONS

34 Allo MD, Thompson NW: Rationale for the operative management of substernal goiters. Surgery **94:**969-977, 1983.
35 Katlic MR, Wang C, Grillo HC: Substernal goiter. Ann Thorac Surg **39:**391-399, 1985.
36 Murphy MN, Glennon PG, Diocee MS, Wick MR, Cavers DJ: Nonsecretory parathyroid carcinoma of the mediastinum. Light microscopic, immunocytochemical, and ultrastructural features of a case, and review of the literature. Cancer **58:**2468-2476, 1986.

THYMUS
Normal anatomy

37 Bach JF: Physiology of the endocrine function of the thymic epithelium. In Yamamura Y, Tada T (eds): Progress in immunology. vol. 5, Tokyo, 1984, Academic Press Japan, Inc.
38 Barthélémy H, Pelletier M, Landry D, Lafontaine M, Perreault C, Tautu C, Montplaisir S: Demonstration of OKT6 antigen on human thymic dendritic cells in culture. Lab Invest **55:**540-545, 1986.
39 Dourov N: Thymic atrophy and immune deficiency in malnutrition. In Müller-Hermelink HK (ed): Current topics in pathology. The human thymus. Histophysiology and pathology. vol. 75, New York, 1986, Springer-Verlag, pp. 127-150.
40 Goldstein G, Mackay IR: The human thymus. St. Louis, 1969, Warren H. Green, Inc.
41 Hsu S-M, Jaffe ES: Phenotypic expression of T lymphocytes in thymus and peripheral lymphoid tissues. Am J Pathol **121:**69-78, 1985.
42 Janossy G, Bofill M, Trejdosiewicz LK, Willcox HNA, Chilosi M: Cellular differentiation of lymphoid subpopulations and their microenvironments in the human thymus. In Müller-Hermelink HK (ed): Current topics in pathology. The human thymus. Histophysiology and pathology. vol. 75, New York, 1986, Springer-Verlag, pp. 89-125.
43 Kendall MD, Van de Wijngaert FP, Schuurman H-J, Rademakers LHPM, Kater L: Heterogeneity of the human thymus epithelial microenvironment at the ultrastructural level. In Klause GCB (ed): Microenvironments in the lymphoid system. Advances in experimental medicine and biology. vol. 186, New York, 1985, Plenum Press.
44 Sharp JG, Crouse DA, Purtilo DT: Ontogeny and regulation of the immune system. Arch Pathol Lab Med **111:**1106-1113, 1987.
45 Smith SM, Ossa-Gomez LJ: A quantitative histologic comparison of the thymus in 100 healthy and diseased adults. Am J Clin Pathol **76:**657-665, 1981.
46 Steinmann GG: Changes in the human thymus during aging. In Müller-Hermelink HK (ed): Current topics in pathology. The human thymus. Histophysiology and pathology. vol. 75, New York, 1986, Springer-Verlag, pp. 43-88.
47 Van Ewijk W: Immunohistology of lymphoid and non-lymphoid cells in the thymus in relation to T lymphocyte differentiation. Am J Anat **170:**311-330, 1984.
48 von Gaudecker B: The development of the human thymus microenvironment. In Müller-Hermelink HK (ed): Current topics in pathology. The human thymus. Histophysiology and pathology. vol. 75, New York, 1986, Springer-Verlag, pp. 1-41.
49 Willcox N, Schluep M, Ritter MA, Schuurman HJ, Newsom-Davis J, Christensson B: Myasthenic and nonmyasthenic thymoma. An expansion of a minor cortical epithelial cell subset? Am J Pathol **127:**447-460, 1987.

Cysts

50 Bleger RC, McAdams AJ: Thymic cysts. Arch Pathol **82:**535-541, 1966.
51 Dyer NH: Cystic thymomas and thymic cysts. A review. Thorax **22:**408-421, 1967.

52 Leong AS-Y, Brown JH: Malignant transformation in a thymic cyst. Am J Surg Pathol **8**:471-475, 1984.

53 McCafferty MH, Bahnson HT: Thymic cyst extending into the pericardium. A case report and review of thymic cysts. Ann Thorac Surg **33**:503-506, 1982.

54 Sanusi ID, Carrington PR, Adams DN: Cervical thymic cyst. Arch Dermatol **118**:122-124, 1982.

55 Ratnesar P: Unilateral cervical thymic cyst. J Laryngol Otol **85**:293-298, 1971.

Primary immunodeficiencies

56 Nezelof C: Pathology of the thymus in immunodeficiency states. In Müller-Hermelink HK (ed): Current topics in pathology. The human thymus. Histophysiology and pathology. vol. 75, New York, 1986, Springer-Verlag, pp. 151-177.

Other non-neoplastic diseases

57 Askin FB, McCann BG, Kuhn C: Reactive eosinophilic pleuritis. A lesion to be distinguished from pulmonary eosinophilic granuloma. Arch Pathol Lab Med **101**:187-191, 1977.

58 Balcom RJ, Hakanson DO, Werner A, Gordon LP: Massive thymic hyperplasia in an infant with Beckwith-Wiedemann syndrome. Arch Pathol Lab Med **109**:153-155, 1985.

59 Bofill M, Janossy G, Willcox N, Chilosi M, Trejdosiewicz LK, Newsom-Davis J: Microenvironments in the normal thymus and the thymus in myasthenia gravis. Am J Pathol **119**:462-473, 1985.

60 Bramwell NH, Burns BF: Histiocytosis X of the thymus in association with myasthenia gravis. Am J Clin Pathol **86**:224-227, 1986.

61 Carmosino L, DiBenedetto A, Feffer S: Thymic hyperplasia following successful chemotherapy. A report of two cases and review of the literature. Cancer **56**:1526-1528, 1985.

62 Havlíček F, Rosai J: Histioeosinophilic granulomas in the thymuses of 29 myasthenic patients. A complication of pneumomediastinum. Hum Pathol **15**:1137-1144, 1984.

63 Jessurun J, Azevedo M, Saldana M: Allergic angiitis and granulomatosis (Churg-Strauss syndrome). A report of a case with massive thymic involvement in a nonasthmatic patient. Hum Pathol **17**:637-639, 1986.

64 Joshi VV, Oleske JM, Saad S, Gadol C, Connor E, Bobila R, Minnefor AB: Thymus biopsy in children with acquired immunodeficiency syndrome. Arch Pathol Lab Med **110**:837-842, 1986.

65 Karcher DS, Pearson CE, Butler WM, Hurwitz MA, Cassell PF: Giant lymph node hyperplasia involving the thymus with associated nephrotic syndrome and myelofibrosis. Am J Clin Pathol **77**:100-104, 1982.

66 Katz SM, Chatten J, Bishop HC, Rosenblum H: Massive thymic enlargement. Report of a case of gross thymic hyperplasia in a child. Am J Clin Pathol **63**:786-790, 1977.

67 Kornstein MJ, Brooks JJ, Anderson AO, Levinson AI, Lisak RP, Zweiman B: The immunohistology of the thymus in myasthenia gravis. Am J Pathol **117**:184-194, 1984.

68 Lau HT, Barlow BA, Gandhi RP: Ectopic thymus presenting as neck mass. J Pediatr Surg **19**:197, 1984.

69 Linder J: The thymus gland in secondary immunodeficiency. Arch Pathol Lab Med **111**:1118-1122, 1987.

70 Löning T, Caselitz J, Otto HF: The epithelial framework of the thymus in normal and pathological conditions. Virchows Arch [Pathol Anat] **392**:7-20, 1981.

71 Okabe H: Thymologic lymph follicles. A histopathological study of 1,356 autopsy cases. Acta Pathol Jpn **16**:109-130, 1966.

72 Seemayer TA, Laroche AC, Russo P, Malebranche R, Arnoux E, Guérin J-M, Pierre G, Dupuy J-M, Gartner JG, Lapp WS, Spira TJ, Elie R: Precocious thymic involution manifest by epithelial injury in the acquired immune deficiency syndrome. Hum Pathol **15**:469-474, 1984.

73 Siegal GP, Dehner LP, Rosai J: Histiocytosis X (Langerhans' cell granulomatosis) of the thymus. A clinicopathologic study of four childhood cases. Am J Surg Pathol **9**:117-124, 1985.

74 Wekerle H, Müller-Hermelink HK: The thymus in myasthenia gravis. In Müller-Hermelink HK (ed): Current topics in pathology. The human thymus. Histophysiology and pathology. vol. 75, New York, 1986, Springer-Verlag, pp. 179-206.

75 Wolff M, Rosai J, Wright DH: Sebaceous glands within the thymus. Report of three cases. Hum Pathol **15**:341-343, 1984.

Thymoma
General features

76 Chatten J, Katz SM: Thymoma in a 12-year-old boy. Cancer **37**:953-957, 1976.

77 Dahlgren S, Sandstedt B, Sundström C: Fine needle aspiration cytology of thymic tumors. Acta Cytol [Baltimore] **27**:1-6, 1983.

78 Dehner LP, Martin SA, Sumner HW: Thymus related tumors and tumor-like lesions in childhood with rapid clinical progression and death. Hum Pathol **8**:53-66, 1977.

79 Furman WL, Buckley PJ, Green AA, Stokes DC, Chien LT: Thymoma and myasthenia gravis in a 4-year-old child. Case report and review of the literature. Cancer **56**:2703-2706, 1985.

80 Göthlin J, Jonsson K, Lunderquist A, Rausing A, Alburquerque LM: The angiographic appearance of thymic tumors. Radiology **124**:47-52, 1977.

81 Green WR, Pressoir R, Gumbs RV, Warner O, Naab T, Qayumi M: Intrapulmonary thymoma. Arch Pathol Lab Med **111**:1074-1076, 1987.

82 Hofmann W, Möller P, Manke H-G, Otto HF: Thymoma. A clinicopathologic study of 98 cases with special reference to three unusual cases. Pathol Res Pract **179**:337-353, 1985.

83 Keen SJ, Libshitz HI: Thymic lesions. Experience with computed tomography in 24 patients. Cancer **59**:1520-1523, 1987.

84 Kung I, Loke SL, So SY, Lam WK, Mok CK, Khin MA: Intrapulmonary thymoma. Report of two cases. Thorax **40**:471-474, 1985.

85 Levine GD, Rosai J: Thymic hyperplasia and neoplasia. A review of current concepts. Hum Pathol **9**:495-515, 1978.

86 Martin JME, Randhawa G, Temple WJ: Cervical thymoma. Arch Pathol Lab Med **110**:354-357, 1986.

87 Müller-Hermelink HK, Marino M, Palestro G: Pathology of thymic epithelial tumors. In Müller-Hermelink HK (ed): Current topics in pathology. The human thymus. Histophysiology and pathology. vol. 75, New York, 1986, Springer-Verlag, pp. 207-268.

88 Rosai J, Levine GD: Tumors of the thymus. In Atlas of tumor pathology, Second Series, Fasc. 13. Washington, D.C., 1975, Armed Forces Institute of Pathology.

89 Tao L-C, Pearson FG, Cooper JD, Sanders DE, Weisbrod G, Donat EE: Cytopathology of thymoma. Acta Cytol [Baltimore] **28**:165-170, 1984.

90 Wick MR, Scheithauer BW, Dines DE: Thymic neoplasia in two male siblings. Mayo Clin Proc **57**:653-656, 1982.

91 Yamashita H, Murakami N, Noguchi S, Noguchi A, Yokoyama S, Moriuchi A, Nakayama I: Cervical thymoma and incidence of cervical thymus. Acta Pathol Jpn **33**:189-194, 1983.

Pathologic features

92 Battifora H, Sunn TT, Bahu RM, Rao S: The use of antikeratin antiserum as a diagnostic tool. Thymoma versus lymphoma. Hum Pathol **11**:635-641, 1980.

93 Chan WC, Zaatari GS, Tabei S, Bibb M, Brynes RK: Thymoma. An immunohistochemical study. Am J Clin Pathol **82**:160-166, 1984.

94 Chilosi M, Iannucci A, Menestrina F, Lestani M, Scarpa A, Bonetti F, Fiore-Donati L, Dipasquale B, Pizzolo G, Palestro G, Tridente G, Janossy G: Immunohistochemical evidence of active thymocyte proliferation in thymoma. Am J Pathol **128**:464-470, 1987.

95 Eimoto T, Teshima K, Shirakusa T, Takeshita M, Okamura H, Naito H, Mitsui T, Kikuchi M: Heterogeneity of epithelial cells and reactive components in thymomas. An ultrastructural and immunohistochemical study. Ultrastruct Pathol **10**:157-173, 1986.

96 Gray GF, Gutowski WT III: Thymoma. Am J Surg Pathol **3**:235-249, 1979.

96a Katzin WE, Linden MD, Fishleder AJ, Tubbs RR: Thymomas lack detectable T-cell receptor beta chain gene rearrangements (abstract). Lab Invest **56**:36A, 1987.

97 Kornstein MJ, Hoxie JA, Levinson AI, Brooks JJ: Immunohistology of human thymomas. Arch Pathol Lab Med **109**:460-463, 1985.

98 Lauriola L, Maggiano N, Marino M, Carbone A, Piantelli M, Musiani P: Human thymoma. Immunologic characteristics of the lymphocytic component. Cancer **48**:1992-1995, 1981.

99 Lauriola L, Michetti F, Stolfi VM, Tallini G, Cocchia D: Detection by S-100 immunolabelling of interdigitating reticulum cells in human thymomas. Virchows Arch [Cell Pathol] **45**:187-195, 1984.

100 LeGolvan DP, Abell MR: Thymomas. Cancer **39**:2142-2157, 1977.

101 Levine GD, Bensch KG: Epithelial nature of spindle-cell thymoma. An ultrastructural study. Cancer **30**:500-511, 1972.

102 Levine GD, Rosai J, Bearman RM, Polliack A: The fine structure of thymoma, with emphasis on its differential diagnosis. A study of ten cases. Am J Pathol **81**:49-66, 1975.

103 Mokhtar N, Hsu S-M, Lad RP, Haynes BF, Jaffe ES: Thymoma. Lymphoid and epithelial components mirror the phenotype of normal thymus. Hum Pathol **15**:378-384, 1984.

104 Müller-Hermelink HK, Marino M, Palestro G, Schumacher U, Kirchner T: Immunohistologic evidences of cortical and medullary differentiation in thymoma. Virchows Arch [Pathol Anat] **408**:143-161, 1985.

105 Osborne B, Mackay B, Battifora H: Thymoma. A clinicopathologic study of 23 cases. Pathol Annu **20**(Pt 2):289-315, 1985.

106 Otto HF: Pathologie des thymus. New York, 1984, Springer-Verlag.
107 Palestro G, Valente G, Botto Micca F, Novero D, Arisio R: Detection and distribution of alfa-naphthyl acetate esterase activity in thymocytes of normal, myasthenic thymus and thymoma. Histochemical and cytochemical study in relation to E-Rosetting. Virchows Arch [Cell Pathol] **35**:33-43, 1980.
108 Rosai J: The pathology of thymic neoplasia. International Academy of Pathology Monograph No. 29, Baltimore, 1987, Williams & Wilkins.
109 Rosai J, Levine GD: Tumors of the thymus. In Atlas of tumor pathology, Second Series, Fasc. 13. Washington, D.C., 1975, Armed Forces Institute of Pathology.
110 Salyer WR, Eggleston JC: Thymoma. A clinical and pathological study of 65 cases. Cancer **37**:229-249, 1976.
111 Sato Y, Watanabe S, Mukai K, Kodama T, Upton MP, Goto M, Shimosato Y: An immunohistochemical study of thymic epithelial tumors. Am J Surg Pathol **10**:862-870, 1986.
112 Savino W, Durand D, Dardenne M: Immunohistochemical evidence for the expression of the carcinoembryonic antigen by human thymic epithelial cells in vitro and in neoplastic conditions. Am J Pathol **121**:418-425, 1985.
113 Savino W, Manganella G, Verley J-M, Wolff A, Berrih S, Levasseur P, Binet J-P, Dardenne M, Bach J-F: Thymoma epithelial cells secrete thymic hormone but do not express class II antigens of the major histocompatibility complex. J Clin Invest **76**:1140-1146, 1985.
114 van der Kwast TH, van Vliet E, Cristen E, van Ewijk W, van der Heul RO: An immunohistologic study of the epithelial and lymphoid components of six thymomas. Hum Pathol **16**:1001-1008, 1985.
115 Watanabe H: A pathological study of thymomas. Acta Pathol Jpn **16**:323-358, 1966.
116 Willcox N, Schluep M, Ritter MA, Schuurman HJ, Newsom-Davis J, Christensson B: Myasthenic and nonmyasthenic thymoma. An expansion of a minor cortical epithelial cell subset? Am J Pathol **127**:447-460, 1987.
117 Woda BA, Bain K, Salm TV: The phenotype of lymphocytes in a thymoma as studied with monoclonal antibodies. Clin Immunol Immunopathol **30**:197-201, 1984.

Myasthenia gravis

118 Alpert LI, Papatestas A, Kark A, Osserman RS, Osserman K: A histologic reappraisal of the thymus in myasthenia gravis. A correlative study of thymic pathology and response to thymectomy. Arch Pathol **91**:55-61, 1971.
119 Azer MS, Zikria E, Ford WB: Myasthenia gravis appearing after removal of a thymoma. Report of a case and review of the literature. Am Surg **37**:109-113, 1971.
120 Butler WM, Diehl LF, Taylor HG, Weltz MD: Metastatic thymoma with myasthenia gravis. Complete remission with combination chemotherapy. Cancer **50**:419-422, 1982.
121 Dardenne M, Savino W, Bach J-F: Thymomatous epithelial cells and skeletal muscle share a common epitope defined by a monoclonal antibody. Am J Pathol **126**:194-198, 1987.
122 Drachman DB: Myasthenia gravis. N Engl J Med **298**:136-142; 186-193, 1978.
123 Drachman DB (ed): Myasthenia gravis. Biology and clinical aspects. Ann NY Acad Sci (In press.)
124 Drachman DB: Present and future treatment of myasthenia gravis (editorial). N Engl J Med **316**:743-745, 1987.
125 Genkins G, Papatestas AE, Horowitz SH, Kornfeld P: Studies in myasthenia gravis. Early thymectomy. Electrophysiologic and pathologic correlations. Am J Med **58**:517-524, 1975.
126 Gilhus NE, Aarli JA, Christensson B, Matre R: Rabbit antiserum to a citric acid extract of human skeletal muscle staining thymomas from myasthenia gravis patients. J Neuroimmunol **7**:55-64, 1984.
127 Gutmann L: Myasthenia gravis. Current concepts. Arch Pathol **100**:401-404, 1976.
127a Kim YI, Neher E: IgG from patients with Lambert-Eaton syndrome blocks voltage-dependent calcium channels. Science **239**:405-408, 1988.
127b Kirchner T, Tzartos S, Hoppe F, Schalke B, Wekerle H, Müller-Hermelink HK: Pathogenesis of myasthenia gravis. Acetylcholine receptor-related antigenic determinants in tumor-free thymuses and thymic epithelial tumors. Am J Pathol **130**:268-280, 1988.
128 Koeda T: Immunopathological study related to myoglobin in myasthenic and non-myasthenic thymuses. Acta Pathol Jpn **36**:209-223, 1986.
129 Lewis JE, Wick MR, Scheithauer BW, Bernatz PE, Taylor WF: Thymoma. A clinicopathologic review. Cancer **60**:2727-2743, 1987.
130 Monden Y, Nakahara K, Fujii Y, Hashimoto J, Ohno K, Masaoka A, Kawashima Y: Myasthenia gravis in elderly patients. Ann Thorac Surg **39**:433-440, 1985.
131 Monden Y, Nakahara K, Kagotani K, Fujii Y, Masaoka A, Kawashima Y: Myasthenia gravis with thymoma. Analysis of and postoperative prognosis for 65 patients with thymomatous myasthenia gravis. Ann Thorac Surg **38**:46-52, 1984.
132 Monden Y, Nakahara K, Nanjo S, Fujii Y, Matsumura A, Masaoka A, Kawashima Y: Invasive thymoma with myasthenia gravis. Cancer **54**:2513-2518, 1984.
133 Monden Y, Uyama T, Nakahara K, Fujii Y, Hashimoto J, Ohno K, Masaoka A, Kawashima Y: Clinical characteristics and prognosis of myasthenia gravis with other autoimmune diseases. Ann Thorac Surg **41**:189-192, 1984.
134 Namba T, Brunner NG: Myasthenia gravis in patients with thymoma, with particular reference to onset after thymectomy. Medicine [Baltimore] **57**:411-433, 1978.
135 Newsom-Davis J, Willcox N, Calder L: Thymus cells in myasthenia gravis selectively enhance production of anti-acetylcholine-receptor antibody by autologous blood lymphocytes. N Engl J Med **305**:1313-1318, 1981.
136 Rosenberg M, Jauregui WO, De Vega ME, Herrera MR, Roncoroni AJ: Recurrence of thymic hyperplasia after thymectomy in myasthenia gravis. Its importance as a cause of failure of surgical treatment. Am J Med **74**:78-82, 1983.
137 Scadding GK, Havard CWH, Lange MJ, Domb I: The long-term experience of thymectomy for myasthenia gravis. J Neurol Neurosurg Psychiatry **48**:401-406, 1985.
138 Schluep M, Willcox N, Vincent A, Dhoot GK, Newsom-Davis J: Acetylcholine receptors in human thymic myoid cells in situ. An immunohistological study. Ann Neurol (In press.)
139 Schumm F, Wiethölter H, Fateh-Moghadam A, Dichgans J: Thymectomy in myasthenia with pure ocular symptoms. J Neurol Neurosurg Psychiatry **48**:332-337, 1985.
140 Slater G, Papatestas AE, Genkins G, Kornfeld P, Horowitz SH, Bender A: Thymomas in patients with myasthenia gravis. Ann Surg **188**:171-174, 1978.
141 Vincent A: Immunology of acetylcholine receptors in relation to myasthenia gravis. Physiol Rev **60**:756-824, 1980.
142 Wekerle H, Ketelsen U-P: Intrathymic pathogenesis and dual genetic control of myasthenia gravis. Lancet **1**:678-680, 1977.
143 Wekerle H, Müller-Hermelink HK: The thymus in myasthenia gravis. In Müller-Hermelink HK (ed): Current topics in pathology. The human thymus. Histophysiology and pathology. vol. 75, New York, 1986, Springer-Verlag.
144 Weltfriend S, David M, Ginzburg A, Sandbank M: Generalized hair follicle hamartoma. The third case report in association with myasthenia gravis. Am J Dermatopathol **9**:428-432, 1987.
145 Wilins EW Jr, Edmunds LH Jr, Castleman B: Cases of thymoma at the Massachusetts General Hospital. J Thorac Cardiovasc Surg **52**:322-330, 1966.
146 Willcox N, Schluep M, Ritter MA, Schuurman HJ, Newsom-Davis J, Christensson B: Myasthenic and nonmyasthenic thymoma. An expansion of a minor cortical epithelial cell subset? Am J Pathol **127**:447-460, 1987.
147 Youssef S: Thymectomy for myasthenia gravis in children. J Pediatr Surg **18**:537-541, 1983.

Other associated diseases

147a Ackland SP, Bur ME, Adler SS, Robertson M, Baron JM: White blood cell aplasia associated with thymoma. Am J Clin Pathol **89**:260-263, 1988.
148 Griffin JD, Aisenberg AC, Long JC: Lymphocytic thymoma associated with T-cell lymphocytosis. Am J Med **64**:1075-1079, 1978.
149 Hirst E, Robertson TT: The syndrome of thymoma and erythroblastopenic anemia. A review of 56 cases including 3 case reports. Medicine [Baltimore] **46**:225-264, 1967.
150 Kirkpatrick CH, Windhorst DB: Mucocutaneous candidiasis and thymoma. Am J Med **66**:939-945, 1979.
151 Levin L, Sealy R, Barron J: Syndrome of inappropriate antidiuretic hormone secretion following cis-dichlorodiammineplatinum II in a patient with malignant thymoma. Cancer **50**:2279-2282, 1982.
152 Palestine RF, Su WPD, Liesegang TJ: Late-onset chronic mucocutaneous and ocular candidiasis and malignant thymoma. Arch Dermatol **119**:580-586, 1983.
153 Skinnider LF, Alexander S, Horsman D: Concurrent thymoma and lymphoma. A report of two cases. Hum Pathol **13**:163-166, 1982.
154 Souadjian JV, Silverstein MN, Titus JL: Thymoma and cancer. Cancer **22**:1221-1225, 1968.
155 Stoll DB, Lublin F, Brodovsky H, Laucius F, Patchefsky A, Cooper H: Association of subacute motor neuronopathy with thymoma. Cancer **54**:770-772, 1984.
156 Thomas J, De Wolf-Peeters C, Tricot G, Bekaert J, Broeckaert-van Orshoven A: T-cell chronic lymphocytic leukemia in a patient with invasive thymoma in remission with chemotherapy. Cancer **52**:313-317, 1983.

Ectopic hamartomatous variant

157 Rosai J, Limas C, Husband EM: Ectopic hamartomatous thymoma. A distinctive benign lesion of lower neck. Am J Surg Pathol **8**:501-513, 1984.

Malignant thymoma

158 Baud M, Stamenkovic I, Kapanci Y: Malignant thymomas. Clinicopathologic study of 13 cases. Prog Surg Pathol **3**:129-146, 1981.

159 Guillan RA, Zelman S, Smalley RL, Iglesias PA: Malignant thymoma associated with myasthenia gravis, and evidence of extrathoracic metastases. An analysis of published cases and report of a case. Cancer **27**:823-830, 1971.

160 Henry K: An unusual thymic tumour with a striated muscle (myoid) component (with a brief review of the literature on myoid cells). Br J Dis Chest **66**:291-299, 1972.

161 Lattes R: Thymoma and other tumors of the thymus. An analysis of 107 cases. Cancer **15**:1224-1260, 1962.

162 Levine GD, Rosai J: Thymic hyperplasia and neoplasia. A review of current concepts. Hum Pathol **9**:495-515, 1978.

163 Lewis JE, Wick MR, Scheithauer BW, Bernatz PE, Taylor WF: Thymoma. A clinicopathologic review. Cancer **60**:2727-2743, 1987.

164 Leyvraz S, Henle W, Chahinian AP, Perlman C, Klein G, Gordon RE, Rosenblum M, Holland JF: Association of Epstein-Barr virus with thymic carcinoma. N Engl J Med **312**:1296-1299, 1985.

164a Mukai K, Sato Y, Hirohashi S, Shimosato Y: Expression of *RAS* P21 protein by thymoma (abstract). Lab Invest **58**:65A, 1988.

165 Murakami S, Shamoto M, Miura K, Takeuchi J: A thymic tumor with massive proliferation of myoid cells. Acta Pathol Jpn **34**:1375-1383, 1984.

165a Nomori H, Horinouchi H, Kaseda S, Ishihara T, Torikata C: Evaluation of the malignant grade of thymoma by morphometric analysis. Cancer **61**:982-988, 1988.

166 Sato Y, Watanabe S, Mukai K, Kodama T, Upton MP, Goto M, Shimosato Y: An immunohistochemical study of thymic epithelial tumors. Am J Surg Pathol **10**:862-870, 1986.

167 Shimosato Y, Kameya T, Nagai K, Suemasu K: Squamous cell carcinoma of the thymus. An analysis of eight cases. Am J Surg Pathol **1**:109-121, 1977.

168 Snover DC, Levine GD, Rosai J: Thymic carcinoma. Five distinctive histologic variants. Am J Surg Pathol **6**:451-470, 1982.

169 Stephens M, Khalil J, Gibbs AR: Primary clear cell carcinoma of the thymus gland. Histopathology **11**:763-765, 1987.

170 Tanaka M, Shimokawa R, Matsubara O, Aoki N, Kamiyama R, Kasuga T, Hatakeyama S: Mucoepidermoid carcinoma of the thymic region. Acta Pathol Jpn **32**:703-712, 1982.

171 Wick MR, Nichols WC, Ingle JN, Bruckman JE, Okazaki H: Malignant, predominantly lymphocytic thymoma with central and peripheral nervous system metastases. Cancer **47**:2036-2043, 1981.

172 Wick MR, Scheithauer BW, Weiland LH, Bernatz PE: Primary thymic carcinomas. Am J Surg Pathol **6**:613-630, 1982.

173 Wolfe JT III, Wick MR, Banks PM, Scheithauer BW: Clear cell carcinoma of the thymus. Mayo Clin Proc **58**:365-370, 1983.

Treatment and prognosis

174 Chahinian AP, Bhardwaj S, Meyer RJ, Jaffrey IS, Kirschner PA, Holland JF: Treatment of invasive or metastatic thymoma. Report of eleven cases. Cancer **47**:1752-1761, 1981.

175 Fechner RE: Recurrence of noninvasive thymomas. Report of four cases and review of the literature. Cancer **23**:1423-1427, 1969.

176 Maggi G, Giaccone G, Donadio M, Ciuffreda L, Dalesio O, Leria G, Trifletti G, Casadio C, Palestro G, Mancuso M, Calciati A: Thymomas. A review of 169 cases, with particular reference to results of surgical treatment. Cancer **58**:765-776, 1986.

177 Masaoka A, Monden Y, Nakahara K, Tanioka T: Follow-up study of thymomas with special reference to their clinical stages. Cancer **48**:2485-2492, 1981.

178 Uematsu M, Kondo M: A proposal for treatment of invasive thymoma. Cancer **58**:1979-1985, 1986.

179 Verley JM, Hollmann KH: Thymoma. A comparative study of clinical stages, histologic features, and survival in 200 cases. Cancer **55**:1074-1086, 1985.

180 Wick MR, Scheithauer BW, Weiland LH, Bernatz PE: Primary thymic carcinomas. Am J Surg Pathol **6**:613-630, 1982.

Carcinoid tumor and oat cell carcinoma

181 Baker J, Holdaway IM, Jagusch M, Kerr AR, Donald RA, Pullan PT: Ectopic secretion of ACTH and met-enkephalin from a thymic carcinoid. J Endocrinol Invest **5**:33-37, 1982.

182 Fetissof F, Boivin F, Jobard P, Arbeille-Brassart B, Romet JL, Maillet M: Microfilamentous carcinoid of the thymus. Correlation of ultrastructural study with Grimelius stain. Ultrastruct Pathol **3**:9-15, 1982.

183 Herbst WM, Kummer W, Hofmann W, Otto H, Heym C: Carcinoid tumors of the thymus. An immunohistochemical study. Cancer **60**:2465-2470, 1987.

184 Ho FCS, Ho JCI: Pigmented carcinoid tumour of the thymus. Histopathology **1**:363-369, 1977.

185 Lagrange W, Dahm H-H, Karstens J, Feichtinger J, Mittermayer C: Melanocytic neuroendocrine carcinoma of the thymus. Cancer **59**:484-488, 1987.

186 Levine GD, Rosai J: A spindle cell variant of thymic carcinoid tumor. A clinical, histologic, and fine structural study with emphasis on its distinction from spindle cell thymoma. Arch Pathol **100**:293-300, 1976.

187 Penman E, Wass JAH, Besser GM, Rees LH: Somatostatin secretion by lung and thymic tumours. Clin Endocrinol **13**:613-620, 1980.

188 Rosai J, Higa E: Mediastinal endocrine neoplasm, of probable thymic origin, related to carcinoid tumor. Clinicopathologic study of 8 cases. Cancer **29**:1061-1074, 1972.

189 Rosai J, Higa E, Davie JM: Mediastinal endocrine neoplasm in patients with multiple endocrine adenomatosis. A previously unrecognized association. Cancer **29**:1075-1083, 1972.

190 Rosai J, Levine G, Weber WR, Higa E: Carcinoid tumors and oat cell carcinomas of the thymus. Pathol Annu **11**:201-226, 1976.

191 Salyer WR, Salyer DC, Eggleston JC: Carcinoid tumors of the thymus. Cancer **37**:958-973, 1976.

192 Snover DC, Levine GD, Rosai J: Thymic carcinoma. Five distinctive histological variants. Am J Surg Pathol **6**:451-470, 1982.

193 Vener JD, Zuckerbraun L, Goodman D: Carcinoid tumor of the thymus associated with a parathyroid adenoma. Arch Otolaryngol **108**:324-326, 1982.

194 Wick MR, Carney JA, Bernatz PE, Brown LR: Primary mediastinal carcinoid tumors. Am J Surg Pathol **6**:195-205, 1982.

195 Wick MR, Scheithauer BW: Oat-cell carcinoma of the thymus. Cancer **49**:1652-1657, 1982.

196 Wick MR, Scheithauer BW: Thymic carcinoid. A histologic, immunohistochemical and ultrastructural study of 12 cases. Cancer **53**:475-484, 1984.

Thymolipoma and other stromal tumors

197 Havlíček F, Rosai J: A sarcoma of thymic stroma with features of liposarcoma. Am J Clin Pathol **82**:217-224, 1984.

198 Otto HF, Löning TH, Lachenmayer L, Janzen RW Ch, Gürtler KF, Fischer K: Thymolipoma in association with myasthenia gravis. Cancer **50**:1623-1628, 1982.

199 Valderrama E, Kahn LB, Wind E: Extraskeletal osteosarcoma arising in an ectopic hamartomatous thymus. Report of a case and review of the literature. Cancer **51**:1132-1137, 1983.

GERM CELL TUMORS

200 Burns BF, McCaughey WTE: Unusual thymic seminomas. Arch Pathol Lab Med **110**:539-541, 1986.

201 Bush SE, Martinez A, Bagshaw MA: Primary mediastinal seminoma. Cancer **48**:1877-1882, 1981.

202 Carter D, Bibro MC, Touloukian RJ: Benign clinical behavior of immature mediastinal teratoma in infancy and childhood. Report of two cases and review of the literature. Cancer **49**:398-402, 1982.

203 Cox JD: Primary malignant germ cell tumors of the mediastinum. A study of 24 cases. Cancer **36**:1162-1168, 1975.

204 DeMent SH, Eggleston JC, Spivak JL: Association between mediastinal germ cell tumors and hematologic malignancies. Report of two cases and review of the literature. Am J Surg Pathol **9**:23-30, 1985.

205 Fox RM, Woods RL, Tattersall MHN, McGovern VJ: Undifferentiated carcinoma in young men. The atypical teratoma syndrome. Lancet **1**:1316-1318, 1979.

206 Gooneratne S, Keh P, Sreekanth S, Recant W, Talerman A: Anterior mediastinal endodermal sinus (yolk sac) tumor in a female infant. Cancer **56**:1430-1433, 1985.

207 Greco FA, Oldham RK, Fer MF: The extragonadal germ cell cancer syndrome. Semin Oncol **9**:448-455, 1982.

208 Greenwood SM, Goodman JR, Schneider G, Forman BH, Kress SG, Gelb AF: Choriocarcinoma in a man—the relationship of gynecomastia to chorionic somatomammotropin and estrogens. Am J Med **51**:416-422, 1971.

209 Hurt RD, Bruckman JE, Farrow GM, Bernatz PE, Hahn RG, Earle JD: Primary anterior mediastinal seminoma. Cancer **49**:1658-1663, 1982.

210 Irie T, Watanabe H, Kawaoi A, Takeuchi J: Alpha-fetoprotein (AFP), human chorionic gonadotropin (HCG), and carcinoembryonic antigen (CEA) demon-

strated in the immature glands of mediastinal teratocarcinoma. A case report. Cancer 50:1160-1165, 1982.

211 Kuzur ME, Cobleigh MA, Greco FA, Einhorn LH, Oldham RK: Endodermal sinus tumor of the mediastinum. Cancer 50:766-774, 1982.

212 Lachman MF, Kim K, Koo B-C: Mediastinal teratoma associated with Klinefelter's syndrome. Arch Pathol Lab Med 110:1067-1071, 1986.

213 Laipply TC, Shipley RA: Extragenital choriocarcinoma in the male. Am J Pathol 21:921-933, 1945.

214 Larsen M, Evans WK, Shepherd FA, Phillips MJ, Bailey D, Messner H: Acute lymphoblastic leukemia. Possible origin from a mediastinal germ cell tumor. Cancer 53:441-444, 1984.

215 Lee YM, Jackson SM: Primary seminoma of the mediastinum. Cancer Control Agency of British Columbia experience. Cancer 55:450-452, 1985.

216 Levine GD: Primary thymic seminoma. A neoplasm ultrastructurally similar to testicular seminoma and distinct from epithelial thymoma. Cancer 31:729-741, 1973.

217 Luna MA, Valenzuela-Tamril J: Germ cell tumors of the mediastinum. Postmortem findings. Am J Clin Pathol 65:450-454, 1976.

218 Manivel C, Wick MR, Abenoza P, Rosai J: The occurrence of sarcomatous components in primary mediastinal germ cell tumors. Am J Surg Pathol 10:711-717, 1986.

219 McNeil MM, Leong AS-Y, Sage RE: Primary mediastinal embryonal carcinoma in association with Klinefelter's syndrome. Cancer 47:343-345, 1981.

220 Mukai K, Adams WR: Yolk sac tumor of the anterior mediastinum. Am J Surg Pathol 3:77-83, 1979.

221 Oberman HA, Libcke JH: Malignant germinal neoplasms of the mediastinum. Cancer 17:498-507, 1964.

222 Parker D, Holford CP, Begent RHJ, Newlands ES, Rustin GJS, Makey AR, Bagshawe KD: Effective treatment for malignant mediastinal teratoma. Thorax 38:897-902, 1983.

223 Sandhaus L, Strom RL, Mukai K: Primary embryonal-choriocarcinoma of the mediastinum in a woman. A case report with immunohistochemical study. Am J Clin Pathol 75:573-578, 1981.

224 Schlumberger HG: Teratoma of the anterior mediastinum in the group of military age. A study of sixteen cases and a review of theories of genesis. Arch Pathol 41:398-444, 1946.

225 Shantz A, Sewall W, Castleman B: Mediastinal germinoma. A study of 21 cases with an excellent prognosis. Cancer 30:1189-1194, 1972.

226 Sickels EA, Belliveau RE, Wiernik PH: Primary mediastinal choriocarcinoma in the male. Cancer 33:1196-1203, 1974.

227 Southgate J, Slade PR: Teratodermoid cyst of the mediastinum with pancreatic enzyme secretion. Thorax 37:476-477, 1982.

228 Suda K, Mizuguchi K, Hebisawa A, Wakabayashi T, Saito S: Pancreatic tissue in teratoma. Arch Pathol Lab Med 108:835-837, 1984.

229 Teilmann I, Kassis H, Pietra G: Primary germ cell tumor of the anterior mediastinum with features of endodermal sinus tumor (mesoblastoma vitellinum). Acta Pathol Microbiol Scand 70:267-278, 1967.

230 Truong LD, Harris L, Mattioli C, Hawkins E, Lee A, Wheeler T, Lane M: Endodermal sinus tumor of the mediastinum. A report of seven cases and review of the literature. Cancer 58:730-739, 1986.

231 Ulbright TM, Loehrer PJ, Roth LM, Einhorn LH, Williams SD, Clark SA: The development of non-germ cell malignancies within germ cell tumors. A clinicopathologic study of 11 cases. Cancer 54:1824-1833, 1984.

232 Wenger ME, Dines DE, Ahmann DL, Good CA: Primary mediastinal choriocarcinoma. Mayo Clin Proc 43:570-575, 1968.

MALIGNANT LYMPHOMA

233 Bonfiglio TA, Dvoretsky PM, Piscioli F, dePapp EW, Patten SF Jr: Fine needle aspiration biopsy in the evaluation of lymphoreticular tumors of the thorax. Acta Cytol [Baltimore] 29:548-553, 1985.

234 Lichtenstein AK, Levine A, Taylor CT, Boswell W, Rossman S, Feinstein DI, Lukes RJ: Primary mediastinal lymphoma in adults. Am J Med 68:509-514, 1980.

235 Van Heerden JA, Harrison EG Jr, Bernatz PE, Kiely JM: Mediastinal malignant lymphoma. Chest 57:518-529, 1970.

Hodgkin's disease

236 Baron RL, Sagel SS, Baglan RJ: Thymic cysts following radiation therapy for Hodgkin disease. Radiology 141:593-597, 1981.

237 Burke WA, Burford TH, Dorfman RF: Hodgkin's disease in the mediastinum. J Thorac Cardiovasc Surg 3:287-296, 1967.

238 Fechner RE: Hodgkin's disease of the thymus. Cancer 23:16-23, 1969.

239 Katz A, Lattes R: Granulomatous thymoma or Hodgkin's disease of thymus? A clinical and histologic study and a re-evaluation. Cancer 23:1-15, 1969.

240 Keller AR, Castleman B: Hodgkin's disease of the thymus gland. Cancer 33:1615-1623, 1974.

241 Kim HC, Nosher J, Haas A, Sweeney W, Lewis R: Cystic degeneration of thymic Hodgkin's disease following radiation therapy. Cancer 55:354-356, 1985.

242 Lowenhaupt E, Brown R: Carcinoma of the thymus of granulomatous type. Cancer 4:1193-1209, 1951.

243 Nickels J, Franssila K, Hjelt L: Thymoma and Hodgkin's disease of the thymus. Acta Pathol Microbiol Scand [A] 81:1-5, 1973.

244 Null JA, LiVolsi VA, Glenn WWL: Hodgkin's disease of the thymus (granulomatous thymoma) and myasthenia gravis. A unique association. Am J Clin Pathol 67:521-525, 1977.

245 Remigio PA: Granulomatous thymoma associated with erythroid hypoplasia. Am J Clin Pathol 55:68-72, 1971.

246 Smith PLC, Jobling C, Rees A: Hodgkin's disease in a large thymic cyst in a child. Thorax 38:392-393, 1983.

247 Van Heerden JA, Harrison EG Jr, Bernatz PE, Kiely JM: Mediastinal malignant lymphoma. Chest 57:518-529, 1970.

Lymphoblastic lymphoma

248 Banerjee D, Silva E: Mediastinal mass with acute leukemia. Myeloblastoma masquerading as lymphoblastic lymphoma. Arch Pathol Lab Med 105:126-129, 1981.

249 Ha K, Minden M, Hozumi N, Gelfand EW: Phenotypic heterogeneity at the DNA level in childhood leukemia with a mediastinal mass. Cancer 56:509-513, 1985.

250 Kubonishi I, Ohtsuki Y, Machida K-I, Agatsuma Y, Tokuoka H, Iwata K, Miyoshi I: Granulocytic sarcoma presenting as a mediastinal tumor. Report of a case and cytological and cytochemical studies of tumor cells in vivo and in vitro. Am J Clin Pathol 82:730-734, 1984.

251 Nathwani BN, Kim H, Rappaport H: Malignant lymphoma, lymphoblastic. Cancer 38:964-983, 1976.

Large cell lymphoma

252 Addis BJ, Isaacson PG: Large cell lymphoma of the mediastinum. A B-cell tumor of probable thymic origin. Histopathology 10:379-390, 1986.

253 Levitt LJ, Aisenberg AC, Harris NL, Linggood RM, Poppema S: Primary non-Hodgkin's lymphoma of the mediastinum. Cancer 50:2486-2492, 1982.

254 Menestrina F, Chilosi M, Bonetti F, Lestani M, Scarpa A, Novelli P, Doglioni C, Todeschini G, Ambrosetti A, Fiore-Donati L: Mediastinal large-cell lymphoma of B-type, with sclerosis. Histopathological and immunohistochemical study of eight cases. Histopathology 10:589-600, 1986.

255 Miller JB, Variakojis D, Bitran JD, Sweet DL, Kinzie JJ, Golomb HM, Ultmann JE: Diffuse histiocytic lymphoma with sclerosis. A clinicopathologic entity frequently causing superior venacaval obstruction. Cancer 47:748-756, 1981.

256 Möller P, Lämmler B, Eberlein-Gonska M, Feichter GE, Hofmann WJ, Schmitteckert H, Otto HF: Primary mediastinal clear cell lymphoma of B-cell type. Virchows Arch [Pathol Anat] 409:79-92, 1986.

257 Perrone T, Frizzera G, Rosai J: Mediastinal diffuse large-cell lymphoma with sclerosis. A clinicopathologic study of 60 cases. Am J Surg Pathol 10:176-191, 1986.

258 Trump DL, Mann RB: Diffuse large cell and undifferentiated lymphomas with prominent mediastinal involvement. A poor prognostic subset of patients with non-Hodgkin's lymphoma. Cancer 50:277-282, 1982.

259 Waldron JA Jr, Dohring EJ, Farber LR: Primary large cell lymphomas of the mediastinum. An analysis of 20 cases, Semin Diagn Pathol 2:281-295, 1985.

260 Yousem SA, Weiss LM, Warnke RA: Primary mediastinal non-Hodgkin's lymphomas. A morphologic and immunologic study of 19 cases. Am J Clin Pathol 83:676-680, 1985.

NEUROGENIC TUMORS

261 Perez CA, Vietti T, Ackerman LV, Eagleton MD, Powers WE: Tumors of the sympathetic nervous system in children. An appraisal of treatment and results. Radiology 88:750-760, 1967.

262 Reed JC, Hallet KK, Feigin DS: Neural tumors of the thorax. Subject review from the AFIP. Radiology 126:9-17, 1978.

263 Schweisguth O, Mathey J, Renault P, Binet JP: Intrathoracic neurogenic tumors in infants and children. A study of forty cases. Am Surg 150:29-41, 1959.

264 Talerman A, Gratama S: Primary ganglioneuroblastoma of the anterior mediastinum in a 61-year-old woman. Histopathology 7:967-975, 1983.

Tumors of sympathetic nervous system

265 Adam A, Hochholzer L: Ganglioneuroblastoma of the posterior mediastinum. A clinicopathologic review of 80 cases. Cancer **47**:373-381, 1981.

266 Carachi R, Campbell PE, Kent M: Thoracic neural crest tumors. A clinical review. Cancer **51**:949-954, 1983.

267 King RM, Telander RL, Smithson WA, Banks PM, Han M-T: Primary mediastinal tumors in children. J Pediatr Surg **17**:512-520, 1982.

268 Schweisguth O, Mathey J, Renault P, Binet JP: Intrathoracic neurogenic tumors in infants and children. A study of forty cases. Am Surg **150**:29-41, 1959.

269 Young DG: Thoracic neuroblastoma/ganglioneuroma. J Pediatr Surg **18**:37-41, 1983.

270 Wahl HR, Craig PE: Multiple tumors of the sympathetic nervous system. Am J Pathol **14**:797-808, 1938.

Tumors of peripheral nerves

271 Ackerman LV, Taylor FH: Neurogenous tumors within the thorax. A clinical pathologic evaluation of forty-eight cases. Cancer **4**:669-691, 1951.

272 Oberman HA, Abell MR: Neurogenous neoplasms of the mediastinum. Cancer **13**:882-898, 1960.

273 Reed JC, Hallet KK, Feigin DS: Neural tumors of the thorax. Subject review from the AFIP. Radiology **126**:9-17, 1978.

TUMORS OF PARAGANGLIA

274 Ogawa J, Inoue H, Koide S, Kawada S, Shohtsu A, Hata J: Functioning paraganglioma in the posterior mediastinum. Ann Thorac Surg **33**:507-510, 1982.

275 Olson JL, Salyer WR: Mediastinal paragangliomas (aortic body tumor). A report of four cases and a review of the literature. Cancer **41**:2405-2412, 1978.

276 Pachter MR: Mediastinal nonchromaffin paraganglioma. A clinicopathological study based on eight cases. J Thorac Cardiovasc Surg **45**:152-160, 1963.

MESENCHYMAL TUMORS

277 Awotwi JD, Zusman J, Waring WW, Beckerman RC: Benign hemangioendothelioma—a rare type of posterior mediastinal mass in children. J Pediatr Surg **18**:581-584, 1983.

278 Brown LR, Reiman HM, Rosenow EC III, Gloviczki PM, Divertie MB: Intrathoracic lymphangioma. Mayo Clin Proc **61**:882-892, 1986.

279 Chen W, Chan CW, Mok CK: Malignant fibrous histiocytoma of the mediastinum. Cancer **50**:797-800, 1982.

280 Dudgeon DL, Haller JA Jr: Pediatric lipoblastomatosis. Two unusual cases. Surgery **95**:371-373, 1984.

281 Gibbs AR, Johnson NF, Giddings JC, Powell DEB, Jasani B: Primary angiosarcoma of the mediastinum. Light and electron microscopic demonstration of factor VIII–related antigen in neoplastic cells. Hum Pathol **15**:687-691, 1984.

282 Gremmel H, Rotthoff F, Willmann KH: Intrathorakale lipome. Thoraxchirurgie **6**:75-85, 1958.

283 Homer MJ, Wechsler RJ, Carter BL: Mediastinal lipomatosis. CT confirmation of a normal variant. Radiology **128**:657-661, 1978.

284 Manivel C, Wick MR, Abenoza P, Rosai J: The occurrence of sarcomatous components in primary mediastinal germ cell tumors. Am J Surg Pathol **10**:711-717, 1986.

285 Pachter MR, Lattes R: Mesenchymal tumors of the mediastinum. Cancer **16**:74-94; 95-107; 108-117, 1963.

286 Standerfer RJ, Armistead SH, Paneth M: Liposarcoma of the mediastinum. Report of two cases and review of the literature. Thorax **36**:693-694, 1981.

287 Sunderrajan EV, Luger AM, Rosenholtz MJ, Maltby JD: Leiomyosarcoma in the mediastinum presenting as superior vena cava syndrome. Cancer **53**:2553-2556, 1984.

288 Svane H, Ottosen P: Cavernous haemangioma of the mediastinum. A rare tumor form. Acta Chir Scand **118**:405-408, 1960.

289 Witkin GB, Rosai J: A biphasic tumor of the mediastinum with features of synovial sarcoma. A report of four cases (abstract). Lab Invest **58**:104A, 1988.

290 Witkin GB, Rosai J: Solitary fibrous tumor of the mediastinum. A report of fourteen cases (abstract). Lab Invest **58**:104A, 1988.

OTHER PRIMARY TUMORS AND TUMORLIKE CONDITIONS

291 Karcher DS, Pearson CE, Butler WM, Hurwitz MA, Cassell PF: Giant lymph node hyperplasia involving the thymus with associated nephrotic syndrome and myelofibrosis. Am J Clin Pathol **77**:100-104, 1982.

292 Keller AR, Hockholzer L, Castleman B: Hyaline-vascular and plasma-cell types of giant lymph node hyperplasia of mediastinum and other locations. Cancer **29**:670-683, 1972.

293 Verani R, Olson J, Moake JL: Intrathoracic extramedullary hematopoiesis. Report of a case in a patient with sickle-cell disease-β-thalassemia. Am J Clin Pathol **73**:133-138, 1980.

294 Wilson AJ, Ratliff JL, Lagios MD, Aguilar MJ: Mediastinal meningioma. Am J Surg Pathol **3**:557-562, 1979.

METASTATIC TUMORS

295 Lindell MM, Doubleday LC, Von Eschenbach AC, Libshitz HI: Mediastinal metastases from prostatic carcinoma. J Urol **128**:331-334, 1982.

296 McLoud TC, Kalisher L, Stark P, Green R: Intrathoracic lymph node metastases from extrathoracic neoplasms. AJR **131**:403-407, 1978.

9 Thyroid gland

NORMAL ANATOMY

The thyroid gland is made up of follicles that vary considerably in size, with an average diameter of 200 μm. They are lined by a single layer of follicular cells whose shape ranges from flattened to cuboidal depending on the degree of activity. The cytoplasm has a pale acidophilic or amphophilic staining quality; the greater the activity of the cell, the greater its amount. Follicular cells with abundant granular acidophilic cytoplasm are referred to as Hürthle cells (a misnomer), Askanazy's cells, oxyphilic cells, or oncocytes. Ultrastructurally, this granularity is due to the accumulation of mitochondria.

The main ultrastructural features of follicular cells are secretory granules containing thyroglobulin and prominent microvilli in the luminal border.[4] The intraluminal colloid is pale staining and has scalloped borders in follicles with active secretory function and is densely eosinophilic in inactive ones. In old age, it tends to be broken up in globular formations. It is variably PAS-positive and alcianophilic, depending on the types and relative amounts of carbohydrate components present.[13] Birefringent calcium oxalate crystals may be found, their number increasing with age.[12] Collections of small follicles protruding into the lumen of larger follicles are commonly seen in actively secreting glands; they are sometimes referred to as Sanderson's polsters.

Immunohistochemically, reactivity for thyroglobulin, T3, and T4 is found both in the colloid and in the cytoplasm of the follicular cells.[3,11,14] Thyroglobulin is the most useful of these three markers, especially when it is searched for with monoclonal antibodies.[5,14] A lesser degree of reactivity is found in Hürthle cells. Follicular cells are also positive for low molecular weight keratin, EMA, and vimentin.[1] The follicles rest on a basement membrane that is positive for laminin and the other components of this structure.[8]

Between and within the follicles are collections of endocrine cells of neural crest derivation known as C-cells or parafollicular cells. They predominate in the central portion of the lateral lobes; in old age, they increase in number and may form small nodules.[10] Under normal conditions, there should be no more than five per follicle. Ultrastructurally, they contain numerous dense-core granules of neurosecretory type.[16] Immunohistochemically, they show reactivity for calcitonin and CEA, although the latter marker seems to be expressed in lesser amounts than in hyperplastic or neoplastic disorders of C-cells[15] (see Color plate I, D).

Focal collections of lymphocytes are seen at autopsy in the thyroid of about one half of females and one fourth of males; this finding is regarded as a subclinical manifestation of focal lymphocytic thyroiditis.[9]

Small solid epithelial nests can occur in the thyroid.[7] Some represent metaplastic follicles, others are small collections of C-cells, and still others may be rests related to the thyroglossal duct or the neighboring branchial arches. Occasionally, thymic or parathyroid tissue is found in an intrathyroid location.[2]

The occasional occurrence of a pitch black thyroid is a rather dramatic gross finding, but this is simply due to the accumulation of melanin-like pigment in the follicular cell cytoplasm in old age or, in its most advanced form, in patients on long-term minocycline therapy.[6]

CONGENITAL ABNORMALITIES

The thyroid anlage appears in the embryo as a midline structure at the site corresponding to the foramen cecum of the adult tongue. From here, the thyroglossal duct descends along the cervical midline to reach its final position in the midneck.[25] Later, the hyoid bone is formed from the second branchial arch. The thyroglossal duct usually passes anteriorly to the bone and is divided by it into a suprahyoid and an infrahyoid portion. In the normal course of events, the thyroglossal duct is obliterated and disappears.[39]

Thyroglossal duct cyst represents a localized persistence of this structure in the midline of the neck, in the region of the hyoid bone [17,22] (Fig. 9-1). It is more common in childhood, but it may assume clinical significance later in life.[20,37] The cystic change develops because of secretion from the lining cells.

The cyst may connect through a sinus tract with the foramen cecum and become infected as a result. Sinuses can also develop from the region of the hyoid bone to the skin at the level of the suprasternal notch.[34] Microscopically, the cyst is lined by pseudostratified ciliated or squamous epithelium (Fig. 9-2). Mucous glands and thyroid follicles are commonly seen in the subjacent stroma. Secondary inflammatory changes are usually present.[38]

Treatment is surgical. It is important to include in the excision the middle third of the hyoid bone to minimize recurrence.[23] If the sinus tract extends to the foramen cecum, it should be removed in its entire length.

The thyroid tissue located in these cysts can undergo neoplastic changes, nearly always in the form of papillary carcinoma.[26,27,29] The prognosis is excellent following local excision; it is not necessary to remove the thyroid gland. Other tumor types have been rarely described, including undifferentiated (anaplastic) carcinoma.[33]

Heterotopic thyroid tissue can be found anywhere along the course of the thyroglossal duct (Fig. 9-3). The most frequent location is the base of the tongue, where it may result in difficulty in swallowing and respiratory obstruction, which in a few cases has proved fatal. At a microscopic

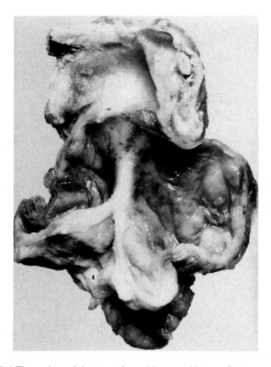

Fig. 9-1 Thyroglossal duct cyst from 62-year-old man. Cyst measured 6 cm × 6 cm.

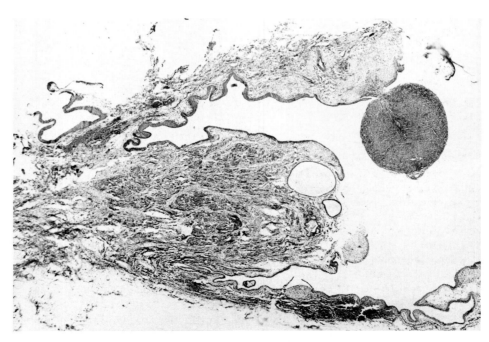

Fig. 9-2 Thyroglossal duct cyst. Note lymphoid tissue, epithelial lining, and cystic spcaes.

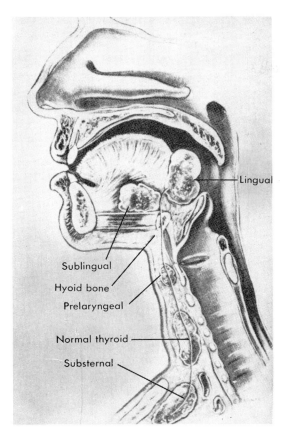

Fig. 9-3 Distribution of heterotopic thyroid tissue. (From Lemmon WT, Paschal GW Jr: Lingual thyroid. Am J Surg **52:**82-85, 1941.)

subclinical level, lingual thyroid is found in 10% of all individuals.[35] Grossly and microscopically, the heterotopic thyroid does not differ from that seen in the main gland. Sometimes a capsule is formed around it; in other instances, the follicles grow between the skeletal muscle of the tongue, a feature that may simulate invasion by tumor.[40] In 70% of the patients with grossly evident lingual thyroid there is absence of the normal thyroid gland. Therefore removal of the heterotopic thyroid tissue will lead to hypothyroidism, requiring subsequent medical therapy.

Other sites of heterotopic thyroid tissue are the anterior tongue, larynx, mediastinum (usually superior but sometimes posterior), and heart.[28] The common denominator in all these sites is their location in or close to the midline, the large majority being found in the so-called Woelfler's area, described by anatomists as an isosceles triangle with the edge of the mandible at its base and the concavity of the aortic arch at its apex. The possible occurrence of heterotopic thyroid tissue in cervical nodes is discussed on p. 434.

Branchial cleft defects are not thyroid-related anomalies but are discussed here because of their close proximity to the gland.[41] They may present as a patent fistula, a simple sinus, a blind cyst, or an island of cartilage[19,31] (Fig. 9-4). They are located in the anterolateral region of the neck, their exact position depending on the specific branchial cleft involved. Those related to the first cleft appear in the preauricular area or beneath the posterior half of the mandible and may be connected to the external auditory canal. Those related to the second cleft appear just anterior to the sternocleidomastoid muscle in the midneck and may have an open tract communicating with the pharynx near the superior fold of the tonsil.[30] Those related to the third and fourth

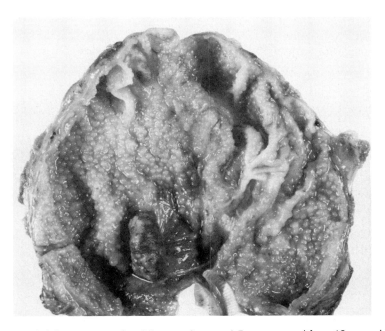

Fig. 9-4 Branchial cleft cyst measuring 4.5 cm × 3 cm × 1.5 cm removed from 18-year-old youth. It has been opened to expose inner surface. This is made irregular by presence of folds and innumerable hyperplastic lymphoid follicles.

arches are typically found in the lower neck, in a supra-sternal or supraclavicular location.

The lining of these cysts and fistulous tracts is usually squamous epithelium, but columnar ciliated epithelium is also common. Abundant lymphoid tissue, often with germinal centers, is observed beneath. Mucinous and sero-mucinous glands can also occur.[36] Infection may complicate the microscopic picture. Epidermoid cancers arising in a branchial cleft cyst probably exist, but they are exceptionally rare.[18] Any cystic mass in the neck containing squamous cancer must be considered a lymph node metastasis with cystic degeneration until proved otherwise.[21,32]

Branchial cleft remnants are sometimes found inside the thyroid in the form of heterotopic cartilage or thymic tissue.[24] Parenthetically, the presence of normal or cystic thymic tissue in the neck also represents a branchial cleft–derived anomaly (see Chapter 8).

THYROIDITIS
Acute thyroiditis

Acute thyroiditis is usually of infectious nature and is often associated with acute infections of the upper aerodigestive tract. *Streptococcus hemolyticus*, *Staphylococcus aureus*, and *Pneumococcus* are the organisms most commonly responsible.[42,43] Grossly and microscopically, nonsuppurative and suppurative forms have been described, the latter sometimes evolving into an abscess.

Medical treatment of acute thyroiditis is usually effective, but abscesses need to be drained surgically.

Granulomatous (de Quervain's) thyroiditis

Granulomatous thyroiditis, also known as de Quervain's or subacute thyroiditis, typically presents in young women with sore throat, painful deglutition, and marked tenderness on palpation in the thyroid region.[44] Once the acute process has subsided, pressure symptoms and/or mild hypothyroidism may develop. Because of these manifestations and the sometimes asymmetric involvement of the gland, the disease may be clinically confused with carcinoma. Elevated serum levels of T4 and T3 in combination with complete suppression of ^{131}I uptake is typical of the initial phase of this disease.

Grossly, the process usually involves the entire gland, but the enlargement is often asymmetric. In a typical case, the gland is enlarged approximately twice its normal size. In the advanced stage, the involved areas are firm (Fig. 9-5). In contrast to Riedel's thyroiditis, there is usually little or no adherence to the surrounding structures.

Microscopically, areas of marked inflammation and foreign body giant cell–containing granulomas are present. It is characteristic for these granulomas to surround follicles and for the giant cells to engulf colloid (Fig. 9-6). The granulomas are not very distinct, and caseation necrosis is consistently absent. Different stages of the same process may be seen in the same gland.[46]

The etiology is not known. Although the disease often follows an infection of the upper aerodigestive tract, the thyroiditis itself is of nonbacterial nature.[45] A viral etiology has been often suggested but not proven.[47]

Other granulomatous inflammations

Tuberculosis as a primary clinical manifestation within the thyroid gland is a pathologic curiosity. In disseminated miliary tuberculosis, it is common for an occasional tubercle to occur within the gland. It is also possible for tuberculosis of cervical lymph nodes or larynx to involve the thyroid gland secondarily. Many of the cases diagnosed in the past as tuberculosis of the thyroid were actually examples of granulomatous (de Quervain's) thyroiditis.

Mycoses of various types have been described. The lesions of actinomycosis are suppurative and characterized by a generally indolent clinical course.[49]

Syphilis of the thyroid may be seen in the tertiary phase of the disease, but the process is extremely rare nowadays. Grossly, the lesion is asymmetric and frequently hard. It may cause fixation of the gland to the surrounding structures

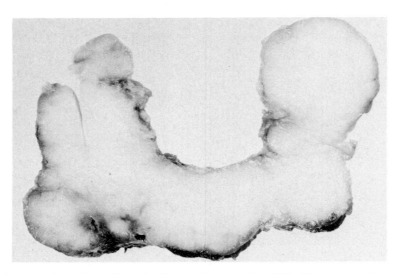

Fig. 9-5 Cross section of thyroid gland with granulomatous thyroiditis. Note preservation of normal symmetry and presence of capsule. Patient had minimal pressure signs and symptoms.

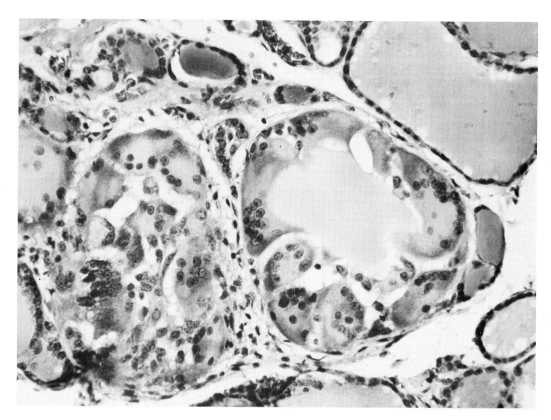

Fig. 9-6 Focus of granulomatous thyroiditis. Note intimate relation and formation of giant cells around colloid.

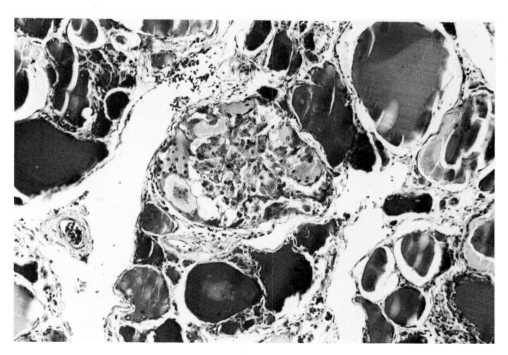

Fig. 9-7 Multifocal granulomatous thyroiditis (so-called palpation thyroiditis). Several small granulomas are present involving individual follicles. They are mainly composed of macrophages and lymphocytes, with occasional multinucleated giant cells.

and even paralysis of the recurrent laryngeal nerve, thus simulating carcinoma clinically. Microscopically, the lesion is a nodular granulomatous reaction rich in plasma cells and multinucleated giant cells, often associated with coagulative ("gummatous") necrosis and vasculitis.

Multifocal granulomatous thyroiditis is the term given to a relatively common, clinically insignificant and grossly inconspicuous thyroid process in which collections of histiocytes (some of them foamy), lymphocytes, and a few multinucleated giant cells are seen within the lumen of scattered thyroid follicles (Fig. 9-7). In some of these follicles, the inflammatory infiltrate disrupts the epithelium and extends into the perifollicular region. These changes bear no relationship to granulomatous (de Quervain's) thyroiditis. Carney et al.[48] believe that they result from rupture of follicles caused by palpation of the gland and therefore also refer to this process as *palpation thyroiditis*.

Lymphocytic thyroiditis

Lymphocytic thyroiditis is a common cause of goiter in children.[51] It can be accurately diagnosed by needle biopsy.[53] Patients with this condition usually present with asymptomatic goiter, often of short duration. A few complain of transient hyperthyroidism,[52] which may result from disruption of the gland by the inflammatory process, with release of stored hormone into the circulation. In contrast with Graves' disease, the radioactive iodine uptake is low.[50]

Grossly, there is diffuse enlargement of the gland and increased consistency (Fig. 9-8). Microscopically, there is extensive lymphocytic infiltration, germinal centers often being present. The feature distinguishing it from Hashimoto's disease is the absence or inconspicuousness of oxyphilic epithelial changes.

It is now generally agreed that lymphocytic and Hashimoto's thyroiditis are different clinicopathologic expressions of the same process. The common occurrence of transitional forms supports this concept. Some authors use the two terms as synonymous, and others lump the two conditions under the term *autoimmune thyroiditis*.

Hashimoto's thyroiditis

Hashimoto's thyroiditis, also known as autoimmune thyroiditis and struma lymphomatosa, is predominantly a disease of women over 40 years of age.[60,66] It presents as diffuse firm thyroid enlargement, sometimes accompanied by signs of tracheal or esophageal compression. Initially the disease may be accompanied by mild hyperthyroidism and later by hypothyroidism. At surgery, the thyroid gland is easily separated from other structures. The fascial attachment between the thyroid gland and the tracheal wall is, at times, slightly thickened, but there is no strong fixation. Because of the firm character of the lesion, it may be confused with carcinoma, but the diffuse involvement without fixation to the surrounding structures should be strong evidence against it.

Grossly, the typical case shows diffuse enlargement of the gland. However, in some instances one lobe is more enlarged than the other, and in others the disease has a distinctly multinodular quality. The consistency is firm but not stony hard as in Riedel's thyroiditis. There is no extension of the process outside the gland. The cut surface is friable, vaguely or distinctly nodular, yellowish gray, and greatly resembles a hyperplastic lymph node (Fig. 9-9). Colloid is not clearly discernible. Necrosis and calcification are absent.

Microscopically, the two main diagnostic criteria are lymphocytic infiltration of the stroma and oxyphilic change of the follicular epithelium. The lymphoid tissue is distributed within and around the lobules, and it invariably exhibits large follicles with prominent germinal centers. Plasma cells, histiocytes, and scattered intrafollicular multinu-

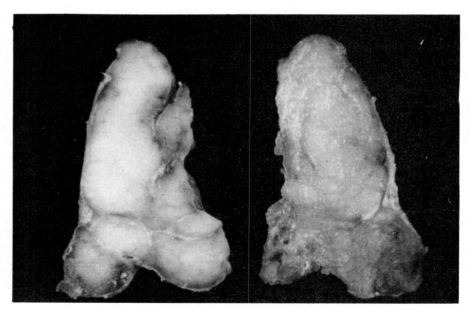

Fig. 9-8 Gross appearance of lymphocytic thyroiditis. Vaguely nodular white appearance of gland is due to replacement of parenchyma by mature lymphocytes.

cleated giant cells can be present. Ultrastructurally, some of the latter have been found to be of epithelial and others of histiocytic nature.[64] The plasma cell population has been found to be polyclonal by immunohistochemical and gene rearrangement techniques.[55,65]

The thyroid follicles are small and atrophic. Most or all of them are lined by variably sized Hürthle cells. The nuclei of these cells may show enlargement and hyperchromasia or, conversely, an optically clear appearance and overlapping quality reminiscent of papillary carcinoma (Fig. 9-10). Squamous nests thought to arise from metaplasia of follic-

ular cells are common and can reach sizable proportions. Rarely, large cysts lined by squamous epithelium and bordered by a row of lymphoid follicles are seen, their appearance being highly reminiscent of branchial cleft cysts.[65a]

In the typical case of Hashimoto's thyroiditis, connective tissue is scanty, with slight or moderate thickening of the interlobular septa. In the *fibrous variant* of this disease, which comprises about 12% of all cases, fibrosis is more extensive. In contrast to Riedel's thyroiditis, this fibrosis is of dense hyaline type (instead of the active proliferative

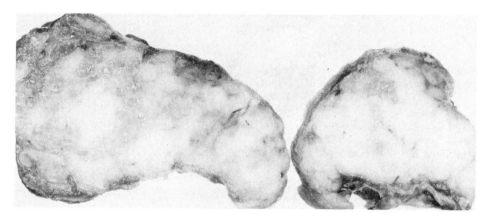

Fig. 9-9 Hashimoto's disease in child demonstrating homogenous yellowish gray areas, representing increased lymphoid tissue.

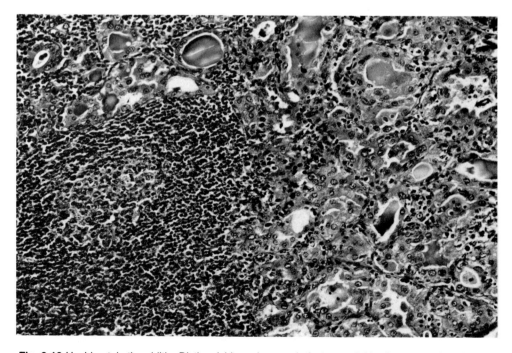

Fig. 9-10 Hashimoto's thyroiditis. Distinguishing microscopic features of this disease are lymphocytic infiltration with germinal center formation and oxyphilic change of follicular epithelium.

fibrosis seen in the latter) and does not extend beyond the thyroid capsule. It can be confused with carcinoma when the fibrosis is associated with epithelial islands showing squamous metaplasia.[63] Clinically, this variant is characterized by a very firm goiter (often with sudden enlargement), severe pressure symptoms, physical signs suggestive of cancer, and markedly elevated tanned red cell antibody titer to thyroglobulin.[63]

The differential diagnosis of the ordinary form of Hashimoto's thyroiditis includes lymphocytic thyroiditis and diffuse hyperplasia. In this regard, it should be remembered that the majority of the follicles should exhibit oxyphilic changes for a diagnosis of Hashimoto's thyroiditis to be made.[68]

The pathogenesis of this disease is clearly immune-mediated, involving humoral and cellular events.[57,71,73] Circulating autoantibodies exist against thyroglobulin and other follicular cell antigens, such as thyrotropin receptors. It has been suggested that the main factor resulting in autoimmune thyroid disease, including Hashimoto's thyroiditis, is an organ-specific defect in suppressor T lymphocytes.[54] The possible role of aberrant HLA-DR antigen expression on the membrane of the follicular cells remains controversial.[54,56] Parenthetically, it should be noted that a milder elevation of antithyroglobulin autoantibodies is also seen in other thyroid diseases associated with lymphocytic infiltration, such as Graves' disease, "toxic" adenoma, and nodular hyperplasia.[67] Indeed, a pathogenetic relationship has been postulated between Graves' disease and Hashimoto's disease, one evolving into the latter through a transition stage sharing features of both disorders (so-called *hashitoxicosis*).[61,72] According to this interpretation, there is an immune-mediated insult that leads initially to diffuse or nodular hyperactivity of the gland and eventually to exhaustion atrophy, manifested by diffuse oxyphilia.[70] Occasionally, Hashimoto's thyroiditis is seen in association with adrenal insufficiency due to adrenalitis, a condition known as *Schmidt's syndrome*.[58]

Complications of Hashimoto's thyroiditis include malignant lymphoma and leukemia[62] (see p. 437), papillary carcinoma (see p. 407), and Hürthle cell neoplasms (see p. 417). Since all three of these conditions evolve gradually from a setting of hyperplasia of the respective cell component, their early identification may be extremely difficult. This probably explains the remarkable difference in the reported figures for these complications, particularly the latter two.[59] In this regard, the occurrence of sometimes striking nuclear clearing and overlapping in the cells of Hashimoto's thyroiditis is of interest; one wonders whether this might not represent a precursor (preneoplastic) stage of papillary carcinoma. Medullary carcinoma has also been described in thyroid glands with Hashimoto's thyroiditis, but the occurrence is probably coincidental.[74]

The treatment of Hashimoto's thyroiditis depends on its severity. In mild cases no therapy is needed. In some, thyroid hormone is given to relieve hypothyroidism. In still others, surgery in the form of subtotal thyroidectomy is performed because of large size and/or pressure symptoms. Actually, many cases of Hashimoto's thyroiditis are treated surgically because they are clinically confused with a neoplastic process.[69]

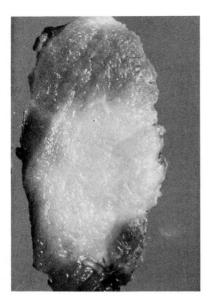

Fig. 9-11 Riedel's thyroiditis. Diffuse fibrotic process involves thyroid gland and surrounding tissues and obliterates anatomic boundaries.

Riedel's thyroiditis

Riedel's thyroiditis, also known as Riedel's struma and invasive thyroiditis, is an extremely rare disorder that affects adult and elderly patients and shows a slight predilection for females.[77,78] Clinically, it presents with ill-defined thyroid enlargement often associated with profound dyspnea. The lesion, which is extremely firm, binds the soft tissues of the neck in an iron collar and may compress the trachea to a slit-like state. Clinically, it is often thought to be carcinoma. In contrast to granulomatous thyroiditis, it is not preceded by an acute inflammatory process or by tenderness of the thyroid gland. The regional lymph nodes are not involved. Grossly, the process is asymmetric and involves only localized areas of the thyroid gland (Fig. 9-11). The affected portion is stony hard and cuts with great resistance. Dense fibrous tracts extend from the thyroid capsule into adjacent muscle, so that at surgery the tissue planes are obliterated. On cross section, areas with complete obliteration of the architecture alternate with others having a nearly normal appearance.

Microscopically, fibrous tissue that is frequently extensively hyalinized completely replaces the area of the gland involved (Fig. 9-12). Muscle cells in the immediate area are often directly infiltrated by this connective tissue. Giant cells are absent. The inflammation present is patchy and of mononuclear type, with a predominance of lymphocytes and plasma cells. IgA-producing cells are abundant among the latter.[76] Collections of eosinophils may also be present. Medium-sized veins encased by the fibrosis may show inflammation of their wall, an important diagnostic feature.[76] The main differential diagnosis is with the fibrous form of Hashimoto's thyroiditis, which is limited to the thyroid, distinctly lobulated, and accompanied by extensive oxyphilic changes of the follicular epithelium.

Riedel's thyroiditis is not related to either Hashimoto's

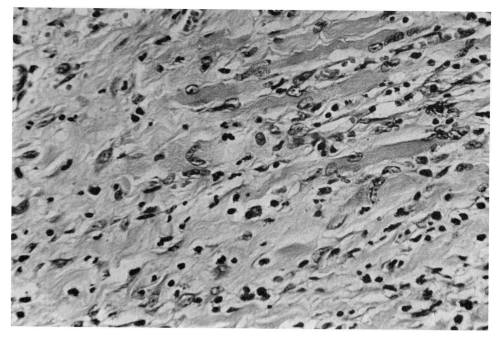

Fig. 9-12 Riedel's thyroiditis with extensive fibrosis and chronic inflammatory cells. No residual thyroid tissue can be identified. (Slide contributed by Dr. L. Woolner, Rochester, MN.)

or granulomatous thyroiditis. It represents instead a manifestation of the group of idiopathic disorders generically known as *inflammatory fibrosclerosis*. As such, it may be seen coexisting with mediastinal or retroperitoneal fibrosis, sclerosing cholangitis, or inflammatory pseudotumor of the orbit.[75]

Steroid therapy has been effective in some cases, but most patients need surgical intervention to relieve the compression symptoms and to rule out the presence of carcinoma. The resection is quite difficult because no plane of cleavage exists. Adjoining muscle must be cut, and large veins may be torn. The incidence of postoperative hypothyroidism is very low.

HYPERPLASIA
Dyshormonogenetic goiter

There are several types of goiter due to enzyme defects in hormone synthesis[79,82] (Figs. 9-13 and 9-14). Kennedy[81] found, in a review of thirty such cases, that in those associated with the formation of an abnormal iodoprotein, the thyroid gland had a characteristic microcystic pattern on gross examination. Microscopically, nodules were often present, formed by trabeculae and small follicles with scanty colloid. Papillary foci and a moderate degree of cellular pleomorphism also were noted. Goiters associated with defective deiodination of monoiodotyrosine and diiodotyrosine were always nodular and showed papillary proliferation and pleomorphism. In some, there was capsular and/or blood vessel invasion. Goiters secondary to defective organification of iodine were also nodular and trabecular/microfollicular but showed only a moderate degree of cellular atypia. Mitotic figures can be seen with any of these forms, as a result of the continuous thyrotropin stimulation.

Cases of thyroid carcinoma have been reported in patients with dyshormonogenetic goiter, but the number of well documented cases is very low.[80] Most have been of follicular type. Since dyshormonogenetic goiter is commonly associated with pleomorphism, hypercellularity, and mitotic activity of the follicular epithelium, one should be particularly strict with the criteria for the diagnosis of follicular cancer in this setting. Specifically, nothing short of clearcut capsular or blood vessel invasion should be accepted.

Diffuse hyperplasia (Graves' disease)

Diffuse hyperplasia of thyroid (also known as Graves' disease, thyrotoxicosis, and exophthalmic goiter) typically presents in young females with muscle weakness, weight loss, exophthalmus, irritability, tachycardia, goiter, and often a great increase of appetite. Atrial fibrillation may occur. Late clinical manifestations are localized pretibial myxedema and so-called thyroid acropachy; the latter is characterized by swelling of the extremities and clubbing of fingers and toes due to periosteal new bone formation.[90] Laboratory tests show elevation of serum protein–bound iodine level and increased radioactive iodine uptake.

Grossly, the gland shows a mild to moderate symmetric diffuse enlargement. It is succulent and reddish and has the consistency of pancreatic tissue. The cut surface is uniformly gray or red depending on the degree of vascularity (Fig. 9-15). In long standing cases, the gland appears friable and dull yellow.

Microscopically, the follicles are markedly hyperplastic, with prominent papillary infolding that may cause confusion with papillary carcinoma (Fig. 9-16). The lining epithelium is columnar, with basally located nuclei and a clear, sometimes foamy cytoplasm that may contain fat and glycogen.

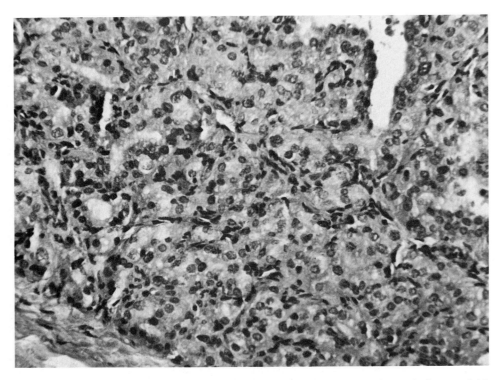

Fig. 9-13 Congenital goiter in 14-day-old male infant. It is a cellular lesion with practically no colloid.

A variable number of oxyphilic cells may be present, suggesting the existence of a link with Hashimoto's thyroiditis. The colloid is pale and finely vacuolated. The stroma contains aggregates of lymphoid tissue with only occasional germinal centers. Immunohistochemically, most of these lymphocytes are of the T-cell type, the cytotoxic-suppressor subtype predominating in the follicles and the helper-induced subtype in the interstitium.[89] Mild fibrosis is present in long-standing cases. The proliferating follicles may surpass the confines of the thyroid gland and grow into the skeletal muscle of the neck, a feature that should not be interpreted as evidence of malignancy (Fig. 9-17).

An incidental carcinoma may be found on pathologic examination of a thyroid gland removed for hyperthyroidism, the incidence varying from less than 1% to 9% in the reported series.[86] Nearly all of the cases have been small papillary carcinomas without clinical significance.

The treatment of Graves' disease may consist of antithyroid drugs such as propylthiouracil, methimazole and carbimazole, destruction of the gland with radioactive iodine, or subtotal thyroidectomy.[93] The latter operation provides the specimen most commonly seen by the pathologist in this disorder. It should be noted that the microscopic changes previously described are rarely seen in their pristine state in these organs because of the changes that supervene as a result of the therapy with antithyroid drugs and iodine or beta blockers, which are given routinely in the preoperative period. The glandular enlargement and the lymphoid infiltrate persist, but most of the hyperplastic changes in the follicles regress.[85] However, thorough sampling will usually reveal residual foci of hyperplasia. Following surgery, the thyroid remnant regenerates so that an euthyroid status can be maintained in most of the patients, especially if the amount of thyroid tissue left is 5 g on each side.[83] The greater the lymphocytic infiltration and the larger the number of oxyphilic cells in the operative specimen, the greater the chances that the patient will develop myxedema postoperatively.[88]

Glands treated with radioactive iodine show initially nuclear abnormalities, dissolution of some of the follicles, and vascular alterations. In later stages, there is glandular atrophy and fibrosis.[84] As a consequence, the long-term incidence of hypothyroidism is very high with this therapy.[93] It should be noted that none of these therapies alters the course of the exophthalmos associated with hyperthyroidism.

Graves' disease is currently included among the autoimmune thyroid diseases, together with Hashimoto's thyroiditis and idiopathic myxedema. Thyrotropin (TSH) does not seem to be involved in the pathogenesis.[87] Long-acting thyroid stimulator (LATS), an IgG immunoglobulin with thyroid-stimulating properties, is present in approximately 70% of the patients with Graves' disease. It is thought to be directed against the TSH receptor on a contiguous site on the thyroid cell membrane.[94] Basement membrane deposits with an appearance consistent with immune complexes are seen ultrastructurally.[91] How this autoimmune process relates to the well known clinical fact that thyrotoxicosis often arises following a psychologic stress remains a mystery.

Amiodarone-associated thyrotoxicosis is an iatrogenically induced form of hyperthyroidism. Amiodarone is a

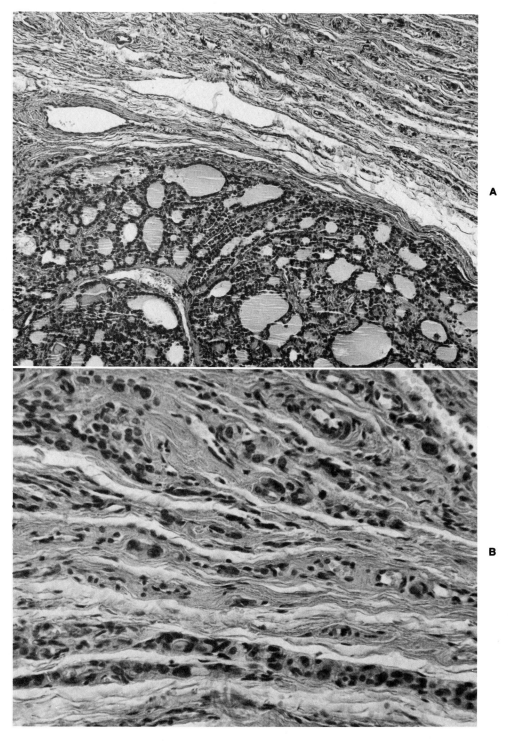

Fig. 9-14 Thyroid gland of cretin showing focal area of glandular proliferation associated with another zone in which follicles are atrophic and nuclei are atypical. (**A** and **B,** slides contributed by Dr. G.H. Moore, Denver, CO.)

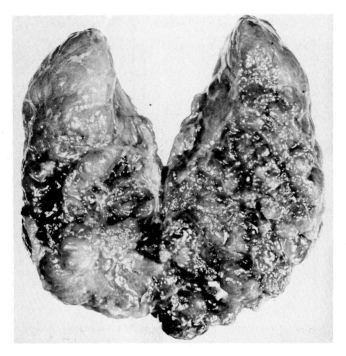

Fig. 9-15 Thyroid gland in diffuse hyperplasia. Gland is diffusely enlarged, hyperemic, and without nodules.

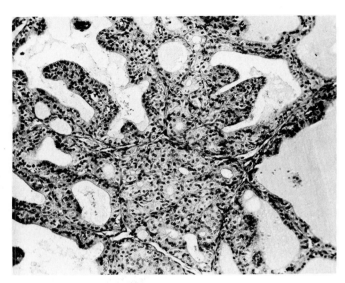

Fig. 9-16 Diffuse hyperplasia of thyroid gland. Note solid masses of cells, high columnar epithelium, and papillary infolding.

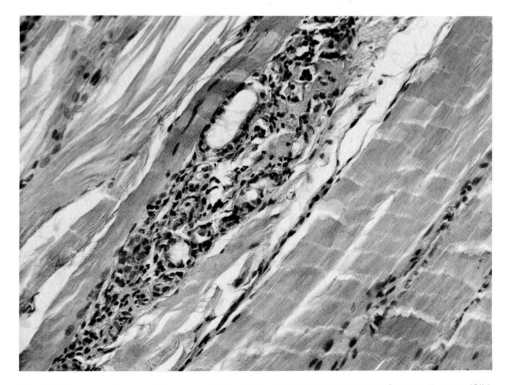

Fig. 9-17 Hyperplastic thyroid tissue invading muscle in 29-year-old man with Graves' disease. (Slide contributed by Dr. J. Glenn, Billings, MT.)

cardiac antiarrhythmia and antiangina agent that contains 37% iodine by weight. The morphologic changes in the thyroid include degenerative and destructive follicular lesions, involutional changes, and fibrosis.[92]

Nodular hyperplasia

Nodular hyperplasia (nodular or multinodular goiter, adenomatoid goiter, adenomatous hyperplasia) is the most common thyroid disease. In the form traditionally known as **endemic goiter**, the disease is due to low iodine content of the water and soil, and it can be largely prevented by the addition of iodine to common salt. The deficiency in thyroid hormone production induced by the iodine deficiency leads to increase in thyrotropin secretion, which results initially in a hyperactive thyroid with tall follicular epithelium and small amounts of colloid (so-called *parenchymatous goiter*) and later in follicular atrophy with massive storage of colloid, with or without nodularity (so-called *diffuse* or *nodular colloid goiter*). In these endemic areas, the frequency of the disease at postmortem examination is virtually 100%.

In the form known as **sporadic nodular goiter**, which is the most common seen in this country, the pathogenesis remains unknown. Mild dietary deficiency of iodine, slight impairment of hormone synthesis, increased iodide clearance by the kidneys, and presence of thyroid-stimulating immunoglobulins have been variously suggested.[95,100] Some

cases are associated with lymphocytic or Hashimoto's thyroiditis and can be viewed as the nodular forms of these immune-mediated inflammatory diseases. In most patients with nodular hyperplasia, the blood levels of thyrotropin are not elevated. The incidence of the disease in the general adult population is 3% to 5% clinically and about 50% at autopsy.[99,101] The morphologic changes are similar to those of the nodular form of endemic goiter.

Clinically, most patients are euthyroid and present with a multinodular gland that may become very large, cause tracheal obstruction, and produce considerable disfigurement. In cases with a single, firm, dominant nodule, the clinical distinction with a true neoplasm becomes impossible. Hemorrhage within a nodule can cause sudden enlargement and pain. A small proportion of patients present with clinical signs of hyperthyroidism, but the exophthalmos of Graves' disease does not occur.

Some cases of thyroid nodular hyperplasia are located substernally and enter in the differential diagnosis of superior mediastinal tumors (Fig. 9-18) (see Chapter 8).

Grossly, the thyroid is enlarged and its shape is distorted, one lobe being frequently larger than the other (Fig. 9-19). The thyroid capsule may be stretched but is intact. On cross section, multiple nodules are seen, some surrounded by a partial or complete capsule. Secondary changes in the form

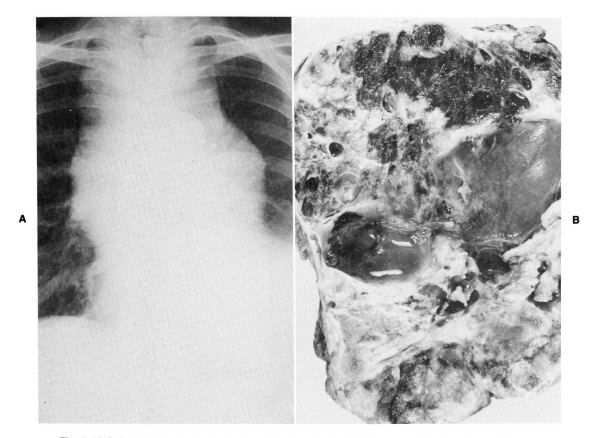

Fig. 9-18 A, Large anterior mediastinal nodular thyroid gland. **B,** Same nodular thyroid gland shown in **A.** Note nodulation, hemorrhage, and cyst formation.

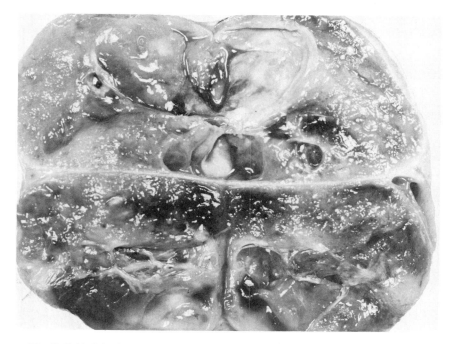

Fig. 9-19 Nodular hyperplasia of thyroid gland with cystic and hemorrhagic areas.

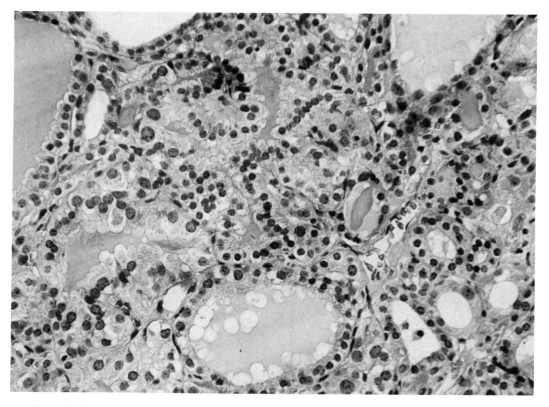

Fig. 9-20 Thyroid gland from 13-year-old Marshallese girl who developed nodular thyroid 10 years after accidental exposure to radioactive fallout. Many nuclei are enlarged and hyperchromatic.

of hemorrhage, calcification, and cystic degeneration are common. Microscopically, there is a wide range of appearances. Some nodules are composed of huge follicles lined by flattened epithelium, others are extremely cellular and hyperplastic, and still others are composed predominantly or exclusively by Hürthle cells. Some of the dilated follicles have a conglomerate of small active follicles at one pole (so-called Sanderson's polsters). Others have papilloid projections facing the lumen of a cystic follicle, a feature that may lead to confusion with papillary carcinoma. Rupture of follicles leads to a granulomatous reaction to the colloid, with appearance of histiocytes and foreign body–type giant cells. Areas of fresh and old hemorrhage, coarse fibrous trabeculation, and foci of calcification are common. Occasionally, osseous metaplasia is seen. Greatly thickened vessels with calcified media may be present at the periphery. A variable number of chronic inflammatory cells are present in the stroma in many of the cases, indicating the existence of a coexisting chronic thyroiditis; the larger their number, the higher the chances of postoperative hypothyroidism.[97,98] Presence of highly atypical nuclei in a case of nodular hyperplasia should raise the possibility of previous exposure to radioactive substances (Fig. 9-20). It is not possible to predict on the basis of the morphologic appearance whether or not the patient has clinical or laboratory evidence of hyperthyroidism.

The differential diagnosis between a dominant nodule from a case of nodular hyperplasia and a true adenoma is based on a set of admittedly arbitrary criteria. The adenoma is usually single, is totally surrounded by a capsule, is dissimilar from the remaining parenchyma, compresses the adjacent tissue, and is composed mainly of follicles that are smaller than those of the normal gland. The lesion of nodular hyperplasia is almost always one of many nodules, its encapsulation is incomplete, the follicular size is variable, some or all of the follicles are larger than those in the surrounding gland, and there is no compression of the adjacent parenchyma. In some cases the distinction becomes impossible, inasmuch as lesions with the morphologic features of adenoma may be multiple and/or occur in a setting of nodular hyperplasia.

A long-standing and still unresolved issue is whether nodular hyperplasia is associated with an increased incidence of carcinoma, particularly of the follicular type.[96] Suffice it to say that if such an increase really exists, it is small enough to be disregarded for practical purposes.

Mild asymptomatic cases of nodular hyperplasia require no treatment. Suppressive medical therapy with exogenous thyroid hormones is only moderately effective. If the enlargement is such that disfigurement of pressure symptoms develop, bilateral subtotal thyroidectomy is carried out.

TUMORS

The large majority of clinically apparent thyroid neoplasms are primary and epithelial. Traditionally, they have been divided into adenomas and carcinomas, the latter group incorporating the medullary carcinomas together with the more common lesions composed of follicular cells. From a histogenetic/differentiation standpoint, it is preferable to divide thyroid neoplasms into three major categories, depending on the cell types involved, and subdivide them into the various benign and malignant categories:

1 Tumors exhibiting follicular differentiation
2 Tumors exhibiting C-cell differentiation
3 Tumors exhibiting follicular and C-cell differentiation

Lesions in the first category comprise well over 95% of the cases, the remainder being largely made up by tumors in the second category.[102]

Epithelial tumors—specific types
Follicular adenoma

Follicular adenoma is defined as a benign encapsulated tumor composed of follicular cells. Most patients are euthyroid adults who present with a thyroid lump, which on scan is usually "cold," sometimes "cool" or "warm," and only rarely "hot." Many patients with thyroid adenomas have elevated circulating levels of thyroglobulin,[116] but few of the tumors are associated with clinical hyperthyroidism (so-called *toxic adenomas*).[115] It has been suggested that these autonomously functioning tumors are more common in regions with iodine deficiency.[103]

Adenomas are usually solitary. They are characteristically surrounded by a capsule that is grossly and microscopically complete (Figs. 9-21 and 9-22). The architectural and cytologic features are different from those of the surrounding gland, which usually shows signs of compression. Adenomas may exhibit a variety of patterns, singly or in combination: normofollicular (simple), macrofollicular (colloid), microfollicular (fetal), and trabecular/solid (embryonal). While the morphologic differences may be striking, they have no apparent clinical significance. Mitoses are rare or absent in the follicular adenomas. They are not necessarily indicators of malignancy, but when present in appreciable numbers one should sample and examine the specimen with particular care. Secondary degenerative changes such as hemorrhage, edema, fibrosis, calcification, bone formation, and cystic degeneration are common, especially among the larger tumors. Like hyperplastic nodules, adenomas may exhibit pseudopapillary structures, which may prompt confusion with papillary carcinoma. Some authors have referred to these tumors as *papillary adenoma*, a diagnosis which we believe should be avoided. In our opinion, encapsulated thyroid tumors with a papillary pattern of growth are either hyperplastic nodules, adenomas with papilloid formations, or encapsulated papillary carcinomas.

Some correlation between the microscopic appearance of a follicular adenoma and its activity as judged by the scan appearance is possible.[104,110] In general, hyperfunctioning ("hot") adenomas are more cellular and their cells have more abundant cytoplasm (and therefore a decreased nucleocytoplasmic ratio) than nonfunctioning ("cold") tumors. The enzyme histochemical and immunohistochemical profile mirrors that of the normal follicle.[107] There is reactivity for low molecular weight keratin and thyroglobulin in the cytoplasm and for laminin and other basement membrane components around the follicles.[114] DNA aneuploidy has been found by flow cytometry in about a quarter of follicular adenomas, but this does not appear to be associated with an aggressive behavior.[112]

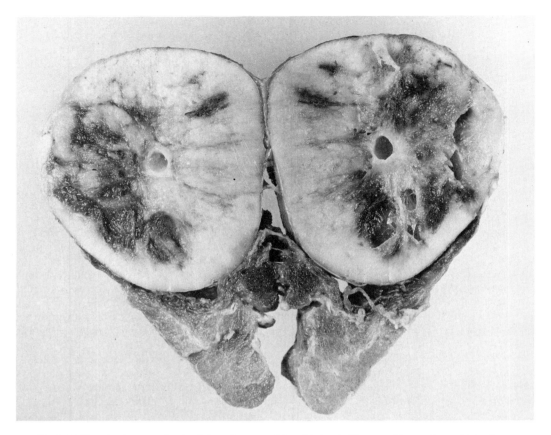

Fig. 9-21 Sharply circumscribed cellular adenoma of thyroid gland with central hemorrhage. Note sharp demarcation between tumor and normal thyroid gland.

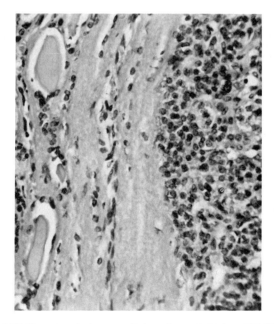

Fig. 9-22 Boundary between cellular adenoma and normal thyroid gland. Note difference in appearance between adenoma and thyroid gland and presence of well-defined capsule.

Several variants of follicular adenoma have been described. *Hürthle cell adenoma* is discussed on p. 417. The term *atypical adenoma* has been proposed for adenomas with pronounced cellular proliferation and less regular cytoarchitectural patterns but still lacking evidence of capsular or blood vessel invasion.[111,113] *Hyalinizing trabecular adenoma* is a term recently proposed for a peculiar type of adenoma exhibiting prominent trabecular arrangement and equally prominent stromal hyalinization. The trabeculae can be straight or curved, resulting in curious organoid formations (Fig. 9-23). The pattern simulates paraganglioma and medullary carcinoma; the occasional presence of nuclear grooves and psammoma bodies may suggest papillary carcinoma, particularly in material from fine needle aspiration.[105] *Adenoma with bizarre nuclei* is characterized by the presence of huge hyperchromatic nuclei, usually in clusters, unaccompanied by other features of malignancy (Fig. 9-24). This phenomenon is analogous to that seen in parathyroid adenomas and other endocrine neoplasms.[106]

Other rare types of follicular adenoma are those with clear cell changes (including the signet-ring, mucin-producing, and lipid-rich types) (see p. 422) and adenomas with adipose metaplasia of the stroma (so-called *adenolipomas*).

The differential diagnosis of follicular adenoma includes a dominant nodule of nodular hyperplasia, minimally in-

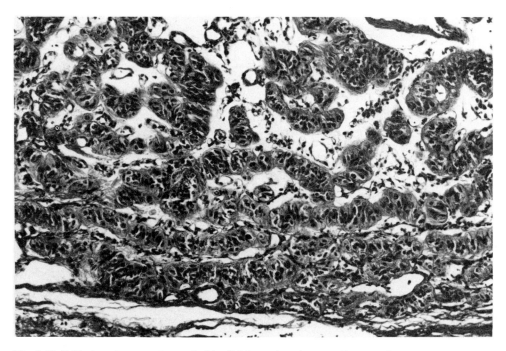

Fig. 9-23 Follicular adenoma of so-called hyalinizing trabecular type. Tumor cells are growing in well-defined trabeculae separated by abundant stroma.

vasive follicular carcinoma, and the follicular variant of papillary carcinoma. Some follicular adenomas may also be confused with vascular tumors because of their high vascularization.

The standard therapy for follicular adenoma is removal by lobectomy. Enucleation of the adenoma should not be attempted. Suppression of the nodule with levothyroxine and treatment of the toxic adenoma with ^{131}I have been employed, but the results have generally been less than satisfactory.[108,109]

Papillary carcinoma

General features. Papillary carcinoma is the most common type of thyroid malignancy. Females are more affected than males. It can present in any age group, the mean age at the time of initial diagnosis being approximately 40 years. Papillary carcinoma makes up over 90% of thyroid malignancies in children. In 5% to 10% of the cases, there is a history of irradiation exposure to the neck, and the nonneoplastic gland may show nuclear aberrations as a result (Fig. 9-25). There is convincing evidence for an increase in the incidence of papillary carcinoma in Hashimoto's thyroiditis, but the wide variation in the figures quoted suggests that the diagnostic criteria vary just as widely.[119] Whether the frequency of papillary carcinoma is increased in Graves' disease remains a controversial subject.[118]

Nearly all patients present with clinically evident disease in the neck. This is localized to the thyroid gland in 67% of the cases, thyroid and lymph nodes in 13%, and lymph nodes alone in 20%.[117]

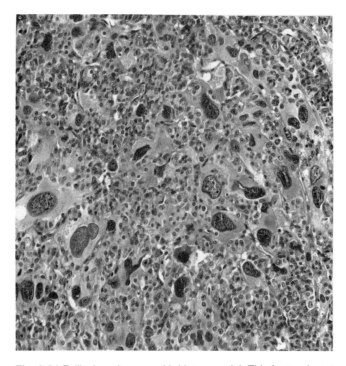

Fig. 9-24 Follicular adenoma with bizarre nuclei. This feature is not a sign of malignancy and is analogous to that seen in many other endocrine tumors.

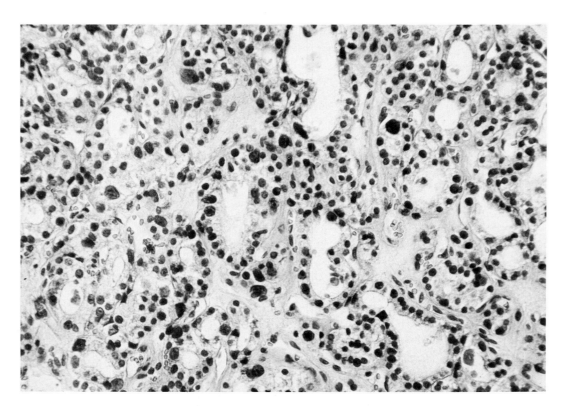

Fig. 9-25 Patient, 20-year-old man, who had received irradiation for "thymic enlargement" at age of 5 months, developed papillary carcinoma of thyroid gland. This photomicrograph was taken from non-tumoral thyroid gland to illustrate nuclear aberrations frequently seen in patients with history of past irradiation.

Pathologic features. The size of the primary tumor ranges from microscopic to huge. A very high proportion of thyroid cancers measuring less than 1 cm in diameter are of papillary type. Grossly, most cases are solid, whitish, firm, and clearly invasive; less than 10% are surrounded by a complete capsule.[124] Marked cystic changes are seen in about 10% of the cases. Sometimes papillary formations are evident to the naked eye (Figs. 9-26, 9-27, and 9-28).

Microscopically, the diagnosis of papillary carcinoma depends on the presence of certain architectural features (mainly in the form of true papillae) and/or characteristic nuclear changes.[125,137,139] The papillae are usually complex, branching, and randomly oriented, with a central fibrovascular core and a single or stratified lining of cuboidal cells (Fig. 9-28, B). The stroma of the papillae may be edematous or hyaline, and it may contain lymphocytes, foamy macrophages, hemosiderin, or—exceptionally—adipose tissue. These papillae are nearly always associated with the formation of follicles, the ratio between the two components varying greatly from case to case. The follicles tend to be irregularly shaped, often tubular. Tumors with a combination of papillary and follicular structures have the biologic behavior of papillary carcinoma and should therefore be classified as such instead of as mixed carcinomas.

The nuclear features of papillary carcinoma, which are as important diagnostically as the presence of papillae, consist of:

1 Ground glass (optically clear) nuclei, which often have a large size and an overlapping quality[127] (Fig. 9-29, A). The nucleolus is usually inconspicuous and pushed against the nuclear membrane, which appears thickened. This change is present in sections obtained from paraffin-embedded material regardless of the fixative used but is less apparent or absent altogether in frozen sections or cytology material. The mechanism of its formation has not yet been ascertained.

2 Nuclear pseudoinclusions. These represent invaginations of the cytoplasm and appear as sharply outlined acidophilic formations.[120,129] In contrast to the ground glass feature, the pseudoinclusions are readily apparent in specimens from frozen section and aspirations (Fig. 9-29, B).

3 Nuclear grooves. This recently described nuclear change is as common as the other changes and may have greater diagnostic significance[126] (Fig. 9-29, C).

It should be pointed out that all three nuclear features may be present only focally or altogether absent in cases that are otherwise typical of papillary carcinoma.[127]

Mitoses are nil or absent.[132] Over half of the cases show extensive fibrosis, usually in the form of bands traversing the tumor; this fibrosis may have a sclerohyaline or a highly cellular appearance.

Psammoma bodies are seen in approximately half of the cases. They may be located in the papillary stalk, fibrous

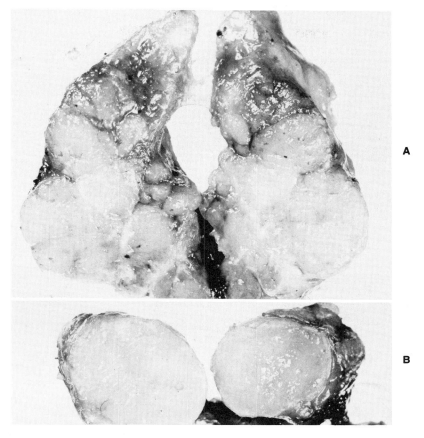

Fig. 9-26 A, Lobe of thyroid gland completely replaced by papillary carcinoma. **B,** Small mass represents complete replacement of lymph nodes.

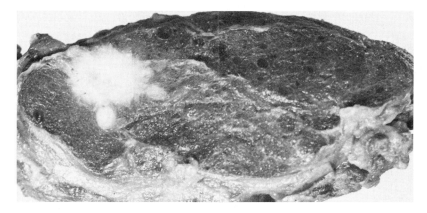

Fig. 9-27 Papillary carcinoma of thyroid gland measuring about 1 cm. Patient had extensive lymph node metastases. Naturally, primary tumor could not be felt.

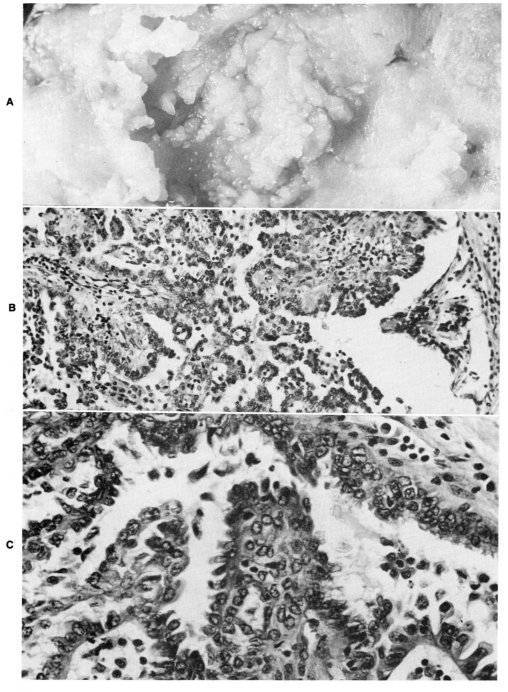

Fig. 9-28 A, Papillary carcinoma. This has been slightly enlarged so that papillary character of tumor can be seen. **B,** Low-power photomicrograph demonstrating papillary character of same tumor. **C,** High-power photomicrograph demonstrating layering of cells in individual papillae of same tumor.

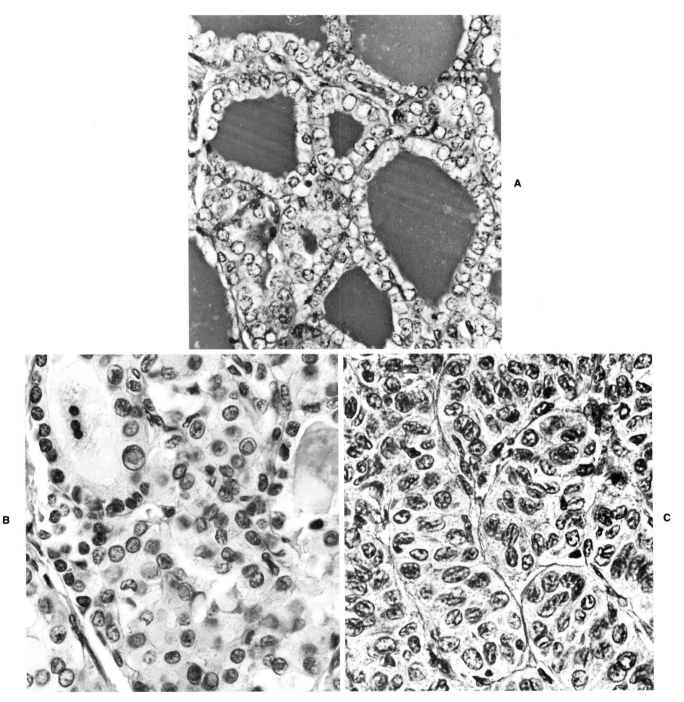

Fig. 9-29 Appearance of nuclei of cells of papillary carcinoma. **A,** Ground glass appearance and overlapping. **B,** Several nuclear pseudoinclusions. **C,** Large number of nuclear grooves.

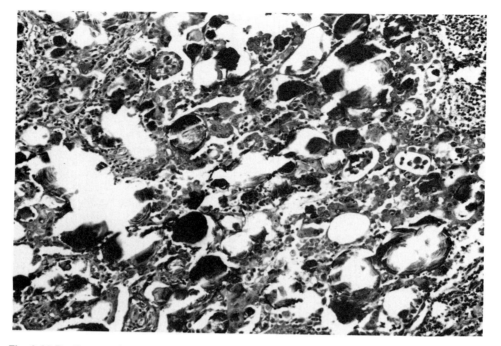

Fig. 9-30 Papillary carcinoma with numerous psammoma bodies. Calcification within these structures often results in artifactual breaks during sectioning. Concentric lamination can be appreciated in several of these structures.

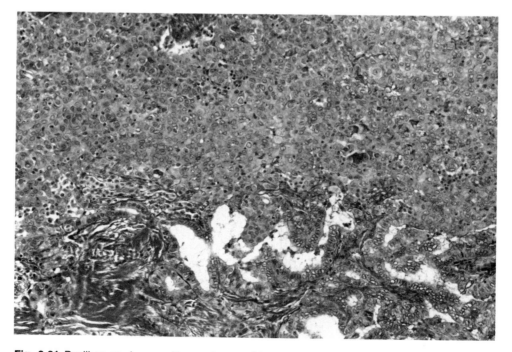

Fig. 9-31 Papillary carcinoma with prominent solid and squamoid metaplasia. This change is not indicative of a more aggressive behavior in this tumor.

stroma, or between tumor cells in solid foci (Fig. 9-30). They are nearly synonymous with the diagnosis of papillary carcinoma, inasmuch as their occurrence in other thyroid lesions is exceptional[134]; Klinck and Winship[131] found them only once in a review of 2,153 benign thyroids. Thus they represent a very important clue to the diagnosis not only in paraffin sections, but also in frozen sections, cytology preparations, and—if numerous enough—in roentgenograms.[133] If present in what is otherwise normal thyroid tissue or lymph nodes from the neck, the chances are high that a papillary carcinoma is present in the immediate vicinity.[131] These laminated basophilic structures stain for mucin, calcium, and iron and appear to arise from necrosis of individual tumor cells[126a,130]; they should be distinguished from other forms of calcification and from the intraluminal foci of inspissated secretion often seen in Hürthle cell tumors.[125]

Areas with a solid/trabecular pattern of growth are present in 20% of the cases and foci of squamous metaplasia in a similar number; these two patterns often merge and are probably related[125] (Fig. 9-31).

Lymphocytic infiltration of the stroma is seen in a fourth of the cases; it is not clear whether this represents a reaction to the tumor or the expression of pre-existing thyroiditis.[136] Many tumors also exhibit a heavy infiltrate of S-100 protein-positive dendritic/Langerhans' cells and lysozyme-positive histiocytes.[135a]

Multiple microscopic foci of tumor are found in about 20% of the cases if a few random sections are taken and in over 75% if step sections of the entire gland are examined.[135] Controversy still exists as to whether this represents multicentricity or intrathyroidal lymphatic permeation. Blood vessel invasion is found in only 5% of the cases.

Ultrastructurally, the most distinctive feature of the cells of papillary carcinoma is the highly indented nuclear membrane, with formation of pseudoinclusions and multilobation.[121,129] Immunohistochemically, these cells are reactive for low and high molecular weight keratin; the latter is of some diagnostic importance, because normal and hyperplastic follicles and follicular neoplasms usually show positivity only for the low molecular weight types.[122] Reactivity for thyroglobulin is the rule, although the intensity is generally less than in follicular neoplasms. There is also positivity for EMA, CEA (occasionally), vimentin, and ceruloplasmin.[138,140] Keratin and vimentin are often expressed in the same tumor cell.[123,128] Laminin and other basement membrane components are also identifiable.

The benign lesion that most closely simulates the appearance of papillary carcinoma is the hyperplastic nodule with central cystic degeneration and papillary or pseudopapillary fronds in the wall (Fig. 9-32). In contrast to papillary carcinomas, these lesions are "hot" on thyroid scan, lack clear nuclei, and are accompanied by a pale, vacuolated colloid. Furthermore, the papillary areas are largely limited

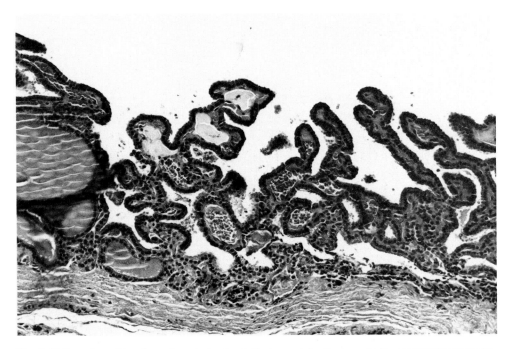

Fig. 9-32 Pseudopapillary formations in benign follicular nodule. Features in favor of benignancy are lack of characteristic nuclear changes of papillary carcinoma and fact that these structures face lumen of a cystically dilated cavity.

to the area facing the cystic cavity.

Variants. The following morphologic variants of papillary carcinoma have been described:

1 *Papillary microcarcinoma.* This is defined as a papillary carcinoma measuring 1 cm or less in diame-

ter (Fig. 9-33, *A* and *B*). Most cases have a stellate configuration and correspond to so-called occult sclerosing carcinoma or non-encapsulated sclerosing tumor,[151,152,154] whereas others show partial or near total encapsulation.[157] This entity is a common incidental

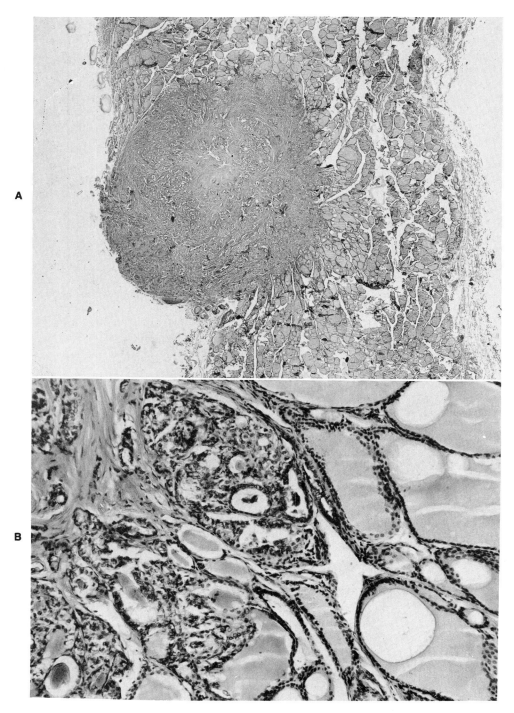

Fig. 9-33 A, Poorly delimited papillary microcarcinoma of thyroid gland discovered incidentally at time of subtotal thyroidectomy for nontoxic nodular goiter. **B,** Same lesion shown in **A.** Tumor is growing in a follicular pattern.

finding in population-based autopsy studies.[141,149] It is associated with cervical node metastases in about one third of the cases,[155] but distant metastases are exceptionally rare,[159] and the prognosis is generally excellent.[152]

2 *Encapsulated variant.* Papillary carcinoma *totally* surrounded by a capsule may still be associated with nodal metastases, but the incidence of distant metastases or tumor death is nearly zero.[148,156] As already indicated, the use of the term papillary adenoma is not recommended.[160]

3 *Follicular variant.* This is a papillary carcinoma composed entirely or almost entirely of follicles (Fig. 9-34).[145,155] The diagnosis is largely based on the presence of the set of nuclear features classically associated with papillary carcinoma (see p. 408). Supportive features for the diagnosis are an invasive pattern of growth, fibrous trabeculation, psammoma bodies, strongly eosinophilic colloid with scalloped edges, and presence of abortive papillae. The mere presence of ground glass nuclei focally in a lesion having otherwise the cytoarchitectural features of follicular adenoma is not sufficient for the diagnosis of this variant in the absence of the supportive features above described. The behavior is analogous to that of conventional papillary carcinoma, particularly in regard to the high incidence of nodal metastases.[143,146] Interestingly, these metastases usually exhibit well developed papillary formations.

4 *Diffuse sclerosing variant.* This variant is characterized by diffuse involvement of one or both thyroid lobes, dense sclerosis, abundant psammoma bodies, extensive solid foci, squamous metaplasia, and heavy lymphocytic infiltration (Fig. 9-35). Nodal metastases are nearly always present, lung metastases are common, and the disease-free survival rate is lower than for conventional papillary carcinoma.[142,144,161]

5 *Oxyphilic variant.* Papillary carcinoma composed of Hürthle cells is discussed on p. 422.

6 *Tall cell and columnar variants.* Tall cell carcinoma is a type of papillary carcinoma characterized by tall cells with abundant eosinophilic cytoplasm.[150,153] The variant recently described as columnar is similar but exhibits nuclear stratification[147,158] (Fig. 9-36). Both types are said to run a more aggressive clinical course.

Spread and metastases. Extrathyroid extension into the soft tissues of the neck is found in about one fourth of the cases.[162,163] Involvement of cervical lymph nodes is very common (particularly in young patients), and it may be the first manifestation of the disease. The nodal metastases have a tendency to undergo cystic changes (see p. 394). These metastases may not be clinically apparent because of their small size and also because their consistency may not differ from that of a normal node. In a study of sixty-seven patients with clinically negative nodes, forty-one (61%) had metastatic tumor on microscopic examination.[164]

Blood-borne metastases are less frequent than with other thyroid carcinomas, but they also occur; the most common site is the lung, but they can also develop in bones, central nervous system, and other organs.[162] The lung metastases

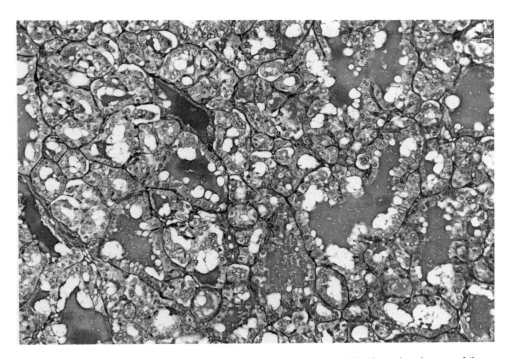

Fig. 9-34 Follicular variant of papillary carcinoma. Follicles are irregularly shaped and some of them show papillary infoldings. Nuclei have ground glass appearance. Colloid has homogeneous dark-staining quality and scalloped edges.

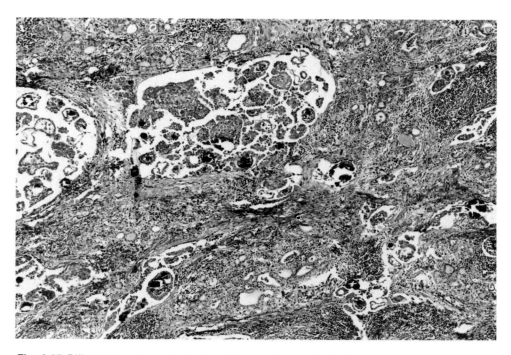

Fig. 9-35 Diffuse sclerosing variant of papillary carcinoma. Much of tumor is located within large endothelial-lined spaces. There are numerous papillary formations and psammoma bodies. There is also extensive fibrosis and chronic inflammation in stroma.

can have a miliary micronodular pattern detectable only on ^{131}I scintiscan, or they can be rounded and macronodular.[165]

Prognosis. The overall outcome of patients with papillary carcinoma is excellent, not significantly different than that of the general population.[168,171] Factors relating to prognosis are the following:

1 *Age.* This is of great importance. Nearly all the deaths from papillary carcinomas occur when the tumor manifests itself after the age of 40 years.[166]

2 *Sex.* Females are said to have a better prognosis than males, although in some series the difference has not been significant.[166]

3 *Extrathyroid extension.* This feature affects adversely the prognosis in a very significant fashion.[166,174]

4 *Microscopic variants* (see p. 414).

5 *History of previous irradiation.* Despite previous statements to the contrary, the prognosis of these tumors does not seem to differ significantly from the others.

6 *Tumor size.* A rough inverse correlation is present between tumor size and prognosis.

7 *Capsule and margins.* Tumors that are encapsulated and/or with pushing margins have a better outcome than the others.[166]

8 *Multicentricity.* Patients in whom this is a prominent feature have a greater incidence of metastasis and a lesser chance of disease-free survival.[166]

9 *Distant metastases.* Metastases to lung have an adverse influence on prognosis; this influence is even greater for distant metastases in other sites, such as the skeletal system.[166,173]

10 *Poorly differentiated (insular), epidermoid, or anaplastic foci.* These features have a markedly detrimental effect on prognosis. Fortunately, they are present in less than 5% of the cases.[166,172]

11 *DNA ploidy.* Some recent studies have shown a good correlation between aneuploidy and aggressive behavior in papillary carcinoma, but it is not yet clear whether this provides information not already obtainable from the above listed clinical and morphologic parameters.[167,169]

12 Factors not generally found to correlate with prognosis are relative proportion of papillae and follicles; presence or amount of fibrosis; and presence or amount of solid areas, squamous metaplasia, or psammoma bodies. Interestingly, presence of cervical node metastases does not worsen the prognosis at all. The effect of the type of therapy on prognosis remains controversial,[170] but we[166] and others have found little if any relation between the two parameters (see p. 436).

Follicular carcinoma

Follicular carcinoma could be defined in a generic sense as any malignant thyroid tumor exhibiting evidence of follicular cell differentiation. However, we prefer not to include in this category the follicular variant of papillary carcinoma (see p. 415), Hürthle cell carcinoma (see p. 420), poorly differentiated (insular) carcinoma (see p. 423), and the exceptionally rare mixed medullary-follicular carcinoma (see

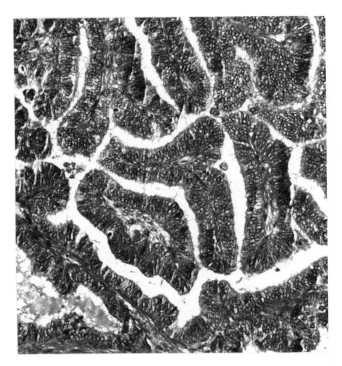

Fig. 9-36 Columnar variant of papillary carcinoma. Papillae are lined by pseudostratified layer of spindle tumor cells.

p. 431). When thus categorized, follicular carcinoma becomes a relatively rare neoplasm. It shares with papillary carcinoma the same predilection for females but it occurs, on the average, in patients who are a decade older. Its microscopic appearance is extremely variable, ranging from well-formed follicles to a predominantly solid growth pattern. Poorly formed follicles, cribriform areas, or trabecular formations may be present, sometimes in combination. Focal or extensive cytoplasmic clear changes can occur. Mitotic activity and nuclear atypia are usually seen but may be entirely lacking. Psammoma bodies are absent, and squamous metaplasia is exceptionally rare.[187]

Immunohistochemically, follicular carcinomas are reactive for thyroglobulin, low molecular weight keratin, EMA, S-100 protein, and basement membrane components such as laminin and type IV collagen.[184,192,193] Their lectin-binding pattern and ultrastructural appearance are not significantly different from those of adenoma.[182,190]

The diagnosis of follicular carcinoma depends largely on the identification of capsular and/or blood vessel invasion. Depending on the extent of the invasiveness, follicular carcinomas have been subdivided into a minimally invasive and a widely invasive form.

Minimally invasive follicular carcinoma is a grossly encapsulated tumor, often with a solid and fleshy cut surface. The pattern of growth usually resembles that of an adenoma of embryonal, fetal, or atypical type. Since the diagnosis of malignancy depends entirely on the demonstration of blood vessel and/or capsular invasion, one should be very strict about these criteria (Fig. 9-37). The blood vessel invasion is only occasionally evident grossly.

Microscopically, the vessels should be of venous caliber, be located in or immediately outside the capsule (rather than within the tumor), and should contain a cluster of tumor cells attached to the wall and protruding into the lumen. Often, these intravascular tumor masses are covered by endothelium, in a fashion similar to that of an ordinary thrombus. We have found elastic tissue stains of only limited utility in identifying these vessels. Immunohistochemical stains for actin are more likely to be positive, but often these peculiar capsular vessels lack an elastico-muscular layer altogether, despite their relatively large size. Search for endothelial markers—such as FVIII-related antigen and *Ulex europaeus* I lectin—is more rewarding,[178,179] although the erratic staining pattern of the former limits somewhat its practical value, rendering *Ulex* the top choice among the two.[179,191] Interruption of the capsule must be full thickness in order for the process to qualify as capsular invasion. Penetration of the inner half or presence of tumor islands embedded within the capsule does not qualify. It follows from the previous comments that thorough sampling of encapsulated follicular lesions is of paramount importance[186] (see Appendix A). Evans[177] has made the interesting observation that the capsule of follicular carcinoma tends to be thicker and more irregular than that of adenoma. Whether this neoplasm represents a malignant transformation of a follicular adenoma or a malignancy *ab initio* is a moot point.

Widely invasive follicular carcinoma shows widespread infiltration of blood vessels and/or adjacent thyroid tissue. It often lacks encapsulation altogether. In our experience, many of these tumors belong to the category of poorly differentiated carcinomas (see p. 423). It has been suggested that grossly encapsulated tumors showing *extensive* blood vessel invasion should be placed in this category because of their similar natural history.

In contrast to papillary carcinomas, follicular carcinomas of either subtype are almost always solitary and practically never occult. Metastases are usually blood borne (particularly to lung and bones) rather than to regional nodes.[188] The skeletal metastases have a predilection for the shoulder girdle, sternum, skull, and iliac bone.[189] Sometimes they pulsate because of their vascularity, a feature they share with metastatic renal cell carcinoma. These metastases have a strong affinity for radioiodine and—curiously— often exhibit a better differentiated appearance than the primary tumor, to the point of looking like normal thyroid as an expression of terminal differentiation (so-called metastasizing adenoma, malignant adenoma, or metastasizing goiter). Immunoglobulin staining is invaluable in confirming the thyroid origin of a metastatic tumor. These metastases are common in the widely invasive type, occur in less than 5% of the minimally invasive tumors *with* blood vessel invasion, and in less than 1% of the tumors diagnosed as carcinoma *only* on the basis of minimal capsular invasion.[175,176,180,185] Whether DNA evaluation will provide information of prognostic significance still needs to be determined.[181,183]

Hürthle cell tumors

Tumors included in this category are those in which more than half of the cell population is made up of Hürthle cells.[203]

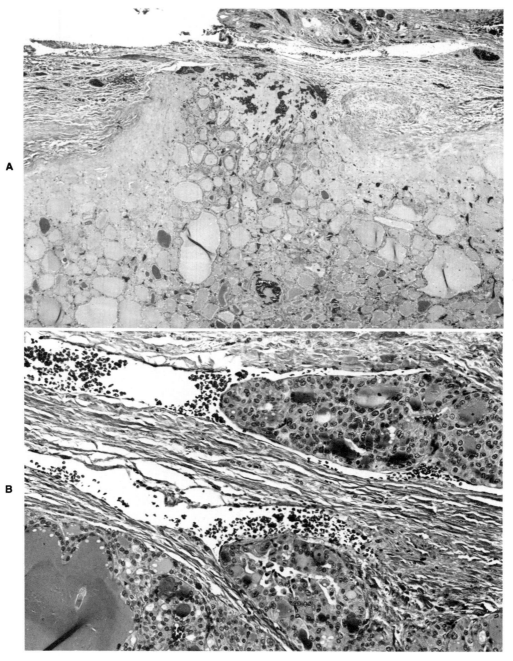

Fig. 9-37 A, Minor capsular invasion in follicular neoplasm. Entire thickness of capsule has been violated by advancing tumor edge. **B,** Vascular invasion in follicular neoplasm. Vessels are of vein caliber and located in capsule. Tumor thrombi are attached to wall and covered by layer of endothelium.

Some authors do not view these tumors as a distinct type and place them into one of the existing tumor types (i.e., follicular or papillary), depending on their pattern of growth. We think that their morphology and natural history are distinctive enough for them to be regarded as a special group. Most patients are adults, and there is a predominance of females.

Grossly, the tumors are characteristically solid, tan, and well-vascularized (Fig. 9-38). Most are well-encapsulated throughout; the invasive tumors tend to grow into the parenchyma in a lobulated fashion. Microscopically, the pattern of growth may be follicular, trabecular/solid, or papillary. The former is by far the most common. The follicles, when large, are separated by thin fibrovascular septa that

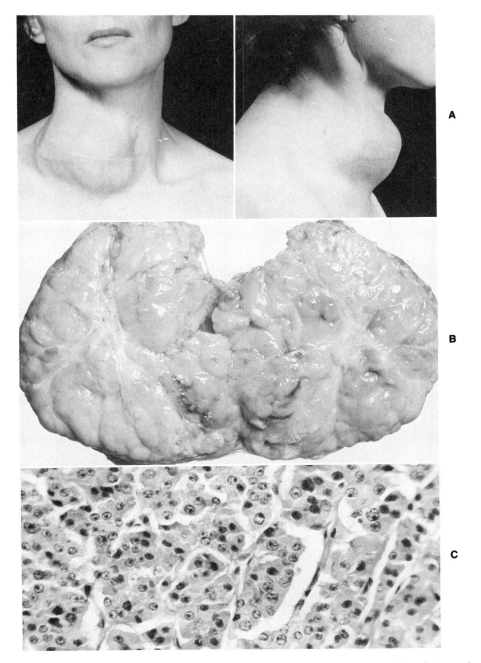

Fig. 9-38 Hürthle cell carcinoma of thyroid gland. **A,** Well-circumscribed thyroid nodule of 2 years' duration in 44-year-old woman. Scar is from operation done 9 years before for hyperthyroidism. **B,** Note relative circumscription and cellularity of tumor. **C,** Note large cells with prominent cytoplasm. Tumor invaded veins. Patient died with bone and lung metastases 6 years after operation.

simulate papillae when cut tangentially. Another diagnostic trap is the presence of inspissated intraluminal colloid with concentric laminations, having an appearance strongly reminiscent of psammoma bodies. The nuclei may show pleomorphism and prominent nucleoli, with occurrence of isolated bizarre form. The cytoplasm has a distinct granular acidophilic quality (Fig. 9-38). Ultrastructurally, the cells are packed with mitochondria showing abnormalities in size, shape, and content[200,208] (Fig. 9-39). Immunohistochemically, there is reactivity for thyroglobulin, although in lesser degree than in conventional follicular lesions; positivity for CEA has also been detected.[207]

We believe that Hürthle cell tumors with follicular or solid/trabecular patterns—which constitute the large majority—should be evaluated and diagnosed using analogous criteria to those employed for follicular neoplasms of non-Hürthle cell types, i.e., the presence of capsular and/or blood vessel invasion should be used as the main criterion for malignancy. We do not adhere to the extreme view that all Hürthle cell neoplasms are to be regarded as malignant or potentially malignant.[213] Actually, the majority behave in a benign fashion and are properly designated as *Hürthle cell adenoma*[196,197,199,206] (Fig. 9-40, *A*). Tumors with clearcut

capsular and/or blood vessel invasion are called *Hürthle cell carcinoma*. As a group, the carcinomas occur in an older age group, show a lesser degree of female predominance, are larger, and tend to have a solid/trabecular rather than a follicular pattern of growth (Fig. 9-40, *B*). Curiously, the cells of carcinoma are often smaller than those of adenoma, a feature also noticeable on cytologic examination. In the presence of any of these features, the search for capsular and/or vascular invasion should be particularly

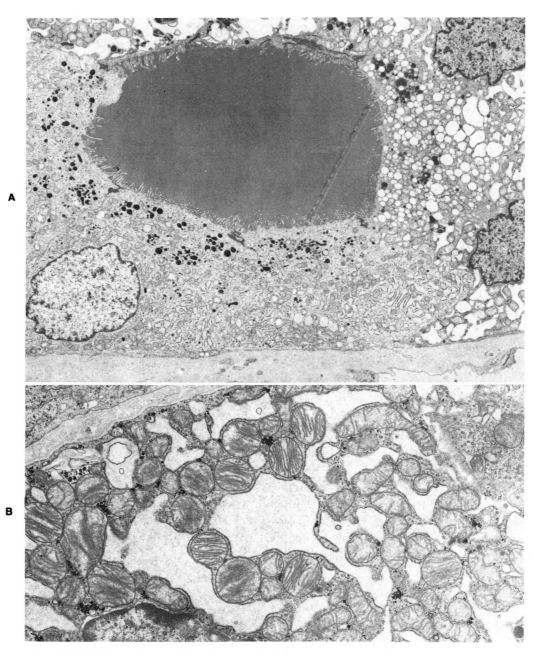

Fig. 9-39 Hürthle cell tumor of thyroid gland. **A,** Cytoplasm is packed with mitochondria. Secretory product is located toward lumen, which is filled with colloid. **B,** Variably sized mitochondria with prominent cristae. (**A,** ×3,840; **B,** ×11,230.)

thorough. We and others have used the noncommittal term *Hürthle cell neoplasm* (biologically indeterminate; of undeterminate malignant potential; borderline) for the tumors that exhibit one or more of these features but lack unequivocal signs of malignancy.[198,209]

The adenomas are almost always cured by excision. The carcinomas are rather aggressive neoplasms, with a 5-year-mortality rate between 20% and 40%.[202,204,205,210] Metastases occur mainly in lungs and bone and less commonly in cervical nodes.[211,214] Analysis of DNA ploidy may prove of some prognostic significance; preliminary observations have shown a high incidence of invasive growth in aneuploid tumors.[195,201]

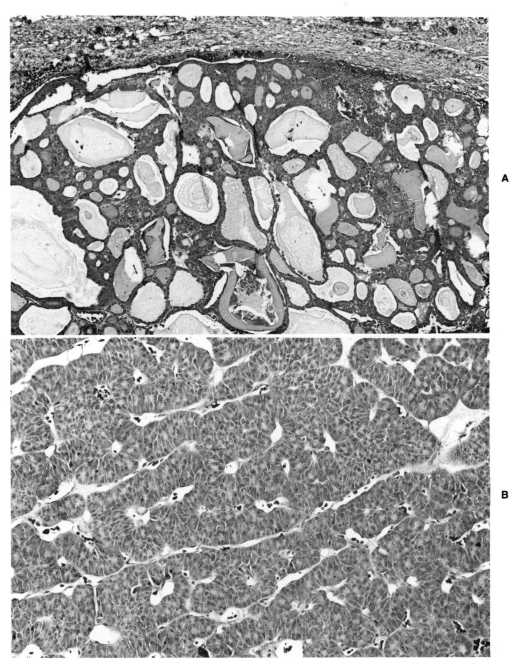

Fig. 9-40 A, Hürthle cell adenoma. Tumor has follicular pattern of growth and is completely surrounded by capsule. There was no evidence of capsular or blood vessel invasion. **B,** Hürthle cell carcinoma. Tumor has solid and trabecular pattern that by itself is suggestive but not diagnostic of cancer. Elsewhere, there were obvious areas of capsular and blood vessel invasion.

An unresolved problem is represented by the rare Hürthle cell tumors composed entirely of papillae (as opposed to the more common pseudopapillary formations previously mentioned).[194,212] In our experience, those that were encapsulated have behaved in a benign fashion. Those that are invasive are said to behave like conventional papillary carcinomas.[194]

Clear cell tumors

Clear cell changes can occur in thyroid neoplasms of various microscopic types (Fig. 9-41). The natural history of these tumors is determined by their basic nature rather than the presence or degree of cytoplasmic clearing in them. Therefore *clear cell carcinoma* should not be viewed as a specific tumor type.[215,222]

The neoplasm most prone to undergo secondary clear cell changes is Hürthle cell tumor, this being the result of vesicular swelling of mitochondria.[221] The oxyphilic and clear cell changes may be seen in adjacent cells or even in different regions of the same cell.[217] Clear cell changes can also occur in follicular adenomas and carcinomas (usually due to vesicles of either mitochondrial or granular endoplasmic reticulum derivation), papillary carcinoma (usually due to glycogen accumulation),[225] undifferentiated carcinoma (also the result of glycogen overload) and—exceptionally—medullary carcinoma.[218] Except for the latter, thyroglobulin stain is usually positive in these neoplasms although sometimes in a focal and faint fashion.[215,216] Although the presence of clear cell change in a follicular neoplasm *per se* is not an indication of malignancy, it occurs more frequently in carcinomas than in adenomas.

A peculiar variant of thyroid tumor with clear cell changes is *signet ring adenoma*, in which the formation of variously sized cytoplasmic vacuoles results in a configuration reminiscent of signet-ring cells or lipoblasts.[219,223] Immunohistochemically, the vacuoles contain intracellular thyroglobulin.[215] The stroma is usually heavily hyalinized and with punctate calcification, suggesting that the signet-ring change may be of degenerative nature and the expression of an arrest of folliculogenesis.[219] Some of this material has been found to react positively with mucin stains.[220]

Another rare form is the *lipid-rich cell adenoma*, in which the cytoplasmic vacuolization is due to the accumulation of neutral fat.[224]

The main differential diagnosis of primary thyroid tumors with clear cells is with parathyroid neoplasms and metastatic renal cell carcinoma[215,222] (see p. 438).

It should be remembered that cytoplasmic clear cell changes can also occur in non-neoplastic thyroid disorders, including Hashimoto's thyroiditis and dyshormonogenetic goiter.[215]

Epidermoid, mucinous, and related tumors

Squamous cells can be found in the thyroid from persistence of thyroglossal duct or branchial cleft structures (such as thymic epithelium) or as an expression of squamous metaplasia in Hashimoto's thyroiditis or papillary carci-

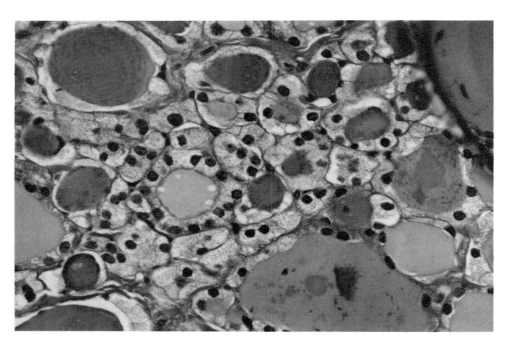

Fig. 9-41 Thyroid follicular tumor with clear cell changes. Note fine cytoplasmic granularity, a feature of importance in differential diagnosis with metastatic renal cell carcinoma.

noma.[230,231] Pure *epidermoid carcinomas* are exceptional.[229] Some have been associated with leukocytosis and hypercalcemia.[235] Most high-grade thyroid tumors with squamous foci blend with areas of undifferentiated (anaplastic) carcinoma and are generally placed in the latter category because of their similar natural history.[226] Indeed, many of them are seen to develop from papillary carcinoma in a fashion analogous to that of undifferentiated carcinoma.[234] In the presence of an obvious epidermoid carcinoma involving the thyroid, the possibility should also be considered of secondary direct involvement from a tumor of larynx or trachea or a metastasis from lung or other sites.

Mucoepidermoid carcinoma has been described as a low-grade thyroid neoplasm combining foci of squamous change with mucin production and lacking immunoreactivity for thyroglobulin[227,233] (Fig. 9-42). The clinical features of the reported cases and the presence in some of these tumors of ground glass nuclei and psammoma bodies suggests to us that they may represent papillary carcinomas with extreme squamous and mucinous metaplasia.

A few cases of *mucinous carcinoma* lacking a squamous component have been described.[238] In this regard, it is opportune to note that the thyroglobulin molecule contains variable amounts of carbohydrates that may result in some degree of alcianophilia.[236]

We have seen four cases of a *sclerosing squamoid tumor* of the thyroid associated with heavy eosinophilic infiltration arising in a background of florid Hashimoto's thyroiditis;

despite the occurrence of extrathyroid extension, the behavior has been favorable.[237]

Miyauchi et al.[232] have described several cases of a nonkeratinizing large cell carcinoma, which they have interpreted as an *intrathyroidal epithelial thymoma;* they base their rather imaginative proposal on the undeniable morphologic similarities of this tumor with thymic carcinoma and the fact that ectopic thymic tissue is occasionally found within the thyroid gland (Fig. 9-43). This tumor is immunoreactive for keratin and negative for thyroglobulin; its prognosis is markedly better than for epidermoid carcinoma.

There also occurs in the thyroid a biphasic tumor composed of spindle cells and mucous cysts, which has also been interpreted as of thymic origin.[228] Finally, we have seen several cases of *thymoma* with a typical microscopic appearance located in a juxtathyroid position.

Poorly differentiated carcinoma

In the traditional scheme of thyroid neoplasia, malignant tumors of follicular cells are divided into a well-differentiated type composed of papillary and follicular carcinoma and an undifferentiated or anaplastic type. There is growing evidence for the existence of a group of tumors that fall in between these two extremes, both in terms of morphologic appearance and behavior.[239-242] We have identified one such type under the descriptive name of *insular carcinoma.*[240] The tumor occurs in an older group than the well-differentiated tumors and is usually grossly invasive. Microscopically, the distinguishing features are a nesting ("in-

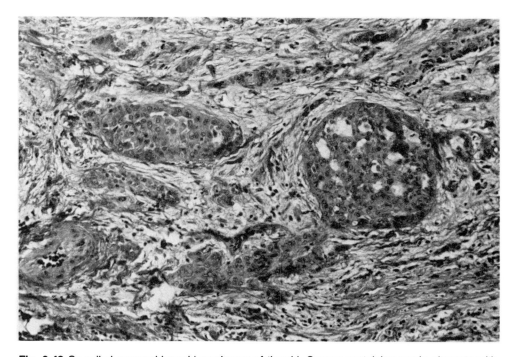

Fig. 9-42 So-called mucoepidermoid carcinoma of thyroid. Spaces containing mucin alternate with solid areas showing squamoid features. This tumor may represent metaplastic change in papillary carcinoma.

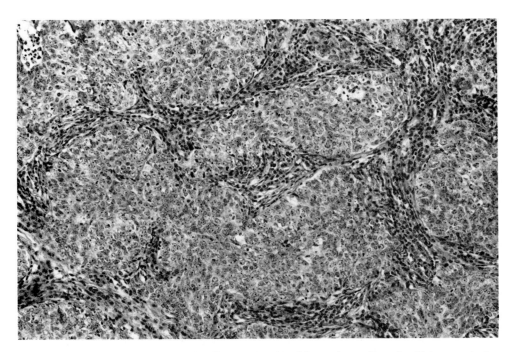

Fig. 9-43 So-called intrathyroid thymoma. Tumor grows in solid nests formed by cells with large vesicular nuclei with prominent nucleoli, giving it a resemblance to lymphoepithelioma. (Courtesy Dr. A. Miyauchi, Kagawa, Japan.)

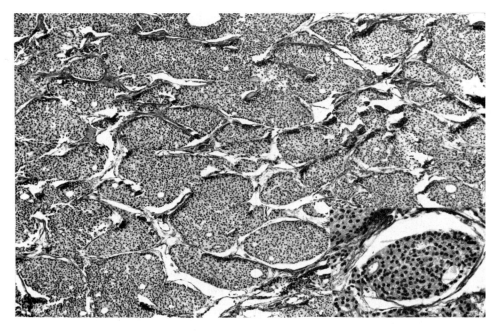

Fig. 9-44 Poorly differentiated (insular) carcinoma of thyroid. Distinctly nesting pattern of growth may induce confusion with medullary carcinoma. **Inset** shows uniformity of small tumor cells and predominantly solid pattern of growth within islets, with occasional formation of small follicles.

sular'') pattern of growth, solid to microfollicular arrangement, small uniform tumor cells, variable mitotic activity, and fresh tumor necrosis resulting in a peritheliomatous pattern (Fig. 9-44). Some of the so-called compact types of undifferentiated small cell carcinoma probably belong to this category. The insular pattern may result in a mistaken

diagnosis of medullary carcinoma. Immunohistochemically, there is reactivity for thyroglobulin but not for calcitonin (see Color plate II, *F*). The behavior is aggressive. Both nodal and blood-borne metastases occur. In our series, the mortality rate was about 60%.[239]

This neoplasm, which is probably analogous to Langhans'

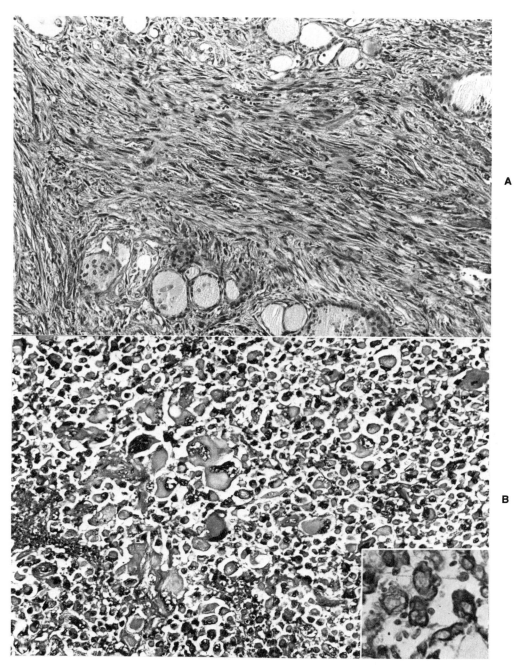

Fig. 9-45 A, Undifferentiated carcinoma of spindle-cell type. Tumor grows in diffuse fashion around thyroid follicles. Appearance closely simulates that of soft tissue sarcoma. **B,** Undifferentiated carcinoma of pleomorphic (giant cell) type. Several giant tumor cells with huge hyperchromatic nuclei are present in solid and myxoid background. **Inset** shows positive immunocytochemical reaction for keratin in a similar case.

wuchernde Struma, has a peculiar geographic distribution, in the sense that it seems to be more common in some parts of Europe and South America than in the United States. We view it as a poorly differentiated variant of either follicular or papillary carcinoma. Indeed, some of our cases coexisted or were preceded by typical papillary carcinoma.[240]

Other authors have also proposed the existence of poorly differentiated tumors, although using different morphologic criteria. French authors[239,243] designate as "less differentiated" follicular carcinomas those exhibiting a trabecular pattern of growth; Sakamoto et al.[242] include in their category of poorly differentiated follicular or papillary carcinomas tumors showing solid, trabecular, and/or scirrhous patterns.

Undifferentiated carcinoma

Undifferentiated carcinoma, also known as anaplastic or sarcomatoid carcinoma, usually presents in elderly patients as a rapidly growing mass associated with hoarseness, dysphagia, and dyspnea.[246] Extrathyroid extension is encountered at the time of initial presentation in most of the cases. Grossly, a highly necrotic and hemorrhagic solid tumor mass is seen replacing large portions of the organ. Microscopically, three major patterns occur, sometimes in combination. In the first, which we designate as *squamoid*, the cells are undifferentiated but retain an unmistakable epithelial appearance.[246] Occasionally, these areas blend with foci of obvious keratinization. The other two patterns are known as *spindle cell* and *giant cell* (Fig. 9-45). They may exhibit a fascicular or storiform pattern of growth, heavy neutrophilic infiltration, prominent vascularization, and cartilaginous/osseous metaplasia. As a result, their appearance may closely simulate a large variety of soft tissue sarcomas, particularly malignant fibrous histiocytoma (including the inflammatory and myxoid variants), angiosarcoma, malignant hemangiopericytoma, and fibrosarcoma.[246] Osteoclast-like multinucleated giant cells may be present, giving the tumor an appearance reminiscent of giant cell tumor of bone or soft tissues.[250,262] It should be kept in mind that nearly all sarcoma-like tumors of the thyroid are in reality undifferentiated carcinoma. Common and diagnostically useful features are palisading at the necrotic edges and tendency for the tumor cells to invade the wall of veins replacing the normal smooth muscle. Ultrastructural examination will reveal markers suggestive of epithelial differentiation in about half of the cases.[246,253,258] Immunohistochemically, the most useful marker is keratin, which will be found to be expressed in 50% to 100% of the cases, according to the different series.[246,251,255,256] Vimentin is consistently present in the spindle-cell component, there is scattered reactivity for laminin,[257] and focal CEA positivity may be found in the squamoid type.[246] We and others have been unable to detect thyroglobulin in the truly undifferentiated cases[246,260] but other authors have been more successful, even in metastatic foci.[244,247,251,255,264] The use of monoclonal as opposed to polyclonal antibodies could explain some of these discrepancies. Also, care should be exercised not to misinterpret areas of entrapped normal thyroid or thyroglobulin diffusion in the tumor.

Most if not all undifferentiated thyroid carcinomas arise as a result of anaplastic transformation of a pre-existing well-differentiated tumor, usually papillary carcinoma (Fig. 9-46).[248,249] In most instances, this transformation takes place in the primary tumor, but it can also occur in a metastatic focus. Thorough sampling may be necessary to detect the residual well-differentiated component.[252] The suggestion that most undifferentiated thyroid carcinomas are of medullary (C-cell) type has not been confirmed.[246]

In older classifications of undifferentiated carcinoma, a small-cell type with either a diffuse or compact pattern of growth was often included. It has become apparent that nearly all of the former are in reality malignant lymphomas and that the majority of the latter represent small-cell variants of medullary carcinomas or insular carcinomas. Therefore the use of the term small-cell thyroid carcinoma without a qualifier should be discouraged.[246,261]

The evolution of undifferentiated thyroid carcinoma is very rapid, with massive growth in the neck, infiltration of the ribbon muscles, esophagus, trachea, skin, and even contiguous bones. Nodal and distant metastases are also common.[259] The mortality rate is nearly 100%, the mean survival less than 6 months, and the immediate cause of death is usually involvement of vital structures in the neck.[246] There is a slightly better chance of cure for those patients in whom the undifferentiated component is only a focal change in an otherwise well-differentiated neoplasm.[245] Isolated successes have been obtained with a combination of surgery, radiation therapy, and chemotherapy.[254,263]

Medullary carcinoma, C-cell hyperplasia, and related tumors

Medullary carcinoma is the name originally given to a distinctive type of thyroid malignancy composed of C (parafollicular) cells; it is also known as solid carcinoma, hyaline carcinoma, and *C-cell carcinoma*.[280,281] Grossly, it is solid, firm, nonencapsulated but relatively well-circumscribed and with a grey cut surface. Most cases are located in the upper half of the gland, corresponding to a greater concentration of C-cells in this region. Microscopically, the typical case is characterized by a solid proliferation of round to polygonal cells of granular amphophilic cytoplasm and medium-sized nucleus, separated by a highly vascular stroma, hyalinized collagen, and amyloid[270] (Fig. 9-47). Coarse calcification is common and can be prominent enough to be detected radiographically.

The number of cytoarchitectural variations on this theme is very large. The pattern of growth can be in the form of distinct carcinoid-like nests, trabecular, glandular (tubular and follicular), or pseudopapillary.[277,279,284] The stroma may be scanty, hemorrhagic, ossified, or edematous. The amyloid deposition may be widespread, limited to small psammomatoid concretions, or absent altogether. Sometimes this amyloid elicits a florid foreign body–type giant cell reaction. True psammoma bodies may be present. A heavy neutrophilic infiltrate is occasionally seen (so-called inflammatory type). The tumor cells may be plasmacytoid (due to nuclear peripheralization), spindle shaped, have an abundant granular acidophilic cytoplasm (thus simulating Hürthle

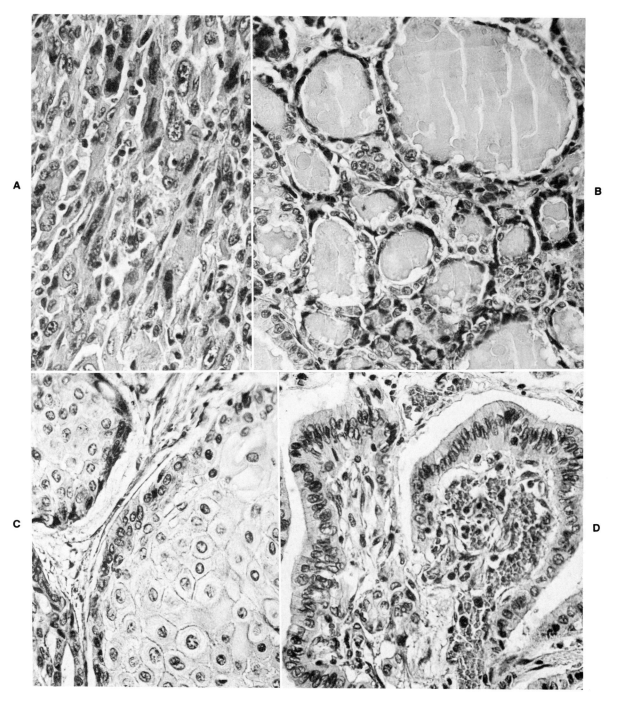

Fig. 9-46 Morphologic variations of thyroid carcinoma in various anatomic sites. The pattern of growth is undifferentiated in the thyroid **(A),** follicular in the kidney **(B),** squamous in the hilar lymph nodes **(C),** and papillary in the lung **(D).** This case could be explained by postulating the existence of a papillary carcinoma that metastasized widely and which subsequently developed anaplastic transformation.

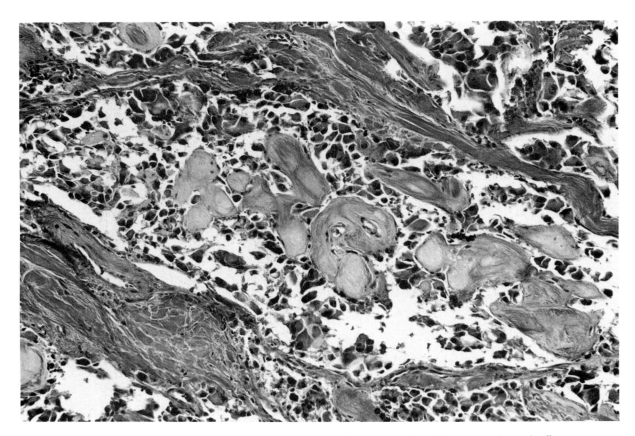

Fig. 9-47 Medullary carcinoma with classic appearance. Tumor grows in solid nests of polygonal cells, accompanied by depositions of large amounts of amyloid.

cells), or exhibit bizarre features (so-called anaplastic type, not to be equated with the real anaplastic carcinoma).[286,296] Unusual varieties of medullary carcinoma include a true papillary form,[287] a type exhibiting mucinous features (mucinous medullary carcinoma),[276] a clear cell variant,[290] a small cell type (see p. 426), and a pigmented (melanin-producing) variant[294] (Fig. 9-48).

Ultrastructurally, cytoplasmic dense-core secretory granules are invariably present. A variability in their sizes has been detected, suggesting the existence of multiple endocrine cell types in this tumor.[269] These granules are usually argyrophilic with the Grimelius stain, expecially if the tissue has been fixed in Bouin's fluid. Mucin stains have been found to be often positive in this neoplasm.[318]

Immunohistochemically, the tumor cells are reactive for epithelial markers such as keratin, for pan-endocrine markers such as neuron-specific enolase, chromogranin A, B, and C (the latter also known as secretogranin II), synaptophysin, and opioid peptides, and for the specific product of C-cells, i.e., calcitonin[267,272,301,303,308] (Fig. 9-49). They are also consistently positive for CEA and dsgenerally negative for thyroglobulin.[271,293,310] Other products that have

been detected in cases of medullary carcinoma include somatostatin, ACTH, calcitonin gene–related peptide, serotonin, MSH, prostaglandins, bombesin, gastrin-releasing peptide, substance P, L-dopa decarboxylase, histaminase, glucagon, insulin, and HCG.*

Conceptually, synthesis of these various peptide hormones by medullary carcinoma points to a histogenetic relation of this neoplasm with carcinoid tumors of other organs, and it raises the possibility that what is now considered a single entity may well represent a family of related but eventually separable "neuroendocrine" neoplasms. Along these lines, we have seen several cases of thyroid carcinoma with a distinctly "neuroendocrine" pattern of growth that were devoid of amyloid, negative for calcitonin and thyroglobulin, and positive for neuron-specific enolase, chromogranin, and CEA. Whether these tumors should be viewed as poorly differentiated variants of medullary carcinoma that have lost the capacity to produce calcitonin, or whether they should be considered as separate "neouroendocrine carci-

*See references 273, 275, 282, 289, 291, 295, 297, 311, 314, and 317.

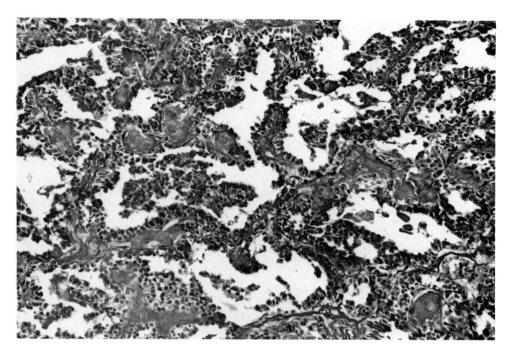

Fig. 9-48 Medullary carcinoma with pseudopapillary pattern of growth, resulting from lack of cohesiveness of tumor cells.

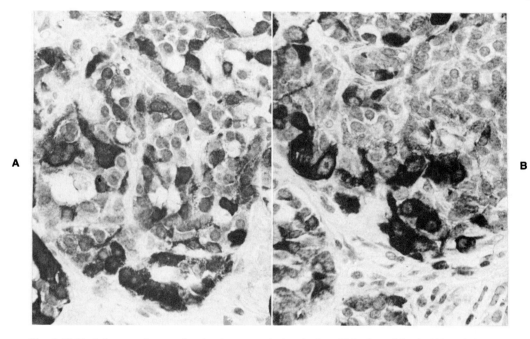

Fig. 9-49 Medullary carcinoma showing immunocytochemical positivity for calcitonin **(A)** and chromogranin **(B).**

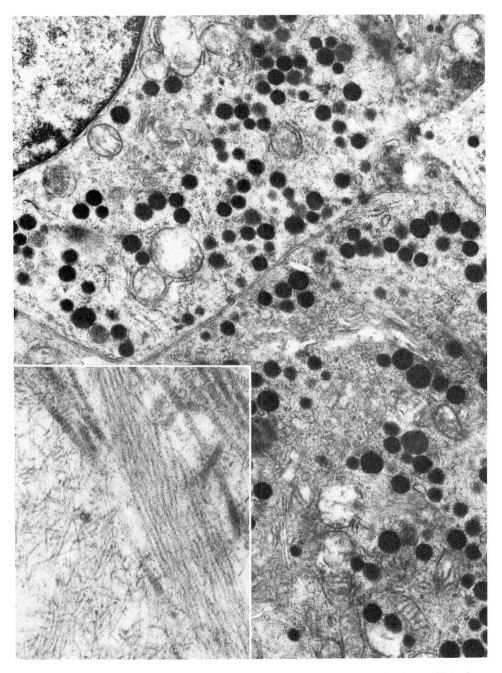

Fig. 9-50 Portions of two cells from medullary carcinoma of thyroid gland showing multiple dense secretory granules in cytoplasm. Each granule is surrounded by single membrane, and dense central portion is separated from it by clear zone. **Inset** shows both oriented and randomly placed amyloid filaments and may be contrasted with larger banded collagen fibers. (Courtesy Dr. J.S. Meyer, St. Louis, MO.)

nomas'' analogous to those seen in many other organs is not clear.

The amyloid of medullary carcinoma reacts with the generic stains for this substance and has a typical microfibrillary appearance ultrastructurally (Fig. 9-50). It also shows reactivity for calcitonin, suggesting that its production may be related to the secretion or degradation of this hormone.[268]

Two forms of medullary carcinoma exist: sporadic and familial. The *sporadic* form comprises about 80% of the cases, affects adult individuals (mean age, 45 yrs) and is almost always solitary.[292] It presents as a thyroid mass which is cold on thyroid scan; in some cases, it is accompanied by intractable diarrhea or Cushing's syndrome.[312] Only rarely is it clinically occult.[316]

The *familial* form becomes clinically apparent in a young age group (mean age, 35 yrs), is often multiple and bilateral, and is invariably accompanied by C-cell hyperplasia in the residual gland. Nearly all cases of medullary thyroid carcinomas occurring in children belong to this type, which is inherited as an autosomal dominant of virtually complete penetrance. In many of the cases, it represents a component of multiple endocrine adenomatosis type II or III, particularly the former[266] (see Chapter 15).

C-cell hyperplasia is the precursor lesion of familial medullary carcinoma. It is particularly pronounced in the central part of the lateral lobes. It may be diffuse or nodular, and the C-cells may be seen in an inter- or intrafollicular location (see Color plate I, *D*). The arbitrary figure of more than six cells per thyroid follicle has been suggested as an indicator of C-cell hyperplasia.[266] As a rule, these cells exhibit greater CEA immunoreativity than normal C-cells and greater calcitonin immunoreactivity than the cells of medullary carcinoma. The differential diagnosis of this preneoplastic disorder includes the C-cell hyperplasia of probable reactive nature recently described in the immediate periphery of thyroid neoplasms of various microscopic types.[265] Monitoring of patients with the familial medullary carcinoma syndrome is carried out by periodic determinations of serum levels of calcitonin and CEA.[315] In medullary carcinoma, there is also serum elevation of chromogranin A.[300]

Medullary carcinoma invades locally and gives rise to metastases in cervical and mediastinal lymph nodes and also in distant organs, particularly lung, liver, and skeletal system.[274] They appear to be more common in sporadic and MEA III–associated tumors than in MEA II–associated neoplasms.[285] These metastases may be the first manifestation of the disease and be a source of confusion to the pathologist.[313] Microscopically, they tend to resemble the primary tumor and—as a result—usually contain amyloid. The resemblance also applies to their immunohistochemical reactivity, although notable exceptions occur.[304]

The primary treatment is surgical, in the form of total thyroidectomy (particularly for the familial form) and cervical lymphadenectomy. Local recurrence supervenes in about 35% of the patients, and the 5-year survival rate varies between 70% and 80%.[270,307] The tumor is not particularly responsive to radioactive iodine, external radiation therapy, or chemotherapy.

Good prognostic factors are young age, female sex, occurrence in a familial setting, and tumor confinement to the gland.[270,307,309] Microscopically, a greater degree of aggressiveness should be expected of tumors with high mitotic activity and/or of the small cell type. It has been claimed that poor immunohistochemical reactivity for calcitonin is an indicator of poor prognosis, particularly if coupled with increased reactivity for CEA.[298,305,306] Persistent or recurrent elevation of serum calcitonin following surgery is a reliable indicator of tumor persistence or relapse.

Medullary (C-cell) adenoma has been suggested as a diagnosis for the encapsulated forms for C-cell tumors, but its existence as an entity separate from medullary carcinoma is doubtful.

Mixed medullary-follicular carcinoma is a controversial entity in which the morphologic features of medullary carcinoma (together with immunoreactivity for calcitonin) coexist with those of a follicular neoplasm (together with immunoreactivity for thyroglobulin).[302] It has been suggested that thyroglobulin-containing medullary carcinoma may be an unusual expression of multihormonal production by this tumor.[283] Although a mixed medullary-follicular carcinoma probably exists, most cases in which this diagnosis has been entertained represent medullary carcinomas with entrapped follicles and/or secondary incorporation of thyroglobulin by the medullary carcinoma cells.

Paraganglioma can occur adjacent to or within the thyroid, sometimes in association with carotid body tumors.[278,288] The differential diagnosis with medullary carcinoma and follicular adenoma can be very difficult, particularly with the former (Fig. 9-51). Paraganglioma reacts immunohistochemically for the panendocrine markers such as chromogranin and opioid peptides but is negative for calcitonin and thyroglobulin. A particularly useful feature is the presence of S-100 protein-positive sustentacular cells at the periphery of the *zellballen* (see Chapter 16). The behavior of all but one of the reported cases has been benign.[299]

Small cell carcinoma morphologically identical to the homonymous lung tumor has been described in the thyroid. Some of these tumors are calcitonin-positive and are therefore regarded as small cell variants of medullary carcinoma. Those which are calcitonin-negative probably represent the most undifferentiated members of the spectrum; their behavior is extremely aggressive.

Epithelial tumors—general features
Geographic distribution

The previously accepted link between iodine deficiency and thyroid carcinoma is now disputed, largely because of the fact that several authors have not found differences in the incidence of thyroid cancer in iodine-deficient areas before and after the introduction of iodized salt.[323] However, most series show that a statistical correlation exists between iodine deficiency and thyroid carcinoma of both follicular and undifferentiated types.[319-322] Papillary carcinoma is the predominant type in areas without iodine deficiency, and its frequency is said to be increased in regions with a high iodine uptake.[324]

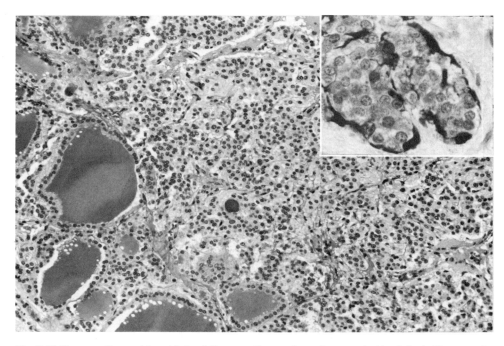

Fig. 9-51 Paraganglioma of thyroid gland. Tumor cells grow in nests separated by delicate fibrovascular stroma and infiltrate between normal follicles. Presence of S-100–positive sustentacular cells, as shown in **inset**, is important feature in differential diagnosis with medullary carcinoma.

Thyroid neoplasia in childhood

Most thyroid tumors developing in childhood are benign and examples of either follicular adenoma or nodular hyperplasia. However, the proportion of carcinomas is much higher than that seen in adults, to the point of surpassing the benign processes in some recent series.[326] Among the malignancies, papillary carcinoma comprises the overwhelming majority of the cases, followed by the familial form of medullary carcinoma and Hürthle cell neoplasms.[325] In older series there is also an important representation of follicular carcinomas, but most of those would now be regarded as papillary carcinomas with predominantly or exclusively follicular pattern of growth.[327,328] Undifferentiated and poorly differentiated carcinomas are exceptionally rare in this age group.

The papillary carcinomas occurring in children tend to have solid and/or squamous areas and are associated with a high frequency of cervical node metastases, but their prognosis is excellent. Some of these children give a history of previous radiation exposure to the neck (see next section).

Thyroid neoplasia and radiation exposure

Exposure of the thyroid gland to low-dose therapeutic radiation (administered for thymic enlargement, tonsillar hypertrophy, or acne to about one million patients in this country) can result in a number of abnormalities later in life. The most common of them are of a *benign* nature — a fact to remember — and consist of nodular hyperplasia, lymphocytic thyroiditis, and fibrosis.[330,332,336] There is also an increased incidence of carcinoma in this population, the large majority of the tumors being of the papillary type.[331,333] Of patients in this population having a thyroid operation, the incidence of carcinoma ranges from 20% to over 50%.[329,337] Despite earlier statements to the contrary, there is no convincing evidence that these tumors behave differently than others. The quoted incidences of multicentricity and nodal metastases have been high, but the long-term prognosis has been very good.

Tumors from other structures of the neck can also develop in individuals with radiation exposure to the area; these include salivary gland, parathyroid, osseous, and neural neoplasms.[334,335] This obviously indicates the need for a continuous surveillance of this population.

High-dose radiation to the region, such as that administered for Hodgkin's disease, can also result in thyroid carcinoma and other abnormalities.

Association with other conditions

Cases of thyroid carcinoma of nonmedullary types (particularly of the papillary variety) have been reported in a familial setting,[340] in patients with ataxia-telangiectasia,[341] and in association with parathyroid tumors,[338] carotid body tumors, and polyposis coli.[342] Whether the co-existence of these diseases is significant or simply a coincidence remains to be determined.[339]

Evaluation of the solitary thyroid nodule

The most common thyroid problem facing the surgeon and the pathologist is the evaluation of the patient with an apparently single thyroid mass. The magnitude of the problem is obvious from the fact that about 4% of the U.S. population between the ages of 30 and 60 years have one or more palpable nodules. Since the large majority of these nodules are benign and most are not even neoplastic, the goal is to be selective in the cases taken to surgery while at the same time including most of the carcinomas in this group. Factors to consider when making this difficult selection process are the following:

1 *Age*. The incidence of malignancy is higher in the two extremes of life.
2 *Sex*. The incidence of malignancy is higher in males.
3 *Number*. Solitary nodules are more likely to be malignant than multiple ones.
4 *Associated ipsilateral adenopathy*. This is the strongest clinical indicator of malignancy if present.
5 *Function*. Nodules that are hyperfunctioning ("toxic") at the clinical level and/or "hot" on thyroid scintiscan are less likely to be malignant than the others.
6 *Ultrasonography*. Cystic nodules are less likely to be malignant than solid ones.
7 *Hashimoto's thyroiditis*. The likelihood of malignancy for a nodule present in Hashimoto's thyroiditis is roughly the same as for that occurring in a normal gland.
8 *Needle biopsy*. In experienced hands, this technique will provide the best predictor of malignancy.[343]

To put these various clinical criteria in perspective, it should be mentioned that even when the nodule is solitary, solid, and cold on scintiscan, it will prove malignant in no more than 10% to 20% of the cases.

Needle biopsy and fine needle aspiration

Core needle biopsy has been used extensively in a few institutions in this country and abroad but has not gained widespread acceptance.[356] It is particularly helpful in diffuse diseases such as Hashimoto's thyroiditis and in confirming the diagnosis of an advanced malignant neoplasm.[362] Most authors have been reluctant to use this technique in the evaluation of the single thyroid nodule not only because of the small but definite risk of complications (bleeding, nerve injury, tracheal perforation, tumor implantation),[350] but also because of the fact that the differential diagnosis between a benign and malignant follicular lesion is impossible with this technique. This is hardly surprising, inasmuch as the two main histologic criteria of malignancy (i.e., capsular and vascular invasion) will not be apparent in most needle biopsies.

Fine needle aspiration has become, in a matter of few years, an extremely popular technique for the evaluation of solitary thyroid nodules. Its appeal is obvious: it is quick, inexpensive, it can be carried out in the physician's office, and the risk of complications (including tumor implantation) is minimal.[346,357a] Published results claim a sensitivity and specificity of over 90%, leading some authors to recommend fine needle aspiration as the initial test in the evaluation of any thyroid nodule.[344,359-361] Most papillary carcinomas and other types of malignancy other than follicular carci-noma can be identified with ease.[345,348,353,357] The same is true for the various types of thyroiditis.[347] The main difficulty, as in the case of the core needle biopsy, resides in the identification of well-differentiated follicular carcinoma, a task which may be impossible with this method in view of the nature of the diagnostic criteria required.[358] In most instances, the cytology report will be one of the following three:

1 *Probably benign nodule*, when the material is composed largely of colloid, histiocytes, and a few normal-looking follicular cells. This will be an indication for a conservative approach unless the clinical data suggest otherwise.
2 *Follicular neoplasm*, when cellularity is higher than that found in the usual hyperplastic nodule but when the nuclear features of papillary carcinoma are absent. The diagnosis of Hürthle cell neoplasm would fall into this category.[352] The diagnosis of follicular neoplasm is an indication for removal of the nodule unless this is contraindicated for medical reasons.
3 *Papillary carcinoma*, when the characteristic cytoarchitectural features of this tumor type are present, such as papillary fronds, psammoma bodies, nuclear pseudoinclusions, and nuclear grooves. It should be remembered that the ground glass nuclear feature is usually not apparent in cytologic preparations, that nuclear pseudoinclusions are not pathognomonic of papillary carcinoma, and that cystic degeneration of the tumor may obscure the cell details.[349,355] The cytologic diagnosis of papillary carcinoma is obviously an indication for therapeutic intervention.

Performance of fine needle aspiration may result in partial or complete infarct of the tumor, with only a thin rim of tissue preserved at the periphery; this complication seems to be more common with Hürthle cell tumors,[351] and it may result in transient elevation of the serum levels of thyroglobulin.[354]

Frozen section

The pathologist is often asked to perform a frozen section at the time of exploration of a thyroid mass.[364] The specimen may be from an area of extrathyroid invasion by carcinoma or from a metastatic cervical node. In these instances, the diagnosis is usually obvious, although Riedel's thyroiditis (p. 398), extrathyroid growth in diffuse hyperplasia (p. 400), and sequestered nodular goiter (p. 434) represent important diagnostic pitfalls.[365] The most common specimen received for frozen section is a lobectomy carried out because of a nodule. A few of these will be found to be examples of granulomatous thyroiditis, Hashimoto's thyroiditis, or malignant lymphoma, each of which may manifest as a apparently single nodule on physical examination. However, in the large majority of the cases the differential diagnosis will be between a dominant nodule of nodular hyperplasia, adenoma, and carcinoma. An experienced pathologist should have no problem in identifying most cases of undifferentiated carcinomas, poorly differentiated carcinomas, widely invasive follicular carcinomas, conventional papillary carcinomas, or medullary carcinomas. The most difficult problem resides in the distinction between a dominant nodule of nodular hyperplasia, follicular adenoma, minimally invasive follicular carcinoma, and the variant of papillary carcinoma that is both follicular and encapsulated. These considerations also apply to the encapsulated Hürthle cell neoplasms. Evidence of capsular and/or blood vessel invasion may not be evident in the samples chosen for frozen sections but become obvious later in the more thorough sampling of permanent sections. The ground glass nuclear feature that is one of the most distinguishing features of papillary carcinoma may not show up at all in the frozen section. For these reasons, the surgeon should accept the fact that a certain percentage of well-differentiated carcinomas will not be identifiable on frozen section examination no matter how experienced and astute the pathologist is. This apparent deficiency does not create serious therapeutic problems because, in our opinion, most if not all of the lesions listed in this paragraph are effectively treated by lobectomy or—at the most—subtotal thyroidectomy. Indeed, the number of cases in which the frozen section results influence significantly the surgical planning is quite small.[363]

Presence of thyroid tissue outside gland

There are several circumstances in which normal or abnormal thyroid tissue may be found in the neck outside the confines of the thyroid gland:

1 Ectopic thyroid tissue resulting from faulty embryogenesis. Thyroglossal duct cyst and lingual thyroid are the most common examples (see p. 392).
2 Extension of hyperplastic thyroid tissue outside the gland in Graves' disease (see p. 400).
3 Mechanical implantation of thyroid tissue in the neck as a result of accidental trauma or surgical intervention.

In the latter instance, suture material may be seen adjacent to the thyroid tissue.

4 So-called *sequestered thyroid nodule*. This refers to the occurrence of a peripherally located thyroid nodule that either loses its anatomic connection with the main gland or this connection is missed by the surgeon, the process being somewhat analogous to that of parasitic uterine leiomyoma.[367,370] The nodule is usually an expression of nodular hyperplasia or nodular Hashimoto's thyroiditis rather than adenoma. The diagnosis requires that the tissue reside in the same fascial plane as the thyroid gland, that it be unassociated with lymph nodes, and that it exhibit the same or similar histology as the main gland, whenever the latter is available. Sequestration also occurs (and it may actually be more common) in thyroid nodular hyperplasia located in the mediastinum.
5 Thyroid tissue within cervical lymph nodes. The determination of the significance of this finding in the presence of an apparently normal thyroid gland can be a very difficult exercise. This phenomenon accounts for most cases of the condition formerly called *lateral aberrant thyroid*.[366] It is now generally accepted that this may be the result of two unrelated processes and that microscopic examination permits their separation in the majority of the instances.[369]

Most cases represent metastases of clinically undetected thyroid carcinomas, nearly always of the papillary variety. It should be emphasized that detection of the primary neoplasm may require extremely careful microscopic study with embedding of the entire thyroid gland and cutting of the blocks at various levels.[371] The metastatic deposits may replace most of the node, al-

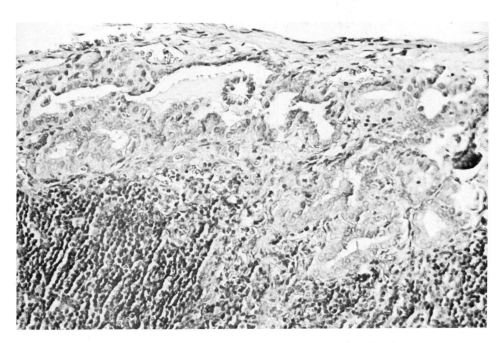

Fig. 9-52 Papillary carcinoma metastatic to cervical lymph node.

though a peripheral rim of residual lymphoid tissue can usually be found (Fig. 9-52). The smaller tumor foci are frequently located within sinuses. The pattern of growth may be so well differentiated as to simulate normal thyroid tissue. However, close inspection will usually reveal the presence of one or more of the cy-

toarchitectural features of papillary carcinoma, such as small papillae, psammoma bodies, follicles with darkly staining colloid, and the characteristic nuclear changes of this tumor type.

The second situation is the occurrence of normal follicles within nodes, a concept originally proposed

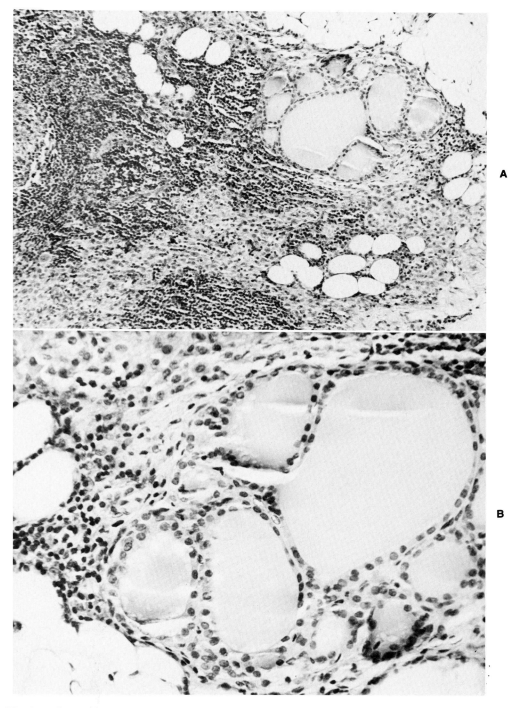

Fig. 9-53 A, Non-neoplastic inclusion consisting of aggregate of ten thyroid follicles at periphery of cervical lymph node. **B,** Similarity of these follicles to normal thyroid tissue is apparent.

by Frantz[366] and which some authors still have difficulties in accepting. The best evidence in its favor is the study performed by Meyer and Steinberg.[368] These authors serially sectioned cervical lymph nodes from 106 autopsies and found thyroid tissue in five of them. Serial section of the whole thyroid gland in these cases failed to reveal carcinoma, except for a probably unrelated microscopic papillary carcinoma in the contralateral lobe of one case.

The ectopic thyroid tissue typically presents as a small conglomerate of follicles lacking all the attributes of papillary carcinoma and limited to the periphery of one or two nodes (Fig. 9-53). Any thyroid tissue replacing most of the node and/or involving several nodes is likely to be metastatic carcinoma.

Treatment

The treatment of most types of thyroid tumors is surgical. In cases in which the nodule is limited to one lobe, lobectomy with isthmusectomy is usually done, with subsequent therapy depending on the nature of the nodule. Nodulectomy is no longer an accepted form of therapy for these lesions. Lobectomy is adequate therapy for follicular adenoma, including Hürthle cell adenoma. We and others believe that lobectomy or—at the most—subtotal thyroidectomy also constitutes adequate therapy for most minimally invasive follicular carcinomas (including minimally invasive Hürthle cell carcinomas) and papillary carcinomas, since it achieves very similar results without the high risk of complications associated with the more radical procedures.[374,376,378,386,387,389] However, the issue remains highly controversial, with several groups recommending total thyroidectomy followed by the administration of radioactive iodine for these patients.[375,379,383,384] We are of the opinion that total thyroidectomy should be reserved for the high-risk group of papillary carcinomas,[374,380] widely invasive follicular carcinomas (including widely invasive Hürthle cell carcinomas), poorly differentiated carcinomas, and medullary carcinomas (particularly those arising in a familial setting). Radical surgery should also be carried out in undifferentiated carcinoma whenever feasible, but most of these tumors are found inoperable.

Radical neck dissection is recommended in cases of medullary carcinoma but no longer in papillary carcinoma.[381] In the cases of the latter tumor associated with obvious nodal metastases, these are taken out without performing a formal *en bloc* lymphadenectomy.

Suppression of thyroid function is carried out routinely by the exogenous administration of thyroid hormone in cases of papillary and follicular carcinoma, although the need for this procedure has been recently questioned.[373]

Another controversial aspect of the therapy regards the

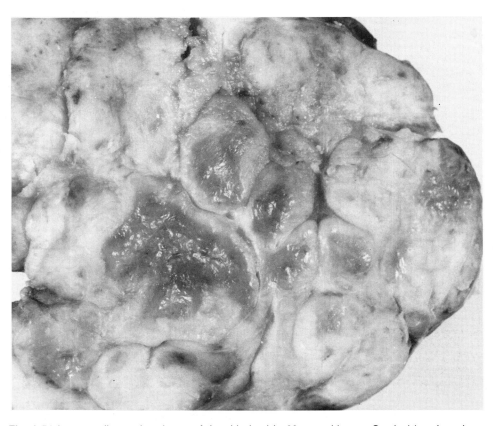

Fig. 9-54 Large malignant lymphoma of thyroid gland in 63-year-old man. Cervical lymph node on same side also was involved.

postoperative administration of radioactive iodine. Some authors recommend it routinely for both papillary and follicular carcinoma.[382,383] We[374] and others[377,389] have not found convincing evidence that its prophylactic administration is needed, even accepting the fact that its effectiveness in the presence of detectable metastases is unquestioned.

External radiation therapy is of limited use in the treatment of thyroid malignancy; its main indication is for incompletely excised tumors.[372,388]

The prognosis following these various forms of therapy is discussed under the different microscopic types. The postoperative monitoring of patients with tumors arising from follicular cells is done with physical examination, chest x-rays, radioiodine scan, and measurements of serum thyroglobulin levels.[385]

Prognostic factors

Most of the clinical and pathologic factors that relate to prognosis have been discussed with the specific tumor types. In general terms, the most important are age and sex of the patient, microscopic type, and tumor stage.[392,394] These and other factors have been sometimes combined in rather complicated prognostic indices.[395] Cady et al.[390] divide their patients with well-differentiated (papillary or follicular) carcinomas into two categories having strikingly different survival rates: low risk (comprised of men under 40 years of age and women under 50 years) and high risk (all older

patients). We confirmed their findings for papillary carcinomas and found that the prognostic difference is even more striking if the low-risk group includes women 60 years and under.[391] The large majority of deaths from thyroid carcinomas result from undifferentiated, poorly differentiated, Hürthle cell, and medullary tumors. It should be realized that in many series several of these tumor types are included among the follicular carcinomas.[393]

Lymphoid tumors and tumorlike conditions

Most cases of primary *malignant lymphoma* of the thyroid are seen in adult or elderly females. The thyroid enlargement is often rapid and can lead to symptoms of tracheal or laryngeal compression.[401,409] Most patients are euthyroid, and the tumor presents as one or more cold nodules on thyroid scan.[403] Grossly, the tumor shows a solid white cut surface with a fish-flesh appearance (Fig. 9-54). Microscopically, the large majority of the cases are of diffuse large cell type and of follicular center cell origin (Fig. 9-55).[401] Sclerosis may be focally prominent. Immunoblastic lymphoma is the second most common type.[398] Lymphomas of poorly differentiated (small cleaved cells) or intermediate type also occur,[399] as well as rare varieties such as signet ring lymphoma.[396] Plasmacytoid features have been detected in many of the cases.[402] Immunohistochemically, they exhibit consistent positivity for leukocyte common antigen.[403a] In addition, nearly all of them show markers indicative of B-cell derivation.[403a,407] An important diagnostic finding is the packing of follicular lumina by lymphoid cells, a feature usually not present in thyroiditis.[402] The differential diagnosis includes the small cell variant of medullary carcinoma and insular carcinoma.

A high proportion of primary thyroid lymphomas arise in a background of lymphocytic or Hashimoto's thyroiditis, perhaps as a result of persistent antigenic stimulation.[401] Accordingly, most of the patients have positive serum tests for antithyroid antibodies.[398] Thyroid lymphoma has been regarded as an example of mucosa-associated lymphoid tissue (MALT).[397] It may be restricted to the thyroid, may spread to the soft tissues by direct extension, or may involve the regional nodes. The prognosis is better for intrathyroid tumors than for those that have extended beyond the thyroid capsule,[413] and for follicular center cell tumors than for immunoblastic lymphomas.[398] It is not uncommon for the recurrence to be located in the gastrointestinal tract.[412]

Primary thyroid lymphoma should be distinguished from generalized lymphoma with thyroid involvement, a somewhat unusual event.

Plasmacytoma of thyroid can be seen as a component of widespread myeloma or as the only manifestation of the disease.[410] Immunoglobulin abnormalities may be present in the serum.[408] The term should be restricted to tumors entirely composed of plasma cells of various degrees of maturity; tumors with a lymphoid component should be placed into the malignant lymphoma category.[400] Plasmacytoma should also be distinguished from *plasma cell granuloma*, a nonneoplastic condition in which a polyclonal infiltrate of mature plasma cells is seen admixed with other inflammatory cells in a fibrotic background.[405]

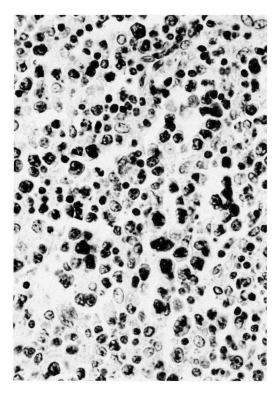

Fig. 9-55 Large cell malignant lymphoma of thyroid gland in adult treated by radiation therapy. Tumor completely disappeared, and patient was still alive more than 7 years after radiation therapy.

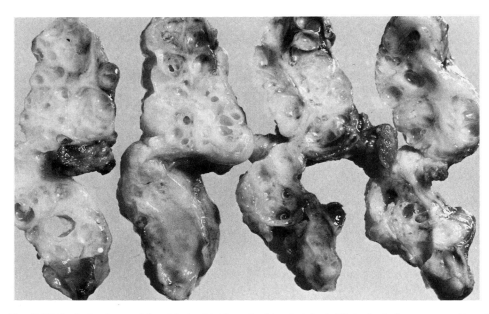

Fig. 9-56 Cystic teratoma of thyroid gland in 4-week-old male infant. Clinically, lesion was considered to be congenital goiter.

Hodgkin's disease involving primarily the thyroid is extremely rare, but its occurrence has been documented. Most of the cases have been of the nodular sclerosis type, and some have shown concomitant involvement of cervical lymph nodes.[404]

Isolated cases of thyroid involvement by *histiocytosis X*[402a,411] and *sinus histiocytosis with massive lymphadenopathy*[406] have been reported.

Mesenchymal tumors

Benign mesenchymal tumors of thyroid are exceptional. Isolated cases of lipoma, hemangioma, and leiomyoma have been reported.

Primary *sarcomas* of the thyroid probably exist, but it should be remembered that most sarcoma-like thyroid tumors are examples of undifferentiated (sarcomatoid) carcinoma[417] (see p. 426). Controversy still exists about the frequency and very existence of thyroid *angiosarcoma*, most examples of which have been reported from Switzerland and other mountainous regions. There is no question that some of these neoplasms exhibit all the attributes of angiosarcoma, such as anastomosing vascular channels, Weibel-Palade bodies on ultrastructural examination, immunoreactivity for FVIII-related antigen and other endothelial cell markers, and tendency to produce hemorrhagic pleuropulmonary metastases.[415,416] The difficulty arises from the fact that sometimes these tumors also display features of carcinoma, either through the simultaneous detection of keratin and FVIII-related antigen[414] or through the presence of obvious areas with an epithelial morphology within the neoplasm. Most cases of this tumor type have arisen in glands with nodular hyperplasia, and the evolution has been almost uniformly fatal.

Other primary tumors

Teratomas of thyroid usually occur in infants or children.[418] The large majority of the cases have been cystic and benign (Fig. 9-56). The few that have been described in adults have been malignant; some of the reported cases and one that we have personally observed were composed of a very primitive neuroepithelial component with rosette formations associated with islands of well-differentiated cartilage,[419] raising some doubts about the truly teratomatous nature of the process.

Metastatic tumors

Direct extension into the thyroid may occur in carcinomas of larynx or trachea.[423] Blood-borne metastases are found in the thyroid at autopsy in about 10% of patients dying of malignant tumors, the most common sites for the primary being skin (melanoma) (39%), breast (21%), kidney (12%), and lung (11%).[422] However, it is rare for these metastases to simulate clinically a primary thyroid neoplasm.[421]

The major exception is renal cell carcinoma, which can present as a thyroid mass in the absence of renal symptoms, years or decades after the removal of the primary tumor.[420] The differential diagnosis is with primary thyroid tumors with clear cell features (see p. 422). Features favoring the diagnosis of metastatic renal cell carcinoma are multiplicity of the nodules, optically clear (as opposed to finely granular) cytoplasm, sinusoidal-type blood vessels, intraluminal fresh hemorrhage, and large amounts of cytoplasmic glycogen and fat[420] (Fig. 9-57). Immunohistochemical stains for thyroglobulin are also helpful, but one should be aware of the fact that diffusion of this marker from entrapped follicles may occur, with subsequent nonspecific absorption by neighboring tumor cells.[420]

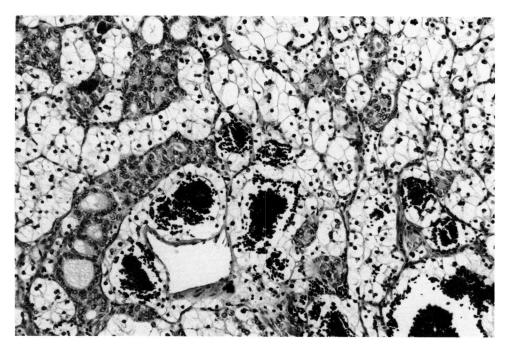

Fig. 9-57 Renal cell carcinoma metastatic to thyroid. Tumor is growing between small thyroid follicles. Presence of totally clear cytoplasm and of extravasated fresh red blood cells in lumina are useful points in differential diagnosis with primary thyroid tumors with clear cell changes.

For adenocarcinomas of other types, mucin stains are also of some utility. Although exceptions certainly occur (see p. 423), the presence of *epithelial* mucin in a malignant tumor located within the thyroid gland points toward a metastatic origin. Similarly, the presence of mucin in a metastatic tumor of unknown source makes very unlikely the possibility that the primary is in the thyroid gland.

REFERENCES
NORMAL ANATOMY

1 Bulley ID, Gatter KC, Hertet A, Mason DY: Expression of intermediate filament proteins in normal and diseased thyroid glands. J Clin Pathol **40**:136-142, 1987.
2 Carpenter JL, Emery GR: Inclusions in the human thyroid. J Anat **122**:77-89, 1976.
3 Kawaoi A, Okano T, Nemoto N, Shikata T: Production of thyroxine (T$_4$) and triiodothyronine (T$_3$) in nontoxic thyroid tumors. An immunohistochemical study. Virchows Arch [Pathol Anat] **390**:249-257, 1981.
4 Klinck GH, Oertel JE, Winship T: Ultrastructure of normal human thyroid. Lab Invest **22**:2-22, 1970.
5 Kurata A, Ohta K, Mine M, Fukuda T, Ikari N, Kanazawa H, Matsunaga M, Izumi M, Nagataki S: Monoclonal antihuman thyroglobulin antibodies. J Clin Endocrinol Metab **59**:573-579, 1984.
6 Landas SK, Schelper RL, Tio FO, Turner JW, Moore KC, Bennett-Gray J: Black thyroid syndrome. Exaggeration of a normal process? Am J Clin Pathol **85**:411-418, 1986.
7 LiVolsi VA, Merino MJ: Squamous cells in the human thyroid gland. Am J Surg Pathol **2**:133-140, 1978.
8 Miettinen M, Virtanen I: Expression of laminin in thyroid gland and thyroid tumors. An immunohistologic study. Int J Cancer **34**:27-30, 1984.
9 Mitchell JD, Kirkham N, Machin D: Focal lymphocytic thyroiditis in Southampton. J Pathol **144**:269-273, 1984.
10 O'Toole K, Fenoglio-Preiser C, Pushparaj N: Endocrine changes associated with the human aging process. III. Effect of age on the number of calcitonin immunoreactive cells in the thyroid gland. Hum Pathol **16**:991-1000, 1985.
11 Permanetter W, Nathrath WBJ, Löhrs U: Immunohistochemical analysis of thyroglobulin and keratin in benign and malignant thyroid tumours. Virchows Arch [Pathol Anat] **398**:221-228, 1982.
12 Reid JD, Choi C-H, Oldroyd NO: Calcium oxalate crystals in the thyroid. Their identification, prevalence, origin, and possible significance. Am J Clin Pathol **87**:443-454, 1987.
13 Rigaud C, Bogomoletz WV: "Mucin secreting" and "mucinous" primary thyroid carcinomas. Pitfalls in mucin histochemistry applied to thyroid tumours. J Clin Pathol **40**:890-895, 1987.
14 Stanta G, Carcangiu ML, Rosai J: The biochemical and immunohistochemical profile of thyroid neoplasia. Pathol Annu **23**(Pt 1):129-157, 1988.
15 Stevenson JC: The structure and function of calcitonin. Invest Cell Pathol **3**:187-193, 1980.
16 Teitelbaum SL, Moore KE, Shieber W: Parafollicular cells in the normal human thyroid. Nature **230**:334-335, 1971.

CONGENITAL ABNORMALITIES

17 Allard RHB: The thyroglossal cyst. Head Neck Surg **5**:134-146, 1982.
18 Bernstein A, Scardino PT, Tomaszewski M-M, Cohen MH: Carcinoma arising in a branchial cleft cyst. Cancer **37**:2417-2422, 1976.
19 Bhaskar SN, Bernier JL: Histogenesis of branchial cysts. A report of 468 cases. Am J Pathol **35**:407-423, 1959.
20 Brintnall ES, Davies J, Huffman WC, Lierle DM: Thyroglossal ducts and cysts. Arch Otolaryngol **59**:282-289, 1954.
21 Compagno J, Hyams VJ, Safavian M: Does branchiogenic carcinoma really exist? Arch Pathol Lab Med **100**:311-314, 1976.
22 Dalgaard JB, Witteland P: Thyroglossal anomalies. A follow-up study of 58 cases. Acta Chir Scand **111**:444-455, 1956.
23 Ein SH, Shandling B, Stephens CA, Mancer K: The problem of recurrent thyroglossal duct remnants. J Pediatr Surg **19**:437-439, 1984.
24 Finkle HI, Goldman RL: Heterotopic cartilage in the thyroid. Arch Pathol **95**:48-49, 1973.
25 Hoyes AD, Kershaw DR: Anatomy and development of the thyroid gland. Ear Nose Throat J **64**:318-333, 1985.
26 Jaques DA, Chambers RG, Oertel JE: Thyroglossal tract carcinoma. A review of the literature and addition of eighteen cases. Am J Surg **120**:439-446, 1970.

27 Joseph TJ, Komorowski RA: Thyroglossal duct carcinoma. Hum Pathol 6:717-729, 1975.

28 Kantelip B, Lusson JR, DeRiberolles C, Lamaison D, Bailly P: Intracardiac ectopic thyroid. Hum Pathol 17:1293-1296, 1986.

29 LiVolsi VA, Perzin KH, Savetsky L: Carcinoma arising in median ectopic thyroid (including thyroglossal duct tissue). Cancer 34:1303-1315, 1974.

30 Lyall D, Stahl WM Jr: Lateral cervical cysts, sinuses, and fistulas of congenital origin. Int Abstr Surg 102:417-434, 1956.

31 Maran AGD, Buchanan DR: Branchial cysts, sinuses and fistulae. Clin Otolaryngol 3:77-92, 1978.

32 Micheau C, Cachin Y, Caillou B: Cystic metastases in the neck revealing occult carcinoma of the tonsil. A report of six cases. Cancer 33:228-233, 1974.

33 Nussbaum M, Buchwald RP, Ribner A, Mori K, Litwins J: Anaplastic carcinoma arising from median ectopic thyroid (thyroglossal duct remnant). Cancer 48:2724-2728, 1981.

34 Rees CE, Brown MJ: Cysts of the thyroglossal duct. Am J Surg 85:597-599, 1953.

35 Sauk JJ Jr: Ectopic lingual thyroid. J Pathol 102:239-243, 1970.

36 Shareef DS, Salm R: Ectopic vestigial lesions of the neck and shoulders. J Clin Pathol 34:1155-1162, 1981.

37 Solomon JR, Rangecroft L: Thyroglossal-duct lesions in childhood. J Pediatr Surg 19:555-561, 1984.

38 Soucy P, Penning J: The clinical relevance of certain observations on the histology of the thyroglossal tract. J Pediatr Surg 19:506-509, 1984.

39 Sugiyama S: The embryology of the human thyroid gland including ultimo-branchial body and others related. Ergeb Anat Entwicklungsgesch 44:3-111, 1971.

40 Wapshaw H: Lingual thyroid. Br J Surg 30:160-165, 1942.

41 Wilson DB: Embryonic development of the head and neck. Part 2. The branchial region. Head Neck Surg 2:59-66, 1979.

THYROIDITIS
Acute thyroiditis

42 Hazard JB: Thyroiditis. A review. Am J Clin Pathol 25:289-298; 399-426, 1955.

43 Volpé R: Etiology, pathogenesis, and clinical aspects of thyroiditis. Pathol Annu 13(Pt 2):399-413, 1978.

Granulomatous (de Quervain's) thyroiditis

44 de Quervain F, Giordanengo G: Die akute und subakute nichteitrige Thyreoiditis. Mitt Grenzgeb Med Chir 44:538-590, 1936.

45 Greene JN: Subacute thyroiditis. Am J Surg 51:97-108, 1971.

46 Stein AA, Hernandez I, McClintock JC: Subacute granulomatous thyroiditis. Ann Surg 153:149-156, 1961.

47 Volpé R: Etiology, pathogenesis, and clinical aspects of thyroiditis. Pathol Annu 13(Pt 2):399-413, 1978.

Other granulomatous inflammations

48 Carney JA, Moore SB, Northcutt RC, Woolner LB, Stillwell GK: Palpation thyroiditis (multifocal granulomatous folliculitis). Am J Clin Pathol 64:639-647, 1975.

49 Leers WD, Dussault J, Mullens JE, Volpé R, Arthurs K: Suppurative thyroiditis. An unusual case caused by *Actinomyces naeslundi*. Can Med Assoc J 101:714-718, 1969.

Lymphocytic thyroiditis

50 Gluck FB, Nusynowitz ML, Plymate S: Chronic lymphocytic thyroiditis, thyrotoxicosis, and low radioactive iodine uptake. Report of four cases. N Engl J Med 293:624-628, 1975.

51 Greenberg AH, Czernichow P, Hung W, Shelley W, Winship T, Blizzard RM: Juvenile chronic lymphocytic thyroiditis. Clinical, laboratory and histological correlations. J Clin Endocrinol Metab 30:293-301, 1970.

52 Nikolai TF, Brosseau J, Kettrick MA, Roberts R, Beltaos E: Lymphocytic thyroiditis with spontaneously resolving hyperthyroidism (silent thyroiditis). Arch Intern Med 140:478-482, 1980.

53 Weitzman JJ, Ling SM, Kaplan SA, Reed GB, Costin G, Landing BH: Percutaneous needle biopsy of goiter in childhood. J Pediatr Surg 5:251-255, 1970.

Hashimoto's thyroiditis

54 Aichinger G, Fill H, Wick G: In situ immune complexes, lymphocyte subpopulations, and HLA-DR-positive epithelial cells in Hashimoto thyroiditis. Lab Invest 52:132-140, 1985.

55 Ben-Ezra J, Wu A, Sheibani K: Absence of clonal lymphoid gene rearrangements in Hashimoto's thyroiditis (abstract). Lab Invest. 58:9A, 1988.

56 Bottazzo GF, Pujol-Borrell R, Hanafusa T, Feldmann M: Role of aberrant HLA-DR expression and antigen presentation in induction of endocrine autoimmunity. Lancet 2:1115-1119, 1983.

57 Burek CL, Rose NR: Cell-mediated immunity in autoimmune thyroid disease. Hum Pathol 17:246-253, 1986.

58 Carpenter CCJ, Solomon N, Silverberg SG, Bledsoe T, Northcutt RC, Klinenberg JR, Bennett IL, Harvey AM: Schmidt's syndrome (thyroid and adrenal insufficiency). A review of the literature and a report of fifteen new cases including ten instances of coexistent diabetes mellitus. Medicine [Baltimore] 43:153-180, 1964.

59 Dailey ME, Lindsay S, Skahen R: Relation of thyroid neoplasms to Hashimoto's disease of the thyroid gland. Arch Surg 70:291-297, 1955.

60 Hashimoto H: Zur Kenntniss der Lymphomatosen Veranderung der Schilddrüse (Struma lymphomatosa). Arch Klin Chir 97:219-248, 1912.

61 Hirota Y, Tamai H, Hayashi Y, Matsubayashi S, Matsuzuka F, Kuma K, Kumagai F, Nagataki S: Thyroid function and histology in forty-five patients with hyperthyroid Graves' disease in clinical remission more than ten years after thionamide drug treatment. J Clin Endocrinol Metab 62:165-169, 1986.

62 Holm L-E, Blomgren H, Löwhagen T: Cancer risks in patients with chronic lymphocytic thyroiditis. N Engl J Med 312:601-604, 1985.

63 Katz SM, Vickery AL: The fibrous variant of Hashimoto's thyroiditis. Hum Pathol 5:161-170, 1974.

64 Knecht H, Hedinger Chr E: Ultrastructural findings in Hashimoto's thyroiditis and focal lymphocytic thyroiditis with reference to giant cell formation. Histopathology 6:511-538, 1982.

65 Knecht H, Saremaslani P, Hedinger Chr E: Immunohistological findings in Hashimoto's thyroiditis, focal lymphocytic thyroiditis and thyroiditis de Quervain. Comparative study. Virchows Arch [Pathol Anat] 393:215-231, 1981.

65a Louis DN, Vickery AL Jr, Rosai J, Wang CA: Multiple branchial cleft-like cysts in Hashimoto's thyroiditis. Am J Surg Pathol, 1988 (In press.)

66 Marshall SF, Meissner WA: Struma lymphomatosa (Hashimoto's disease). Ann Surg 141:737-746, 1955.

67 Schade ROK, Owen SG, Smart GA, Hall R: The relation of thyroid autoimmunity to round-cell infiltration of the thyroid gland. J Clin Pathol 13:499-501, 1960.

68 Spjut HJ, Warren WD, Ackerman LV: A clinical-pathologic study of 76 cases of recurrent Graves' disease, toxic (nonexophthalmic) goiter, and non-toxic goiter. Am J Clin Pathol 27:367-392, 1957.

69 Thomas CG Jr, Rutledge RG: Surgical intervention in chronic (Hashimoto's) thyroiditis. Ann Surg 193:769-776, 1981.

70 Volpé R: Etiology, pathogenesis, and clinical aspects of thyroiditis. Pathol Annu 13(Pt 2):399-413, 1978.

71 Volpé R (ed): Autoimmunity and endocrine disease. New York, 1985, Marcel Dekker, pp. 109-285.

72 Volpé R, Farid NR, Von Westarp C, Row VV: The pathogenesis of Graves' disease and Hashimoto's thyroiditis. Clin Endocrinol 3:239-261, 1974.

73 Weetman AP, McGregor AM: Autoimmune thyroid disease. Developments in our understanding. Endocr Rev 5:309-355, 1984.

74 Weiss LM, Weinberg DS, Warhof MJ: Medullary carcinoma arising in a thyroid with Hashimoto's disease. J Clin Pathol 80:534-538, 1983.

Riedel's thyroiditis

75 Comings DE, Skubi KB, Van Eyes J, Motulsky AG: Familial multifocal fibrosclerosis. Ann Intern Med 66:884-892, 1967.

76 Harach HR, Williams ED: Fibrous thyroiditis. An immunopathological study. Histopathology 7:739-751, 1983.

77 Riedel H: Die chronische, die Bildung eisenharter Tumoren führende Entzündung der Schilddrüse. Verh Dtsch Ges Chir, 1896.

78 Woolner LB, McConaher WM: Beahrs OH: Invasive fibrous thyroiditis. J Clin Endocrinol Metab 17:201-220, 1957.

HYPERPLASIA
Dyshormonogenetic goiter

79 Batsakis JG, Nishiyama RH, Schmidt RW: Sporadic goiter syndrome. A clinicopathologic analysis. Am J Clin Pathol 39:241-251, 1963.

80 Cooper DS, Axelrod L, DeGroot LJ, Vickery AL Jr, Maloof F: Congenital goiter and the development of metastatic follicular carcinoma with evidence for a leak of nonhormonal iodide. Clinical, pathological, kinetic, and biochemical studies and a review of the literature. J Clin Endocrinol Metab 52:294-306, 1981.

81 Kennedy JS: The pathology of dyshormonogenetic goiter. J Pathol 99:251-264, 1969.

82 Moore GH: The thyroid in sporadic goitrous cretinism. Arch Pathol **74**:35-46, 1962.

Diffuse hyperplasia (Graves' disease)

83 Bradley EL III, Liechty RD: Modified subtotal thyroidectomy for Graves' disease. A two-institution study. Surgery **94**:955-958, 1983.

84 Curran RC, Eckert H, Wilson GM: The thyroid gland after treatment of hyperthyroidism by partial thyroidectomy or iodine 131. J Pathol Bacteriol **76**: 541-560, 1958.

85 Eggen PC, Seljelid R: The histological appearance of hyperfunctioning thyroids following various pre-operative treatments. Acta Pathol Microbiol Scand [A] **81**:16-20, 1973.

86 Farbota LM, Calandra DB, Lawrence AM, Paloyan E: Thyroid carcinoma in Graves' disease. Surgery **98**:1148-1152, 1985.

87 Hall R: Hyperthyroidism—pathogenesis and diagnosis. Br Med J **1**:743-745, 1970.

88 Hargreaves AW, Garner A: The significance of lymphocytic infiltration of the thyroid gland in thyrotoxicosis. Br J Surg **55**:543-545, 1968.

89 Margolick JB, Hsu S-M, Volkman DJ, Burman KD, Fauci AS: Immunohistochemical characterization of intrathyroid lymphocytes in Graves' disease. Interstitial and intraepithelial populations. Am J Med **76**:815-821, 1984.

90 Nixon DW, Samols E: Acral changes associated with thyroid diseases. JAMA **212**:1175-1181, 1970.

91 Pfaltz M, Hedinger CE: Abnormal basement membrane structures in autoimmune thyroid disease. Lab Invest **55**:531-539, 1966.

92 Smyrk TC, Goellner JR, Brennan MD, Carney JA: Pathology of the thyroid in amiodarone-associated thyrotoxicosis. Am J Surg Pathol **11**:197-204, 1987.

93 Sridama V, McCormick M, Kaplan EL, Fauchet R, DeGroot LJ: Long-term follow-up study of compensated low-dose ^{131}I therapy for Graves' disease. N Engl J Med **311**:426-432, 1984.

94 Volpé R: The pathogenesis of Graves' disease. An overview. Clin Endocrinol Metab **7**:3-29, 1978.

Nodular hyperplasia

95 Brown RS, Pohl SL, Jackson IMD, Reichlin S: Do thyroid-stimulating immunoglobulins cause non-toxic and toxic multinodular goitre? Lancet **1**:904-906, 1978.

96 Doniach I: Etiological consideration of thyroid carcinoma. In Smithers D (ed): Tumors of the thyroid gland. Monographs on neoplastic disease at various sites, vol. 6. Edinburgh and London, 1970, E. & S. Livingstone.

97 Greene R: Lymphadenoid change in the thyroid gland and its relation to post-operative hypothyroidism. Mem Soc Endocrinol **1**:16-20, 1953.

98 Hargreaves AW, Garner A: The significance of lymphocytic infiltration of the thyroid gland in thyrotoxicosis. Br J Surg **55**:543-545, 1968.

99 Mortensen JD, Woolner LB, Bennett WA: Gross and microscopic findings in clinically normal thyroid glands. J Clin Endocrinol Metab **15**:1270-1280, 1955.

100 Studer H, Ramelli F: Simple goiter and its variants. Euthyroid and hyperthyroid multinodular goiters. Endocr Rev **3**:40-61, 1982.

101 Tunbridge WMG, Evered DC, Hall R, Appleton D, Brewis M, Clark F, Evans JG: The spectrum of thyroid disease in a community. The Whickham survey. Clin Endocrinol **7**:481-493, 1977.

TUMORS

102 Zampi G, Carcangiu ML, Rosai J (eds): Thyroid tumor pathology. Proceedings of an international workshop, San Miniato, Italy, October 1984. Semin Diagn Pathol **2**:87-146, 1985.

Epithelial tumors–specific types
Follicular adenoma

103 Belfiore A, Sava L, Runello F, Tomaselli L, Vigneri R: Solitary autonomously functioning thyroid nodules and iodine deficiency. J Clin Endocrinol Metab **56**:283-287, 1983.

104 Campbell WL, Santiago HE, Perzin KH, Johnson PM: The autonomous thyroid nodule. Correlation of scan appearance and histopathology. Radiology **107**:133-138, 1973.

105 Carney JA, Ryan J, Goellner JR: Hyalinizing trabecular adenoma of the thyroid gland. Am J Surg Pathol **11**:583-591, 1987.

106 Carcangiu ML, Rosai J: Follicular adenoma of thyroid with bizarre nuclei. (In preparation.)

107 Cohen MB, Miller TR, Beckstead JH: Enzyme histochemistry and thyroid neoplasia. Am J Clin Pathol **85**:668-673, 1986.

108 Gharib H, James EM, Charboneau JW, Naessens JM, Offord KP, Gorman CA: Suppressive therapy with levothyroxine for solitary thyroid nodules. A double-blind controlled clinical study. N Engl J Med **317**:70-75, 1987.

109 Goldstein R, Hart IR: Follow-up of solitary autonomous thyroid nodules treated with [131]I. N Engl J Med **309**:1473-1476, 1983.

110 Hamburger JI: Solitary autonomously functioning thyroid lesions. Diagnosis, clinical features and pathogenetic considerations. Am J Med **58**:740-748, 1975.

111 Hazard JB, Kenyon R: Atypical adenoma of the thyroid. Arch Pathol **58**:554-563, 1954.

112 Joensuu H, Klemi P, Eerola E: DNA aneuploidy in follicular adenomas of the thyroid gland. Am J Pathol **124**:373-376, 1986.

113 Lang W, Georgii A, Stauch G, Kienzle E: The differentiation of atypical adenomas and encapsulated follicular carcinomas in the thyroid gland. Virchows Arch [Pathol Anat] **385**:125-141, 1980.

114 Miettinen M, Virtanen I: Expression of laminin in thyroid gland and thyroid tumors. An immunohistologic study. Int J Cancer **34**:27-30, 1984.

115 Panke TW, Croxson MS, Parker JW, Carriere DP, Rosoff L Sr, Warner NE: Triiodothyronine-secreting (toxic) adenoma of the thyroid gland. Light and electron microscopic characteristics. Cancer **41**:528-537, 1978.

116 Shlossberg AH, Jacobson JC, Ibbertson HK: Serum thyroglobulin in the diagnosis and management of thyroid carcinoma. Clin Endocrinol **10**:17-27, 1979.

Papillary carcinoma
General features

117 Carcangiu ML, Zampi G, Pupi A, Castagnoli A, Rosai J: Papillary carcinoma of the thyroid. A clinicopathologic study of 241 cases treated at the University of Florence, Italy. Cancer **55**:805-828, 1985.

118 Farbota LM, Calandra DB, Lawrence AM, Paloyan E: Thyroid carcinoma in Graves' disease. Surgery **98**:1148-1152, 1985.

119 Ott RA, Calandra DB, McCall A, Shah KH, Lawrence AM, Paloyan E: The incidence of thyroid carcinoma in patients with Hashimoto's thyroiditis and solitary cold nodules. Surgery **98**:1202-1206, 1985.

Pathologic features

120 Albores-Saavedra J, Altamirano-Dimas M, Alcorta-Anguizola B, Smith M: Fine structure of human papillary thyroid carcinoma. Cancer **28**:763-774, 1971.

121 Beaumont A, Ben Othman S, Fragu P: The fine structure of papillary carcinoma of the thyroid. Histopathology **5**:377-388, 1981.

122 Bennett WP, Bhan AK, Vickery AL Jr: Keratin expression as a diagnostic adjunct in thyroid tumors with papillary architecture (abstract). Lab Invest **58**:9A, 1988.

123 Buley ID, Gatter KC, Heryet A, Mason DY: Expression of intermediate filament proteins in normal and diseased thyroid glands. J Clin Pathol **40**:136-142, 1987.

124 Carcangiu ML, Zampi G, Pupi A, Castagnoli A, Rosai J: Papillary carcinoma of the thyroid. A clinicopathologic study of 241 cases treated at the University of Florence, Italy. Cancer **55**:805-828, 1985.

125 Carcangiu ML, Zampi G, Rosai J: Papillary thyroid carcinoma. A study of its many morphologic expressions and clinical correlates. Pathol Annu **20**(Pt 1):1-44, 1985.

126 Chan JKC, Saw D: The grooved nucleus. A useful diagnostic criterion of papillary carcinoma of the thyroid. Am J Surg Pathol **10**:672-679, 1986.

126a Chan JKC, Tse CCH: Mucin production in metastatic papillary carcinoma of the thyroid. Hum Pathol **19**:195-200, 1988.

127 Gray A, Doniach I: Morphology of the nuclei of papillary carcinoma of the thyroid. Br J Cancer **23**:49-51, 1969.

128 Henzen-Logmans SC, Mullink H, Ramaekers FCS, Tadema T, Meijer CJLM: Expression of cytokeratins and vimentin in epithelial cells of normal and pathologic thyroid tissue. Virchows Arch [Pathol Anat] **410**:347-354, 1987.

129 Johannessen JV, Gould VE, Jao W: The fine structure of human thyroid cancer. Hum Pathol **9**:385-400, 1978.

130 Johannessen JV, Sobrinho-Simões M: The origin and significance of thyroid psammoma bodies. Lab Invest **43**:287-296, 1980.

131 Klinck GH, Winship T: Psammoma bodies and thyroid cancer. Cancer **12**:656-662, 1959.

132 Lee TK, Myers RT, Marshall RB, Bond MG, Kardon B: The significance of mitotic rate. A retrospective study of 127 thyroid carcinomas. Hum Pathol **16**:1042-1046, 1985.

133 Margolin FR, Winfield J, Steinbach HL: Patterns of thyroid calcifications. Roentgenologic-histologic study of excised specimens. Invest Radiol **2**:208-212, 1967.

134 Patchefsky AS, Hoch WS: Psammoma bodies in diffuse toxic goiter. Am J Clin Pathol **57**:551-556, 1972.

135 Russell WO, Ibanez ML, Clark RL, White EC: Thyroid carcinoma. Classification, intraglandular dissemination and clinicopathological study based upon whole organ sections of 80 glands. Cancer **16**:1425-1460, 1963.

135a Schröder S, Schwarz W, Rehpenning W, Loning T, Bocker W: Dendritic/ Langerhans cells and prognosis in patients with papillary thyroid carcinomas. Immunocytochemical study of 106 thyroid neoplasms correlated to follow-up data. Am J Clin Pathol **89:**295-300, 1988.

136 Selzer G, Kahn LB, Albertyn L: Primary malignant tumors of the thyroid gland. A clinicopathologic study of 254 cases. Cancer **40:**1501-1510, 1977.

137 Tscholl-Ducommun J, Hedinger CE: Papillary thyroid carcinomas. Morphology and prognosis. Virchows Arch [Pathol Anat] **396:**19-39, 1982.

138 Tuccari G, Barresi G: Immunohistochemical demonstration of ceruloplasmin in follicular adenomas and thyroid carcinomas. Histopathology **11:**723-731, 1987.

139 Vickery AL Jr: Thyroid papillary carcinoma. Am J Surg Pathol **7:**797-807, 1983.

140 Wilson NW, Pambakian H, Richardson TC, Stokoe MR, Makin CA, Heyderman E: Epithelial markers in thyroid carcinoma. An immunoperoxidase study. Histopathology **10:**815-829, 1986.

Variants

141 Bondeson L, Ljungberg O: Occult papillary thyroid carcinoma in the young and the aged. Cancer **53:**1790-1791, 1984.

142 Carcangiu ML, Bianchi S, Rosai J: Diffuse sclerosing papillary carcinoma. Report of 8 cases of a distinctive variant of thyroid malignancy (abstract). Lab Invest **56:**10A, 1987.

143 Carcangiu ML, Zampi G, Pupi A, Castagnoli A, Rosai J: Papillary carcinoma of the thyroid. A clinicopathologic study of 241 cases treated at the University of Florence, Italy. Cancer **55:**805-828, 1985.

144 Chan JKC, Tsui MS, Tse CH: Diffuse sclerosing variant of papillary carcinoma of the thyroid. A histological and immunohistochemical study of three cases. Histopathology **11:**191-201, 1987.

145 Chen KTK, Rosai J: Follicular variant of thyroid papillary carcinoma. A clinicopathologic study of six cases. Am J Surg Pathol **1:**123-130, 1977.

146 Evans HL: Follicular neoplasms of the thyroid. Cancer **54:**535-540, 1984.

147 Evans HL: Columnar-cell carcinoma of the thyroid. A report of two cases of an aggressive variant of thyroid carcinoma. Am J Clin Pathol **85:**77-80, 1986.

148 Evans HL: Encapsulated papillary neoplasms of the thyroid. A study of 14 cases followed for a minimum of 10 years. Am J Surg Pathol **11:**592-597, 1987.

149 Harach HR, Franssila KO, Wasenius V-M: Occult papillary carcinoma of the thyroid. A "normal" finding in Finland. A systematic autopsy study. Cancer **56:**531-538, 1985.

150 Hawk WA, Hazard JB: The many appearances of papillary carcinoma of the thyroid. Cleve Clin Q **43:**207-216, 1976.

151 Hazard JB: Small papillary carcinoma of the thyroid. A study with special reference to so-called nonencapsulated sclerosing tumor. Lab Invest **9:**86-97, 1960.

152 Hubert JP Jr, Kiernan PD, Beahrs OH, McConahey WM, Woolner LB: Occult papillary carcinoma of the thyroid. Arch Surg **115:**394-398, 1980.

153 Johnson TL, Lloyd RV, Thompson NW, Beierwaltes WH, Sisson JC: Prognostic implications of the tall cell variant of papillary thyroid carcinoma. Am J Surg Pathol **12:**22-27, 1988.

154 Klinck GH, Winship T: Occult sclerosing carcinoma of the thyroid. Cancer **8:**701-706, 1955.

155 Rosai J, Zampi G, Carcangiu ML: Papillary carcinoma of the thyroid. A discussion of its several morphologic expressions, with particular emphasis on the follicular variant. Am J Surg Pathol **7:**809-817, 1983.

156 Schröder S, Böcker W, Dralle H, Kortman K-B, Stern C: The encapsulated papillary carcinoma of the thyroid. A morphologic subtype of the papillary thyroid carcinoma. Cancer **54:**90-93, 1984.

157 Schröder S, Pfannschmidt N, Böcker W, Muller HW, De Heer K: Histopathologic types and clinical behaviour of occult papillary carcinoma of the thyroid. Pathol Res Pract **179:**81-87, 1984.

158 Sobrinho-Simões M, Nesland JM, Johannessen JV: Columnar-cell carcinoma. Another variant of poorly differentiated carcinoma of the thyroid. Am J Clin Pathol **89:**264-267, 1988.

159 Strate SM, Lee EL, Childers JH: Occult papillary carcinoma of the thyroid with distant metastases. Cancer **54:**1093-1100, 1984.

160 Vickery AL Jr: Thyroid papillary carcinoma. Am J Surg Pathol **7:**797-807, 1983.

161 Vickery AL Jr, Carcangiu ML, Johannessen JV, Sobrinho-Simões M: Papillary carcinoma. Semin Diagn Pathol **2:**90-100, 1985.

Spread and metastases

162 Carcangiu ML, Zampi G, Pupi A, Castagnoli A, Rosai J: Papillary carcinoma of the thyroid. A clinicopathologic study of 241 cases treated at the University of Florence, Italy. Cancer **55:**805-828, 1985.

163 Cody HS III, Shah JP: Locally invasive, well-differentiated thyroid cancer. Am J Surg **142:**480-483, 1981.

164 Frazell EL, Foote FW Jr: Papillary thyroid carcinoma. Pathological findings in cases with and without clinical evidence of cervical node involvement. Cancer **8:**1165-1166, 1955.

165 Hoie J, Stenwig AE, Kullmann G, Lindegaard M: Distant metastases in papillary thyroid cancer. A review of 91 patients. Cancer **61:**1-6, 1988.

Prognosis

166 Carcangiu ML, Zampi G, Pupi A, Castagnoli A, Rosai J: Papillary carcinoma of the thyroid. A clinicopathologic study of 241 cases treated at the University of Florence, Italy. Cancer **55:**805-828, 1985.

167 Cohn K, Bäckdahl M, Forsslund G, Auer G, Lundell G, Löwhagen T, Tallroth E, Willems J-S, Zetterberg A, Granberg P-O: Prognostic value of nuclear DNA content in papillary thyroid carcinoma. World J Surg **8:**474-480, 1984.

168 Crile G Jr: Changing end results in patients with papillary carcinoma of the thyroid. Surg Gynecol Obstet **132:**460-468, 1971.

169 Joensuu H, Klemi P, Eerola E, Tuominen J: Influence of cellular DNA content on survival in differentiated thyroid cancer. Cancer **58:**2462-2467, 1986.

170 Mazzaferri EL, Young RL: Papillary thyroid carcinoma. A 10 year follow-up report of the impact of therapy in 576 patients. Am J Med **70:**511-518, 1980.

171 McConahey WM, Hay ID, Woolner LB, Van Heerden JA, Taylor WF: Papillary thyroid cancer treated at the Mayo Clinic, 1946 through 1970. Initial manifestations, pathologic findings, therapy, and outcome. Mayo Clin Proc **61:**978-996, 1986.

172 Motoyama T, Watanabe H: Simultaneous squamous cell carcinoma and papillary adenocarcinoma of the thyroid gland. Hum Pathol **14:**1009-1010, 1983.

173 Schlumberger M, Tubiana M, De Vathaire F, Hill C, Gardet P, Travagli J-P, Fragu P, Lumbroso J, Caillou B, Parmentier C: Long-term results of treatment of 283 patients with lung and bone metastases from differentiated thyroid carcinoma. J Clin Endocrinol Metab **63:**960-967, 1986.

174 Torres J, Volpato RD, Power EG, Lopez EC, Dominguez ME, Maira JL, Ugarte JA, Martinez VC: Thyroid cancer. Survival in 148 cases followed for 10 years or more. Cancer **56:**2298-2304, 1985.

Follicular carcinoma

175 Cady B, Rossi R, Silverman M, Wool M: Further evidence of the validity of risk group definition in differentiated thyroid carcinoma. Surgery **98:**1171-1178, 1985.

176 Elsner B, Curutchet HP, Bellotti MS, Degrossi OJ, Kerman A: Carcinoma folicular de la glándula tiroides. Estudio clinicopatológico. Medicina [Buenos Aries] **40:**501-510, 1980.

177 Evans HL: Follicular neoplasms of the thyroid. A study of 44 cases followed for a minimum of 10 years, with emphasis on differential diagnosis. Cancer **54:**535-540, 1984.

178 González-Cámpora R, Montero C, Martin-Lacave I, Galera H: Demonstration of vascular endothelium in thyroid carcinomas using *Ulex europaeus* I agglutinin. Histopathology **10:**261-266, 1986.

179 Harach HR, Jasani B, Williams ED: Factor VIII as a marker of endothelial cells in follicular carcinoma of the thyroid. J Clin Pathol **36:**1050-1054, 1983.

180 Iida F: Surgical significance of capsule invasion of adenoma of the thyroid. Surg Gynecol Obstet **144:**710-712, 1977.

181 Joensuu H, Klemi P, Eerola E, Tuominen J: Influence of cellular DNA content on survival in differentiated thyroid cancer. Cancer **58:**2462-2467, 1986.

182 Johannessen JV, Sobrinho-Simões M: Well differentiated thyroid tumors. Problems in diagnosis and understanding. Pathol Annu **18**(Pt 1):255-285, 1983.

183 Johannessen JV, Sobrinho-Simões M, Lindmo T, Tangen KO: The diagnostic value of flow cytometric DNA measurements in selected disorders of the human thyroid. Am J Clin Pathol **77:**20-25, 1982.

184 Kendall CH, Sanderson PR, Cope J, Talbot IC: Follicular thyroid tumours. A study of laminin and type IV collagen in basement membrane and endothelium. J Clin Pathol **38:**1100-1105, 1985.

185 Lang W, Choritz H, Hundeshagen H: Risk factors in follicular thyroid carcinomas. A retrospective follow-up study covering a 14-year period with emphasis on morphological findings. Am J Surg Pathol **10:**246-255, 1986.

186 Lang W, Georgii A, Stauch G, Kienzle E: The differentiation of atypical adenomas and encapsulated follicular carcinomas in the thyroid gland. Virchows Arch [Pathol Anat] **385:**125-141, 1980.

187 Mahoney JP, Saffos RO, Rhatigan RM: Follicular adenoacanthoma of the thyroid gland. Histopathology **4:**547-557, 1980.

188 Massin J-P, Savoie J-C, Garnier H, Guiraudon G, Leger FA, Bacourt F: Pulmonary metastases in differentiated thyroid carcinoma. Study of 58 cases with implications for the primary tumor treatment. Cancer **53:**982-992, 1984.

189 Nagamine Y, Suzuki J, Katakura R, Yoshimoto T, Matoba N, Takaya K: Skull metastasis of thyroid carcinoma. Study of 12 cases. J Neurosurg 63:526-531, 1985.

190 Sobrinho-Simões M, Damjanov I: Lectin histochemistry of papillary and follicular carcinoma of the thyroid gland. Arch Pathol Lab Med 110:722-729, 1986.

191 Stephenson TJ, Griffiths DWR, Mills PM: Comparison of Ulex europaeus I lectin binding and factor VIII-related antigen as markers of vascular endothelium in follicular carcinoma of the thyroid. Histopathology 10:251-260, 1986.

192 Vanstapel MJ, Gatter KC, De Wolf-Peeters C, Mason DY, Desmet VD: New sites of human S-100 immunoreactivity detected with monoclonal antibodies. Am J Clin Pathol 85:160-168, 1986.

193 Wilson NW, Pameakian H, Richardson TC, Stokoe MR, Makin CA, Heyderman E: Epithelial markers in thyroid carcinoma. An immunoperoxidase study. Histopathology 10:815-829, 1986.

Hürthle cell tumors

194 Beckner M, Oertel J: Papillary carcinomas of the oxyphil cell subtype (abstract). Lab Invest 56:5A, 1987.

195 Bondeson L, Azavedo E, Bondeson A-G, Caspersson T, Ljungberg O: Nuclear DNA content and behavior of oxyphil thyroid tumors. Cancer 58:672-675, 1986.

196 Bondeson L, Bondeson A-G, Ljungberg O, Tibblin S: Oxyphil tumors of the thyroid. Follow-up of 42 surgical cases. Ann Surg 194:677-680, 1981.

197 Bronner MP, LiVolsi VA: Oxyphilic (Askanazy/Hürthle cell) tumors of the thyroid. Microscopic features predict biologic behavior. Surg Pathol 1:137-150, 1988.

198 Bruni F, Batsakis JG, Luna MA, Remmler D: Hürthle cell tumors of the thyroid gland (abstract). Am J Clin Pathol 88:528, 1987.

199 Caplan RH, Abellera M, Kisken WA: Hürthle cell tumors of the thyroid gland. A clinicopathologic review and long-term follow-up. JAMA 251:3114-3117, 1984.

200 Feldman PS, Horvath E, Kovacs K: Ultrastructure of three Hürthle cell tumors of the thyroid. Cancer 30:1279-1285, 1972.

201 Flint A, Davenport RD, Lloyd RV, Beckwith AL, Thompson NW: Cytophotometric measurements of Hürthle cell tumors of the thyroid gland. Correlation with pathologic features and clinical behavior. Cancer 61:110-113, 1988.

202 Frazell EL, Duffy BJ Jr: Hürthle-cell cancer of the thyroid. A review of forty cases. Cancer 4:952-956, 1951.

203 Gardner L: Hürthle-cell tumors of the thyroid. Arch Pathol 59:372-381, 1955.

204 Gundry SR, Burney RE, Thompson NW, Lloyd R: Total thyroidectomy for Hürthle cell neoplasm of the thyroid. Arch Surg 118:529-532, 1983.

205 Har-El G, Hadar T, Segal K, Levy R, Sidi J: Hürthle cell carcinoma of the thyroid gland. A tumor of moderate malignancy. Cancer 57:1613-1617, 1986.

206 Horn RC Jr: Hürthle-cell tumors of the thyroid. Cancer 7:234-244, 1954.

207 Johnson TL, Lloyd RV, Burney RE, Thompson NW: Hürthle cell thyroid tumors. An immunohistochemical study. Cancer 59:107-112, 1987.

208 Nesland JM, Sobrinho-Simões MA, Holm R, Sambade MC, Johannessen JV: Hürthle-cell lesions of the thyroid. A combined study using transmission electron microscopy, scanning electron microscopy and immunocytochemistry. Ultrastruct Pathol 8:269-290, 1985.

209 Rosai J, Carcangiu ML: Pathology of thyroid tumors. Some recent and old questions. Hum Pathol 15:1008-1012, 1984.

210 Ruchti C, Komor J, König MP: Grosszellige Tumoren (sogenannte Hürthlezell-Tumoren) der Schilddrüse. Helv Chir Acta 43:129-132, 1976.

211 Samaan NA, Schultz PN, Haynie TP, Ordonez NG: Pulmonary metastasis of differentiated thyroid carcinoma. Treatment results in 101 patients. J Clin Endocrinol Metab 65:376-380, 1985.

212 Sobrinho-Simões MA, Nesland JM, Holm R, Sambade MC, Johannessen JV: Hürthle cell and mitochondrion-rich papillary carcinomas of the thyroid gland. An ultrastructural and immunocytochemical study. Ultrastruct Pathol 8:131-142, 1985.

213 Thompson NW, Dunn EL, Batsakis JG, Nishiyama RH: Hürthle cell lesions of the thyroid gland. Surg Gynecol Obstet 139:555-560, 1974.

214 Watson RG, Brennan MD, Goellner JR, van Heerden JA, McConahey WM, Taylor WF: Invasive Hürthle cell carcinoma of the thyroid. Natural history and management. Mayo Clin Proc 59:851-855, 1984.

Clear cell tumors

215 Carcangiu ML, Sibley RK, Rosai J: Clear cell change in primary thyroid tumors. A study of 38 cases. Am J Surg Pathol 9:705-722, 1985.

216 Civantos F, Albores-Saavedra J, Nadji M, Morales AR: Clear cell variant of thyroid carcinoma. Am J Surg Pathol 8:187-192, 1984.

217 Dickersin GR, Vickery AL Jr, Smith SB: Papillary carcinoma of the thyroid, oxyphil cell type, "clear cell" variant. A light- and electron-microscopic study. Am J Surg Pathol 4:501-509, 1980.

218 Landon G, Ordóñez NG: Clear cell variant of medullary carcinoma of the thyroid. Hum Pathol 16:844-847, 1985.

219 Mendelsohn G: Signet-cell–simulating microfollicular adenoma of the thyroid. Am J Surg Pathol 8:705-708, 1984.

220 Rigaud C, Peltier F, Bogomoletz WV: Mucin producing microfollicular adenoma of the thyroid. J Clin Pathol 38:277-280, 1985.

221 Saleiro JV, Faria V, Oliveira MC: Clear cell tumor of the thyroid gland. J Submicrosc Cytol 13:75-77, 1981.

222 Schröder S, Böcker W: Clear-cell carcinomas of thyroid gland. A clinicopathological study of 13 cases. Histopathology 10:75-89, 1986.

223 Schröder S, Böcker W: Signet-ring–cell thyroid tumors. Follicle cell tumors with arrest of folliculogenesis. Am J Surg Pathol 9:619-629, 1985.

224 Schröder S, Hüsselmann H, Böcker W: Lipid-rich cell adenoma of the thyroid gland. Report of a peculiar thyroid tumour. Virchows Arch [Pathol Anat] 404:105-108, 1984.

225 Variakojis D, Getz ML, Paloyan E, Straus FH II: Papillary clear cell carcinoma of the thyroid gland. Hum Pathol 6:384-390, 1975.

Epidermoid, mucinous, and related tumors

226 Carcangiu ML, Steeper T, Zampi G, Rosai J: Anaplastic thyroid carcinoma. A study of 70 cases. Am J Clin Pathol 83:135-158, 1985.

227 Franssila KO, Harach HR, Wasenius V-M: Mucoepidermoid carcinoma of the thyroid. Histopathology 8:847-860, 1984.

228 Harach HR, Day ES, Franssila KO: Thyroid spindle-cell tumor with mucous cysts. An intrathyroid thymoma? Am J Surg Pathol 9:525-530, 1985.

229 Huang T-Y, Assor D: Primary squamous cell carcinoma of the thyroid gland. A report of four cases. Am J Clin Pathol 55:93-98, 1971.

230 Klinck GH, Menk KF: Squamous cells in the human thyroid. Milit Surg 109:406-414, 1951.

231 LiVolsi VA, Merino MJ: Squamous cells in the human thyroid gland. Am J Surg Pathol 2:133-140, 1978.

232 Miyauchi A, Kuma K, Matsuzuka F, Matsubayashi S, Kobayashi A, Tamai H, Katayama S: Intrathyroidal epithelial thymoma. An entity distinct from squamous cell carcinoma of the thyroid. World J Surg 9:128-135, 1985.

233 Mizukami Y, Matsubara F, Hashimoto T, Haratake J, Terahata S, Noguchi M, Hirose K: Primary mucoepidermoid carcinoma in the thyroid gland. A case report including an ultrastructural and biochemical study. Cancer 53:1741-1745, 1984.

234 Motoyama T, Watanabe H: Simultaneous squamous cell carcinoma and papillary adenocarcinoma of the thyroid gland. Hum Pathol 14:1009-1010, 1983.

235 Riddle PE, Dincsoy HP: Primary squamous cell carcinoma of the thyroid associated with leukocytosis and hypercalcemia. Arch Pathol Lab Med 111:373-374, 1987.

236 Rigaud C, Bogomoletz WV: "Mucin secreting" and "mucinous" primary thyroid carcinomas. Pitfalls in mucin histochemistry applied to thyroid tumours. J Clin Pathol 40:890-895, 1987.

237 Rosai J, Albores-Saavedra J, Battifora H: A sclerosing squamous tumor of the thyroid with eosinophilic infiltration arising in Hashimoto's thyroiditis. Report of 4 cases of a distinctive tumor entity (abstract). Lab Invest 56:66A, 1987.

238 Sobrinho-Simões MA, Nesland JM, Johannessen JV: A mucin-producing tumor in the thyroid gland. Ultrastruct Pathol 9:277-281, 1985.

Poorly differentiated carcinoma

239 Cabanne F, Gérard-Marchant R, Heimann R, Williams ED: Tumeurs malignes du corps thyroïde. Problèmes de diagnostic histopathologique. A propos de 692 lésions recueillies par le groupe coopérateur des cancers du corps thyroïde de l'OERTC. Ann Anat Pathol [Paris] 19:129-148, 1974.

240 Carcangiu ML, Zampi G, Rosai J: Poorly differentiated ("insular") thyroid carcinoma. A reinterpretation of Langhans' "wuchernde Struma." Am J Surg Pathol 8:655-668, 1984.

241 Rosai J, Saxén EA, Woolner L: Undifferentiated and poorly differentiated carcinoma. Semin Diagn Pathol 2:123-136, 1985.

242 Sakamoto A, Kasai N, Sugano H: Poorly differentiated carcinoma of the thyroid. A clinicopathologic entity for a high risk group of papillary and follicular carcinomas. Cancer 52:1849-1855, 1983.

243 Tubiana M, Schlumberger M, Rougier P, Laplanche A, Benhamou E, Gardet P, Caillou B, Travagli J-P, Parmentier C: Long-term results and prognostic factors in patients with differentiated thyroid carcinoma. Cancer 55:794-804, 1985.

Undifferentiated carcinoma

244 Albores-Saavedra J, Nadji M, Civantos F, Morales AR: Thyroglobulin in carcinoma of the thyroid. An immunohistochemical study. Hum Pathol 14:62-66, 1983.

245 Aldinger KA, Samaan NA, Ibanez M, Hills CS Jr: Anaplastic carcinoma of the thyroid. A review of 84 cases of spindle and giant cell carcinoma of the thyroid. Cancer 41:2267-2275, 1978.

246 Carcangiu ML, Steeper T, Zampi G, Rosai J: Anaplastic thyroid carcinoma. A study of 70 cases. Am J Clin Pathol 83:135-158, 1985.

247 De Micco C, Ruf J, Carayon P, Chrestian M-A, Henry J-F, Toga M: Immunohistochemical study of thyroglobulin in thyroid carcinomas with monoclonal antibodies. Cancer 59:471-476, 1987.

248 Fisher ER, Gregorio R, Shoemaker R, Horvat B, Hubay C: The derivation of so-called "giant-cell" and "spindle-cell" undifferentiated thyroidal neoplasms. Am J Clin Pathol 61:680-689, 1974.

249 Harada T, Ito K, Shimaoka K, Hosoda Y, Yakumaru K: Fatal thyroid carcinoma. Anaplastic transformation of adenocarcinoma. Cancer 39:2588-2596, 1977.

250 Hashimoto H, Koga S, Watanabe H, Enjoji M: Undifferentiated carcinoma of the thyroid gland with osteoclast-like giant cells. Acta Pathol Jpn 30:323-334, 1980.

251 Hurlimann J, Gardiol D, Scazziga B: Immunohistology of anaplastic thyroid carcinoma. A study of 43 cases. Histopathology 11:567-580, 1987.

252 Hutter RVP, Tollefsen HR, DeCosse JJ, Foote FW Jr, Frazell EL: Spindle and giant cell metaplasia in papillary carcinoma of the thyroid. Am J Surg 110:660-668, 1965.

253 Johannessen JV, Gould VE, Jao W: The fine structure of human thyroid cancer. Hum Pathol 9:385-400, 1978.

254 Kim JH, Leeper RD: Treatment of anaplastic giant and spindle cell carcinoma of the thyroid gland with combination adriamycin and radiation therapy. Cancer 52:954-957, 1983.

255 LiVolsi VA, Brooks JJ, Arendash-Durand B: Anaplastic thyroid tumors. Immunohistology. Am J Clin Pathol 87:434-442, 1987.

256 Miettinen M, Franssila K, Kehto V-P, Paasivuo R, Virtanen I: Expression of intermediate filament proteins in thyroid gland and thyroid tumors. Lab Invest 50:262-270, 1984.

257 Miettinen M, Virtanen I: Expression of laminin in thyroid gland and thyroid tumors. An immunohistologic study. Int J Cancer 34:27-30, 1984.

258 Newland JR, Mackay B, Hill CS Jr, Hickey RC: Anaplastic thyroid carcinoma. An ultrastructural study of 10 cases. Ultrastruct Pathol 2:121-129, 1981.

259 Nishiyama RH, Dunn EL, Thompson NW: Anaplastic spindle-cell and giant-cell tumors of the thyroid gland. Cancer 30:113-127, 1972.

260 Ryff-de Lèche A, Staub JJ, Kohler-Faden R, Müller-Brand J, Heitz PU: Thyroglobulin production by malignant thyroid tumors. An immunocytochemical and radioimmunoassay study. Cancer 57:1145-1153, 1986.

261 Schmid KW, Kroll M, Hofstadter F, Ladurner D: Small cell carcinoma of the thyroid. A reclassification of cases originally diagnosed as small cell carcinomas of the thyroid. Pathol Res Pract 181:540-543, 1986.

262 Silverberg SG, DeGiorgi LS: Osteoclastoma-like giant cell tumor of the thyroid. Cancer 31:621-625, 1973.

263 Spanos GA, Wolk D, Desner MR, Khan A, Platt N, Khafif RA, Cortes EP: Preoperative chemotherapy for giant cell carcinoma of the thyroid. Cancer 50:2252-2256, 1982.

264 Wilson NW, Pambakian H, Richardson TC, Stokoe MR, Makin CA, Heyderman E: Epithelial markers in thyroid carcinoma. An immunoperoxidase study. Histopathology 10:815-829, 1986.

Medullary carcinoma, C-cell hyperplasia, and related tumors

265 Albores-Saavedra J, Monforte H, Nadji M, Morales AR: C-cell hyperplasia in thyroid tissue adjacent to follicular cell tumors. Hum Pathol, 19:795-799, 1988.

266 Bigner S, Mendelsohn G, Wells SA Jr, Cox EB, Baylin SB, Eggleston JC: Medullary carcinoma of the thyroid in the multiple endocrine neoplasia IIA syndrome. Am J Surg Pathol 5:459-472, 1981.

267 Bishop AE, Polak JM, Facer P, Ferri GL, Marangos PJ, Pearse AG: Neuron specific enolase. A common marker for the endocrine cells and innervation of the gut and pancreas. Gastroenterology 83:902-915, 1982.

268 Butler M, Khan S: Immunoreactive calcitonin in amyloid fibrils of medullary carcinoma of the thyroid gland. An immunogold staining technique. Arch Pathol Lab Med 110:647-649, 1986.

269 Capella C, Bordi C, Monga G, Buffa R, Fontana P, Bonfanti S, Bussolati G, Solcia E: Multiple endocrine cell types in thyroid medullary carcinoma. Evidence for calcitonin, somatostatin, ACTH, 5HT and small granule cells. Virchows Arch [Pathol Anat] 377:111-128, 1978.

270 Chong GC, Beahrs OH, Sizemore GW, Woolner LH: Medullary carcinoma of the thyroid gland. Cancer 35:695-704, 1975.

271 DeLellis RA, Rue AH, Spiler I, Nathanson L, Tashjian AH Jr, Wolfe HJ: Calcitonin and carcinoembryonic antigen as tumor markers in medullary thyroid carcinoma. Am J Clin Pathol 70:587-594, 1978.

272 DeLellis RA, Wolfe H: Calcitonin immunohistochemistry. In DeLellis RA (ed): Diagnostic immunohistochemistry, New York, 1981, Masson Publishing USA, Inc., pp. 61-74.

273 Engbaek F: Serotonin (5-hydroxytryptamine) in medullary thyroid carcinoma with or without pheochromocytoma. Eur J Cancer Clin Oncol 21:469-473, 1985.

274 Fletcher JR: Medullary (solid) carcinoma of the thyroid gland. A review of 249 cases. Arch Surg 100:257-262, 1970.

275 Ghatei MA, Springall DR, Nicholl CG, Polak JM, Bloom SR: Gastrin-releasing peptide-like immunoreactivity in medullary thyroid carcinoma. Am J Clin Pathol 84:581-586, 1985.

276 Golouh R, Us-Krasovec M, Auersperg M, Jancar J, Bondi A, Eusebi V: Amphicrine—composite calcitonin and mucin-producing—carcinoma of the thyroid. Ultrastruct Pathol 8:197-206, 1985.

277 Gordon PR, Huvos AG, Strong EW: Medullary carcinoma of the thyroid gland. A clinicopathologic study of 40 cases. Cancer 31:915-924, 1973.

278 Haegert DG, Wang NS, Farrer PA, Seemayer TA, Thelmo W: Non-chromaffin paragangliomatosis manifesting as a cold thyroid nodule. Am J Clin Pathol 61:561-570, 1974.

279 Harach HR, Williams ED: Glandular (tubular and follicular) variants of medullary carcinoma of the thyroid. Histopathology 7:83-97, 1983.

280 Hazard JB: The C cells (parafollicular cells) of the thyroid gland and medullary thyroid carcinoma. A review. Am J Pathol 88:214-250, 1977.

281 Hazard JB, Hawk WA, Crile G Jr: Medullary (solid) carcinoma of the thyroid. A clinicopathologic entity. J Clin Endocrinol Metab 19:152-161, 1959.

282 Holm R, Sobrinho-Simões M, Nesland JM, Gould VE, Johannessen JV: Medullary carcinoma of the thyroid gland. An immunocytochemical study, Ultrastruct Pathol 8:25-41, 1985.

283 Holm R, Sobrinho-Simões M, Nesland JM, Sambade C, Johannessen JV: Medullary thyroid carcinoma with thyroglobulin immunoreactivity. A special entity? Lab Invest 57:258-268, 1987.

284 Horvath E, Kovacs K, Ross RC: Medullary cancer of the thyroid gland and its possible relations to carcinoids. An ultrastructural study. Virchows Arch [Pathol Anat] 356:281-292, 1972.

285 Kakudo K, Carney JA, Sizemore GW: Medullary carcinoma of thyroid. Biologic behavior of the sporadic and familial neoplasm. Cancer 55:2818-2821, 1985.

286 Kakudo K, Miyauchi A, Ogihara T, Takai SI, Kitamura H, Kosaki G, Kumahara Y: Medullary carcinoma of the thyroid. Giant cell type. Arch Pathol Lab Med 102:445-447, 1978.

287 Kakudo K, Miyauchi A, Takai S, Katayama S, Kuma K, Kitamura H: C cell carcinoma of the thyroid. Papillary type. Acta Pathol Jpn 29:653-659, 1979.

288 Kay S, Montague JW, Dodd RW: Nonchromaffin paraganglioma (chemodectoma) of thyroid region. Cancer 36:582-585, 1975.

289 Krisch K, Krisch I, Horvat G, Neuhold N, Ulrich W, Srikanta S: The value of immunohistochemistry in medullary thyroid carcinoma. A systematic study of 30 cases. Histopathology 9:1077-1089, 1985.

290 Landon G, Ordóñéz NG: Clear cell variant of medullary carcinoma of the thyroid. Hum Pathol 16:844-847, 1985.

291 Lippmann SM, Mendelsohn G, Trump DL, Wells SA Jr, Baylin SB: The prognostic and biological significance of cellular heterogeneity in medullary thyroid carcinoma. A study of calcitonin, L-DOPA decarboxylase, and histaminase, J Clin Endocrinol Metab 54:233-240, 1982.

292 Ljungberg O: On medullary carcinoma of the thyroid. Acta Pathol Microbiol Scand [A] 231[Suppl]:1-57, 1972.

293 Lloyd RV, Sisson JC, Marangos PJ: Calcitonin, carcinoembryonic antigen and neuron-specific enolase in medullary thyroid carcinoma. An immunohistochemical study. Cancer 51:2234-2239, 1983.

294 Marcus JN, Dise CA, LiVolsi VA: Melanin production in a medullary thyroid carcinoma. Cancer 49:2518-2526, 1982.

295 Matsubayashi S, Yanaihara C, Ohkubo M, Fukata S, Hayashi Y, Tamai H, Nakagawa T, Miyauchi A, Kuma K, Abe K: Gastrin-releasing peptide immunoreactivity in medullary thyroid carcinoma. Cancer 53:2472-2477, 1984.

296 Mendelsohn G, Bigner SH, Eggleston JC, Baylin SB, Wells SA Jr: Anaplastic variants of medullary thyroid carcinoma. Am J Surg Pathol 4:333-341, 1980.

297 Mendelsohn G, Eggleston JC, Weisburger WR, Gann DS, Baylin SB: Calcitonin and histaminase in C-cell hyperplasia and medullary thyroid carcinoma. A light microscopic and immunohistochemical study. Am J Pathol 92:35-52, 1978.

298 Mendelsohn G, Wells SA Jr, Baylin SB: Relationship of tissue carcinoembryonic antigen and calcitonin to tumor virulence in medullary thyroid carcinoma. An immunohistochemical study in early, localized, and virulent disseminated stages of disease. Cancer 54:657-662, 1984.

299 Mitsudo SM, Grajower MM, Balbi H, Silver C: Malignant paraganglioma of the thyroid gland. Arch Pathol Lab Med 111:378-380, 1987.

300 O'Connor DT, Deftos LJ: Secretion of chromogranin A by peptide-producing endocrine neoplasms. N Engl J Med 314:1145-1151, 1986.

301 Ohashi M, Yanase T, Fujio N, Ibayashi H, Kinjo M, Matsuo H: Alpha-neoendorphin-like immunoreactivity in medullary carcinoma of the thyroid. Cancer 59:277-280, 1987.

302 Pfaltz M, Hedinger Chr E, Mühlethaler JP: Mixed medullary and follicular carcinoma of the thyroid. Virchows Arch [Pathol Anat] 400:53-59, 1983.

303 Roth KA, Bensch KG, Hoffman AR: Characterization of opioid peptides in human thyroid medullary carcinoma. Cancer 59:1594-1598, 1987.

304 Ruppert JM, Eggleston JC, DeBustros A, Baylin SB: Disseminated calcitonin-poor medullary thyroid carcinoma in a patient with calcitonin-rich primary tumor. Am J Surg Pathol 10:513-518, 1986.

305 Saad MF, Fritsche HA Jr, Samaan NA: Diagnostic and prognostic values of carcinoembryonic antigen in medullary carcinoma of the thyroid. J Clin Endocrinol Metab 58:889-894, 1984.

306 Saad MF, Ordoñéz NG, Guido JJ, Samaan NA: The prognostic value of calcitonin immunostaining in medullary carcinoma of the thyroid. J Clin Endocrinol Metab 59:850-856, 1984.

307 Saad MF, Ordoñéz NG, Rashid RK, Guido JJ, Hill CS Jr, Hickey RC, Samaan NA: Medullary carcinoma of the thyroid. A study of the clinical features and prognostic factors in 161 patients. Medicine [Baltimore] 63:319-342, 1984.

308 Schmid KW, Fischer-Colbrie R, Hagn C, Jasani B, Williams ED, Winkler H: Chromogranin A and B and secretogranin II in medullary carcinomas of the thyroid. Am J Surg Pathol 11:551-556, 1987.

309 Schröder S, Böcker W, Baisch H, Bürk CG, Arps H, Meiners I, Kastendieck H, Heitz PU, Klöppel G: Prognostic factors in medullary thyroid carcinomas. Survival in relation to age, sex, stage, histology, immunocytochemistry, and DNA content. Cancer 61:806-816, 1988.

310 Schröder S, Klöppel G: Carcinoembryonic antigen and nonspecific cross-reacting antigen in thyroid cancer. An immunocytochemical antigen in thyroid cancer. An immunocytochemical study using polyclonal and monoclonal antibodies. Am J Surg Pathol 11:100-108, 1987.

311 Sikri KL, Varndell IM, Hamid QA, Wilson BS, Kameya T, Ponder BAJ, Lloyd RV, Bloom SR, Polak JM: Medullary carcinoma of the thyroid. An immuno-cytochemical and histochemical study of 25 cases using eight separate markers. Cancer 56:2481-2491, 1985.

312 Steinfeld CM, Moertel CG, Woolner LB: Diarrhea and medullary carcinoma of the thyroid. Cancer 31:1237-1239, 1973.

313 Sweeney EC, McDonnell L, O'Brien C: Medullary carcinoma of the thyroid presenting as tumours of the pharynx and larynx. Histopathology 5:263-275, 1981.

314 Uribe M, Grimes M, Fenoglio-Preiser CM, Feind C: Medullary carcinoma of the thyroid gland. Clinical, pathological, and immunohistochemical features with review of the literature. Am J Surg Pathol 9:577-594, 1985.

315 Wells SA Jr, Baylin SB, Leight GS, Dale JK, Dilley WG, Farndon JR: The importance of early diagnosis in patients with hereditary medullary thyroid carcinoma. Ann Surg 195:595-599, 1982.

316 White IL, Vimadalal SD, Catz B, Van de Velde R, La Gange T: Occult medullary carcinoma of thyroid. An unusual clinical and pathologic presentation. Cancer 47:1364-1368, 1981.

317 Wurzel JM, Kourides IA, Brooks JSJ: Medullary carcinomas of the thyroid contain immunoreactive human chorionic gonadotropin alpha subunit. Horm Metab Res 16:677, 1984.

318 Zaatari GS, Saigo PE, Huvos AG: Mucin production in medullary carcinoma of the thyroid. Arch Pathol Lab Med 107:70-74, 1983.

Epithelial tumors—general features
Geographic distribution

319 Cuello C, Correa P, Eisenberg H: Geographic pathology of thyroid carcinoma. Cancer 23:230-239, 1969.

320 Franssila K, Saxén E, Teppo L, Bjarnason O, Tulinius H, Normann T, Ringertz N: Incidence of different morphological types of thyroid cancer in the nordic countries. Acta Pathol Microbiol Scand [A] 89:49-55, 1981.

321 Hedinger Chr E: Geographic pathology of thyroid disease. Pathol Res Pract 171:285-292, 1981.

322 Hofstädter F: Frequency and morphology of malignant tumors of the thyroid before and after the introduction of iodine-prophylaxis. Virchows Arch [Pathol Anat] 385:263-270, 1980.

323 Pendergrast WJ, Milmore BK, Marcus SC: Thyroid cancer and thyrotoxicosis in the United States. Their relation to endemic goiter. J Chronic Dis 13:22-38, 1961.

324 Williams ED, Doniach I, Bjarnason O, Michie W: Thyroid cancer in an iodine rich area. A histopathological study. Cancer 39:215-222, 1977.

Thyroid neoplasia in childhood

325 Hayles AB, Kennedy RLJ, Beahrs OH, Woolner LB: Carcinoma of the thyroid gland in children. Am J Dis Child 90:705-715, 1955.

326 Raju U, Kini S: Neoplasms of thyroid follicular epithelium in children and adolescents (abstract). Lab Invest 58:8P, 1988.

327 Root AW: Cancer of the thyroid in childhood and adolescence. Am J Med Sci 246:734-749, 1963.

328 Winship T, Rosvoll RV: Childhood thyroid carcinoma. Cancer 14:734-743, 1961.

Thyroid neoplasia and radiation exposure

329 Calandra DB, Shah KH, Lawrence AM, Paloyan E: Total thyroidectomy in irradiated patients. A twenty-year experience in 206 patients. Ann Surg 202:356-360, 1985.

330 Hanson GA, Komorowski RA, Cerletty JM, Wilson SD: Thyroid gland morphology in young adults. Normal subjects versus those with prior low-dose neck irradiation in childhood. Surgery 96:984-988, 1984.

331 Hempelmann LH, Hall WJ, Phillips M, Cooper RA, Ames WR: Neoplasms in persons treated with x-rays in infancy. Fourth survey in 20 years. J Natl Cancer Inst 55:519-530, 1975.

332 Komorowski RA, Hanson GA: Morphologic changes in the thyroid following low-dose childhood radiation. Arch Pathol Lab Med 101:36-39, 1977.

333 Schneider AB, Pinsky S, Bekerman C, Ryo UY: Characteristics of 108 thyroid cancers detected by screening in a population with a history of head and neck irradiation. Cancer 46:1218-1227, 1980.

334 Schneider AB, Shore-Freedman E, Ryo UY, Bekerman C, Favus M, Pinsky S: Radiation-induced tumors of the head and neck following childhood irradiation. Prospective studies. Medicine [Baltimore] 64:1-15, 1985.

335 Schneider AB, Shore-Freedman E, Weinstein RA: Radiation-induced thyroid and other head and neck tumors. Occurrence of multiple tumors and analysis of risk factors. J Clin Endocrinol Metab 63:107-112, 1986.

336 Spitalnik PF, Straus FH II: Patterns of human thyroid parenchymal reaction following low-dose childhood irradiation. Cancer 41:1098-1105, 1978.

337 Wilson SD, Komorowski R, Cerletty J, Majewski JT, Hooper M: Radiation-associated thyroid tumors. Extent of operation and pathology technique influence the apparent incidence of carcinoma. Surgery 94:663-669, 1983.

Association with other conditions

338 Hedman I, Tisell L-E: Associated hyperparathyroidism and nonmedullary thyroid carcinoma. The etiologic role of radiation. Surgery 95:392-397, 1984.

339 Lever EG, Refetoff S, Straus FH II, Nguyen M, Kaplan EL: Coexisting thyroid and parathyroid disease—are they related? Surgery 94:893-900, 1983.

340 Lote K, Andersen K, Nordal E, Brennhovd IO: Familial occurrence of papillary thyroid carcinoma. Cancer 46:1291-1297, 1980.

341 Narita T, Takagi K: Ataxia-telangiectasia with dysgerminoma of right ovary, papillary carcinoma of thyroid, and adenocarcinoma of pancreas. Cancer 54:1113-1116, 1984.

342 Plail RO, Bussey HJR, Glazer G, Thomson JPS: Adenomatous polyposis. An association with carcinoma of the thyroid. Br J Surg 74:377-380, 1987.

Evaluation of the solitary thyroid nodule

343 Lo Gerfo P, Starker P, Weber C, Moore D, Feind C: Incidence of cancer in surgically treated thyroid nodules based on method of selection. Surgery 98:1197-1201, 1985.

Needle biopsy and fine needle aspiration

344 Åkerman M, Tennvall J, Biörklund A, Måartensson H, Möller T: Sensitivity and specificity of fine needle aspiration cytology in the diagnosis of tumors of the thyroid gland. Acta Cytol [Baltimore] 29:850-855, 1985.

345 Droese M: Cytological aspiration biopsy of the thyroid gland. Stuttgart, 1980, F.K. Schattauer Verlag.

346 Frable WJ, Frable MA: Fine-needle aspiration biopsy of the thyroid. Histo-pathologic and clinical correlations. In Fenoglio CM, Wolff M (eds): Progress in surgical pathology, vol. 1. New York, 1980, Masson Publishing USA, Inc., pp. 105-118.

347 Friedman M, Shimaoka K, Rao U, Tsukada Y, Gavigan M, Tamura K: Diagnosis of chronic lymphocytic thyroiditis (nodular presentation) by needle aspiration. Acta Cytol [Baltimore] 25:513-522, 1981.

348 Geddie WR, Bedard YC, Strawbridge HTG: Medullary carcinoma of the thyroid in fine-needle aspiration biopsies. Am J Clin Pathol **82:**552-558, 1984.

349 Goellner JR, Johnson DA: Cytology of cystic papillary carcinoma of the thyroid. Acta Cytol [Baltimore] **26:**797-799, 1982.

350 Hawk WA, Crile G Jr, Hazard JB, Barrett DL: Needle biopsy of thyroid gland. Surg Gynecol Obstet **122:**1053-1065, 1966.

351 Kini SR, Miller JM, Abrash MP, Gaba A, Johnson T: Post fine needle aspiration biopsy infarction in thyroid nodules (abstract). Lab Invest **58:**48A, 1988.

352 Kini SR, Miller JM, Hamburger JI: Cytopathology of Hürthle cell lesions of the thyroid gland by fine needle aspiration. Acta Cytol [Baltimore] **25:**647-652, 1981.

353 Kini SR, Miller JM, Hamburger JI, Smith MJ: Cytopathologic features of medullary carcinoma of the thyroid. Arch Pathol Lab Med **108:**156-159, 1984.

354 Lever EG, Refetoff S, Scherberg NH, Carr K: The influence of percutaneous fine needle aspiration on serum thyroglobulin, J Clin Endocrinol Metab **56:**26-29, 1983.

355 Lew W, Orell S, Henderson DW: Intranuclear vacuoles in nonpapillary carcinoma of the thyroid. A report of three cases. Acta Cytol [Baltimore] **28:**581-586, 1984.

356 Lo Gerfo P, Colacchio T, Caushaj F, Weber C, Feind C: Comparison of fine-needle and coarse-needle biopsies in evaluating thyroid nodules. Surgery **92:**835-838, 1982.

357 Miller JM, Hamburger JI, Kini SR: The needle biopsy diagnosis of papillary thyroid carcinoma. Cancer **48:**989-993, 1981.

357a Miller JM, Kini SR, Hamburger JI: Needle biopsy of the thyroid. New York, 1983, Praeger, p. 171.

358 Miller JM, Kini SR, Hamburger JI: The diagnosis of malignant follicular neoplasms of the thyroid by needle biopsy. Cancer **55:**2812-2817, 1985.

359 Ramacciotti CE, Pretorius HT, Chu EW, Barsky SH, Brennan MF, Robbins J: Diagnostic accuracy and use of aspiration biopsy in the management of thyroid nodules. Arch Intern Med **144:**1169-1173, 1984.

360 Silverman JF, West RL, Larkin EW, Park HK, Finley JL, Swanson MS, Fore WW: The role of fine-needle aspiration biopsy in the rapid diagnosis and management of thyroid neoplasm. Cancer **57:**1164-1170, 1986.

361 Suen KC, Quenville NF: Fine needle aspiration biopsy of the thyroid gland. A study of 304 cases. J Clin Pathol **36:**1036-1045, 1983.

362 Vickery AL Jr: Needle biopsy pathology. Clin Endocrinol Metab **10:**275-293, 1981.

Frozen section

363 Hamburger JI, Hamburger SW: Declining role of frozen section in surgical planning for thyroid nodules. Surgery **98:**307-312, 1986.

364 Kraemer BB: Frozen section diagnosis and the thyroid. Semin Diagn Pathol **4:**169-189, 1987.

365 Rosai J, Carcangiu ML: Pitfalls in the diagnosis of thyroid tumors. Pathol Res Pract **182:**169-179, 1987.

Presence of thyroid tissue outside gland

366 Frantz VK, Forsythe R, Hanford JM, Rogers WM: Lateral aberrant thyroids. Ann Surg **115:**161-183, 1942.

367 Hathaway BM: Innocuous accessory thyroid nodules. Arch Surg **90:**222-227, 1965.

368 Meyer JS, Steinberg LS: Microscopically benign thyroid follicles in cervical lymph nodes. Serial section study of lymph node inclusions and entire thyroid gland in 5 cases. Cancer **24:**302-311, 1969.

369 Roth LM: Inclusions of non-neoplastic thyroid tissue within cervical lymph nodes. Cancer **18:**105-111, 1965.

370 Sisson JC, Schmidt RW, Beierwaltes WH: Sequestered nodular goiter. N Engl J Med **270:**927-932, 1964.

371 Wozencraft P, Foote FW Jr, Frazell EL: Occult carcinomas of the thyroid. Their bearing on the concept of lateral aberrant thyroid cancer. Cancer **1:**574-583, 1948.

Treatment

372 Ampil FL: Postoperative external irradiation in thyroid carcinoma. A clinical experience of 20 treated patients and literature radiotherapy review. J Surg Oncol **30:**83-90, 1985.

373 Cady B, Cohn K, Rossi RL, Sedgwick CE, Meissner WA, Werber J, Gelman RS: The effect of thyroid hormone administration upon survival in patients with differentiated thyroid carcinoma. Surgery **94:**978-983, 1983.

374 Carcangiu ML, Zampi G, Pupi A, Castagnoli A, Rosai J: Papillary carcinoma of the thyroid. A clinopathologic study of 241 cases treated at the University of Florence, Italy. Cancer **55:**805-828, 1985.

375 Clark OH: Total thyroidectomy. The treatment of choice for patients with differentiated thyroid cancer. Ann Surg **196:**361-370, 1982.

376 Cohn KH, Bäckdahl M, Forsslund G, Auer G, Zetterberg A, Lundell G, Granberg P-O, Löwhagen T, Willems J-S, Cady B: Biologic considerations and operative strategy in papillary thyroid carcinoma. Arguments against the routine performance of total thyroidectomy. Surgery **96:**957-971, 1984.

377 Crile G Jr: Changing end results in patients with papillary carcinoma of the thyroid. Surg Gynecol Obstet **132:**460-468, 1971.

378 Crile G Jr, Antunez AR, Esselstyn CB, Hawk WA, Skillern PG: The advantages of subtotal thyroidectomy and suppression of TSH in the primary treatment of papillary carcinoma of the thyroid. Cancer **55:**2691-2697, 1985.

379 Harness JK, Thompson NW, McLeod MK, Eckhauser FE, Lloyd RV: Follicular carcinoma of the thyroid gland. Trends and treatment. Surgery **96:**972-980, 1984.

380 Hay ID, Grant CS, Taylor WF, McConahey WM: Ipsilateral lobectomy versus bilateral lobar resection in papillary thyroid carcinoma. A retrospective analysis of surgical outcome using a novel prognostic scoring system. Surgery **102:**1088-1095, 1987.

381 Hutter RVP, Frazell EL, Foote FW Jr: Elective radical neck dissection. An assessment of its use in the management of papillary thyroid cancer. CA **20:**87-93, 1970.

382 Maheshwari YK, Hill CS Jr, Haynie TP III, Hickey RC, Samaan NA: [131]I Therapy in differentiated thyroid carcinoma. M.D. Anderson hospital experience. Cancer **47:**664-671, 1981.

383 Mazzaferri EL, Young RL: Papillary thyroid carcinoma. A 10 year follow-up report of the impact of therapy in 576 patients. Am J Med **70:**511-518, 1981.

384 Mazzaferri EL, Young RL, Oertel JE, Kemmerer WT, Page CP: Papillary thyroid carcinoma: the impact of therapy in 576 patients. Medicine [Baltimore] **56:**171-196, 1977.

385 Ramanna L, Waxman AD, Brachman MB, Sensel N, Tanasescu DE, Berman DS, Catz B, Braunstein GD: Correlation of thyroglobulin measurements and radioiodine scans in the follow-up of patients with differentiated thyroid cancer. Cancer **55:**1525-1529, 1985.

386 Schroder DM, Chambors A, France CJ: Operative strategy for thyroid cancer. It total thyroidectomy worth the price? Cancer **58:**2320-2328, 1986.

387 Starnes HF, Brooks DC, Pinkus GS, Brooks JR: Surgery for thyroid carcinoma. Cancer **55:**1376-1381, 1985.

388 Tubiana M, Haddad E, Schlumberger M, Hill C, Rougier P, Sarrazin D: External radiotherapy in thyroid cancers. Cancer **55:**2062-2071, 1985.

389 Vickery AL Jr, Wang C-A, Walker AM: Treatment of intrathyroidal papillary carcinoma of the thyroid. Cancer **60:**2587-2595, 1987.

Prognostic factors

390 Cady B, Rossi R, Silverman M, Wool M: Further evidence of the validity of risk group definition in differentiated thyroid carcinoma. Surgery **98:**1171-1178, 1985.

391 Carcangiu ML, Zampi G, Pupi A, Castagnoli A, Rosai J: Papillary carcinoma of the thyroid. A clinicopathologic study of 241 cases treated at the University of Florence, Italy. Cancer **55:**805-828, 1985.

392 Franssila KO: Prognosis in thyroid carcinoma. Cancer **36:**1138-1146, 1975.

393 Heitz P, Moser H, Staub JJ: Thyroid cancer. A study of 573 thyroid tumors and 161 autopsy cases observed over a thirty-year period. Cancer **37:**2329-2337, 1976.

394 Ito J, Noguchi S, Murakami N, Noguchi A: Factors affecting the prognosis of patients with carcinoma of the thyroid. Surg Gynecol Obstet **150:**539-544, 1980.

395 Tennvall J, Biörklund A, Möller T, Ranstam J, Åkerman M: Is the EORTC prognostic index of thyroid cancer valid in differentiated thyroid carcinoma? Retrospective multivariate analysis of differentiated thyroid carcinoma with long follow-up. Cancer **57:**1405-1414, 1986.

Lymphoid tumors and tumorlike conditions

396 Allevato PA, Kini SR, Rebuck JW, Miller JM, Hamburger JI: Signet ring cell lymphoma of the thyroid. A case report. Hum Pathol **16:**1066-1068, 1985.

397 Anscombe AM, Wright DH: Primary malignant lymphoma of the thyroid—a tumour of mucosa-associated lymphoid tissue. Review of seventy-six cases. Histopathology **9:**81-97, 1985.

398 Aozasa K, Inoue A, Tajima K, Miyauchi A, Matsuzuka F, Kuma K: Malignant lymphomas of the thyroid gland. Analysis of 79 patients with emphasis on histologic prognostic factors. Cancer **58:**100-104, 1986.

399 Aozasa K, Inoue A, Yoshimura H, Katagiri S, Katayama S, Matsuzuka F, Yonezawa T: Intermediate lymphocytic lymphoma of the thyroid. An immunologic and immunohistologic study. Cancer **57:**1762-1767, 1986.

400 Aozasa K, Inoue A, Yoshimura H, Miyauchi A, Matsuzuka F, Kuma K: Plasmacytoma of the thyroid gland. Cancer **58**:105-110, 1986.

401 Burke JS, Butler JJ, Fuller LM: Malignant lymphomas of the thyroid. A clinical pathologic study of 35 patients including ultrastructural observations. Cancer **39**:1587-1602, 1977.

402 Compagno J, Oertel JE: Malignant lymphoma and other lymphoproliferative disorders of the thyroid gland. A clinopathologic study of 245 cases. Am J Clin Pathol **74**:1-11, 1980.

402a Coode PE, Shaikh MU: Histocytosis X of the thyroid masquerading as thyroid carcinoma. Hum Pathol **19**:239-241, 1988.

403 Devine RM, Edis AJ, Banks PM: Primary lymphoma of the thyroid. A review of the Mayo Clinic experience through 1978. World J Surg **5**:33-38, 1981.

403a Fauré P, Chittal S, Woodman-Memeteau W, Caveriviere P, Gorguet B, Voigt J-J, Delsol G: Diagnostic features of primary malignant lymphomas of the thyroid with monoclonal antibodies. Cancer **61**:1852-1861, 1988.

404 Feigin GA, Buss DH, Paschal B, Woodruff RD, Myers RT: Hodgkin's disease manifested as a thyroid nodule. Hum Pathol **13**:774-776, 1982.

405 Holck S: Plasma cell granuloma of the thyroid. Cancer **48**:830-832, 1981.

406 Larkin DFP, Dervan PA, Munnelly J, Finucane J: Sinus histiocytosis with massive lymphadenopathy simulating subacute thyroiditis. Hum Pathol **17**:321-324, 1986.

407 Maurer R, Taylor CR, Terry R, Lukes RJ: Non-Hodgkin lymphomas of the thyroid. A clinico-pathological review of 29 cases applying the Lukes-Collins classification and an immunoperoxidase method. Virchows Arch [Pathol Anat] **383**:293-317, 1979.

408 Ottó S, Péter I, Végh S, Juhos E, Besznyák I: Gamma-chain heavy-chain disease with primary thyroid plasmacytoma. Arch Pathol Lab Med **110**:893-896, 1986.

409 Rasbach DA, Mondschein MS, Harris NL, Kaufman DS, Wang C-A: Malignant lymphoma of the thyroid gland. A clinical and pathologic study of twenty cases. Surgery **98**:1166-1170, 1985.

410 Shimaoka K, Gailani S, Tsukada Y, Barcos M: Plasma cell neoplasm involving the thyroid. Cancer **41**:1140-1146, 1978.

411 Teja K, Sabio H, Langdon DR, Johanson AJ: Involvement of the thyroid gland in histiocytosis X. Hum Pathol **12**:1137-1139, 1981.

412 Williams ED: Malignant lymphoma of the thyroid. Clin Endocrinol Metab **10**:379-389, 1981.

413 Woolner LB, McConahey WM, Beahrs OH, Black BM: Primary malignant lymphoma of the thyroid. Review of forty six cases. Am J Surg **111**:502-523, 1966.

Mesenchymal tumors

414 Mills SE, Stallings RG, Austin MB: Angiomatoid carcinoma of the thyroid gland. Anaplastic carcinoma with follicular and medullary features mimicking angiosarcoma. Am J Clin Pathol **86**:674-678, 1986.

415 Pfaltz M, Hedinger Chr E, Saremaslani P, Egloff B: Malignant hemangioendothelioma of the thyroid and factor VIII–related antigen. Virchows Arch [Pathol Anat] **401**:177-184, 1983.

416 Ruchti C, Gerber HA, Schaffner T: Factor VIII–related antigen in malignant hemangioendothelioma of the thyroid. Additional evidence for the endothelial origin of this tumor. Am J Clin Pathol **82**:474-480, 1984.

417 Shin W, Aftalion B, Hotchkiss E, Schenkman R, Berkman J: Ultrastructure of a primary fibrosarcoma of the human thyroid gland. Cancer **44**:584-591, 1979.

Other primary tumors

418 Bale GF: Teratoma of the neck in the region of the thyroid gland. A review of the literature and report of four cases. Am J Pathol **26**:565-580, 1950.

419 Kimler SC, Muth WF: Primary malignant teratoma of the thyroid. Case report and literature review of cervical teratomas in adults. Cancer **42**:311-317, 1978.

Metastatic tumors

420 Carcangiu ML, Sibley RK, Rosai J: Clear cell change in primary thyroid tumors. A study of 38 cases. Am J Surg Pathol **9**:705-722, 1985.

421 Horace KI: Cancer metastatic to the thyroid. A diagnostic problem. Mayo Clin Proc **59**:856-859, 1984.

422 Shimaoka K, Sokal JE, Pickren JW: Metastatic neoplasms in the thyroid gland. Pathological and clinical findings. Cancer **15**:557-565, 1962.

423 Zirkin HJ, Tovi F: Tracheal carcinoma presenting as a thyroid tumor. J Surg Oncol **26**:268-271, 1984.

10 Parathyroid glands

GROSS ANATOMY AND EMBRYOLOGY

Normally, there are four oval, resilient parathyroid glands, each averaging 4 × 3 × 1.5 mm. In rare cases, more than four glands are present. In a study of 527 autopsy cases, Gilmour and Martin[2] found two instances in which there were six glands and thirty-one in which there were five. Variations in the weights of the normal glands were studied by the same authors,[2] who found that in 189 cases the mean weight of all four glands was 117.6 ± 4 mg in men and 131.3 ± 5.8 mg in women. The color varies from reddish brown to light tan to yellow, depending on fat content, which, in turn, depends on age, nutrition, and activity of the individual.

Parathyroid glands are arranged in two pairs. The upper pair arises from the fourth branchial cleft and descends into the neck with the thyroid gland during embryonic life. The lower pair arises from the third branchial cleft and descends into the neck with the thymus. Normally, the upper pair is located on the middle third of the posterolateral border of the thyroid gland, and the lower pair is close to the lower pole of the thyroid gland, in close proximity to the inferior thyroid artery. It has been pointed out that the parathyroid glands usually have a symmetric distribution—when one superior parathyroid gland is located in one place, the opposite parathyroid gland will be in a similar area.[1]

The vascular supply of the lower parathyroid glands comes from branches of the inferior thyroid arteries. This supply is usually independent, a circumstance that may be helpful in locating abnormally placed glands. If one of these arteries is ligated, infarction of the parathyroid gland may result.

Faulty migration of the glands during embryonic life may result in anomalous positions. The upper glands may be found inside the carotid sheath or behind the cervical or thoracic esophagus. The lower glands may continue their descent with the thymus into the anterior portion of the mediastinum. They may also be located inside the thyroid gland or in the pharynx.[3] Wang[4] has pointed out that despite the wide distribution patterns that parathyroid glands may exhibit, these fall into an orderly scheme and can be uncovered by the experienced surgeon in the great majority of cases.

HISTOLOGY

In the past, a rigid division of cell types has been applied to the normal parathyroid gland; however, evidence suggests that this organ is made up of a basic cell type, the *chief cell*, and that all the other cells that have been described represent morphologic variations of the former that are caused by differences in physiologic activity[10] (Fig. 10-1).

The chief cell measures 6 to 8 μm in diameter, has a centrally located nucleus, a moderate amount of pale granular cytoplasm, and ill-defined cell margins. Ultrastructurally, there are variable amounts of glycogen particles and secretory droplets, an inverse relationship being present in the amount of these two components.[10] Parathormone secretion can be demonstrated immunohistochemically.[9]

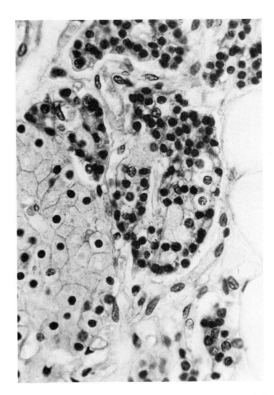

Fig 10-1 Normal parathyroid gland. Note lack of encapsulation and persistence of fat. Cells with deep-staining nuclei are chief cells, and those with prominent granular cytoplasm are oxyphil cells.

There is also cytoplasmic reactivity for various types of keratin, but not for vimentin, glial fibrillary acidic protein, or neurofilament.[8]

The *oxyphil cell* has a more abundant cytoplasm, which is deeply granular and acidophilic. Ultrastructurally, there are many mitochondria but few secretory granules. A rich content of oxidative enzymes can be demonstrated histochemically. *Transitional oxyphil cells* have an appearance that is intermediate between chief cells and oxyphil cells. The *water-clear cell* is characterized by abundant optically clear cytoplasm and sharply defined cell membranes. *Transitional water-clear cells* have an appearance that is intermediate between chief cells and water-clear cells. Both types of transitional cells are more common in hyperfunctioning than in normal glands.

The frequency distribution of the different cells varies with the age of the patient. Until puberty, the gland is composed wholly of chief cells that contain cytoplasmic glycogen but not fat. The latter appears in these cells as very fine droplets soon after puberty at about the same time that the oxyphil cells appear. They appear first singly, then in pairs, and after 40 years of age, in the form of sharply outlined but not encapsulated islands, which may be large.

Following puberty, mature adipose tissue appears in the stroma and increases in amount until about 40 years of age, to remain relatively constant thereafter. Gilmour[6] has shown that when a parathyroid gland in an adult is smaller than normal, this decrease in size is caused by a decrease in the amount of fat, whereas the parenchymal cell volume remains constant.

A few follicles and cysts of varying sizes are observed in about half of the parathyroid glands beyond puberty. They may be filled with granular and cellular debris or with a dark blue–staining, finely granular material that is morphologically indistinguishable from thyroid colloid.[5] This material, which sometimes is positive with amyloid stains, is thought to be a result of a conformational change in the stored parathormone polypeptide.[7] When these follicles are present, the distinction between thyroid and parathyroid tissue may become difficult. Presence of sizable amounts of cytoplasmic glycogen favors a parathyroid nature. If doubts persist, immunohistochemical stains for thyroglobulin, parathormone, and chromogranin should dispel them.[9]

PHYSIOLOGY

The parathyroid glands mediate their endocrine function through the production of parathormone.[12] There are several forms of circulating parathormone. The relationship among them is not clear, but it is known that the structural requirements for the biologic activity reside in the first thirty-four amino acid residues.[13] The chief cells are most critically sensitive to calcium concentrations in vivo and in vitro.

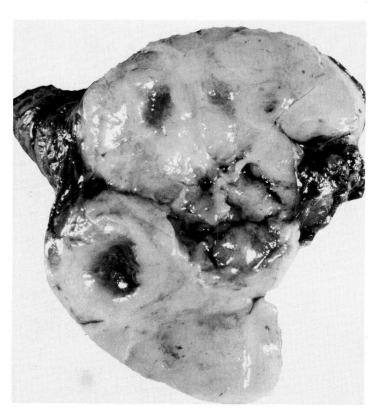

Fig. 10-2 Functioning parathyroid adenoma. Note encapsulation and cystic change. (From Black BK, Ackerman LV: Tumors of the parathyroid. A review of twenty-three cases. Cancer **3:**415-444, 1950.)

Roth and Raisz[14] have shown marked ultrastructural changes corresponding to enhanced production of parathormone secretion when calcium concentration was reduced. These active cells contain abundant secretory granules, a prominent Golgi apparatus, and very little glycogen. Under conditions of elevated calcium concentration, the cells are nearly devoid of secretion, have an inconspicuous Golgi apparatus, and contain abundant glycogen. These observations provide objective proof of the role of ionized serum calcium in regulating chief cell function and parathormone production. The most important physiologic actions of parathormone are increased renal excretion of phosphate, increased renal tubular reabsorption of calcium, increased intestinal absorption of calcium, and direct effects in bone. The latter are mainly manifested by an increase in the number of osteoclasts and an apparent increase in their phagocytic activity, with a resulting resorption of bone tissue.

A single hormone is probably responsible for both renal and osseous effects. It has been postulated that the mechanism of action of parathormone in the receptor tissues is a rapid stimulation of adenyl-cyclase, a membrane-bound enzyme, with a resulting increase in the intracellular concentration of cyclic 3', 5' AMP.[11]

ADENOMA

Parathyroid adenomas occur in women and men in a ratio of 3:1. They can develop at almost any age, but most occur in patients in the fourth decade. A few cases have been reported in children,[25] and some have been seen following radiation therapy to the head and neck region.[30] The large majority are single. Cases of double or triple adenomas exist,[34,37] but some of them would be reinterpreted today as examples of chief cell hyperplasia. Their size and weight vary greatly, the majority being too small to allow detection on palpation of the neck. Some may be recognizable only microscopically ("microadenomas")[23,29]; however, many of them will still cause radiographically detectable deformities in the esophagus or trachea.[38] Adenomas are usually oval, may show slight lobulation, and usually have a thin connective tissue capsule. On section, they are often grayish brown (Fig. 10-2). Foci of hemorrhage and calcification may occur.

In terms of location, about 75% involve one of the inferior glands, 15% one of the superior glands, and 10% occur in anomalous positions. Of the latter, 70% are in the mediastinum, 20% within the thyroid gland, and the remainder in the soft tissues behind the esophagus or—in rare cases—the esophageal wall itself.[26,32]

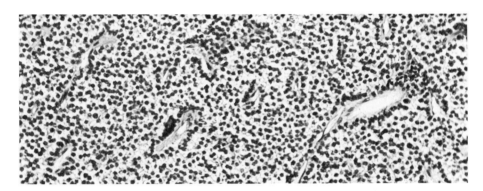

Fig. 10-3 Functioning parathyroid adenoma. Note difference in microscopic pattern from adenoma shown in Fig. 10-5. Patient has survived 11 years.

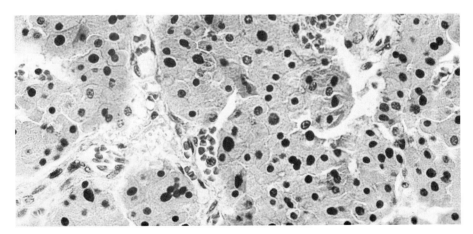

Fig. 10-4 Characteristic cells in oxyphil adenoma. The cytoplasm is abundant, granular, and deeply oxyphilic.

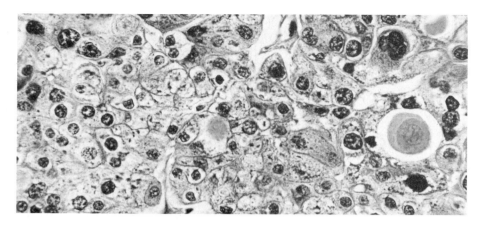

Fig. 10-5 Functioning parathyroid adenoma with extreme variation in nuclear size. Patient has survived 18 years following operation. (From Black BK, Ackerman LV: Tumors of the parathyroid. A review of twenty-three cases, Cancer **3:**415-444, 1950.)

Microscopically, the tumor is encapsulated and very cellular (Figs. 10-3 and 10-4). A rim of compressed nonneoplastic parathyroid tissue can be identified in about 60% of the cases. The adenoma itself may be composed of any of the various cell types that make up the normal parathyroid gland, but chief cells usually predominate. Combinations of chief cells, oxyphil cells, water-clear cells, and transitional elements are common. Variation in nuclear size may be conspicuous, with the appearance of cells with isolated or clustered huge hyperchromatic nuclei (Fig. 10-5). Presence of these nuclei does not indicate malignancy; on the contrary, it favors a benign diagnosis. Mitoses are usually absent, but an occasional one may be found. The pattern of growth is generally diffuse, but it may be nesting, follicular, or pseudopapillary.[29a] The follicles may contain a colloid-like material. This material sometimes stains for amyloid, as in the normal gland.[21]

The ultrastructural appearance of the tumor cells is indicative of hyperfunction and not substantially different from that seen in primary or secondary chief cell hyperplasia. Secretory granules, prominent Golgi apparatus, abundant cisternae of granular endoplasmic reticulum, annulate lamellae, numerous ribosomes, and interdigitating cytoplasmic membranes are the main features[15,19] (Fig. 10-6). In contrast to normal chief cells, large quantities of glycogen and secretory vacuoles can be seen simultaneously. Immunohistochemically, there is reactivity for parathormone and various types of keratin.[24] Miettinen et al.[24] found that some tumor cells do express neurofilament, an intermediate filament not found in normal parathyroid cells. In other studies, immunoreactivity for neuron-specific enolase, chromogranin, a number of peptide hormones, and opioid peptides has been encountered.[16a,35] The other parathyroid glands have a normal or atrophic appearance. To summarize, a typical parathyroid adenoma is single, surrounded by a rim of atrophic parathyroid tissue, and the other glands are normal or atrophic. The presence of a *microscopically normal* second gland is the best evidence that a given parathyroid lesion is an adenoma.

The large majority of parathyroid adenomas are functionally active, at least at the biochemical level.

The term *oxyphil adenoma* should be restricted to parathyroid adenomas composed entirely or almost entirely of oxyphil cells, inasmuch as a component of oxyphil cells can be found in many adenomas. When thus defined, most oxyphil adenomas are nonfunctioning; however, cases associated with hyperparathyroidism have been reported, with secretion of parathormone and proparathormone being documented ultrastructurally, immunohistochemically, and biochemically.[16,27,28,31] The main ultrastructural feature of these cells is the packing of the cytoplasm by mitochondria.[31]

Lipoadenoma is an unusual morphologic variant of parathyroid adenoma in which the glandular elements are associated with abundant mature adipose tissue (Fig. 10-7). This lesion also has been reported as parathyroid lipohyperplasia, parathyroid hamartoma, and parathyroid adenoma with myxoid stroma.[22,33,36] Most cases are functioning.[17,18,20]

CHIEF CELL HYPERPLASIA

Chief cell hyperplasia, a condition accompanied by increased production of parathormone, can be primary or secondary to impairment of renal function or chronic malabsorption.[48]

Primary chief cell hyperplasia is a constant finding in patients with multiple endocrine adenomatosis (MEA) types I and IIa. In contrast, patients with MEA type IIb (also known as type III) exhibit normal parathyroid histology during childhood and only a minimal degree of chief cell hyperplasia (consistent with absence of normal involution) during adulthood.[45]

In a *classic* case of primary chief cell hyperplasia, all glands are enlarged (up to 10 g or more) and have a tan to reddish color.[39,46] The superior glands tend to be larger than the inferior ones, but the difference is not as striking as with water-clear cell hyperplasia. In other instances, only one gland is visibly enlarged and nodular, whereas the others

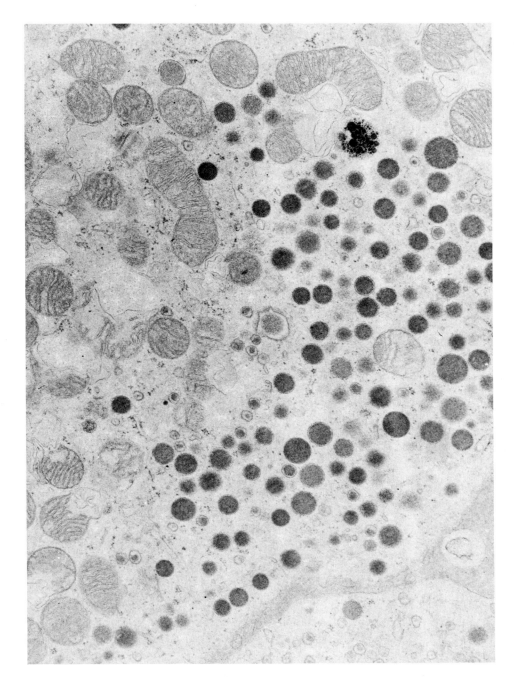

Fig. 10-6 Membrane-limited secretory granules are far more numerous in this cell from parathyroid adenoma than in normal chief cells. Granules vary in size depending on their stages of maturity. (Uranyl acetate; approximately ×12,000.)

are nearly normal in size. This latter variant can be confused grossly with an adenoma and is therefore referred to as *pseudoadenomatous*. In still other cases (designated as *occult*) all four glands appear normal in size to the surgeon but appear hyperplastic on histologic examination.[41]

Microscopically, the predominant element is the chief cell, but other cell types are also present in most instances. Those cells are often grouped in nodules, hence the alter-

native term *primary nodular hyperplasia*. This is particularly true in early lesions, in which they appear as small dispersed islands of hyperplastic tissue separated by intervening areas containing abundant fat[46] (Figs. 10-8 and 10-9). Fibrous septa, acinar formations, and cells with giant hyperchromatic nuclei may be present.[39] The ultrastructural features are qualitatively similar to those seen in adenoma and are indicative of a hyperfunctioning state. Their pres-

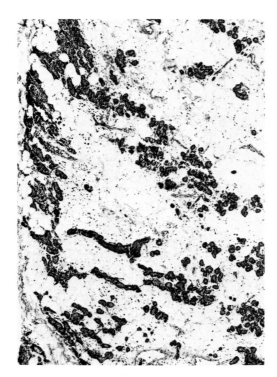

Fig. 10-7 Lipoadenoma of parathyroid gland. Elongated cords of parathyroid chief cells of normal cytologic appearance are widely separated by abundant mature adipose tissue.

ence may establish the hyperplastic state of a gland that is debatable by light microscopy.[40]

Exceptionally, innumerable microscopic foci of hyperplastic parathyroid tissue are found in the neck in association with primary chief cell hyperplasia of the four glands, in the absence of previous surgery.[50] This phenomenon, called *parathyromatosis*, may be responsible for some cases of recurrent hyperparathyroidism following adequate surgical therapy.

Another rare entity is that of chief cell hyperplasia associated with *chronic parathyroiditis*, interpreted as a possible parathyroid equivalent of Hashimoto's thyroiditis.[43]

In *secondary chief cell hyperplasia*, all gradations are seen. At one end is the normal-sized gland that is recognized as hyperplastic only because of its tan to reddish color and the microscopic replacement of adipose tissue by chief cells; at the other, there is the gland measuring up to 2 cm and weighing up to 6 g. In general, there is an inverse correlation between the size of the glands and the mean serum calcium level.[52] Chief cells predominate, but there may also be increased numbers of oxyphil and transitional oxyphil cells that form hyperplastic nodular collections.

The distinction between primary and secondary chief cell hyperplasia cannot be made on morphologic grounds with any certainty.[51,53] As a rule, nodularity, fibrous septation, acinar formation, and giant nuclei are more prominent in the primary form, whereas the number of oxyphil cells is higher in the secondary form. However, in the final analysis, the differential diagnosis is made on the basis of the historical, chemical, and laboratory findings.[39]

Another difficult and more pressing problem is the morphologic distinction between chief cell hyperplasia and ad-

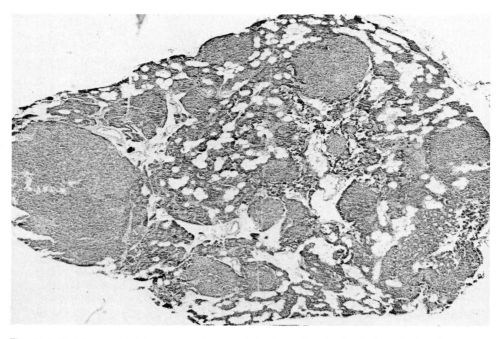

Fig. 10-8 Nodular chief cell hyperplasia in normal-sized parathyroid gland. Some fat is still present. This illustration demonstrates that parathyroid gland may not be enlarged but still, because of its cellular population, may be hyperplastic.

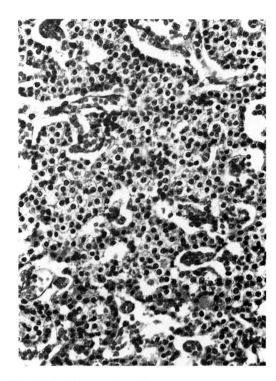

Fig. 10-9 Chief cell hyperplasia of parathyroid gland. Cells are uniform, have pale granular cytoplasm, and are supported by abundant vascular stroma. Adipose tissue is absent.

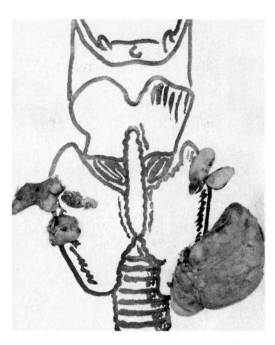

Fig. 10-10 Distribution of parathyroid tissue in water-clear cell hyperplasia in 48-year-old woman. Total weight of tissue removed was 125 g. Patient died 35 months after first operation, and equal amount of parathyroid tissue was again found. There was generalized diminished bone density and only mild hyperparathyroidism.

enoma. Size, shape, color, consistency, the cell types present and their relative frequency are of no help in this regard. The presence of a rim of normal parenchyma around the mass and the identification of at least a normal parathyroid gland are the only definite criteria by which a diagnosis of adenoma can be made over that of chief cell hyperplasia, but these criteria may be difficult to evaluate. It may well be, as Black and Utley[42] have suggested, that adenoma and chief cell hyperplasia merely represent different morphologic manifestations of the same process. This view is supported by a study in which four lesions classified morphologically as adenomas in patients heterozygous for G-6-P dehydrogenase were found to contain both A and B isoenzymes in proportions similar to those observed in normal tissues.[49]

Despite these observations, we believe that for practical reasons it is still worthwhile to distinguish adenomas from chief cell hyperplasias on morphologic grounds, using the criteria previously outlined. It remains to be seen whether special techniques such as DNA ploidy evaluation with flow cytometry[44] or determination of ABO(H) cell surface antigens[54] will allow a sharper distinction between these entities. Preliminary results with the former technique seem to indicate that this is not the case.[44]

WATER-CLEAR CELL HYPERPLASIA

In contrast to chief cell hyperplasia, water-clear cell hyperplasia shows no familial incidence and is not associated with multiple endocrine adenomatosis. It is characterized by extreme enlargement of all parathyroid tissue so that the total weight of the glands may exceed 100 g (Fig. 10-10).

Grossly, the superior glands are distinctly larger than the inferior. Moreover, glands may coalesce so that two glands appear as one. They are soft and have a typical chocolate brown color. Cysts and hemorrhages have been observed. Another common gross feature is the formation of pseudopods that may extend a considerable distance from the main mass of the gland.

Microscopically, the most characteristic feature is the presence of cells with optically clear cytoplasm throughout the lesion. These cells vary markedly in size, from some not larger than normal parathyroid cells to others that measure up to 40 μm (Fig. 10-11). Thus there is a combination of hyperplasia and hypertrophy. In most regions, the cytoplasm of the cell is water-clear, but in some cells small eosinophilic granules are present. High-power examination of thin sections reveals that the clarity of the cytoplasm is the result of a conglomerate of spherical clear vacuoles that are surrounded by thin portions of eosinophilic cytoplasmic material. This is confirmed by ultrastructural examination, which reveals numerous membrane-bound vacuoles, 0.2 to 2 μm in diameter, presumably derived from the Golgi apparatus.[58]

The nuclei average 6 to 7 μm and are basally oriented, a very distinctive feature. Although their size may vary, giant forms are not seen.

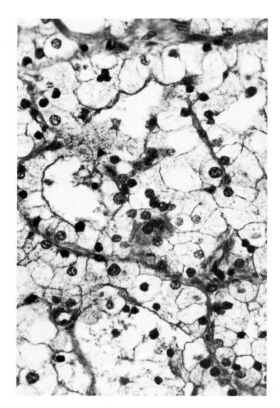

Fig. 10-11 Water-clear cell hyperplasia. Note increase in size and number of water-clear cells.

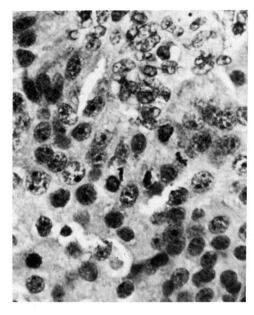

Fig. 10-12 Carcinoma of parathyroid gland in which nerve invasion and tumor thrombi occurred. Mitotic figures were numerous.

The pattern of growth may be alveolar (pseudoglandular) or compact. The connective tissue is delicate and sparse for the most part, but in some areas it may be dense. A chief cell component is occasionally present.

Water-clear cell hyperplasia results in primary hyperparathyroidism, a close correlation existing between the weight of the parathyroid tissue and the severity of the symptoms.[55] This disorder has all but disappeared in the past few decades; the reason for this phenomenon is unknown.[56] A case has been reported associated with a similar vacuolated clear cell appearance in the submaxillary gland.[57]

CARCINOMA

Parathyroid carcinoma typically presents with hyperparathyroidism; in one series, skeletal disease was present in 73% of the patients and renal disease in 26%.[64] A few convincing nonfunctioning cases are on record, and these are said to be more aggressive.[59,67,70] The absence of function may be caused by the lack of conversion of the preparathormone to the biologically active compound.[60] Parathyroid carcinoma may coexist with chief cell hyperplasia.[62,63] and with adenoma.[71]

Clinical features suggestive of parathyroid carcinoma in a hyperparathyroid patient include very high values of serum calcium, a palpable cervical mass, vocal cord paralysis, and recurrence of hyperparathyroidism a short time following surgery.[61,69,73] At operation, a parathyroid tumor should be

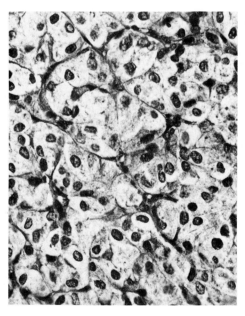

Fig. 10-13 Carcinoma of parathyroid gland. Note trabecular pattern. Lesion recurred after operation and invaded mediastinum widely.

suspected of being carcinoma if it is hard, surrounded by a dense fibrous reaction, and adherent to or infiltrating adjacent structures.

Microscopically, carcinomas differ from adenomas mainly because of a trabecular arrangement, dense fibrous bands (present in 90% of the cases), spindle shape of the tumor cells, presence of mitotic figures (in 81%), capsular invasion (in 6%), and blood vessel invasion (in 12%)[68] (Figs. 10-12 and 10-13). Some caveats are in order. A certain degree of fibrous banding can also occur in adenoma and in chief cell hyperplasia, particularly the primary form of the latter. Nests of tumor cells may be present within the capsule of a benign tumor. For tumor in a vein to be of significance, it must be attached to the wall. The presence of an occasional mitotic figure in a parathyroid lesion does not necessarily indicate that the lesion in question is a carcinoma. Snover and Foucar[72] found mitoses by exhaustive search in 71% of adenomas and 80% of the chief cell hyperplasias that they examined. Exceptionally, parathyroid carcinoma is composed of oxyphil cells.[65] If the parathyroid origin of the tumor is questionable—particularly in the absence of function—immunochemical demonstration of parathormone should be carried out.[66]

In a follow-up of forty-three patients with parathyroid carcinoma reported by Holmes et al.,[64] it was found that thirty (65%) of the patients were dead, five were living with persistent tumor, and eight were living without evidence of recurrent disease. Of thirty-nine patients studied by Shantz and Castleman,[68] 41% were alive and well, 13% were alive with disease, and 46% were dead of carcinoma. Local recurrence within the first 2 years after surgery was found to be an ominous prognostic sign.

OTHER LESIONS

Parathyroid cysts usually arise from the inferior glands but can be located in the upper region of the neck or the mediastinum.[74] In most cases, they cause no symptoms other than those related to pressure.[76] Their mean diameter is 4 cm.[74] They are lined by cuboidal or low columnar epithelial cells and contain parathyroid tissue in their wall.[77] The cyst fluid contains assayable parathormone.[79] The few reported cases of parathyroid cysts associated with hyperparathyroidism most likely represent adenomas with cystic degeneration.[78]

Amyloidosis often involves the parathyroid gland, both in primary and "reactive" forms of the disease.[75]

HYPERPARATHYROIDISM

The term *hyperparathyroidism* is applied to any condition associated with the persistent production of parathyroid hormone. It is divided into primary, secondary, and tertiary, according to the presumed mechanism of production.

Primary hyperparathyroidism

In primary hyperparathyroidism, there is no evidence of previous parathyroid stimulation by chronic renal or intestinal disease. The pathologic changes in the gland may be those of adenoma, chief cell hyperplasia, carcinoma, or water-clear cell hyperplasia. Carcinoma constitutes less than 4% of the cases, and water-clear cell hyperplasia has essentially disappeared; therefore, the large majority of cases are caused by either adenoma or chief cell hyperplasia. An interesting argument has developed over the years about the relative incidence of these two processes. Traditionally, adenoma had been regarded as the more frequent of the two. A series of articles written during the past 25 years[82,86,88,93,99] challenged that view and proposed that chief cell hyperplasia was actually the commonest pathologic change. In retrospect, it seems that these conclusions may have been influenced by the inclusion of many familial cases (which tend to show hyperplasia, see discussion following), by a perhaps liberal interpretation of minimal hyperplastic changes in the other glands, and possibly because chief cell hyperplasia and adenoma are truly interrelated and merging processes. Be that as it may, the pendulum is now back to its original position, i.e., with adenoma being held responsible for over 80% of the cases.[97]

Primary hyperparathyroidism is said to be present in 2.5 per 1,000 individuals. It is usually seen in adults but can also be found in children.[96] When seen in a familial setting, the abnormality is usually chief cell hyperplasia, although exceptions occur.[80,84] It may also be seen, again in a familial form, as a component of MEA types I or IIa[81,84] (see Chapter 15). In this syndrome the parathyroid change is practically always chief cell hyperplasia, perhaps humorally induced.[83] In MEA type IIa, it is not uncommon for the surgeon to find parathyroid chief cell hyperplasia and medullary carcinoma of the thyroid gland during the same exploration. In about 10% of the cases of sporadic primary hyperparathyroidism not associated with MEA, a nonmedullary thyroid carcinoma—usually of the papillary type—is found incidentally at operation.[90] Whether this represents more than a fortuitous association remains to be determined. An association between primary hyperparathyroidism and sarcoidosis also has been encountered.[101] Finally, a definite increase in the incidence of hyperparathyroidism following irradiation to the neck has been documented.[92,98]

The typical case of primary hyperparathyroidism is biochemically characterized by hypercalcemia, hypophosphatemia, lowering of the renal phosphate threshold, hypercalciuria, elevated levels of immunoreactive parathormone, elevated concentrations of 1,25-dihydroxyvitamin D, and enhanced excretion of nephrogenous cyclic AMP.[94] Another associated, albeit inconstant, chemical finding is elevation of serum alkaline phosphatase level. Although hypercalcemia has traditionally been one of the most constant biochemical markers of parathyroid hyperfunction, well-documented instances of normocalcemic primary hyperparathyroidism have been reported.[100] In a series on eighty-four patients with this variant, parathyroid adenomas were found in nineteen, chief cell hyperplasia in thirty-nine, and normal parathyroid glands in twenty-six; no morphologic differences were detected between patients in this group and patients with primary hyperparathyroidism associated with hypercalcemia.[87]

According to the clinical presentation, patients with primary hyperparathyroidism may be classified into (1) those with osseous manifestations, (2) those with renal manifestations, and (3) those with neither of the foregoing. With

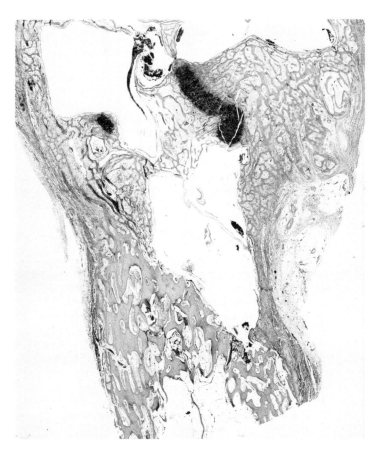

Fig. 10-14 Osteitis fibrosa cystica. Note bone production and destruction with cyst formation. Dark areas represent hemorrhage and giant cell formation (brown tumor).

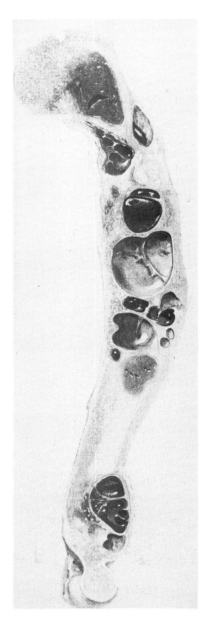

Fig. 10-15 Extreme osteitis fibrosa cystica. Note deformity of bone with numerous cysts and brown tumors. (From Hunter D, Turnbull HN: Hyperparathyroidism. Generalized osteitis fibrosa, with observations upon bones, parathyroid tumours, and normal parathyroid glands. Br J Surg **19**:203-284, 1931.)

the routine use of the serum analyzer in most hospital centers, there has been a sharp increase in the incidence of the latter group, sometimes referred to as "occult."[88]

The *skeletal changes* of hyperparathyroidism are always generalized, although they may appear localized clinically or radiographically. The initial lesions show merely a decrease in bone density. In time, they may become very extensive and lead to deformities and fractures. The full-blown osseous manifestations of hyperparathyroidism have been traditionally known as Recklinghausen's disease (not to be confused with neurofibromatosis, which also carries this eponym) (Figs. 10-14, 10-15, and 10-16). The seemingly localized lesions are those more likely to be misinterpreted. They present radiographically as expansile, multilocular masses. The jaw is the preferred location, and this may be the first clinical manifestation of the disease. Grossly, there is an alternation of solid and cystic areas; the latter often have a brown color because of the accumulation of abundant hemosiderin, hence the term *brown tumor* sometimes used for them. Microscopically, there is a combination of osteoblastic and osteoclastic activity, often associated with cyst formation and clusters of hemosiderin-laden macrophages. It is this combination of findings that should suggest the diagnosis.

The differential diagnosis with central giant cell reparative granulomas may be impossible on morphologic grounds because both lesions have a predilection for the jaw, and their microscopic appearances are essentially the same; therefore the distinction is based on the laboratory findings. The other differential diagnosis is with giant cell tumor, with which brown tumor has often been confused in the past. In giant cell tumor, the osteoclasts are more evenly spaced, the stromal cells are plumper, and osteoblastic activity is less conspicuous.

Removal of the hyperfunctioning gland is usually followed by a spectacular reversal of the bone changes, sometimes in a remarkably short time (Figs. 10-17 and 10-18); however, some of the cystic lesions may persist indefinitely (Fig. 10-19).

The *renal changes* of primary hyperparathyroidism include renal stones, nephrocalcinosis, polyuria, polydipsia, and impairment of renal function. It is now recognized that renal stones are the most common clinical manifestation of hyperparathyroidism.[95] These renal lesions are frequently associated with hypertension and are the most important cause of death. In contrast to the skeletal changes, the renal abnormalities may still progress following the removal of the parathyroid lesion.

Other manifestations of hyperparathyroidism include hypertension, peptic ulcer, acute and chronic pancreatitis, and mental disturbances. The peptic ulcer is usually in the duodenum and is more common in males[89]; it often heals following removal of the hyperfunctioning gland. Dent et al.[85] found elevated levels of plasma gastrin in ten of twenty patients with hyperparathyroidism without achlorhydria. These levels fell after removal of the diseased parathyroid, together with the serum calcium and the parathyroid hormone concentration.

Rarely, acute gastrointestinal, cardiovascular, or central nervous system symptoms develop because of very high serum calcium levels. This condition, designated as *parathyroid crisis*, is fatal unless the offending gland or glands are rapidly excised.[91]

Secondary hyperparathyroidism

Secondary hyperparathyroidism occurs as a consequence of chronic renal disease or intestinal malabsorption, usually the former. The renal insufficiency leads to elevation of the serum phosphorus level and reciprocal decrease of serum calcium concentrations, with the resulting stimulation of the parathyroid glands.[102] Vitamin D resistance is a characteristic feature of advanced renal disease and also may play a role by contributing to a reduction in serum calcium con-

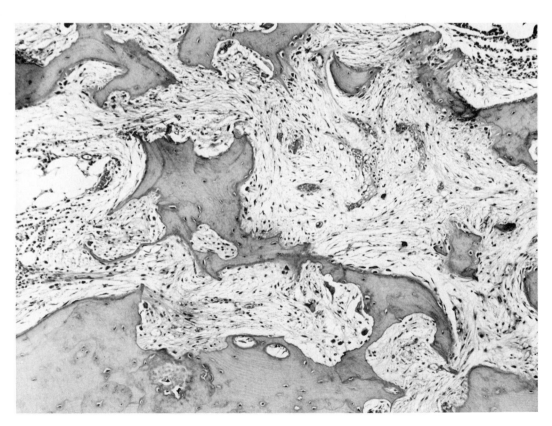

Fig. 10-16 Bone changes in hyperparathyroidism. There is marrow fibrosis, extreme osteoclastic resorption, and some bone production. Patient had extensive bone disease with normal renal function.

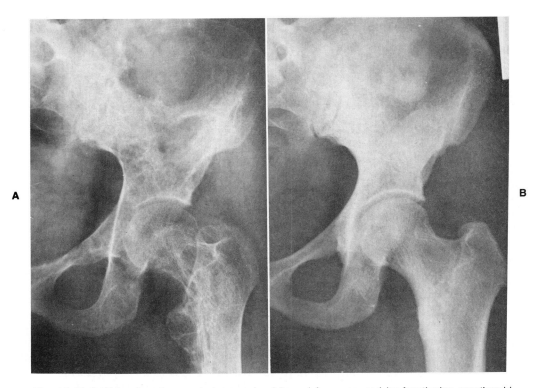

Fig. 10-17 A, Extensive changes in bones of pelvis and femur caused by functioning parathyroid adenoma. **B,** Same pelvis and femur 8 years following removal of adenoma. Note complete reversion to normal. (**A** and **B,** from Black BK, Ackerman LV: Tumors of the parathyroid. A review of twenty-three cases. Cancer **3:**415-444, 1950.)

centrations.[103] Radioimmunoassay determinations of circulating parathormone levels have shown these to be roughly proportional to the severity of renal failure. It also has been found that these levels are higher in renal failure than in any form of primary hyperparathyroidism.[105]

The parathyroid abnormality in secondary hyperparathyroidism is *chief cell hyperplasia.* The bone changes are similar to those seen in primary hyperparathyroidism. They are usually milder in degree, but sometimes extensive changes with cyst formation occur.[104]

"Tertiary" hyperparathyroidism

The term *"tertiary" hyperparathyroidism* is applied to patients with hyperparathyroidism secondary to chronic renal disease or intestinal malabsorption, in whom one or more of the stimulated parathyroid glands seem to become autonomous.[108] Most cases have been detected after correction of the renal disease by hemodialysis or homotransplantation.[111] The existence of such an entity is still debated. Follow-up studies seem to indicate that if enough time is given, the parathyroid glands will revert to a normal state in the large majority of cases.[107,109] In some cases, the microscopic appearance of these "nonsuppressable" or "autonomous" parathyroid glands is that of chief cell hyperplasia and is not substantially different from that seen in the usual "suppressible" or "responsive" form of secondary hyperparathyroidism,[110] but in others a well-defined nodule

with an adenomatous appearance is seen superimposed on the diffuse hyperplastic lesion. In rare cases, this nodule is entirely composed of oxyphil cells[112]; even in cases with diffuse hyperplastic changes, morphometric studies have suggested that the nuclear size is larger than that of secondary hyperplasia and approaching that seen in adenomas.[106]

Differential diagnosis

Primary hyperparathyroidism needs to be distinguished clinically from a relatively large number of conditions associated with hypercalcemia, such as sarcoidosis, hyperthyroidism, multiple myeloma, milk-alkali syndrome, vitamin D and vitamin A intoxication, and the condition known as *familial hypercalcemic hypocalciuria*.[114,116] The latter should be suspected in young patients presenting with a presumptive diagnosis of hyperparathyroidism, especially if there is a family history. The determination of the calcium : creatinine clearance ratio is the most useful test for the identification of this disorder. Microscopically, the parathyroid glands may appear normal or exhibit a mild degree of chief cell hyperplasia, sometimes with a prominent clear cell component.[120]

Nonparathyroid tumors may induce hypercalcemia by producing widespread metastases in the skeletal system. In addition, symptoms and signs suggestive of hyperparathyroidism may be seen in malignant tumors of nonparathyroid

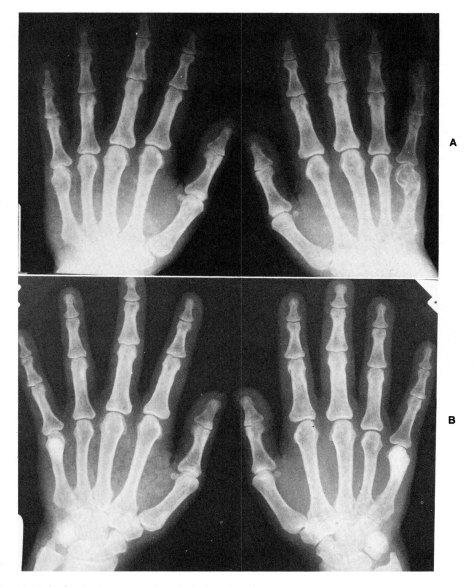

Fig. 10-18 A, Cystic changes and cortical alterations in bones of hands of patient with functioning parathyroid adenoma. **B,** Dramatic change evident 9 months after removal of adenoma.

origin in the absence of significant osseous metastases. Omenn et al.[117] have reviewed seventy-three cases of this condition, sometimes known as pseudohyperparathyroidism. Renal cell carcinoma and epidermoid carcinoma of the lung account for 60% of the cases.[115] The parathyroid glands appear morphologically normal or perhaps minimally hyperplastic,[113,118] but the serum biochemical parameters clearly indicate a state of suppressed parathyroid function. The mechanism for the hypercalcemia is not clear and may differ among the various tumor types. Some of the postulated factors include parathormone or a parathormone-like substance, a parathyrotrophic factor, vitamin D metabolites, prostaglandins, osteoclast-activating factor, and cyclic AMP-stimulating factor.[114a,116a,118,119]

Therapy

The surgeon embarking on the therapy of hyperparathyroidism should have a thorough knowledge of parathyroid physiology and of the variations in the appearance and anatomic locations of the parathyroid glands[145,146,148] and the tumors arising from them. Wang[145] reoperated on 112 patients for persistent hyperparathyroidism following surgery. In cervical re-explorations the missing glands were most frequently found in the posterosuperior portion of mediastinum at the thoracic inlet (38%); in mediastinal re-explorations, they were found in the anteroposterior portion of the mediastinum (67%). He estimated that the reasons for the initial unsuccessful surgery were (1) lack of knowledge by the surgeon of the normal location of the glands

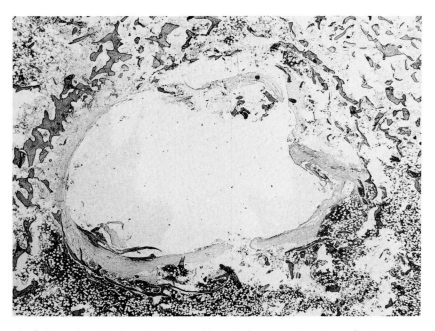

Fig. 10-19 Failure of repair of cystic lesions of bone in hyperparathyroidism. Section was made 23 months after removal of functioning parathyroid adenoma. This man, who died of renal insufficiency, was the first patient in whom a functioning adenoma of parathyroid gland was successfully diagnosed and surgically treated (1928). (Reported by Barr DP, Bulger HA: Clinical syndromes of hyperparathyroidism. Am J Med Sci **179:**449-476, 1930.)

and the way they may be displaced when diseased, (2) misdiagnosis of cases of chief cell hyperplasia as adenomas, resulting in insufficient surgery, and (3) technical incompetence.

Several techniques have been used to localize the abnormal gland preoperatively. These include ultrasonography, CT scan, radioactive scan, and selective venous catheterization, the latter being the most sensitive.[124] These techniques have been found to be particularly useful in cases of recurrent hyperparathyroidism.

Surgical identification of *all four* parathyroid glands remains the most popular approach, although dissenting voices exist.[144] If a thorough examination of the neck reveals only three normal parathyroid glands, some authors advocate the performance of a hemithyroidectomy on the side of the missing gland, since 2% of all adenomas are found in this location.[132] If this also proves negative, sternotomy and mediastinal exploration should be considered 2 or 3 weeks later. The majority of the mediastinal parathyroid adenomas can be removed from the neck, through a low collar thyroid incision.[135,140] If all four identified glands appear normal, the possibility should be considered of an abnormal fifth (supernumerary) gland being present, whether in the neck or—more commonly—in the mediastinum.[141] Roth et al.[138] devised a flow sheet that should be very helpful to the surgeon who undertakes surgery for primary hyperparathyroidism as well as to the pathologist who will assist him. We agree with their recommendations, except that we are in favor of an exploration of the second side of the neck even if an abnormal gland has been found on one side.

Adenomas are adequately treated by local excision of the tumor.[139] It is imperative *to excise or biopsy at least one other parathyroid gland* in order to rule out the possibility of chief cell hyperplasia.

Primary chief cell hyperplasia and the exceptionally rare water-clear cell hyperplasia are conventionally treated by subtotal parathyroidectomy, i.e., total excision of three glands and partial excision of the fourth, leaving 30 to 50 mg of viable tissue.[147]

Some surgeons have recommended the performance of the latter procedure as the routine treatment for primary hyperparathyroidism regardless of the underlying abnormality, in view of the difficulty that sometimes exists in distinguishing chief cell hyperplasia from adenoma.[136,137] We do not subscribe to this extreme form of treatment, not only because of the increased risk of hypoparathyroidism, but also because it represents unnecessarily radical surgery in the majority of the cases. Many large recent series document the fact that the patient with a *single* enlarged parathyroid gland is adequately treated by removal of that gland plus an additional one for diagnostic purposes. This procedure is nearly 100% effective if the enlarged gland is the harbinger of an adenoma and is also effective in a good number of cases on a long-term basis if the patient has a "pseudoadenomatous" form of chief cell hyperplasia *as long as the other glands are identified and are found to be normal in size.* The reason seems to be that even if the other glands have microscopic chief cell hyperplasia, the degree of this hyperplasia is such as to be of functional insignificance in the large majority of the cases.[121,122,126,128] In other words, the *amount* of abnormal parathyroid tissue removed and left in place seems to represent the most important prognostic determinator.

A novel and somewhat controversial approach to the treatment of chief cell hyperplasia has been the performance of total parathyroidectomy with autotransplantation of parathyroid tissue into the forearm muscle.[142,149]

Parathyroid carcinoma is best treated by excision of the tumor and surrounding soft tissues and removal of the ipsilateral thyroid lobe; the indication for ipsilateral node dissection remains controversial.[125,134] Surgical resection of isolated metastases is justified because of its marked palliative effect.[129]

The large majority of patients with secondary and "tertiary" hyperparathyroidism respond well to medical treatment[123,131]; however, if bone lesions are severe and if the hypercalcemia is excessive, subtotal parathyroidectomy may become necessary.[103]

It is not clear whether asymptomatic individuals who are found to have mild hypercalcemia (less than 11 mg%) on routine screening should be operated upon.[127,130,133] A group of such patients was followed on a long-term basis to determine their outcome. At the end of a 10-year period, 26% of the patients had had surgery because of increased serum calcium levels, decreased renal function, renal stones, psychologic considerations, or bone disease; the authors were unable to define criteria that would predict which patients with asymptomatic hyperparathyroidism would eventually require surgery.[143]

Frozen section

The main role of the pathologist at the time of surgery, as pedestrian as this may sound, is to determine by frozen section whether a given nodule is, in reality, parathyroid tissue.[163] Nodules of thyroid gland, small lymph nodes, aberrant thymic tissue, and even fat may be mistaken grossly for parathyroid tissue. This determination can also be made in imprints stained with polychrome methylene blue, a technique which saves considerable surgical time.[156,164]

As far as the pathologist providing a specific diagnosis is concerned, most cases of carcinoma and water-clear cell hyperplasia should be identifiable by frozen section, particularly if the carcinoma has invaded local tissues; however, this comprises a very small proportion of cases. The two most common—and unfortunately most difficult—situations faced by the pathologist are to decide whether a gland is normal or abnormal and, if abnormal, whether it is involved by chief cell hyperplasia or adenoma. The differential features between the two latter entities have already been discussed on p. 455. Suffice it to say that if the pathologist is given a single gland, such a distinction will be impossible in most instances. In regard to the decision about whether a small gland is normal or hyperplastic, estimation of the amount of stromal fat has been used, but the value of this estimate is very limited.[151,155,157,162] Some residual fat can be present in hyperplastic glands; conversely, parathyroid glands of young patients may have a very small amount. Furthermore, the distribution of stromal fat varies considerably from area to area; therefore, the validity of a subjective evaluation of a few microscopic sections can be seriously questioned, as studies using image-analyzing computer techniques have shown.[158]

Presence of distinct nodularity and/or more than occasional acinar formations are features favoring a diagnosis of hyperplasia.[150] Performance of stains for lipid (such as Sudan IV, Oil red O, or osmium carmine) have been recommended, the rationale being that the chief cells of a normal or suppressed gland have cytoplasmic lipid droplets, whereas those of adenoma or chief cell hyperplasia do not.[152,154,159,161] Although there is an undeniable inverse relationship between functional activity and fat content, the number of discordant results is high enough to call for caution in its interpretation.[153,160]

REFERENCES
GROSS ANATOMY AND EMBRYOLOGY

1 Akerström G, Malmacus J, Bergström R: Surgical anatomy of human parathyroid glands. Surgery **95**:14-21, 1984.
2 Gilmour JR, Martin WJ: The weight of the parathyroid glands. J Pathol Bacteriol **44**:431-462, 1937.
3 Herrold KM, Rabson AS, Ketcham AS: Aberrant parathyroid gland in pharyngeal submucosa. Arch Pathol **73**:60-62, 1962.
4 Wang C: The anatomic basis of parathyroid surgery. Ann Surg **183**:271-275, 1976.

HISTOLOGY

5 Boquist L: Follicles in human parathyroid glands. Lab Invest **28**:313-320, 1973.
6 Gilmour JR: The parathyroid glands and skeleton in renal diseases. London, 1947, Oxford University Press.
7 Lieberman A, DeLellis RA: Intrafollicular amyloid in normal parathyroid glands. Arch Pathol **95**:422-423, 1973.
8 Miettinen M, Clark R, Lehto V-P, Virtanen I, Damjanov I: Intermediate-filament proteins in parathyroid glands and parathyroid adenomas. Arch Pathol Lab Med **109**:986-989, 1985.
9 Ordoñez NG, Ibañez ML, Samaan NA, Hickey RC: Immunoperoxidase study of uncommon parathyroid tumors. Report of two cases of nonfunctioning parathyroid carcinoma and one intrathyroid parathyroid tumor–producing amyloid. Am J Surg Pathol **7**:535-542, 1983.
10 Roth SI, Capen CC: Ultrastructural and functional correlations of the parathyroid gland. Int Rev Exp Pathol **13**:161-221, 1974.

PHYSIOLOGY

11 Chase LR, Aurbach GD: Parathyroid function and the renal excretion of 3'5'-adenylic acid. Proc Natl Acad Sci USA **58**:518-525, 1967.
12 Habener JF, Rosenblatt M, Potts JT Jr: Parathyroid hormones. Biochemical aspects of biosynthesis, secretion, action, and metabolism. Physiol Rev **64**:985-1053, 1984.
13 Martin KJ, Hruska KA, Freitag JJ, Klahr S, Slatopolsky E: The peripheral metabolism of parathyroid hormone. N Engl J Med **301**:1092-1098, 1979.
14 Roth SI, Raisz LG: The course and reversibility of the calcium effect on the ultrastructure of the rat parathyroid gland in organ culture. Lab Invest **15**:1187-1211, 1966.

ADENOMA

15 Aguilar-Parada E, Gonzalez-Angulo A, Del Peon L, Mravko E: Functioning microvillous adenoma of the parathyroid gland containing nuclear pores and annulate lamellae. Hum Pathol **16**:511-516, 1985.
16 Bedetti CD, Dekker A, Watson CG: Functioning oxyphil cell adenoma of the parathyroid gland. A clinicopathologic study of ten patients with hyperparathyroidism. Hum Pathol **15**:1121-1126, 1984.
16a Bostwick DG, Null WE, Holmes D, Weber E, Barchas JD, Bensch KG: Expression of opioid peptides in tumors. N Engl J Med **317**:1439-1443, 1987.
17 Daroca PJ Jr, Landau RL, Reed RJ, Kappelman MD: Functioning lipoadenoma of the parathyroid gland. Arch Pathol Lab Med **101**:28-30, 1977.
18 Ducatman BS, Wilkerson SY, Brown JA: Functioning parathyroid lipoadenoma. Report of a case diagnosed by intraoperative touch preparations. Arch Pathol Lab Med **110**:645-647, 1986.
19 Faccini JM: The ultrastructure of parathyroid glands removed from patients with primary hyperparathyroidism. A report of 40 cases, including four carcinomata. J Pathol **102**:189-199, 1970.
20 Geelhoed GW: Parathyroid adenolipoma. Clinical and morphologic features. Surgery **92**:806-810, 1982.
21 Leedham PW, Pollock DJ: Intrafollicular amyloid in primary hyperparathyroidism. J Clin Pathol **23**:811-818, 1970.

22 Legolvan DP, Moore BP, Nishiyama RH: Parathyroid hamartoma. Report of two cases and review of the literature. Am J Clin Pathol **67**:31-35, 1977.

23 Liechty RD, Teter A, Suba EJ: The tiny parathyroid adenoma. Surgery **100**:1048-1052, 1986.

24 Miettinen M, Clark R, Lehto V-P, Virtanen I, Damjanov I: Intermediate-filament proteins in parathyroid glands and parathyroid adenomas. Arch Pathol Lab Med **109**:986-989, 1985.

25 Nolan RB, Hayles AB, Woolner LB: Adenoma of the parathyroid gland in children. Report of case and brief review of the literature. Am J Dis Child **99**:622-627, 1960.

26 Norris EH: Parathyroid adenoma. Study of 322 cases. Int Abstr Surg **84**:1-41, 1947; in Surg Gynecol Obstet, Jan. 1947.

27 Ordoñez NG, Ibañez ML, Mackay B, Samaan NA, Hickey RC: Functioning oxyphil cell adenomas of parathyroid gland. Immunoperoxidase evidence of hormonal activity in oxyphil cells. Am J Clin Pathol **78**:681-689, 1982.

28 Poole GV, Albertson DA, Marshall RB, Myers RT: Oxyphil cell adenoma and hyperparathyroidism. Surgery **92**:799-805, 1982.

29 Rasbach DA, Monchik JM, Geelhoed GW, Harrison TS: Solitary parathyroid microadenoma. Surgery **96**:1092-1098, 1984.

29a Sahin A, Robinson RA: Papillae formation in parathyroid adenoma. A source of possible diagnositc error. Arch Pathol Med **112**:99-100, 1988.

30 Schachner SH, Hall A: Parathyroid adenoma and previous head-and-neck irradiation. Ann Intern Med **88**:804, 1978.

31 Selzman HM, Fechner RE: Oxyphil adenoma and primary hyperparathyroidism. Clinical and ultrastructural observations. JAMA **199**:359-361, 1967.

32 Sloane JA, Moody HC: Parathyroid adenoma in submucosa of esophagus. Arch Pathol Lab Med **102**:242-243, 1978.

33 Straus FH II, Kaplan EL, Nishiyama RH, Bigos ST: Five cases of parathyroid lipohyperplasia. Surgery **94**:901-905, 1983.

34 Verdonk CA, Edis AJ: Parathyroid "double adenomas." Fact or fiction? Surgery **90**:523-526, 1981.

35 Weber CJ, Marangos PJ, Richardson S, LoGerfo P, Hardy MA, Feind C, Reemtsma K: Presence of neuron-specific enolase and somatostatin in human parathyroid tissues. Surgery **98**:1008-1012, 1985.

36 Weiland LH, Garrison RC, ReMine WH, Scholz DA: Lipoadenoma of the parathyroid gland. Am J Surg Pathol **2**:3-7, 1978.

37 Woolner LB, Keating FR Jr, Black BM: Tumors and hyperplasia of the parathyroid glands. A review of the pathological findings in 140 cases of primary hyperparathyroidism. Cancer **5**:1069-1088, 1952.

38 Wyman SM, Robbins LL: Roentgen recognition of parathyroid adenoma. Am J Roentgenol Radium Ther Nucl Med **71**:777-784, 1954.

CHIEF CELL HYPERPLASIA

39 Adams PH, Chalmers TM, Peters N, Rack JH, Truscott B McN: Primary chief cell hyperplasia of the parathyroid glands. Ann Intern Med **63**:454-467, 1965.

40 Black WC III: Correlative light and electron microscopy in primary hyperparathyroidism. Arch Pathol **88**:225-241, 1969.

41 Black WC III, Haff RC: The surgical pathology of parathyroid chief cell hyperplasia. Am J Clin Pathol **53**:565-579, 1970.

42 Black WC III, Utley JR: The differential diagnosis of parathyroid adenoma and chief cell hyperplasia. Am J Clin Pathol **49**:761-775, 1968.

43 Bondeson A-G, Bondeson L, Ljungberg O: Chronic parathyroiditis associated with parathyroid hyperplasia and hyperparathyroidism. Am J Surg Pathol **8**:211-215, 1984.

44 Bowlby LS, DeBault LE, Abraham SR: Flow cytometric DNA analysis of parathyroid glands. Relationship between nuclear DNA and pathologic classifications. Am J Pathol **128**:338-344, 1987.

45 Carney JA, Roth SI, Heath H III, Sizemore GW, Hayles AB: The parathyroid glands in multiple endocrine neoplasia type 2b. Am J Pathol **99**:387-398, 1980.

46 Castleman B, Schantz A, Roth SI: Parathyroid hyperplasia in primary hyperparathyroidism. A review of 85 cases. Cancer **38**:1668-1675, 1976.

47 Cope, O: Hyperparathyroidism. Diagnosis and management. Am J Surg **99**:394-403, 1960.

48 Cope O, Keynes WM, Roth SI, Castleman B: Primary chief-cell hyperplasia of the parathyroid glands. A new entity in the surgery of hyperparathyroidism. Ann Surg **148**:375-388, 1958.

49 Fialkow PJ, Jackson CE, Block MA, Greenawald KA: Multicellular origin of parathyroid "adenomas." N Engl J Med **297**:696-698, 1977.

50 Reddick RL, Costa JC, Marx SJ: Parathyroid hyperplasia and parathyromatosis [letter]. Lancet **1**:549, 1977.

51 Roth SI: Pathology of the parathyroids in hyperparathyroidism. Arch Pathol **73**:495-510, 1962.

52 Roth SI, Marshall RB: Pathology and ultrastructure of the human parathyroid glands in chronic renal failure. Arch Intern Med **124**:397-407, 1969.

53 Roth SI, Munger BL: The cytology of the adenomatous, atrophic, and hyperplastic parathyroid glands of man. A light- and electron-microscopic study, Virchows Arch [Pathol Anat] **335**:389-410, 1962.

54 Wolfering EA, Emmott RC, Javadpour N, Marx SJ, Brennan MF: ABO(H) cell surface antigens in parathyroid adenoma and hyperplasia. Surgery **90**:1-9, 1981.

WATER-CLEAR CELL HYPERPLASIA

55 Albright F, Sulkowitch HW, Bloomberg E: Hyperparathyroidism due to idiopathic hypertrophy (hyperplasia?) of parathyroid tissue. Follow-up report of 6 cases. Arch Intern Med **62**:199-215, 1938.

56 Castleman B, Schantz A, Roth SI: Parathyroid hyperplasia in primary hyperparathyroidism. A review of 85 cases. Cancer **38**:1668-1675, 1976.

57 Dorado AE, Hensley G, Castleman B: Water clear cell hyperplasia of parathyroid. Autopsy report of a case with supernumerary glands. Cancer **38**:1676-1683, 1976.

58 Roth SI: The ultrastructure of primary water-clear cell hyperplasia of the parathyroid glands. Am J Pathol **61**:233-240, 1970.

CARCINOMA

59 Aldinger KA, Hickey RC, Ibanez ML, Samaan NA: Parathyroid carcinoma. A clinical study of seven cases of functioning and two cases of nonfunctioning parathyroid cancer. Cancer **49**:388-397, 1982.

60 Baba H, Kishihara M, Tohmon M, Fukase M, Kizaki T, Okada S, Matsuzuka F, Kobayashi A, Kuma K, Fujita T: Identification of parathyroid hormone messenger ribonucleic acid in an apparently nonfunctioning parathyroid carcinoma transformed from a parathyroid carcinoma with hyperparathyroidism. J Clin Endocrinol Metab **62**:247-252, 1986.

61 Cohn K, Silverman M, Corrado J, Sedgewick C: Parathyroid carcinoma. The Lahey Clinic experience. Surgery **98**:1095-1100, 1985.

62 Dinnen JS, Greenwood RH, Jones JH, Walker DA, Williams ED: Parathyroid carcinoma in familial hyperparathyroidism. J Clin Pathol **30**:966-975, 1977.

63 Haghighi P, Astarita RW, Wepsic T, Wolf PL: Concurrent primary parathyroid hyperplasia and parathyroid carcinoma. Arch Pathol Lab Med **107**:349-350, 1983.

64 Holmes EC, Morton DL, Ketcham AS: Parathyroid carcinoma. A collective review. Ann Surg **169**:631-640, 1969.

65 Obara T, Fujimoto Y, Yamaguchi K, Takanashi R, Kino I, Sasaki Y: Parathyroid carcinoma of the oxyphil cell type. A report of two cases, light and electron microscopic study. Cancer **55**:1482-1489, 1985.

66 Ordóñez NG, Ibañez ML, Samaan NA, Hickey RC: Immunoperoxidase study of uncommon parathyroid tumors. Report of two cases of nonfunctioning parathyroid carcinoma and one intrathyroid parathyroid tumor-producing amyloid. Am J Surg Pathol **7**:535-542, 1983.

67 Pachter MR, Lattes R: Uncommon mediastinal tumors. Report of two parathyroid adenomas, one nonfunctional parathyroid carcinoma and one "bronchial-type-adenoma." Dis Chest **43**:519-528, 1963.

68 Schantz A, Castleman B: Parathyroid carcinoma. Cancer **31**:600-605, 1973.

69 Shane E, Bilezikian JP: Parathyroid carcinoma. A review of 62 patients. Endocr Rev **3**:218-226, 1982.

70 Sieracki JC, Horn RC Jr: Nonfunctional carcinoma of the parathyroid. Cancer **13**:502-506, 1960.

71 Smith JF, Coombs RRH: Histological diagnosis of carcinoma of the parathyroid gland. J Clin Pathol **37**:1370-1378, 1984.

72 Snover DC, Foucar K: Mitotic activity in benign parathyroid disease. Am J Clin Pathol **75**:345-347, 1981.

73 van Heerden JA, Weiland LH, ReMine H, Walls JT, Purnell DC: Cancer of the parathyroid glands. Arch Surg **114**:475-480, 1979.

OTHER LESIONS

74 Calandra DB, Shah KH, Prinz RA, Sullivan H, Hofmann C, Oslapas R, Ernst K, Lawrence AM, Paloyan E: Parathyroid cysts. A report of eleven cases including two associated with hyperparathyroid crisis. Surgery **94**:887-892, 1984.

75 Ellis HA, Mawhinney WHB: Parathyroid amyloidosis. Arch Pathol Lab Med **108**:689-690, 1984.

76 Gordon A, Harcourt-Webster JN: Parathyroid cysts. A report of two cases. J Pathol Bacteriol **89**:374-377, 1965.

77 Maxwell DB, Horn RC Jr, Rhoads JE: Cysts of the parathyroid. Report of three cases clinically simulating nodular goiter. Arch Surg **64**:208-213, 1952.

78 Rogers LA, Fetter BF, Peete WPJ: Parathyroid cyst and cystic degeneration of parathyroid adenoma. Arch Pathol **88**:476-479, 1969.

79 Silverman JF, Khazanie PG, Norris HT, Fore WW: Parathyroid hormone (PTH) assay of parathyroid cysts examined by fine-needle aspiration biopsy. Am J Clin Pathol **86**:776-780, 1986.

HYPERPARATHYROIDISM
Primary hyperparathyroidism

80 Allo M, Thompson NW: Familial hyperparathyroidism caused by solitary adenomas. Surgery **92**:486-490, 1982.

81 Ballard HS, Frame B, Hartsock RJ: Familial multiple endocrine adenoma-peptic ulcer complex. Medicine [Baltimore] **43**:481-516, 1964.

82 Black WC III, Utley JR: The differential diagnosis of parathyroid adenoma and chief cell hyperplasia. Am J Clin Pathol **49**:761-775, 1968.

83 Brandi ML, Aurbach GD, Fitzpatrick LA, Quarto R, Spiegel AM, Bliziotes MM, Norton JA, Doppman JL, Marx SJ: Parathyroid mitogenic activity in plasma from patients with familial multiple endocrine neoplasia type 1. N Engl J Med **314**:1287-1293, 1986.

84 Cutler RE, Reiss E, Ackerman LV: Familial hyperparathyroidism. A kindred involving eleven cases with a discussion of primary chief cell hyperplasia. N Engl J Med **270**:859-865, 1964.

85 Dent RI, James HJ, Wang C, Deftos LJ, Talamo R, Fischer JE: Hyperparathyroidism. Gastric acid secretion and gastrin. Ann Surg **176**:360-369, 1972.

86 Ghandur-Mnaymneh L, Kimura N: The parathyroid adenoma. A histopathologic definition with a study of 172 cases of primary hyperparathyroidism. Am J Pathol **115**:70-83, 1984.

87 Grimelius L, Ejerblad S, Johansson H, Werner I: Parathyroid adenomas and glands in normocalcemic hyperparathyroidism. A light microscopic study. Am J Pathol **83**:475-484, 1976.

88 Haff RC, Black WC III, Ballinger WF II: Primary hyperparathyroidism. Changing clinical, surgical and pathological aspects. Ann Surg **171**:85-92, 1970.

89 Hellström J, Ivemark BI: Primary hyperparathyroidism. Clinical and structural findings in 138 cases. Acta Chir Scand **294**[Suppl]:1-113, 1962.

90 LiVolsi VA, Feind CR: Parathyroid adenoma and nonmedullary thyroid carcinoma. Cancer **38**:1391-1393, 1976.

91 MacLeod WAJ, Holloway CK: Hyperparathyroid crisis. A collective review. Ann Surg **166**:1012-1015, 1967.

92 Netelenbos C, Lips P, Van Der Meer C: Hyperparathyroidism following irradiation of benign diseases of the head and neck. Cancer **52**:458-461, 1983.

93 Paloyan E, Lawrence AM: The rationale for subtotal parathyroidectomy. In Varco RL, Delaney JP (eds): Controversy in surgery. Philadelphia, 1976, W.B. Saunders Co.

94 Potts JT Jr, Murray TM, Peacock M, Niall HD, Tregear GW, Keutmann HT, Powell D, Deftos LJ: Parathyroid hormone. Sequence, synthesis, immunoassay studies. Am J Med **50**:639-649, 1971.

95 Pyrah LN, Hodgkinson A, Anderson CK: Critical review. Primary hyperparathyroidism. Br J Surg **53**:245-316, 1966.

96 Rapaport D, Ziv Y, Rubin M, Huminer D, Dintsman M: Primary hyperparathyroidism in children. J Pediatr Surg **21**:395-397, 1986.

97 Smith JF, Coombs RRH: Histological diagnosis of carcinoma of the parathyroid gland. J Clin Pathol **37**:1370-1378, 1984.

98 Tisell L-E, Carlsson S, Fjalling M, Hansson G, Lindberg S, Lundberg L-M, Oden A: Hyperparathyroidism subsequent to neck irradiation. Risk factors. Cancer **56**:1529-1533, 1985.

99 Utley JR III, Black WC III: Hyperparathyroidism. A clinicopathologic evaluation. Am J Surg **114**:788-795, 1967.

100 Wills MR: Normocalcaemic primary hyperparathyroidism. Lancet **1**:849-853, 1971.

101 Winnacker JL, Becker KL, Friedlander M, Higgins GA Jr, Moore CF: Sarcoidosis and hyperparathyroidism. Am J Med **46**:305-312, 1969.

Secondary hyperparathyroidism

102 Breslau NA: Update on secondary forms of hyperparathyroidism. Am J Med Sci **294**:120-131, 1987.

103 Bricker NS, Slatopolsky E, Reiss E, Avioli LV: Calcium, phosphorus, and bone in renal disease and transplantation. Arch Intern Med **123**:543-553, 1969.

104 Morgan AD, Maclagan NF: Renal disease in hyperparathyroidism. Am J Pathol **30**:1141-1168, 1954.

105 Reiss E, Canterbury JM, Egdahl RH: Experience with radioimmunoassay of PTH in human sera. Trans Assoc Am Physicians **81**:104-115, 1968.

"Tertiary" hyperparathyroidism

106 Banerjee SS, Faragher B, Hasleton PS: Nuclear diameter in parathyroid disease. J Clin Pathol **36**:143-148, 1983.

107 Black WC III, Slatopolsky E, Elkan I, Hoffsten P: Parathyroid morphology in suppressible and nonsuppressible renal hyperparathyroidism. Lab Invest **23**:497-509, 1970.

108 Davies DR, Dent CE, Watson L: Tertiary hyperparathyroidism. Br Med J **3**:395-399, 1968.

109 Johnson JW, Hattner RS, Hampers CL, Bernstein DS, Merrill JP, Sherwood LM: Secondary hyperparathyroidism in chronic renal failure. Effects of renal homotransplantation. JAMA **215**:478-480, 1971.

110 Krause MW, Hedinger CE: Pathologic study of parathyroid glands in tertiary hyperparathyroidism. Hum Pathol **16**:772-784, 1985.

111 McIntosh DA, Peterson EW, McPhaul JJ Jr: Autonomy of parathyroid function after renal homotransplantation. Ann Intern Med **65**:900-907, 1966.

112 Misonou J, Ishikura H, Aizawa M, Ohira S: Functioning oxyphil cell adenoma in a patient with secondary hyperparathyroidism. Acta Pathol Jpn **37**:1357-1366, 1987.

Differential diagnosis

113 Dufour DR, Marx SJ, Spiegel AM: Parathyroid gland morphology in nonparathyroid hormone-mediated hypercalcemia. Am J Surg Pathol **9**:43-51, 1985.

114 Falko JM, Maeder MC, Conway C, Mazzaferri EL, Skillman TG: Primary hyperparathyroidism. Analysis of 220 patients with special emphasis on familial hypocalciuric hypercalcemia. Heart Lung **13**:124-131, 1984.

114a Horiuchi N, Caulfield MP, Fisher JE, Goldman ME, McKee RL, Reagan JE, Levy JJ, Nutt RF, Rodan SB, Schofield TL, Clemens TL, Rosenblatt M: Similarity of synthetic peptide from human tumor to parathyroid hormone in vivo and in vitro. Science **238**:1566-1568, 1987.

115 Lafferty FW: Pseudohyperparathyroidism. Medicine [Baltimore] **45**:247-260, 1966.

116 Marx SJ, Spiegel AM, Levine MA, Rizzoli RE, Lasker RD, Santora AC, Downs RW Jr, Aurbach GD: Familial hypocalciuric hypercalcemia. The relation to primary parathyroid hyperplasia. N Engl J Med **307**:416-426, 1982.

116a Mundy, GR, Ibbotson KJ, D'Souza SM, Simpson EL, Jacobs JW, Martin TJ: The hypercalcemia of cancer. Clinical implications and pathogenic mechanisms. N Engl J Med **310**:1718-1727, 1984.

117 Omenn GS, Roth SI, Baker WH: Hyperparathyroidism associated with malignant tumors of nonparathyroid origin. Cancer **24**:1004-1012, 1969.

118 Sharp CF Jr, Rude RK, Terry R, Singer FR: Abnormal bone and parathyroid histology in carcinoma patients with pseudohyperparathyroidism. Cancer **49**:1449-1455, 1982.

119 Stewart AF, Horst R, Deftos LJ, Cadman EC, Lang R, Broadus AE: Biochemical evaluation of patients with cancer-associated hypercalcemia. Evidence for humoral and nonhumoral groups. N Engl J Med **303**:1377-1383, 1980.

120 Thorgeirsson U, Costa J, Marx SJ: The parathyroid glands in familial hypocalciuric hypercalcemia. Hum Pathol **12**:229-237, 1981.

Therapy

121 Attie JN, Wise L, Mir R, Ackerman LV: The rationale against routine subtotal parathyroidectomy for primary hyperparathyroidism. Am J Surg **136**:437-444, 1978.

122 Badder EM, Graham III WP, Harrison TS: Functional insignificance of microscopic parathyroid hyperplasia. Surg Gynecol Obstet **145**:863-868, 1977.

123 Bricker NS, Slatopolsky E, Reiss E, Avioli LV: Calcium, phosphorus, and bone in renal disease and transplantation. Arch Intern Med **123**:543-553, 1969.

124 Clark OH, Okerlund MD, Moss AA, Stark D, Norman D, Newton TH, Duh QY, Arnaud CD, Harris S, Gooding GAW: Localization studies in patients with persistent or recurrent hyperparathyroidism. Surgery **98**:1083-1094, 1985.

125 Cohn K, Silverman M, Corrado J, Sedgewick C: Parathyroid carcinoma. The Lahey Clinic experience. Surgery **98**:1095-1100, 1985.

126 Cooke TJC, Boey JH, Sweeney EC, Gilbert JM, Taylor S: Parathyroidectomy. Extent of resection and late results. Br J Surg **64**:153-157, 1977.

127 Corlew DS, Bryda SL, Bradley EL, DiGirolamo M: Observations on the course of untreated primary hyperparathyroidism. Surgery **98**:1064-1071, 1985.

128 Edis AJ, Beahrs OH, van Heerden JA, Akwari OE: "Conservative" versus "liberal" approach to parathyroid neck exploration. Surgery **82**:466-473, 1977.

129 Flye MW, Brennan MF: Surgical resection of metastatic parathyroid carcinoma. Ann Surg **193**:429-435, 1981.

130 Gaz RD, Wang C: Management of asymptomatic hyperparathyroidism. Am J Surg **147**:124-131, 1984.

131 Goldsmith RS, Furszyfer J, Johnson WJ, Fournier AE, Arnaud CD: Control of secondary hyperparathyroidism during long-term hemodialysis. Am J Med **50**:692-699, 1971.

132 Goodman ML, Egdahl RH, Kemp A, Carey LC: Hyperparathyroidism from intrathyroid parathyroid adenomas. Arch Pathol **87**:418-422, 1969.

133 Graham JJ, Harding PE, Hoare LL, Thomas DW, Wise PH: Asymptomatic hyperparathyroidism. An assessment of operative intervention. Br J Surg **67**:115-118, 1980.

134 Holmes EC, Morton DL, Ketcham AS: Parathyroid carcinoma. A collective review. Ann Surg **169**:631-640, 1969.

135 Nathaniels EK, Nathaniels AM, Wang C: Mediastinal parathyroid tumors. A clinical and pathological study of 84 cases. Ann Surg **171:**165-170, 1970.

136 Paloyan E, Lawrence AM: The rationale for subtotal parathyroidectomy. In Varco RL, Delaney JP (eds): Controversy in surgery. Philadelphia, 1976, W.B. Saunders Co.

137 Paloyan E, Paloyan D, Pickleman JR: Hyperparathyroidism today. Surg Clin North Am **53:**211-220, 1973.

138 Roth SI, Wang C, Potts JT Jr: The team approach to primary hyperparathyroidism. Hum Pathol **6:**645-648, 1975.

139 Rudberg C, Akerström G, Palmér M, Ljunghall S, Adami HO, Johansson H, Grimelius L, Thorén L, Bergström R: Late results of operation for primary hyperparathyroidism in 441 patients. Surgery **99:**643-651, 1986.

140 Russell CF, Edis AJ, Scholz DA, Sheedy PF, van Heerden JA: Mediastinal parathyroid tumors. Experience with 38 tumors requiring mediastinotomy for removal. Ann Surg **193:**805-809, 1981.

141 Russell CF, Grant CS, van Heerden JA: Hyperfunctioning supernumerary parathyroid glands. An occasional cause of hyperparathyroidism. Mayo Clin Proc **57:**121-124, 1982.

142 Saxe A: Parathyroid transplantation. A review. Surgery **95:**507-526, 1984.

143 Scholz DA, Purnell DC: Asymptomatic primary hyperparathyroidism. 10-year prospective study. Mayo Clin Proc **56:**473-478, 1981.

144 Tibblin S, Bondeson A-G, Bondeson L, Ljungberg O: Surgical strategy in hyperparathyroidism due to solitary adenoma. Ann Surg **200:**776-784, 1984.

145 Wang C: Parathyroid re-exploration. A clinical and pathological study of 112 cases. Ann Surg **186:**140-145, 1977.

146 Wang C: Surgical management of primary hyperparathyroidism. Curr Probl Surg **22:**1-50, 1985.

147 Wang C, Castleman B, Cope O: Surgical management of hyperparathyroidism due to primary hyperplasia. A clinical and pathologic study of 104 cases. Ann Surg **195:**384-392, 1982.

148 Wang C, Gaz RD: Natural history of parathyroid carcinoma. Diagnosis, treatment, and results. Am J Surg **149:**522-527, 1985.

149 Wells SA Jr, Ellis GJ, Gunnells JC, Schneider AB, Sherwood LM: Parathyroid autotransplantation in primary parathyroid hyperplasia. N Engl J Med **295:**57-62, 1976.

Frozen section

150 Akerstrom G, Rudberg C, Grimelius L, Bergstrom R, Johansson H, Ljunghall S, Rastad J: Histologic parathyroid abnormalities in an autopsy series. Hum Pathol **17:**520-527, 1986.

151 Allen TB, Thorburn KM: The oxyphil cell in abnormal parathyroid glands. A study of 114 cases. Arch Pathol Lab Med **105:**421-427, 1981.

152 Bondeson A-G, Bondeson L, Ljungberg O, Tibblin S: Fat staining in parathyroid disease. Diagnostic value and impact on surgical strategy. Clinicopathologic analysis of 191 cases. Hum Pathol **16:**1255-1263, 1985.

153 Dekker A, Watson CG, Barnes EL Jr: The pathologic assessment of primary hyperparathyroidism and its impact on therapy. A prospective evaluation of 50 cases with oil-red-O stain. Ann Surg **190:**671-675, 1979.

154 Dufour DR, Durkowski C: Sudan IV stain. Its limitations in evaluating parathyroid functional status. Arch Pathol Lab Med **106:**224-227, 1982.

155 Dufour DR, Wilkerson SY: The normal parathyroid revisited. Percentage of stromal fat. Hum Pathol **13:**717-721, 1982.

156 Geelhoed GW, Silverberg SG: Intraoperative imprints for the identification of parathyroid tissue. Surgery **96:**1124-1130, 1984.

157 Ghandur-Mnaymneh L, Cassady J, Hajianpour MA, Paz J, Reiss E: The parathyroid gland in health and disease. Am J Pathol **125:**292-299, 1986.

158 Grimelius L, Akerström G, Johansson H, Lundqvist H: Estimation of parenchymal cell content of human parathyroid glands using the image analyzing computer technique. Am J Pathol **93:**793-800, 1978.

159 Kasdon EJ, Rosen S, Cohen RB, Silen W: Surgical pathology of hyperparathyroidism. Usefulness of fat stain and problems in interpretation. Am J Surg Pathol **5:**381-384, 1981.

160 Monchik JM, Farrugia R, Teplitz C, Teplitz J, Brown S: Parathyroid surgery. The role of chief cell intracellular fat staining with osmium carmine in the intraoperative management of patients with primary hyperparathyroidism. Surgery **94:**877-886, 1983.

161 Roth SI, Gallagher MJ: The rapid identification of "normal" parathyroid glands by the presence of intracellular fat. Am J Pathol **84:**521-527, 1976.

162 Saffos RO, Rhatigan RM, Urgulu S: The normal parathyroid and the borderline with early hyperplasia. A light microscopic study. Histopathology **8:**407-422, 1984.

163 Saxe AW, Baier R, Tesluk H, Toreson W: The role of the pathologist in the surgical treatment of hyperparathyroidism. Surg Gynecol Obstet **161:**101-105, 1985.

164 Silverberg SG: Imprints in the intraoperative evaluation of parathyroid disease. Arch Pathol **99:**375-378, 1975.

11 Gastrointestinal tract

Esophagus
Stomach
Small bowel
Appendix
Large bowel
Anus

Esophagus

ATRESIA AND RELATED ANOMALIES

The esophagus of a 3-week-old embryo is an annular constriction between the pharynx and the stomach. With growth of lung beds and elongation of the neck, it becomes tubular. At first, the cephalad portions of the esophagus and the trachea form a single channel. Later, a septum grows in and separates them.

Five major types of tracheoesophageal anomalies have been described[4] (Fig. 11-1). The most common, referred to as type C, is esophageal atresia with fistula between the lower portion of the esophagus and the respiratory tree.[2,3,5] In this type, the hypertrophied and dilated upper portion of the esophagus ends blindly at a variable distance below the larynx, whereas the lower portion communicates with the trachea (usually about 0.5 cm above the bifurcation) or

the right main stem bronchus. Striated muscle is present in the upper portion of the esophagus but not in the lower, which may contain instead cartilaginous rings near its fistulous end.[6]

There also can be defects of the esophagus alone, such as congenital narrowing, stenosis, or an occluding diaphragm of mucous membrane.[1] Successful surgical repair can be accomplished for most of these abnormalities.[5]

HETEROTOPIA

Heterotopic gastric mucosa can occur at any point in the esophagus but appears most frequently in the postcricoid region.[11] It is found in approximately 4% of patients who undergo esophagoscopic examinations and is sometimes referred to as the "inlet patch."[9] Rarely, it results in a filling defect in the midportion of the esophagus[7] (Fig. 11-2, *A*). It is usually asymptomatic, but it may produce dysphagia and simulate clinically and radiographically a malignant neoplasm.

Grossly, the surface resembles gastric mucosa (Fig. 11-2, *B*). It is sharply delineated, and the border with the normal stratified epithelium is apparent. At times, ulceration occurs.

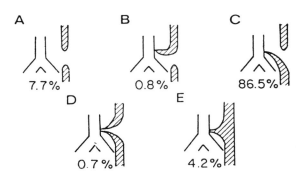

Fig. 11-1 Types of tracheoesophageal anomalies and their relative frequencies. (Adapted from Holder TM, Ashcraft KW: Ann Thorac Surg **9**:445-467, 1970.)

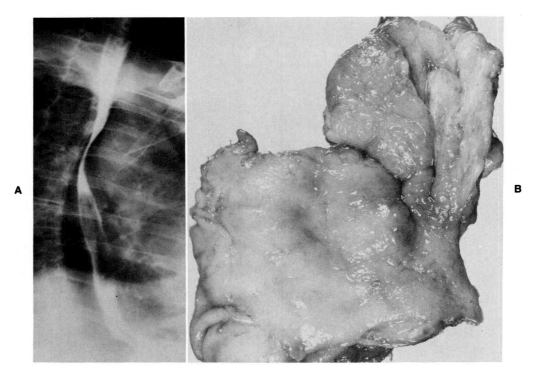

Fig. 11-2 A, Esophagogram showing smooth filling defect with compression. **B,** Resected esophagus illustrated in **A** showing smooth heterotopic gastric mucosa containing area of ulceration.

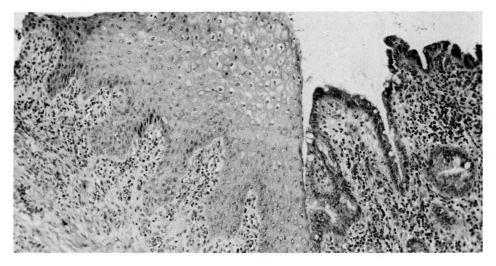

Fig. 11-3 Heterotopic gastric mucosa demonstrating abrupt transition between gastric and squamous epithelium.

Microscopically, this gastric mucosa is usually made up of long, typical gastric glands that are almost entirely mucin secreting (Fig. 11-3). Parietal and chief cells are rare. There often is an extensive inflammatory reaction that may induce reactive proliferation and architectural distortion of the glands and lead to a mistaken diagnosis of malignancy. True

instances of adenocarcinoma of the upper esophagus in heterotopic gastric mucosa have been described in which normal lining squamous epithelium was present both proximal and distal to the lesion.[8]

Heterotopic sebaceous glands are rarely seen in the mid or distal portion of the esophagus.[10]

DIVERTICULA

The diverticula appearing in the upper portion of the esophagus (Zenker's diverticula) are the result of outpouching esophageal mucosa at points of weakness in the wall of the esophagus, at the junction with the pharynx. They are more properly designated as pharyngoesophageal and are classified as *pulsion diverticula*. They occur at this point because of the relationship between the inferior constrictor muscle and the obliquely passing fibers of the cricopharyngeal muscles as they descend on the posterior wall of the esophagus to become longitudinal.[14]

In the lower third of the esophagus and in the region of the hilum of the lung, inflammatory lymph nodes (usually tuberculous) can become firmly attached to the esophagus and produce *traction diverticula.*

Just above the diaphragm, so-called *epiphrenic* diverticula of the pulsion variety occur rarely.[13] These outpouchings contain mucosa, submucosa, and often muscularis mucosae. They are lined by squamous epithelium and may be associated with considerable inflammation. Complications include obstruction, infection with perforation and mediastinitis, hemorrhage, and even malignancy. Carcinomas can arise within esophageal diverticula of both the pharyngoesophageal and epiphrenic varieties[15]; in one series, the incidence of malignancy in pharyngoesophageal diverticula was 0.3%.[17]

An altogether different type of esophageal diverticular process has been designated *diffuse intramural esophageal diverticulosis.*[12] Dysphagia may be the presenting symptom. Roentgenography and endoscopy reveal innumerable 1 to 3 mm flask-shaped diverticula, with a pinpoint mouth, more numerous in the upper third of the organ. The lining is predominantly squamous. A short stricture is usually present in the region. It has been suggested that these formations represent cystically dilated ducts of submucosal glands.[16] The etiology remains undetermined.

CYSTS

Esophageal cysts are classified into inclusion cysts (lined by squamous or columnar epithelium, sometimes ciliated), retention cysts or mucoceles (arising from cystic dilatation of submucosal glands), and developmental cysts (of esophageal, bronchial, or gastric origin).[19] Their microscopic distinction may be very difficult. A case of epidermoid carcinoma arising in such a cyst was reported by McGregor et al.[18]

RINGS AND WEBS

Esophageal shadows with a configuration resembling rings and webs are often described by radiologists in patients complaining of dysphagia. Those located in the upper esophagus of women and associated with iron-deficient anemia are a component of the Plummer-Vinson or Paterson-Kelly syndrome, in which an increased incidence of carcinoma has been described. Those located in the lower esophagus are commonly referred as "Schatzki's ring" or "lower esophageal ring." The nature of the morphologic structure behind these shadows has been unclear because of the lack of correlative roentgenographic and microscopic studies. Goyal et al.[21] partially corrected this deficiency by examining 100 autopsy specimens both roentgenographically and microscopically. They found two structurally different types of rings, which could be separated on roentgenographic examination. Nine were formed by a transverse circumferential fold of the mucosa; they were located at the squamocolumnar junction and produced a thin weblike shadow on roentgenograms. Five were formed by a localized annular thickening of the muscle. They were proximal to the site of the mucoscal ring, were covered by squamous epithelium, and produced a wide constriction when examined roentgenographically.

Clements et al.,[20] in a similar study, have shown that the cervical esophageal (pharyngoesophageal) webs also represent transverse folds of normal mucosa and submucosa.

ACHALASIA AND RELATED MOTOR DISORDERS

Achalasia (cardiospasm; megaesophagus) is due to a failure of the cardiac mechanism to open when peristaltic waves conveying food through the esophagus reach it.[32] A nearly complete loss of myenteric ganglion cells has been found in the upper thickened segment. Ganglion cells with varying degrees of degeneration were present in the lower segment in half of the cases studied by Adams et al.[22] Misiewicz et al.[30] performed pharmacologic and histologic studies on strips of muscle removed at surgery for achalasia. They found loss of the beta-adrenergic activity, which mediates the relaxation of the muscle. Ganglion cells in this strip were either absent or abnormal. Some authors have suggested that the primary disorder is in the preganglionic neuron,[23] but this seems rather unlikely.[22]

In the early stages, achalasia is reversible. With the passage of time, however, chronic inflammation and ulceration supervene, and fibrotic stricture results. Esophagomyotomy and pneumatic dilation remain the major treatment modalities.[24] Rarely, cancer is associated with long-standing achalasia[27,29] (Fig. 11-4). Wychulis et al.[33] observed seven cases in a group of 1,318 patients. Achalasia had been present for an average of 28 years before the diagnosis of carcinoma. The tumors arose at all levels of the esophagus but were more common in the middle third; they were of epidermoid type in all but one patient.

Cricopharyngeal dysphagia (achalasia, spasm) is a well-recognized entity with prominent clinical symptoms but only meager microscopic findings.[31] Cruse et al.[25] found degeneration and regeneration of the fibers of the cricopharyngeal muscle, accompanied by interstitial fibrosis.

Chagas' disease, an endemic parasitosis of South America, can be associated with alterations of Auerbach's plexus and megaesophagus.

Giant muscular hypertrophy (diffuse spasm; corkscrew esophagus; diffuse leiomyomatosis) is a motor disorder of the esophagus characterized clinically by dysphagia and pain and pathologically by focal or diffuse hypertrophy of the muscular layer, up to a thickness of 1 cm.[28] Ferguson et al.[26] reported fourteen cases of this disorder and pointed out that surgical therapy is not so successful as in achalasia.

LYE STRICTURES

Lye strictures of the esophagus are most common at the level of bifurcation of the trachea.[38] The mean age of the

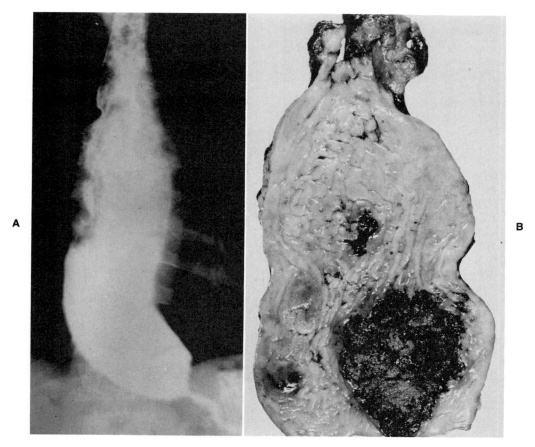

Fig. 11-4 A, Achalasia with superimposed ulcerating squamous carcinoma. **B,** Same lesion shown in **A.**

patients at the time of lye ingestion is about 6 years. Once the lesion is well established, the only method of cure is surgical resection.[36,37] Carcinoma of the esophagus may develop at the site.[34,35] The mean latent time is about 40 years; the later in life the lye is ingested, the shorter the interval.

REFLUX ESOPHAGITIS

As the name indicates, this form of esophagitis is the result of reflux of gastroduodenal contents into the esophagus. It is often associated with a sliding hiatal hernia, although it should be stressed that it is the reflux and not the hernia that is the cause of the abnormality.[51] Esophageal reflux and the complications arising from it have also been described as a result of scleroderma[48] and Zollinger-Ellison syndrome.[47]

Esophageal reflux is accompanied by regurgitation, heartburn, pain, and dysphagia. Massive bleeding and perforation almost never occur. The early microscopic lesions are those of epithelial hyperplasia and infiltration by neutrophils and eosinophils, sometimes accompanied by focal epithelial necrosis.[43,46] The papillary height of the lamina propria and the degree of basal cell proliferation are substantially higher than in the control subjects.[41] Dilated and congested venules are seen high up in the top of the lengthened papillae be-

tween the epithelial layers.[44,45] According to Brown et al.[43] intraepithelial eosinophils are the most frequent abnormality; they were noted in over half of the cases and correlate best with the gross endoscopic features. However, Tummala et al.[53] have shown that in human volunteers without evidence of esophageal reflux occasional eosinophils are found in one third of the esophageal biopsies; therefore, they are not by themselves a reliable criterion in the evaluation of this disorder.

Reflux esophagitis may progress to superficial ulceration, spread of inflammation to the wall, and circumferential fibrosis with stricture formation and fixation to the surrounding structures.[49,54] Sometimes, a lesion develops in this background that has gross and microscopic features identical to those of a gastric ulcer (''Barrett's ulcer'').[39,40,42] It is often large, oval, and well circumscribed, with elevated borders and deep craters (Fig. 11-5) and may result in massive bleeding or perforation. Microscopic examination of the short tubular segment distal to the ulcer, anatomically resembling the esophagus, shows the segment to be lined by gastric mucosa.[52] As such, this is to be regarded as an expression of Barrett's esophagus, an alteration associated with reflux esophagitis that is discussed in the next section. Occasionally, the inflammatory reaction associated with the

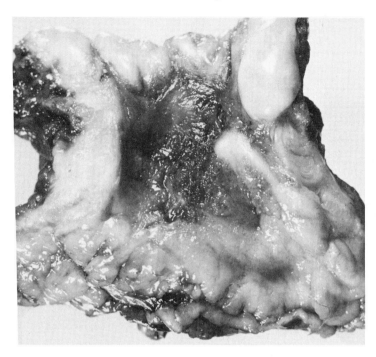

Fig. 11-5 Resected terminal third of esophagus demonstrating chronic peptic ulceration with deep penetration into wall.

esophagitis may be of such a degree as to result in a pseudolymphomatous appearance.[50]

Barrett's esophagus

The occurrence of columnar epithelium lining a segment of distal esophagus, with or without an associated peptic ulcer, is referred to as *Barrett's esophagus*.[66,70] Most patients are adults, but the disorder also occurs in children.[58,62] It has been debated for years whether this represents a congenital or acquired abnormality[63] and whether this segment should be regarded as belonging to the esophagus because of its shape and mobility or to the stomach because of its lining. Lack of a precise definition on the nature and location of the gastroesophageal junction and the microscopic variations at this junction complicate the issue.[61,73] Most clinical and experimental evidence, however, favors the interpretation that this change is acquired and is the result of ulceration and subsequent reepithelization by gastric cells of what originally was esophageal squamous mucosa.[55,57,60] The ulceration is nearly always induced by reflux, but it may also result from chemotherapy effect.[57a] This mucosal extension may be circumferential or in the form of finger-like projections or islands[64] (Fig. 11-6). Microscopically, the epithelium can have one or a combination of three distinct appearances: (1) atrophic fundal type (with parietal and chief cells), (2) cardiac or junctional type (mainly composed of mucous glands), and (3) specialized columnar. The last is the most common type encountered in adults and is regarded as a form of incomplete intestinal metaplasia; as such, it exhibits a villiform surface and crypts, with a mixed population of columnar, goblet, Paneth, and endocrine cells[67,72] (Fig. 11-7). Most of the mucin present is of neutral type, but in over 70% of the cases there are also sialomucins and sulfomucins.[65,68] Endocrine cells are demonstrated by argyrophilic stains in 90% of the biopsies, irrespective of the type of epithelium; serotonin, somatostatin, secretin, and pancreatic polypeptide have been detected immunohistochemically in them.[59]

The diagnosis of Barrett's esophagus is usually first suggested by the barium swallow. Manometric examinations, intraesophageal pH monitoring, and other techniques are useful as supporting evidence, but confirmation of the diagnosis requires endoscopic examination and biopsy.[72] It is essential that the biopsy be taken above the lower esophageal sphincter; it is generally agreed that the diagnosis of Barrett's esophagus is justified when velvety red mucosa with the microscopic appearance of columnar epithelium is seen to involve 3 cm or more of the distal tubular esophagus.[72] Microscopically the presence of specialized columnar epithelium with submucosal glands beneath can be regarded as pathognomonic of the condition. The treatment can be medical or surgical, in the form of esophagogastroplasty, fundoplication, or posterior gastroplexy. There is controversy as to how often these procedures will result in microscopic regression of the changes, but most studies suggest that this phenomenon does indeed occur.[56,69,71]

Dysplasia and carcinoma in Barrett's esophagus

One of the most important complications that can supervene in a Barrett's esophagus is carcinoma, which is nearly always accompanied and preceded by dysplasia. The dys-

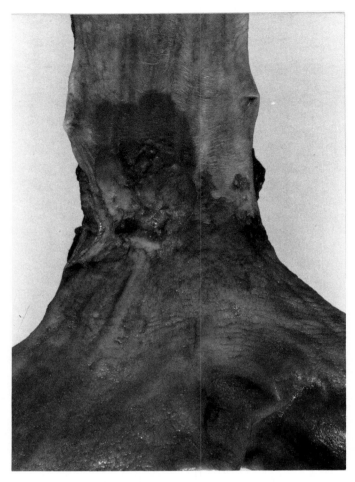

Fig. 11-6 Barrett's esophagus with superimposed polypoid adenocarcinoma. Areas of Barrett's change are identifiable on right of tumor as irregular protrusions of gastric-type mucosa into terminal esophagus.

plasia has been observed in all three types of Barrett's epithelium but seems more frequent in the specialized columnar type.[78] It should be distinguished from the reactive hyperplasia seen secondarily to inflammatory injury and should be graded according to its severity.[89a] In *reactive hyperplasia,* the glands are regular and the nuclei—although mildly hyperchromatic and crowded—retain their basal location. In *low-grade dysplasia,* the glands are still regular, but the nuclei are more hyperchromatic and crowded, with some degree of pleomorphism and elongation. In *high-grade dysplasia* (which merges with and is probably synonymous with carcinoma in situ), there is glandular distortion and marked nuclear changes, which extend into the upper portions of the epithelium. In dysplasia there is also a depletion of mucous granules and disappearance of mature goblet cells. In some cases of dysplasia, the architecture of the lesion and the crowding and stratification of the hyperchromatic nuclei are similar to those seen in adenomas of the large bowel,[86] whereas other cases resemble the pattern of dysplasia seen in the large bowel as a complication of ulcerative colitis[90,93]; it has been suggested that carcinoma

is associated more often with the latter pattern[83,90] (Figs. 11-8 and 11-9).

Dysplasia, as thus defined, is found in Barrett's esophagus in the absence of carcinoma in 5% to 10% of the cases and in association with carcinoma in 68% to 100% of the cases.* The risk for the development of invasive carcinoma in partients with dysplasia in Barrett's esophagus is certainly elevated, at least for the high-grade type,[87] but the magnitude of this risk remains to be determined.[96] It has been suggested that cytology and flow cytometry may be useful in the detection of dysplasia in Barrett's esophagus.[81a,90a]

Invasive carcinoma developing in Barrett's esophagus is nearly always of the adenocarcinoma type.[82,84,97] The risk is said to be thirty-fold to forty-fold above that of the general population.[77,95] It has been estimated that Barrett-associated adenocarcinoma accounts for 5% to 10% of all esophageal cancers.[81] The main features used to suggest an origin of adenocarcinoma from a Barrett's esophagus are the asso-

---

*See references 75, 79, 81, 89, 90, and 93.

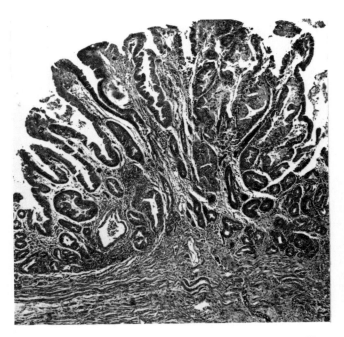

Fig. 11-7 Microscopic appearance of Barrett's esophagus. Metaplastic glandular epithelium is seen covering what was originally squamous eosphageal mucosa.

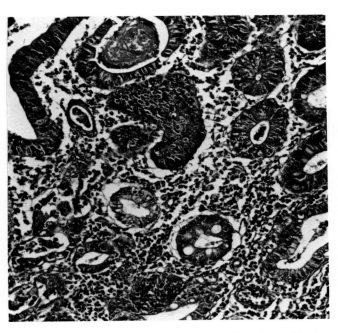

Fig. 11-8 Mild dysplasia in Barrett's esophagus. There is stratification of surface epithelium and glands, but only mild degree of atypia.

ciation with a dysplastic or nondysplastic Barrett's mucosa and the location of more than half of the tumor mass in the esophagus. Adenocarcinomas of the gastroesophageal junction have essentially similar morphologic and epidemiologic features, whether an associated Barrett's metaplasia can be detected in the specimen or not.[80,84,85,88,98] The tumor may be multicentric and is often far advanced at the time of diagnosis, with extension into the wall and nodal metastases.[94] Most patients are white males, and the average age at diagnosis is 57 years.[95] Microscopically, there is a wide range of glandular differentiation, sometimes in the same tumor[74]; unusual varieties include adenocarcinoid and adenosquamous carcinoma.[94]

The prognosis is poor, with a 5-year survival rate of 14.5% in one of the largest published series.[92] Stage by stage, this prognosis seems to be similar to that of conventional epidermoid carcinoma of the esophagus.[91] Surgical resection is the primary treatment.

OTHER TYPES OF ESOPHAGITIS

Herpes simplex esophagitis is a frequent autopsy finding in immunosuppressed hosts and is being detected with increasing frequency[99,107,108]; the diagnosis should be suspected in the presence of "volcano ulcers" at endoscopy and discrete diffusely scattered shallow ulcers on double-contrast esophagogram.[99]

Candida esophagitis can complicate the ulcers of herpes esophagitis or appear in the absence of viral infection, usually in immunosuppressed individuals. It may also be seen secondarily to esophageal stricture or in children as mu-

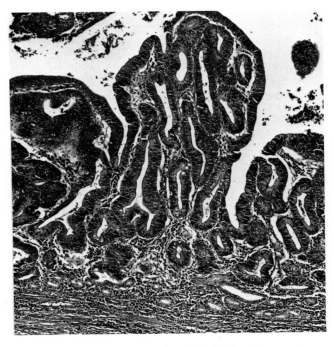

Fig. 11-9 Moderate-to-severe dysplasia in Barrett's esophagus. There is marked pseudostratification and proliferation of glandular epithelium, resulting in polypoid configuration of mucosa.

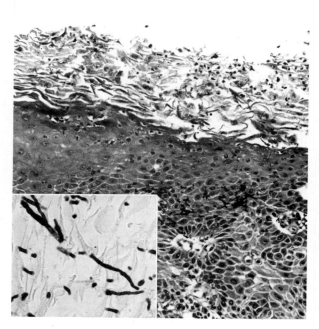

Fig. 11-10 Candidiasis of esophagus. Organisms are growing on the surface, mixed with desquamated squamous cells and neutrophils. **Inset** demonstrates fungi with Grocott's stain.

cocutaneous candidiasis, an expression of an immunologic deficiency.[111] The diagnosis can be made by brush cytology[112] (Fig. 11-10).

Crohn's disease can involve the esophagus, usually in association with gastric and/or intestinal disease.[102,104]

Idiopathic eosinophilic esophagitis has been described as an unusual variant of the presumably allergic eosinophilic infiltrations that can involve any portion of the gastrointestinal tract.[106] This very rare condition should be distinguished from the much more common eosinophilic infiltration of esophageal mucosa seen in patients with reflux (see p. 470).

Other types of esophagitis include those caused by tuberculosis,[100] blastomycosis,[109] cytomegalovirus,[103] Behcet's disease,[110] and those that are drug-related, post-irradiation, and seen secondarily to ingestion of corrosive chemicals.[101] Primarily dermatologic diseases that can involve the esophagus include scleroderma, pemphigus vulgaris, and epidermolysis bullosa.[105] Inflammation and sometimes perforation of the esophagus may result from instrumentation, intubation, or the ingestion of foreign bodies.[101]

EPIDERMOID CARCINOMA
General features

Epidermoid carcinoma of the esophagus occurs more frequently in men over 50 years of age. It is relatively common in China and other Oriental countries and is the most common tumor of the alimentary tract in the African Bantus.[121] In the United States it is distinctly less common than carcinoma of the large bowel but affects a disproportionately large number of blacks.[122a]

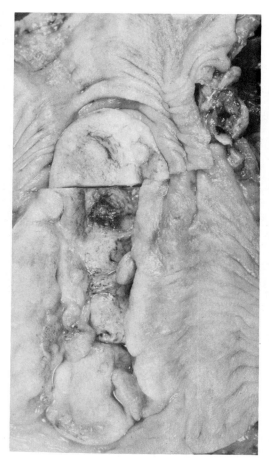

Fig. 11-11 Epidermoid carcinoma of terminal third of esophagus demonstrating well-delineated mass with central ulceration.

Epidermoid carcinoma of the esophagus has been reported in association with lye strictures, achalasia, Plummer-Vinson syndrome, and diverticula (see respective sections in this chapter). Some authors have also found an increased incidence of esophagitis[114,116,119] and history of previous gastrectomy[117] in patients with esophageal epidermoid carcinoma. However, the disease does not seem to be related to leukoplakia. In this regard, it should be pointed out that most lesions diagnosed endoscopically or grossly as "leukoplakia" of the esophagus have no microscopic resemblance to the lesions so designated in the oral cavity. They represent, instead, focal thickening of the epithelium due to a marked increase in cytoplasmic glycogen content ("glycogenic acanthosis").[120]

Cases of carcinoma have been reported following irradiation to the area.[115] Another known association is with cancer in other sites, particularly the oropharynx and larynx; in one autopsy series, this combination was found in 12% of the cases.[118] Multicentricity in the esophagus may occur either synchronously or metachronously, but it is rare.[113]

The main symptom of esophageal cancer—dysphagia—is related to the local spread of the tumor and is usually the

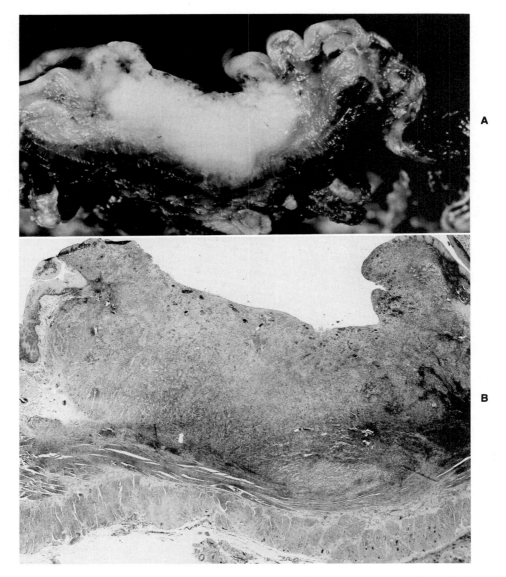

Fig. 11-12 A Cross section of specimen of tumor shown in Fig. 11-11. Tumor is still confined to esophageal wall. **B** Same tumor as shown in **A**. Patient died 18 years later of unrelated disorder.

expression of advanced disease; a few cases of esophageal cancer have been reported in association with humoral hypercalcemia.[122]

Morphologic features and local spread

Epidermoid carcinoma can occur in any portion of the esophagus but is most common in the middle and lower thirds, in areas of normal anatomic constrictions.[125,129] Grossly, the tumor usually is circumferential, often ulcerated, with sharply demarcated margins (Fig. 11-11). Polypoid forms occur but are much less common than in adenocarcinoma.[129] On cut section, a grayish white tumor is seen to invade part or all of the muscular wall, from which it may extend into the surrounding soft tissues and trachea (Figs. 11-12 and 11-13). Intraluminar growth also occurs and eventually leads to total obstruction. Distally located

tumors often invade the stomach.[132] Submucosal spread, not appreciable grossly, is also common, sometimes up to 5 or more cm beyond the gross margins of the tumor.[123] Intraepithelial spread is even more frequent, with or without involvement of the glandular ducts.[127,131]

Microscopically, the degree of squamous differentiation is variable, but most tumors are well or moderately differentiated. Occasionally, detachment of tumor cells results in a pseudoglandular configuration.[124] With extensive search, true glandular and/or mucus-secreting components are found focally in one fifth of the cases[126]; when these are extensive, the tumors are designated *adenosquamous carcinomas*. The occasional presence of an intraepithelial component with the appearance of Paget's disease has also been described.[133]

Poor microscopic differentiation is associated with a

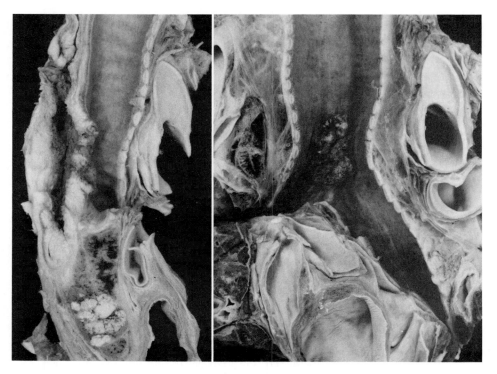

Fig. 11-13 Carcinoma of esophagus involving entire circumference of organ, invading trachea, and producing intratracheal polypoid mass. This may result in mistaken diagnosis of primary tracheal carcinoma. There are metastases in mediastinal lymph nodes. (Courtesy Dr. E.F. Lascano, Buenos Aires, Argentina.)

high DNA ploidy in microspectrophotometric determinations[130]; the latter determination may prove of prognostic utility.[128]

In situ and superficial spreading carcinoma

Epidermoid carcinoma in situ is found at the periphery of invasive cancer in 30% of the cases, the incidence being much higher when no preoperative irradiation has been given and when the main lesion is superficial[135]; sometimes, the in situ lesion is found anatomically separate from the main tumor and associated with foci of dysplasia, supporting the concept of a field effect[134,135,138] (Figs. 11-14 to 11-16).

Carcinoma in situ and dysplasia of the esophagus in the absence of an invasive component are being recognized with increasing frequency, particularly in areas with a high incidence of esophageal carcinoma[134]; biopsies taken in asymptomatic individuals in these high-risk groups have shown an increased degree of epithelial proliferation by tritiated thymidine labeling.[136]

The term *superficial spreading carcinoma* has been proposed, in analogy with the similarly named gastric lesion, for an esophageal tumor having an intramucosal extension of carcinoma 2 cm or more from the invasive lesion.[137] These superficial lesions are still associated with a high incidence of permeation of lymphatic channels and lymph node metastases and therefore with a poor prognosis.[137]

Metastases

The abundant lymphatic supply of the esophagus is responsible for the high frequency of lymph node metastases in the periesophageal area, below the diaphragm, and upward into the cervical nodes.[139] These nodal metastases occur early in the course of the disease and are the main reason for treatment failure. In a series of 40 patients without incidence of metastatic disease by conventional techniques, laparotomy with celiac lymph node biopsy showed involvement in 40%.[141] Metastases to distant organs are also frequent, particularly to liver, lung, and the adrenal glands.[140] The tumor may also metastasize to the submucosa of the stomach, probably through the submucosal lymphatic plexus.[142]

Diagnosis

Exfoliative cytology in experienced hands is an extremely accurate technique for the evaluation of esophageal lesions.[148] It is clearly superior to roentgenology or endoscopy, as shown in the classic study of MacDonald et al.,[146] involving 166 patients with pathologically proven lesions of the esophagus or the cardiac portion of the stomach. In seventy two cases of carcinoma, the false negative rate was 6% for cytology, 25% for roentgenography, and 40% for esophagoscopy; of 94 patients with benign lesions, the false positive rate was 0% for cytology, 18% for roentgenology, and 28% for esophagoscopy.[146]

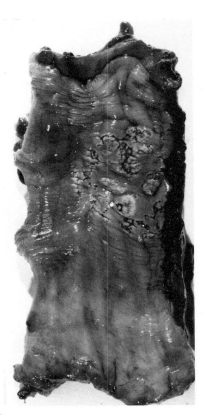

Fig. 11-14 Gross appearance of esophagus with foci of dysplasia, carcinoma in situ, and microinvasive carcinoma. (Courtesy Dr. J. Costa, Lausanne, Switzerland.)

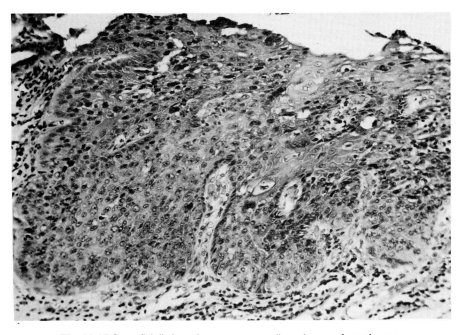

Fig. 11-15 Superficially invasive squamous cell carcinoma of esophagus.

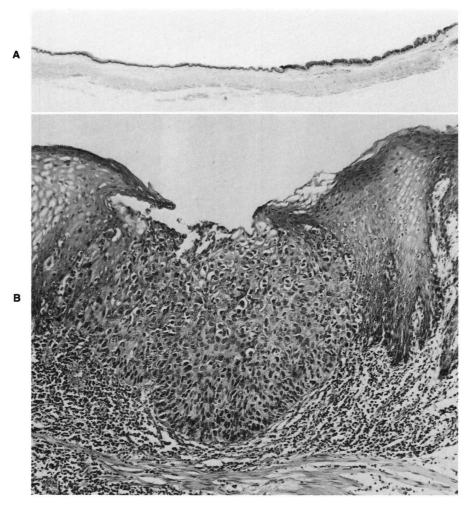

Fig. 11-16 A, Low-power view of segment of esophagus removed from Chinese patient following positive cytology. Areas of thickened mucosa contain multicentric foci of carcinoma in situ. There was no invasion beyond muscularis mucosae. **B,** High-power view of one of many foci of carcinoma in situ, sharply demarcated from surrounding squamous epithelium (From Ackerman LV, Weinstein IB, Kaplan HS, other members of Delegation: Cancer of the esophagus. In Kaplan HS, Tsuchitani PJ (eds): Cancer in China. New York, 1978, Alan R. Liss, Inc.)

With the introduction of the flexible fiberoptic endoscope, the diagnostic accuracy of direct-vision biopsy has become as high as that of cytology.[144] Prolla et al.[147] compared the results of direct-vision endoscopic biopsy with brush cytology performed in 183 patients with proved carcinoma of the esophagus and stomach: 95% were diagnosed correctly by cytology and 79% by biopsy. The combined biopsy and cytology approach provided a positive diagnosis in 95%. In the experience of Kasugai et al.[145] with 116 cases of esophageal carcinoma, the diagnostic accuracy was 97% for brush cytology using a fiberscope, 90% for direct-vision biopsy, and 99% for combined cytology and biopsy.

Diagnostic cytology is particularly rewarding in countries with a high incidence of esophageal carcinoma, such as China. Positive results have been obtained in asymptomatic patients with negative roentgenograms. Surgical resection has shown in situ or superficially invasive lesion, often with multiple foci of origin (Fig. 11-16). A high percentage of these patients have survived for 5 years.[143]

Treatment and prognosis

Radiation therapy is the treatment of choice for carcinoma of the upper two thirds of the esophagus, and surgery is usually performed for carcinoma of the lower third.[158,159] Several groups are presently advocating a combined modality consisting of preoperative radiation therapy followed by surgery[152,161] or preoperative chemotherapy, surgery, and irradiation.[155] Smithers[160] reviewed the world literature in 1957 and found seventy-four 5-year survivors among patients treated by surgery who had carcinoma of the lower third of the esophagus and sixty-one 5-year survivors among patients treated by radiotherapy who had carcinoma of the upper third of the esophagus. Earlam and Cunha-Melo[149] reviewed data from 83,783 patients with epidermoid car-

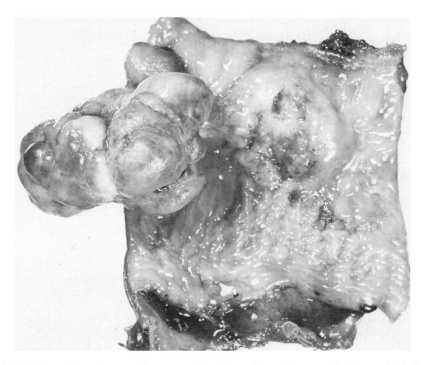

Fig. 11-17 Epidermoid carcinoma with sarcoma-like stroma ("pseudosarcoma") of upper third of esophagus in 66-year-old man. Note typical polypoid configuration. There were no metastases, and tumor had not extended through wall.

cinoma of the esophagus reported in 122 articles. Of these, 58% were explored and 39% had the tumor resected; 13% died in the hospital. Of the 26% leaving the hospital with the tumor excised, 18% survived for 1 year, 9% for 2 years, and 4% for 5 years. The operative mortality, still inordinately high, is mainly due to pyothorax, pulmonary complications, suture leak, and hemorrhage.[150,151,154]

In inoperable cases, considerable palliation can still be achieved by well-planned irradiation.[153,156,157]

OTHER TYPES OF CARCINOMA

Epidermoid carcinoma with spindle-cell stroma (pseudosarcoma; carcinosarcoma; spindle cell carcinoma; polypoid carcinoma) usually presents as a large polypoid neoplasm[170,170a] (Fig. 11-17). The epithelial-appearing component can be very inconspicuous and is usually limited to a few areas of in situ or superficially invasive epidermoid carcinoma and/or adenocarcinoma. The bulk of the tumor has a pleomorphic sarcoma-like appearance (Fig. 11-18). It usually resembles malignant fibrous histiocytoma of soft tissues, and sometimes it exhibits focal differentiation toward cartilage, bone, or skeletal muscle.[171] Most evidence suggests that this component is also of epithelial derivation, although the longstanding controversy about its nature still persists.[163,168,182] Ultrastructurally, *some* of these sarcoma-like cells in *some* of the tumors retain epithelial markers, such as desmosomes and tonofibrils. Most others have the appearance of myofibroblasts or other mesenchymal cells.[177,178] Immunohistochemically, keratin can be consistently demonstrated in the epithelial-appearing component, and in a high proportion of cases also in some of the sarcoma-like cells. The latter also exhibit strong reactivity for vimentin but are negative for S-100 protein.[176,195] Metastases or recurrences supervene in about 20% of the patients undergoing surgery, and the overall survival rate is in the neighborhood of 50%.[184] The nodal metastases usually contain epithelial elements alone or a mixture of epithelial and spindle elements; occasionally, the entire metastatic focus is made up of the spindle-cell element, giving further credence to the interpretation that this component is indeed neoplastic and not a stromal reaction to the tumor.[180]

Verrucous carcinoma, morphologically identical to its more common counterpart in the oral cavity, has been described in the esophagus.[162,183] It is grossly polypoid and well-differentiated throughout microscopically.

Adenocarcinoma of esophagus can arise from Barrett's metaplastic mucosa (discussed on p. 471), from a focus of heterotopic gastric mucosa (see p. 467), or—theoretically—from esophageal glands (Fig. 11-19). Adenocarcinomas make up about 10% of esophageal cancers, but their relative frequency seems to be on the rise in this country.[194] A very small proportion of primary esophageal adenocarcinomas have *signet ring cell* features[165a]; in these cases, esophageal extension of a gastric carcinoma should be ruled out.

Adenosquamous carcinoma shows evidence of both squamous and glandular differentiation. For all practical purposes, this rare high-grade tumor should be equated with the conventional epidermoid carcinoma. It should be distinguished from both the low-grade *mucoepidermoid carcinoma,* possibly arising in salivary-type submucosal esoph-

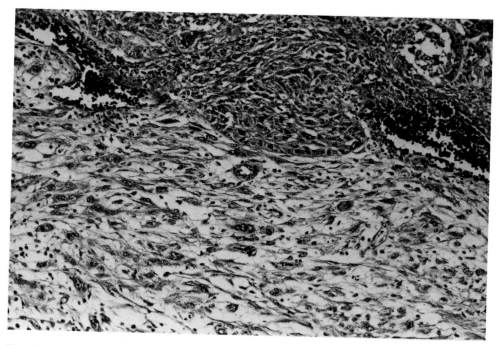

Fig. 11-18 Epidermoid carcinoma with sarcoma-like stroma. Island of clearly identifiable squamous cell carcinoma is sharply separated from component with pleomorphic sarcoma-like appearance.

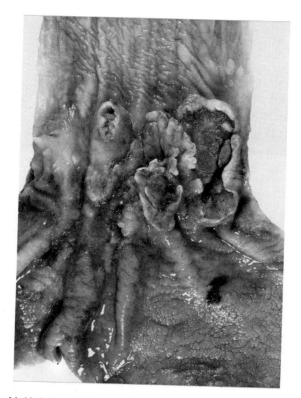

Fig. 11-19 Adenocarcinoma of cardia region, presenting as multiple ulcerating nodules that connect with each other submucosally. (Courtesy Dr. J. Costa, Lausanne, Switzerland.)

ageal glands,[167,196] and the equally rare *collision tumor*, represented by a merging of two originally separate neoplasms, i.e., epidermoid carcinoma and adenocarcinoma.[179,189]

Basaloid carcinoma is probably the best term for a highly malignant esophageal neoplasm often reported as adenoid cystic carcinoma.[175] Although this tumor has been viewed as the esophageal counterpart of adenoid cystic carcinoma of the salivary glands, it exhibits both morphologic and behavioral differences from the latter. It should be regarded primarily as an epidermoid tumor exhibiting focal and sometimes extensive differentiation towards a certain type of glandular structure.[169] Peripheral palisading, round glandular lumina, and abundant basal lamina material are the most important features (Fig. 11-20). The behavior is extremely aggressive. Similar tumors occur in the oral cavity, pharynx, larynx, and anal canal.[193]

Small cell carcinoma (neuroendocrine carcinoma; anaplastic carcinoma) is a highly malignant esophageal tumor composed of anaplastic small cells, having morphologic features very similar to those of its pulmonary counterpart. Grossly, it usually exhibits a fungating pattern of growth.[181] Occasionally, multiple foci are found.[186] Microscopically, small cells with dark nuclei of round or oval shape and very scanty cytoplasm are seen growing in a predominantly diffuse fashion. As in small cell carcinoma of the lung, there may be rosette formation and focal mucin secretion. Argyrophilic granules can be demonstrated by the Sevier-Munger or Grimelius technique, and dense-core granules are consistently found by electron microscopy.[174,181,185] Some cases have been associated with ACTH and serotonin production.[173,191] Some tumors, presumably lesser differentiated, lack these ultrastructural and histochemical markers but are otherwise identical morphologically and behaviorally.[165] The prognosis is very poor; most patients die quickly with generalized metastases.[187] This tumor probably arises from the same multipotent epithelial basal cells that give rise to conventional epidermoid carcinoma.[172] Supporting this contention is the fact that it may be found closely intermingled with in situ or invasive epidermoid carcinoma.[166,188]

Small cell carcinoma should be clearly separated from the better differentiated *carcinoid tumor*.[164,190] This vanishingly rare neoplasm probably arises from the endocrine cells ordinarily present in the normal esophageal mucosa and apparently representing a different population from basal melanocytes.[192]

SMOOTH MUSCLE TUMORS

Leiomyoma is the most common benign tumor of the esophagus.[202] In careful autopsy cases, the frequency of this tumor has been found to be almost 8%.[203] Half of the surgically excised cases are asymptomatic; dysphagia and vague thoracic pain are the main complaints in the others.[201] The majority arise from the inner circular muscle and are more common in the distal third.[203] Multiple leiomyomas occur and need to be distinguished from giant muscular hypertrophy (see p. 469). Grossly, leiomyomas from well-defined masses in the esophageal wall and have a solid, grayish white appearance on cross section. When they grow intraluminally, they encroach on the mucosa and appear as a sessile or pedunculated polyp. Ulceration of the overlying mucosa is a rare event, in contrast to its common occurrence in gastric leiomyomas.

Esophageal leiomyomas can encircle the entire esophagus in its lower third and constrict it.[198] Microscopically, they have the usual characteristics of a benign smooth muscle tumor. Local resection or enucleation is usually successful.[199]

Leiomyosarcomas are quite unusual in the esophagus, in contrast to the lower gastrointestinal tract.[197] Grossly, they may be indistinguishable from leiomyoma, although they tend to be larger and softer and often are associated with areas of hemorrhage and necrosis.[200] The presence of a large number of mitotic figures is the main microscopic criterion by which they are separated from their benign counterpart.

OTHER TUMORS AND TUMORLIKE CONDITIONS

Benign *fibrovascular polyps* (inflammatory fibrous polyps; inflammatory pseudotumors) of the esophagus usually are pedunculated and solitary. They may attain giant proportions.[225] Patients present with dysphagia and sometimes with intermittent regurgitation of a fleshy mass in the mouth. Death from asphyxia can result from laryngeal impaction. Most of the fifty-three cases reviewed by Jang et al.[213] occurred in adults. About 85% were located in the upper third of the esophagus. Microscopically, they are composed of fibrous tissue and numerous blood vessels, with stromal edema and occasional lymphocytic infiltration.[227a] The overlying mucosa often is ulcerated. These polyps most likely represent a reactive condition. Local excision is curative.[214]

Squamous papillomas rarely occur in the esophagus.[210]

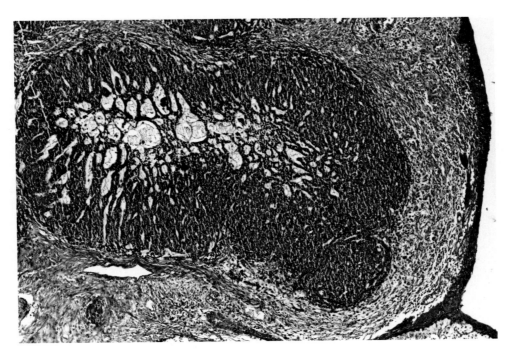

Fig. 11-20 Basaloid carcinoma of esophagus. Surface epithelium was involved by squamous carcinoma in situ. Invasive component grows in form of islands, which contain cystic spaces with mucin. There is vague resemblance to adenoid cystic carcinoma.

Winkler et al.[227] detected in some of these papillomas and in smaller esophageal lesions that they called *focal epithelial hyperplasia* evidence of human papilloma virus infection, both on microscopic and immunohistochemical grounds.

Granular cell tumors have been described in the esophagus, as either solitary or multiple nodules; sometimes, they are associated with similar lesions in the stomach.[207,226] As in other sites, they can induce a pseudoepitheliomatous hyperplasia of the overlying epithelium. A malignant example has also been recorded.[219]

Other reported benign esophageal tumors include lobular capillary hemangioma,[221] neurofibroma,[224] and a peculiar benign pigmented tumor of probably neural origin.[205]

Localized *amyloidosis* (so-called amyloid tumor) can present as an intramural esophageal mass; in a case reported by Heitzman et al.[212] it resulted in perforation and hematemesis.

Sclerotherapy for bleeding esophageal varices may be complicated by superficial and deep mucosal ulceration, extensive fibrosis, and sometimes the formation of hematomas.[209,223]

Malignant melanoma as a primary esophageal neoplasm has been fully documented.[208] The tumor can be located at any level in the esophagus, with a predilection for the lower third.[218] Grossly, the tumor is usually large and has a prominent polypoid appearance.[215] Microscopically, epithelioid, spindle-cell, and pleomorphic areas may be seen singly or in combination. The amount of melanin produced is highly variable. S-100 protein positivity is the rule.[208] Search for a lateral intraepidermal component ("junctional activity") should be made in order to rule out a metastatic neoplasm. In some cases, the melanoma has been associated with focal or diffuse melanosis of the esophageal mucosa.[222] The prognosis is exceedingly poor.

Malignant lymphoma[216,220] and *plasmacytoma*[204] occasionally present with dysphagia because of diffuse esophageal involvement.

There have been isolated reports of *mesenchymal neoplasms* other than of smooth muscle origin, such as hemangiopericytoma[206] and osteosarcoma.[217]

Metastatic carcinoma in the esophagus usually represents extension from lung, larynx, or stomach tumors, either directly or via periesophageal nodes. Rarely, blood-borne metastases occur from carcinomas of distant sites, such as the prostate[211] or the endometrium.[228]

REFERENCES

ATRESIA AND RELATED ANOMALIES

1 Aprigliano F: Esophageal stenosis in children. Ann Otol Rhinol Laryngol **89:**391-396, 1980.

2 Clatworthy HW Jr: Esophageal atresia. Importance of early diagnosis and adequate treatment illustrated by a series of patients. Pediatrics **16:**122-128, 1955.

3 Holden MP, Wooler GH: Tracheooesophageal fistula and oesophageal atresia. Results of 30 years' experience. Thorax **25:**406-412, 1970.

4 Holder TM, Ashcraft KW: Esophageal atresia and tracheoesophageal fistula. Ann Thorac Surg **9:**445-467, 1970.

5 Holder TM, Cloud DT, Lewis JE Jr, Pilling GP IV: Esophageal atresia and tracheoesophageal fistula. A survey of its members by the Surgical Section of the American Academy of Pediatrics. Pediatrics **34:**542-549, 1964.

6 Rosenthal AH: Congenital atresia of the esophagus with tracheo-esophageal fistula. Arch Pathol **12:**756-772, 1931.

HETEROTOPIA

7 Bosher LH Jr, Taylor FH: Heterotopic gastric mucosa in the esophagus with ulceration and stricture formation. J Thorac Surg **21:**306-312, 1951.

8 Christensen WN, Sternberg SS: Adenocarcinoma of the upper esophagus arising in ectopic gastric mucosa. Two case reports and review of the literature. Am J Surg Pathol **11:**397-402, 1987.

9 Jabbari M, Goresky CA, Lough J, Yaffe C, Daly D, Côté C: The inlet patch. Heterotopic gastric mucosa in the upper esophagus. Gastroenterology **89:**352-356, 1985.

10 Merino MJ, Brand M, LiVolsi VA, McCallum RW: Sebaceous glands in the esophagus diagnosed in a clinical setting. Arch Pathol Lab Med **106:**47-48, 1982.

11 Rector LE, Connerley ML: Aberrant mucosa in the esophagus in infants and children. Arch Pathol **31:**285-294, 1941.

DIVERTICULA

12 Graham DY, Goyal RK, Sparkman J, Cogan ME, Pogonowska MJ: Diffuse intramural esophageal diverticulosis. Gastroenterology **68:**781-785, 1975.

13 Janes RM: Diverticula of the lower thoracic esophagus. Ann Surg **124:**637-652, 1946.

14 Lahey FH: Pharyngoesophageal diverticulum. Its management and complications. Ann Surg **124:**617-652, 1946.

15 Pierce WS, Johnson J: Squamous cell carcinoma in a pharyngoesophageal diverticulum. Cancer **24:**1068-1070, 1969.

16 Umlas J, Sakhuja R: The pathology of esophageal intramural pseudodiverticulosis. Am J Clin Pathol **65:**314-320, 1976.

17 Wychulis AR, Gunnlaugsson GH, Claggett OT: Carcinoma occurring in pharyngoesophageal diverticulum. Report of three cases. Surgery **66:**976-979, 1969.

CYSTS

18 McGregor DH, Mills G, Boudet RA: Intramural squamous cell carcinoma of the esophagus. Cancer **37:**1556-1561, 1976.

19 Ming SC: Tumors of the esophagus and stomach. In Atlas of tumor pathology, Second Series, Fasc. VII. Washington DC, 1971, Armed Forces Institute of Pathology, pp. 19-22.

RINGS AND WEBS

20 Clements JL Jr, Cox GW, Torres WE, Weens HS: Cervical esophageal webs—a roentgenanatomic correlation. Observations on the pharyngoesophagus. Am J Roentgenol Radium Ther Nucl Med **121:**221-231, 1974.

21 Goyal RK, Bauer JL, Spiro HM: The nature and location of lower esophageal ring. N Engl J Med **284:**1175-1180, 1971.

ACHALASIA AND RELATED MOTOR DISORDERS

22 Adams CWM, Brain RHF, Trounce JR: Ganglion cells in achalasia of the cardia. Virchows Arch [Pathol Anat] **372:**75-79, 1976.

23 Cassella RR, Brown AL Jr, Sayre GP, Ellis FJ Jr: Achalasia of the esophagus. Ann Surg **160:**474-487, 1964.

24 Cohen S: Motor disorders of the esophagus. N Engl J Med **301:**184-192, 1979.

25 Cruse JP, Edwards DAW, Smith JF, Wyllie JH: The pathology of a cricopharyngeal dysphagia. Histopathology **3:**223-232, 1979.

26 Ferguson TB, Woodbury JD, Roper CL, Burford TH: Giant muscular hypertrophy of the esophagus. Ann Thorac Surg **8:**209-218, 1969.

27 Hankins JR, McLaughlin JS: The association of carcinoma of the esophagus with achalasia. J Thorac Cardiovasc Surg **69:**355-360, 1975.

28 Heald J, Moussalli H, Hasleton PS: Diffuse leiomyomatosis of the oesophagus. Histopathology **10:**755-759, 1986.

29 Just-Viera JO, Haight C: Achalasia and carcinoma of the esophagus. Surg Gynecol Obstet **128:**1081-1095, 1969.

30 Misiewicz JJ, Waller SL, Anthony PP, Gummer JWP: Achalasia of the cardia. Pharmacology and histopathology of isolated cardiac sphincteric muscle from patients with and without achalasia. Q J Med **149:**17-30, 1969.

31 Palmer ED: Disorders of the cricopharyngeus muscle. A review. Gastroenterology **71:**510-519, 1976.

32 Puppel ID: The role of esophageal motility in the surgical treatment of megaesophagus. J Thorac Surg **19:**371-390, 1950.

33 Wychulis AR, Woolam GL, Andersen HA, Ellis FH Jr: Achalasia and carcinoma of the esophagus. JAMA **215:**1638-1641, 1971.

LYE STRICTURES

34 Appelqvist P, Salmo M: Lye corrosion carcinoma of the esophagus. A review of 63 cases. Cancer **45:**2655-2658, 1980.

35 Bigelow NH: Carcinoma of the esophagus developing at the site of lye stricture. Cancer 6:1159-1164, 1953.

36 Bosher LH Jr, Burford TH, Ackerman LV: The pathology of experimentally produced lye burns and strictures of the esophagus. J Thorac Surg 21:483-489, 1951.

37 Burford T, Webb WR, Ackerman LV: Caustic burns of the esophagus and their surgical management. Ann Surg 138:453-460, 1953.

38 Kiviranta UK: Corrosion of esophagus and stomach. Sequels and therapy. Clinical studies and follow-up examination of 379 patients. Acta Otolaryngol [Suppl] [Stockh] 81:1-128, 1949.

REFLUX ESOPHAGITIS

39 Allison PR: Peptic ulcer of the esophagus. Thorax 3:20-42, 1948.

40 Barrett NR: Chronic peptic ulcer of the oesophagus and "oesophagitis." Br J Surg 38:175-182, 1950.

41 Behar J, Sheahan DC: Histologic abnormalities in reflux esophagitis. Arch Pathol 99:387-391, 1975.

42 Belsey R: Peptic ulcer of the esophagus. Ann R Coll Surg Engl 14:303-322, 1954.

43 Brown LF, Goldman H, Antonioli DA: Intraepithelial eosinophils in endoscopic biopsies of adults with reflux esophagitis. Am J Surg Pathol 8:899-905, 1984.

44 Collins BJ, Elliott H, Sloan JM, McFarland RJ, Love AHG: Oesophageal histology in reflux oesophagitis. J Clin Pathol 38:1265-1272, 1985.

45 Geboes K, Desmet V, Vantrappen G: Esophageal histology in the early stage of gastroesophageal reflux [letter]. Arch Pathol Lab Med 103:205, 1979.

46 Ismail-Beigi F, Horton PF, Pope CE II: Histological consequences of gastroesophageal reflux in man. Gastroenterology 58:163-174, 1970.

47 Karl TR, Pindyck F, Sicular A: Zollinger-Ellison syndrome with esophagitis and Barrett mucosa. Am J Gastroenterol 78:611-614, 1983.

48 McKinley M, Sherlock P: Barrett's esophagus with adenocarcinoma in scleroderma. Am J Gastroenterol 79:438-440, 1984.

49 Sandry RJ: Pathology of reflux esophagitis. In Skinner DB, Belsey RHR, Hendrix TR, Zuidema GD (eds): Gastroesophageal reflux in hiatal hernia. Boston, 1972, Little, Brown & Co.

50 Sheahan DG, West AB: Focal lymphoid hyperplasia (pseudolymphoma) of the esophagus. Am J Surg Pathol 9:141-147, 1985.

51 Skinner DB: Pathophysiology of gastroesophageal reflux. Ann Surg 202:546-556, 1985.

52 Trier JS: Morphology of the epithelium of the distal esophagus in patients with midesophageal peptic strictures. Gastroenterology 58:444-461, 1970.

53 Tummala V, Barwick KW, Sontag SJ, Vlahcevic RZ, McCallum RW: The significance of intraepithelial eosinophils in the histologic diagnosis of gastroesophageal reflux. Am J Clin Pathol 87:43-48, 1987.

54 Yardley JH: Biopsy findings in low-grade reflux esophagitis. In Skinner DB, Belsey RHR, Hendrix TR, Zuidema GD (eds): Gastroesophageal reflux and hiatal hernia. Boston, 1972, Little, Brown & Co.

Barrett's esophagus

55 Berenson MM, Herbst JJ, Freston JW: Enzyme and ultrastructural characteristics of esophageal columnar epithelium. Am J Dig Dis 19:895-907, 1974.

56 Brand DL, Ylvisaker JT, Gelfand M, Pope CE II: Regression of columnar esophageal (Barrett's) epithelium after antireflux surgery. N Engl J Med 302:844-848, 1980.

57 Bremner CG, Lynch VP, Ellis FH Jr: Barrett's esophagus. Congenital or acquired? An experimental study of esophageal mucosal regeneration in the dog. Surgery 68:209-216, 1970.

57a Dahms BB, Greco MA, Strandjord SE, Rothstein FC: Barrett's esophagus in three children after antileukemia chemotherapy. Cancer 60:2896-2900, 1987.

58 Dahms BB, Rothstein FC: Barrett's esophagus in children. A consequence of chronic gastroesophageal reflux. Gastroenterology 86:318-323, 1984.

59 Griffin M, Sweeney EC: The relationship of endocrine cells, dysplasia and carcinoembryonic antigen in Barrett's mucosa to adenocarcinoma of the oesophagus. Histopathology 11:53-62, 1987.

60 Hamilton SR, Yardley JA: Regeneration of cardiac type mucosa and acquisition of Barrett mucosa after esophagogastrostomy. Gastroenterology 72:669-675, 1977.

61 Harrison CP: Where is the gastroesophageal junction? [letter]. Can Med Assoc J 99:867-868, 1968.

62 Hassall E, Weinstein WM, Ament ME: Barrett's esophagus in childhood. Gastroenterology 89:1331-1337, 1985.

63 Heitmann P, Csendes A, Strauszer T: Esophageal strictures and low esophagus lined with columnar epithelium. Am J Dig Dis 16:307-320, 1971.

64 Herlihy KJ, Orlando RC, Bryson JC, Bozymski EM, Carney CN, Powell DW: Barrett's esophagus. Clinical, endoscopic, histologic, manometric, and electrical potential difference characteristics. Gastroenterology 86:436-443, 1984.

65 Lee RG: Mucins in Barrett's esophagus. A histochemical study. Am J Clin Pathol 81:500-503, 1984.

66 Mossberg SM: The columnar-lined esophagus (Barrett's syndrome). An acquired condition? Gastroenterology 50:671-676, 1966.

67 Paull A, Trier JS, Dalton MD, Camp RC, Loeb P, Goyal RK: The histologic spectrum of Barrett's esophagus. N Engl J Med 295:476-480, 1976.

68 Peuchmaur M, Potet F, Goldfain D: Mucin histochemistry of the columnar epithelium of the oesophagus (Barrett's oesophagus). A prospective biopsy study. J Clin Pathol 37:607-610, 1984.

69 Pope CE II: Regression of Barrett's epithelium. In Spechler SJ, Goyal RK (eds): Barrett's esophagus. Pathophysiology, diagnosis, and management. New York, 1985, Elsevier Science, pp. 224-229.

70 Sjogren RW Jr, Johnson LF: Barrett's esophagus. A review. Am J Med 74:313-321, 1984.

71 Skinner DB, Walther BC, Riddell RH, Schmidt H, Iascone C, DeMeester TR: Barrett's esophagus. Ann Surg 198:554-566, 1983.

72 Spechler SJ, Goyal RK: Barrett's esophagus. N Engl J Med 315:362-371, 1986.

73 Takubo K: Squamous metaplasia with reserve cell hyperplasia in the esophagogastric junction zone. Acta Pathol Jpn 31:349-359, 1981.

Dysplasia and carcinoma in Barrett's esophagus

74 Banner, BF, Memoli VA, Warren WH, Gould VE: Carcinoma with multidirectional differentiation arising in Barrett's esophagus. Ultrastruct Pathol 4:205-217, 1983.

75 Berenson MM, Riddell RH, Skinner DB, Freston JW: Malignant transformation of esophageal columnar epithelium. Cancer 41:554-561, 1978.

76 Bozymski EM, Herlihy KJ, Orlando RC: Barrett's esophagus. Ann Int Med 97:103-107, 1982.

77 Cameron AJ, Ott BJ, Payne WS: The incidence of adenocarcinoma in columnar-lined (Barrett's) esophagus. N Engl J Med 313:857-859, 1985.

78 Chejfec G: Atypias, dysplasias, and neoplasias of the esophagus and stomach. Semin Diagn Pathol 2:31-41, 1985.

79 Cho KJ, Hunter TB, Whitehouse WM: The columnar-lined lower esophagus and its association with adenocarcinoma of the esophagus. Radiology 115:563-586, 1975.

80 Fein R, Kelsen DP, Geller N, Bains M, McCormack P, Brennan MF: Adenocarcinoma of the esophagus and gastroesophageal junction. Prognostic factors and results of therapy. Cancer 56:2512-2518, 1985.

81 Haggitt RC, Dean PJ: Adenocarcinoma in Barrett's epithelium. In Spechler SJ, Goyal RK (eds): Barrett's esophagus. Pathophysiology, diagnosis, and management. New York, 1985, Elsevier Science, pp. 153-166.

81a Haggitt RC, Reid BJ, Rabinovitch PS, Rubin CE: Barrett's esophagus. Correlation between mucin histochemistry, flow cytometry, and histologic diagnosis for predicting increased cancer risk. Am J Pathol 131:53-61, 1988.

82 Haggitt RC, Tryzelaar J, Ellis FH, Colcher H: Adencarcinoma complicating columnar epithelium–lined (Barrett's) esophagus. Am J Clin Pathol 70:1-5, 1978.

83 Hamilton SR, Smith RRL: The relationship between columnar epithelial dysplasia and invasive adenocarcinoma arising in Barrett's esophagus. Am J Clin Pathol 87:301-312, 1987.

84 Harle IA, Finley RJ, Belsheim M, Bondy DC, Booth M, Lloyd D, McDonald JWD, Sullivan S, Valberg LS, Watson WC, Frei JV, Slinger R, Troster M, Meads GE, Duff JH: Management of adenocarcinoma in a columnar-lined esophagus. Ann Thorac Surg 60:330-336, 1985.

85 Kalish RJ, Clancy PE, Orringer MB, Appelman HD: Clinical, epidemiologic, and morphologic comparison between adenocarcinomas arising in Barrett's esophageal mucosa and in the gastric cardia. Gastroenterology 86:461-467, 1984.

86 Lee RG: Adenomas arising in Barrett's esophagus. Am J Clin Pathol 85:629-632, 1986.

87 Lee RG: Dysplasia in Barrett's esophagus. A clinicopathologic study of six patients. Am J Surg Pathol 9:845-852, 1985.

88 MacDonald WC, MacDonald JB: Adenocarcinoma of the esophagus and/or gastric cardia. Cancer 60:1094-1098, 1987.

89 Neal AP, Savary M, Ozzello L: Columnar-lined lower esophagus. An acquired lesion with malignant predisposition. J Thorac Cardiovasc Surg 70:826-835, 1975.

89a Reid BJ, Haggitt RC, Rubin CE, Roth G, Surawicz CM, Van Belle G, Lewin K, Weinstein WM, Antonioli DA, Goldman H, MacDonald W, Owen D: Observer variation in the diagnosis of dysplasia in Barrett's esophagus. Hum Pathol 19:166-178, 1988.

90 Riddell RH: Dysplasia and regression in Barrett's epithelium. In Spechler SJ, Goyal RK (eds): Barrett's esophagus. Pathophysiology, diagnosis, and management. New York, 1985, Elsevier Science, pp. 143-152.

90a Robey SS, Hamilton SR, Gupta PK, Erozan YS: Diagnostic value of cytopathology in Barrett esophagus and associated carcinoma. Am J Clin Pathol **89**:493-498, 1988.

91 Rosenberg JC, Budev H, Edwards RC, Singal S, Steiger Z, Sundareson AS: Analysis of adenocarcinoma in Barrett's esophagus utilizing a staging system. Cancer **55**:1353-1360, 1985.

92 Sanfey H, Hamilton SR, Smith RRL, Cameron JL: Carcinoma arising in Barrett's esophagus. Surg Gynecol Obstet **161**:570-574, 1985.

93 Schmidt HG, Riddell RH, Walther B, Skinner DB, Riemann JF: Dysplasia in Barrett's esophagus. Cancer Res Clin Oncol **110**:145-152, 1985.

94 Smith RRL, Hamilton SR, Boitnott JK, Rogers EL: The spectrum of carcinoma arising in Barrett's esophagus. A clinicopathologic study of 26 patients. Am J Surg Pathol **8**:563-573, 1984.

95 Spechler SJ, Goyal RK: Barrett's esophagus. N Engl J Med **315**:362-371, 1986.

96 Spechler SJ, Robbins AH, Rubins HB, Vincent ME, Heeren T, Doos WG, Colton T, Schimmel EM: Adenocarcinoma and Barrett's esophagus. An overrated risk? Gastroenterology **87**:927-933, 1984.

97 Stillman AE, Selwyn JI: Primary adenocarcinoma of the esophagus arising in a columnar-lined esophagus. Am J Dig Dis **20**:557-582, 1975.

98 Thompson, JJ, Zinsser KR, Enterline HT: Barrett's metaplasia and adenocarcinoma of the esophagus and gastroesophageal junction. Hum Pathol **14**:42-61, 1983.

OTHER TYPES OF ESOPHAGITIS

99 Agha FP, Lee HH, Nostrant TT: Herpetic esophagitis. A diagnostic challenge in immunocompromised patients. Am J Gastroenterol **81**:246-253, 1986.

100 Dow CJ: Oesophageal tuberculosis. Four cases. Gut **22**:234-236, 1981.

101 Enterline H, Thompson J: Pathology of the esophagus. New York, 1984, Springer-Verlag.

102 Freedman PG, Dieterich DT, Balthazar EJ: Crohn's disease of the esophagus. Case report and review of the literature. Am J Gastroenterol **79**:835-838, 1984.

103 Freedman PG, Weiner BC, Balthazar EJ: Cytomegalovirus esophagogastritis in a patient with acquired immunodeficiency syndrome. Am J Gastroenterol **80**:434-437, 1985.

104 Haggitt RC, Meissner WA: Crohn's disease of the upper gastrointestinal tract. Am J Clin Pathol **59**:613-622, 1973.

105 Kaneko F, Mori M, Tsukinaga I, Miura Y: Pemphigus vulgaris of esophageal mucosa. Arch Dermatol **121**:272-273, 1985.

106 Lee RG: Marked eosinophilia in esophageal mucosal biopsies. Am J Surg Pathol **9**:475-479, 1985.

107 McDonald GB, Sharma P, Hackman RC, Meyers JD, Thomas ED: Esophageal infections in immunosuppressed patients after marrow transplantation. Gastroenterology **88**:1111-1117, 1985.

108 McKay JS, Day DW: Herpes simplex oesophagitis. Histopathology **7**:409-420, 1983.

109 McKenzie R, Khakoo R: Blastomycosis of the esophagus presenting with gastrointestinal bleeding. Gastroenterology **88**:1271-1273, 1985.

110 Mori S, Yoshihira A, Kawamura H, Takeuchi A, Hashimoto T, Inaba G: Esophageal involvement in Behcet's disease. Am J Gastroenterol **78**:548-553, 1983.

111 Orringer MB, Sloan H: Monilial esophagitis—an increasingly frequent cause of esophageal stenosis. Ann Thorac Surg **26**:364-374, 1978.

112 Young JA, Elias E: Gastro-oesophageal candidiasis. Diagnosis by brush cytology. J Clin Pathol **38**:293-296, 1985.

EPIDERMOID CARCINOMA
General features

113 Burkett FE, Johnson RL: Carcinoma of the esophagus twelve years after curative resection for carcinoma of the esophagus. Cancer **51**:2237-2331, 1983.

114 Crespi M, Muñoz N, Grassi A, Qiong S, Jing WK, Jien LJ: Precursor lesions of oesophageal cancer in a low-risk population in China. Comparison with high-risk populations. Int J Cancer **34**:599-602, 1984.

115 Goffman TE, McKeen EA, Curtis RE, Schein PS: Esophageal carcinoma following irradiation for breast cancer. Cancer **52**:1808-1809, 1983.

116 Kuylenstierna R, Munck-Wikland E: Esophagitis and cancer of the esophagus. Cancer **56**:837-839, 1985.

117 Maeta M, Koga S, Andachi H, Yoshioka H, Wakatsuki T: Esophageal cancer developed after gastrectomy. Surgery **95**:87-91, 1986.

118 Mandard AM, Chasle J, Marnay J, Villedieu B, Bianco C, Roussel A, Elie H, Vernhes JC: Autopsy findings in 111 cases of esophageal cancer. Cancer **48**:329-335, 1981.

119 Oettlé GJ, Paterson AC, Leiman G, Segal I: Esophagitis in a population at risk for esophageal carcinoma. Cancer **57**:2222-2229, 1986.

120 Rywlin AM, Ortega R: Glycogenic acanthosis of the esophagus. Arch Pathol **90**:439-443, 1970.

121 Schottenfeld D: Epidemiology of cancer of the esophagus, Semin Oncol **11**:92-100, 1984.

122 Stephens RL, Hansen HH, Muggia FM: Hypercalcemia in epidermoid tumors of the head and neck and esophagus. Cancer **31**:1487-1491, 1973.

122a Yang PC, Davis S: Incidence of cancer of the esophagus in the U.S. by histologic type. Cancer **61**:612-617, 1988.

Morphologic features and local spread

123 Burgess HM, Baggentoss AH, Moersch HJ, Clagett OT: Carcinoma of the esophagus. A clinical pathologic study. Surg Clin North Am **31**:965-976, 1951.

124 Drut R: Acantholytic squamous-cell carcinoma of the esophagus. Patología **15**:81-90, 1977.

125 Gunnlaugsson Gh, Wychulis AR, Roland C, Ellis FH Jr: Analysis of the records of 1,657 patients with carcinoma of the esophagus and cardia of the stomach. Surg Gynecol Obstet **130**:997-1005, 1970.

126 Kuwano H, Ueo H, Sugimachi K, Inokuchi K, Toyoshima S, Enjoji M: Glandular or mucus-secreting components in squamous cell carcinoma of the esophagus. Cancer **56**:514-518, 1985.

127 Mandard AM, Marnay J, Gignoux M, Segol P, Blanc L, Ollivier JM, Borel B, Mandard JC: Cancer of the esophagus and associated lesions. Detailed pathologic study of 100 esophagectomy specimens. Hum Pathol **15**:660-669, 1984.

128 Matsuura H, Sugimachi K, Ueo H, Kuwano H, Koga Y, Okamura T: Malignant potentiality of squamous cell carcinoma of the esophagus predictable by DNA analysis. Cancer **57**:1810-1814, 1986.

129 Sons HU, Borchard F: Esophageal cancer. Autopsy findings in 171 cases. Arch Pathol Lab Med **108**:983-988, 1984.

130 Sugimachi K, Koga Y, Mori M, Huang GJ, Yang K, Zhang RG: Comparative data on cytophotometric DNA in malignant lesions of the esophagus in the Chinese and Japanese. Cancer **59**:1947-1950, 1987.

131 Takubo K, Takai A, Takayama S, Sasajima K, Yamashita K, Fujita K: Intraductal spread of esophageal squamous cell carcinoma. Cancer **59**:1751-1757, 1987.

132 Tanner NC, Smithers DW (eds): Tumours of the oesophagus. In Smithers DW (gen ed): Neoplastic disease at various sites, vol. IV. London, 1961, E. & S. Livingstone Ltd.

133 Yates DR, Ross LG: Paget's disease of the esophageal epithelium. Arch Pathol **86**:447-452, 1968.

In situ and superficial spreading carcinoma

134 Ackerman LV, Weinstein IB, Kaplan HS, other members of Delegation: Cancer of the esophagus. In Kaplan HS, Tsuchitani PJ (eds): Cancer in China, New York, 1978, Alan R. Liss, Inc., pp. 111-136.

135 Kuwano H, Matsuda H, Matsuoka H, Kai H, Okudaira Y, Sugimachi K: Intraepithelial carcinoma concomitant with esophageal squamous cell carcinoma. Cancer **59**:783-787, 1987.

136 Muñoz N, Lipkin M, Crespi M, Wahrendorf J, Grassi A, Shih-Hsien L: Proliferative abnormalities of the oesophageal epithelium of Chinese populations at high and low risk for oesophageal cancer. Int J Cancer **36**:187-189, 1985.

137 Soga J, Tanaka O, Sasaki K, Kawaguchi M, Muto T: Superficial spreading carcinoma of the esophagus. Cancer **50**:1641-1645, 1982.

138 Ushigome S, Spjut HJ, Noon GP: Extensive dysplasia and carcinoma in situ of esophageal epithelium. Cancer **20**:1023-1029, 1967.

Metastases

139 Akiyama H, Tsurumaru M, Kawamura T, Ono Y: Principles of surgical treatment for carcinoma of the esophagus. Analysis of lymph node involvement. Ann Surg **194**:438-446, 1981.

140 Anderson LL, Lad TE: Autopsy findings in squamous-cell carcinoma of the esophagus. Cancer **50**:1587-1590, 1982.

141 Guernsey JM, Knudsen DF: Abdominal exploration in the evaluation of patients with carcinoma of the thoracic esophagus. J Thorac Cardiovasc Surg **59**:62-66, 1970.

142 Saito T, Iizuka T, Kato H, Watanabe H: Esophageal carcinoma metastatic to the stomach. A clinicopathologic study of 35 cases. Cancer **56**:2235-2241, 1985.

Diagnosis

143 Ackerman LV, Weinstein IB, Kaplan HS, other members of Delegation: Cancer of the esophagus. In Kaplan HS, Tsuchitani PJ (eds): Cancer in China. New York, 1978, Alan R. Liss, Inc., pp. 111-136.

144 Goldman H, Antonioli DA: Mucosal biopsy of the esophagus, stomach, and proximal duodenum. Hum Pathol **13**:423-448, 1982.
145 Kasugai T, Kobayashi S, Kuno N: Endoscopic cytology of the esophagus, stomach and pancreas. Acta Cytol [Baltimore] **22**:327-330, 1978.
146 MacDonald WC, Brandburg LL, Taniguchi L, Rubin CE: Esophageal exfoliative cytology. Ann Intern Med **59**:332-337, 1963.
147 Prolla JC, Reilly RW, Kirsner JB, Cockerham L: Direct vision endoscopic cytology and biopsy in the diagnosis of esophageal and gastric tumors. Current experience. Acta Cytol [Baltimore] **21**:399-402, 1977.
148 Prolla JC, Taebel DW, Kirsner JB: Current status of exfoliative cytology in diagnoses of malignant neoplasms of the esophagus. Surg Gynecol Obstet **121**:743-752, 1965.

Treatment and prognosis

149 Earlam R, Cunha-Melo JR: Oesophageal squamous cell carcinoma. I. A critical review of surgery. Br J Surg **67**:381-390, 1980.
150 Galandiuk S, Hermann RE, Cosgrove DM, Gassman JJ: Cancer of the esophagus. The Cleveland Clinic experience. Ann Surg **203**:101-108, 1986.
151 Giuli R, Sancho-Garnier H: Diagnostic, therapeutic, and prognostic features of cancers of the esophagus. Results of the international prospective study conducted by the OESO group (790 patients). Surgery **99**:614-622, 1986.
152 Hambraeus GM, Mercke CE, Hammar E, Landberg TG, Wang-Andersen W: Surgery alone or combined with radiation therapy in esophageal carcinoma. Cancer **48**:63-68, 1981.
153 Hancock SL, Glatstein E: Radiation therapy of esophageal cancer. Semin Oncol **11**:144, 1984.
154 Isono K, Onoda S, Ishikawa T, Sato H, Nakayama K: Studies on the causes of deaths from esophageal carcinoma. Cancer **49**:2173-2179, 1982.
155 Kelsen DP, Ahuja R, Hopfan S, Bains MS, Kosloff C, Martini N, McCormack P, Golbey RB: Combined modality therapy of esophageal carcinoma. Cancer **48**:131-137, 1981.
156 Marcial VA, Tomé JM, Ubiñas J, Bosch A, Correa JN: The role of radiation therapy in esophageal cancer. Radiology **87**:231-239, 1966.
157 Pearson JG: The value of radiotherapy in the management of squamous oesophageal cancer. Br J Surg **58**:794-798, 1971.
158 Pearson JG: The present status and future potential of radiotherapy in the management of esophageal cancer. Cancer **39**:882-890, 1977.
159 Skinner DB: Surgical treatment for esophageal carcinoma. Semin Oncol **11**:136-143, 1984.
160 Smithers DW: The treatment of carcinoma of the oesophagus. Ann R Coll Surg Engl **20**:36-49, 1957.
161 van Andel JG, Dees J, Dijkhuis CM, Fokkens W, van Houten H, de Jong PC, van Woerkom-Eykenboom WM: Carcinoma of the esophagus. Results of treatment. Ann Surg **190**:684-689, 1979.

OTHER TYPES OF CARCINOMA

162 Agha FP, Weatherbee L, Sams JS: Verrucous carcinoma of the esophagus. Am J Gastroenterol **79**:844-849, 1984.
163 Battifora H: Spindle cell carcinoma. Ultrastructural evidence of squamous origin and collagen production by the tumor cells. Cancer **37**:2275-2282, 1976.
164 Brenner S, Heimlich H, Widman M: Carcinoid of esophagus. NY State J Med **69**:1337-1339, 1969.
165 Briggs JC, Ibrahim NBN: Oat cell carcinoma of the oesophagus. A clinicopathological study of 23 cases. Histopathology **7**:261-277, 1983.
165a Chejfec G, Jablokow VR, Gould VE: Linitis plastica carcinoma of the esophagus. Cancer **51**:2139-2143, 1983.
166 Cook MG, Eusebi V, Betts CM: Oat-cell carcinoma of the oesophagus. A recently recognized entity. J Clin Pathol **29**:1068-1073, 1976.
167 Drut R: Carcinoma mucoepidermoide del esofago. Presentación de dos casos y revisión de la literatura. Patología **15**:163-169, 1977.
168 Du Boulay CEH, Isaacson P: Carcinoma of the oesophagus with spindle cell features. Histopathology **5**:403-414, 1981.
169 Epstein JI, Sears DL, Tucker RS, Eagan JW Jr: Carcinoma of the esophagus with adenoid cystic differentiation. Cancer **53**:1131-1136, 1984.
170 Fraser GM, Kinley CE: Pseudosarcoma with carcinoma of the esophagus. Arch Pathol **85**:325-330, 1968.
170a Gal AA, Martin SE, Kernen JA, Patterson MJ: Esophageal carcinoma with prominent spindle cells. Cancer **60**:2244-2250, 1987.
171 Hanada M, Nakano K, Ii Y, Yamashita H: Carcinosarcoma of the esophagus with osseous and cartilagenous production. A combined study of keratin immunohistochemistry and electron microscopy. Acta Pathol Jpn **34**:669-678, 1984.

172 Ho K-J, Herrera GA, Jones JM, Alexander CB: Small cell carcinoma of the esophagus. Evidence for a unified histogenesis. Hum Pathol **15**:460-468, 1984.
173 Horai T, Nishihara H, Tateishi R, Matsuda M, Hattori S: Oat-cell carcinoma of the lung simultaneously producing ACTH and serotonin. J Clin Endocrinol Metab **37**:212-219, 1973.
174 Imai T, Sannohe Y, Okano H: Oat cell carcinoma (apudoma) of the esophagus. A case report. Cancer **41**:358-364, 1978.
175 Kabuto T, Taniguchi K, Iwanaga T, Terasawa T, Sano M, Tateishi R, Taniguchi H: Primary adenoid cystic carcinoma of the esophagus. Report of a case. Cancer **43**:2452-2456, 1979.
176 Kuhajda FP, Sun T-T, Mendelsohn G: Polypoid squamous carcinoma of the esophagus. A case report with immunostaining for keratin. Am J Surg Pathol **7**:495-499, 1983.
177 Lagacé R, Schurch W, Seemayer TA: Carcinome polypoïde pseudosarcomateux. Histogènese. Evidence d'une réponse myofibroblastique. Ann Pathol **1**:27-37, 1981.
178 Linder J, Stein RB, Roggli VL, Vollmer RT, Croker BP, Postlethwait RW, Shelburne JD: Polypoid tumor of the esophagus. Hum Pathol **18**:692-700, 1987.
179 Majmudar B, Dillard R, Susann PW: Collision carcinoma of the gastric cardia. Hum Pathol **9**:471-473, 1978.
180 Martin MR, Kahn LB: So-called pseudosarcoma of the esophagus. Nodal metastases of the spindle cell element. Arch Pathol Lab Med **101**:604-609, 1977.
181 Matsusaka T, Watanabe H, Enjoji M: Anaplastic carcinoma of the esophagus. Report of three cases and their histogenetic consideration. Cancer **37**:1352-1358, 1976.
182 Matsusaka T, Watanabe H, Enjoji M: Pseudosarcoma and carcinosarcoma of the esophagus. Cancer **37**:1546-1555, 1976.
183 Minielly JA, Harrison EG Jr, Fontana RS, Payne WS: Verrucous squamous cell carcinoma of the esophagus. Cancer **20**:2078-2087, 1967.
184 Osamura RY, Shimamura K, Hata J, Tamaoki N, Watanabe K, Kubota M, Yamazaki S, Mitomi T: Polypoid carcinoma of the esophagus. A unifying term for "carcinosarcoma" and "pseudosarcoma." Am J Surg Pathol **2**:201-208, 1978.
185 Reyes CV, Chejfec G, Jao W, Gould VE: Neuroendocrine carcinomas of the esophagus. Ultrastruct Pathol **1**:367-376, 1980.
186 Rosenthal SN, Lemkin JA: Multiple small cell carcinomas of the esophagus. Cancer **51**:1944-1946, 1983.
187 Sabanathan S, Graham GP, Salama FD: Primary oat cell carcinoma of the oesophagus. Thorax **41**:318-321, 1986.
188 Sato T, Mukai M, Ando N, Tashiro Y, Iri H, Abe O, Watanabe Y: Small cell carcinoma (non-oat cell type) of the esophagus concomitant with invasive squamous cell carcinoma and carcinoma in situ. A case report. Cancer **57**:328-332, 1986.
189 Spagnolo DV, Heenan PJ: Collision carcinoma at the esophagogastric junction. Report of two cases. Cancer **46**:2702-2708, 1980.
190 Tanoue S, Shimoda T, Suzuki M, Ikegami M, Ishikawa E, Sano T: Anaplastic carcinoma of the esophagus. Acta Pathol Jpn **33**:831-841, 1983.
191 Tateishi R, Taniguchi K, Horai T, Iwanaga T, Taniguchi H, Kabuto T, Sano M, Ishiguro S, Wada A: Argyrophil cell carcinoma (apudoma) of the esophagus. A histopathologic entity. Virchows Arch [Pathol Anat] **371**:283-294, 1976.
192 Tateishi R, Taniguchi H, Wada A, Horai T, Taniguchi K: Argyrophil cells and melanocytes in esophageal mucosa. Arch Pathol **98**:87-89, 1974.
193 Wang HH, Antonioli DA, Goldman H: Comparative features of esophageal and gastric adenocarcinomas. Recent changes in type and frequency. Hum Pathol **17**:482-487, 1986.
194 Wain SL, Kier R, Vollmer RT, Bossen EH: Basaloid-squamous carcinoma of the tongue, hypopharynx, and larynx. Report of 10 cases. Hum Pathol **17**:1158-1166, 1986.
195 Weidner N: Sarcomatoid carcinoma of the upper aerodigestive tract. Semin Diagn Pathol **4**:157-168, 1987.
196 Woodard BH, Shelburn JD, Vollmer RT, Postlethwait RW: Mucoepidermoid carcinoma of the esophagus. A case report. Hum Pathol **9**:352-354, 1978.

SMOOTH MUSCLE TUMORS

197 Athanasoulis CA, Aral IM: Leiomyosarcoma of the esophagus. Gastroenterology **54**:271-274, 1968.
198 Harrington SW: Surgical treatment of benign and secondarily malignant tumors of the esophagus. Arch Surg **58**:646-661, 1949.
199 Lewis B, Maxfield RG: Leiomyoma of the esophagus. Case report and review of the literature. Int Abstr Surg **99**:2, 105-128, 1954.
200 Rainer WG, Brus R: Leiomyosarcoma of the esophagus. Review of the literature and report of 3 cases. Surgery **50**:343-350, 1965.
201 Seremetis MG, Lyons WS, deGuzman VC, Peabody JW Jr: Leiomyomata of the esophagus. An analysis of 838 cases. Cancer **38**:2166-2177, 1976.

202 Solomon MP, Rosenblum H, Rosato FE: Leiomyoma of the esophagus. Ann Surg **199:**246-248, 1984.

203 Takubo K, Nakagawa H, Tsuchiya S, Mitomo Y, Sasajima K, Shirota A: Seedling leiomyoma of the esophagus and esophagogastric junction zone. Hum Pathol **12:**1006-1010, 1981.

OTHER TUMORS AND TUMORLIKE CONDITIONS

204 Ahmed N, Ramos S, Sika J, LeVeen HH, Piccone VA: Primary extramedullary esophageal plasmacytoma. First case report. Cancer **38:**943-947, 1976.

205 Assor D: A melanocytic tumor of the esophagus. Cancer **35:**1438-1443, 1975.

206 Burke JS., Ranchod M: Hemangiopericytoma of the esophagus. Hum Pathol **12:**96-97, 1981.

207 de S Coutinho DS, Soga J, Yoshikawa T, Miyashita K, Tanaka O, Sasaki K, Muto T, Shimizu T: Granular cell tumors of the esophagus. A report of two cases and review of the literature. Am J Gastroenterol **80:**758-762, 1985.

208 DiCostanzo DP, Urmacher C: Primary malignant melanoma of the esophagus. Am J Surg Pathol **11:**46-52, 1987.

209 Evans DMD, Jones DB, Cleary BK, Smith PM: Oesophageal varices treated by sclerotherapy. A histopathological study. Gut **23:**615-620, 1982.

210 Goldman H, Antonioli DA: Mucosal biopsy of the esophagus, stomach, and proximal duodenum, Hum Pathol **13:**423-448, 1982.

211 Gore RM, Sparberg M: Metastatic carcinoma of the prostate to the esophagus. Am J Gastroenterol **77:**358-359, 1982.

212 Heitzman EJ, Heitzman GC, Elliott CF: Primary esophageal amyloidosis. Arch Intern Med **109:**595-600, 1962.

213 Jang GC, Clouse ME, Fleischner FG: Fibrovascular polyp—a benign intraluminal tumor of the esophagus. Radiology **92:**1196-1200, 1969.

214 LiVolsi VA, Perzin KH: Inflammatory pseudotumors (inflammatory fibrous polyps) of the esophagus. A clinicopathologic study. Am J Dig Dis **20:**475-481, 1975.

215 Ludwig ME, Shaw R, de Suto-Nagy G: Primary malignant melanoma of the esophagus. Cancer **48:**2528-2534, 1981.

216 Matsuura H, Saito R, Nakajima S, Yoshihara W, Enomoto T: Non-Hodgkin's lymphoma of the esophagus. Am J Gastroenterol **80:**941-946, 1985.

217 McIntyre M, Webb JN, Browning GCP: Osteosarcoma of the esophagus. Hum Pathol **13:**680-682, 1982.

218 Mills SE, Cooper PH: Malignant melanoma of the digestive system. Pathol Annu **18**(Pt 2):1-26, 1983.

219 Ohmori T, Arita N, Uraga N, Tabei R, Tani M, Okamura H: Malignant granular cell tumor of the esophagus. A case report with light and electron microscopic, histochemical, and immunohistochemical study. Acta Pathol Jpn **37:**775-783, 1987.

220 Okerbloom JA, Armitage JO, Zetterman R, Linder J: Esophageal involvement by non-Hodgkin's lymphoma, Am J Med **77:**359-361, 1984.

221 Okumura T, Tanoue S, Chiba K, Tanaka S: Lobular capillary hemangioma of the esophagus. A case report and review of the literature. Acta Pathol Jpn **33:**1303-1308, 1983.

222 Piccone VA, Klopstock R, LeVeen HH, Sika J: Primary malignant melanoma of the esophagus associated with melanosis of the entire esophagus. First case report. J Thorac Cardiovasc Surg **59:**865-870, 1970.

223 Pushpanathan C, Idikio H: Pathological findings in the esophagus after endoscopic sclerotherapy for variceal bleeding. Am J Gastroenterol **81:**9-13, 1986.

224 Saitoh K, Nasu M, Kamiyama R, Hatakeyama S, Maruyama M, Tsuruta K, Takeshita K: Solitary neurofibroma of the esophagus. Acta Pathol Jpn **35:**527-531, 1985.

225 Totten RS, Stout AP, Humphreys GH II, Moore RL: Benign tumors and cysts of the esophagus. J Thorac Surg **25:**606-622, 1953.

226 Vuyk HD, Snow GB, Tiwari RM, van Velzen D, Veldhuizen RW: Granular cell tumor of the proximal esophagus. A rare disease. Cancer **55:**445-449, 1985.

227 Winkler B, Capo V. Reumann W, Ma A, La Porta R, Reilly S, Green PMR, Richart RM, Crum CP: Human papillomavirus infection of the esophagus. A clinicopathologic study with demonstration of papillomavirus antigen by the immunoperoxidase technique. Cancer **55:**149-155, 1985.

227a Wolf BC, Khettry U, Leonardi HK, Neptune WB, Bhattacharyya AK, Legg MA: Benign lesions mimicking malignant tumors of the esophagus. Hum Pathol **19:**148-154, 1988.

228 Zarian LP, Berliner L, Redmond P: Metastatic endometrial carcinoma to the esophagus. Am J Gastroenterol **78:**9-11, 1983.

Stomach

NORMAL ANATOMY

The stomach is divided grossly into three regions: cardia, fundus, and antrum. These correspond roughly but not exactly to the three major microscopic types of gastric mucosa: cardiac, fundic, and pyloric (antral), with transitional areas in between.[1,2,4] Cardiac and pyloric mucosa are similar: foveolae (crypts, pits) occupy the upper half and mucus-secreting glands occupy the lower half. Looser packing of the glands and presence of occasional cysts in cardiac mucosa are the only two minor microscopic differences that exist compared with the pyloric mucosa. Fundic mucosa is characterized by foveolae, which occupy only one fourth of the thickness, and straight glands of composite cell distribution, including chief cells (pepsin-secreting), parietal cells (acid-secreting), and mucous neck cells. Endocrine cells of a variety of types also exist throughout the stomach; G-cells (gastrin-secreting) predominate in the pyloric mucosa and enterochromaffin-like (ECL) cells in the fundic mucosa. Silver stains, immunohistochemistry, or electron microscopy are needed for their identification.[3] The foveola is the most important area in the genesis of gastric carcinoma, in particular the layer of generative cells located at the base.[2]

HETEROTOPIC TISSUES

Heterotopic pancreas can present clinically as a gastric mass or is found incidentally at autopsy or at laparotomy.[6] Grossly, it may form a hemispheric mass, a symmetric cone, or a short cylindric nipple-like projection. In the latter instance, one or more ducts are usually seen emptying on the gastric lumen; this feature constitutes an important diagnostic sign radiographically (Fig. 11-21). Approximately 85% of these lesions occur in the submucosa and most of the others in the muscular layer. Most of these are located in the antrum (61%) or pylorus (24%).[6] Grossly, the cut surface looks like normal pancreas except for the occasional occurrence of cystic structures. Microscopically, pancreatic acini and ducts are always present, but islets are seen in only one third of the cases. Some cases of intramural gastric carcinoma are said to have arisen in these heterotopic tissues.[5]

The lesion described as **gastric adenomyoma** is closely related to heterotopic pancreas. It is probably a hamartoma rather than a true neoplasm, the usual components being large ducts, Brunner's glands, and prominent smooth muscle bundles.[7]

HYPERTROPHIC PYLORIC STENOSIS

This is one of the most common congenital anomalies. Most patients are males, and the most common age of onset is between 3 and 12 weeks. The gross appearance is that of a greatly thickened pyloric muscle, which occludes the pyloric channel and partially obstructs the gastric outflow. The etiology remains obscure; a ganglion dysfunction similar to that of esophageal achalasia has been postulated. The operation of choice is the Fredet-Ramstedt pyloromyotomy, which basically consists of a linear incision through the hypertrophic muscle, leaving the mucosa intact. Usually no tissue is resected in this procedure. The few microscopic studies that have been done on this condition have shown no alterations of note.[8]

Hypertrophy of the pylorus in the adult is a rare condition. Approximately 80% of the cases have occurred in males.

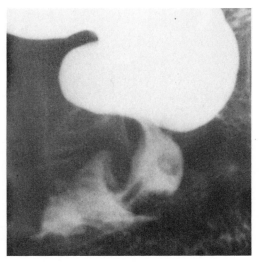

Fig. 11-21 Heterotopic pancreatic tissue presenting as small round nodule with central umbilication in antrum.

Roentgenographically and clinically, a tumor may be suspected. In rare instances, the stomach is resected because of an erroneous diagnosis of neoplasm. Grossly and microscopically, all that is found is hypertrophy of the pyloric circular muscle fibers that ends abruptly at the duodenum, sometimes accompanied by a mild degree of fibrosis. Chronic gastritis is usually present.[9,10,12]

The presence of pyloric hypertrophy in an adult in the absence of another gastric abnormality is exceptional.[11] Although it is possible that some of the cases represent a

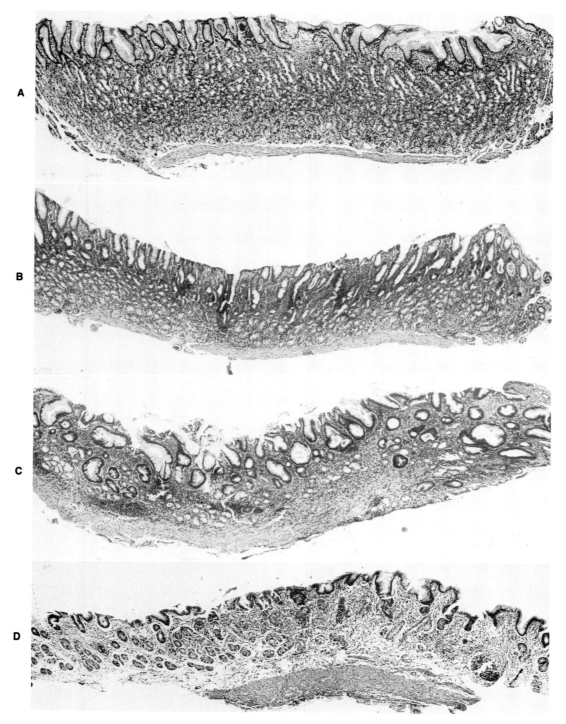

Fig. 11-22 Panoramic view of normal gastric mucosa, **A,** and of chronic gastritis with mild, **B,** moderate, **C,** and severe, **D,** degrees of atrophy. All of these biopsies were taken from fundic region.

persistence of the infantile form into adult life, in most instances the process is probably secondary to antral gastritis or peptic ulcer of the pyloric channel, which may have healed by the time of surgery. It is also well to remember that the gross appearance of pyloric hypertrophy can be simulated by linitis plastica.

CHRONIC GASTRITIS

The concept of chronic gastritis has been greatly clarified by the systematic use of endoscopic gastric biopsy.[21,25] The two main features of this disease are infiltration of the lamina propria by inflammatory cells and atrophy of the glandular epithelium. Plasma cells and lymphocytes (with occasional formation of follicles) predominate among the inflammatory cells, but eosinophils and neutrophils may also be present. If an inflammatory infiltrate limited to the foveolar region is the only abnormality seen, the condition is designated as **chronic superficial gastritis.** When the inflammation is more extensive and accompanied by glandular atrophy, the condition is termed **chronic atrophic gastritis** and is further categorized as mild, moderate, or severe by roughly estimating the thickness of the glandular portion in relation to the thickness of the whole mucosa[37,38] (Fig. 11-22). Naturally, a properly oriented biopsy containing muscularis mucosae is needed to make this estimation. If thinning of the mucosa is seen in the absence of inflammatory changes, the condition is designated **gastric atrophy,** although in most cases this probably represents the end stage of a chronic atrophic gastritis. Increasing degrees of atrophy are commonly associated with cystic dilatation of glands and metaplasia.

Two types of **metaplastic changes** can occur in chronic gastritis, sometimes together: pyloric metaplasia of the fundic mucosa and intestinal metaplasia. The latter refers to the progressive replacement of the gastric mucosa by epithelium having light and electron microscopic features of intestinal epithelium, including goblet cells, absorptive (brush border) cells, Paneth cells, and a variety of endocrine cells[14,28,32,34] (Fig. 11-23). In advanced cases, structures resembling small bowel villi are formed. Intestinal metaplasia has been further divided into complete or type I and incomplete or type II. In the latter, absorptive cells are absent whereas columnar cells with the appearance of gastric foveolar cells are retained.[13,27,31] Subnuclear vacuolization of mucous cells sometimes occurs and should not be misinterpreted as an expression of metaplasia.[35a]

Histochemically, the predominant mucin present in complete intestinal metaplasia is sialomucin, with small amounts of sulphomucins and/or neutral mucins; in the incomplete form, there may be predominance of either neutral mucins (type IIA) or sulphomucins (type IIB).[24] Intestinal metaplasia is also accompanied by increased immunoreactivity for the secretory component of immunoglobulins.[36] Type IIB intestinal metaplasia is said to show a closer association with gastric carcinoma than the other types.[19,23,33]

Endoscopically and grossly, well-developed atrophic gastritis produces a thin, smooth mucosa with undue prominence of submucosal vessels. In most cases, the disease seems to begin in the antrum and progress proximally, so that the fundic-pyloric border rises up gradually.[17] This

form, by far the most frequent, is referred to as *type B* or *nonimmune gastritis* in some classification schemes.[35] It has been further subdivided into a type that is restricted to the antrum and is associated with hyperchlorhydria and often duodenal peptic ulceration *(hypersecretory gastritis)* and one that involves both antrum and fundus in an initially patchy and eventually diffuse distribution *(environmental gastritis).*[16,25,26] It is the latter that shows an epidemiologic and pathogenetic relationship with gastric carcinoma.

The other major form of gastritis, designated at *type A* or *immune,*[35] usually affects the fundus in a diffuse manner, spares the antrum, and is associated with antibodies to parietal cells, hypochlorhydria or achlorhydria, and high serum gastrin levels; this form may evolve into pernicious anemia.

There is an excellent correlation between the degree of gastric atrophy as estimated by endoscopic biopsy and the results of acid secretory tests. Conversely, the correlation of histology with symptomatology, radiology, and gastroscopy has been disappointing. We have found severe atrophic gastritis in asymptomatic individuals and a normal gastric mucosa in patients with persistent dyspepsia.

Chronic atrophic gastritis is the rule in cases of gastric cancer and in general its severity is proportional to the extent of the tumor.[22] Most cases of gastric peptic ulcer are associated with antral and fundic gastritis, whereas in duodenal ulcer the gastritis, if present at all, is restricted to the antrum. Morson[29] has studied the incidence and extent of intestinal metaplasia and found it greatest in stomachs removed for carcinoma, least in those with duodenal ulcer, and intermediate in cases of gastric ulcer.

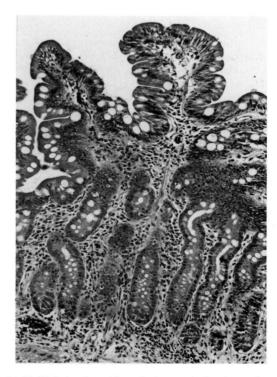

Fig. 11-23 Well-developed intestinal metaplasia of complete type. Numerous goblet cells are present.

The etiology of chronic gastritis is complex and probably multifactorial. Agents found to be associated with this disorder include alcohol, tobacco, duodenal reflux, allergy to foods, various drugs (particularly anti-inflammatory agents), and the already-mentioned immunologic factors.[13,30] The etiologic role of *Campylobacter pyloridis*, a curved spirochete-like organism, remains controversial, although most authors favor a direct relationship.[15,18,38a] This organism can be identified with a Giemsa or with silver technique similar to that used for other spirochetes.[20]

OTHER TYPES OF GASTRITIS

Acute gastritis may result from the ingestion of alcohol, salicylates and other anti-inflammatory drugs, or by the reflux of bile salts. Endoscopic biopsies, rarely taken in this condition, may show hyperemia, focal fresh hemorrhage, focal necrosis of surface and foveolar cells, and neutrophilic infiltration of the foveolar and glandular lumina.[46]

The common *acute infectious nonbacterial gastroenteritis* (induced by the Norwalk agent) is not associated with a histologically detectable gastric mucosal lesion, at least in its mild form.[60]

In *allergic gastroenteritis*, gastric biopsy shows infiltration of the lamina propria by eosinophils, which in severe cases is diffuse and accompanied by degenerative and regenerative changes of the surface and foveolar epithelium.[47]

Hemorrhagic gastritis is an acute life-threatening condition usually engrafted on a background of chronic gastritis.[62] Alcoholism, anti-inflammatory drugs, and stress have been implicated as precipitating factors.[43] The appearance of the stomach at surgery is characterized by multiple, minute areas of hemorrhage throughout the entire mucosa. The microscopic appearance is not as dramatic as the surgical findings would anticipate. In some cases, multiple superficial erosions are found (and the term *erosive gastritis* is therefore used), but in many others the only abnormality seen in the biopsy is a chronic atrophic gastritis, with perhaps some extravasation of blood in the lamina propria. In Lulu and Dragstedt's series,[51] the overall mortality was 55%. They advocated vagotomy and high subtotal gastrectomy as the treatment of choice.

The diffuse gastric condition often seen as a complication of portal hypertension and sometimes leading to severe hemorrhage is often reported as a form of hemorrhagic gastritis, but the microscopic changes are more consistent with mucosal vascular ectasia ("congestive gastropathy"), with secondary and usually mild inflammatory changes.[52]

Diffuse eosinophilic gastroenteritis involves the distal portion of the stomach and proximal portion of the duodenum and can cause pyloric obstruction.[49,50,54] It may be associated with allergic phenomena and extreme eosinophilia.[57] Microscopically, edema and diffuse infiltration by eosinophils are prominent. Necrotizing angiitis has been observed in some cases.[53] The lesion probably represents in most cases a local reaction to ingested allergens. Ashby et al.[39] concluded that many of their cases were secondary to infestation by *Eustoma rotundatum*, a parasite of the North Sea herring. In other instances, the disease may be a manifestation of a collagen-vascular disease, such as scleroderma, polymyositis, or polyarteritis.[42] Diffuse eosinophilic gastroenteritis should be distinguished from other disorders in which eosinophils may be numerous, such as inflammatory fibroid polyp (see p. 497), malignant lymphoma, and even carcinoma. There is no evidence that diffuse eosinophilic gastroenteritis and inflammatory fibroid polyp are related conditions.

Granulomatous gastritis can be caused by tuberculosis,[41] mycosis, sarcoidosis,[58] or Crohn's disease.[44,48]

Syphilis of the stomach, now extremely rare, begins as an erosive or ulcerative lesion in the pyloric portion.[40] In later stages, the stomach is shrunken and fibrotic, with a leather bottle appearance that simulates radiographically and grossly linitis plastica.[56,61] Microscopically, there is ulceration, chronic inflammation rich in plasma cells, and fibrosis; endarteritis obliterans may also be present.

Malakoplakia can present as a focal gastric lesion. As in other sites, the disease is characterized microscopically by a predominantly histiocytic inflammatory infiltrate containing Michaelis-Guttman bodies.[45,55]

Cytomegalovirus infection has been diagnosed in gastric biopsies of bone marrow transplant recipients and other immunocompromised patients; the finding is indicative of generalized disease.[59]

PEPTIC AND OTHER BENIGN ULCERS

Peptic ulcer can occur wherever mucosa is bathed by gastric secretion. This includes stomach, duodenum, lower third of esophagus, the margin of a gastrojejunostomy, and Meckel's diverticulum with ectopic gastric mucosa. Acid peptic digestion is the ultimate cause for ulceration, but the mechanism that renders the mucosa susceptible to this digestion is poorly understood.[66,69] Duodenal ulcers (which are more common than gastric ulcers, although their relative incidence seems to be decreasing) are classically associated with acid hypersecretion, but most patients with gastric ulcer secrete either low normal or below normal amounts of acid. Thus it would seem that the initial event in gastric ulcer is mucosal injury, which renders it more susceptible to acid peptic damage. This injury may be mediated in some instances by reflux of bile and pancreatic juice and is manifested anatomically by the presence of gastritis, an almost invariable finding in patients with peptic ulcer disease.

Acute gastric ulcer is a common finding at autopsy and is usually a terminal event. It may also be seen during life in any debilitating illness, in sepsis, following surgery or trauma (stress ulcer), in patients with central nervous injury of disease (Cushing's ulcer), as a complication of long-term steroid therapy (steroid ulcer), in association with aspirin ingestion, in patients with extensive burns (Curling's ulcer), as a complication of radiation therapy or hepatic arterial chemotherapy, and following the introduction of tubes into the stomach.[64,68,72,74,75] If the ulcer involves only the mucosa (a process usually designated as *erosion*), it can heal completely, but if part of the muscle is destroyed, it is replaced by fibrotic tissue leaving a depressed pit. Any of these ulcers, if deep enough, may perforate; this complication is particularly common in those induced by radiation therapy (Fig. 11-24).

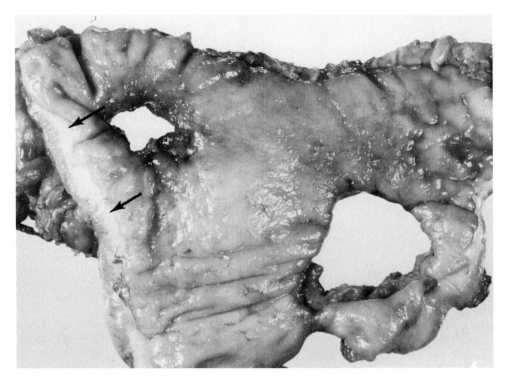

Fig. 11-24 Subtotal resection of stomach showing two large well-delimited ulcers. Arrows indicate prominent submucosal fibrosis elsewhere in stomach. Patient had received intensive irradiation for Hodgkin's disease.

Chronic peptic ulcer always occurs in an achlorhydric zone of mucosa, i.e., an area of stomach lined by antral type of mucosa. Up 95% of the ulcers are located on the lesser curvature (so-called *Magenstrasse*) near the incisura angularis; however, since chronic gastritis is accompanied by antral metaplasia of the fundal mucosa that progresses proximally from the pylorus, peptic ulcer can be found anywhere in the stomach, although always surrounded by antral-type mucosa.

The average age at the time of diagnosis is 50 years, but the disease can occur in any age group, including children. A male predilection exists but seems to be decreasing. About 5% of the ulcers are multiple. The radiographic diagnosis is about 95% accurate, but atypical cases cannot be distinguished with certainty from carcinoma. Although some controversy persists, most authors believe that ulcers of giant size (over 3 cm) or located in the greater curvature do not indicate a high likelihood of malignancy, as formerly believed.[67] The diagnosis of peptic ulcer has been greatly facilitated by the introduction of fiberoptic gastroscopy, which allows the endoscopist to have a direct view of the ulcer, to photograph it, and to obtain biopsies from the edges; multiple (about ten) biopsies are recommended for the standard-size ulcer.

Grossly, an active lesion is sharply delineated, usually oval or round but sometimes linear, with converging mucosal folds extending to its margin (Figs. 11-25 and 11-26). The proximal margin tends to have overhanging edges, whereas the distal margin usually has sloping borders. On section, there is undermining of the edges (especially on the proximal side) and complete replacement of the muscle wall by grayish-white fibrous tissue (Fig. 11-27). On the serosal side, one often sees subserosal fibrosis and inflammatory enlargement of the regional lymph nodes. Prominent marginal nodularity about the ulcer should suggest the presence of carcinoma; however, it should be remembered that in some instances it is impossible to distinguish grossly a peptic ulcer from an ulcerated carcinoma. As a matter of fact, about 10% to 15% of gastric carcinomas appear grossly to be benign ulcers.

Microscopically, an active, well-developed, chronic peptic ulcer will show four more or less distinct layers: (1) a surface coat of purulent exudate, bacteria, and necrotic debris; (2) fibrinoid necrosis; (3) granulation tissue; and (4) fibrosis replacing the muscle wall and extending into the subserosa. At the edges, the muscularis mucosae is seen to fuse with the muscularis externa. Other common features in the ulcer bed include thickening of vessels due to subendothelial fibrous proliferation (Fig. 11-28) and hypertrophy of nerve bundles; both of these changes are probably secondary events. The necrotic surface may show superimposed infection by *Candida albicans*.[70]

Peptic ulcers can be classified according to their shape and size (round-oval, giant, linear), activity (open ulcers or ulcer scars), depth of penetration (submucosa, muscularis externa, or beyond), or a combination of these criteria.[73]

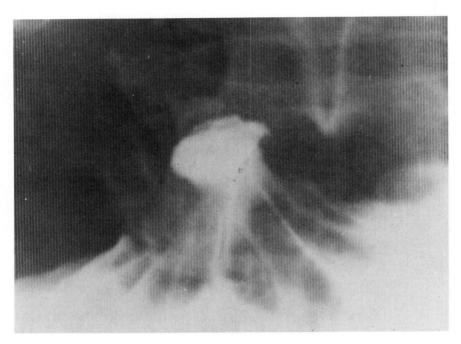

Fig. 11-25 Converging mucosal folds, so well seen in chronic ulcer shown in Fig. 11-26, can also be seen roentgenographically.

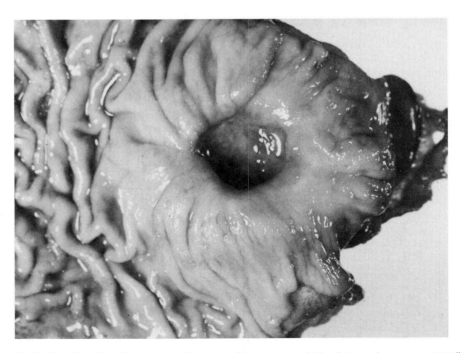

Fig. 11-26 Sharply delimited chronic gastric ulcer with converging folds of stomach mucosa extending right to margin of ulcer. Ulcer occurred in 53-year-old man.

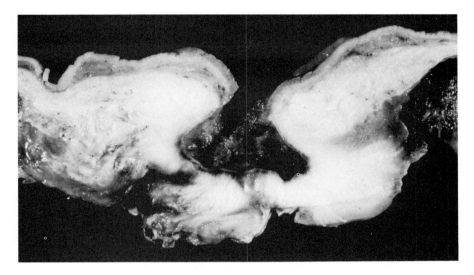

Fig. 11-27 Typical gross appearance of chronic peptic ulcer. Entire thickness of muscular layer has been destroyed.

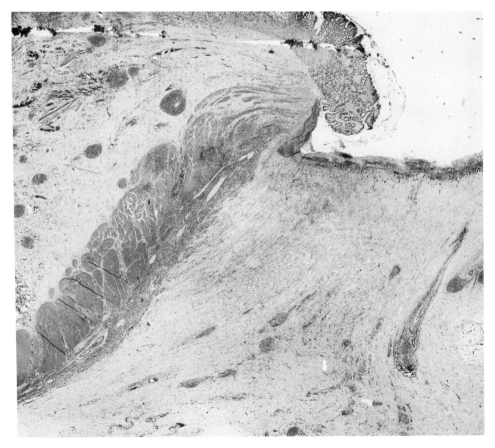

Fig. 11-28 Chronic ulcer of stomach. Base is completely replaced by fibrous tissue, proximal area has overhanging mucosal borders, and muscle has been displaced because of fibrosis.

In the healing process of a peptic ulcer, regenerating epithelium grows over the surface. Any epithelium growing above an area where the muscularis mucosae is interrupted is to be regarded as regenerating. This epithelium often exhibits features of intestinal metaplasia and may contain chief and parietal cells when the ulcer is located in the fundic area[73]; presence of irregularities in its deep portion should not be misinterpreted as carcinoma. The danger of overdiagnosis is particularly great in the ulcers due to arterial infusion chemotherapy because of the marked epithelial atypia that may be present.[75] The problem of the possible malignant transformation of peptic ulcer is discussed in the carcinoma section (see p. 504)

The medical treatment of gastric ulcer consists of antacids and/or H_2-blockers.[71] The usual criterion for adequate healing is a reduction in crater size of at least 50% over a 6- to 8-week period of intensive medical management. Failure to pass this test, development of complications (hemorrhage, perforation, obstruction), or recurrence of the ulcer are indications for surgery. Giant ulcer size (over 3 cm) is another quoted indication, although medical therapy can also be successful in these cases.[63] It should be remembered that as many as 15% of gastric carcinomas may pass the "healing test" and that some benign ulcers may actually enlarge during the test. The surgical procedures in general use for peptic ulcer are subtotal gastric resection without vagotomy, truncal vagotomy and drainage (either gastroenterostomy or pyloroplasty), and truncal vagotomy plus antrectomy. When a portion of stomach is removed, continuity is reestablished through a gastroduodenostomy (Billroth I) or gastrojejunostomy (Billroth II). The long-term results of surgery are good to excellent in over 80% of the patients.[65]

OTHER NON-NEOPLASTIC LESIONS

Duplication of the stomach, a very rare anomaly, presents as a unilocular or multilocular cyst lined by gastric mucosa. It may communicate with the lumen of the normal stomach; usually it does not, the result being distension with fluid causing obstruction and a palpable mass.[82,93]

Diverticula occur for the most part in a juxtacardiac position and are probably the result of anatomically weak areas. The remaining lesions can occur anywhere else in the stomach and are commonly associated with an acquired disease, such as peptic ulcer.[79]

Cysts may be found in a mucosal or submucosal location. Intramucosal cysts, which are the most common, have been classified into various types according to their lining; they appear to be associated with intestinal metaplasia. Submucosal cysts have also been designated as *gastritis cystica profunda*.[81] Both of these are said to be more common in patients with gastric carcinoma.[84,86,96,99] Although some may be an expression of heterotopia,[98] it seems likely that the majority are acquired.[84]

Bezoars are foreign bodies in the stomach and are occasionally seen as surgical specimens. The great majority fall into two categories: *trichobezoar*, composed of hair, and *phytobezoar*, composed of vegetable matter.[83] More than 85% of the latter are caused by ingestion of unripened

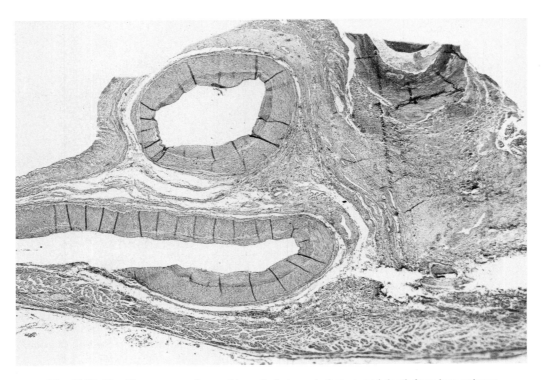

Fig. 11-29 Cirsoid aneurysm of vessel in wall of stomach that caused death from hemorrhage.

persimmons.[78] Factors favoring the development of bezoars include lack of teeth, vagotomy, and obstructing lesions of the gastric outlet.[76]

Aneurysms of gastric vessels (Dieulafoy's disease; caliber-persistent artery) are thought to be of malformative rather than degenerative origin.[90,91] They are usually single, located in the submucosa, usually high on the lesser curvature, and characterized by a large tortuous vessel surmounted by a small defect in the overlying mucosa[91] (Fig. 11-29). Amyloid may deposit in the vessel wall.[97] When the lesion perforates, massive and sometimes fatal hemorrhage may result.[89]

Antral vascular ectasia ("watermelon stomach") has been described as an acquired vascular disease of the stomach that may result in blood loss and iron deficient anemia. Endoscopically, one sees parallel red stripes at the crest of the mucosal folds in the antrum, resembling the stripes of a watermelon. The microscopic changes on gastric biopsy are minimal and consist of an increase in the number and caliber of vessels, fibrin thrombi, and fibromuscular hyperplasia.[96a] It remains to be seen whether this is a real entity.

Xanthoma (xanthelasma) of the stomach appears as a small yellow intramucosal lesion characterized by the accumulation of neutral fat in foamy histiocytes in the lamina propria. This clinically insignificant lesion, which seems to be relatively common in Japan and was described many years ago by German pathologists as *Lipoidinsel der Magenschleinhaut,* should not be confused microscopically with early carcinoma or signet ring carcinoma.[95]

Other rare non-neoplastic gastric disorders include *pseudoxanthoma elasticum* (which can result in severe hemorrhage),[77] *elastofibroma* (accompanied by similar lesions in their usual soft tissue location),[80] *hyalinization* (severe hyaline thickening of the submucosa),[88,94] *amyloidosis* (diffuse or localized, sometimes complicated by bleeding),[85] *barium granuloma* (developing in the gastric wall following radiographic examination),[87] and isolated *histiocytosis X.*[92]

POLYPS

The nomenclature of gastric polyps is confusing, one of the reasons being that in the past they have often been regarded as analogous to colorectal polyps in microscopic appearance and natural history.[113,117] This is unfortunate because most types of gastric polyps do not have an exact counterpart in the large bowel.

Hyperplastic polyps (also known as regenerative, inflammatory, hyperplasiogenic, hamartomatous, and types I and II polyps of Japanese authors) comprise approximately 75% of all gastric polyps.[118] Use of the term *hamartomatous polyp* for these lesions should be discouraged because it elicits confusion with the different type of polyp seen as a component of the Peutz-Jeghers syndrome. Hyperplastic polyps are randomly distributed in the stomach; they are generally small, sessile, and multiple, with a smooth or slightly lobulated contour. Microscopically, they show elongation, tortuosity, and dilatation (often cystic) of the gastric foveolae, with a component of pyloric or—less commonly—fundic type glands in the deeper portion. The stroma, usually prominent, is characterized by edema, patchy fibrosis, inflammatory cells, and scattered smooth muscle bundles from the muscularis mucosae (Fig. 11-30). Atypia is either absent or minimal, of a regenerative type, and limited to the tips of the foveolae. Some authors separate hyperplastic from inflammatory polyps on the basis of relative amounts of glandular and stromal changes, but the presence of a continuous spectrum suggests that these are different stages of the same process.[110] Rarely atypical reactive cells appear in the stroma and simulate a malignant process.[101]

The gastric lesion designated by Menétrier as *polyadenomes polypeux* probably corresponds to multiple hyperplastic polyps[114] (see p. 497). The polypoid lesion sometimes developing on the gastric side of gastroenterostomy stomas may also have a microscopic appearance similar to that of a hyperplastic polyp, except for its more diffuse nature; adenomatous and dysplastic changes can also occur at this site.[103,123]

Hyperplastic polyps have been found to coexist frequently with carcinoma elsewhere in the stomach,[116,124] but these figures are biased due to the fact that most of the specimens studied had been removed because of carcinoma. The incidence of gastric carcinoma developing after endoscopic removal of hyperplastic polyps is low and probably more related to the atrophic gastritis that often accompanies the polyp than to the polyp itself; in a recent study from Germany with up to 7 years' follow-up, this incidence was only 1.4%.[120]

Neoplastic polyps or *adenomas* (types III and IV polyps of Japanese authors) are usually antral in location, generally single and large, either sessile or pedunculated (Figs. 11-31 and 11-32). Microscopically, they are composed of *atypical* glands with pseudostratified epithelium showing nuclear abnormalities and high mitotic count.[118,124] These polyps are analogous in appearance and natural history to those in the colorectum and are thought to arise on the basis of intestinal metaplasia.[107] Like their large bowel counterparts, they can be divided into adenomatous polyps (tubular adenomas), villoglandular polyps (tubulovillous adenomas), and villous adenomas.[115] Scattered endocrine cells positive for serotonin and a variety of peptide hormones have been found in them. CEA reactivity is usually found in the cytologically most atypical areas.[107] Many neoplastic polyps have been described in stomachs that contain an independent carcinoma, but a selection bias is obviously operating[124]; however, there is no question that the polyps themselves can undergo malignant transformation, along similar lines to those of their colorectal counterparts.[109] The exact incidence of this complication is not known, but it seems to be relatively low. In a recent series from Germany with up to 7 years' follow-up, it was 3.4%.[120]

Mixed (hyperplastic and neoplastic) polyps are also recognized. These should be distinguished from the more common regenerative changes commonly seen focally at the surface of hyperplastic polyps.[105]

Fundic gland polyps (fundic gland hyperplasia, hamartomatous cystic polyps, polyps with fundic glandular cysts)

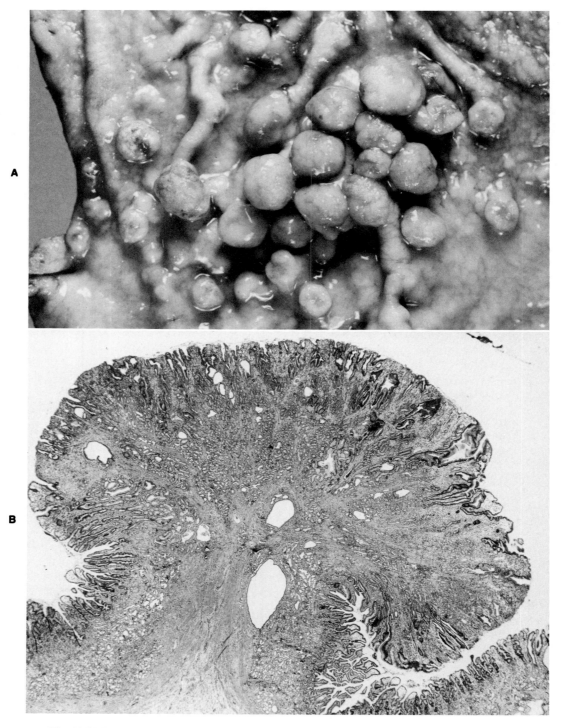

Fig. 11-30 Gastric polyps of hyperplastic type occurring in 65-year-old woman. **A,** Large sessile polyps of firm consistency occupy large portion of gastric mucosa. **B,** Panoramic microscopic view of one of polyps. Note cystic dilatation of glands and bundles of smooth muscle between glands.

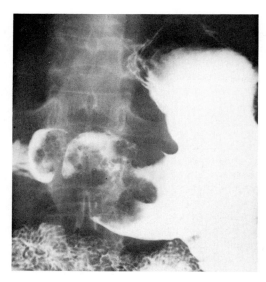

Fig. 11-31 Large polypoid lesion with filling defect in region of pylorus.

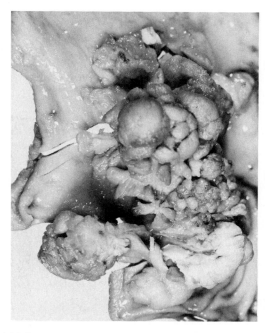

Fig. 11-32 Same lesion shown in Fig. 11-31. Subtotal gastric resection demonstrated polypoid lesion with focal carcinoma. There was no tumor in stalk and no lymph node metastases. Patient remained well over 5 years.

present as multiple small polypoid projections in the gastric fundus or body. Their distinguishing microscopic feature is the presence of microcysts lined by fundic epithelium, including oxyphilic cells; the overlying foveolae are usually shortened.[102,111,121]

Other types of gastric epithelial polypoid lesions that have been described include foveolar or focal hyperplasia (which may well be an early stage of hyperplastic polyp), antral gland hyperplasia, the true hamartomatous polyp associated with the Peutz-Jeghers syndrome, and retention (juvenile) polyps.[122]

It should be stated that polyps of different types can coexist in the same stomach and that occasional lesions cannot be properly placed in a specific category, especially if the only material available is a small biopsy.

Polyposis syndromes of the gastrointestinal tract often involve the stomach. In familial colonic polyposis and related Gardner's syndrome, gastric involvement occurs in over 50% of the cases; the gastric polyps can be adenomatous, hyperplastic, or of the fundic gland hyperplasia type.[106a,122,125,126]

The latter type seems to be particularly common, but it is certainly not specific for this disorder, as previously claimed. Other gastric tumors described in the familial colonic polyposis are adenocarcinoma and carcinoid tumor.[125,126] In Peutz-Jeghers syndrome, hamartomatous gastric polyps have been found in about 20% of the cases and gastric adenocarcinomas occasionally.[104] In generalized juvenile polyposis and the related Cronkhite-Canada syndrome, the incidence of gastric retention (juvenile) polyps is very high.[112] Cowden's syndrome (multiple hamartoma syndrome) can also be accompanied by small sessile gastric polyps, most of which seem to be of the hyperplastic type.[122]

Inflammatory fibroid polyp of the stomach is probably the best name for a lesion also described under names such as eosinophilic granuloma, granuloblastoma, neurofibroma, and hemangiopericytoma.[100,108] It is frequently associated with hypochlorhydria or achlorhydria and is usually located in the antrum.[106] It is probably not a true neoplasm. The gross appearance is somewhat similar to a pyogenic granuloma. Microscopically, this lesion is centered in the submucosa and is characterized by vascular and fibroblastic proliferation (often in a whorl-like arrangement simulating the pattern of a peripheral nerve tumor) and a polymorphic inflammatory response, usually dominated by eosinophils (Fig. 11-33). Ultrastructurally, many of the proliferating cells have a myofibroblastic appearance, in keeping with the presumed reactive nature of the process.[119]

MENÉTRIER'S DISEASE AND ZOLLINGER-ELLISON SYNDROME

In 1888, Menétrier described two different gastric diseases under the common term *polyadenomes*.[130,131] The first, *polyadenomes polypeux*, is probably equivalent to multiple hyperplastic polyps (see p. 495). The second, *polyadenomes en nappe*, is the form to which the term *Menétrier's disease* is usually applied at present (Fig. 11-34). It is also known as hypertrophic or hyperplastic gastropathy, giant hypertrophic gastritis, and giant hypertrophy of gastric rugae.[127] It is accompanied by hypochlorhydria or achlorhydria and often by impressive hypoproteinemia. Chronicity and severity are the rule in adults, but in the few pediatric cases reported, the disease has usually been self-limited.[129] Roentgenographically and grossly, the condition can be confused with malignant lymphoma and carcinoma. It is often centered along the greater curvature of the stomach and is characterized grossly by markedly hypertrophic rugae re-

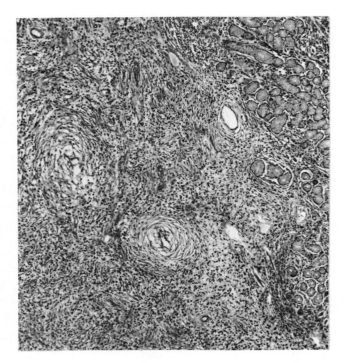

Fig. 11-33 Inflammatory fibroid polyp of stomach. Whorls of spindle cells around blood vessels and heavy inflammatory infiltrate rich in eosinophils are characteristic of this lesion.

sembling cerebral convolutions. The transition between normal and diseased mucosa is always abrupt. A lack of antral involvement is characteristic of the disease. Microscopically, there is a striking *foveolar hyperplasia*, accompanied by tortuosity, some degree of cystic dilatation, and extension into the base of the glands and sometimes even beyond the muscularis mucosae. The glandular component is diminished, and the stroma is edematous and inflamed. It should be mentioned here that many cases diagnosed by radiologists and gastroscopists as ''hypertrophic gastritis'' will show normal or atrophic mucosa on biopsy.

Carcinoma may develop in a stomach affected by Menétrier's disease, but the incidence does not seem higher than that seen in the ordinary atrophic gastritis.[132]

Zollinger-Ellison syndrome may be accompanied by gastric changes radiographically and grossly similar to those of Menétrier's disease; however, microscopic examination will reveal hyperplasia primarily of the glandular rather than the foveolar portion of the fundic gland, even if the latter may also participate. This hyperplasia mainly involves the parietal cells, but there may also be an increase in the number of enterochromaffin-like (ECL) cells, both of these phenomena presumably the result of gastrin stimulation. In some of these patients, the Zollinger-Ellison syndrome is part of multiple endocrine adenomatosis.[128] We have seen two cases of this syndrome associated with multicentric carcinoid tumors, mainly located in the fundus and seem-

ingly arising from ECL cells (see p. 508).

The occurrence of cases with features similar to those of Zollinger-Ellison syndrome but without hypergastrinemia, some of them associated with protein loss, suggests the existence of clinicopathologic variations among these poorly understood disorders.[133]

DYSPLASIA

It is now widely acknowledged that most carcinomas of the stomach are accompanied—and often preceded—by a phase of *dysplasia;* therefore, the recognition of dysplasia in biopsy specimens is of great importance in giving warning of the possibility of a coexisting carcinoma and in indicating that the patient may be at a higher risk for the subsequent development of gastric cancer. Several grading systems of dysplasia have been suggested over the years; recently, an International Pathology Panel has proposed uniform criteria for the recognition and grading of this process.[137] Dysplasia should be clearly separated from the *regenerative hyperplasia* that often occurs in areas of mucosal injury, such as gastritis and peptic ulceration. Regenerative hyperplasia can be divided into simple and atypical forms. In *simple* hyperplasia, the cells are immature, with basophilic cytoplasm, hyperchromatic nuclei, and reduced or absent mucous secretion. These cells are uniform in size and shape, with basally or centrally located nuclei arranged in a row; pseudostratification is slight or absent. Maturation and differentiation toward the surface are present. There may also be glandular dilatation and some degree of intraglandular papillary growth. In *atypical* hyperplasia, there is more pseudostratification and compression and less maturation and differentiation, but the cytologic features are not substantially different. There is usually an accompanying inflammatory reaction, sometimes intense, and focal erosive changes are common.

In *dysplasia*, there is increased cell proliferation, accompanied by abnormalities in cell size, configuration, and orientation. Mucous secretion is reduced or absent, and there is an increase in the nucleocytoplasmic ratio, loss of nuclear polarity, and pseudostratification. Mitoses are numerous, and some of them are atypical.[139] These cellular abnormalities are accompanied by architectural derangement of the glands, resulting in cellular crowding, intraluminal folding, and glandular budding and branching. Sometimes the appearance is reminiscent of the mucosa lining colonic polyps.[136] The dysplasia can be divided into two grades (moderate or severe) or three (mild, moderate, or severe)[134,137,138] (Figs. 11-35 to 11-38). Severe dysplasia is essentially synonymous with carcinoma in situ and needs to be distinguished from intramucosal carcinoma, in which the process has broken through the basement membrane (see p. 507). The risk for invasive carcinoma is small for mild and moderate dysplasia and high for severe dysplasia–carcinoma in situ, to the extent that the performance of a gastrectomy should be considered whenever the latter change is found.[139a]

It remains to be seen whether morphometric analysis will provide a more objective and useful way of evaluating these abnormalities.[135]

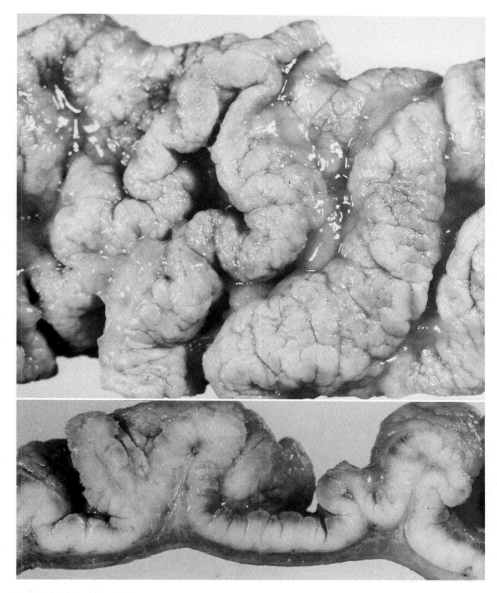

Fig. 11-34 Menétrier's disease in 65-year-old woman. This gross pattern could easily be confused with malignant lymphoma.

CARCINOMA
General features

The pathogenesis of gastric carcinoma is closely related to environmental factors; its incidence has markedly decreased in recent years in some countries, such as the United States and England.[144,157] It remains inordinately high in others, such as Japan, Chile, and Italy.

Most patients are over 50 years of age,[142] but cases in younger individuals and even children are on record.[143,152,156]

Practically all gastric carcinomas arise from the generative or basal cells of the foveolae,[155] in most instances on a background of chronic atrophic gastritis with intestinal metaplasia and preceded by various stages of dysplasia, carcinoma in situ, and early (superficial) carcinoma.[146] Some cases have been said to originate in heterotopic pancreatic tissue or other epithelial-lined submucosal cysts in the gastric wall,[148,150] but this is an exceptional event.

Gastric cancer is accompanied by hypochlorhydria in 85% to 90% of the cases, and it has been shown that hypochlorhydria may precede gastric cancer by several years. It has been postulated that high intragastric pH promotes the growth of bacteria that reduce dietary nitrate to nitrite and then convert dietary amines, in the presence of this nitrite, into carcinogenic N-nitroso compounds.[145] The coexistence

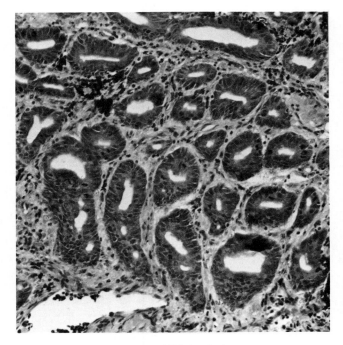

Fig. 11-35 Mild dysplasia.

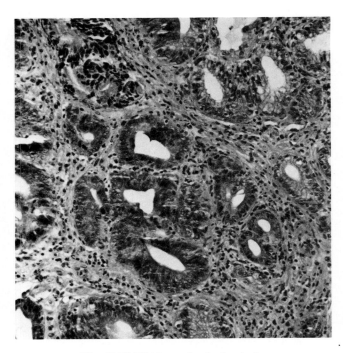

Fig. 11-36 Mild to moderate dysplasia.

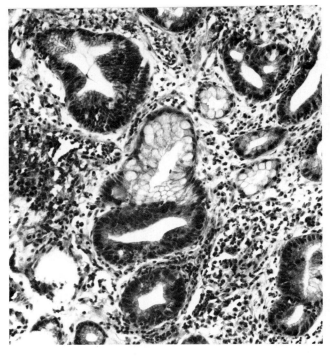

Fig. 11-37 Moderate to severe dysplasia.

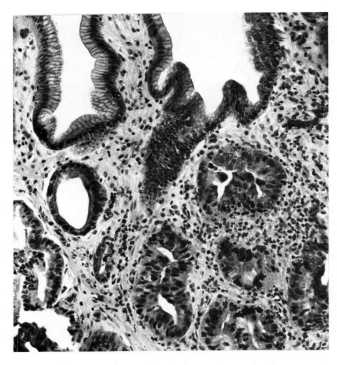

Fig. 11-38 Severe dysplasia—carcinoma in situ.

of chronic atrophic gastritis and carcinoma is common, but the etiopathogenic link between the two and the relative risk for malignancy in the former condition remain controversial.[147,153,154] The same could be said for pernicious anemia; the rate of carcinoma development, although statistically increased, is not high enough to justify surveillance in asymptomatic patients.[151]

It has been postulated that the tumor characterized by the epidemiologic and sequential features described previously represents one type of gastric carcinoma, albeit the most common one; it has been referred to as *intestinal-type adenocarcinoma* by Lauren.[149] The other, designated as the *diffuse type*, does not show these associations and seems to be less related to environmental influences. Thus it has been shown that in high-risk areas the intestinal-type carcinoma predominates; furthermore, when a population shows a decline in the incidence of gastric cancer, the fall is primarily in that microscopic type.[141]

Other factors thought to be involved in the pathogenesis of gastric cancer are gastric polyps, Menétrier's disease, gastric peptic ulcer, and gastric stump (see respective sections in this chapter).

Cases of gastric carcinoma in young patients following irradiation and chemotherapy for other malignancies have been reported.[140]

Morphologic features and classification

There is wide variation in the gross appearance of carcinoma of the stomach. Many intermediate stages exist between the two extremes represented by the fungating tumor growing mainly into the lumen and the flat, ulcerated, and deeply invasive tumor growing through the wall of the stomach[163] (Fig. 11-39). Borrman[160] based his classic gross classification of gastric carcinoma on the relative proportions of exophytic and endophytic components. Depending on the relative amounts of mucin secreted and desmoplastic reaction elicited, the tumors may have a fleshy, fibrous, or gelatinous gross appearance. In terms of location, any area of the stomach can be affected: anterior and posterior walls, lesser curvature, and greater curvature (in that order of frequency).[186] Multiple independent tumors may also be present.[164]

Microscopically, nearly all gastric cancers are of the adenocarcinoma type and are composed of one or more of the following four major cell types: foveolar, mucopeptic, intestinal columnar, and goblet cell.[165] As already indicated, two major categories exist, which have been designated *intestinal* (53%) and *diffuse* (33%) by Lauren[171]; the remainder are heterogeneous in composition.

Intestinal-type adenocarcinomas are thought to arise from metaplastic epithelium, an assumption supported by electron microscopic studies.[175] Their degree of differentiation ranges widely. In the better differentiated tumors, most of the cells are columnar and mucin-secreting. Poorly differentiated variants have a predominantly solid pattern.[176] The secretion is usually an acid mucosubstance, easily detected with Alcian blue or colloidal iron stains and having immunohistochemical features analogous to those of intestinal-type mucins.[172,173] The amount of mucin production is highly variable; when abundant, it is often accompanied by calcification.

Reactivity of the tumor cells for keratin, epithelial membrane antigen, and CEA is the rule.[158,177] Scattered endocrine cells may be demonstrated with silver or immunohistochemical stains (see p. 503). The occurrence of easily identifiable Paneth cells is less common but has been well

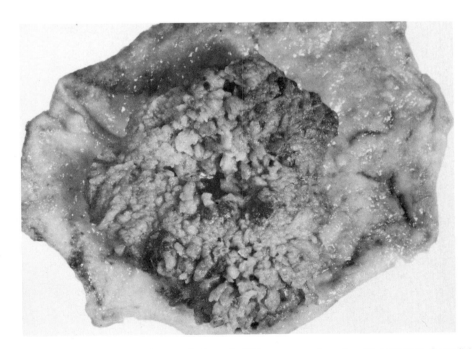

Fig. 11-39 Polypoid adenocarcinoma of stomach. Villous areas alternate with solid foci. Superficial stromal invasion was present.

documented[167]; the reactivity that has been detected for lysozyme in about one third of gastric carcinomas may be an abortive expression of Paneth cell differentiation.[161] Immunohistochemical positivity for alpha-1-antitrypsin, alpha-1-antichymotrypsin, and alpha-2-macroglobulin are also common, particularly in advanced tumors.[183] Gastric proteases such as pepsinogen I, pepsinogen II, and chymosin have also been demonstrated.[164a,185] HCG reactivity is found in scattered tumor cells in about 10% of the cases[169]; the microscopic appearance of these tumors is usually not different from others, and therefore this phenomenon should not be equated with the rare entity of gastric choriocarcinoma, whether pure or associated with adenocarcinoma (see p. 514).

The diffuse type of gastric carcinoma is best represented by the tumor type classically known as *linitis plastica*.[180] It represents a disproportionately high percentage of cases of gastric cancers occurring in the young,[166,184] and its *relative* incidence seems to be on the rise in this country.[159] The gross alterations usually begin in the prepyloric area. Pyloric obstruction often develops, as the wall of the stomach becomes thickened and rigid (Fig. 11-40). Sections of the wall show marked submucosal fibrosis, with or without mucosal ulceration. The muscle is hypertrophic and segmented by the presence of thin, parallel, grayish white,

longitudinal lines that give it a comb-like appearance. These lines are continuous with foci of subserosal thickening. Lymph node involvement is usually present.

Microscopically, a diffuse growth of malignant cells is seen, associated with extensive fibrosis and inflammation. Often, the entire wall is involved. Although an *intramucosal* type of signet ring carcinoma occurs,[187] in many cases of this entity the mucosa is less affected than the deeper layers. Glandular formations are rare and most tumor cells grow individually. Most of the mucin produced is intracytoplasmic, resulting in the typical signet ring appearance, which is particularly well demonstrated with a mucicarmine stain. Pools of extracellular mucin may also be present, but as long as signet ring cells are present this tumor should be categorized as signet ring carcinoma rather than mucinous (mucoid) carcinoma (see p. 503).

There are few malignant tumors in the human body that are more likely to be missed on microscopic examination than this type of gastric cancer. Over the years, we have seen specimens from stomach wall, lymph nodes, omentum, mesentery, pelvic peritoneum, and ovary that were initially misinterpreted as some benign process due to the inconspicuousness of the tumor cells and the marked degree of inflammatory and desmoplastic reaction. The tumor may also closely simulate malignant lymphoma because of its

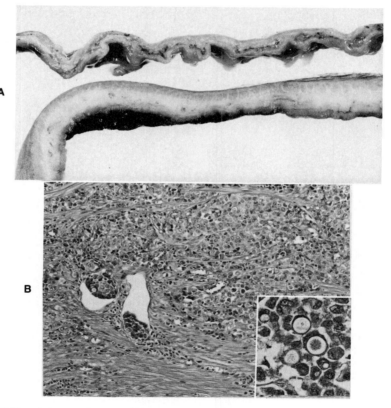

Fig. 11-40 Signet ring carcinoma of stomach. **A,** Typical gross appearance which is compared with thickness of normal stomach on top. **B,** Microscopic appearance of tumor, growing in diffuse fashion in muscle wall and permeating vascular channels. **Inset** shows classic appearance of signet-ring cells, some of which contain granular mucinous material in intracellular lumen.

diffuse pattern of growth and the round shape of the cells and their nuclei. Special stains that are particularly helpful in localizing the isolated tumor cells and identifying them as epithelial are Mayer's mucicarmine, Alcian blue–PAS, CEA, and keratin, the latter two at the immunocytochemical level. It should be noted that the mucin secreted by this tumor may be of either acidic or neutral type, the latter predominating in some of the cases.[162]

The most important classifications that have been proposed for gastric carcinoma, including the one already mentioned, are listed in the box below.

The differential diagnosis of gastric carcinoma in a biopsy specimen includes severe dysplasia and a variety of reactive or otherwise non-neoplastic conditions that may simulate malignancy—such as bizarre epithelial atypia associated with arterial infusion chemotherapy,[179] degenerative changes associated with erosion and regeneration (characterized by a striking background eosinophilia),[168] plump reactive mesenchymal cells related to granulation tissue,[168] and gastric ''xanthoma'' (sometimes confused with signet ring carcinoma) (see p. 495).

Other microscopic types

Endocrine differentiation can be seen in a wide range of gastric neoplasms, in terms of both morphologic and behavioral features. Although admixtures and overlaps occur, most of the gastric tumors with endocrine differentiation can be placed into one of the following categories:

1 Well-differentiated and slow-growing *carcinoid tumors,* composed of any of the endocrine cells of the gastric mucosa (see p. 508).

CLASSIFICATIONS OF GASTRIC CARCINOMA

Stout (Atlas of Tumor Pathology) 1953[181]
  Fungating
  Penetrating
  Spreading
    Superficial spreading
    Linitis plastica
  No special type
Lauren 1965[171]
  Intestinal
  Diffuse
Ming 1977[174]
  Expanding
  Infiltrative
World Health Organization 1977[178]
  Papillary
  Tubular
  Mucinous
  Signet ring
Japenese Society for Gastric Cancer 1981[170]
  Papillary
  Tubular
  Poorly differentiated
  Mucinous
  Signet ring

---

2 Tumors with obvious morphologic features of endocrine differentiation (trabecula, rosettes, insulae; dense-core secretory granules ultrastructurally; immunoreactivity for neuron-specific enolase) but equally obvious atypical morphologic features (marked invasiveness, necrosis, mitotic activity). These neoplasms have been designated by some as *atypical carcinoids* and are found to have a better prognosis than conventional adenocarcinoma, although not nearly as good as classic carcinoid.[197,199] Some of these atypical carcinoids are admixed with areas of conventional adenocarcinoma.

3 *Small cell carcinomas* that are morphologically analogous to their more common pulmonary counterpart and characterized by a very aggressive clinical course.

4 Otherwise typical *adenocarcinomas* of either diffuse or intestinal type (particularly the former) having cells that exhibit argyrophilia or some other attribute of endocrine cells.[189,194,200] These tumors do not behave differently from ordinary adenocarcinoma.

Most of the gastric tumors described in the literature as *neuroendocrine carcinomas* belong to the second and third categories. Admixtures occur, particularly between the third and fourth types. Adenocarcinomas or early carcinomas occurring concurrently but independently from carcinoids have also been described.[188,201a,202]

Adenosquamous and *squamous cell (epidermoid) carcinomas* comprise less than 1% of all gastric cancers.[191,198] Only cases surrounded on all sides by gastric mucosa can be accepted, particularly for the pure squamous cell carcinomas. Those also involving the lower end of the esophagus should be interpreted as primary esophageal carcinomas with gastric extension. The behavior of gastric adenosquamous carcinomas is largely determined by the degree of differentiation of the glandular component, which varies widely.[195] Careful sectioning of tumors originally thought to be squamous cell carcinoma will show a minute glandular component in most of them.[196]

Mucinous (mucoid) carcinoma is characterized by prominent glandular formations and abundant mucin deposition, nearly all of which is extracellular. In contrast to signet ring carcinoma, the prognosis of this exceedingly rare form of gastric carcinoma is good.[190]

Hepatoid adenocarcinoma is a recently described type of gastric cancer having both glandular and hepatocellular differentiation, with frequent admixtures between the two components.[193] These tumors produce large amounts of alpha-fetoprotein and are characterized by a nodular or massive pattern of growth, extensive venous invasion, and poor prognosis.

Parietal gland carcinoma is yet another newly recognized variant of gastric cancer.[192] The tumor grows in a solid fashion and is composed of cells with abundant eosinophilic granular cytoplasm that stains for PTAH and Luxol fast blue. The most distinctive features are seen ultrastructurally—abundant mitochondria, tubulovesicles, intracellular canaliculi, and intercellular lumina filled with undulating microvilli. It is possible that immunohistochemical evaluation of gastric tumors with parietal cell antibodies obtained from patients with type A gastritis will allow the detection of this cell type in additional cases.[201]

Diagnosis—biopsy and cytology

Symptoms from gastric carcinoma usually indicate advanced disease. If the tumor is located in the cardiac or pyloric areas, it may produce obstruction relatively early; otherwise the symptoms are vague and nonspecific, consisting of dyspepsia, weight loss, and anemia. Sometimes, the first sign of gastric carcinoma is the detection of a nodal, hepatic, or pulmonary metastasis. Isolated nodal metastasis in the left supraclavicular region is sometimes referred to as Trousseau's sign or Virchow's node.

Roentgenographic examination of the stomach will demonstrate the lesion in most cases, but in about 10% it will be impossible to determine whether it is benign or malignant.

In countries with a high incidence of gastric carcinoma, particularly Japan, the increased use of mass screening, endoscopy, cytology, and biopsy has resulted in the identification of a large percentage (up to a third) of early cases, with a corresponding increase in survival rates* (see p. 508).

The technique traditionally used for cytologic examination of the stomach has been vigorous lavage by saline or Ringer's solution in patients who had been prepared with overnight fasting, proper hydration, and overnight suction in the presence of gastric obstruction to ensure a completely empty stomach at the time of the test. This method has provided very accurate results over the years for symptomatic patients, as good as or better than with the use of mucolytic agents or abrasive methods[205,216]; however, this rather involved procedure precludes its use as a general screening method for unselected patients. Furthermore, even in high risk patients such as those with pernicious anemia or low hydrochloric acid, the results of screening tests have been disappointing.[203,213] MacDonald et al.[213] screened 500 patients with these conditions and found only three cases of carcinoma, only one of which was potentially curable.

With the introduction of the flexible fiberoptic gastroscope, the results of direct-vision gastric biopsy and brush cytology have improved dramatically.[204,207] In sixty-three patients with carcinoma of the stomach studied by Kasugai et al.[212] the accuracy was 78% for direct-vision cytology, 85% for biopsy, and 94% for both used in combination. In 119 patients with carcinomas of the cardia, a positive diagnosis was obtained by cytology in 78%, by biopsy in 73%, and by both in 89%. The same authors obtained extremely high accuracy (96%) by gastric lavage cytology under direct vision in 512 patients with gastric carcinoma, both in early (95%) and advanced (97%) cases. Yamada et al.[218] described an improved selective chymotrypsin lavage method under fluoroscopy. This method was applied to 420 selected patients suspected of having small carcinoma on radioscopy and/or endoscopy. In sixteen patients, small (<1 cm) and "point" (<0.3 cm) cancers were found by combined cytology and biopsy.

False negative diagnoses with biopsy specimens are most

---

*See references 206, 208, 209, 211, 214, 215, and 217.

often seen with the ulcerating types and are inversely related to the number of specimens obtained.[210] There is also a greater rate of false negative results with diffuse as compared with intestinal-type carcinomas, a finding not surprising in view of the predominantly submucosal distribution of this tumor[208] (see p. 501).

The suggestion has been recently made that immunocytochemical straining for *ras* oncogene p21 may prove of utility in the cytologic diagnosis of gastric carcinoma.[204a]

Relationship with peptic ulcer

The possibility of malignant transformation of chronic peptic ulcer of the stomach has been argued for years. Stout,[237] Gömöri,[223] and others have accepted it, whereas equally prominent authorities such as Mallory[229] and Palmer[232] have denied it. It seems to us that the problem should be analyzed from two different perspectives.

The first approach is pathogenetic and can be proposed in the following way: Are there any pathologic criteria by which a gastric cancer can be assumed to have arisen from a peptic ulcer? Malignant tumors with central ulceration without steep overhanging margins, with neoplastic cells at the base, and with preservation of the muscle should be considered primary ulcerating carcinomas (Fig. 11-41). Presence of carcinoma on both margins of an ulcer is also suggestive that the ulceration is secondary to the neoplasm. The main problem of interpretation resides with lesions having all the typical features of chronic peptic ulcer in which carcinoma is found *in only one margin* after subserially sectioning the lesion. In these cases, did the carcinoma arise from the mucosa at one edge of the ulcer, or did the ulcer arise because of the carcinoma in an area of diminished resistance? There is simply no way to answer this question with the data presently available.

The second approach dealing with a possible relationship is a practical one and regards the management of patients with symptoms and roentgenologic signs suggestive of peptic ulcer. Fortunately, there is now enough information to satisfactorily answer the three basic questions in this regard[225]:

1 How reliable are our diagnostic methods in distinguishing a benign peptic ulcer from a carcinoma? The differential diagnosis between peptic ulcer and ulcerated carcinoma by roentgenographic examination is subject to error.[230] In a published series of patients with lesions diagnosed roentgenographically as benign who were subsequently operated upon, carcinoma was found in 6% to 15%[225]; however, by combining radiographic, endoscopic, and pathologic (biopsy and/or cytology) techniques, the degree of accuracy in making this distinction approaches 100%.

2 Of patients with a clinical and roentgenographic diagnosis of peptic ulcer who have been treated medically, how many will later be found to have gastric cancer? Of 473 cases followed for a minimum of 10 years by Ihre et al.,[225] gastric cancer developed in only five (1.1%). In Jordan's series[226] of 111 patients who were followed for a minimum of 5 years, only two developed carcinoma.

3 Is the risk of developing gastric cancer greater among

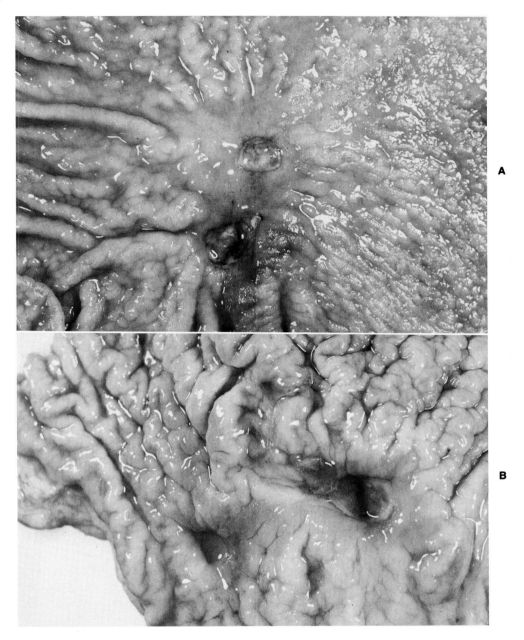

Fig. 11-41 Gross appearance of ulcers demonstrating difficulty in determining whether they are benign or malignant. **A,** Two sharply demarcated benign ulcers with converging mucosal folds. **B,** Two ulcers that do not look too dissimilar but in reality represent primary ulcerating carcinoma.

patients who have had surgical treatment for benign peptic ulcer than among the general population? This remains a controversial question.[236] The incidence of gastric cancer in this group has been variously reported as higher than,[220-222,231,235] similar to, or even lower than[225,227,234,238] the frequency of gastric cancer in the general population. Chronic atrophic gastritis with intestinal metaplasia and some degree of atypia is common in the gastric stump, especially in the anastomotic area,[218a,219,233,235] and this has been said to be responsible for the alleged increase in incidence of cancer; however, it should be concluded that if there is indeed an increased risk in these patients, it must be very small. Thus it would not seem that prophylactic endoscopic examination of these patients is indicated.[224] Interestingly, some of the cancers that have developed at the site of old gastrojejunostomy stomas have been associated with prominent polypoid cystic mucosal changes of hyperplastic type (see p. 495).

Parenthetically, it should be mentioned that the coexistence of *duodenal* peptic ulcer and gastric cancer is very rare, to the extent that the presence of an active duodenal ulcer has been thought to protest against the development of gastric cancer; however, cases showing this combination certainly occur and the natural history of the gastric cancer

developing under these circumstances is not significantly different from others.[228]

"Early" carcinoma

"Early" gastric cancer is defined by the Japanese authors as a carcinoma confined to the mucosa or to the mucosa

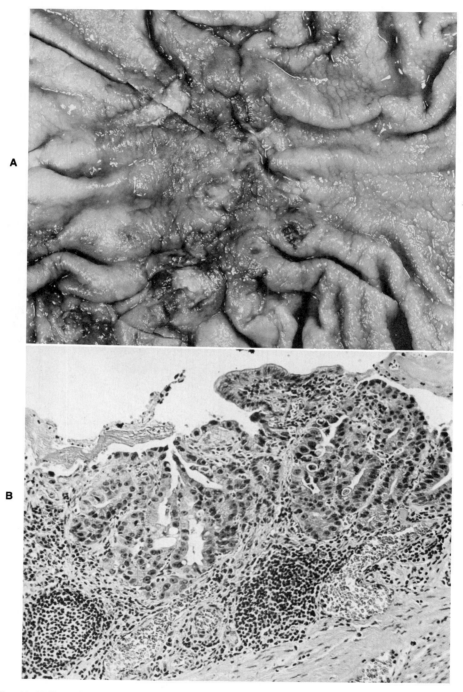

Fig. 11-42 Superficial spreading type of carcinoma. **A,** Margins are indistinct. **B,** Note complete disorganization of lining glands. There was no penetration of muscular coat of stomach. Patient was alive and well 13 years following gastrectomy.

and submucosa (not extending into the muscularis externa), regardless of the status of the regional lymph nodes.[242,246,247,252] Despite the name, the concept is not related to size or duration of the lesion but exclusively to depth of penetration. Other terms that have been used for this entity include *surface, superficial, superficial spreading,* and *mucoinvasive cancer*[243,245] (Fig. 11-42). The form limited to the mucosa, known as *intramucosal carcinoma,* needs to be separated from severe dysplasia–carcinoma in situ. This is based on the presence of invasion through the glandular basement membrane into the lamina propria, a determination that is not always easy to make.

Most cases of early carcinoma are of Lauren's intestinal type but a diffuse form also exists, composed almost purely of signet ring cells.[257] The degree of microscopic differentiation varies widely. The deep mucosal component underlying the cancer often shows cystic dilatation of the glands.[255] Early carcinoma can coexist with peptic ulcer, pseudolymphoma, and carcinoid tumor.[239,240]

The relative incidence of early carcinoma is clearly related to the magnitude of the diagnostic efforts of fiberoptic gastroscopy and double-contrast barium meal examination, which, when combined with histologic-cytologic evaluation, allows diagnosis of lesions measuring 5 mm or less in diameter.[248,254] In Japan, the proportion of early cancer cases has risen from 5.7% in 1961 to 34% in 1969.[242] Variations in gross appearance of early carcinoma at endoscopy mirror those of its larger counterpart—protruding or type I (polypoid, nodular, or villous), superficial or type II (elevated, flat, or depressed), and excavated or type III. Combinations are common.[253] Most cases are located in the distal third of the stomach, but they also occur at the gastric cardia[251]; multicentricity is seen in about 10% of the cases, although the reported incidence varies widely.[241,242] Abnormalities in DNA ploidy are just as common in early as in advanced carcinomas.[250] Czerniak et al.[244] made the interesting observation that most intestinal-type early cancers are diploid whereas the majority of diffuse-type cancers are aneuploid, a pattern that mirrors that of advanced cancers.

On the average, lymph node metastases are seen in about 5% of the intramucosal tumors and in 10% to 20% of those invading the submucosa[243]; the incidence seems higher in those tumors that invade the submucosa in an expansile fashion with complete destruction of the muscularis mucosae.[249]

The 5-year survival rate following resection is between 80% and 95% and remains remarkably high even when nodal metastases are present.[243] The natural evolution of cases not treated by gastrectomy is to progress to advanced cancer.[256]

Spread

Distal carcinomas of the stomach invade the duodenum in about 50% of the cases.[262] Similarly, carcinomas of the proximal stomach often involve the esophagus, to the point that a distinction between them and the tumors arising from Barrett's esophagus is not always possible or warranted. Local extension also occurs in the omentum, colon, pancreas, and spleen. The rich mucosal and submucosal (Borrman's) lymphatic plexus of the stomach is often invaded;

from here, the tumor can spread to perigastric, periaortic, and celiac axis–related lymph nodes.[261] Tumor cells can also permeate diffusely the lymphatic plexus of the bowel, more often at the level of the upper duodenum but sometimes down into the distal ileum and even the large bowel; the latter feature is seen almost exclusively in carcinomas of the diffuse type.[259] The most frequent sites of distant metastases are liver (often found unexpectedly at operation), peritoneum, lung, adrenal gland, and ovary. Bilateral ovarian metastases from stomach cancer constitute the majority of the cases referred to as *Krukenberg's tumor.*

The diffuse type of gastric carcinoma shows a wider pattern of dissemination than the intestinal type, with more frequent involvement of peritoneum, lungs, and ovary.[258] On the other hand, liver metastases are more common with intestinal-type tumors, particularly if they are highly cellular (''medullary'').[260]

Treatment

The standard treatment for gastric carcinoma is gastrectomy, the type of surgery being largely dependent on the extent of tumor and status of the rest of the mucosa.[263,265a] In this country, the resectability rate is around 50%. The operations most commonly performed are subtotal gastrectomy, radical subtotal gastrectomy, and total gastrectomy. The operative mortality following total gastrectomy is low, but the morbidity remains high. This operation is most often performed for cancers located at the cardia or high on the lesser curvature. For most of the others, subtotal resections are most popular because of the lower morbidity, despite occasional tumor recurrence in the gastric stump.[264,265] Gastric cancer responds little to radiation therapy and is also relatively unresponsive to chemotherapy.[263a]

Frozen section

The need for frozen section in a gastric ulcer of debatable nature depends a great deal on its location. If it is situated in the midportion of the distal half of the stomach and no evidence of neoplastic spread beyond the stomach exists, it is probably better to perform a resection directly, without gastrotomy and biopsy, since the extent of the excision will not differ significantly regardless of whether the lesion is benign or malignant. If the lesion is located instead in the cardiac region, not only are the chances of its being malignant increased, but the type of surgical therapy will vary considerably according to the nature of the process; therefore, frozen section biopsy is indicated, despite the theoretic possibility of tumor spread. Frozen sections may also be performed at the edge of perforated ulcers, surgical margins, enlarged regional nodes, and liver nodules or peritoneal implants.

Diagnosis of diffuse carcinoma is one of the most difficult problems that the surgical pathologist will ever encounter in frozen section material. The small size of the tumor cells, lack or inconspicuousness of glandular formations, and marked inflammatory and fibroblastic reaction that accompany this neoplasm all combine to render its determination a very difficult one. We have had some success in demonstrating intracytoplasmic mucin in the tumor cells at the time of frozen section by staining the ethanol-fixed frozen sections in 1% Alcian blue at pH 2.5 for 1 minute, using nuclear-fast red as counterstain. The tumor cells, which often show a distinct cytoplasmic staining, should be distinguished from mast cells, which also stain with this technique.

Prognosis

The overall prognosis for gastric carcinoma in this country remains disappointingly poor. The overall survival rate for all patients admitted is between 4% and 13%.[266,269,275,278] The rate is substantially better (over 40%) in countries like Japan, largely as a result of earlier detection.[278] Different criteria in the differential diagnosis between severe dysplasia and carcinoma between Japanese and Western authors may also account for some of the differences.[278]

The prognosis for gastric carcinoma has been found to be related to several other factors:

1 *Patient's age.* Gastric cancers in the young have traditionally been associated with a grim prognosis, this being the result of both delay in diagnosis and a higher percentage of diffuse cases in this age group.[270,283]

2 *Location within the stomach.* In 80% of the 5-year survivors the lesion is in the distal half of the stomach. In a series of 1,497 cases reported by Dupont et al.,[269] there were practically no long-term survivors among those with lesions of the cardia, fundus, or esophagogastric junction.

3 *Depth of invasion.* As already indicated, this is a feature of great prognostic significance, for the deeper the penetration, the greater the chance of metastases.[280] This feature is directly related to the gross appearance of the tumors—polypoid, largely intraluminal neoplasms have a much lower incidence of metastases than those growing primarily within the wall.[267] In tumors with serosal involvement, there seems to be a relation between prognosis and the surface area of serosal invasion.[273]

4 *Tumor margins.* The presence of a pushing or expanding border is a favorable prognostic sign, whereas diffuse infiltration is associated with a decreased survival rate.[271,276,279,281,285] Consequently, prognosis for the expanding type of gastric carcinoma in Ming's classification is better than for the infiltrative type.[277]

5 *Tumor size.* Small tumor size is associated with a better prognosis, but this is closely linked to the depth of penetration.

6 *Microscopic type and grading.* The intestinal-type tumors in Lauren's classification behave relatively better than the diffuse types.[277,282] Within each category, there is very little correlation between microscopic grading and prognosis once the special types of gastric cancer have been excluded.

7 *Inflammatory reaction.* The finding of a cellular infiltrate at the interface between the tumor and normal tissue, often associated with degenerative changes in the tumor, is a good prognostic sign.[285] This has also been claimed for the presence of abundant S-100 protein–positive Langerhans' cells in advanced cancers.[284]

8 *Surgical margins.* When carcinoma is found at the limit of the excision, early recurrence and death are to be expected.

9 *Regional lymph node involvement.* If lymph nodes are found to be negative on a thorough pathologic examination, over 50% of the patients may be expected to survive for 5 years. With nodal involvement, the figure drops to less than 10%.[268,271]

10 *Type of surgery.* In one large series, subtotal gastrectomy was the procedure performed most frequently, but radical subtotal gastrectomy resulted in the best survival (22.1%).[269]

11 *DNA ploidy.* Preliminary results suggest that determination of DNA ploidy with flow cytometry may provide a reliable indicator of prognosis in gastric carcinoma.[272,274]

CARCINOID TUMORS

Gastric carcinoid tumors tend to be small, well-defined, and covered by a flattened mucosa.[299] They may present endoscopically as gastric polyps.[292] Microscopically, the predominant pattern of growth may be microglandular, trabecular, or—rarely—insular. The nuclei are regular and normochromatic, mitoses are scanty, necrosis is usually absent, and vascularization is florid. Focal mucin positivity may be present. Immunohistochemically, there is consistent positivity for neuron-specific enolase, chromogranin, and keratin[295] (see Color plate 1, *C*). Ultrastructurally, dense-core secretory granules are found in the cytoplasm, usually in abundance. The rate of growth of these tumors is very slow. Metastases are usually restricted to regional lymph nodes and liver, and their presence does not rule out long-term survival.[299,309]

It should be realized that *carcinoid tumor* is a generic term, which can be properly applied to any neoplasm comprised of any of several types of endocrine cells known to be present in the normal human stomach.[300,301,305] This histogenetic diversity is already suggested by the variety of products that these tumors have been found to secrete, such as 5-hydroxytryptophan, serotonin, epinephrine, norepinephrin, somatostatin, VIP, PP, YY peptide, ACTH, beta-MSH, and alpha-1-antitrypsin.[286,294,296,306-308]

A combined morphologic, ultrastructural, and immunohistochemical approach has allowed the identification of at least two definite subtypes of carcinoid. The first is a tumor composed of *G-cells* (gastrinoma), analogous to its most common pancreatic or duodenal counterpart; this is usually solitary, located in the antrum, non-argentaffin and non-argyrophilic, immunoreactive for gastrin, and sometimes associated with peptic ulcer.[297] Parenthetically, gastric G-cell tumor should be clearly separated from the disputed entity of *primary G-cell hyperplasia*, in which an increased number of G-cells in the antrum is accompanied by hypergastrinemia and an ulcerogenic syndrome resembling the Zollinger-Ellison syndrome.[302]

The second form, which probably constitutes the most common type of gastric carcinoid tumor, is composed of *enterochromaffin-like (ECL) cells.* The tumors are usually multiple, often polypoid, distributed throughout the fundus; they are nonargentaffin but strongly argyrophilic, nonreactive for any of the standard gastroduodenopancreatic hor-

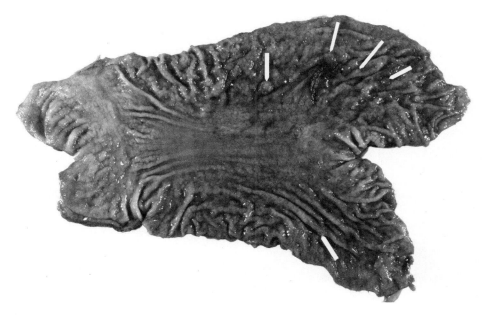

Fig. 11-43 Gross appearance of multiple carcinoid tumors of stomach. Neoplasms are small, covered by gastric mucosa, and located exclusively in fundic portion. Microscopically, these were composed of ECL-like cells. (Courtesy Dr. J. Costa, Lausanne, Switzerland.)

mones, and accompanied by diffuse hyperplasia of similar argyrophilic cells in the surrounding mucosa[288,289] (Fig. 11-43). These tumors usually occur on a background of atrophic gastritis with intestinal metaplasia, with or without pernicious anemia.[291,303,310] They have also seen them in association with the Zollinger-Ellison syndrome, either alone or as a component of multiple endocrine adenomatosis.[287,304] Since the common denominator for these disorders is hypergastrinemia and since gastrin is known to have a trophic influence on ECL cells, it has been postulated that these tumors are the direct result of a continuous stimulation by gastrin.[290,293,298,304a] Although no secretory product has yet been identified in these tumor cells, it is pertinent to mention that murine ECL cells produce histamine and that histamine-producing carcinoid tumors composed of argyrophilic ECL-like cells are very common in the stomach of the South African rodent, *Mastomys natalensis*.

Carcinoid tumors with an atypical histology and adenocarcinomas with focal endocrine features are discussed in the section on gastric carcinoma (see p. 503).

SMOOTH MUSCLE TUMORS

Gastric leiomyomas are common as an incidental autopsy finding; Meissner[321] found forty-four leiomyomas in twenty-three of fifty consecutive autopsies. They are often multiple, small, and subserosal. Leiomyomas occur much less frequently clinically than carcinomas but are the most common benign neoplasm of the stomach. They may arise from the muscularis propria, muscularis mucosae, or the muscle present in the blood vessel wall. They appear most commonly in the region of the pars media (40%) and antrum (25%).[322]

Although 20% occur near the pylorus, obstruction is rare. They usually are submucosal (about 60%) and grow toward the lumen of the stomach, where they make a smooth projection (Fig. 11-44). In time, a central ulceration occurs that may penetrate deeply into the tumor and may result in hematemesis. The smooth outline of the tumor and the central niche result in a highly characteristic roentgenographic appearance. Leiomyomas also may grow out from the serosal surface (30%). They have a characteristic gross appearance and may attain a very large size. On section, they are well circumscribed and have a smooth, lobulated or whorled-silk appearance. An hourglass defect may occur at the cardia or pylorus if the tumor encircles the stomach.

Microscopically, most smooth muscle tumors show well-differentiated smooth muscle cells with a variable degree of hyalinized connective tissue.[317] However, a relatively large number show a wide variation from the classic pattern. Peculiar features sometimes seen in gastric leiomyomas include extreme cellularity, presence of occasional large cells with bizarre hyperchromatic nuclei, marked diffuse vascularity, regimentation of nuclei (palisading), and cells with round shape and clear cytoplasm (see the following discussion).

Electron microscopic studies have shown that myofibrils are very sparse or even absent in many of the cases, in contrast to those found in normal smooth muscle cells and uterine smooth muscle tumors.[319a,335,336] As a result, special stains at a light microscopic level, such as Masson's trichrome or Mallory's phosphotungstic acid–hematoxylin, are usually of no help. This may result in a smooth muscle

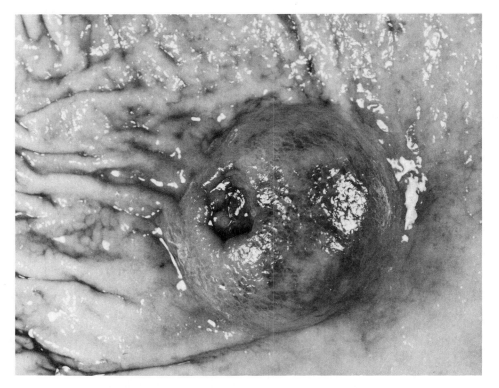

Fig. 11-44 Leiomyoma of stomach with characteristic central ulceration.

tumor being misdiagnosed as neurilemoma, fibroma, or some other neoplasm.

There is now fairly general agreement that the single most important criterion for distinguishing a leiomyoma from a leiomyosarcoma is the number of mitotic figures present.[316] Cellularity, hemorrhage, bizarre nuclei, necrosis, large size, and mucosal ulceration are common accompanying features of malignant tumors, but they are not diagnostic per se. For instance, of forty-nine *very cellular* smooth muscle tumors that had a low mitotic count studied by Appelman and Helwig,[313] only one metastasized. Myxoid changes, hyalinization, and calcification are more common in benign types of tumors, whereas hemorrhage and fresh tumor necrosis are more frequent with malignant types.[325] We have seen examples of myxoid leiomyosarcoma of the stomach, similar to those reported in the female genital tract (see Chapter 19).

Unfortunately, correlation between mitotic activity and behavior is not nearly as good as for uterine smooth muscle tumors. Ranchod and Kempson[325] found that all tumors with five or more mitoses per ten high-power fields behaved aggressively, but they also found that as many as 40% of the gastrointestinal leiomyosarcomas had fewer than five mitoses per ten high-power fields. The proposal has been made to designate as ''*s*mooth muscle *t*umors of *u*ndeterminate *m*alignant *p*otential (STUMP)'' those neoplasms that are suspected of being malignant because of high cellularity, atypia, and/or tumor cell necrosis but that have fewer than five mitoses per ten high-power fields.

Gastric smooth muscle tumors are very rare in children and in adolescents, the majority being malignant.[338]

At the time of operation, the surgeon and pathologist can easily make a gross diagnosis of smooth muscle tumor, but it is often impossible to tell with certainty whether the tumor is benign or malignant. This dilemma may still persist after a frozen section has been carried out. Fortunately, this does not influence the surgical decision much. Simple enucleation of the tumor should be discouraged in every instance. Local excision of the neoplasm and stomach wall is the least that should be undertaken. Depending on the site and size of the tumor, this may involve performing a subtotal gastrectomy. Since this tumor tends to spread distantly without involvement of lymph nodes, wide resection of any lymph node area does not appear indicated.

The two organs most commonly involved by metastatic tumor are liver and lungs[327]; these metastases can develop 10 years or more after the removal of the primary tumor. The overall 5-year survival rate for gastric leiomyosarcoma is 56%; large tumor size, invasion of adjacent organs, and higher microscopic grade affect the prognosis adversely.[330] The microscopic grade largely depends on mitotic count and has proved to be a very powerful prognostic indicator.[316] Preliminary data suggest that determination of DNA ploidy by flow cytometry may also provide information of prognostic value in leiomyosarcoma, even if it cannot be used to distinguish benign from malignant smooth muscle tumors.[333]

A reasonably distinct variety of gastric smooth muscle tu-

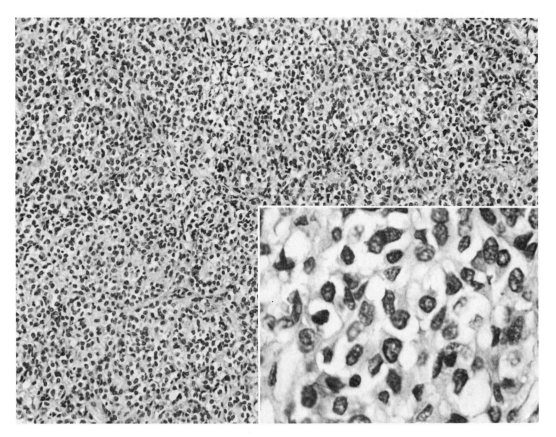

Fig. 11-45 Leiomyoblastoma of stomach. Tumor has indistinct lobular configuration. **Inset** shows clear cytoplasm and well-defined cell margins.

mor is the *leiomyoblastoma* (bizarre smooth muscle tumor; clear cell or epithelioid leiomyoma and leiomyosarcoma). It is characterized by round cells with a central nucleus and abundant clear cytoplasm[311,323] (Fig. 11-45). The latter is probably an artifact of fixation.[326] Areas of transition with typical spindle cells are often present. The diagnosis of leiomyoblastoma should be restricted to those tumors that have a marked predominance of clear or epithelioid cells. The large majority of these neoplasms follow a benign clinical course.[315,325,331,332] The malignant tumor may metastasize to the liver and other sites, sometimes many years (30 years or more) after the original excision. The criteria for distinguishing the benign from the less common malignant type are similar to those of spindle-cell tumors and just as difficult to apply. Appelman and Helwig[311] found that most benign tumors were located in the anterior wall, whereas the malignant ones occurred more frequently in the posterior wall. In addition to having more mitotic figures, the malignant leiomyoblastomas had cells of smaller size, anaplasia, alveolar arrangement, and less reticulin. Although malignant leiomyoblastomas are rare, they constitute the most common variant of gastric sarcoma exclusive of lymphoma.[312]

A multiple malignant type of gastric leiomyoblastoma has been seen as a component of a syndrome that also in-

cludes pulmonary chondromas and extra-adrenal paraganglioma.[314,324,337]

The interpretation of leiomyoblastomas as smooth muscle tumors is based on their occasional transition with typical smooth muscle elements and the fact that about half of these tumors will show ultrastructural and/or immunohistochemical evidence of smooth muscle differentiation in the form of pinocytotic vesicles, subplasmalemmal dense patches, cytoplasmic microfilaments with focal densities, and desmin positivity.[319,321a,328,335] These features have been detected even in some gastric tumors developing in patients with Recklinghausen's disease[329]; however, there are tumors with a similar light microscopic appearance that are immunohistochemically negative for smooth muscle markers but positive for S-100 protein.[320] This percentage is low (around 5%) in the largest published series, but it still suggests that some of these tumors may be of peripheral nerve rather than smooth muscle origin.[315a,318] Because of this uncertainty, some authors have employed the noncommittal term *gastric stromal tumors* for this group of neoplasms.[320] Related to this problem and further compounding the issue is the recent description of spindle-cell tumors of the stomach compatible with smooth muscle origin on light microscopy but having features suggestive of autonomic nerve plexus derivation at the ultrastructural level.[334]

LYMPHOID TUMORS AND TUMORLIKE CONDITIONS

Malignant lymphoma of the stomach may represent a primary or a secondary manifestation of the disease.[338b,379] The primary type makes up only a small percentage of all malignant tumors of the stomach.[356,370,377] The patients are usually over 50 years old; some may have a large palpable mass and still be in excellent physical condition. The clinical symptoms often simulate those of gastritis or benign peptic ulcer. At times, free perforation into the abdominal cavity occurs. Typically, the tumor arises from the lymphoid tissue of the lamina propria and presents grossly either as a giant convolution mimicking hypertrophic gastritis, or as a large lobulated, sometimes polypoid, mass with areas of superficial or deep ulceration (Fig. 11-46). Although most cases are located in the distal half of the stomach, the pylorus is involved only rarely. The roentgenographic or gross distinction from carcinoma is very difficult. There is direct extension to adjacent organs and involvement of regional lymph nodes but only late in the course of the disease.

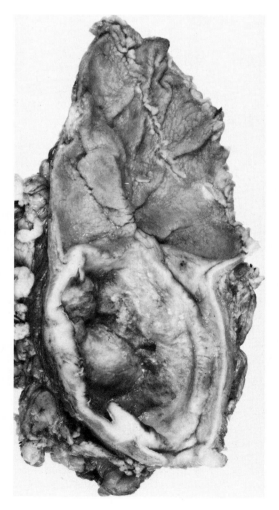

Fig. 11-46 Malignant lymphoma of stomach resulting in large infiltrating and ulcerating mass in distal portion.

Microscopically, nearly all primary malignant lymphomas of the stomach are of non-Hodgkin's type, and the large majority are of B-cell derivation.[348,352,358,383] Most belong to the diffuse large cell type category, followed by small cleaved (poorly differentiated) and mixed cell types.[364,383] The pattern of growth may be nodular or diffuse, the latter being the most frequent (Fig. 11-47). It should be pointed out that the presence of follicles in a gastric lymphoid lesion does not rule out the possibility of malignant lymphoma, especially if these follicles are located at the periphery of the tumor. The reported high incidence of "true histiocytic" lymphomas of stomach in some series may have been due to overinterpretation of results using lysozyme and other histiocytic markers.[348,361] A few of the gastric lymphomas have a signet ring configuration due to intracellular immunoglobulin accumulation and thus may simulate signet ring carcinoma.[349] It is common for gastric lymphomas to exhibit focal or extensive plasmacytoid differentiation; although some of these have been designated as *plasmacytomas*, it is better to reserve this term for the rare neoplasms *entirely composed* of mature and immature plasma cells[347,369,373]; it is very rare for these tumors to be associated with the presence of an M protein in the serum.[363]

Isaacson et al.[353,354] have commented that mucosa-associated lymphoid tissue (MALT) such as that present in the stomach is of a specific type and that the lymphoma arising from it is also distinctive. The slow evolution of these lymphomas, their tendency to remain localized for a long time, and their propensity to involve other mucosal sites when they spread has been explained by the normal homing pattern of MALT lymphocytes; as part of this scheme, a particular tendency of lymphoma of the Waldeyer's ring to develop following gastrointestinal lymphoma has been described.[368]

The prognosis for gastric lymphoma is substantially better than for gastric carcinoma. Following a biopsy diagnosis of lymphoma, exploratory laparotomy with gastric resection and surgical staging is indicated.[342,346,355] Controversy still exists as to whether postoperative radiation therapy and/or chemotherapy should be given in cases of apparently limited disease, but many authors have recommended adjuvant radiation for stage IE and adjuvant radiation plus chemotherapy for stage IIE.[362,376,384] The tumor may also be treated with radiation therapy alone following a biopsy diagnosis, but danger of gastric perforation exists if the tumor involvement is transmural.[346] Distant disease is the most common form of treatment failure.[375] The overall 5-year disease-free survival rate is approximately 60%.[340,358,360] Favorable prognostic signs are small tumor size, superficial mural invasion, nodular versus diffuse pattern, low-grade histologic type, and absence of regional lymph node involvement.[340,345,359,375] Tumors located in the lesser curvature have a significantly worse prognosis than those located elsewhere.[375] Perhaps determination of DNA content will add information of prognostic utility.[354a]

Occasionally, gastric lymphoma is seen adjacent to an adenocarcinoma, as an expression of collision tumor.[357] In other instances, the lymphoma precedes a carcinoma by several years, raising the possibility that the latter might have been related to the therapy for the former.[338a,374]

The diagnosis of gastric lymphoma can be made with

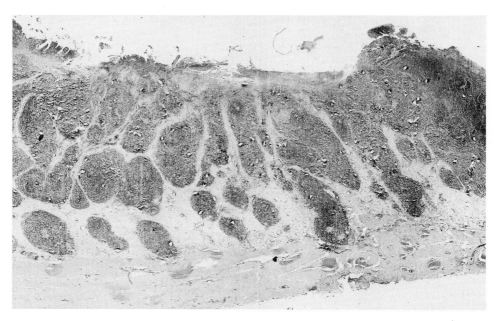

Fig. 11-47 Malignant lymphoma of stomach that has spread through wall and ulcerated surface.

biopsy or cytology; with the latter technique, the detection rate is between 40% and 60%.[366,381]

The differential diagnosis of malignant lymphoma includes undifferentiated carcinoma, pseudolymphoma, and plasma cell granuloma. Features favoring a diagnosis of lymphoma over carcinoma are the lack of continuity between epithelium and tumor cells, lack of suggestion of an acinar pattern, and preservation of muscularis mucosae fibers. If uncertainties remain, they can be eliminated in nearly every instance with the performance of mucin and immunocytochemical stains or with those for leukocyte common antigen, low molecular weight keratin, and CEA.[341a]

The distinction between malignant lymphoma and *pseudolymphoma (lymphoid hyperplasia)* can be much more difficult to make, not only radiographically but also grossly and microscopically.[344,367] Pseudolymphoma presents in most cases in association with a gastric ulceration or erosion and is accompanied by extensive fibrosis.[350,365] This form is variously referred to as inflammatory, ulcerative, or erosive.[339,382] In other instances, one or more submucosal nodules are present, sometimes in association with similar lesions in the intestine.[339] Microscopically, the features favoring the diagnosis of pseudolymphoma are the presence of clearly reactive germinal centers throughout the lesions, a mixed population of inflammatory cells (including mature lymphocytes and plasma cells), and proliferation of blood vessels. Immunohistochemical stains for immunoglobulins will usually show a polyclonal pattern[371] (Fig. 11-48). Occasionally, the lymphoid nodules present in the lesion have the morphologic features of progressively transformed germinal centers[350] or of those seen in giant lymph node hyperplasia (Castleman's disease).[339]

Traditionally, pseudolymphoma has been regarded as a reactive condition, arising in most cases as an exaggerated inflammatory reaction to peptic ulcer; however, the presence in some cases of monotypic cytoplasmic immunoglobulin,[343] the occasional coexistence with malignant lymphoma,[372] and the fact that some patients with this lesion have subsequently developed gastric lymphoma[339,385] would seem to indicate the need for caution in the interpretation of this process (particularly in its nodular form) and the necessity for careful follow-up of these patients.

Plasma cell granuloma is a localized reactive condition rich in plasma cells, which should be distinguished from plasmacytoma and from malignant lymphoma with plasmacytoid differentiation.[351,378] The plasma cells are mature and are accompanied by other inflammatory elements and fibrosis. Immunoglobulin production is polyclonal. Some of these cases have occurred in association with gastric carcinoma.[380]

Granulocytic sarcomas can occasionally present initially as gastric tumors in the absence of bone marrow involvement and be confused with malignant lymphoma or carcinoma.[341]

OTHER TUMORS

Glomus tumors have been described in the stomach.[387,396] Microscopically, they are composed of clear epithelioid cells arranged around dilated vessels. By electron microscopy, the cytoplasm is packed with myofilaments exhibiting focal condensations.[395] This tumor is closely related morphologically and perhaps histogenetically to leiomyoblastoma, to such an extent that a sharp distinction between the two is not always possible.[398] All of the reported cases have followed a benign clinical course.[386]

Lipomas arise within the wall and may protrude into the lumen, resulting in a typical filling defect on roentgeno-

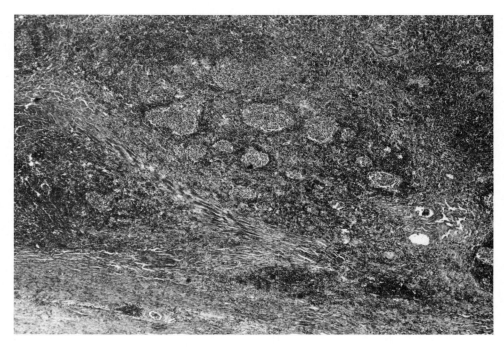

Fig. 11-48 Pseudolymphoma of stomach. Lymphoid infiltrate containing numerous reactive germinal centers infiltrates wall of stomach.

graphic examination.[400] Sometimes they mimic peptic ulcer in their clinical presentation.

Granular cell tumors can occur beneath the gastric mucosa; they can be either solitary or multiple and can be associated with similar tumors in other portions of the gastrointestinal tract.[394]

The possible existence of *peripheral nerve tumors* in the stomach has already been discussed (see p. 511). We have seen a classic schwannoma in the stomach of a patient with Recklinghausen's disease. A case of primary melanocytic gastric schwannoma, positive for S-100 protein and glial fibrillary acidic protein, has also been reported.[388]

We have seen an apparently benign gastric *fibrous histiocytoma* associated with severe anemia, and a similar case has been reported.[386] *Malignant fibrous histiocytoma* has also been observed.[400a]

The existence of *fibroma* and *myxofibroma* in the stomach is doubtful. A few reasonably convincing cases have been reported,[392] but most tumors reported under these rubrics represent in all likelihood smooth muscle neoplasms with secondary changes.

Primary gastric *choriocarcinomas* occur, either in pure form or mixed with adenocarcinoma.[393] Some of them have been associated with signs of excessive human chorionic gonadotropin secretion, and the hormone has been detected in the tumor cells immunohistochemically.[399,401] *Yolk sac tumor (endodermal sinus tumor)* has also been reported as a primary gastric neoplasm, either alone[397] or in combination with choriocarcinoma.[391] *Metastatic carcinoma* may occur in the stomach from any widely disseminated

neoplasm, particularly from the breast.[389] When the primary breast tumor is a lobular carcinoma, the gross appearance of the stomach may be that of linitis plastica.[390] Another malignancy that may metastasize to the stomach as part of its systemic spread is malignant melanoma.

REFERENCES
NORMAL ANATOMY

1 Joske RA, Finckh ES, Wood IJ: Gastric biopsy. A study of 1,000 consecutive successful gastric biopsies. Q J Med **95:**269-294, 1955.

2 Owen DA: Normal histology of the stomach. Am J Surg Pathol **10:**48-61, 1986.

3 Rubin W, Ross LL, Sleisenger MJ, Jeffries GH: The normal human gastric epithelia. A fine structural study. Lab Invest **19:**598-626, 1968.

4 Whitehead R: Intrepretation of mucosal biopsies from the gastrointestinal tract. In Dyke SC (ed): Recent advances in clinical pathology, Series 5, London, 1968, A. & A. Churchill, Ltd., pp. 375-400.

HETEROTOPIC TISSUES

5 Goldfarb WB, Bennett D, Monafo W: Carcinoma in heterotopic gastric pancreas. Ann Surg **158:**56-58, 1963.

6 Palmer ED: Benign intramural tumors of the stomach. A review with special reference to gross pathology. Medicine [Baltimore] **30:**81-181, 1951.

7 Stewart MJ, Taylor AL: Adenomyoma of the stomach. J Pathol Bacteriol **28:**195-202, 1925.

HYPERTROPHIC PYLORIC STENOSIS

8 Batcup G, Spitz L: A histopathological study of gastric mucosal biopsies in infantile hypertrophic pyloric stenosis. J Clin Pathol **32:**625-628, 1979.

9 Bateson EM, Talerman A, Walrond ER: Radiological and pathological observations in a series of seventeen cases of hypertrophic pyloric stenosis of adults. Br J Radiol **42:**1-8, 1969.

10 Du Plessis DJ: Primary hypertrophic pyloric stenosis in the adult. Br J Surg **53:**485-492, 1966.

11 Lumsden K, Truelove SC: Primary hypertrophic pyloric stenosis in the adult. Br J Radiol **31:**261-266, 1955.

12 Wellman KF, Kagan A, Fang H: Hypertrophic pyloric stenosis in adults. Gastroenterology **46:**601-608, 1964.

CHRONIC GASTRITIS

13 Barwick KW: Chronic gastritis. The pathologist's role. Pathol Annu **22**(Pt 2):223-251, 1987.

14 Bordi C, Gabrielli M, Missale G: Pathological changes of endocrine cells in chronic atrophic gastritis. An ultrastructural study on peroral gastric biopsy specimens. Arch Pathol Lab Med **102:**129-135, 1978.

15 Buck GE, Gourley WK, Lee WK, Subramanyam K, Latimer JM, DiNuzzo AR: Relation of *Campylobacter pyloridis* to gastritis and peptic ulcer. J Infect Dis **153:**664-669, 1986.

16 Correa P: The epidemiology and pathogenesis of chronic gastritis. Three etiologic entities. Fron Gastointest Res **6:**98-108, 1980.

17 Correa P: Clinical implications of recent developments in gastric carcinoma pathology and epidemiology. Semin Oncol **12:**2-10, 1985.

18 Drumm B, Sherman P, Cutz E, Karmali M: Association of *Campylobacter pylori* on the gastric mucosa with antral gastritis in children, N Engl J Med **316:**1557-1561, 1987.

19 Filipe MI, Potet F, Bogomoletz WV, Dawson PA, Fabiani B, Chauveinc P, Fenzy A, Gazzard B, Goldfain D, Zeegen R: Incomplete sulphomucin-secreting intestinal metaplasia for gastric cancer. Preliminary data from a prospective study from three centres. Gut **26:**1319-1326, 1985.

20 Garvey W, Fathi A, Bigelow F: Modified Steiner for the demonstration of spirochetes. J Histotechnol **8:**15-17, 1985.

21 Goldman H, Antonioli DA: Mucosal biopsy of the esophagus, stomach, and proximal duodenum. Hum Pathol **13:**423-448, 1982.

22 Hebbel R: Chronic gastritis, its relation to gastric and duodenal ulcer and to gastric carcinoma. Am J Pathol **19:**43-71, 1943.

23 Iida F, Kusama J: Gastric carcinoma and intestinal metaplasia. Significance of types of intestinal metaplasia upon development of gastric carcinoma. Cancer **50:**2854-2858, 1982.

24 Jass JR, Filipe MI: The mucin profiles of normal gastric mucosa, intestinal metaplasia and its variants and gastric carcinoma. Histochem J **13:**931-939, 1981.

25 Joske RA, Finckh ES, Wood IJ: Gastric biopsy. A study of 1,000 consecutive successful gastric biopsies. Q J Med **95:**269-294, 1955.

26 Kekki M, Villako K: Dynamic behavior of gastritis in various populations and subpopulations, Ann Clin Res **13:**119-122, 1981.

27 Matsukura N, Suzuki K, Kawachi T, Aoyagi M, Sugimura T, Kitaoka H, Numajiri H, Shirota A, Itabashi M, Hirota T: Distribution of marker enzymes and mucin in intestinal metaplasia in human stomach and relation of complete and incomplete types of intestinal metaplasia to minute gastric carcinoma. J Natl Cancer Inst **65:**231-240, 1980.

28 Mingazzini P, Carlei F, Malchiodi-Albedi F, Lezoche E, Covotta A, Speranza V, Polak JM: Endocrine cells in intestinal metaplasia of the stomach. J Pathol **144:**171-178, 1984.

29 Morson BC: Intestinal metaplasia of the gastric mucosa. Br J Cancer **9:**365-376, 1955.

30 Parl FF, Lev R, Thomas E, Pitchumoni CS: Histologic and morphometric study of chronic gastritis in alcoholic patients. Hum Pathol **10:**45-56, 1979.

31 Rothery GA, Day DW: Intestinal metaplasia in endoscopic biopsy specimens of gastric mucosa. J Clin Pathol **38:**613-621, 1985.

32 Rubin W: Proliferation of endocrine-like (enterochromaffin) cells in atrophic gastric mucosa. Gastroenterology **57:**641-648, 1969.

33 Segura DI, Montero C: Histochemical characterization of different types of intestinal metaplasia in gastric mucosa. Cancer **52:**498-503, 1983.

34 Stockton M, McColl I: Comparative electron microscopic features of normal intermediate and metaplastic pyloric epithelium. Histopathology **7:**859-871, 1983.

35 Strickland RG, MacKay IR: A reappraisal of the nature and significance of chronic atrophic gastritis. Am J Dig Dis **18:**426-440, 1973.

35a Thompson IW, Day DW, Wright NA: Subnuclear vacuolated mucous cells. A novel abnormality of simple mucin-secreting cells of nonspecialized gastric mucosa and Brunner's glands. Histopathology **11:**1067-1081, 1987.

36 Tsutsumi YT, Nagura H, Watanabe K: Immune aspects of intestinal metaplasia of the stomach. An immunohistochemical study. Virchows Arch [Pathol Anat] **403:**345-359, 1984.

37 Whitehead R: Gastritis—clinical and pathological aspects. In Truelove SC, Jewell DP (eds): Topics in gastroenterology. Oxford, 1973, Blackwell Scientific Publications, pp. 45-57, chap. 4.

38 Whitehead R, Truelove SC, Gear MWL: The histological diagnosis of chronic gastritis in fibreoptic gastroscope biopsy specimens. J Clin Pathol **25:**1-11, 1972.

38a Yardley JH, Pauli G: Campylobacter pylori. A newly recognized infectious agent in the gastrointestinal tract. Am J Surg Pathol **12:**89-99, 1988.

OTHER TYPES OF GASTRITIS

39 Ashby BS, Appleton PJ, Dawson I: Eosinophilic granuloma of gastro-intestinal tract caused by herring parasite, *Eustoma rotundatum.* Br Med J **1:**1141-1145, 1964.

40 Butz WC, Watts JC, Rosales-Quintana S, Hicklin MD: Erosive gastritis as a manifestation of secondary syphilis. Am J Clin Pathol **63:**895-900, 1975.

41 Clagett OT, Walters W: Tuberculosis of the stomach. Arch Surg **37:**505-520, 1938.

42 DeSchryver-Kecskemeti K, Clouse RE: A previously unrecognized subgroup of "eosinophilic gastroenteritis." Association with connective tissue diseases. Am J Surg Pathol **8:**171-180, 1984.

43 Editorial: Erosive gastritis. Br Med J **2:**211-212, 1974.

44 Fahimi HD, Deren JJ, Gottlieb LS, Zamcheck N: Isolated granulomatous gastritis. Its relationship to disseminated sarcoidosis and regional enteritis. Gastroenterology **45:**161-175, 19863.

45 Flint A, Murad TM: Malakoplakia amd malakoplakia like lesions of the upper gastrointestinal tract. Ultrastruct Pathol **7:**167-176, 1984.

46 Goldman H, Antonioli DA: Mucosal biopsy of the esophagus, stomach and proximal duodenum. Hum Pathol **13:**423-448, 1982.

47 Goldman H, Proujansky R: Allergic proctitis and gastroenteritis in children. Clinical and mucosal biopsy features in 53 cases. Am J Surg Pathol **10:**75-86, 1986.

48 Haggitt RC, Meissner WA: Crohn's disease of the upper gastrointestinal tract. Am J Clin Pathol **59:**613-622, 1973.

49 Heddle SB, Parrott KB, Paloschi GPG, Prentice RSA, Persyko L, Beck IT: Diffuse eosinophilic gastroenteritis. Can Med Assoc J **100:**554-559, 1969.

50 Johnstone JM, Morson BC: Eosinophilic gastroenteritis. Histopathology **2:**335-348, 1978.

51 Lulu DJ, Dragstedt LR II: Massive bleeding due to acute hemorrhagic gastritis. Arch Surg **101:**550-554, 1970.

52 McCormack TT, Sims J, Eyre-Brook I, Kennedy H, Goepel J, Johnson AG, Triger DR: Gastric lesions in portal hypertension. Inflammatory gastritis or congestive gastropathy? Gut **26:**1226-1232, 1985.

53 McCune WS, Gusack M, Newman W: Eosinophilic gastroduodenitis with pyloric obstruction. Ann Surg **142:**510-518, 1955.

54 McNabb PC, Fleming CR, Higgins JA, Davis GL: Transmural eosinophilic gastroenteritis with ascites. Mayo Clin Proc **54:**119-122, 1979.

55 Nakabayashi H, Ito T, Izutsu K, Yatani R, Ishida K: Malakoplakia of the stomach. Report of a case and review of the literature. Arch Pathol Lab Med **102:**136-139, 1978.

56 Palmer WL, Schindler R, Templeton FE, Humphreys EM: Syphilis of the stomach. Case report. Ann Intern Med **18:**393-406, 1943.

57 Salmon PR, Paulley JW: Eosinophilic granuloma of the gastro-intestinal tract. Gut **8:**8-14, 1967.

58 Sirak HD: Boeck's sarcoid of the stomach simulating linitis plastica. Arch Surg **69:**769-776, 1954.

59 Strayer DS, Phillips GB, Barker KH, Winokur T, DeSchryver-Kecskemeti K: Gastric cytomegalovirus infection in bone marrow transplant patients. An indication of generalized disease. Cancer **48:**1478-1483, 1981.

60 Widerlite L, Trier JS, Blacklow NR, Schreiber S: Structure of the gastric mucosa in acute infectious nonbacterial gastroenteritis. Gastroenterology **68:**425-430, 1975.

61 Williams C, Kimmelstiel P: Syphilis of the stomach. JAMA **115:**578-582, 1940.

62 Winawer SJ, Bejar J, McCray RS, Zamcheck N: Hemorrhagic gastritis. Importance of associated chronic gastritis. Arch Intern Med **127:**120-131, 1971.

PEPTIC AND OTHER BENIGN ULCERS

63 Barragry TP, Blacthford JW III, O'Connor Allen M: Giant gastric ulcers. A review of 49 cases. Ann Surg **203:**255-259, 1986.

64 Börsch G, Schmidt G: What's new in steroid and nonsteroid drug effects on gastroduodenal mucosa? Pathol Res Pract **180:**437-444, 1985.

65 Davis Z, Verheyden CN, Van Heerden JA: The surgically treated chronic gastric ulcer. An extended followup. Ann Surg **185:**205-209, 1977.

66 Dragstedt LR: The pathogenesis of duodenal and gastric ulcers. Am J Surg **136:**286-301, 1978.

67 Elliott GV, Wald SM, Benz RI: A roentgenologic study of ulcerating lesions of the stomach. Am J Roentgenol Radium Ther Nucl Med **77:**612-622, 1957.

68 Fitts CD, Cathcart RS III, Artz CP, Spicer SS: Acute gastrointestinal tract ulceration. Cushing's ulcer, steroid ulcer, Curling's ulcer and stress ulcer. Am J Surg **37:**218-223, 1971.

69 Isenberg JI, Johansson C (eds): Peptic ulcer disease. Clin Gastroenterol 13:287-654, 1984.

70 Katzenstein AL, Maksem J: Candidal infection of gastric ulcers. Am J Clin Pathol 71:137-141, 1979.

71 Kelly KA, Malagelada JR: Medical and surgical treatment of chronic gastric ulcer. Clin Gastroenterol 13:621-634, 1984.

72 Langman MJS: Epidemiological evidence for the association of aspirin and acute gastrointestinal bleeding. Gut 11:627-634, 1970.

73 Oohara T, Tohma H, Aono G, Ukawa S, Kondo Y: Intestinal metaplasia of the regenerative epithelia in 549 gastric ulcers. Hum Pathol 14:1066-1071, 1983.

74 Pruitt BA Jr, Foley FD, Moncrief JA: Curling's ulcer. A clinical-pathology study of 323 cases. Am Surg 172:523-539, 1970.

75 Weidner N, Smith JG, LaVanway JM: Peptic ulceration with marked epithelial atypia following hepatic arterial infusion chemotherapy. A lesion initially misinterpreted as carcinoma. Am J Surg Pathol 7:261-268, 1983.

OTHER NON-NEOPLASTIC LESIONS

76 Buchholz RR, Haisten AS: Phytobezoars following gastric surgery for duodenal ulcer. Surg Clin North Am 52:341-352, 1972.

77 Cunningham JR, Lippman SM, Renie WA, Francomano CA, Maumenee IH, Pyeritz RE: Pseudoxanthoma elasticum. Treatment of gastrointestinal hemorrhage by arterial embolization and observations on autosomal dominant inheritance. Johns Hopkins Med J 147:168-173, 1980.

78 Delia CW: Phytobezoars (diospyrobezoars). A clinicopathologic correlation and review of six cases. Arch Surg 82:579-583, 1961.

79 Eells RW, Simril WA: Gastric diverticula. Report of thirty-one cases. Am J Roentgenol Radium Ther Nucl Med 68:8-14, 1952.

80 Enjoji M, Sumiyoshi K, Sueyoshi K: Elastofibromatous lesion of the stomach in a patient with elastofibroma dorsi. Am J Surg Pathol 9:233-237, 1985.

81 Franzin G, Novelli P: Gastritis cystica profunda. Histopathology 5:535-547, 1981.

82 Goon CD: Duplication of the stomach with extension into the chest. Am Surg 19:721-727, 1953.

83 Holloway WD, Lee SP, Nicholson GI: The composition and dissolution of phytobezoars. Arch Pathol Lab Med 104:159-161, 1980.

84 Iwanaga T, Koyama H, Takahashi Y, Taniguchi H, Wada A: Diffuse submucosal cysts and carcinoma of the stomach. Cancer 36:606-614, 1975.

85 Jensen K, Raynor S, Rose SG, Bailey ST, Schenken JR: Amyloid tumors of the gastrointestinal tract. A report of two cases and review of the literature. Am J Gastroenterol 80:784-786, 1985.

86 Kato Y, Sugano H, Rubio CA: Classification of intramucosal cysts of the stomach. Histopathology 7:931-938, 1983.

87 Marek J, Jurek K: Comparative light microscopical and x-ray microanalysis study of barium granuloma. Pathol Res Pract 171:293-302, 1981.

88 McGregor DH, Haque AU: Gastric hyalinization associated with peptic ulceration. Arch Pathol Lab Med 106:472-475, 1982.

89 Millard M: Fatal rupture of gastric aneurysm. Arch Pathol 59:363-371, 1955.

90 Molnár P, Mikó T: Multiple arterial caliber persistence resulting in hematomas and fatal rupture of the gastric wall. Am J Surg Pathol 6:83-86, 1982.

91 Mower GA, Whitehead R: Gastric hemorrhage due to ruptured arteriovenous malformation (Dieulafoy's disease). Pathology 18:54-57, 1986.

92 Nihei K, Terashima K, Aoyama K, Imai Y, Sato H: Benign histiocytosis X of stomach. Previously undescribed lesion. Acta Pathol Jpn 33:577-588, 1983.

93 Parker BC, Guthrie J, France NE, Atwell JD: Gastric duplications in infancy. J Pediatr Surg 7:294-298, 1972.

94 Parrott NR, Sunter JP, Taylor RMR, Johnston IDA: Gastric hyalinization presenting in life and mimicking gastric cancer. Arch Pathol Lab Med 110:155-156, 1986.

95 Pieterse AS, Rowland R, Labrooy JT: Gastric xanthomas. Pathology 17:455-457, 1985.

96 Rubio CA, Öhman U: The intramucosal cysts of the stomach. I. In Swedish subjects with gastric or duodenal ulcers. Acta Pathol Microbiol Immunol Scand [A] 90:363-366, 1982.

96a Suit PF, Petras RE, Bauer TW, Petrini JL Jr: Gastric antral vascular ectasia. A histologic and morphometric study of "the watermelon stomach." Am J Surg Pathol 11:750-757, 1987.

97 Walley VM: Amyloid deposition in a gastric arteriovenous malformation. Arch Pathol Lab Med 110:69-71, 1986.

98 Yamagiwa H, Matsuzaki O, Ishihara A, Yoshimura H: Heterotopic gastric glands in the submucosa of the stomach. Acta Pathol Jpn 29:347-350, 1979.

99 Zhu-F-G, Deng X-J, Cheng N-J: Intramucosal cysts in gastric mucosa adjacent to carcinoma and peptic ulcer. A histochemical study. Histopathology 11:631-638, 1987.

POLYPS

100 Bolck F, Katenkamp D: Granuloblastomas of the stomach (so-called eosinophilic granulomas)—a variant of fibrous histiocytomas? Pathol Res Pract 171:336-344, 1981.

101 Dirschmid K, Walser J, Hügel H: Pseudomalignant erosion in hyperplastic gastric polyps. Cancer 54:2290-2293, 1984.

102 Elster K: Histologic classification of gastric polyps. Curr Topics Pathol 63:77-93, 1976.

103 Griffel B, Engleberg M, Reiss R, Saba H: Multiple polypoid cystic gastritis in old gastroenteric stoma. Arch Pathol 97:316-318, 1974.

104 Halbert RE: Peutz-Jeghers syndrome with metastasizing gastric adenocarcinoma. Report of a case. Arch Pathol Lab Med 106:517-520, 1982.

105 Hattori T: Morphological range of hyperplastic polyps and carcinomas arising in hyperplastic polyps of the stomach. J Clin Pathol 38:622-630, 1985.

106 Helwig EB, Ranier A: Inflammatory fibroid polyps of the stomach. Surg Gynecol Obstet 96:355-367, 1953.

106a Iida M, Yao T, Itoh H, Watanabe H, Matsui T, Iwashita A, Fujishima M: Natural history of gastric adenomas in patients with familial adenomatosis coli/Gardner's syndrome. Cancer 61:605-611, 1988.

107 Ito H, Hata J, Yokozaki H, Nakatani H, Oda N, Tahara E: Tubular adenoma of the human stomach. An immunohistochemical anaylsis of gut hormones, serotonin, carcinoembryonic antigen, secretory component, and lysozyme. Cancer 58:2264-2272, 1986.

108 Johnstone JM, Morson BC: Inflammatory fibroid polyp of the gastrointestinal tract. Histopathology 2:349-361, 1978.

109 Kamiya T, Morishita T, Asakura H, Miura S, Munakata Y, Tsuchiya M: Long-term follow-up study of gastric adenoma and its relation to gastric protruded carcinoma. Cancer 50:2496-2503, 1982.

110 Laxén F, Sipponen P, Ihamáki T, Hakkiluoto A, Dortscheva A: Gastric polyps. Their morphological and endoscopical characteristics and relation to gastric carcinoma. Acta Pathol Microbiol Immunol Scand [A] 90:221-228, 1982.

111 Lee RG, Burt RW: The histopathology of fundic gland polyps of the stomach. Am J Clin Pathol 86:498-503, 1986.

112 Lipper S, Kahn LB: Superficial cystic gastritis with alopecia. A forme fruste of the Cronkhite-Canada syndrome. Arch Pathol Lab Med 101:432-436, 1977.

113 Marshak RH, Feldman F: Gastric polyps. Am J Dig Dis 10:909-935, 1965.

114 Menétrier P: Des polyadenomes gastriques et de leures rapports avec le cancer de l'estomac. Arch Physiol Norm Pathol 1:32-55, 236-262, Pl. III, 1888.

115 Miller JH, Gisvold JJ, Weiland LH, Mellrath DC: Upper gastrointestinal tract villous tumors. AJR 134:933-936, 1980.

116 Ming SC, Goldman H: Gastric polyps. Histogenetic classification and its relation to carcinoma. Cancer 18:721-726, 1965.

117 Monaco AP, Roth SI, Castleman B, Welch CE: Adenomatous polyps of the stomach. A clinical and pathological study of one hundred and fifty-three cases. Cancer 15:456-467, 1962.

118 Nakamura T, Nakano G-I: Histopathological classification and malignant change in gastric polyps. J Clin Pathol 38:754-764, 1985.

119 Navas-Palacios JJ, Colina-Ruizdelgado F, Sanchez-Larrea MD, Cortes-Cansino J: Inflammatory fibroid polyps of the gastrointestinal tract. An immunohistochemical and electron microscopic study. Cancer 51:1682-1690, 1983.

120 Seifert E, Gail K, Weismuller J: Gastric polypectomy. Long term results (survey of 23 centres in Germany). Endoscopy 15:8-11, 1983.

121 Sipponen P, Laxén F, Seppälä K: Cystic "hamartomatous" gastric polyps. A disorder of oxyntic glands. Histopathology 7:729-737, 1983.

122 Snover DC: Benign epithelial polyps of the stomach. Pathol Annu 20(Pt 1):303-329, 1985.

123 Stemmermann GN, Hayashi T: Hyperplastic polyps of the gastric mucosa adjacent of gastroenterostomy stomas. Am J Clin Pathol 71:341-345, 1979.

124 Tomasulo J: Gastric polyps. Histologic types and their relationship to gastric carcinoma. Cancer 27:1346-1355, 1971.

125 Utsunomiya J, Maki T, Iwama T, Hamaguchi E, Aoki M: Gastric lesion of familial polyposis coli. Cancer 34:745-754, 1974.

126 Watanabe H, Enjoji M, Yao T, Ohsato K: Gastric lesions in familial adenomatosis coli. Their incidence and histologic analysis. Hum Pathol 9:269-283, 1978.

MENÉTRIER'S DISEASE AND ZOLLINGER-ELLISON SYNDROME

127 Bartlett JP, Adams WE: Generalized giant hypertrophic gastritis simulating neoplasm. Arch Surg 60:543-588, 1950.

128 Kenney FD, Dockerty MB, Waugh JM: Giant hypertrophy of gastric mucosa. Cancer 7:671-681, 1954.

129 Kraut JR, Powell R, Hruby MA, Lloyd-Still JD: Menétrier's disease in childhood. Report of two cases and a review of the literature. J Pedriatr Surg 16:707-711, 1981.

130 Menétrier P: Des polyadenomes gastriques et de leures rapports avec le cancer de l'estomac. Arch Physiol Norm Pathol **1**:32-55, 236-262, Pl III, 1888.

131 Palmer ED: What Menétrier really said. Gastrointest Endosc **15**:83-90, 1968.

132 Scharschmidt BF: The natural history of hypertropic gastropathy (Menétrier's disease). Report of a case with 16 year follow-up and review of 120 cases from the literature. Am J Med **63**:644-652, 1977.

133 Solcia E, Capella C, Buffa R, et al.: Pathology of the Zollinger-Ellison syndrome. In Fenoglio CM, Wolff M (eds): Progress in surgical pathology. New York, 1980, Masson Publishing Co.

DYSPLASIA

134 Grundmann E: Classification and clinical consequences of precancerous lesions in the digestive and respiratory tracts. Acta Pathol Jpn **33**:195-217, 1983.

135 Jarvis LR, Whitehead R: Morphometric anaylsis of gastric dysplasia. J Pathol **147**:133-138, 1985.

136 Jass JR: A classification of gastric dysplasia. Histopathology **7**:181-193, 1983.

137 Ming S-C, Bajtai A, Correa P, Elster K, Jarvi OH, Munoz N, Nagayo T, Stemmerman GN: Gastric dysplasia. Significance and pathologic criteria. Cancer **54**:1794-1801, 1984.

138 Morson BC, Sobin LH, Grundmann E, Johansen A, Nagoya T, Serck-Hanssen A: Precancerous conditions and epithelial dysplasia in the stomach. J Clin Pathol **33**:711-721, 1980.

139 Rubio CA, Hirota T, Itabashi T: Atypical mitoses in elevated dysplasias of the stomach. Pathol Res Pract **180**:372-376, 1985.

139a Saraga E-P, Gardiol D, Costa J: Gastric dysplasia. A histological follow-up study. Am J Surg Pathol **11**:788-796, 1987.

CARCINOMA
General features

140 Brumback RA, Gerber JE, Hicks DG, Strauchen JA: Adenocarcinoma of the stomach following irradiation and chemotherapy of lymphoma in young patients. Cancer **54**:994-998, 1984.

141 Correa P: Clinical implications of recent developments in gastric carcinoma pathology and epidemiology. Semin Oncol **12**:2-10, 1985.

142 Dupont JB Jr, Lee JR, Burton GR, Cohn I Jr: Adenocarcinoma of the stomach. Review of 1,497 cases. Cancer **41**:941-947, 1978.

143 Grabiec J, Owen DA: Carcinoma of the stomach in young persons. Cancer **56**:388-396, 1985.

144 Grundmann E (ed): Gastric carcinogenesis. Pathol Res Pract **164**:1-355, 1979.

145 Hall CN, Darkin D, Brimblecombe R, Cook AJ, Kirkham JS, Northfield TC: Evaluation of the nitrosamine hypothesis of gastric carcinogenesis in precancerous conditions. Gut **27**:491-498, 1986.

146 Hattori T: Development of adenocarcinomas in the stomach. Cancer **57**:1528, 1534, 1986.

147 Hill MJ: Etiology of gastric carcinoma. Clin Oncol **3**:237-249, 1984.

148 Iwanaga T, Koyama H, Takahashi Y, Taniguchi H, Wada A: Diffuse submucosal cysts and carcinoma of the stomach. Cancer **36**:606-614, 1975.

149 Lauren P: The two histological main types of gastric carcinoma. Diffuse and so-called intestinal type carcinoma. Acta Pathol Microbiol Scand **64**:31-49, 1965.

150 Pillay I, Petrelli M: Diffuse cystic glandular malformation of the stomach associated with adenocarcinoma. Case report and review of the literature. Cancer **38**:915-920, 1976.

151 Schafer LW, Larson DE, Melton LJ III, Higgins JA, Zinsmeister AR: Risk of development of gastric carcinoma in patients with pernicious anemia. A population-based study in Rochester, Minnesota. Mayo Clin Proc **60**:444-448, 1985.

152 Siegel SM, Hays DM, Romansky S, Issacs H: Carcinoma of the stomach in childhood. Cancer **38**:1781-1784, 1976.

153 Sipponen P, Kekki M, Haapakoski J, Ihamäki T, Siurala M: Gastric cancer risk in chronic atrophic gastritis. Statistical calculations of cross-sectional data. Int J Cancer **35**:173-177, 1985.

154 Sipponen P, Kekki M, Siurala M: Atrophic chronic gastritis and intestinal metaplasia in gastric carcinoma. Comparison with a representative population sample. Cancer **52**:1062-1068, 1983.

155 Taki K, Kuwabara N: Studies of histogenesis of the gastric carcinoma using minute cancers. Pathol Res Pract **172**:176-190, 1981.

156 Tso PL, Bringaze WL III, Dauterive AH, Correa P, Cohn I Jr: Gastric carcinoma in the young. Cancer **59**:1362-1365, 1987.

157 Whitehead R, Skinner JM, Heenan PJ: Incidence of carcinoma of stomach and tumour type. Br J Cancer **30**:370-372, 1974.

Morphologic features and classification

158 Altmannsberger M, Weber K, Hölscher A, Schauer A, Osborn M: Antibodies to intermediate filaments as diagnostic tools. Human gastrointestinal carcinomas express prekeratin. Lab Invest **46**:520-526, 1982.

159 Antonioli DA, Goldman H: Changes in the location and type of gastric adenocarcinoma. Cancer **50**:775-781, 1982.

160 Borrman R: Geschwülste des Magens und Duodenums. In Henske F, Lubarsch O (eds): Handbuch der Speziellen Pathologischen Antomie und Histologie. Berlin, 1926, Julius Springer, pp. IV-L, 864-871.

161 Capella C, Cornaggia M, Usellini L, Bordi C, Bondi A, Cook MG, Eusebi V: Neoplastic cells containing lysozyme in gastric carcinomas. Pathology **16**:87-92, 1984.

162 Cook HC: Neutral mucin content of gastric carcinomas as a diagnostic aid in the identification of secondary deposits. Histopathology **6**:591-599, 1982.

163 Correa P: Pathology of gastric cancer. Clin Oncol **3**:251-257, 1984.

164 Esaki Y, Hirokawa K, Yamashiro M: Multiple gastric cancers in the aged with special reference to intramucosal cancers. Cancer **59**:560-565, 1987.

164a Fiocca R, Cornaggia M, Villani L, Capella C, Solcia E, Samloff IM: Expression of pepsinogen II in gastric cancer. Its relationship to local invasion and lymph node metastases. Cancer **61**:956-962, 1988.

165 Fiocca R, Villani L, Tenti P, Solcia E, Cornaggia M, Frigerio B, Capella C: Characterization of four main cell types in gastric cancer. Foveolar, mucopeptic, intestinal columnar and goblet cells. An histopathologic, histochemical and ultrastructural study of "early" and "advanced" tumours. Pathol Res Pract **182**:308-325, 1987.

166 Grabiec J, Owen DA: Carcinoma of the stomach in young persons. Cancer **56**:388-396, 1985.

167 Heitz PU, Wegmann W: Identification of neoplastic Paneth cells in an adenocarcinoma of the stomach using lysozyme as a marker and electron microscopy. Virchows Arch [Pathol Anat] **386**:107-116, 1980.

168 Isaacson P: Biopsy appearances easily mistaken for malignancy in gastrointestinal endoscopy. Histopathology **6**:377-389, 1982.

169 Ito H, Tahara E: Human chorionic gonadotropin in human gastric carcinoma. A retrospective immunohistochemical study. Acta Pathol Jpn **33**:287-296, 1983.

170 Kaibara N, Kimura O, Nishidoi H, Makino M, Kawasumi H, Koga S: High incidence of liver metastasis in gastric cancer with medullary growth pattern. J Surg Oncol **28**:195-198, 1985.

171 Lauren P: The two histological main types of gastric carcinoma—diffuse and so-called intestinal type carcinoma. Acta Pathol Microbiol Scand **64**:31-49, 1965.

172 Lev R: The mucin histochemistry of normal and neoplastic gastric mucosa. Lab Invest **14**:2080-2100, 1965.

173 Ma J, De Boer WGRM, Nayman J: Intestinal mucinous substances in gastric intestinal metaplasia and carcinoma studied by immunofluorescence. Cancer **49**:1664-1667, 1982.

174 Ming SC: Gastric carcinoma. A pathobiological classification. Cancer **39**:2475-2485, 1977.

175 Ming SC, Goldman H, Freiman DG: Intestinal metaplasia and histogenesis of carcinoma in human stomachs. Light and electron microscopic study. Cancer **20**:1418-1429, 1967.

176 Murayama H, Imai T, Kikuchi J: Solid carcinomas of the stomach. A combined histochemical, light and electron microscopic study. Cancer **51**:1673-1681, 1983.

177 Nielsen K, Teglbjaerg PS: Carcino-embryonic antigen (CEA) in gastric adenocarcinomas. Morphologic patterns and their relationship to a histogenetic classification. Acta Pathol Microbiol Immunol Scand [A] **90**:393-396, 1982.

178 Oota R, Sobin J: Histological typing of gastric and oesophageal tumors. Geneva, 1977, WHO.

179 Petras RE, Hart WR, Bukowski RM: Gastric epithelial atypia associated with heptic arterial infusion chemotherapy. Its distinction from early gastric carcinoma. Cancer **56**:745-750, 1985.

180 Saphir O: Linitis plastica type of carcinoma. Surg Gynecol Obstet **76**:206-213, 1943.

181 Stout AP: Tumors of the stomach. In Atlas of tumor pathology, Sect. VI, Fasc. 21, Washington, DC, 1953, Armed Forces Institute of Pathology.

182 Tahara E, Ito H, Shimamoto F, Iwamoto T, Nakagami K, Niimoto H: Lysozyme in human gastric carcinoma. A retrospective immunohistochemical study. Histopathology **6**:409-421, 1982.

183 Tahara E, Ito H, Taniyama K, Yokozaki H, Hata J: Alpha₁-antitrypsin, alpha₁-antichymotrypsin, and alpha₂-macroglobulin in human gastric carcinomas. A retrospective immunohistochemical study. Hum Pathol **15**:957-964, 1984.

184 Tso PL, Bringaze WL III, Dauterive AH, Correa P, Cohn I Jr: Gastric carcinoma in the young. Cancer **59**:1362-1365, 1987.

185 Warner TF, Donnelly WJ, Hafez GR, Renwick B, Engstrand D, Barsness L:

Immunocytochemical evidence of gastric proteases in adenocarcinoma of the stomach. Cancer **58:**1328-1332, 1986.

186 Yamagiwa H, Yoshimura H, Tomiyama H, Onishi T, Matsuzaki O: Clinicopathological study of gastric cancers in the greater curvature. Acta Pathol Jpn **34:**519-527, 1984.

187 Yamashina M: A variant of early gastric carcinoma. Histologic and histochemical studies of early signet ring cell carcinomas discovered beneath preserved surface epithelium. Cancer **58:**1333-1339, 1986.

Other microscopic types

188 Ambe K, Mori M, Enjoji M: Early gastric carcinoma with multiple endocrine cell micronests. Am J Surg Pathol **11:**310-315, 1987.

189 Bonar SF, Sweeney EC: The prevalence, prognostic significance and hormonal content of endocrine cells in gastric cancer. Histopathology **10:**53-63, 1986.

190 Brander WL, Needham PRG, Morgan AD: Indolent mucoid carcinoma of stomach. J Clin Pathol **27:**536-541, 1974.

191 Callery CD, Sanders MM, Pratt S, Turnbull AD: Squamous cell carcinoma of the stomach. A study of four patients with comments on histogenesis. J Surg Oncol **29:**166-172, 1985.

192 Capella C, Frigerio B, Cornaggia M, Solcia E, Pinzon-Trujillo Y, Chejfcc G: Gastric parietal cell carcinoma—a newly recognized entity. Light microscopic and ultrastructural features. Histopathology **8:**813-824, 1984.

193 Ishikura H, Kirimoto K, Shamoto M, Miyamoto Y, Yamagiwa H, Itoh T, Aizawa M: Hepatoid adenocarcinomas of the stomach. An analysis of seven cases. Cancer **58:**119-126, 1986.

194 Kubo T, Watanabe H: Neoplastic argentaffin cells in gastric and intestinal carcinomas. Cancer **27:**447-454, 1971.

195 Mori M, Iwashita A, Enjoji M: Adenosquamous carcinoma of the stomach. A clinicopathologic analysis of 28 cases. Cancer **57:**333-339, 1986.

196 Mori M, Iwashita A, Enjoji M: Squamous cell carcinoma of the stomach. Report of three cases. Am J Gastroenterol **81:**339-342, 1986.

197 Rogers LW, Murphy RC: Gastric carcinoid and gastric carcinoma. Am J Surg Pathol **3:**195-202, 1979.

198 Straus R, Heschel S, Fortmann DJ: Primary adenosquamous carcinoma of the stomach. A case report and review. Cancer **24:**985-995, 1969.

199 Sweeney EC, McDonnell LM: Atypical gastric carcinoids. Histopathology **4:**215-224, 1980.

200 Tahara E, Ito H, Nakagami K, Shimamoto F, Yamamoto M, Sumii K: Scirrhous argyrophil cell carcinoma of the stomach with multiple production of polypeptide hormones, amine, CEA, lysozyme, and HCG. Cancer **49:**1904-1915, 1982.

201 Tsutsumi Y, Hara M: Application of parietal cell autoantibody to histopathological studies. Acta Pathol Jpn **35:**823-829, 1985.

201a Ulich TR, Kollin M, Lewin KJ: Composite gastric carcinoma. Report of a tumor of the carcinoma-carcinoid spectrum. Arch Pathol Lab Med **112:**91-93, 1988.

202 Yamashina M, Flinner RA: Concurrent occurrence of adenocarcinoma and carcinoid tumor in the stomach. A composite tumor or collision tumors? Am J Clin Pathol **83:**233-236, 1985.

Diagnosis—biopsy and cytology

203 Boon TH, Schade ROK, Middleton GD, Reece M: An attempt at presymptomatic diagnosis of gastric carcinoma in pernicious anaemia. Gut **5:**269-270, 1964.

204 Chambers LA, Clark WE II: The endoscopic diagnosis of gastroesophageal malignancy. A cytologic review. Acta Cytol [Baltimore] **30:**110-114, 1986.

204a Czerniak B, Herz F, Koss LG, Schlom J: *ras* oncogene p21 as a tumor marker in the cytodiagnosis of gastric and colonic carcinomas. Cancer **60:**2432-2436, 1987.

205 Foushee JHS, Kalnins ZA, Dixon FR, Girsh S, Morehead RP, O'Brien TF, Pribor H, Tattory C: Gastric cytology. Evaluation of methods and results in 1,670 cases. Acta Cytol [Baltimore] **13:**339-406, 1969.

206 Fujita S: Biology of early gastric carcinoma. Pathol Res Pract **163:**297-309, 1978.

207 Gupta RK, Rogers KE: Endoscopic cytology and biopsy in the diagnosis of gastroesophageal malignancy. Acta Cytol [Baltimore] **27:**17-22, 1983.

208 Hayashida T, Kidokoro T: End results of early gastric carcinoma collected from 22 institutions. Stomach and Intestine **4:**1077-1085, 1969.

209 Iishi H, Yamamoto R, Tatsuta M, Okuda S: Evaluation of fine-needle aspiration biopsy under direct vision gastrofiberscopy in diagnosis of diffusely infiltrating carcinoma of the stomach. Cancer **57:**1365-1369, 1986.

210 Jorde R, Østensen H, Bostad LH, Burhol PG, Langmark FT: Cancer detection in biopsy specimens taken from different types of gastric lesions. Cancer **58:**376-382, 1986.

211 Kasugai T: Prognosis in early gastric carcinoma. Gastroenterology **58:**429-431, 1970.

212 Kasugai T, Kobayashi S, Kuno N: Endoscopic cytology of the esophagus, stomach and pancreas. Acta Cytol [Baltimore] **22:**327-330, 1978.

213 MacDonald WC, Brandborg LL, Taniguchi L, Beh JE, Rubin CE: Exfoliative cytologic screening for gastric cancer. Cancer **17:**163-169, 1964.

214 Nagata T, Ikeda M, Nakayama F: Changing state of gastric cancer in Japan. Histologic perspective of the past 76 years. Am J Surg **145:**226-233, 1983.

215 Prolla JC, Kobayashi S, Kirsner JB: Gastric cancer. Arch Intern Med **124:**238-246, 1969.

216 Schade ROK: Gastric cytology. Principles, methods and results. London, 1960, Edward Arnold, Ltd., pp. 38-40.

217 Shiratori Y, Nakagawa S, Kikuchi A, Ishii M, Ueno M, Miyashita T, Sakurai T, Negami J, Suzuki T, Sato I: Significance of a gastric mass screening survey. Am J Gastroenterol **80:**831-835, 1985.

218 Yamada T, Murochisa B, Muto Y, Okubo H, Okamoto K, Doi K, Fujimori I: Point, minute and small cancers of the stomach at the early developmental stage detected by improved chymotrypsin lavage method for diagnostic cytology. Acta Cytol [Baltimore] **22:**460-469, 1978.

218a Bedossa P, Lemaigre G, Martin ED: Histochemical study of mucosubstances in carcinoma of the gastric remnant. Cancer **60:**2224-2227, 1987.

Relationship with peptic ulcer

219 Bogomoletz WV, Potet F, Barge J, Molas G, Qizilbash AH: Pathological features and mucin histochemistry of primary gastric stump carcinoma associated with gastritis cystica polyposa. A study of six cases. Am J Surg Pathol **9:**401-410, 1985.

220 Côté R, Dockerty MB, Cain JC: Cancer of the stomach after gastric resection for peptic ulcer. Surg Gynecol Obstet **107:**200-204, 1958.

221 Domellof L, Janunger K-G: The risk for gastric carcinoma after partial gastrectomy. Am J Surg **134:**581-584, 1977.

222 Giarelli L, Melato M, Stanta G, Bucconi S, Manconi R: Gastric resection. A cause of high frequency of gastric carcinoma. Cancer **52:**1113-1116, 1983.

223 Gömöri G: Carcinoma arising from chronic gastric ulcer. Surg Gynecol Obstet **57:**439-450, 1933.

224 Graem N, Fischer AB, Beck H: Dysplasia and carcinoma in the Billroth II resected stomach. 27-35 years postoperatively. Acta Pathol Microbiol Immunol Scand [A] **92:**185-188, 1984.

225 Ihre BJE, Barr H, Havermark G: Ulcer-cancer of the stomach. A follow-up study of 473 cases of gastric ulcer. Gastroenterologia [Basel] **102:**78-91, 1964.

226 Jordan S: The relationship of gastric ulcer to gastric carcinoma. Cancer **3:**515-552, 1950.

227 Krag E: Long-term prognosis in medically treated peptic ulcer. A clinical, radiographical and statistical follow-up study. Acta Med Scand **180:**657-670, 1966.

228 Lewis JH, Woods M III: Gastric carcinoma in patients with unoperated duodenal ulcer disease. Am J Gastroenterol **77:**368-373, 1982.

229 Mallory TB: Carcinoma in situ of the stomach and its bearing on the histogenesis of malignant ulcers. Arch Pathol **30:**348-362, 1940.

230 Nelson SW: The discovery of gastric ulcers and the differentiated diagnosis between benignancy and malignancy. Radiol Clin North Am **7:**5-25, 1969.

231 Nicholls JC: Carcinoma of the stomach following partial gastrectomy for benign gastroduodenal lesions. Br J Surg **61:**244-249, 1974.

232 Palmer WL: Benign and malignant gastric ulcers. Their relation and clinical differentiation. Ann Intern Med **13:**317-338, 1939.

233 Savage A, Jones S: Histological appearances of the gastric mucosa 15-27 years after partial gastrectomy. J Clin Pathol **32:**179-186, 1979.

234 Schafer LW, Larson DE, Melton LJ III, Higgins JA, Ilstrup DM: The risk of gastric carcinoma after surgical treatment for benign ulcer disease. A population-based study of Olmsted County, Minnesota. N Engl J Med **309:**1210-1213, 1983.

235 Schrumpf E, Stadaas J, Myren J, Serck-Hanssen A, Aune S, Osnes M: Mucosal changes in the gastric stump 20-25 years after partial gastrectomy. Lancet **2:**467-469, 1977.

236 Stalsberg H, Taksdal S: Stomach cancer following gastric surgery for benign conditions. Lancet **2:**1175-1177, 1971.

237 Stout AP: The relationship of gastric ulcer to gastric carcinoma. Cancer **3:**515-552, 1950.

238 Tokudome S, Kono S, Ikeda M, Kuratsune M, Sano C, Inokuchi K, Kodama Y, Ichimiya H, Nakayama F, Kaibara N, Koga S, Yamada H, Ikejiri T, Oka N, Tsurumaru H: A prospective study of primary gastric stump cancer following partial gastrectomy for benign gastroduodenal diseases. Cancer Res **44:**2208-2212, 1984.

"Early" carcinoma

239 Adachi Y, Mori M, Enjoji M, Saku M: Coexistence of pseudolymphoma and early carcinoma in the stomach. Arch Pathol Lab Med **110:**1080-1082, 1986.

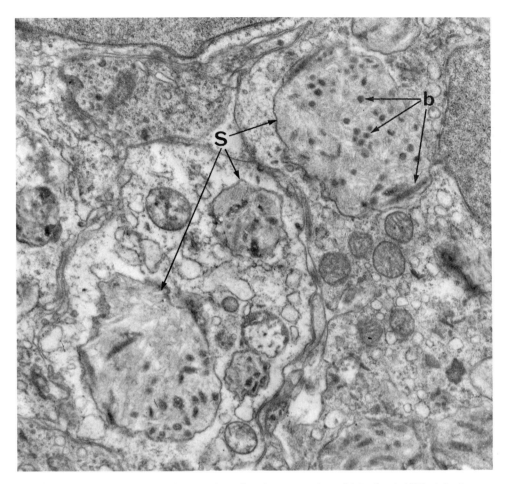

Fig. 11-53 Electron micrograph of macrophage in submucosa of small intestine in Whipple's disease. Cytoplasm contains membrane-limited sacs, *S,* that are filled with dense spherical and rod-shaped bodies, **b,** intermixed with fine membranous profiles. These rods hae been shown to have fine structural morphology of bacteria and may be responsible for disease. Material in these sacs is periodic acid—Schiff positive (× 15,000.)

or a common organism in a host with impaired immunity remains to be determined.[30a]

Other diseases associated with malabsorption in which small bowel biopsy may be of value include *abeta-lipo-proteinemia* (acanthocytosis) in which the apical villous cytoplasm shows striking vacuolation as a result of inability to synthesize beta-lipoprotein,[41] *agammaglobulinemic sprue* characterized by total absence of plasma cells in the lamina propria,[46] *intestinal lymphangiectasia* in which a protein-losing enteropathy develops probably as a result of the entrance of protein-rich fluid into the extracellular space of the lamina propria from the dilated lymphatic channels and subsequent drainage into the gut lumen[70] (Fig. 11-54), *amyloidosis, scleroderma,*[49] and *parasitic infestation,* such as giardiasis,[63,77] hookworm disease,[66] strongyloidiasis,[76] and capillariasis.[74]

Pena and Whitehead[60] studied the small bowel morphology in different types of disaccharide deficiencies. They found no detectable abnormality in isolated lactase deficiency. Whenever morphologic changes are present, *all* the

disaccharidases measured—i.e., lactase, maltases, and sucrase—were found to be depressed.

ULCERS

Duodenal peptic ulcer remains a very common disease although its incidence seems to be decreasing.[86] Its pathogenesis is related to the interplay of aggressive factors (gastric juice eroding and digesting its way into the mucosa) and defensive factors (bicarbonate and intact epithelium). Gastric acid hypersecretion is the rule in these patients.

Grossly, this chronic lesion is usually single and within 2 cm of the pylorus (Fig. 11-55), although it may also occur in the second portion of the duodenum. When the ulcer is in the latter position, it may be the source of upper abdominal pain and bleeding yet not be discernible roentgenographically. When duodenal ulcers are multiple and randomly distributed in the proximal and distal portions of the duodenum, the possibility of Zollinger-Ellison syndrome should be ruled out.

Peptic ulcer has well-defined margins sharply set off from

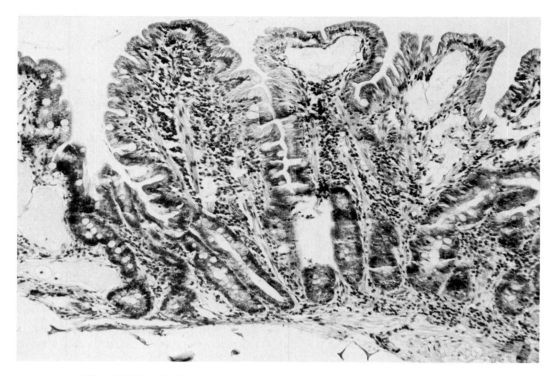

Fig. 11-54 Intestinal lymphangiectasia responsible for protein-losing enteropathy.

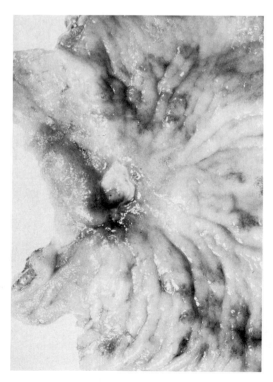

Fig. 11-55 Penetrating chronic peptic ulcer of first portion of duodenum.

the surrounding mucosa. Most of its microscopic features are analogous to those of its gastric counterpart (see section on stomach in this chapter). At times, a large vessel with an open lumen may be seen at the base of the ulcer. Fibrosis of a healed ulcer may produce secondary diverticula and considerable shortening of the duodenum. Chronic duodenitis is regularly present.[82] Peptic ulcer of the duodenum does not become malignant.

With modern medical treatment using cimetidine or other drugs, 80% of the ulcers heal within a month. The refractory ulcers tend to occur in younger patients, to be larger, and to be associated with more severe duodenitis.[83] About one in five duodenal peptic ulcers requires surgical therapy. Indications for surgery are complications such as hemorrhage, perforation, and obstruction, and lack of response to medical therapy.[87] The two standard surgical techniques currently performed are vagotomy with antrectomy and gastroenterostomy and vagotomy with pyloroplasty. The gastric resection may not include the ulcer and only in a few instances is complete excision of the ulcer performed.

Marginal ulcer is a type of peptic ulcer that appears at the site of a gastrojejunostomy opening. Although the ulcer may be at the stoma itself, in most instances it is located on the jejunum at some distance from the opening. It was a common complication at the time when gastroenterostomy for duodenal peptic ulcer was being done without a concomitant gastric resection. It is still seen, although rarely, following gastroenteromastomosis with gastric resection (Billroth II operation) for duodenal ulcer, especially if the entire antrum is not removed, or if the afferent jejunal loop is of excessive length.[81] Occasionally, marginal ulcer develops following gastric resection for peptic ulcer or cancer of the stomach.

Small bowel ulcer not related to gastroduodenal pathology is an uncommon lesion. Most cases seen in the early 1960s were due to the ingestion of enteric-coated tablets of potassium chloride. Grossly, a transverse area of ulceration is seen surrounded by congestion, hemorrhage, or edema.[78] Obstruction, perforation, and hemorrhage are the commonest presenting signs. Microscopically, the changes are nonspecific and indistinguishable from those seen in the "idiopathic" form, i.e., in those ulcers in which no demonstrable etiology can be found.[80] Diseases to be considered in the differential diagnosis include congenital abnormalities, mechanical disorders, vascular occlusions,[84,85] specific inflammations, radiation effect, celiac disease, endometriosis, and tumors.[80] As is sometimes the case with peptic ulcers, idiopathic ulcers of the small bowel can be accompanied by a prominent lymphocytic and histiocytic reaction, which can be confused with malignant lymphoma.[79]

VASCULAR DISEASES

The consequences of mesenteric vascular occlusion are discussed in Chapter 27, but a few points regarding small bowel changes will be made here. These changes can closely mimic Crohn's disease, both clinically and roentgenologically.[93] They range from complete gangrene to foci of mucosal ulceration, accompanied by extensive submucosal edema.[94,95] Perforation may develop. Healing may lead to severe stenosis.

The vascular alterations in the bowel that lead to these complications are usually the result of atherosclerosis but can also be secondary to postoperative adhesions from radiation therapy (see p. 535), rheumatoid arthritis,[90] periarteritis nodosa, oral contraceptives,[92] or cocaine ingestion.[91] Anticoagulant therapy can be complicated by the development of massive hemorrhage in the wall of small and large bowel.[88,89]

CROHN'S DISEASE (REGIONAL ILEITIS)

Crohn's disease occurs with equal frequency in both sexes. Most patients are in their twenties or thirties,[101,119] but it can first manifest at any age, including childhood[99,134] and old age.[107] White individuals of Anglo-Saxon extraction are more susceptible to the disease, the incidence of which seems to be on the increase.[122] The etiology remains unknown. The isolation of a transmissible agent has been claimed on several occasions,[97] but the significance of this finding is not clear.

Grossly, the ileum is the usual site of the disease, although any portion of the small bowel can be involved. As a matter of fact, Crohn's disease can affect any segment of the digestive tract, including oral cavity, minor salivary glands, esophagus, stomach, duodenum, large bowel, and anus.[109,126,137] Of the eleven cases of Crohn's disease of duodenum reported by Wise et al.,[144] all but one were accompanied by involvement of the distal small bowel. Large bowel involvement is discussed later in this chapter.

In a series of 297 cases of Crohn's disease studied by Morson,[126] 66% of the cases were restricted to the small bowel, 17% to the large bowel, and 17% had involvement of both segments. In more recent series, in only one third of the cases have lesions been limited to the small bowel.

Crohn's disease can also involve sites outside the alimentary system, such as skin (particularly around ileostomy or colostomy stomas),[139] vulva,[103] bone and joints,[128] skeletal muscle,[124] larynx, and spleen. The overall incidence of extraintestinal involvement is about 25%.[132] Nonspecific complications of the disease include arthritis, hydronephrosis, osteoporosis, amyloidosis, pyoderma gangrenosum, and various ocular disorders.[113]

Grossly, in the early stages of the disease the involved small bowel has a soggy feeling. The mucosa is reddish purple, and it may show pinpoint ulcers known as "aphthoid ulcers." In later stages, ulceration becomes prominent. These ulcers are linear or serpiginous and often have a longitudinal disposition, arranged in parallel and connected by short transverse ulcerations.[131] Rarely, the mucosa has a polypoid configuration because of granulation tissue formation or nodular lymphangiectasia.[118] The gross changes in the wall evolve from edema to fibrosis, with marked narrowing of the lumen accompanied by dilatation and hypertrophy of the proximal segment (Figs. 11-56 and 11-57). At this stage, the impression on palpation has been imaginatively likened to an eel in rigor mortis. The serosa may be focally or diffusely thickened; rarely, it is found to have multiple ("miliary") white nodules composed of either lymphoid aggregates or granulomas.[102] The mesentery becomes fibrosed and shortened, resulting in a corrugated bowel contour and piling up of mesenteric fat. Regional lymph nodes are moderately enlarged.

Two of the most distinctive features of Crohn's disease, partially alluded to, are the predilection for the terminal portion of the small bowel and the often segmental nature of the process, with sharply outlined foci separated by seemingly normal bowel ("skip areas").

Local complications of Crohn's disease include the development of intramural abscesses and the formation of fistulae connecting the small bowel with other loops of small bowel or with large bowel, abdominal wall, or bladder. At times, free perforation occurs.[125]

Microscopically, submucosal lymphedema is one of the earliest changes. This is accompanied by lymphoid hyperplasia in the lamina propria and submucosa and a scattering of chronic inflammatory cells, including plasma cells (containing IgG, IgM, and IgA, some of the plasma cells being binucleated), lymphocytes, eosinophils, histiocytes (some containing prominent lysosomal inclusions),[141] and mast cells.[105,129] The ulcerations are often seen to begin at the very top of the lymphoid follicles and are preceded by epithelial patchy necrosis, as detected by light microscopy[104] or ultrastructural examination.[121]

The most typical ulcers are referred to as *fissures*. These are seen in about 30% of the cases and are defined as slit-like formations with sharp edges and narrow lumina, arranged perpendicularly to the mucosa and extending deeply in to the submucosa and even the muscularis externa. The nonulcerated mucosa usually shows a combination of atro-

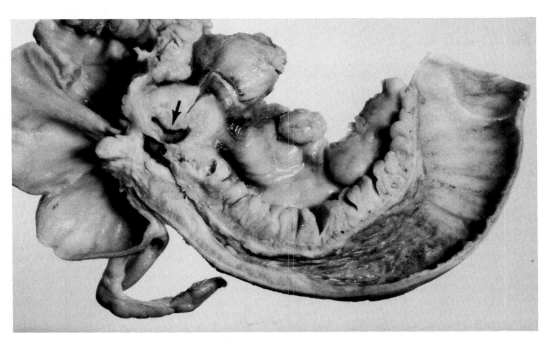

Fig. 11-56 Typical gross appearance of Crohn's disease involving terminal ileum. There are extensive ulceration, marked narrowing of lumen, and thickening of wall. Subserosal fat is prominent. Fistula is beginning to form (arrow). Disease stops abruptly at ileocecal valve.

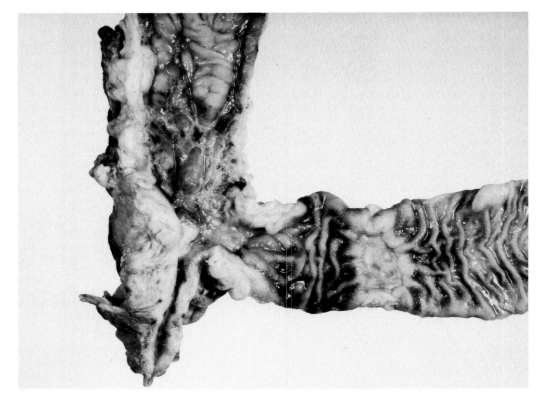

Fig. 11-57 Crohn's disease involving small bowel, cecum, appendix, and ascending colon. Longitudinal ulcerations and "skin areas" are two common features of this disease.

phy and regenerative hyperplasia. Foci of pyloric metaplasia may also be present.[133]

In well-developed Crohn's disease, there is always microscopic evidence of ***transmural involvement***, although the changes are much more severe in the submucosa and subserosa than in the muscularis externa (Fig. 11-58). There is edema, lymphatic dilatation, hyperemia, hyperplasia of the muscularis mucosae, and fibrosis.[133] The hyperemia is usually of mild to moderate degree. The inflammatory changes can involve the walls of veins and arteries.[111] The submucosal and myenteric nerve plexuses are often prominent, and electron microscopy has shown severe and extensive axonal necrosis,[106] but these are generally regarded as representing secondary phenomena related to the intense inflammation. Exceptionally, cystically dilated glands are seen in the wall of the bowel, an abnormality known as *enteritis cystica profunda*.[108]

Another important microscopic change of Crohn's disease, seen in about 60% of the cases, is the presence of ***granulomas.*** These have been described as sarcoid-like and are often seen to arise from within the centers of the lymphoid follicles. They are largely composed of epithelioid cells and multinucleated giant cells, with necrosis being usually absent or limited to a small central area. If necrosis is extensive, the alternative possibility of tuberculosis and other infectious processes should be ruled out with the appropriate techniques. The granulomas of Crohn's disease may be found anywhere in the wall of the bowel (including serosa), in the regional lymph nodes (which also show sinusal dilatation and lymphoid hyperplasia), and at any other site of involvement (Fig. 11-59).

Of all the microscopic features described above, those with greater diagnostic significance are transmural involvement, fissures, and granulomas.

Crohn's disease has an undulating yet progressive course. Complete regression is rare. Occasionally, this disorder is complicated by the development of small bowel carcinoma, most of the reported cases being of adenocarcinoma type and located in the ileum.[100,127,136,142] Sometimes the tumors are very small and detected only at the time of pathologic examination.[140] Some have been identified at the in situ stage, in association with dysplastic changes of the adjacent mucosa.[130,138] The carcinomas always develop in inflamed portions of bowel; in about one third of the cases they have arisen in a surgically bypassed segment.[110] Anaplastic carcinomas and carcinosarcomas have also been reported.[117]

The initial treatment of Crohn's disease is medical (immunosuppression, elemental diet, total parenteral nutrition);

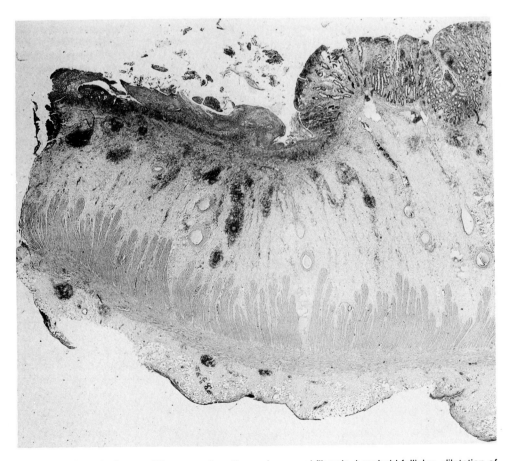

Fig. 11-58 Crohn's disease. There are ulceration, submucosal fibrosis, lymphoid follicles, dilatation of lymphatics, and subserosal fibrosis.

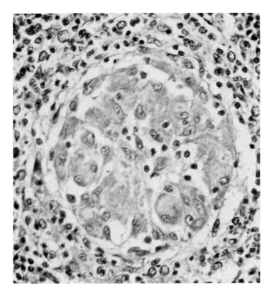

Fig. 11-59 Sarcoid-like granuloma in mesenteric lymph node of patient with Crohn's disease.

influences the prognosis after surgery, the risk of recurrence being higher in ileocolonic disease than in pure ileal or colonic disease.[114,120,143] Recurrence rates are the lowest in patients with the longest preoperative duration.[135]

In general, the type and extent of the pathologic features bear little relationship to prognosis.[115] No statistical relationship has been found between involvement of the surgical margins as determined by frozen section at the time of surgery and recrudescence.[116] Claims have been made that the presence of granulomas is associated with a better prognosis,[112] at least for Crohn's disease of the large bowel,[98] but more recent studies have shown no statistically significant differences between the two groups.[145]

OTHER INFLAMMATORY DISEASES

Duodenitis is a common microscopic finding in patients with dyspepsia, which correlates well with the endoscopic appearance.[161] Mild cases show increase in the number of plasma cells, edema, and some degree of intra-epithelial neutrophilic infiltration; more severe cases are accompanied by a more pronounced neutrophilic response and villous atrophy but a decrease in the number of plasma cells,[153] Since the evaluation of the milder changes is difficult and subjective, the suggestion has been made to use as control a biopsy of endoscopically normal mucosa from the lower duodenum taken at the same time.[158]

Acute (phlegmonous) jejunitis is a rare entity of unknown etiology that occurs with equal frequency in men and women past 55 years of age.[147] Grossly, the involved loop of bowel is sharply demarcated. The inflammation is mainly in the mucosa, but there may be pus on the serosal surface. The bowel wall is edematous and frequently slightly distended. This process may also involve the jejunum or the duodenum. Microscopically, there is frequently a widespread lymphangitis and regional lymphadenitis, accompanied by lymph node enlargement. The mesentery has a somewhat glassy appearance. Abscesses between folds of the mesentery have been observed.

however, because of the limitations and hazards of these therapies, more aggressive surgical intervention has been carried out in recent years.[96] Operation is also indicated with the development of partial or complete intestinal obstruction, internal or external fistulas, perforation with abscess, hemorrhage, and intractability despite medical management.

Specific surgical procedures to be used in these patients should be individualized; however, resection of the involved small bowel seems preferable to bypass procedures when the condition of the patient is not critical, unless there is extensive disease with several stenotic segments. The reason for this is that bypass surgery is associated with the highest reoperation rate.[123] The initial location of the disease also

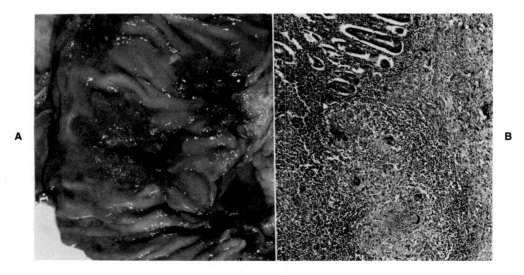

Fig. 11-60 A, Gross appearance of tuberculosis of small bowel. Several areas of flat ulceration are present. **B,** Microscopic appearance of tuberculosis of small bowel. Several caseating granulomas are seen adjacent to ulcerated mucosa. (**A,** Courtesy Dr. J. Costa, Lausanne, Switzerland.)

Tuberculosis of the small bowel, still frequent in some parts of the world, can be confused with Crohn's disease both on gross and microscopic examination.[159] In contrast with Crohn's disease, tuberculous ulcers are multiple and circumferential rather than linear and serpiginous.[166] Destruction of the muscularis externa is common. Microscopically, the tuberculous granulomas tend to be confluent and often have a caseous center and a peripheral lymphocytic ring (Fig. 11-60). Obviously, special stains for acid-fast bacilli are in order whenever this differential diagnosis is entertained.

Atypical mycobacteriosis in immunocompromised patients may result in an appearance similar to Whipple's disease. The lamina propria of the bowel and the regional lymph nodes are infiltrated by plump, foamy, PAS-positive macrophages containing myriads of organisms.[151,157]

Cryptosporidiosis results from a coccidial protozoan in immunocompromised hosts, most of the reported cases being in AIDS patients. In sections, the organisms appear as 2 to 5 μm basophilic spherical structures attached to the luminal surface of the epithelium. Their appearance can be simulated by cellular debris or mucin. The organisms stain well with Giemsa, silver methenamine, and PAS, but are not acid-fast. Their ultrastructural appearance is characteristic. They do not result in identifiable light microscopic changes in the mucosa.[152,155,162]

Giardiasis may result in malabsorption (see earlier discussion) and be associated with nodular lymphoid hyperplasia (see p. 546). The mucosa is usually intact, but there may be blunting of villi and increase in the number of inflammatory cells. The organisms have a teardrop shape, with paired nuclei ("owl-eye" appearance) and a central longitudinal axostyle[165] (Fig. 11-61).

Sarcoidosis may involve the small bowel as part of a disseminated disease, but the occurrence is exceptional.[163] The large majority of cases containing sarcoid-like granulomas in the bowel wall or mesenteric lymph nodes are the result of Crohn's disease.

Yersinia enterocolitica infection may result in an ulcerative enteritis, enterocolitis, acute appendicitis, and/or mesenteric lymphadenitis. The small bowel changes resemble somewhat those of typhoid fever. Elongated ulcerations with underlying lymphoid hyperplasia are seen together with small punctate aphthoid ulcers.[150] Although the microscopic appearance is suggestive, the correct diagnosis depends on proper identification of the organism in cultures.[146]

Necrotizing enterocolitis, a disease predominantly affecting premature infants, is discussed in the section on the large bowel.

Eosinophilic enteritis and *gastroenteritis* often are accompanied by marked peripheral eosinophilia and allergic symptoms. The gastrointestinal manifestations include nausea, vomiting, diarrhea, pain, steatorrhea, and protein-losing enteropathy. Morphologically, the main change is a diffuse eosinophilic infiltration of the intestinal wall, accompanied by other inflammatory cells, increased vascularity, and, in some cases, necrotizing granulomas and vasculitis.[164] The involvement may be predominantly in the muscle or subserosa; in the latter instance, it is often associated with eosinophilic peritonitis and ascites. Although some cases may be the result of undetected parasitic infestation and others are secondary to collagen vascular disease,[149] the pathogenesis of most remains obscure.[164]

Inflammatory fibroid polyp (inflammatory pseudotumor) has a similar microscopic composition to eosinophilic enteritis but appears grossly as a localized submucosal ses-

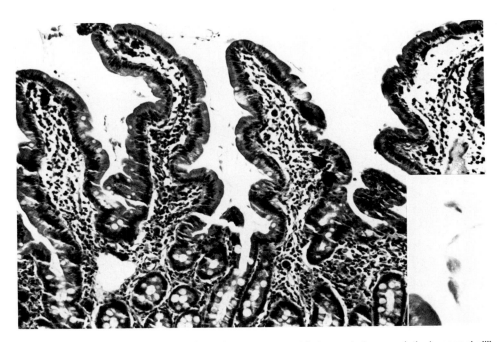

Fig. 11-61 Giardiasis of small bowel. Organisms are present in lumen between relatively normal villi and are shown better in **inset.** (Courtesy Dr. J.B. Atkinson, Nashville, TN.)

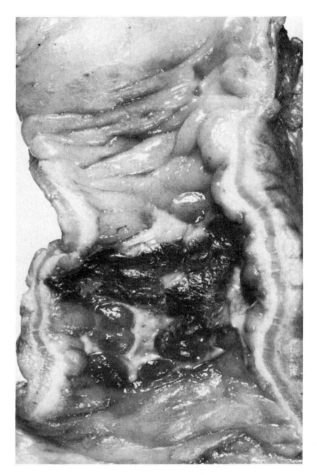

Fig. 11-62 Stenosing lesion of bowel with ulceration due to irradiation. Submucosal fibrosis is present, and muscular layer is well defined. (From Perkins DE, Spjut HJ: Intestinal stenosis following radiation therapy. Am J Roentgenol Radium Ther Nucl Med **88**:953-966, 1962.)

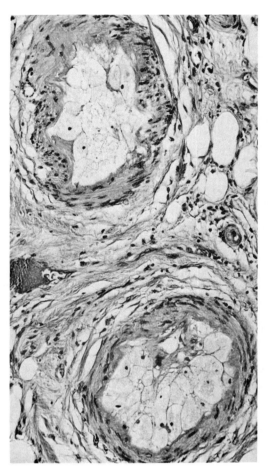

Fig. 11-63 Irradiation effect in two small mesenteric arteries. Subintimal foam cells are present, changes that are almost specific for irradiation effect. (From Perkins DE, Spjut HJ: Intestinal stenosis following radiation therapy. Am J Roentgenol Radium Ther Nucl Med **88**:953-966, 1962.)

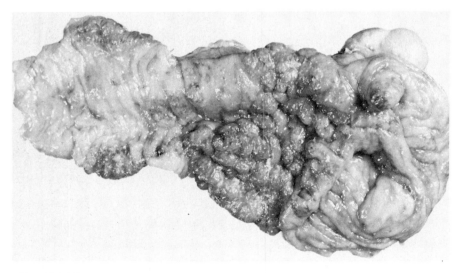

Fig. 11-64 Extreme lymphoid hyperplasia of ileum with intussusception in 4-year-old child.

sile polypoid mass sometimes leading to obstruction or intussusception.[148,154,156,160] The two entities are probably not related. The appearance of this intestinal polyp is similar to that of the homonymous gastric lesion, except that the neural-like features commonly seen in the latter are less common. By electron microscopy, the principal mesenchymal cell has the features of a myofibroblast. The lesion is benign and the pathogenesis is unknown.[160] Multiple and recurrent cases in a familial setting have been described.[145a]

IRRADIATION EFFECT

Roentgentherapy of malignant tumors within the peritoneal cavity may cause damage to the intestinal tract, the amount of which depends on many factors.[169] Damage occurs most frequently in patients treated for carcinoma of the cervix, but there is an increased number of cases in children who had been treated for Wilms' tumor, malignant lymphoma, or other tumors.[167]

Grossly, the small bowel appears thickened. The wall may be partially replaced by fibrous tissue, particularly in the submucosa. This is often accompanied by mucosal ulceration.[170]

Microscopically, early irradiation effect is manifested by an increased production of mucus and by nuclear changes in the lining epithelium.[171] Later, submucosal edema that may be completely reversible occurs. If the damage is severe, fibrosis of the muscular wall and ulceration develop (Fig. 11-62). Vascular changes are prominent; they are characterized by subendothelial accumulation of lipid-laden macrophages, calcification, and thrombosis[168,169] (Fig. 11-63).

Frozen section is a reliable method in determining the degree of radiation damage and in assessing whether or not the ends of the intestine after resection and anastomosis can be expected to heal.

INTUSSUSCEPTION

In intussusception, a length of intestine (the intussuscipiens) literally swallows part of the bowel just proximal to it. This swallowed portion (the intussusceptum) is drawn down within the intussuscipiens until it can go no farther because of the traction of the mesentery. The specimen has a curved sausage-like form, with concavity toward the root of the mesentery. Increasing traction and compression shut off circulation to the intussusceptum so that it becomes necrotic and sloughs. The upper ends of the intussuscipiens and the intussusceptum may become firmly united. In exceptional instances, the end result has been spontaneous cure in the form of a naturally occurring equivalent of a surgical end-to-end anastomosis.

Most cases of intussusception are seen during the first 5 years of life, with over one half occurring during the first year. This is probably related to the fact that the amount of lymphoid tissue in the ileocecal region and the degree of projection of the valve into the cecum are at their maximum during this period and that both decrease substantially after the second year[174] (Fig. 11-64). There is now general agreement that the lymphoid hyperplasia precedes and is often the cause of the intussusception rather than the result, although secondary inflammatory changes do certainly occur. This lymphoid hyperplasia, which is limited to the mucosa and submucosa, is probably of viral etiology in many instances, as indicated by the finding of intranuclear inclusion bodies in one third of the cases[175] and the fact that viruses (particularly adenoviruses) have often been isolated from these children.[172]

In early uncomplicated cases, a barium enema may be used to reduce the intussusception.[173] Surgery is otherwise needed. If performed early enough, manual reduction of the intussusception is possible; resection is necessary when reduction is not feasible. Mortality is directly related to the time that elapses between onset and surgery. In children there is a rapid rise in mortality after the second day.

In older children and in adults, intussusception is frequently the result of a pedunculated intraluminal tumor such as lipoma or leiomyoma.

OTHER NON-NEOPLASTIC DISEASES

Endometriosis may result in a mass-like effect and cause obstruction.[179] Microscopically, endometrial glands and stroma, foci of fresh and old hemorrhage, and bundles of hypertrophic smooth muscle (which may constitute the bulk of the process) are seen.

The *brown bowel syndrome* is characterized by a prominent brown discoloration of the bowel wall, seen from the serosal side and on cut section, and often associated with malabsorption. Microscopically, large amounts of lipofuscin granules are seen in the cytoplasm of smooth muscle cells. The pathogenesis is unknown but the suggestion that it may be due to vitamin E deficiency has been advanced[177]; a primary abnormality of smooth muscle mitochondria has also been postulated.[176]

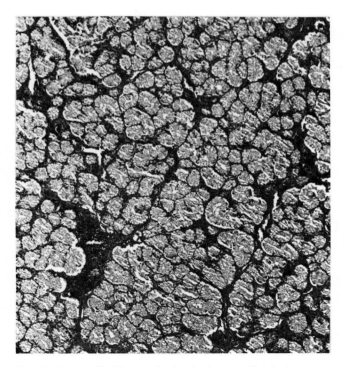

Fig. 11-65 So-called Brunner's gland adenoma. Cytologic appearance is relatively normal, and there is vague lobular configuration.

Amyloidosis may involve the vessels or the stroma of the small bowel, either as part of generalized disease or—rarely—as a localized finding.[178,180]

Graft-versus-host disease following bone marrow transplantation affects primarily skin, gastrointestinal tract, and liver. Involvement of small bowel is manifested clinically by diarrhea and microscopically by a variety of changes, of which single epithelial cell necrosis is the most consistent.[181]

TUMORS
Benign epithelial tumors

So-called *Brunner's gland adenoma* (polypoid hamartoma; brunneroma) is characterized by a nodular prolifer-ation of histologically normal Brunner's glands, accompanied by ducts and scattered stromal elements (Fig. 11-65). It is probably not a true neoplasm but rather an expression of nodular hyperplasia or hamartoma.[199] The most common location is the posterior wall of the duodenum at the junction between the first and second portions. It can be the cause of melena or duodenal obstruction.[197]

Adenomas similar to those of the large bowel can develop in the small bowel, but their frequency is minuscule.[195] The duodenum and jejunum are involved more often than the ileum. They can be single or multiple, pedunculated or sessile, and have the microscopic appearance of an adenomatous polyp (tubular adenoma), villoglandular polyp

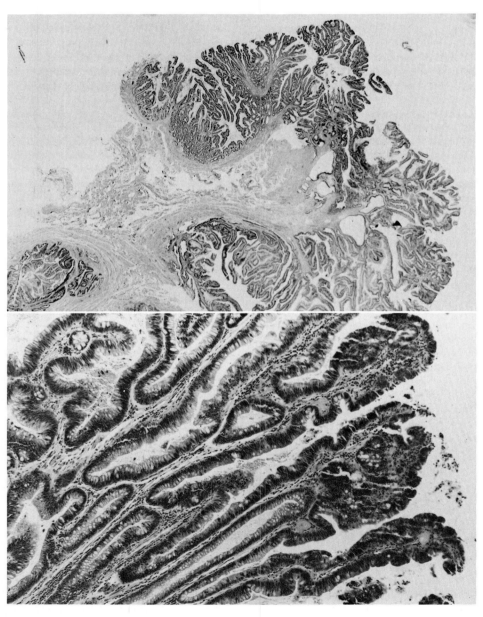

Fig. 11-66 Villous tumor of duodenum. Appearance is analogous to that of villous adenoma of large bowel. There was no invasive cancer in resected specimen.

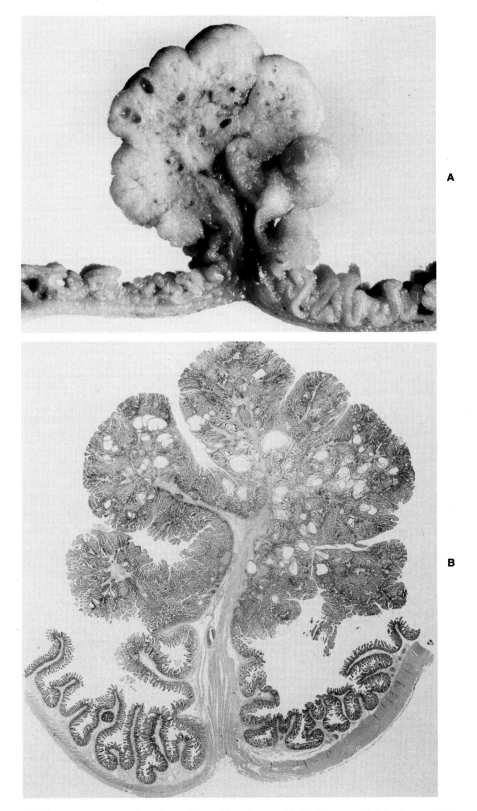

Fig. 11-67 Hamartomatous polyp of small bowel in 12-year-old girl. Tumor, which had caused intussusception, was not associated with other features of Peutz-Jeghers syndrome. **A,** Gross appearance of tumor, showing distinct lobulation, short stalk, and multiple small cysts. **B,** Panoramic view of microscopic section, Ramifying central stalk containing numerous muscle bundles supports florid epithelial proliferation. Many of glands show cystic dilatation.

(tubulo-villous adenoma), or villous adenoma[185,192] (Fig. 11-66). Malignant transformation can occur in them; as for their colorectal counterparts, the incidence of this complication is greater if the lesions are villous, large, or multiple. Villous adenomas of the duodenum have been reported with increasing frequency in recent years, undoubtedly as a result of the widespread use of endoscopy. Many of them are located at the level of the ampulla of Vater and are further discussed in Chapter 15. Their morphologic appearance and natural history are entirely similar to those of villous adenomas of large bowel: they are often large, sessile, with tendency to recur, and with a high incidence of malignant transformation.[190,195] Thorough sampling at endoscopy is of importance for detection of the latter.[183]

Hamartomatous polyps of the jejuno-ileum are usually seen as a component of the *Peutz-Jeghers syndrome*. This is a familial disorder transmitted as a mendelian autosomal dominant trait with variable degrees of penetrance.[188] Similar polyps can also be present in the stomach, duodenum, and large bowel, and the patients have a typical pigmentation of the lips, oral mucosa, digits, palms, and soles[182,198] Grossly these polyps do not differ from the usual adenomatous polyp (Fig. 11-67), but microscopically they are much different. The glands are supported by broad bands of smooth muscle fibers, thick in the center of the lesion and thinner on the periphery. The intimate intermingling of glands and smooth muscle fibers may simulate the appearance of invasion and lead to a mistaken diagnosis of carcinoma.[193]

Several types of epithelial cells are present, as demonstrated by light and electron microscopy.[187] Columnar and goblet cells predominate in the superficial portion, whereas Paneth's and endocrine cells are seen at the base next to the muscular framework. This microscopic architecture is similar for polyps occurring elsewhere in the gastrointestinal tract, but the cytologic composition depends on the location.[188]

Some hamartomatous polyps occur in the absence of the other features of the syndrome. Some are associated with mucosal glands and mucinous cysts deeply embedded in the submucosa, a change designated as *enteritis cystica profunda*.[191,200] Several cases of adenocarcinoma of the gastrointestinal tract have been reported in patients with Peutz-Jeghers syndrome. They have been located in the stomach, small bowel, or large bowel.[189] The prognosis is poor, probably because of the lateness of the diagnosis.[186] In some of these cases, the invasive carcinoma is seen to coexist with areas of carcinoma in situ and adenomatous change.[194,196] Patients with Peutz-Jeghers syndrome may also develop the distinctive ovarian neoplasm known as sex cord tumor with annular tubules (see Chapter 19), so-called adenoma malignum of uterine cervix (see Chapter 19), ovarian mucinous tumors, breast carcinoma (often bilateral), and other types of malignancy.[184,201]

Adenocarcinoma

Adenocarcinoma of the small bowel is forty to sixty times less common than its counterpart in the large bowel. Most patients are elderly, and there is no sex predilection.[203] It can develop in any segment but is more common in the upper portions.[208,210a] Approximately 40% of the cases occur in the duodenum; an increasing number of cases in this location are being reported with the use of fiberoptic endoscopy.[213,214] Most cases of duodenal carcinomas arise from the mucosa in the region of the ampulla. They are described in Chapter 15, in the section on carcinoma of the periampullary region exclusive of the pancreas.

Duodenal cancer tends to have a papillary configuration. Those lesions located more distally usually have a napkin ring appearance and produce partial intestinal obstruction with marked dilatation of the proximal bowel (Fig. 11-68); about 20% have a predominantly polypoid or fungating appearance, perhaps due in some instances to their origins in pre-existing adenomatous polyps or villous adenomas.[208] Occasionally, these carcinomas present as multiple tumors[215] or in association with primary malignant neoplasms in other sites.[206]

Microscopically, these tumors are usually moderately well-differentiated adenocarcinomas. Mucin production and CEA reactivity are the rule[207]; there may also be immunoreactivity for lysozyme, suggesting focal differentiation toward Paneth cells.[212] In addition, it is common to find a scattering of endocrine cells, particularly in ileal tumors. These cells are positive for chromogranin and serotonin and may show immunoreactivity for a variety of peptide hormones, including somatostatin, YY peptide, neurotensin, glucagon, and glycentin.[210] Ultrastructurally, there is a prominent development of microvilli.[215a]

At the time of diagnosis, the majority of the tumors have extended deeply into the wall and may have already metastasized to regional lymph nodes. The prognosis mainly depends on the presence or absence of regional lymph node involvement. In the series of Bridge and Perzin,[208] 88% of the patients with positive nodes died of tumor as contrasted with 45% of those with negative nodes.

Small bowel adenocarcinomas can develop as a complication of Peutz-Jeghers syndrome and Crohn's disease as already indicated (see p. 531). They have also been described in bowel duplication,[202] at ileostomy sites,[205,209] in surgically bypassed duodenum,[211] and in association with Recklinghausen's disease.[204]

Other types of carcinoma

Small cell carcinoma (oat cell carcinoma) is a rare type of small bowel malignancy composed of small, round, or oval cells of scanty cytoplasm and hyperchromatic nucleus.[218] The appearance is very similar to that of pulmonary small cell carcinoma. As in the latter, dense core granules of neurosecretory type can be identified ultrastructurally and neuroendocrine markers immunohistochemically.[217] These tumors can present in a pure form or mixed with ordinary adenocarcinoma. They are deeply invasive, highly prone to metastasize, and associated with a very poor prognosis.

Adenosquamous carcinoma has been reported on a few occasions, with either the glandular or the squamous component predominating.[216]

Anaplastic (sarcomatoid) carcinoma is composed of highly bizarre tumor cells, some of them multinucleated, with abundant cytoplasm and no signs of glandular differentiation. The behavior is extremely aggressive.[216a]

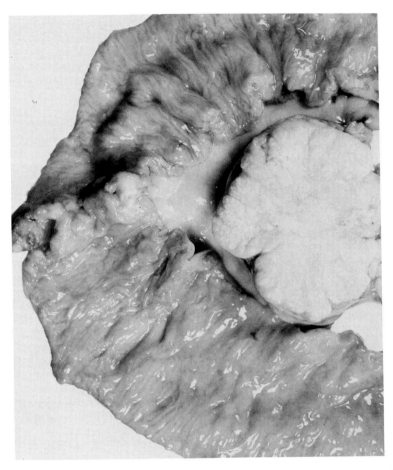

Fig. 11-68 Classic constricting adenocarcinoma of small bowel with large metastasis. This case, although hopeless, was found at time of exploratory laparotomy for gallbladder disease.

Carcinoid tumors and related endocrine tumors

Carcinoid tumor is the generic term applied to low-grade malignant neoplasms originating from the diffuse endocrine system outside of the pancreas and the thyroid C-cell.[230] It is now acknowledged that they represent a group of neoplasms rather than a single pathologic entity.[247,271] This stems from the fact that the digestive tract in general, and the small bowel in particular, contain a large number of endocrine types, any of which can be represented in these neoplasms, singly or in combination.[247,248,260,267] The most common form of carcinoid tumor is known as classical or insular; this is the type usually referred to when the designation "carcinoid tumor" is used for a neoplasm of the small bowel without a qualifier. It comprises about one third of all neoplasms of this organ.[239] The majority occur in adults, but they have also been documented in children.[227] Most are located in the ileum (including Meckel's diverticulum), followed in frequency by the jejunum and distal duodenum. They have also been described in small bowel affected by celiac disease,[238] in bowel duplication,[268] and in association with Recklinghausen's disease.[243] These tumors are multiple in 15% to 35% of the cases and are sometimes associated with malignant gastrointestinal tumors of other microscopic types[246] or with tumors of endocrine differentiation in other locations.[277] Because of these factors, thorough exploration of the gastrointestinal tract is indicated whenever a carcinoid tumor of the small bowel is identified at surgery.

The mucosa is often intact over the tumor. Infiltration of the submucosa is the rule, and infiltration of the muscularis externa is common. The tumor invasion and the accompanying fibrosis may "buckle" the bowel wall (Fig. 11-69). Following formalin fixation, the tumor acquires a bright yellow color that is not evident in the fresh state. Microscopically, the pattern is that of solid masses of monotonous-appearing cells with small nuclei, inconspicuous cytoplasm, and fine nucleoli (Fig. 11-70). Mitotic figures are scanty. Tumor emboli in lymphatic vessels are often seen. It is also common to find tumor cells within submucosal nerves.

The very distinctive profile of classic carcinoid tumor can be demonstrated by a variety of special techniques. At the histochemical level, it is argentaffin (and therefore also argyrophilic), positive for the diazo reaction, and generally negative for mucin stains. Ultrastructurally, there are numerous dense-core pleomorphic secretory granules scattered

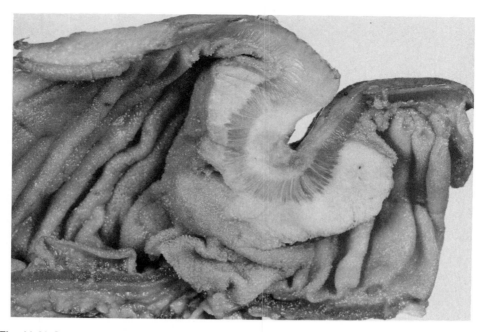

Fig. 11-69 Carcinoid tumor of small bowel. Note "buckling" of bowel wall with hypertrophy of muscle. Bulk of tumor lies above muscle. (Specimen contributed by Dr. W. Hall, Chambersburg, PA.)

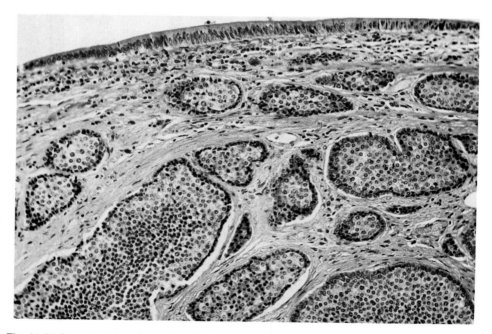

Fig. 11-70 Characteristic pattern of carcinoid tumor growing just beneath thinned overlying epithelium.

throughout the cytoplasm. Immunohistochemically, there is reactivity indicative both of epithelial and neuroendocrine differentiation. The first is manifested by keratin and—in the tumors with a glandular component—by apical or luminal CEA[254,258]; the second is brought forward by a series of "pan-endocrine" markers, such as neuron-specific en-

olase, chromogranin, synaptophysin, Leu 7, and serotonin.[253,265,276] The latter can also be demonstrated by formalin-induced fluorescence, both in sections and in smears.[279] A variety of peptide hormones has also been demonstrated in these tumors. This includes gastrin, somatostatin, glucagon, glycentin, substance P, pancreatic polypeptide, bombesin, gastrin-releasing peptide (GRP), and growth hormone–releasing factor (GRF).* Peptide YY is found only rarely, in contrast to its consistent presence in rectal carcinoids.[243,272] Staining for S-100 protein is negative, in contrast to the usual positivity encountered in carcinoid tumors of the appendix; this may be related to the alleged difference in the origin of these tumors: endocrine cells from Lieberkuhn's crypts for the carcinoid tumors of small bowel, and subepithelial endocrine cells related to nerves for those in the appendix.[249,251] Curiously, some carcinoid tumors have also been found to be immunoreactive for prostatic acid phosphatase[269] and human prealbumin.[224]

Most of the metastatic foci react immunohistochemically in a fashion identical to that of the primary tumor, but some produce either additional or fewer hormones.[281] Some of the above-mentioned substances (serotonin, chromogranin, substance P, and—rarely—neuron-specific enolase) can be elevated in the serum of these patients and thus serve as circulatory markers for these tumors.[235]

Many variations within this basic theme exist.[280] Trabecular and glandular (tubular) formations may be present, the latter sometimes containing intraluminal mucin. Carcinoid tumors with a predominantly glandular pattern are referred to as *adenocarcinoids* and are further subdivided into tubular and signet ring types.[242] On occasion, features of endocrine and exocrine secretion can be seen in the same cell (so-called amphicrine cell).[226,232] The existence of these and other variations has led to a division of carcinoid tumors into several types largely based on their patterns of growth: A, B, C, D, E,[270] or insular, trabecular, glandular, undifferentiated, and mixed,[244] these various types correlating with behavioral differences; however, most of these varieties are much less common than in the appendix. Sometimes a typical carcinoid pattern is seen in association with an adenocarcinomatous pattern, whether in the primary tumor or in metastases. Finally, Carstens et al.[225] reported an intestinal tumor with the light microscopic features of a carcinoid tumor (but negative with silver stains) that had electron microscopic features (cytoplasmic filaments, fibrils, and caveolae) similar to those of the recently described intestinal caveolated cell.

Classic carcinoid tumors are malignant neoplasms that have a slow growth rate but also highly invasive and metastasizing properties. Metastases occur most commonly in regional lymph nodes and liver. The liver metastases are usually multiple and solid but occasionally have a prominent cystic component.[233] The overall 5-year relative survival rate of small bowel carcinoid is between 50% and 65%,[239] a marked difference existing between the patients in whom the tumors are confined to the wall (85% 5-year survival) and those in whom the lesions invade the serosa or beyond (5% 5-year survival).[282] Resection of the primary tumor is worthwhile even in the presence of extensive liver metastasis because prolonged survival is possible under these circumstances.[257]

Carcinoid tumor may be associated with the *carcinoid syndrome*.[235a] Nearly all of the reported cases have occurred in tumors that have metastasized to the liver, presumably

because of the liver's capacity to inactivate biologically active substances released into the portal circulation[263,273,274]; however, exceptions occur.[236] The syndrome is characterized by cyanosis of the face and anterior part of the chest, intermittent hypertension, palpitation, and frequent watery stools. Traditionally, it has been assumed that the syndrome was due to serotonin (5-hydroxytryptanin), an indolamine regularly secreted by the tumor cells and easily detectable in the urine in the form of its catabolite 5-hydroxyindolacetic acid[266]; however, there is little relation between the serum levels of this marker and the occurrence of the syndrome, especially in regard to its vasodilatation component. Other substances known to be secreted by carcinoid tumor—such as tachykinins, prostaglandins, and histamine—have been postulated, but the issue remains unresolved.[234,259,264] It is also apparent that the cells of carcinoid tumor must secrete some material that elicits the deposition of extracellular connective tissue around the tumor and sometimes at a distance. Manifestations of this phenomenon include extensive fibrosclerosis often seen in the tumor itself, fibrosclerosis of the right-sided cardiac valves that results in so-called carcinoid heart disease,[274] obliterative elastic sclerosis of mesenteric blood vessels that may lead to small bowel gangrene[221,262] (Fig. 11-71), and dermal sclerosis that results in scleroderma-like lesions.[237] A few carcinoid tumors have resulted in spontaneous hypoglycemia,[256] apparently because of insulin production by the tumor cells.[261]

Endocrine tumors of the proximal small bowel (especially duodenum) rarely have the features of classic carcinoids. Many of the reported cases have been composed of either G- or D-cells, as demonstrated by their immunoreactivity for gastrin and somatostatin, respectively.[219,231,245] The G-cell tumors (gastrinomas) may be associated with the Zollinger-Ellison syndrome,[231,275] whereas D-cell tumors (somatostatinomas) are hormonally silent at the clinical level. A high percentage of duodenal tumors predominantly composed of D-cells have occurred in patients with Recklinghausen's disease.[229] Immunohistochemistry is needed to identify conclusively the specific cell types; however, the nature of these tumors can already be suspected in routinely stained sections by the fact that both of them tend to have a well-developed glandular component and that D-cell tumors have, in addition, numerous psammoma bodies, usually located within glandular lumina.[228,241,252] It should be noted, however, that psammoma bodies are not specific for D-cell tumors; they can also be seen in carcinoid tumors of other types and B-cell tumors of the pancreas.[240] Exceptionally, duodenal endocrine tumors are of pancreatic B-cell type.[255]

Gangliocytic paraganglioma

Gangliocytic paraganglioma (nonchromaffin paraganglioma; paraganglioneuroma) is a peculiar benign tumor occurring almost exclusively in the second portion of the duodenum, especially in the proximity of the ampulla of Vater.[286,291] A few cases have been reported in a more distal location, including jejuno-ileum.[289] Occasionally, the lesion is multiple[285] or seen in association with Recklinghausen's disease and carcinoid tumors.[287,290a] Most lesions are small, pedunculated, and submucosal, with frequent ulceration of

---

*See references 220, 222, 223, 250, 258, 278, and 281.

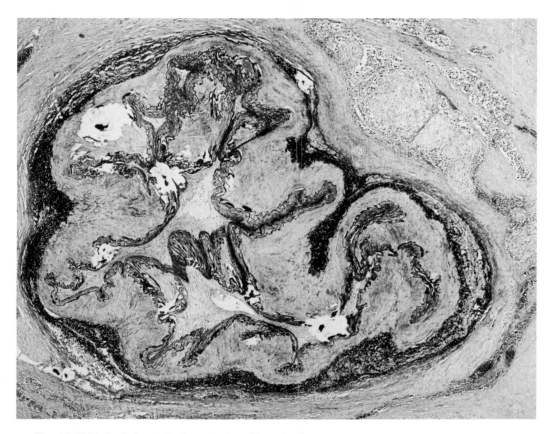

Fig. 11-71 Marked elasatotic degeneration of branch of mesenteric artery associated with carcinoid tumor, which can be seen surrounding vessel. Both elastic laminae are affected. Patient was operated on because of gangrene of small bowel. (Verhoeff–van Gieson.)

the overlying mucosa and bleeding. The microscopic appearance is distinctive, with no exact counterpart elsewhere in the body. Three cell components are present: endocrine cells with a carcinoid-like appearance arranged in compact nests and trabeculae containing dense-core granules ultrastructurally and exhibiting immunoreactivity for a variety of markers, particularly pancreatic polypeptide (PP); isolated ganglion cells, immunoreactive for neuron-specific enolase and other neural markers; and spindle-shaped Schwann cells and/or sustentacular cells, immunoreactive for S-100 protein[283,288,290] (Fig. 11-72). Somatostatin may be present in both ganglion cells and endocrine cells.[284] In one series, three of six cases contained amyloid.[289] The peculiar location of this tumor, its highly organoid arrangement, and the striking predominance of PP cells suggest that this lesion may represent a hamartomatous process derived from the ventral primordium of the pancreas.[288] All cases so far published have followed a benign clinical course.[282a]

Smooth muscle tumors

Smooth muscle tumors of the bowel may occur in any segment but predominate in the distal portions. Of 421 reported cases of small bowel leiomyosarcomas, 10% were in the duodenum, 37% in the jejunum, and 53% in the ileum.[301] The distribution of leiomyomas is roughly the same. Most cases occur in adults, but pediatric examples are also on record.[293] The proportion of malignant tumors is much higher for smooth muscle tumors of the small bowel than for those located in the esophagus or stomach.[298] These smooth muscle tumors may arise from any of the muscular layers, including the muscularis mucosae. Grossly, they are fairly well circumscribed, and their pattern of growth may be predominantly intraluminar or extraluminal. The former may have a central ulcer niche similar to that more often seen in the gastric counterparts. Those growing toward the mesentery can reach huge dimensions. The symptoms depend on their growth pattern. They may be detected because of occult or massive bleeding, pain, obstruction, intussusception, or perforation.[292] They should be suspected of being malignant if large and/or with necrosis or hemorrhage.

Microscopically, the majority of these tumors are spindle-shaped and easily identifiable as of smooth muscle derivation on both light and electron microscopic grounds.[294,300] Immunohistochemically, there is positivity for vimentin in all cases and for actin in the majority, but desmin is almost always undetectable.[298a] The leiomyoblastoma category, which makes for a high percentage of smooth muscle tumors of the stomach and omentum, is very uncommon in this location.[300]

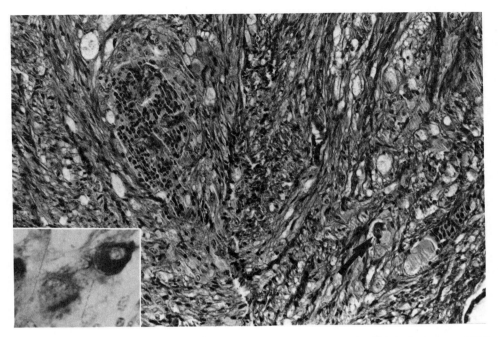

Fig. 11-72 Gangliocytic paraganglioma of duodenum. The three components of this lesion are prominent nests of neuroendocrine cells, diffuse proliferation of spindle-shaped Schwann cells, and scattered mature ganglion cells (arrow). **Inset** shows strong immunocytochemical positivity for pancreatic polypeptide (PP) in neuroendocrine component.

The microscopic differentiation between benign and malignant tumors may be extremely difficult (Fig. 11-73). The guidelines detailed in the discussion of smooth muscle tumors of stomach can also be applied to the small bowel lesion. High mitotic activity is the single most important microscopic feature, both to place tumors in the leiomyosarcoma category and to further divide them into low and high grades.[295,298] Any smooth muscle tumor of the small bowel should be regarded as malignant or at least of indeterminate malignant potential if *any* of these features are present: large size (over 5 cm), fresh tumor necrosis, extensive hemorrhage unrelated to surgery, extreme cellularity, marked atypia, or—most importantly—mitotic activity (five or more mitoses per ten high power fields).[296]

A few cases have been reported associated with human chorionic gonadotropin production.[297] Leiomyosarcomas may invade adjacent structures such as pancreas by direct extension.[299] They also tend to invade the bloodstream and metastasize distantly. Staging and microscopic grading of tumor closely correlates with prognosis.[298a,299] Of twenty patients studied by Ranchod and Kempson,[298] fifteen developed metastases (usually to liver and peritoneum) and four others developed intra-abdominal tumor with prominent retroperitoneal spread; only one patient was found to be alive and free of disease at the time of the last follow-up.

Malignant lymphoma and related disorders

The large majority of malignant lymphomas involving the small bowel can be divided into one of three categories*:

*See references 302, 303, 328, 332, 339, and 344.

(1) lymphomas arising on the basis of long-standing celiac sprue or related malabsorption syndromes, (2) lymphomas arising on the basis of diffuse plasma cell proliferation associated with increase in serum levels of IgA, and (3) lymphomas arising *de novo,* whether localized to the bowel or part of a generalized process. To these, one should add the malignant lymphomas developing in patients with AIDS or other immunocompromised hosts[314,347] and the type rarely complicating Crohn's disease.[331]

The first group is characteristically a large cell lymphoma mixed with a variety of inflammatory cells. It would be classified as histiocytic lymphoma in Rappaport's classification and as centroblastic lymphoma in Kiel's classification.[337,341] It has been regarded by some as a form of malignant histiocytosis,[323] a theory no longer accepted. This tumor has been discussed earlier in this chapter under the topic of malabsorption.

The second type of lymphoma is also known as *Mediterranean lymphoma* and *immunoproliferative small intestine disease*.[322,338,345] It is relatively common among non-European Jews and Arabs in the Middle East and in the black population of South Africa.[310] Patients often have a short history of malabsorption, but the mucosa is not completely flat in most cases. Once the lymphoma has developed, the clinical course is rapidly fatal in the majority of patients. Biopsies of the bowel and regional lymph nodes taken before the development of the malignancy or in areas away from the tumor show a heavy infiltration by plasma cells that appear mature or only slightly immature at both the light and electron microscopic level.[309,343] This is associated with the presence of monoclonal alpha heavy chains

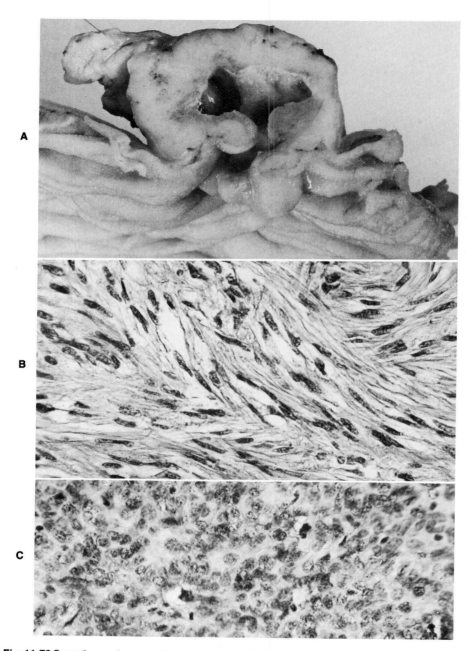

Fig. 11-73 Smooth muscle tumor of jejunum of long clinical duration that was grossly and microscopically thought to be benign. Note classic central excavation. **B,** Same tumor as in **A** showing well-differentiated smooth muscle cells. Mitotic figures were rare. **C,** Two years later, tumor recurred locally and metastasized to liver. Tumor was highly undifferentiated in liver, but other areas showed smooth muscle origin.

of immunoglobulins in the cytoplasm of the plasma cells,[321] as well as in the serum and urine, hence the designation "alpha chain disease." It has been speculated that this plasma cell infiltration is originally reactive in nature, representing a response to a continuous antigenic stimulus of possible infectious nature. The initially polyclonal nature of the proliferation and the fact that some cases have responded to tetracycline supports this contention.[305]

The involvement centers in the distal portions of the duodenum and the upper jejunum. Grossly, the lesions appear as diffusely thickened folds with small nodules or as discrete tumor growths.[329]

Microscopically, the malignant tumor is a highly pleomorphic large cell lymphoma with immunoblastic and plasmacellular features, to the point that it has also been designated as *(malignant) plasmacytoma*. Pangalis and

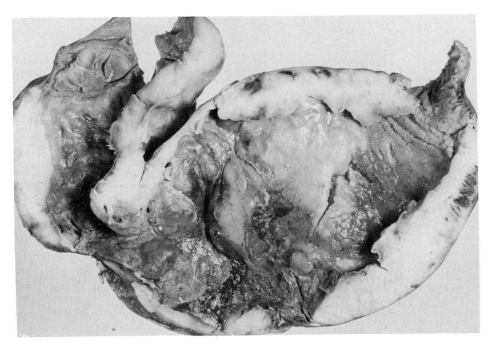

Fig. 11-74 Large malignant lymphoma of small bowel that replaced all layers.

Rappaport[340] have shown that the tumor cells exhibit an immunochemical staining for alpha chain similar to that of the mature plasma cell infiltrate, suggesting that they represent a clone of highly malignant elements originating from the pre-existing infiltrate. A prominent ''starry sky'' pattern may be present, as well as intense follicular lymphoid hyperplasia.[316,338] The diagnosis can usually be made by endoscopic biopsy, especially if areas with an infiltrating pattern are sampled.[317] According to Isaacson et al.,[326] Mediterranean lymphoma is a tumor of follicle center cell origin that undergoes plasma cell differentiation as a result of exposure to lumenal antigen. Isaacson has also pointed out that the intestinal lymphoma that so commonly affects patients in Middle Eastern countries is not always of the Mediterranean type; some cases are of the Western type discussed in the following section.[325]

Small bowel lymphomas not belonging to either of the first two categories but presenting primarily in this organ tend to be solitary (80% to 90% of the cases), although sometimes the formation of multiple small polypoid masses throughout the bowel (to the extent of simulating lymphoid hyperplasia) has been observed. The ileum is more commonly affected, followed by the jejunum and duodenum.[336,350] Grossly, the tumors can show a diffusely infiltrating mass with a garden hose appearance, a bulky tumor mass with extensive ulceration, or a predominantly polypoid growth (Fig. 11-74). Microscopically, most of the cases are of the large cell type,[333] followed by the poorly differentiated lymphocytic type (Fig. 11-75). Some of the former can be quite pleomorphic and simulate Hodgkin's disease. Other lymphomas show evidence of plasmacytoid differentiation,[318] others have a signet ring appearance,[320] and still others have the features of undifferentiated (Burkitt's or non-Burkitt's type) lymphoma. Sometimes the tumors are associated with an intense eosinophilic infiltration that may obscure the diagnosis.[346] Although many of these tumors have been regarded as histiocytic on morphologic grounds and on the basis of their alleged immunohistochemical positivity for lysozyme and alpha-1-antitrypsin, cell marker studies performed on fresh frozen sections have shown that the vast majority are of B-cell origin.[315] The suggestion has been made that these tumors arise from a special type of mucosa-associated lymphoid tissue (MALT), which also includes the lymphoid tissue of other portions of gastrointestinal tract, salivary gland, lung, and thyroid.[324] A small proportion of intestinal lymphomas are of T-cell types,[312] and these are said to be associated with a greater morbidity and worse prognosis.[327] The regional lymph nodes are involved in about half of the patients with bowel lymphoma. In the series of Lewin et al.[333] the 2-year actuarial survival was 42%, lower than for malignant lymphomas of the stomach or rectum. The survival rate is related both to histologic typing and clinical staging.[311]

Although the gastrointestinal tract is the commonest site of primary extranodal lymphoma,[313] the possibility of disease being present elsewhere should always be investigated, inasmuch as 10% of patients with non-Hodgkin's lymphomas have involvement of some part of the gastrointestinal tract at the time of initial evaluation.[333] Occasionally, malignant lymphoma is seen to coexist with adenocarcinoma.[351]

Gastrointestinal lymphoma in children occurs almost exclusively in the ileum and ileocecal region; diffuse large cell and Burkitt's lymphomas are the most common categories.

Table 11-1 Major differences* between small bowel lymphoma arising *de novo* (so-called Western type) and Mediterranean lymphoma

Features	Small bowel lymphoma arising *de novo*	Mediterranean small bowel lymphoma
Average age	25-30 years	40-45 years
Commonest presentation	Malabsorption and abdominal pain	Obstruction
Commonest location	Distal bowel	Proximal bowel
Gross appearance	Bulky mass	Diffuse infiltration
Usual histology	Monomorphic (histiocytic or poorly differentiated lymphocytic)	Pleomorphic
Lymph node involvement	Nodular or massive	With preservation of architecture
Adjacent bowel mucosa and regional nodes	Unremarkable	Massive infiltration by mature plasma cells
Serum and urine	Unremarkable	Increase in IgA

*Differences are valid only at a statistical level; numerous exceptions occur.

The major differences between bowel lymphomas arising *de novo* and the Mediterranean type are given in Table 11-1.

Hodgkin's disease is extremely rare. Only two cases were found by Lewin et al.[333] in a review of 117 lymphomas of the gastrointestinal tract.

Lymphoid hyperplasia may present as a focal process, also known as *pseudolymphoma*.[342,349] The variety leading to intussusception in young children has been discussed previously (see p. 535). In other cases *(nodular lymphoid hyperplasia)*, the entire small bowel is studded with well-circumscribed nodes of lymphoid tissue (Fig. 11-76). *Giardia lamblia* is often present in the latter condition, and some of the patients have low or absent IgA and IgM levels, decreased IgG level, susceptibility to infection, and diarrhea with or without steatorrhea.[319,342,348] In children, this condition is often associated with viral infection.[306] Presence of germinal centers, numerous cell types, and prominent vascularity are the main features in the differential diagnosis with malignant lymphoma. In some reported cases of "pseudolymphoma,"[304] a pleomorphic infiltrate containing atypical cells was described; whether these are indeed inflammatory lesions or early stages of true lymphomas is difficult to decide.

Other cases of lymphoid hyperplasia have a diffuse quality and may lead to intestinal pseudo-obstruction. The in-

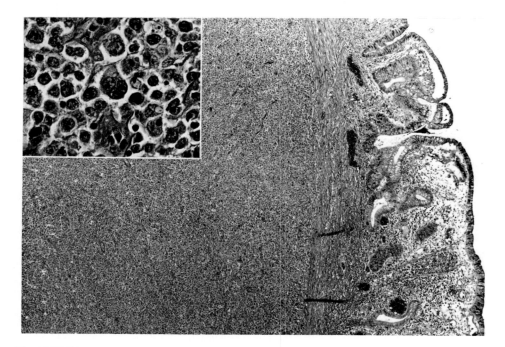

Fig. 11-75 Primary malignant lymphoma of small bowel. Tumor diffusely infiltrates the submucosa and is also present in lamina propria. **Inset** shows large size of cells and presence of occasional multinucleated elements.

filtrate is usually polyclonal on immunohistochemical evaluation,[335] but in some cases it exhibits light chain restriction, raising suggestions about the nature of the lymphoid hyperplasia and its malignant potential.[308a] Cases of nodular lymphoid hyperplasia have been seen in association with malignant lymphoma, but the nature of the pathogenetic relationship between the two processes is unknown.[334]

Granulocytic sarcoma can present initially as a small bowel mass, preceding the development of acute granulocytic leukemia.[307] This condition may be simulated by bacterial infection since macrophages that have phagocytosed large numbers of bacteria may appear strongly positive with the Leder stain.[330]

Other tumors and tumorlike conditions

Lipomas of the small bowel characteristically grow in the submucosa.[361,367] Grossly, they are bright yellow, round, encapsulated tumors that bulge upward into the mucosa surface. They have a very characteristic radiographic appearance.[358] The large majority are solitary. About 5% are multiple; these should be distinguished from the rare condition known as *lipomatosis*, in which a segment of bowel (on occasions the entire organ) is infiltrated by mature fat, sometimes in association with diverticulosis or intussusception.[353] Complications of lipoma include ulceration and intussusception.

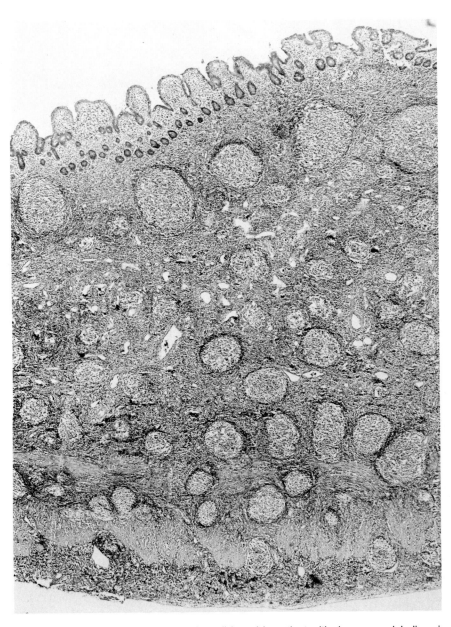

Fig. 11-76 Striking lymphoid hyperplasia of small bowel in patient with dysgammaglobulinemia. Involvement is mainly submucosal.

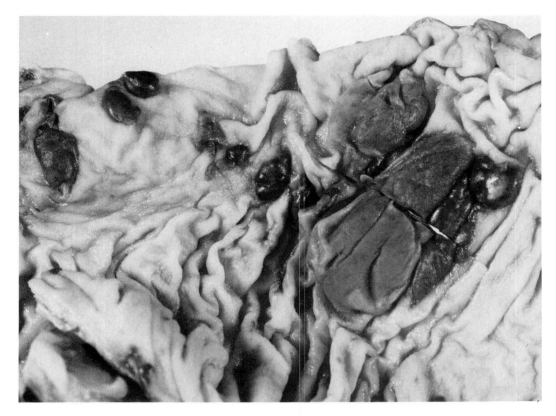

Fig. 11-77 Multiple hemangiomas of small bowel. Microscopically, they were of cavernous variety. (Courtesy Dr. W.C. Black, Albuquerque, NM.)

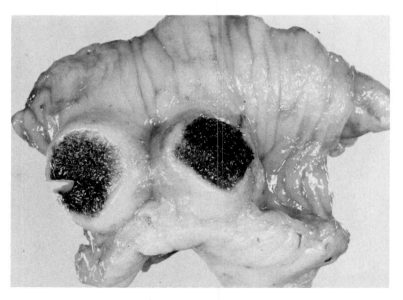

Fig. 11-78 Metastatic carcinoma involving small bowel. Tumor metastasis appeared first in submucosa and finally ulcerated surface. Note how normal mucosa extends to edge of ulceration. This finding helps to differentiate it from primary carcinoma.

Hemangiomas of the small bowel may be single or multiple and may be associated with similar lesions in other organs.[357,365] They may bleed or perforate. Grossly, the lesions are soft, elevated, reddish, and not well defined. The midjejunum is the most common location, but they can also occur in the duodenum and other sites. Microscopically, cavernous hemangioma is the most common variety (Fig. 11-77). *Lymphangiomas* often occur, particularly in children, in association with similar tumors in other sites. They should be distinguished from the *lymphatic cysts (lacteal cysts)* commonly found incidentally in the elderly.[352]

In *hereditary telangiectasia*, there are vascular lesions of the mucous membrane and skin. These lesions are multiple, and severe gastrointestinal hemorrhage can occur from them. Smith et al.[366] reported 159 patients, 21 of whom had significant hemorrhage. Demonstration of these lesions at surgery is difficult, and surgical resection is usually not successful.

Other reported vascular tumors of small bowel are *glomus tumor*,[356] *Kaposi's sarcoma*, and *angiosarcoma*. The two latter tumors are characteristically multiple.[363]

Neurofibroma and *ganglioneuroma* may occur as isolated neoplasms or as components of Recklinghausen's disease or multiple endocrine adenomatosis.[364a] *Plexosarcoma* is a recently described submucosal tumor composed of large epithelioid cells and a fascicular spindle-cell component. Evidence of neural differentiation can be detected ultrastructurally and immunohistochemically. Metastases are common.[358a]

Congenital fibromatosis may result in a solitary intestinal mass leading to intestinal obstruction in the neonate.[355]

Primary malignant tumors other than those already described are rare. Isolated examples of rhabdomyosarcoma, liposarcoma, fibrosarcoma, malignant schwannoma, extraskeletal osteosarcoma, malignant mesenchymoma, and primary choriocarcinoma have been reported.[360,364]

Metastatic tumors can involve the small bowel, often in the form of multiple polypoid tumors (Fig. 11-78). The lesions may result in obstruction or perforation, necessitating palliative resection.[354,369] The most common sites for the primary tumor are malignant melanoma, carcinoma from lung and breast, and choriocarcinoma.[359,362] Willbanks and Fogelman[368] performed palliative surgery on eighteen patients with *malignant melanoma* metastatic to the small and/or large bowel. All fourteen patients with multiple tumors died within 1 year, whereas among the four with an apparently solitary metastasis, there was a 5-year survivor.

REFERENCES
CONGENITAL DEFECTS
Heterotopic pancreas

1 de Castro Barbosa JJ, Dockerty MB, Waugh JM: Pancreatic heterotopia. Surg Gynecol Obstet **82:**527-542, 1946.

Heterotopic gastric mucosa

2 Franzin G, Musola R, Negi A, Mencarelli R, Fratton A: Heterotopic gastric (fundic) mucosa in the duodenum. Endoscopy **14:**166-167, 1982.

3 Lessels AM, Martin DF: Heterotopic gastric mucosa in the duodenum. J Clin Pathol **35:**591-595, 1982.

4 Russin V, Krevsky B, Caroline DF, Tang C-K, Ming S-C: Mixed hyperplastic and adenomatous polyp arising from ectopic gastric mucosa of the duodenum. Arch Pathol Lab Med **110:**556-558, 1986.

5 Spiller RC, Shousha S, Barrison IG: Heterotopic gastric tissue in the duodenum. A report of eight cases. Dig Dis Sci **27:**880-883, 1982.

Duplication, atresia, and related defects

6 Adair HM, Trowell JE: Squamous cell carcinoma arising in a duplication of the small bowel. J Pathol **133:**25-31, 1981.

7 Alvarez SP, Greco MA, Genieser NB: Small intestinal atresia and segmental absence of muscle coats. Hum Pathol **13:**948-951, 1982.

8 Halles JA Jr: Atresia of the small intestine. Current concepts in diagnosis and treatment. Clin Pediatr [Phila] **3:**257-262, 1964.

9 Litwin A, Avidor I, Schujman E, Grunebaum M, Wilunsky E, Wolloch Y, Reisner SH: Neonatal intestinal perforation caused by congenital defects of the intestinal musculature. Am J Clin Pathol **81:**77-80, 1984.

10 Lynn HB, Espinas EE: Intestinal atresia. An attempt to relate location to embryologic processes. Arch Surg **79:**357-361, 1959.

11 Smith DW: Recognizable patterns of human malformation. Genetic, embryologic, and clinical aspects, ed. 3, Philadelphia, 1982, W.B. Saunders Co.

Meckel's diverticulum

12 Bloch T, Tejada E, Brodhecker C: Malignant melanoma in Meckel's diverticulum. Am J Clin Pathol **86:**231-234, 1986.

13 Haugen OA, Pegg CS, Kyle J: Leiomyosarcoma of Meckel's diverticulum. Cancer **26:**929-934, 1970.

14 Mackey WC, Dineen P: A fifty year experience with Meckel's diverticulum. Surg Gynecol Obstet **156:**56-64, 1983.

14a Pfalzgraf, RR, Zumwalt RE, Kenny MR: Mesodiverticular band and sudden death in children. A report of two cases. Arch Pathol Lab Med **112:**182-184, 1988.

15 Söderlund S: Meckel's diverticulum. A clinical and histologic study. Acta Chir Scand [Suppl] **248:**1-233, 1959.

16 Steck WD, Helwig EB: Cutaneous remnants of the omphalomesenteric duct. Arch Dermatol **90:**463-470, 1964.

17 Weitzner S: Carcinoid of Meckel's diverticulum. Report of a case and review of the literature. Cancer **23:**1436-1440, 1969.

Other diverticula

18 Cooke WT, Cox EV, Fone DJ, Meynell MJ, Gaddie R: The clinical and metabolic significance of jejunal diverticula. Gut **4:**115-131, 1963.

19 Fleming CR, Newcomer AD, Stephens DH, Carlson HC: Intraluminal duodenal diverticulum. Report of two cases and review of the literature. Mayo Clin Proc **50:**244-248, 1975.

20 Juler JL, List JW, Stemmer EA, Connolly JE: Duodenal diverticulitis. Arch Surg **99:**572-578, 1969.

21 Krishnamurthy S, Kelly MM, Rohrmann CA, Schuffler MD: Jejunal diverticulosis. A heterogenous disorder caused by a variety of abnormalities of smooth muscle or myenteric plexus. Gastroenterology **85:**538-547, 1983.

22 Nobles ER Jr: Jejunal diverticula. Arch Surg **102:**172-174, 1971.

23 Suda K, Mizuguchi K, Matsumoto M: A histopathological study on the etiology of duodenal diverticulum related to the fusion of the pancreatic anlage. Am J Gastroenterol **78:**335-338, 1983.

24 Zakhour HD, Clark RG: Intramural gas cysts in a case of diverticular disease of the jejunum. Histopathology **6:**363-369, 1982.

Other congenital defects

25 Beighton PH, Murdoch JL, Votteler T: Gastrointestinal complications of the Ehlers-Danlos syndrome. Gut **10:**1004-1008, 1969.

26 Walker AW, Kempson RL, Ternberg JL: Aganglionosis of the small intestine. Surgery **60:**449-457, 1966.

MALABSORPTION

27 Bhagavan BS, Hofkin GA, Cochran BA: Whipple's disease. Morphologic and immunofluorescence characterization of bacterial antigens. Hum Pathol **12:**930-936, 1981.

28 Boitnott JK, Margolis S: Mineral oil in human tissues. II. Oil droplets in lymph nodes of the porta hepatis. Bull Hopkins Hosp **118:**414-422, 1966.

29 Comer GM, Brandt LJ, Abissi CJ: Whipple's disease. A review. Am J Gastroenterol **78:**107-114, 1983.

30 Denholm RB, Mills PR, More IAR: Electron microscopy in the long-term follow-up of Whipple's disease. Effect of antibiotics. Am J Surg Pathol **5:**507-516, 1981.

30a Dobbins WO: Whipple's disease. Springfield, Ill., 1987, Charles C Thomas.

31 Du Boulay CEH: An immunohistochemical study of Whipple's disease using the immunoperoxidase technique. Hum Pathol **13**:925-929, 1982.

32 Ekuan JH, Hill RB Jr: Colonic histiocytosis. Clinical and pathological evaluation. Gastroenterology **55**:619-625, 1968.

33 Enzinger FM, Helwig EB: Whipple's disease. A review of the literature and report of fifteen patients. Virchows Arch [Pathol Anat] **336**:238-269, 1963.

34 Evans DJ, Ali MH: Immunocytochemistry in the diagnosis of Whipple's disease. J Clin Pathol **38**:372-374, 1985.

35 Grody WW, Magidson JG, Weiss LM, Hu E, Warnke RA, Lewin KJ: Gastrointestinal lymphoma. Immunohistochemical studies on the cell of origin. Am J Surg Pathol **9**:328-377, 1985.

36 Guerra R, Wheby MS, Bayless TM: Long-term antibiotic therapy in tropical sprue. Ann Intern Med **63**:619-634, 1965.

37 Halter SA, Greene HL, Helinek G: Gluten-sensitive enteropathy. Sequence of villous regrowth as viewed by scanning electron microscopy. Hum Pathol **13**:811-818, 1982.

38 Harris OD, Cooke WT, Thompson H, Waterhouse JAH: Malignancy in adult coeliac disease and idiopathic steatorrhoea. Am J Med **42**:899-912, 1967.

39 Isaacson P, Wright DH: Intestinal lymphoma associated with malabsorption. Lancet **1**:67-70, 1978.

40 Isaacson P, Wright DH: Malignant histiocytosis of the intestine. Its relationship to malabsorption and ulcerative jejunitis. Hum Pathol **9**:661-667, 1978.

41 Isselbacher KJ, Scheig R, Plotkin GR, Caulfield JB: Congenital β lipoprotein deficiency. An hereditary disorder involving a defect in the absorption and transport of lipids. Medicine [Baltimore] **43**:347-361, 1964.

42 Jeffries GH, Weser E, Steisenger MH: Malabsorption. Gastroenterology **56**:777-797, 1969.

43 Keinath RD, Merrell DE, Vlietstra R, Dobbins WO III: Antibiotic treatment and relapse in Whipple's disease. Long-term followup of 88 patients. Gastroenterology **88**:1867-1873, 1985.

44 Klipstein FA: Tropical sprue in travelers and expatriates living abroad. Gastroenterology **80**:590-600, 1981.

45 Klipstein FA, Baker SJ: Regarding the definition of tropical sprue. Gastroenterology **58**:717-721, 1970.

46 Kopp WL, Trier JS, Stiehm ER, Foroozan P: ''Acquired'' agammaglobulinemia with defective delayed hypersensitivity. Ann Intern Med **69**:309-317, 1968.

47 Kuhajda FP, Belitsos NJ, Keren DF, Hutchins GM: A submucosal variant of Whipple's disease. Gastroenterology **82**:46-50, 1982.

48 Kumar PJ: The enigma of celiac disease. Gastroenterology **89**:214-216, 1985.

49 Levinson JD, Kirsner JB: Infiltrative diseases of the small bowel and malabsorption. Am J Dig Dis **15**:741-766, 1970.

50 MacDermott RP: Cell-mediated immunity in gastrointestinal disease. Hum Pathol **17**:219-233, 1986.

51 Maizell H, Ruffin JM, Dobbins WO III: Whipple's disease. A review of 19 patients from one hospital and a review of the literature since 1950. Medicine [Baltimore] **49**:175-205, 1970.

52 Marsh MN (ed): Immunopathology of the small intestine. New York, 1987, John Wiley & Sons.

53 Mead GM, Whitehouse JM, Thompson J, Sweetenham JW, Williams CJ, Wright DH: Clinical features and management of malignant histiocytosis of the intestine. Cancer **60**:2791-2796, 1987.

54 Menendez-Corrada R: Current views on tropical sprue and a comparison to nontropical sprue. Med Clin North Am **52**:1367-1385, 1968.

55 Modigliani R, Poitras P, Galian A, Messing B, Guyet-Rousset P, Libeskind M, Piel-Desruisseaux JL, Rambaud JC: Chronic non-specific ulcerative duodenojejunoileitis. Report of four cases. Gut **20**:318-328, 1979.

56 Morningstar WA: Whipple's disease. An example of the value of the electron microscope in diagnosis, follow-up, and correlation of pathologic process. Hum Pathol **6**:443-454, 1975.

57 Nielsen K: Coeliac disease. Alpha-1-antitrypsin contents in jejunal mucosa before and after gluten-free diet. Histopathology **8**:759-764, 1984.

58 Nielsen SNJ, Wold LE: Adenocarcinoma of jejunum in association with nontropical sprue. Arch Pathol Lab Med **110**:822-824, 1986.

59 O'Brien CJ, Saverymuttu S, Hodgson HJF, Evans DJ: Coeliac disease, adenocarcinoma of jejunum and in situ squamous carcinoma of oesophagus. J Clin Pathol **36**:62-67, 1983.

60 Peña AS, Whitehead R: Quoted by Whitehead.[76]

61 Perera DR, Weinstein WM, Rubin CE: Small intestinal biopsy. Hum Pathol **6**:157-217, 1975.

62 Petreshock EP, Pessah M, Menachemi E: Adenocarcinoma of the jejunum associated with nontropical sprue. Am J Dig Dis **20**:796-799, 1975.

63 Rosekrans PCM, Lindeman J, Meijer CJLM: Quantitative histological and im-

munohistochemical findings in jejunal biopsy specimens in giardiasis. Virchows Arch [Pathol Anat] **393**:145-151, 1981.

64 Rubin CE, Eidelman S, Weinstein WM: Spruc by any other name. Gastroenterology **58**:409-413, 1970.

65 Rubin W, Ross LL, Sleisenger MH, Weser E: An electron microscopic study of adult celiac disease. Lab Invest **15**:1720-1747, 1966.

66 Sheehy TW, Meroney WH, Cox RS, Soler JE: Hookworm disease and malabsorption. Gastroenterology **42**:148-156, 1962.

67 Thompson H: Necropsy studies on adult coeliac disease. J Clin Pathol **27**:710-721, 1974.

68 Trier JS, Browning TH: Epithelial-cell renewal in cultured duodenal biopsies in celiac sprue. N Engl J Med **283**:1245-1250, 1970.

69 Variend S, Placzek M, Raafat F, Walker-Smith JA: Small intestinal mucosal fat in childhood enteropathies. J Clin Pathol **37**:373-377, 1984.

70 Waldmann TA: Protein-losing enteropathy. Gastroenterology **50**:422-443, 1966.

71 Watson JHL, Haubrich WS: Bacilli bodies in the lumen and epithelium of the jejunum in Whipple's disease. Lab Invest **21**:347-357, 1969.

72 Weinstein WM, Saunders DR, Tytgat GN, Rubin CE: Collagenous sprue. An unrecognized type of malabsorption. N Engl J Med **283**:1297-1301, 1970.

73 Weser E, Jeffries GH, Sleisenger MH: Malabsorption. Gastroenterology **50**:811-828, 1966.

74 Whalen GE, Rosenberg EB, Strickland GT, Gutman RA, Cross JH, Watten RH, Uylangeo C, Dizou JJ: Intestinal capillariasis. A new disease in man. Lancet **1**:13-16, 1969.

75 Whitehead R: Primary lymphadenopathy complicating idiopathic steatorrhoea. Gut **9**:569-575, 1968.

76 Whitehead R: The interpretation and significance of morphological abnormalities in jejunal biopsies. J Clin Pathol **24** [Suppl 5, R Coll Pathol]:108-124, 1971.

77 Yardley JH, Takano J, Hendrix TR: Epithelial and other mucosal lesions of the jejunum in giardiasis. Jejunal biopsy studies. Bull Hopkins Hosp **115**:389-406, 1964.

ULCERS

78 Allen AC, Boley SJ, Schultz L, Schwartz S: Potassium-induced lesions of the small bowel. JAMA **193**:85-90, 1965.

79 Artinian B, Lough JO, Palmer JD: Idiopathic ulcer of small bowel with pseudolymphomatous reactions. A clinicopathological study of six cases. Arch Pathol **91**:327-333, 1971.

80 Davies DR, Brightmore T: Idiopathic and drug-induced ulceration of the small intestine. Br J Surg **57**:134-139, 1970.

81 Dean ACB, Mason MK: The distribution of pyloric mucosa in partial gastrectomy specimens. Gut **5**:64-67, 1964.

82 McCallum RW, Singh D, Wollman J: Endoscopic and histologic correlations of the duodenal bulb. Arch Pathol Lab Med **103**:169-172, 1979.

83 Pounder RE: Duodenal ulcers that will not heal. Gut **25**:697-702, 1984.

84 Raf LE: Ischaemic stenosis of the small intestine. Acta Clin Scand **135**:253-259, 1969.

85 Saito K, Shimizu H, Yokoyama T, Kawata K, Matsumura T, Morioka Y: Annular ulcer of the stagnant ileum. A clinicopathological study on the morphogenesis. Acta Pathol Jpn **33**:257-263, 1983.

86 Szabo S: Pathogenesis of duodenal ulcer disease. Lab Invest **51**:121-147, 1984.

87 Thompson JC, Wiener I: Evaluation of surgical treatment for duodenal ulcer. Acute and long-term effects. Clin Gastroenterol **13**:569-600, 1984.

VASCULAR DISEASES

88 Gilbert AE, Jorgenson NC: Small bowel obstruction due to hemorrhage secondary to anticoagulant therapy. Am J Surg **99**:945-948, 1960.

89 Levine S, Whelan TJ Jr: Small bowel infarction due to intramural hematoma during anticoagulant therapy. Arch Surg **95**:245-248, 1967.

90 McCurley TL, Collins RD: Intestinal infarction in rheumatoid arthritis. Three cases due to unusual obliterative vascular lesions. Arch Pathol Lab Med **108**:125-128, 1984.

91 Nalbandian H, Sheth N, Dietrich R, Georgiou J: Intestinal ischemia caused by cocaine ingestion. Report of two cases. Surgery **97**:374-376, 1985.

92 Ottinger LW: Mesenteric ischemia. N Engl J Med **307**:535-537, 1982.

93 Wang CC, Reeves JD: Mesenteric vascular disease. Am J Roentgenol Radium Ther Nucl Med **83**:895-908, 1960.

94 Whitehead R: The pathology of ischemia of the intestines. Pathol Annu **11**:1-52, 1976.

95 Williams LF Jr: Vascular insufficiency of the intestines. Gastroenterology **61**:757-777, 1971.

CROHN'S DISEASE (REGIONAL ILEITIS)

96 Aufses AH Jr: The surgery of granulomatous inflammatory bowel disease. In Current problems in surgery. Chicago, 1983, Year Book Medical Publishers, Inc.

97 Cave DR, Mitchell DN, Brooke BN: Experimental animal studies of the etiology and pathogenesis of Crohn's disease. Gastroenterology **69**:618-624, 1975.

98 Chambers TJ, Morson BC: The granuloma in Crohn's disease. Gut **20**:269-274, 1979.

99 Chong SKF, Blackshaw AJ, Boyle S, Williams CB, Walker-Smith JA: Histological diagnosis of chronic inflammatory bowel disease in childhood. Gut **326**:55-59, 1985.

100 Collier PE, Turowski P, Diamond DL: Small intestinal adenocarcinoma complicating regional enteritis. Cancer **55**:516-521, 1985.

101 Crohn BR, Ginzburg L, Oppenheimer GD: Regional ileitis. JAMA **99**:1323-1329, 1932.

102 Daum F, Boley SJ, Cohen MI: Miliary Crohn's disease. Gastroenterology **67**:527-530, 1974.

103 Devroede G, Schlaeder G, Sanchez G, Haddad H: Crohn's disease of the vulva. Am J Clin Pathol **63**:348-358, 1975.

104 Dourmashkin RR, Davies H, Wells C, Shah D, Price A, O'Morain C, Levi J: Epithelial patchy necrosis in Crohn's disease. Hum Pathol **14**:643-648, 1983.

105 Dvorak AM, Monahan RA: Crohn's disease—mast cell quantitation using one micron plastic sections for light microscopic study. Pathol Annu **18**(Pt 1):181-190, 1983.

106 Dvorak AM, Silen W: Differentiation between Crohn's disease and other inflammatory conditions by electron microscopy. Ann Surg **201**:53-63, 1985.

107 Fabricius PJ, Gyde SN, Shouler P, Keighley MRB, Alexander-Williams J, Allan RN: Crohn's disease in the elderly. Gut **26**:461-465, 1985.

108 Faul SH, Wong LK, Zinsser KR: Enteritis cystica profunda. Association with Crohn's disease. Hum Pathol **17**:600-603, 1986.

109 Fielding JF, Toye DKM, Benton DC, Cooke WT: Crohn's disease of the stomach and duodenum. Gut **11**:1001-1006, 1970.

110 Fresko D, Lazarus SS, Dotan J, Reingold M: Early presentation of carcinoma of the small bowel in Crohn's disease ("Crohn's carcinoma"). Case reports and review of the literature. Gastroenterology **82**:783-789, 1982.

111 Geller SA, Cohen A: Arterial inflammatory-cell infiltration in Crohn's disease. Arch Pathol Lab Med **107**:473-475, 1983.

112 Glass RE, Baker WNW: Role of the granuloma in recurrent Crohn's disease. Gut **17**:75-77, 1976.

113 Greenstein AJ, Janowitz HD, Sacher DB: The extraintestinal complications of Crohn's disease and ulcerative colitis. A study of 700 patients. Medicine [Baltimore] **55**:401-412, 1976.

114 Greenstein AJ, Sachar DB, Pasternack BS, Janowitz HD: Reoperation and recurrence in Crohn's colitis and ileocolitis. Crude and cumulative rates. N Engl J Med **293**:685-690, 1975.

115 Gump FE, Sakellariadis P, Wolff M, Broell JR: Clinical-pathological investigation of regional enteritis as a guide to prognosis. Ann Surg **176**:233-242, 1972.

116 Hamilton SR: Pathologic features of Crohn's disease associated with recrudescence after resection. Pathol Annu **18**(Pt 1):191-203, 1983.

117 Hawker PC, Gyde SN, Thompson H, Allan RN: Adenocarcinoma of the small intestine complicating Crohn's disease. Gut **23**:188-193, 1982.

118 Kahn E, Daum F: Pseudopolyps of the small intestine in Crohn's disease. Hum Pathol **15**:84-86, 1984.

119 Kirsner JB, Shorter RG: Recent developments in nonspecific inflammatory bowel disease. N Engl J Med **306**:837-848, 1982.

120 Lock MR, Farmer RG, Fazio VW, Jagelman DG, Lavery IC, Weakley FL: Recurrence and reoperation for Crohn's disease. The role of disease location in prognosis. N Engl J Med **304**:1586-1588, 1981.

121 Marin ML, Geller SA, Greenstein AJ, Marin RH, Gordon RE, Aufses AH Jr: Ultrastructural pathology of Crohn's disease. Correlated transmission electron microscopy, scanning electron microscopy, and freeze fracture studies. Am J Gastroenterol **78**:355-364, 1983.

122 Mayberry JF: Epidemiological aspects of Crohn's disease. A review of the literature. Gut **25**:886-899, 1984.

123 Mekhjian HS, Switz DM, Watts HD, Deren JJ, Katon RM, Beman FM: National Cooperative Crohn's Disease Study. Factors determining recurrence of Crohn's disease after surgery. Gastroenterology **77**:907-913, 1979.

124 Menard DB, Haddad H, Blain JG, Beaudry R, Devroede G, Massé S: Granulomatous myositis and myopathy associated with Crohn's colitis. N Engl J Med **295**:818-819, 1976.

125 Mogadam M, Priest RJ: Necrotizing enteritis in Crohn's disease of the small bowel. Gastroenterology **56**:337-341, 1969.

126 Morson B: Crohn's disease. Lecture 2. Trans Med Soc Lond **86**:177-192, 1970.

127 Nesbit RR Jr, Elbadawi NA, Norton JH, Cooper RA Jr: Carcinoma of the small bowel. A complication of regional enteritis. Cancer **37**:2948-2959, 1976.

128 Nugent FW, Glaser D, Fernandez-Herlihy L: Crohn's colitis associated with granulomatous disease. N Engl J Med **294**:262-263, 1976.

129 Otto HF, Gebbers J-O: Electron microscopic, ultracytochemical and immunohistological observations in Crohn's disease of the ileum and colon. Virchows Arch [Pathol Anat] **391**:189-205, 1981.

130 Perzin KH, Peterson M, Castiglione CL, Fenoglio CM, Wolff M: Intramucosal carcinoma of the small intestine arising in regional enteritis (Crohn's disease). Report of a case studied for carcinoembryonic antigen and review of the literature. Cancer **54**:151-162, 1984.

131 Price AB, Morson BC: Inflammatory bowel disease. The surgical pathology of Crohn's disease and ulcerative colitis. Hum Pathol **6**:7-29, 1975.

132 Rankin GB, Watts D, Melnyk CS, Kelley ML Jr: National Cooperative Crohn's Disease Study. Extraintestinal manifestations and perianal complications. Gastroenterology **77**:914-920, 1979.

133 Rappaport H, Bourgoyne FH, Smetana HF: The pathology of regional enteritis. Milit Surg **109**:463-502, 1951.

134 Rubin S, Lambie RW, Chapman J: Regional ileitis in childhood. Am J Dis Child **114**:106-110, 1967.

135 Sachar DB, Wolfson DM, Greenstein AJ, Goldberg J, Styezynski R, Janowitz HD: Risk factors for postoperative recurrence of Crohn's disease. Gastroenterology **85**:917-921, 1983.

136 Savage RA, Farmer RG, Hawk WA: Carcinoma of the small intestine associated with transmural ileitis (Crohn's disease). Am J Clin Pathol **63**:168-178, 1975.

137 Schnitt SJ, Antonioli DA, Jaffe B, Peppercorn MA: Granulomatous inflammation of minor salivary gland ducts. A new oral manifestation of Crohn's disease. Hum Pathol **18**:405-407, 1987.

138 Simpson S, Traube J, Riddell RH: The histologic appearance of dysplasia (precarcinomatous change) in Crohn's disease of the small and large intestine. Gastroenterology **81**:492-501, 1981.

139 Sutphen JL, Cooper PH, Mackel SE, Nelson DL: Metastatic cutaneous Crohn's disease. Gastroenterology **86**:941-944, 1984.

140 Thompson EM, Clayden G, Price AB: Cancer in Crohn's disease—an "occult" malignancy. Histopathology **7**:365-376, 1983.

141 Thyberg J, Graf W, Klingenström P: Intestinal fine structure in Crohn's disease. Lysosomal inclusions in epithelial cells and macrophages. Virchows Arch [Pathol Anat] **391**:141-152, 1981.

142 Valdes-Dapena A, Rudolph I, Hidayat A, Roth JLA, Laucks RB: Adenocarcinoma of the small bowel in association with regional enteritis. Four new cases. Cancer **37**:2938-2947, 1976.

143 Whelan G, Farmer RG, Fazio VW, Goormastic M: Recurrence after surgery in Crohn's disease. Relationship to location of disease (clinical pattern) and surgical indication. Gastroenterology **88**:1826-1833, 1985.

144 Wise L, Kyriakos M, McCown A, Ballinger WF: Crohn's disease of the duodenum. Am J Surg **121**:184-194, 1971.

145 Wolfson DM, Sachar DB, Cohen A, Goldberg J, Styczynski R, Greenstein AJ, Gelernt IM, Janowitz HD: Granulomas do not affect postoperative recurrence rates in Crohn's disease. Gastroenterology **83**:405-409, 1982.

OTHER INFLAMMATORY DISEASES

145a Anthony PP, Morris DS, Vowles KDJ: Multiple and recurrent inflammatory fibroid polyps in three generations of a Devon family. A new syndrome. Gut **23**:854-862, 1984.

146 Bradford WD, Noce PS, Gutman LT: Pathologic features of enteric infection with *Yersinia enterocolitica*. Arch Pathol **98**:17-22, 1974.

147 Brynjulfsen BC: Jejunitis acuta—ileitis regionalis acuta. Acta Chir Scand **96**:361-388, 1948.

148 Campbell WL, Green WM, Seaman WB: Inflammatory pseudotumor of the small intestine. Am J Roentgenol Radium Ther Nucl Med **121**:305-311, 1974.

149 DeSchryver-Kecskemeti K, Clouse RE: A previously unrecognized subgroup of "eosinophilic gastroenteritis." Association with connective tissue diseases. Am J Surg Pathol **8**:171-180, 1984.

150 Gleason TH, Patterson SD: The pathology of *Yersinia enterocolitica* ileocolitis. Am J Surg Pathol **6**:347-355, 1982.

151 Grillin JS, Urmacher C, West R, Shike M: Disseminated *Mycobacterium avium*–intracellulare infection in acquired immunodeficiency syndrome mimicking Whipple's disease. Gastroenterology **85**:1187-1191, 1983.

152 Guarda LA, Stein SA, Cleary KA, Ordonez NG: Human cryptosporidiosis in the acquired immunodeficiency syndrome. Arch Pathol Lab Med **107**:562-566, 1983.

153 Jenkins D, Goodall A, Gillet FR, Scott BB: Defining duodenitis. Quantitative histological study of mucosal responses and their correlations. J Clin Pathol **38**:1119-1126, 1985.

154 Johnstone JM, Morson BC: Inflammatory fibroid polyp of the gastrointestinal tract. Histopathology **2**:349-361, 1978.

155 Lefkowitch JH, Krumholz S, Feng-Chen K-C, Griffin P, Despommier D, Brasitus TA: Cryptosporidiosis of the human small intestine. A light and electron microscopic study. Hum Pathol **15**:746-752, 1984.

156 Nkanza NK, King M, Hutt MSR: Intussusception due to inflammatory fibroid polyps of the ileum. A report of 12 cases from Africa. Br J Surg **67**:271-274, 1980.

157 Roth RI, Owen RL, Keren DF: AIDS with *Mycobacterium avium*–intracellulare lesions resembling those of Whipple's disease. N Engl J Med **309**:1324-1325, 1983.

158 Schmitz-Moormann P, Pittner PM, Reichmann L, Massarat S: Quantitative histological study of duodenitis in biopsies. Pathol Res Pract **178**:499-507, 1984.

159 Schulze K, Warner HA, Murray D: Intestinal tuberculosis. Experience at a Canadian teaching institution. Am J Med **63**:735-745, 1977.

160 Shimer GR, Helwig EB: Inflammatory fibroid polyps of the intestine. Am J Clin Pathol **81**:708-714, 1984.

161 Shousha S, Spiller RC, Parkins RA: The endoscopically abnormal duodenum in patients with dyspepsia. Biopsy findings in 60 cases. Histopathology **7**:23-34, 1983.

162 Soave R, Danner RL, Honig CL, Ma P, Hart CC, Nash T, Roberts RB: Cryptosporidiosis in homosexual men. Ann Intern Med **100**:504-511, 1984.

163 Sprague R, Harper P, McClain S, Trainer T, Beeken W: Disseminated gastrointestinal sarcoidosis. Case report and review of the literature. Gastroenterology **87**:421-425, 1984.

164 Suen KC, Burton JD: The spectrum of eosinophilic infiltration of the gastrointestinal tract and its relationship to other disorders of angiitis and granulomatosis. Hum Pathol **10**:31-43, 1979.

165 Sun T: The diagnosis of giardiasis. Am J Surg Pathol **4**:265-271, 1980.

166 Tandon HD, Prakash A: Pathology of intestinal tuberculosis and its distinction from Crohn's disease. Gut **13**:260-269, 1972.

IRRADIATION EFFECT

167 Donaldson SS, Jundt S, Ricour C, Sarrazin D, Lemerle J, Schweisguth O: Radiation enteritis in childrern. A retrospective review, clinicopathologic correlation, and dietary management. Cancer **35**:1167-1178, 1975.

168 Hasleton PS, Carr N, Schofield PF: Vascular changes in radiation bowel disease. Histopathology **9**:517-534, 1985.

169 Perkins DE, Spjut JH: Intestinal stenosis following radiation therapy. Am J Roentgenol Radium Ther Nucl Med **88**:953-966, 1962.

170 Sugg WL, Lawler WH, Ackerman LV, Butcher HR Jr: Operative therapy for severe irradiational injury in the enteral and urinary tracts. Ann Surg **157**:62-70, 1963.

171 Warren S, Friedman NB: Pathology and pathologic diagnosis of radiation lesions in the gastro-intestinal tract. Am J Pathol **18**:499-513, 1942.

INTUSSUSCEPTION

172 Bell TM, Steyn JH: Viruses in lymph nodes of children with mesenteric adenitis and intussusception. Br Med J **1**:700-702, 1962.

173 Ravitch MM, McCune RM Jr: Reduction of intussusception by barium enema. Clinical and experimental study. Ann Surg **128**:904-917, 1948.

174 Sarason EL, Prior JT, Prowda RL: Recurrent intussusception associated with hypertrophy of Peyer's patches. N Engl J Med **253**:905-908, 1955.

175 Yunis EJ, Atchison RW, Michaels RH, DeCicco FA: Adenovirus and ileocecal intussusception. Lab Invest **33**:347-351, 1975.

OTHER NON-NEOPLASTIC DISEASES

176 Foster CS: The brown bowel syndrome. A possible smooth muscle mitochondrial myopathy? Histopathology **3**:1-17, 1979.

177 Hosler JP, Kimmel KK, Moeller DD: The "brown bowel syndrome." A case report. Am J Gastroenterol **77**:854-855, 1982.

178 Johnson DH, Guthrie TH, Tedesco FJ, Griffin JW, Anthony HF Jr: Amyloidosis masquerading as inflammatory bowel disease with a mass lesion simulating a malignancy. Am J Gastroenterol **77**:141-145, 1982.

179 Kinder CH: Acute small-bowel obstruction due to endometriosis. Br J Surg **41**:550-552, 1953.

180 Smith TR, Cho KC: Small intestine amyloidosis producing a stippled punctate mucosal pattern. Radiological-pathological correlation. Am J Gastroenterol **81**:477-479, 1986.

181 Snover DC, Weisdorf SA, Vercellotti GM, Rank B, Hutton S, McGlave P: A histopathologic study of gastric and small intestinal graft-versus-host disease following allogeneic bone marrow transplantation. Hum Pathol **16**:387-392, 1985.

TUMORS
Benign epithelial tumors

182 Bartholomew LG, Moore CE, Dahlin DC, Waugh JM: Intestinal polyposis associated with mucocutaneous pigmentation. Surg Gynecol Obstet **115**:1-11, 1962.

183 Blackman E, Nash SV: Diagnosis of duodenal and ampullary epithelial neoplasms by endoscopic biopsy. A clinicopathologic and immunohistochemical study. Hum Pathol **16**:901-910, 1985.

184 Chen KTK: Female genital tract tumors in Peutz-Jeghers syndrome. Hum Pathol **17**:858-861, 1986.

185 Cooperman M, Clausen KP, Hecht C, Lucas JG, Keith LM: Villous adenomas of the duodenum. Gastroenterology **74**:1295-1297, 1978.

186 Dozois RR, Judd ES, Dahlin DC, Bartholomew LG: The Peutz-Jeghers syndrome. Is there a predisposition to the development of intestinal malignancy? Arch Surg **98**:509-517, 1969.

187 Estrada R, Spjut HJ: Hamartomatous polyps in Peutz-Jeghers syndrome. A light-histochemical, and electron-microscopic study. Am J Surg Pathol **7**:747-754, 1983.

188 Haggitt RC, Reid BJ: Hereditary gastrointestinal polyposis syndromes. Am J Surg Pathol **10**:871-887, 1986.

189 Halbert RE: Peutz-Jeghers syndrome with metastasizing gastric adenocarcinoma. Report of a case. Arch Pathol Lab Med **106**:517-520, 1982.

190 Komorowski RA, Cohen EB: Villous tumors of the duodenum. A clinicopathologic study. Cancer **47**:1377-1386, 1981.

191 Kyriakos M, Condon SC: Enteritis cystica profunda. Am J Clin Pathol **69**:77-85, 1978.

192 Miller JH, Gisvold JJ, Weiland LH, McIlrath DC: Upper gastrointestinal tract. Villous tumors. AJR **134**:933-936, 1980.

193 Morson BC: Some peculiarities in the histology of intestinal polyps. Dis Colon Rectum **5**:337-344, 1962.

194 Narita T, Eto T, Ito T: Peutz-Jeghers syndrome with adenomas and adenocarcinomas in colonic polyps. Am J Surg Pathol **11**:76-81, 1987.

195 Perzin KH, Bridge MF: Adenomas of the small intestine. A clinicopathologic review of 51 cases and a study of their relationship to carcinoma. Cancer **48**:799-819, 1981.

196 Perzin KH, Bridge MF: Adenomatous and carcinomatous changes in hamartomatous polyps of the small intestine (Peutz-Jeghers syndrome). Report of a case and review of the literature. Cancer **49**:971-983, 1982.

197 ReMine WH, Brown PW Jr, Gomes MMR, Harrison EG Jr: Polypoid hamartomas of Brunner's glands. Report of six surgical cases. Arch Surg **100**:313-316, 1970.

198 River L, Silverstein J, Tope JW: Benign neoplasms of the small intestine. Surg Gynecol Obstet **102**:1-38, 1956.

199 Rüfenacht H, Kasper M, Heitz PU, Streule K, Harder F: "Brunneroma." Hamartoma or tumor? Pathol Res Pract **181**:107-109, 1986.

200 Spjut HJ, Helgason AH, Trabanino JG II: Jejunitis cystica profunda in a hamartomatous polyp. Report of a case. Am J Surg Pathol **11**:328-332, 1987.

201 Trau H, Schewach-Millet M, Fisher BK, Tsur H: Peutz-Jeghers syndrome and bilateral breast carcinoma. Cancer **50**:788-792, 1982.

Adenocarcinoma

202 Adair HM, Trowell JE: Squamous cell carcinoma arising in a duplication of the small bowel. J Pathol **133**:25-31, 1981.

203 Adler SN, Lyon DT, Sullivan PD: Adenocarcinoma of the small bowel. Clinical features, similarity to regional enteritis, and analysis of 338 documented cases. Am J Gastroenterol **77**:326-330, 1982.

204 Albores-Saavedra J, Alcántara-Vazquez A, Cruz-Ortiz H, Olvera-Rabiela J, Rodriguez-Martínez, A: Association of neurofibromatosis and adenocarcinoma of the small intestine. Patologia **12**:89-98, 1974.

205 Baciewicz F, Sparberg M, Lawrence JB, Poticha SM: Adenocarcinoma of an ileostomy site with skin invasion. A case report. Gastroenterology **84**:168-170, 1983.

206 Barclay THC, Schapira DV: Malignant tumors of the small intestine. Cancer **51**:878-881, 1983.

207 Blackman E, Nash SV: Diagnosis of duodenal and ampullary epithelial neoplasms by endoscopic biopsy. A clinicopathologic and immunohistochemical study. Hum Pathol **16**:901-910, 1985.

208 Bridge MF, Perzin KH: Primary adenocarcinoma of the jejunum and ileum. A clinicopathologic study. Cancer **36:**1876-1887, 1975.

209 Cuesta MA, Donner R: Adenocarcinoma arising at an ileostomy site. Report of a case. Cancer **37:**949-952, 1976.

210 Iwafuchi M, Watanabe H, Ishihara N, Enjoji M, Iwashita A, Yanaihara N, Ito S: Neoplastic endocrine cells in carcinomas of the small intestine. Histochemical and immunohistochemical studies of 24 tumors. Hum Pathol **18:**185-194, 1987.

210a Lien G-S, Mori M, Enjoji M: Primary carcinoma of the small intestine. A clinicopathologic and immunohistochemical study. Cancer **61:**316-323, 1988.

211 Lipper S, Graves GV Jr: Villous adenocarcinoma arising in the bypassed duodenum 18 years after a Billroth II subtotal gastrectomy. Report of a case and review of the literature. Am J Gastroenterol **80:**174-176, 1985.

212 Lundqvist M, Wilander E: Exocrine and endocrine cell differentiation in small intestinal adenocarcinomas, Acta Pathol Microbiol Immunol Scand [A] **91:**469-474, 1983.

213 Rudan N, Nola P, Popovic S: Primary adenocarcinoma of the duodenum. Report of two cases. Cancer **54:**1105-1109, 1984.

214 Spira IA, Ghazi A, Wolff WI: Primary adenocarcinoma of the duodenum. Cancer **39:**1721-1726, 1977.

215 Wagner KM, Thompson J, Herlinger H, Caroline D: Thirteen primary adenocarcinomas of the ileum and appendix. A case report. Cancer **49:**797-801, 1982.

215a Yamashina M: Primary adenocarcinoma of the small intestine with emphasis on microvillous differentiation. Acta Pathol Jpn **37:**1061-1070, 1987.

Other types of carcinoma

216 Griesser GH, Schumacher U, Elfeldt R, Horny H-P: Adenosquamous carcinoma of the ileum. Report of a case and review of the literature. Virchows Arch [Pathol Anat] **406:**483-487, 1985.

216a Silva EG: Anaplastic and sarcomatoid carcinomas of jejunum and ileum (abstract). Am J Clin Pathol **81:**805, 1984.

217 Swanson PE, Dykoski D, Wick MR, Snover DC: Primary duodenal small-cell neuroendocrine carcinoma with production of vasoactive intestinal polypeptide. Arch Pathol Lab Med **110:**317-320, 1986.

218 Toker C: Oat cell tumor of the small bowel. Am J Gastroenterol **61:**481-483, 1974.

Carcinoid tumors and related endocrine tumors

219 Alumets J, Ekelund G, Hakanson R, Ljundberg O, Ljungquist U, Sundler F, Tibblin S: Jejunal endocrine tumour composed of somatostatin and gastrin cells and associated with duodenal ulcer disease. Virchows Arch [Pathol Anat] **378:**17-22, 1978.

220 Alumets J, Håkanson R, Ingemansson S, Sundler F: Substance P and 5-HT in granules isolated from an intestinal argentaffin carcinoid. Histochemistry **52:**217-222, 1977.

221 Anthony PP: Gangrene of the small intestine—a complication of argentaffin carcinoma. Br J Surg **57:**118-122, 1970.

222 Bostwick DG, Quan R, Hoffman AR, Webber RJ, Chang J-K, Bensch KG: Growth hormone–releasing factor immunoreactivity in human endocrine tumors. Am J Pathol **117:**167-170, 1984.

223 Bostwick DG, Roth KA, Barchas JD, Bensch KG: Gastrin-releasing peptide immunoreactivity in intestinal carcinoids. Am J Clin Pathol **82:**428-431, 1984.

224 Bussolati G, Papotti M, Sapino A: Binding of antibodies to human prealbumin to intestinal and bronchial carcinoids and to pancreatic endocrine tumours. Virchows Arch [B] (In press.)

225 Carstens PHB, Broghamer WL Jr, Hire D: Malignant fibrillo-caveolated cell carcinoma of the human intestinal tract. Hum Pathol **7:**505-517, 1976.

226 Chejfec G, Capella C, Solcia E, Jao W, Gould VE: Amphicrine cells, dysplasias, and neoplasias. Cancer **56:**2683-2690, 1985.

227 Chow CW, Sane S, Campbell PE, Carter RF: Malignant carcinoid tumors in children. Cancer **49:**802-811, 1982.

228 Dayal Y, Doos WG, O'Brien MJ, Nunnemacher G, DeLellis RA, Wolfe HJ: Psammomatous somatostatinomas of the duodenum. Am J Surg Pathol **7:**653-665, 1983.

229 Dayal Y, Tallberg KA, Nunnemacher G, DeLellis RA, Wolfe HJ: Duodenal carcinoids in patients with and without neurofibromatosis. A comparative study. Am J Surg Pathol **10:**348-357, 1986.

230 DeLellis RA, Dayal Y, Wolfe HJ: Carcinoid tumors. Changing concepts and new perspectives. Am J Surg Pathol **8:**295-300, 1984.

231 DeLellis RA, Gagel RF, Kaplan MM, Curtis LE: Gastrinoma of duodenal G-cell origin. Cancer **38:**201-208, 1976.

232 DeLellis RA, Tischler AS, Wolfe HJ: Multidirectional differentiation in neuroendocrine neoplasms. J Histochem Cytochem **32:**899-904, 1984.

233 Dent GA, Feldman JM: Pseudocystic liver metastases in patients with carcinoid tumors. Report of three cases. Am J Clin Pathol **82:**275-279, 1984.

234 Dollinger MR, Gardner B: Newer aspects of the carcinoid spectrum. Surg Gynecol Obstet **122:**1335-1349, 1966.

235 Emson PC, Gilbert RFT, Martensson H, Nobin A: Elevated concentrations of substance P and 5-HT in plasma in patients with carcinoid tumors. Cancer **54:**715-718, 1984.

235a Feldman JM: Carcinoid tumors and syndrome. Semin Oncol **14:**237-246, 1987.

236 Feldman JM, Jones RS: Carcinoid syndrome from gastrointestinal carcinoids without liver metastasis. Ann Surg **196:**33-37, 1982.

237 Fries JF, Lindgren JA, Bull JM: Scleroderma-like lesions and the carcinoid syndrome. Arch Intern Med **131:**550-553, 1973.

238 Gardiner GW, Van Patter T, Murray D: Atypical carcinoid tumor of the small bowel complicating celiac disease. Cancer **56:**2716-2722, 1985.

239 Godwin JD II: Carcinoid tumors. An analysis of 2837 cases. Cancer **36:**560-569, 1975.

240 Greider MH, DeSchryver-Kecskemeti K, Kraus FT: Psammoma bodies in endocrine tumors of the gastroenteropancreatic axis. A rather common occurrence. Semin Diagn Pathol **1:**19-29, 1984.

241 Griffiths DFR, Jasani B, Newman GR, Williams ED, Williams GT: Glandular duodenal carcinoid—a somatostatin rich tumour with neuroendocrine associations. J Clin Pathol **37:**163-169, 1984.

242 Höfler H, Klöppel G, Heitz PU: Combined production of mucus, amines and peptides by goblet-cell carcinoids of the appendix and ileum. Pathol Res Pract **178:**555-561, 1984.

243 Iwafuchi M, Watanabe H, Ishihara N, Shimoda T, Iwashita A, Ito S: Peptide YY immunoreactive cells in gastrointestinal carcinoids. Immunohistochemical and ultrastructural studies of 60 tumors. Hum Pathol **17:**291-296, 1986.

244 Johnson LA, Lavin P, Moertel CG, Weiland L, Dayal Y, Doos WG, Geller SA, Cooper HS, Nime F, Massé S, Simson IW, Sumner H, Fölsch E, Engstrom P: Carcinoids. The association of histologic growth pattern and survival. Cancer **51:**882-889, 1983.

245 Krejs GJ, Orci L, Conlon JM, Ravazzola M, Davis GR, Raskin P, Collins SM, McCarthy DM, Baetens D, Rubenstein A, Aldor TAM, Unger RH: Somatostinoma syndrome. Biochemical, morphologic and clinical features. N Engl J Med **301:**285-292, 1979.

246 Kuiper DH, Gracie WA Jr, Pollard HM: Twenty years of gastrointestinal carcinoids. Cancer **25:**1424-1430, 1970.

247 Lewin KJ: The endocrine cells of the gastrointestinal tract. The normal endocrine cells and their hyperplasias. Part I. Pathol Annu **21**(Pt 1):1-27, 1986.

248 Lewin KJ, Ulich T, Yang K, Layfield L: The endocrine cells of the gastrointestinal tract tumors. Part II. Pathol Annu **21**(Pt 2):181-215, 1986.

249 Lundqvist M, Wilander E: A study of the histopathogenesis of carcinoid tumors of the small intestine and appendix. Cancer **60:**201-206, 1987.

250 Lundqvist M, Wilander E: Somatostatin-like immunoreactivity in mid-gut carcinoids. Acta Pathol Microbiol Scand [A] **89:**335-337, 1981.

251 Lundqvist M, Wilander E: Subepithelial neuroendocrine cells and carcinoid tumours of the human small intestine and appendix. A comparative immunohistochemical study with regard to serotonin, neuron-specific enolase and S-100 protein reactivity. J Pathol **148:**141-147, 1986.

252 Marcial MA, Pinkus GS, Skarin A, Hinrichs HR, Warhol MJ: Ampullary somatostatinoma. Psammomatous variant of gastrointestinal carcinoid tumor—an immunohistochemical and ultrastructural study. Report of a case and review of the literature. Am J Clin Pathol **80:**755-761, 1983.

253 Martin JME, Maung RT: Differential immunohistochemical reactions of carcinoid tumors, Hum Pathol **18:**941-945, 1987.

254 Miettinen M, Lehto V-P, Dahl D, Virtanen I: Varying expression of cytokeratin and neurofilaments in neuroendocrine tumors of human gastrointestinal tract. Lab Invest **52:**429-436, 1985.

255 Miyazaki K, Funakoshi A, Nishihara S, Wasada T, Koga A, Ibayashi H: Aberrant insulinoma in the duodenum. Gastroenterology **90:**1280-1285, 1986.

256 Modhi G, Nicolis G: Hypoglycemia associated with carcinoid tumors. A case report and review of the literature. Cancer **53:**1804-1806, 1984.

257 Moertel CG, Sauer WG, Dockerty MB, Baggenstoss AH: Life history of the carcinoid tumor of the small intestine. Cancer **14:**901-912, 1961.

258 Nash SV, Said JW: Gastroenteropancreatic neuroendocrine tumors. A histochemical and immunohistochemical study of epithelial (keratin proteins, carcinoembryonic antigen) and neuroendocrine (neuron-specific enolase, bombesin and chromogranin) markers in foregut, midgut, and hindgut tumors. Am J Clin Pathol **86:**415-422, 1986.

259 Oates JA: The carcinoid syndrome. N Engl J Med **315:**702-703, 1986.

260 Pearse AGE: The APUD cell concept and its implications in pathology. Pathol Annu **9:**27-41, 1974.

261 Pelletier G, Cortot A, Launay J-M, Debons-Guillemain M-C, Nemeth J, Le Charpentier Y, Celerier M, Modigliani R: Serotonin-secreting and insulin-secreting ileal carcinoid tumor and the use of in vitro culture of tumoral cells. Cancer **54**:319-322, 1984.

262 Qizilbash AH: Carcinoid tumors, vascular elastosis, and ischemic disease of the small intestine. Dis Colon Rectum **20**:554-560, 1977.

263 Sanders RJ, Axtell HK: Carcinoids of the gastrointestinal tract. Surg Gynecol Obstet **119**:369-380, 1964.

264 Sandler M, Williams ED, Karim SMM: The occurrence of prostaglandins in amine-peptide–secreting tumours. In Mantegazza P, Horton EW (eds): Prostaglandins, peptides and amines. London and New York, 1969, Academic Press, Inc., pp. 3-7.

265 Simpson S, Vinik AI, Marangos PJ, Lloyd RV: Immunohistochemical localization of neuron-specific enolase in gastroenteropancreatic neuroendocrine tumors. Correlation with tissue and serum levels of neuron-specific enolase. Cancer **54**:1364-1369, 1984.

266 Sjoerdsma A, Weissbach H, Udenfriend S: Simple test for diagnosis of metastatic carcinoid (argentaffinoma). JAMA **159**:397, 1955.

267 Sjölund K, Sandén G, Håkanson R, Sundler F: Endocrine cells in human intestine. An immunocytochemical study. Gastroenterology **85**:1120-1130, 1983.

268 Smith JHF, Hope PG: Carcinoid tumor arising in a cystic duplication of the small bowel, Arch Pathol Lab Med **109**:95-96, 1985.

269 Sobin LH, Hjermstad BM, Sesterhenn IA, Helwig EB: Prostatic acid phosphatase activity in carcinoid tumors. Cancer **58**:136-138, 1986.

270 Soga J: Carcinoids. Their changing concepts and a new histologic classification. In Fujita T (ed): Gastro-entero-pancreatic endocrine system. Stuttgart, 1974, Thieme.

271 Solcia E, Capella C, Buffa R, Usellini L, Fiocca R, Sessa F, Tortora O: The contribution of immunohistochemistry to the diagnosis of neuroendocrine tumors. Semin Diagn Pathol **2**:285-296, 1984.

272 Takatoh H, Iwamoto H, Ikezu M, Katoh N, Ito S, Kaneko H: Immunohistochemical demonstration of peptide YY in gastrointestinal endocrine tumors. Acta Pathol Jpn **37**:737-746, 1987.

273 Thorson AH: Studies on carcinoid disease. Acta Med Scand **161**[Suppl 334]:1-132, 1958.

274 Thorson AH, Biorck G, Bjorkman G, Waldenstrom J: Malignant carcinoid of the small intestine with metastases to the liver, valvular disease of the right side of the heart (pulmonary stenosis and tricuspid regurgitation without septal defects), peripheral vasomotor symptoms, bronchoconstriction, and an unusual type of cyanosis. Am Heart J **47**:795-817, 1954.

275 Vesoulis Z, Petras RE: Duodenal microgastrinoma producing the Zollinger-Ellison syndrome. Arch Pathol Lab Med **109**:40-42, 1985.

276 Walts AE, Said JW, Shintaku IP, Lloyd RV: Chromogranin as a marker of neuroendocrine cells in cytologic material—an immunocytochemical study. Am J Clin Pathol **84**:273-277, 1985.

277 Wick MR, Stanley M, Cherwitz DL, Savage JE: Concomitant neuropeptide-producing endometrial carcinomas and ileal carcinoid tumors. Am J Clin Pathol **85**:406-410, 1986.

278 Wilander E, El-Salhy M: Immuno-cyto-chemical staining of mid-gut carcinoid tumours with sequence-specific gastrin antisera. Acta Pathol Microbiol Scand [A] **89**:247-250, 1981.

279 Wilander E, Lundqvist M, El-Salhy M: Serotonin in fore-gut carcinoids. A survey of 60 cases with regard to silver stains, formalin-induced fluorescence and serotonin immunocytochemistry. J Pathol **145**:251-258, 1985.

280 Williams ED, Sandler M: The classification of carcinoid tumours. Lancet **1**:238-239, 1963.

281 Yang K, Ulich T, Cheng L, Lewin KJ: The neuroendocrine products of intestinal carcinoids. An immunoperoxidase study of 35 carcinoid tumors stained for serotonin and eight polypeptide hormones. Cancer **51**:1918-1926, 1983.

282 Zakariai YM, Quan SHQ, Hajdu SI: Carcinoid tumors of the gastrointestinal tract. Cancer **35**:588-591, 1975.

Gangliocytic paraganglioma

282a Burke AP, Heiwig EB: Gangliocytic paraganglioma of the small intestine (abstract). Lab Invest **58**:13A, 1988.

283 Guarda LA, Ordóñez NG, del Junco GW, Luna MA: Gangliocytic paraganglioma of the duodenum. An immunocytochemical study. Am J Gastroenterol **78**:794-798, 1983.

284 Hamid QA, Bishop AE, Rode J, Dhillon AP, Rosenberg BF, Reed RJ, Sibley RK, Polak JM: Duodenal gangliocytic paragangliomas. A study of 10 cases with immunocytochemical neuroendocrine markers. Hum Pathol **17**:1151-1157, 1986.

285 Kawaguchi K, Takizawa T, Koike M, Tabata I, Goseki N: Multiple paraganglioneuromas. Virchows Arch [Pathol Anat] **406**:373-380, 1985.

286 Kepes JJ, Zacharias DL: Gangliocytic paragangliomas of the duodenum. Report of two cases with light and electron microscopic examination. Cancer **27**:61-70, 1971.

287 Kheir SM, Halpern NB: Paraganglioma of the duodenum in association with congenital neurofibromatosis. Possible relationship. Cancer **53**:2491-2496, 1984.

288 Perrone T, Sibley RK, Rosai J: Duodenal gangliocytic paraganglioma. An immunohistochemical and ultrastructural study and a hypothesis concerning its origin. Am J Surg Pathol **9**:31-41, 1985.

289 Reed RJ, Daroca PJ Jr, Harkin JC: Gangliocytic paraganglioma. Am J Surg Pathol **1**:207-216, 1977.

290 Scheithauer BW, Nora FE, Lechago J, Wick MR, Crawford BG, Weiland LH, Carney JA: Duodenal gangliocytic paraganglioma. Clinicopathologic and immunocytochemical study of 11 cases. Am J Clin Pathol **86**:559-565, 1986.

290a Stephens M, Williams GT, Jasani B, Williams ED: Synchronous duodenal neuroendocrine tumours in von Recklinghausen's disease. A case report of co-existing gangliocytic paraganglioma and somatostatin-rich glandular carcinoid. Histopathology **11**:1331-1340, 1987.

291 Taylor HB, Helwig EB: Benign nonchromaffin paragangliomas of the duodenum. Virchows Arch [Pathol Anat] **335**:356-366, 1962.

Smooth muscle tumors

292 Akwari OE, Dozois RR, Weiland LH, Beahrs OH: Leiomyosarcoma of the small and large bowel. Cancer **42**:1375-1384, 1978.

293 Angerpointner TA, Weitz H, Haas RJ, Hecker WC: Intestinal leiomyosarcoma in childhood. Case report and review of the literature. J Pediatr Surg **16**:491-495, 1981.

294 Appelman HD: Stromal tumors of the esophagus, stomach, and duodenum. In Appelman HD (ed): Pathology of the esophagus, stomach and duodenum. New York, 1984, Churchill-Livingstone, pp. 195-242.

295 Evans HL: Smooth muscle tumors of the gastrointestinal tract. A study of 56 cases followed for a minimum of 10 years. Cancer **56**:2242-2250, 1985.

296 Filippa DA, Decosse JJ, Lieberman PH, Bretsky SS, Weingrad DN: Primary lymphomas of the gastrointestinal tract. Analysis of prognostic factors with emphasis on histological type. Am J Surg Pathol **7**:363-372, 1983.

297 Meredith RF, Wagman LD, Piper JA, Mills AS, Neifeld JP: Beta-chain human chorionic gonadotropin–producing leiomyosarcoma of the small intestine. Cancer **58**:131-135, 1986.

298 Ranchod M, Kempson RL: Smooth muscle tumors of the gastrointestinal tract and retroperitoneum. A pathologic analysis of 100 cases. Cancer **39**:255-262, 1977.

298a Ricci A Jr, Ciccarelli O, Cartun RW, Newcomb P: A clinicopathologic and immunohistochemical study of 16 patients with small intestinal leiomyosarcoma. Limited utility of immunophenotyping. Cancer **60**:1790-1799, 1987.

299 Shiu MH, Farr GH, Egeli RA, Quan SHG, Hajdu SI: Myosarcomas of the small and large intestine. A clinicopathologic study. J Surg Oncol **24**:67-72, 1983.

300 Weiss RA, Mackay B: Malignant smooth muscle tumors of the gastrointestinal tract. An ultrastructural study of 20 cases. J Ultrastruct Pathol **2**:231-240, 1981.

301 Wilson JM, Melvin DB, Gray GF, Thorbjarnarson B: Primary malignancies of the small bowel. A report of 96 cases and review of the literature. Ann Surg **180**:175-179, 1974.

Malignant lymphoma and related disorders

302 Al-Bahrani ZR, Al-Mondhiry H, Bakir F, Al-Saleem T: Clinical and pathologic subtypes of primary intestinal lymphoma. Experience with 132 patients over a 14-year period. Cancer **52**:1666-1672, 1983.

303 Appelman HD, Hirsch SD, Schnitzer B, Coon WW: Clinicopathologic overview of gastrointestinal lymphomas. Am J Surg Pathol **9**:71-83, 1985.

304 Artinian B, Lough JO, Palmer JD: Idiopathic ulcer of small bowel with pseudolymphomatous reactions. A clinicopathological study of six cases. Arch Pathol **91**:327-333, 1971.

305 Asselah F, Slavin G, Sowter G, Asselah H: Immunoproliferative small intestinal disease in Algerians. I. Light microscopic and immunochemical studies. Cancer **52**:227-237, 1983.

306 Atwell JD, Burge D, Wright D: Nodular lymphoid hyperplasia of the intestinal tract in infancy and childhood. J Pediatr Surg **20**:25-29, 1985.

307 Brugo EA, Larkin E, Molina-Escobar J, Costanzi J: Primary granulocytic sarcoma of the small bowel. Cancer **35**:1333-1340, 1975.

308 Burke JS, Sheibani K, Nathwani BN, Winberg CD, Rappaport H: Monoclonal small (well-differentiated) lymphocytic proliferations of the gastrointestinal tract

resembling lymphoid hyperplasia. A neoplasm of uncertain malignant potential. Hum Pathol **18**:1238-1245, 1987.

308a Burke JS, Sheibani K, Nathwani BN, Winberg CD, Rappaport H: Monoclonal small (well-differentiated) lymphocytic proliferations of the gastrointestinal tract resembling lymphoid hyperplasia. A neoplasm of uncertain malignant potential. Hum Pathol **18**:1238-1245, 1987.

309 Crow J, Asselah F: Immunoproliferative small intestinal disease in Algerians. II. Ultrastructural studies in alpha-chain disease. Cancer **54**:1908-1913, 1984.

310 Eidelman S, Parkins RA, Rubin CE: Abdominal lymphoma presenting as malabsorption. A clinico-pathologic study of nine cases in Israel and a review of the literature. Medicine [Baltimore] **45**:111-137, 1966.

311 Filippa DA, Lieberman PH, Weingrad DN, Decosse JJ, Bretsky SS: Primary lymphomas of the gastrointestinal tract. Analysis of prognostic factors with emphasis on histological type. Am J Surg Pathol **7**:363-372, 1983.

312 Foucar K, Foucar E, Mitros F, Clamon G, Goeken J, Crossett J: Epitheliotropic lymphoma of the small bowel. Report of a fatal case with cytotoxic/suppressor T-cell immunotype. Cancer **54**:54-60, 1984.

313 Freeman C, Berg JW, Cotlow SJ: Occurrence and prognosis of extra-nodal lymphomas. Cancer **29**:252-260, 1972.

314 Gonzalez-Vitale JC, Gomez LG, Goldblum RM, Goldman AS, Patterson M: Immunoblastic lymphoma of small intestine complicating late-onset immunodeficiency. Cancer **49**:445-449, 1982.

315 Grody WW, Weiss LM, Warnke RA, Magidson JG, Hu E, Lewin KJ: Gastrointestinal lymphomas. Immunohistochemical studies on the cell of origin. Am J Surg Pathol **9**:328-337, 1985.

316 Haghighi P, Kharazmi A, Gerami C, Haghshenass M, Abadi P, Omidi H, Mostafavi N: Primary upper small intestinal lymphoma and alpha-chain disease. Report of 10 cases emphasizing pathological aspects. Am J Surg Pathol **2**:147-157, 1978.

317 Halphen M, Najjar T, Jaafoura H, Cammoun M, groupe Trufali: Diagnostic value of upper intestinal fiber endoscopy in primary small intestinal lymphoma. A prospective study by the Tunisian-French Intestinal Lymphoma Group. Cancer **58**:2140-2145, 1986.

318 Henry K, Farrer-Brown G: Primary lymphomas of the gastrointestinal tract. I. Plasma cell tumors. Histopathology **1**:53-76, 1977.

319 Hermans PE, Huizenga KA, Hoffman HN, Brown AL, Markowitz H: Dysgammaglobulinemia associated with nodular lymphoid hyperplasia of the small intestine. Am J Med **40**:78-89, 1966.

320 Hernandez JA, Sheehan WW: Lymphomas of the mucosa-associated lymphoid tissue. Signet ring cell lymphomas presenting in mucosal lymphoid organs. Cancer **55**:592-597, 1985.

321 Isaacson P: Middle East lymphoma and α-chain disease. An immunohistochemical study. Am J Surg Pathol **3**:431-441, 1979.

322 Isaacson P: Primary gastrointestinal lymphoma. Virchows Arch [Pathol Anat] **391**:1-8, 1981.

323 Isaacson P, Jones DB, Sworn MJ, Wright DH: Malignant histiocytosis of the intestine. Report of three cases with immunological and cytochemical analysis. J Clin Pathol **35**:510-516, 1982.

324 Isaacson P, Wright DH: Malignant lymphoma of mucosa-associated lymphoid tissue. A distinctive type of B-cell lymphoma. Cancer **52**:1410-1416, 1983.

325 Isaacson PG: Middle Eastern intestinal lymphoma. Semin Diagn Pathol **2**:210-223, 1985.

326 Isaacson PG, Price SK: Light chains in Mediterranean lymphoma. J Clin Pathol **38**:601-607, 1985.

327 Isaacson PG, Spencer J: Malignant lymphoma of mucosa-associated lymphoid tissue. Histopathology **11**:445-462, 1987.

328 Kahn LB, Mir R: Gastrointestinal lymphoid neoplasms. Semin Diagn Pathol **2**:197-209, 1985.

329 Khojasteh A, Haghshenass M, Haghighi P: Immunoproliferative small intestinal disease. A "third-world lesion." N Engl J Med **308**:1401-1405, 1983.

330 Kraemer BB, Foucar K, Osborne B, Butler JJ: Bacterial infection simulating granulocytic sarcoma of the small bowel. Am J Clin Pathol **76**:227-231, 1981.

331 Kwee WS, Wils JAMJ, van den Tweel JG: Malignant lymphoma, immunoblastic with plasmacytic differentiation, complicating Crohn's disease. Histopathology **9**:1115-1120, 1985.

332 Lewin KJ, Kahn LB, Novis BH: Primary intestinal lymphoma of "Western" and "Mediterranean" type, alpha chain disease and massive plasma cell infiltration. A comparative study of 37 cases. Cancer **38**:2511-2528, 1976.

333 Lewin KJ, Ranchod M, Dorfman RF: Lymphomas of the gastrointestinal tract. A study of 117 cases presenting with gastrointestinal disease. Cancer **42**:693-707, 1978.

334 Matuchansky C, Touchard G, Lemaire M, Babin P, Demeocq F, Fonck Y, Meyer M, Preud'homme J-L: Malignant lymphoma of the small bowel associated with diffuse nodular lymphoid hyperplasia. N Engl J Med **313**:166-171, 1985.

335 McDonald GB, Schuffler MD, Kadin ME, Tytgat GNJ: Intestinal pseudoobstruction caused by diffuse lymphoid infiltration of the small intestine. Gastroenterology **89**:882-889, 1985.

336 Najem AZ, Porcaro JL, Rush BF Jr: Primary non-Hodgkin's lymphoma of the duodenum. Case report and literature review. Cancer **54**:895-898, 1984.

337 Nash JRG, Gradwell E, Day DW: Large-cell intestinal lymphoma occurring in coeliac disease. Morphological and immunohistochemical features. Histopathology **10**:195-205, 1986.

338 Nassar VH, Salem PA, Shahid MJ, Alami SY, Balikian JB, Salem AA, Nasrallah SM: "Mediterranean abdominal lymphoma" or immunoproliferative small intestinal disease. II. Pathological aspects. Cancer **41**:1340-1354, 1978.

339 Otto HF, Bettmann I, Weltzien Jv, Gebbers J-O: Primary intestinal lymphomas. Virchows Arch [Pathol Anat] **391**:9-31, 1981.

340 Pangalis GA, Rappaport H: Common clonal origin of lymphoplasmacytic proliferation and immunoblastic lymphoma and intestinal alpha-chain disease. Lancet **2**:880, 1977.

341 Ramot B, Shahin N, Bubis JJ: Malabsorption syndrome in lymphoma of small intestine. A study of 13 cases. ISR J Med Sci **52**:221-226, 1965.

342 Ranchod M, Lewin KJ, Dorfman RF: Lymphoid hyperplasia of the gastrointestinal tract. A study of 26 cases and review of the literature. Am J Surg Pathol **2**:383-400, 1978.

343 Rappaport H, Ramot B, Hulu N, Park JK: The pathology of so-called Mediterranean abdominal lymphoma with malabsorption. Cancer **29**:1502-1511, 1972.

344 Salem P, El-Hashimi L, Anaissie E, Geha S, Habboubi N, Ibrahim N, Khalyl M, Allam C: Primary small intestinal lymphoma in adults. A comparative study of IPSID versus non-IPSID in the Middle East. Cancer **59**:1670-1676, 1987.

345 Salem PA, Nassar VH, Shahid MJ, Hajj AA, Alami SY, Balikian JB, Salem AA: "Mediterranean abdominal lymphoma," or immunoproliferative small intestinal disease. I. Clinical aspects. Cancer **40**:2941-2947, 1977.

346 Shepherd NA, Blackshaw AJ, Hall PA, Bostad L, Coates PJ, Lowe DG, Levison DA, Morson BC, Stansfeld AG: Malignant lymphoma with eosinophilia of the gastrointestinal tract. Histopathology **11**:115-130, 1987.

347 Steinberg JJ, Bridges N, Feiner HD, Valensi Q: Small intestinal lymphoma in three patients with acquired immune deficiency syndrome. Am J Gastroenterol **80**:21-26, 1985.

348 Ward H, Jalan KN, Maitra TK, Agarwal SK, Mahalanabis D: Small intestinal nodular lymphoid hyperplasia in patients with giardiasis and normal serum immunoglobulins. Gut **24**:120-126, 1983.

349 Weaver DK, Batsakis JG: Pseudolymphomas of the small intestine. Am J Gastroenterol **44**:374-381, 1965.

350 Weingrad DN, Decosse JJ, Sherlock P, Straus D, Lieberman PH, Filippa DA: Primary gastrointestinal lymphoma. A 30-year review. Cancer **49**:1258-1265, 1982.

351 Williamson RCN, Welch CE, Malt RA: Adenocarcinoma and lymphoma of the small intestine. Distribution and etiologic associations. Ann Surg **197**:172-178, 1983.

Other tumors and tumorlike conditions

352 Aase S, Gundersen R: Submucous lymphatic cysts of the small intestine. An autopsy study. Acta Pathol Microbiol Immunol Scand [A] **91**:191-194, 1983.

353 Climie ARW, Wylin RF: Small intestinal lipomatosis. Arch Pathol Lab Med **105**:40-42, 1981.

354 de Castro CA, Dockerty MB, Mayo CW: Metastatic tumors of the small intestine. Surg Gynecol Obstet **105**:159-165, 1957.

355 Gonzalez-Crussi F, Noronha R: Solitary intestinal fibromatosis in the newborn. Rare cause of neonatal intestinal obstruction. Arch Pathol Lab Med **109**:97-99, 1985.

356 Hamilton CW, Shelburne JD, Bossen EH, Lowe JE: A glomus tumor of the jejunum masquerading as a carcinoid tumor. Hum Pathol **13**:859-861, 1982.

357 Hansen PS: Hemangioma of the small intestine. Am J Clin Pathol **18**:14-42, 1948.

358 Hurwitz MM, Redleaf PD, Williams HJ, Edwards JE: Lipomas of the gastrointestinal tract. An analysis of 72 tumors. AJR **99**:84-89, 1967.

358a Jones J, Sack J, Grizzle W, Pollack WJ, Lott RL, Herrera GA, Cerezo L: Intestinal plexosarcoma (abstract). Lab Invest **58**:44A, 1988.

359 Jorge E, Harvey HA, Simmonds MA, Lipton A, Joehl RJ: Symptomatic malignant melanoma of the gastrointestinal tract. Operative treatment and survival. Ann Surg **193**:328-331, 1985.

360 Matthews TH, Heaton GE, Christopherson WM: Primary duodenal choriocarcinoma. Arch Pathol Lab Med **110**:550-552, 1986.

361 Mayo CW, Pagtalunan RJG, Brown CJ: Lipoma of the alimentary tract. Surgery **53:**598-603, 1963.

362 McNeill PM, Wagman LD, Neifeld JP: Small bowel metastases from primary carcinoma of the lung. Cancer **59:**1486-1489, 1987.

363 Ordóñez NG, del Junco GW, Ayala AG, Ahmed N: Angiosarcoma of the small intestine. An immunoperoxidase study. Am J Gastroenterol **78:**218-221, 1983.

364 Sato N, Zaloudek C, Geelhoed GW, Orenstein JM: Malignant mesenchymoma of the small intestine. Arch Pathol Lab Med **108:**164-167, 1984.

364a Shekitka KM, Sobin LH, Helwig EB: Neurofibromas and ganglioneuromas of the GI tract. Their relation to von Recklinghausen's disease and other multiple tumor syndromes (abstract). Lab Invest **58:**84A, 1988.

365 Shepherd JA: Angiomatous conditions of the gastrointestinal tract. Br J Surg **40:**409-421, 1953.

366 Smith CR Jr, Bartholomew LG, Cain JC: Hereditary hemorrhagic telangiectasia and gastrointestinal hemorrhage. Gastroenterology **44:**1-6, 1963.

367 Weisberg T, Feldman M Sr: Lipomas of the gastrointestinal tract. Am J Clin Pathol **25:**272-281, 1955.

368 Willbanks OL, Fogelman MJ: Gastrointestinal melanosarcoma. Am J Surg **120:**602-606, 1970.

369 Winchester DP, Merrill JR, Victor TA, Scanlon EF: Small bowel perforation secondary to metastatic carcinoma of the lung. Cancer **40:**410-415, 1977.

Appendix

ACUTE APPENDICITIS
Epidemiology and pathogenesis

Acute appendicitis is predominantly a disease of the Western world. It is particularly common in Great Britain and the United States and very rare in Asia and Africa. The difference has been explained on the basis of a dietary variance, the highest risk occurring when the diet is reduced in bulk, with diminished cellulose and a high protein intake.[4]

Many cases of acute appendicitis develop as a result of obstruction, the resulting secretion under pressure impairing the resistance of the appendiceal mucosa to invasion by microorganisms, as shown by Wagensteen's pioneer studies in humans[21] and in experimental animal models. Mucosal injury develops in one area, ulceration occurs, and the inflammation spreads from that point.[7,10a,18] An obstructed appendix that was previously normal is more susceptible to infection than one affected by fibrous obliteration of the lumen. The most common cause of obstruction is a fecalith, but it may be a foreign body, a true calculus, a gallstone, a tumor of the cecum, or a primary tumor of the appendix[6,9,14,24] (Fig. 11-79). In children from the age of 10 years to young adults, diffuse lymphoid hyperplasia is another cause of obstruction[12] (Figs. 11-80 and 11-81). Nonobstructive appendicitis can be secondary to a generalized infection, usually of viral etiology.[15]

Clinical features

Acute appendicitis is seen most frequently in young men but can occur in either sex and at any age. Those occurring in young children[13] and in the elderly[3,20,23] are more likely to be mishandled because of failure to consider the diagnosis and because the clinical findings are often atypical.

The usual presentation of acute appendicitis is with periumbilical colicky pain and vomiting, with the pain later localizing in the right lower abdominal quadrant. These are often accompanied by fever and leukocytosis. If perforation of the appendix occurs, there may be temporary relief of pain followed by signs of acute peritonitis. The accuracy of the clinical diagnosis is approximately 80%.[10] False positive diagnoses are twice as common in females as in males. The conditions most closely mimicking appendicitis are mesenteric lymphadenitis, gynecologic lesions, acute diverticulitis, and infarction of the greater omentum.[1,10]

The diagnosis of acute appendicitis is supported by the

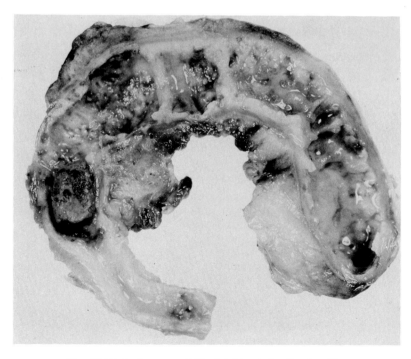

Fig. 11-79 Acute appendicitis distal to obstructing fecalith.

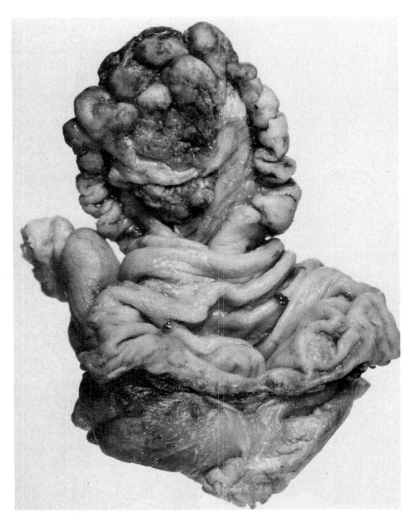

Fig. 11-80 Appendix from 4-year-old child in whom intussusception occurred. There is extreme lymphoid hyperplasia, and cuff of cecum is present.

demonstration of a mass effect on the cecum and nonfilling of the appendix on barium enema, but these radiographic changes are not entirely specific.[8]

Pathology

The mucosa of the normal appendix has a light yellow tint, and the serosa is smooth, glistening, and transparent. Mucosal hemorrhages and hyperemia of surface vessels usually are related to surgical trauma.

Grossly, an appendix with well-developed acute inflammation shows a fibrinous or purulent coating of the serosa, with engorgement of the vessels. The mucosa is markedly hyperemic, with areas of ulceration. Obstruction of the lumen by a fecalith or some other agent is found in about one fourth to one third of the cases.[5] Microscopically, the changes range from minimal focal inflammation to total necrosis of the appendiceal wall, the degree of abnormalities depending on the interval between the onset of symptoms and the operation.

In the early lesion, neutrophils appear at the base of the crypt adjacent to a small defect in the epithelium. After this inflammatory process reaches the submucosa, it spreads quickly to the remaining appendix.[18] In advanced stages, the mucosa is absent and the wall is necrotic. Thrombosed vessels are seen in one fourth of the cases.[16] The various stages of acute appendicitis are sometimes designated as *acute focal, acute suppurative, gangrenous,* and *perforative.*

There is close correlation between the gross and microscopic findings in acute appendicitis. Therkelsen[19] reviewed 154 appendices with microscopic evidence of acute inflammation: 125 demonstrated gross evidence of inflammation, twenty-five showed doubtful evidence of it, and four appeared grossly normal.

The most common complication of acute appendicitis is perforation, which may lead to diffuse peritonitis or to the formation of a periappendiceal abscess or fibrous induration (''ligneous perityphlitis'') (Figs. 11-82 and 11-83).[17] This

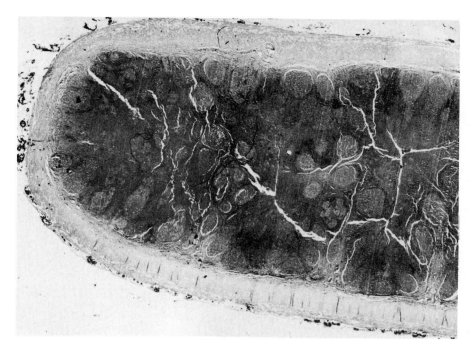

Fig. 11-81 Obliteration of appendiceal lumen by lymphoid tissue.

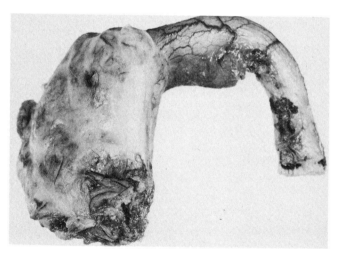

Fig. 11-82 Acute appendicitis with obstruction, perforation, and peri-appendiceal inflammation.

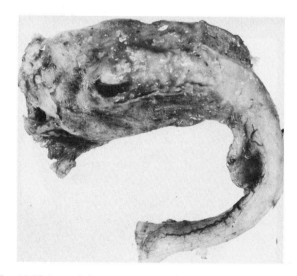

Fig. 11-83 Large inflammatory mass that shows destruction of wall and fecalith in place.

condition, which may clinically simulate a neoplasm, is usually located in the right iliac fossa lateral to the cecum (Figs. 11-84 and 11-85) but can occur in other sites depending on the original location of the appendix. This abscess may perforate into the cecum, ileum, rectum, or even open into the skin surface. Appendicitis with perforation can also result in infertility in women because of obstruction of the fallopian tubes.[11] Another serious complication is the spread of the inflammation via the ileocolic, upper mes-enteric, and portal veins to the liver, with formation of "pylephlebitic" abscesses.

Treatment

In 1886 Fitz demonstrated that the appendix was the origin of the mysterious inflammation of the right iliac fossa previously known as *perityflitis*. Three years later, McBurney emphasized the importance of accurate early diagnosis and prompt surgical intervention. By 1900, the mortality rate

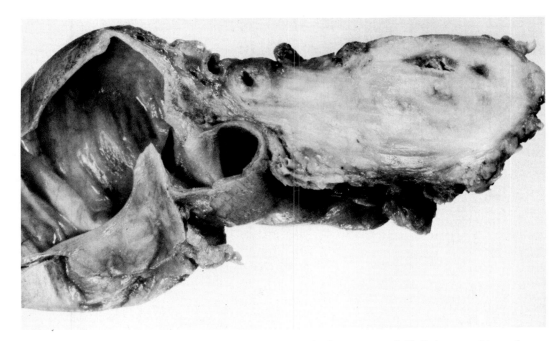

Fig. 11-84 Periappendicular abscess secondary to episode of acute appendicitis that occurred 1 month previously. Abscess was palpable clinically.

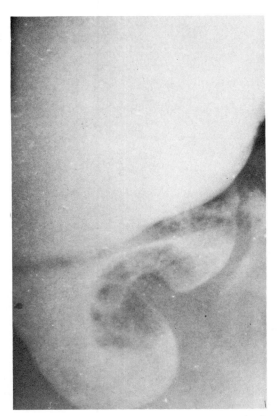

Fig. 11-85 Detailed view of defect in ileocecal area. Lesion was misinterpreted as carcinoma and was radically removed.

had already fallen to 35%.[2,22] During the next three decades, it was further reduced to 5% as a result of better awareness on the part of the patient and the physician concerning the symptoms and signs of acute appendicitis, the need for early surgical intervention, and the dangers of catharsis and morphine for undiagnosed abdominal pain.

In the following 25 years, a combination of improved surgical technique, better preoperative and postoperative care, advances in anesthesiology, and the development of effective antibacterial agents led to further declines in mortality to a fraction of 1%. The later reduction in risk was accomplished mainly in three classes of patients: those with perforation and peritonitis, the very young, and the very old.

CHRONIC APPENDICITIS

The existence of primary chronic appendicitis as a pathologic or clinical entity has been greatly disputed. Its symptoms and signs are as vague and shadowy as its pathology. Unfortunately, in some laboratories the pathologist is a willing accomplice to the surgeon who is liberal in the clinical diagnosis of chronic appendicitis. These pathologists never call an appendix normal. Rough handling and clamping of the appendix may produce mucosal hemorrhage and engorgement of serosal vessels. Normally, there may be collections of lymphocytes in the muscular wall of the appendix, and a rare plasma cell or eosinophil may be seen in the mucosa. In the natural aging process of the appendix, fibrosis beginning at the tip takes place, accompanied by a diminution of lymphoid tissue. Such fibrosis does not cause symptoms. Finally, residual changes may be found in appendices that were the site of an acute appendicitis that

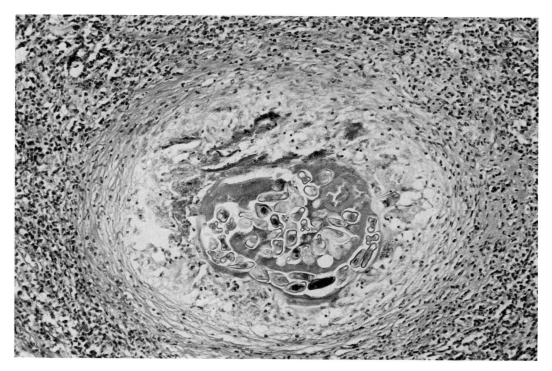

Fig. 11-86 Granulomatous reaction in appendiceal serosa secondary to *Oxyuris vermicularis* infestation in 6-year-old girl. Clinical diagnosis was acute appendicitis.

subsided in the past. If gangrene had occurred, only a stump of the appendix may remain. In other instances in which an inflammatory process has destroyed the muscle, fibrous replacement is present. If the original process was superficial and confined to the mucosa and submucosa, no changes will be found. Just because vague preoperative symptoms disappear following appendectomy is not necessarily evidence that the symptoms were in any way related to the appendix. As Hertzler[25] stated, many years ago, the anatomic structure of appendices commonly removed under the diagnosis of chronic appendicitis shows no variation from the appendices of individuals suffering from no abdominal complaint whatsoever.

PARASITOSES AND OTHER INFLAMMATIONS

In the United States, about 3% of appendices removed show infestation with *Oxyuris vermicularis*.[28] These parasites are most often found in the appendices of children between the ages of 7 and 11 years. The infestation is not a causal agent of appendicitis but occurs with about the same frequency in normal appendices. The parasite wanders widely and frequently invades the lower female genital tract. From there, it may reach the peritoneal cavity by ascending along the uterus and fallopian tubes. Granulomas caused by this organism have been observed in the endometrium, fallopian tubes, ovaries, mesentery, and mesoappendix[39,40] (Fig. 11-86).

Eosinophilic appendicitis is characterized by a diffuse eosinophilic infiltration or by the presence of appendiceal granulomas composed of epithelioid cells, fibroblasts, and a large number of eosinophils having a necrotic center and surrounded by diffuse eosinophilic infiltration. These changes have been correlated by Stemmerman[35] with the presence of *Strongyloides stercoralis* in stool examinations; the larva of the organism is found only exceptionally within the granulomas.[32]

Schistosomiasis can involve the appendix, but its possible role in the pathogenesis of acute appendicitis remains controversial[30,34] (Fig. 11-87).

Campylobacter organisms were found by an immunohistochemical technique in three out of 116 appendectomy specimens studied by van Spreeuwell et al.[38] The histologic changes present in these appendices were similar to those seen in colonic biopsies from patients with *Campylobacter* colitis (see section on large bowel).

Acute necrotizing arteritis may be found in the vessels of the appendix (Fig. 11-88), unaccompanied by systemic involvement.

In the prodromal stage of *measles*, appendicitis may occur. Microscopic examination shows marked lymphoid hyperplasia with the presence of multinucleated giant cells of the Warthin-Finkeldey type, similar to those seen in the tonsil (Fig. 11-89). If the pathologist is astute enough to recognize these changes, he can tell the patient's physician that the child is about to break out into the characteristic rash of measles.[29,31]

Along similar lines, *infectious mononucleosis* can be accompanied by marked hyperplasia of the appendiceal lymphoid tissue, with marked expansion of the lamina propria by a mixed proliferation of small lymphoid cells and im-

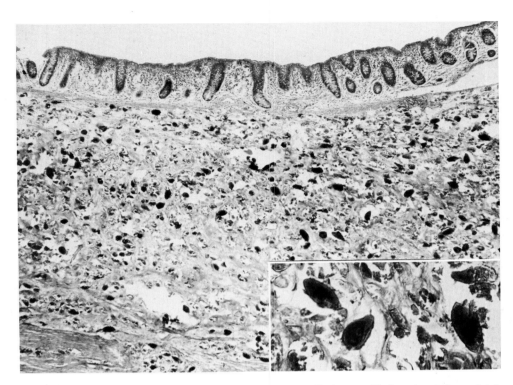

Fig. 11-87 Schistosomiasis of appendiceal submucosa covered by intact epithelium. **Inset** shows detail of parasite eggs. This involvement can cause appendicitis.

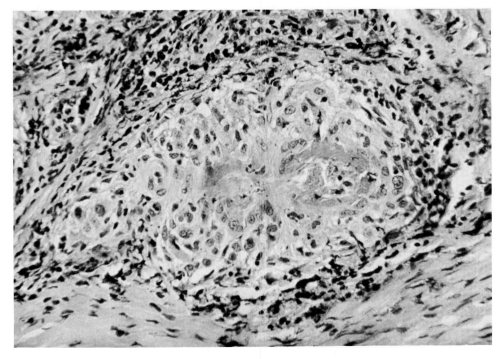

Fig. 11-88 Necrotizing arteritis of appendix in child with possible rheumatic fever.

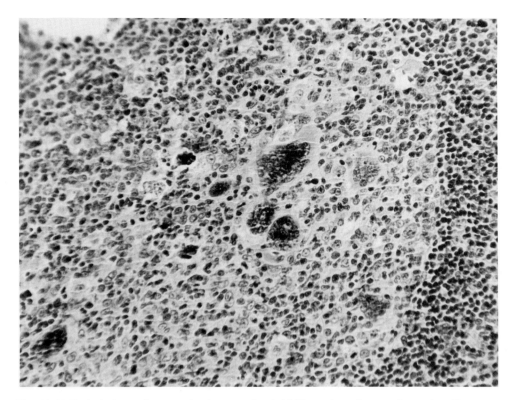

Fig. 11-89 Typical giant cells appearing in appendix of child in prodromal stage of measles. (Courtesy Dr. J.L. Bonenfant, Quebec, Canada.)

munoblasts, some of the latter resembling Reed-Sternberg cells.[33]

Crohn's disease can involve the appendix and simulate acute appendicitis. As a matter of fact, a good number of patients with Crohn's disease give a history of previous appendectomy; however, patients whose removed appendices show granulomatous changes consistent with Crohn's disease very rarely develop disease in other portions of the gastrointestinal tract.[26,27,40] Ariel et al.[27] therefore concluded that so-called Crohn's disease limited to the appendix is a form of granulomatous and follicular appendicitis that is nosologically unrelated in the majority of the cases to true Crohn's disease.

A few cases of granulomatous disease of the appendix are due to involvement by *sarcoidosis*.[37] Others are due to *Yersinia pseudotuberculosis;* these show central necrosis and formation of microabscesses with scanty Langerhans' giant cells. A positive serologic test is necessary to confirm the diagnosis.[36]

TUMORS
So-called mucocele

In the appendiceal disorder classically designated as *mucocele*, the appendix shows localized or diffuse globular enlargement. The lumen is dilated and contains large amounts of glairy mucus (Fig. 11-90). In the past, it has been assumed that the changes are secondary to proximal obstruction of the lumen. Cheng's experimental model[45] is often quoted in this regard. He showed that if the lumen of the rabbit "appendix" is surgically occluded, dilatation of the distal portion with flattening of the epithelium and accumulation of mucus results. If the mucus is transplanted to the rabbit peritoneum, it acts as foreign material and in time is absorbed.

In our opinion, the term *mucocele* embraces a group of conditions having different morphology and pathogenesis.[54] In a few instances, the disease seems indeed to be the result of occlusion of the lumen by endometriosis, carcinoid tumor, or some other process. The epithelium is flat, atrophic, and devoid of any atypical features. In cystic fibrosis, the "mucocele" is due to the accumulation of inspissated mucus. In other cases, a localized focus of *mucosal hyperplasia* is seen, the appearance being indistinguishable from that of a hyperplastic colorectal polyp.[54,73] We believe that the remaining cases, which represent most of the lesions diagnosed as "mucocele," have morphologic, histochemical, and ultrastructural features of mucinous neoplasms of the appendix.[42,54,62,74] The distinction between the hyperplastic and neoplastic cases is in general quite easy, although cases exist that combine features of both.[54,87]

The large majority of these mucinous neoplasms are benign—i.e., *mucinous cystadenomas.* They are lined by *atypical* mucinous epithelium with at least some areas of papillary configuration (Fig. 11-91). It is possible that some of these lesions begin as adenomatous polyps, villoglandular polyps, or villous adenomas[52,53] (Fig. 11-92) and that the progressive accumulation of mucus in the cavity eventually obliterates the diagnostic features of these entities.[47,74] Secondary changes include thinning of the wall, extensive ulceration, and calcification. The latter may be evident roentgenographically. As a result of increased intraluminal pressure, mucus may penetrate into the wall, reach the serosa, and appear as a periappendicular or retroperitoneal mass at operation. Removal of the appendix is curative, even in the presence of the latter complication. A certain proportion of these cases are associated with ovarian mucinous cystadenoma of strikingly similar microscopic appearance.[76] There

is also a high association with synchronous or metachronous neoplasms elsewhere in the colon.[89]

The malignant counterpart—i.e., ***mucinous cystadenocarcinoma***—has the same gross appearance and many microscopic features in common with the benign form[55,90] (Fig. 11-93). It may be associated with a similar independent lesion of the ovary. We have used two criteria for malignancy in these lesions: (1) the identification of invasion of the appendiceal wall by atypical glands, and (2) clearly

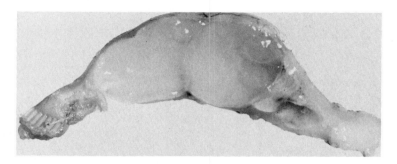

Fig. 11-90 Classic example of so-called mucocele of appendix still confined within lumen but showing extreme distention and thinning of wall. This was incidental finding in woman undergoing cholecystectomy. Microscopically, features were those of mucinous cystadenoma.

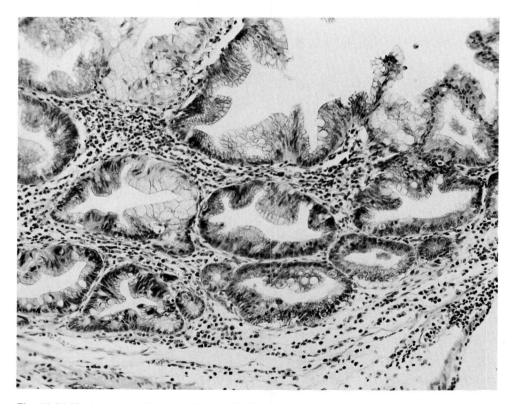

Fig. 11-91 Mucinous cystadenoma of appendix. Glands are of colonic type and have mild degree of atypia and tendency to papillary configuration. Most lesions designated as mucoceles belong to this category.

identifiable epithelial cells (whether atypical or not) in the peritoneal mucinous deposits, when these are present (Fig. 11-94). If one were to use the terminology currently applied to mucinous tumors of the ovary for these appendiceal tumors, many of them would fit into a *borderline* category.

The presence of mucin within the peritoneal cavity has been classically referred to as *pseudomyxoma peritonei*.[63] We believe that this designation should be reserved for those cases in which the condition is widespread (rather than limited to a small pool of mucin around the appendix) and in

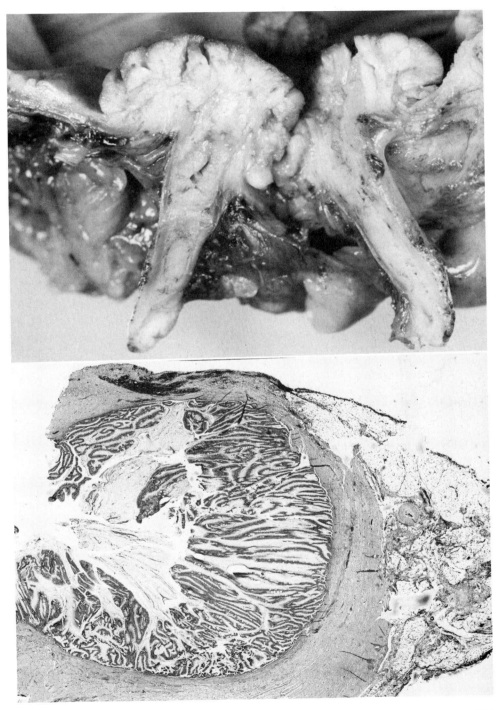

Fig. 11-92 Villous adenoma involving proximal half of appendix and adjacent portion of cecum. With passage of time, this lesion may evolve into a mucinous cystadenoma.

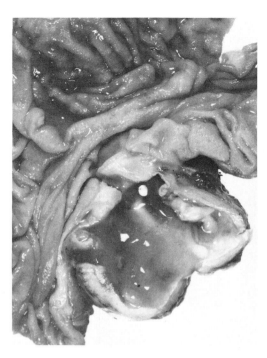

Fig. 11-93 Mucinous cystadenocarcinoma of appendix. Grossly, it would be impossible to distinguish this tumor from mucinous cystadenoma. Microscopically, invasion of wall by malignant glands was identified.

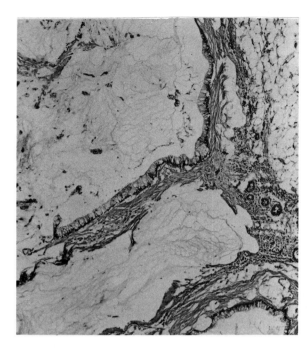

Fig. 11-94 Pseudomyxoma peritonei caused by mucinous cystadenocarcinoma of appendix. Diagnosis is possible because of presence of well-differentiated mucinous epithelium in conjunction with lakes of mucin.

which epithelial tumor cells are identifiable microscopically. Actually, these two features often go together. When thus defined, this process forms gelatinous nodules and in time may cause the death of the patient through infection or intestinal obstruction by invasion of the surrounding structures such as the bladder, abdominal wall, and intestine. Involvement above the diaphragm or metastases to lymph nodes are exceptional. The disease may be first diagnosed through the detection of mucin in a specimen from a herniorrhaphy operation.[43] Radiotherapy may temporarily slow the growth of the metastatic tumor and improve survival figures.[50] Removal of as much of the tumor as possible may be helpful in prolonging life even for several years. However, peritonitis is frequent after such palliative operations. *Pseudomyxoma peritonei* indistinguishable from the one previously described can also be the result of ovarian mucinous cystadenocarcinoma (see Chapter 19).

Adenocarcinoma

It is not uncommon for large carcinomas of the cecum to involve secondarily the base of the appendix. These tumors are sometimes erroneously assumed to be of primary appendiceal origin.

Primary adenocarcinoma of the appendix is a rarity once one eliminates the mucinous cystadenocarcinoma and the carcinoid tumors associated with the production of glands and mucin (adenocarcinoids).[67,81] It can be located in any part of the appendix. The symptoms resemble acute appendicitis; actually, inflammation is often found in addition to

the carcinoma.[88] The microscopic appearance is essentially the same as that of colorectal adenocarcinoma.[75] Right hemicolectomy is the treatment of choice except for very superficial tumors of well-differentiated nature that can be cured by simple appendectomy.[83] The Dukes' staging system correlates with prognosis just as well as it does in the colorectum.[88]

An exceptionally rare type of primary appendiceal tumor is the *signet-ring* or linitis plastica type of carcinoma.[75] This needs to be distinguished from a metastasis of a gastric or mammary tumor (an almost impossible task in the absence of an autopsy) and from mucinous carcinoid tumor (see the following discussion). Signet-ring carcinomas have more extensive mucosal involvement, more nuclear atypia, and a more complex and irregular invasive pattern than mucinous carcinoid tumor, and lack features of neuroendocrine differentiation ultrastructurally and immunohistochemically. It seems to us, though, that the morphologic, histogenetic, and behavioral differences between pure signet-ring carcinoma and mucinous carcinoid tumors with a predominance of signet-ring cells are minimal.

Carcinoid tumor

Carcinoid tumors are found in about one out of every 300 routine appendectomies[71] and represent the most common tumor of the appendix. The peak incidence occurs in the third and fourth decades of life, but they also occur in children.[80] In most of the cases, they are incidental findings, but they may be found associated with acute appendicitis

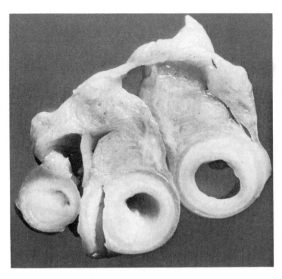

Fig. 11-95 Carcinoid tumor of appendix that blocked lumen and caused acute appendicitis.

as a result of obstruction of the lumen. In the 144 cases reported by Moertel et al.,[71] 71% were located in the tip of the appendix, 22% in the body, and 7% in the base; 70% of the lesions were less than 1 cm in diameter, and only two measured 2 cm or more. Grossly, the tumors are firm, yellow, white, and fairly well circumscribed but not encapsulated (Fig. 11-95). Those located at the tip often result in a typical "bell clapper" configuration.

Microscopically, most carcinoid tumors of the appendix can be roughly divided into three categories. The *classic* type is formed by solid nests of small monotonous cells with occasional acinar or rosette formation[66,82] (Fig. 11-96, *A*). Mitoses are exceedingly rare. A peculiar retraction of the tumor periphery from the stroma is evident. Some of the cells are found within intra-appendiceal nerves.[56] Invasion of muscle and lymphatic vessels is the rule, and spread to the peritoneal surface is not rare. The tumor cells are argentaffin, argyrophilic, positive for the diazo reaction, filled with pleomorphic dense-core secretory granules on ultrastructural examination, and immunohistochemically reactive for neuron-specific enolase, chromogranin, serotonin, and (inconstantly) for a variety of peptide hormones, including somatostatin, substance P, peptide YY, and glucagon.[58a]

A second type of carcinoid tumor, referred to as *tubular type adenocarcinoid* by Warkel et al.,[86] is often misdiagnosed as primary or metastatic carcinoma. It is characterized by glandular formation without solid nests[48] (Fig. 11-96, *B*). Mucin may be present. The argentaffin reaction is positive in 75% of the cases and the argyrophilic reaction in 89%.[86] The lack of mitoses and atypia, orderly arrangement, and origin at the base of the glands with an otherwise normal mucosa should suggest the diagnosis. On occasion, the cytoplasmic granules of these cells are large and acidophilic, simulating those of Paneth cells, a feature also sometimes exhibited by normal Kultschitsky's cells.[69] Elec-

tron microscopic examination is diagnostic even with formalin-fixed material because of the presence of neurosecretory granules.[79]

The third type is variously called *mucinous carcinoid tumor*,[61] *goblet cell carcinoid*,[44,84] *goblet cell type adenocarcinoid*,[86] *microglandular carcinoma*,[88] and *crypt cell carcinoma*.[58] Grossly, it may be found in any portion of the appendix and appears as an area of whitish, sometimes mucoid induration without dilatation of the lumen; acute appendicitis is a common complication. Microscopically, and like the other two carcinoid types, it is characterized by a predominantly submucosal growth. Extension into the muscle and serosa is common, but the mucosa is characteristically spared, except for areas of apparent connection between tumor nests and the base of the crypts. The tumor itself is formed by small uniform nests of signet ring cells, often arranged in a microglandular fashion, and sometimes accompanied by extracellular mucus (Fig. 11-96, *C*). A component of lysozyme-positive cells with features of Paneth cells may also be present[58] as well as foci resembling Brunner glands.[86] Mucicarmine and CEA stains are consistently positive, and argyrophil stains show cytoplasmic granules in about 88% of the cases.[60,86] Electron microscopic studies have shown mucin droplets and neurosecretory type granules, although there is controversy about whether they are located in the same cell.[41,46,78]

The morphologic, immunohistochemical, and ultrastructural features of this carcinoid type indicate that all the cells normally present in the Lieberkuhn's crypt may be represented in it, hence the alternative term *crypt cell carcinoma*.[58]

There is little question that the cells of classic carcinoid tumor have morphologic, immunohistochemical, and ultrastructural features corresponding to those of the Kultschitsky's cell normally located at the base of Lieberkuhn's glands, but there is still debate over whether this tumor arises from these cells or from similar cells located within nerves of the lamina propria, originally identified by Masson.[64,70,77]

Carcinoid syndrome secondary to appendiceal carcinoid tumor is extremely rare and is almost always related to the presence of liver metastases.[65] Occasionally, appendiceal carcinoids are found to secrete ACTH and to result in a clinical picture of Cushing's syndrome.[59] Five (4.2%) of the patients with carcinoid tumor in the series reported by Moertel et al.[71] had an associated carcinoid of the ileum, and nineteen (13%) had a second primary cancer.

The behavior of most classic and tubular carcinoid tumors is very indolent. Metastatic spread is unusual, often limited to the regional lymph nodes and usually restricted to tumors greater than 2 cm in diameter. Although some controversy still persists,[85] we agree with Moertel et al.[71,71a] and Glasser and Bhagavan[51] that simple appendectomy is adequate therapy for this neoplasm even in the presence of serosal invasion, except for the very rare cases measuring 2 cm or more in diameter. The behavior of mucinous carcinoid tumor is much more aggressive than the other two types: metastases have been documented in 8% to 20% of the cases.[49,72,84,86,88] They are particularly common in the ovary, where they can acquire the features of Krukenberg tumor.[57,68] Because of

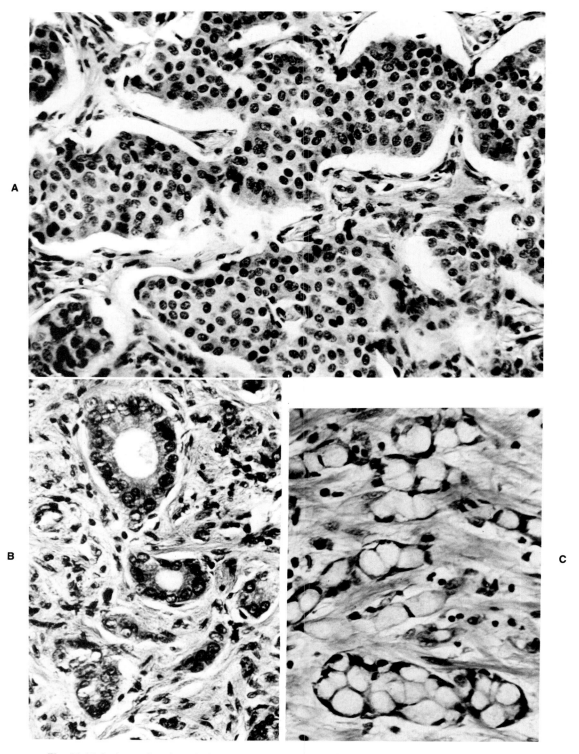

Fig. 11-96 A, Appendiceal carcinoid tumor of classic type. This variety usually contains argentaffin as well as argyrophil cells. **B,** Appendiceal carcinoid tumor forming well-defined glandular structures (tubular type adenocarcinoid). In this variety, cells are often argyrophil but only rarely argentaffin. **C,** Mucinous carcinoid tumor formed by nests of mucin-positive signet-ring cells infiltrating entire wall. There is little stromal reaction to tumor, no cellular atypia, and no individual cell infiltration. Argentaffin and/or argyrophil cells can often be demonstrated.

this, we favor the performance of a right hemicolectomy for this tumor type, especially if the neoplasm has spread beyond the appendix and/or shows a high mitotic count.[86]

OTHER LESIONS

Heterotopic gastric and *esophageal tissue* have been described within the appendix.[94]

Endometriosis and *ectopic decidual reaction* are sometimes seen as incidental findings beneath the serosa[100]; exceptionally, endometriosis may result in appendiceal rupture.

Diverticula of the appendix are usually multiple. They are of the "false" type, arising in a weak area as a result of increased intraluminal pressure. Diverticulitis may occur, resulting in a clinical picture indistinguishable from that of acute appendicitis.[93,103] Diverticulosis of the appendix is relatively common in patients with cystic fibrosis, presumably as a result of increased intraluminal pressure produced by the inspissated mucus.[95]

Inverted appendiceal stump from a previous appendectomy may appear as a filling defect in the cecum on barium examination and simulate a neoplasm.

Intussusception of the appendix into the cecal lumen may develop spontaneously; it may be of the entire appendix or, more commonly, of only the base. The cause is often lymphoid hyperplasia.

Granular cell tumor can involve the appendiceal wall.[97] In about 5% of appendectomy specimens, single or clustered granular cells with an appearance similar to those of granular cell tumor are found in the wall[96]; these seem to represent altered smooth muscle cells rather than Schwann cells.[105]

A case of *paraganglioma* located in the mesoappendix has been described.[92]

Neuroma (neurogenous hyperplasia) of the appendix presenting with the gross appearance of fibrous obliteration was thoroughly described by Masson over 50 years ago[98,99]; recent immunohistochemical and ultrastructural studies have confirmed the correctness of his interpretation.[102,106] Endocrine cells are often found within the hypertrophied nerve bundles, and these may well be the cells of origin for carcinoid tumor.

Neurofibroma of the appendix or mesoappendix has been reported, either as a solitary lesion or as a component of Recklinghausen disease[101] (Fig. 11-97).

Malignant lymphoma can involve the appendix; cases of Burkitt's lymphoma have been seen in children presenting with the clinical picture of appendicitis.[104]

Metastases to the appendix usually originate in carcinomas of the gastrointestinal tract, breast, or female genital tract.[91]

REFERENCES
ACUTE APPENDICITIS

1 Alecce AA, Sullivan SG, Ashworth W: Spontaneous idiopathic segmental infarction of the omentum. Ann Surg **142:**316-320, 1955.

2 Berry J Jr, Malt RA: Appendicitis near its centenary. Ann Surg **200:**567-575, 1984.

3 Boyce FF: Special problems of acute appendicitis in middle and late life. Arch Surg **68:**296-304, 1957.

4 Burkitt DP: The aetiology of appendicitis. Br J Surg **58:**695-699, 1971.

5 Butler C: Surgical pathology of acute appendicitis. Hum Pathol **12:**870-878, 1981.

6 Clark LP: Calculi in the appendix. Br J Surg **40:**272-273, 1946.

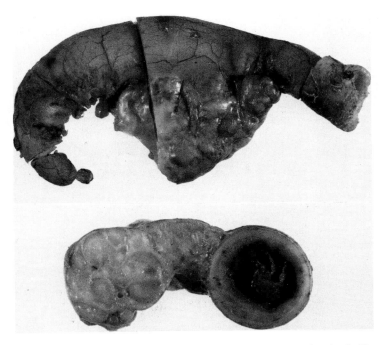

Fig. 11-97 Neurofibroma of appendiceal mesentery. Appendix itself is uninvolved. (Courtesy Dr. J. Costa, Lausanne, Switzerland.)

7 Dymock RB: Pathological changes in the appendix. A review of 1000 cases. Pathology **9:**331-339, 1977.

8 Fedyshin P, Kelvin FM, Rice RP: Nonspecificity of barium enema findings in acute appendicitis. Am J Radiol **143:**99-102, 1984.

9 Forbes GB, Lloyd-Davies RW: Calculous disease of the vermiform appendix. Gut **7:**583-592, 1966.

10 Gilmore OJA, Browett JP, Griffin PH, Ross IK, Brodribb AJM, Cooke TJC, Higgs MJ, Williamson RCN: Appendicitis and mimicking conditions. A prospective study. Lancet **2:**421-424, 1975.

10a Gray GF Jr, Wackym PA: Surgical pathology of the vermiform appendix. Pathol Annu **21**(Pt 2):111-144, 1986.

11 Mueller BA, Daling JR, Moore DE, Weiss NS, Spadoni LR, Stadel BV, Soules MR: Appendectomy and the risk of tubal infertility. N Engl J Med **315:**1506-1508, 1986.

12 Nathans AA, Merenstein H, Brown SS: Lymphoid hyperplasia of the appendix. Pediatrics **12:**516-524, 1955.

13 Packard GB, McLauthlin CH: Acute appendicitis in children. J Pediatr **39:**708-714, 1951.

14 Peltokallio P: Acute appendicitis associated with carcinoma of the colon. Dis Colon Rectum **9:**453-456, 1966.

15 Reif RM: Viral appendicitis. Hum Pathol **12:**193-196, 1981.

16 Remington JH, McDonald JR: Vascular thrombosis in acute appendicitis. Surgery **24:**787-792, 1948.

17 Rex JC, Harrison EG Jr, Priestley JT: Appendicitis and ligneous perityphlitis. Arch Surg **82:**735-745, 1961.

18 Sisson RG, Ahlvin RC, Harlow MC: Superficial mucosal ulceration and the pathogenesis of acute appendicitis in childhood. Am J Surg **122:**378-380, 1971.

19 Therkelsen F: On histologic diagnosis of appendicitis. Acta Chir Scand **94** [Suppl 108]:1-48, 1948.

20 Thorbjarnarson B, Loehr WJ: Acute appendicitis in patients over the age of sixty. Surg Gynecol Obstet **125:**1277-1280, 1967.

21 Wangensteen OH, Dennis C: Experimental proof of the obstructive origin of appendicitis in man. Ann Surg **110:**629-647, 1939.

22 Williams GR: A history of appendicitis. With anecdotes illustrating its importance. Ann Surg **197:**495-506, 1983.

23 Williams JS, Hale HW Jr: Acute appendicitis in the elderly. Review of 83 cases. Ann Surg **162:**208-212, 1965.

24 Zarabi M, LaBach JP: Ganglioneuroma causing acute appendicitis. Hum Pathol **13:**1143-1146, 1982.

CHRONIC APPENDICITIS

25 Hertzler AE: An inquiry into the nature of chronic appendicitis. Am J Obstet Gynecol **11:**155-170, 1926.

PARASITOSES AND OTHER INFLAMMATIONS

26 Allen DC, Biggart JD: Granulomatous disease in the vermiform appendix. J Clin Pathol **36:**632-638, 1983.

27 Ariel I, Vinograd I, Hershlag A, Olsha O, Argov S, Klausner JM, Rabau MY, Freund U, Rosenmann E: Crohn's disease isolated to the appendix. Truths and fallacies. Hum Pathol **17:**1116-1121, 1986.

28 Ashburn LL: Appendiceal oxyuriasis. Am J Pathol **17:**841-856, 1941.

29 Bonenfant JL: Lésions appendiculaires au cours de la rougeole. Arch Fr Pediatr **9:**1-10, 1952.

30 Collins DC: 71,000 human appendix specimens. A final report, summarizing forty years' study. Am J Proctol **14:**265-281, 1963.

31 Galloway WH: Appendicitis in the course of measles. Br Med J **2:**1412-1414, 1957.

32 Noodleman JS: Eosinophilic appendicitis. Demonstration of *Strongyloides stercoralis* as a causative agent. Arch Pathol Lab Med **105:**148-149, 1981.

33 O'Brien A, O'Briain DS: Infectious mononucleosis. Appendiceal lymphoid tissue involvement parallels characteristic lymph node changes. Arch Pathol Lab Med **109:**680-682, 1985.

34 Satti MB, Tamimi DM, Sohaibani MA, Quorain AA: Appendicular schistosomiasis. A cause of clinical acute appendicitis? J Clin Pathol **40:**424-428, 1987.

35 Stemmerman GN: Eosinophilic granuloma of the appendix. A study of its relation to *Strongyloides* infestation. Am J Clin Pathol **36:**524-531, 1961.

36 Timmcke AE: Granulomatous appendicitis. Is it Crohn's disease? Report of a case and review of the literature. Am J Gastroenterol **81:**283-287, 1986.

37 Tinker MA, Viswanathan B, Laufer H, Margolis IB: Acute appendicitis and pernicious anemia as complications of gastrointestinal sarcoidosis. Am J Gastroenterol **79:**868-872, 1984.

38 van Spreeuwel JP, Lindeman J, Bax R, Elbers HJR, Sybrandy R, Meijer CJLM: *Campylobacter*-associated appendicitis. Prevalence and clinicopathologic features. Pathol Annu **22**(Pt 1):55-65, 1987.

39 Vinuela A, Fernandez-Rojo F, Martinez-Merino A: Oxyuris granulomas of pelvic peritoneum and appendicular wall. Histopathology **3:**69-77, 1979.

40 Yang SS, Gibson P, McCaughey RS, Arcari FA, Bernstein J: Primary Crohn's disease of the appendix. Report of 14 cases and review of the literature. Ann Surg **189:**334-339, 1979.

TUMORS

41 Abt AB, Carter SL: Goblet cell carcinoid of the appendix. An ultrastructural and histochemical study. Arch Pathol Lab Med **100:**301-306, 1976.

42 Aho AJ, Heinonen R, Laurén P: Benign and malignant mucocele of the appendix. Acta Chir Scand **139:**392-400, 1973.

43 Campbell, TE: Mucinous neoplasms of the appendix appearing as hernias. Arch Pathol **105:**57-58, 1981.

44 Chen V: Goblet cell carcinoid tumors of the appendix. Arch Pathol Lab Med **103:**180-182, 1979.

45 Cheng KK: An experimental study of mucocele of the appendix and pseudomyxoma peritonei. J Pathol Bacteriol **61:**217-225, 1940.

46 Cooper PH, Warkel RL: Ultrastructure of the goblet cell type of adenocarcinoid of the appendix. Cancer **42:**2687-2695, 1978.

47 Darby AJ, Doctor A: Villous papilloma of the appendix associated with mucocoele and intussusception. Postgrad Med J **50:**650-654, 1974.

48 Dische FE: Argentaffin and non-argentaffin carcinoid tumours of the appendix. J Clin Pathol **21:**60-66, 1968.

49 Edmonds P, Merino MJ, LiVolsi VA, Duray PH: Adenocarcinoid (mucinous carcinoid) of the appendix. Gastroenterology **86:**302-309, 1984.

50 Fernandez RN, Daly JM: Pseudomyxoma peritonei. Arch Surg **115:**409-414, 1980.

51 Glasser CM, Bhagavan BS: Carcinoid tumors of the appendix. Arch Pathol Lab Med **104:**272-275, 1980.

52 Goldfarb WB, Kempson RL: Villous adenomas of the appendix. Surgery **55:**769-772, 1964.

53 Hameed K: Villous adenoma of the vermiform appendix with Cushing's syndrome. Ultrastructural study of a case. Cancer **27:**681-686, 1971.

54 Higa E, Rosai J, Pizzimbono CA, Wise L: Mucosal hyperplasia, mucinous cystadenoma and mucinous cystadenocarcinoma of the appendix. A reevaluation of appendiceal "mucocele." Cancer **33:**1525-1541, 1973.

55 Hilsabeck JR, Judd ES Jr, Woolner LB: Carcinoma of the vermiform appendix. Surg Clin North Am **31:**995-1011, 1951.

56 Hirose T, Sano T, Hizawa K: Ultrastructural study on an appendiceal carcinoid tumor showing intra-nerve fiber growth. Acta Pathol Jpn **36:**123-131, 1986.

57 Hirschfield LS, Kahn LB, Winkler B, Bochner RZ, Gibstein AA: Adenocarcinoid of the appendix presenting as bilateral Krukenberg's tumor of the ovaries. Immunohistochemical and ultrastructural studies and literature review. Arch Pathol Lab Med **109:**930-933, 1985.

58 Isaacson P: Crypt cell carcinoma of the appendix (so-called adenocarcinoid tumor). Am J Surg Pathol **5:**213-224, 1981.

58a Iwafuchi M, Watanabe H, Kijima H, Ajioka Y, Shimoda T, Ito S: Argyrophil, non-argentaffin carcinoids of the appendix vermiformis. Immunohistochemical and ultrastructural studies. Acta Pathol Jpn **37:**1237-1247, 1987.

59 Johnston WH, Waisman J: Carcinoid tumor of the vermiform appendix with Cushing's syndrome. Cancer **27:**681-686, 1971.

60 Klappenbach RS, Kurman RJ, Sinclair CF, James LP: Composite carcinoma—carcinoid tumors of the gastrointestinal tract. A morphologic, histochemical, and immunocytochemical study. Am J Clin Pathol **84:**137-143, 1985.

61 Klein HZ: Mucinous carcinoid tumor of the vermiform appendix. Cancer **33:**770-777, 1974.

62 Klemi PJ, Nevalainen TJ, Aho AJ: The histogenesis of mucinous cystadenoma of the appendix. Arch Pathol **104:**162-163, 1980.

63 Little JM, Halliday JP, Glenn DC: Pseudomyxoma peritonei. Lancet **2:**659-663, 1969.

64 Lundqvist M, Wilander E: A study of the histopathogenesis of carcinoid tumors of the small intestine and appendix. Cancer **60:**201-206, 1987.

65 Markgraf WH, Dunn TM: Appendiceal carcinoid with carcinoid syndrome. Am J Surg **107:**730-732, 1964.

66 Masson P: Carcinoids (argentaffin-cell tumors) and nerve hyperplasia of the appendicular mucosa. Am J Pathol **4:**181-211, 1928.

67 Mauritzen K: Primary adenocarcinoma of the appendix. Report of sixteen cases. Acta Chir Scand **115:**447-456, 1958.

68 Merino MJ, Edmonds P, LiVolsi V: Appendiceal carcinoma metastatic to the ovaries and mimicking primary ovarian tumors. Int J Gynecol Pathol **4:**110-120, 1985.

69 Millikin PD: Eosinophilic argentaffin cells in the human appendix. Arch Pathol **98**:393-395, 1974.

70 Millikin PD: Extraepithelial enterochromaffin cells and schwann cells in the human appendix. Arch Pathol Lab Med **107**:189-194, 1983.

71 Moertel CG, Dockerty MB, Judd ES: Carcinoid tumors of the vermiform appendix. Cancer **21**:270-278, 1968.

71a Moertel CG, Weiland LH, Nagorney DM, Dockerty MB: Carcinoid tumor of the appendix. Treatment and prognosis. N Engl J Med **317**:1699-1701. 1987.

72 Olsson B, Ljungberg O: Adenocarcinoid of the vermiform appendix. Virchows Arch [Pathol Anat] **386**:201-210, 1980.

73 Qizilbash AH: Hyperplastic (metaplastic) polyps of the appendix. Report of 19 cases. Arch Pathol **97**:385-388, 1974.

74 Qizilbash AH: Mucoceles of the appendix. Their relationship to hyperplastic polyps, mucinous cystadenomas, and cystadenocarcinomas. Arch Pathol **99**:548-555, 1975.

75 Qizilbash AH: Primary adenocarcinoma of the appendix. A clinicopathological study of 11 cases. Arch Pathol **99**:556-562, 1975.

76 Ries, E: Pseudomyxoma peritonei. Surg Gynecol Obstet **39**:569-579, 1924.

77 Rode J, Dhillon AP, Papadaki L, Griffiths D: Neurosecretory cells of the lamina propria of the appendix and their possible relationship to the carcinoids. Histopathology **6**:69-79, 1982.

78 Rodriguez FH Jr, Sarma DP, Lunseth JH: Goblet cell carcinoid of the appendix. Hum Pathol **13**:286-288, 1982.

79 Rosai J, Rodriguez HA: Application of electron microscopy to the differential diagnosis of tumors. Am J Clin Pathol **50**:555-562, 1968.

80 Ryden SE, Drake RM, Franciosi RA: Carcinoid tumors of the appendix in children. Cancer **36**:1538-1542, 1975.

81 Sieracki JC, Tesluck H: Primary adenocarcinoma of vermiform appendix. Cancer **9**:997-1011, 1956.

82 Soga J, Tazawa K: Pathologic analysis of carcinoids. Histologic re-evaluation of 62 cases. Cancer **28**:990-998, 1971.

83 Steinberg M, Cohn I Jr: Primary adenocarcinoma of the appendix. Surgery **61**:644-660, 1967.

84 Subbuswamy SG, Gibbs NM, Ross CF, Morson BC: Goblet cell carcinoid of the appendix. Cancer **34**:338-344, 1974.

85 Syracuse DC, Perzin KH, Price JB, Wiedel PD, Mesa-Tejada R: Carcinoid tumors of the appendix. Mesoappendiceal extension and nodal metastases. Ann Surg **190**:58-63, 1979.

86 Warkel RL, Cooper PH, Helwig EB: Adenocarcinoid, a mucin-producing carcinoid tumor of the appendix. A study of 39 cases. Cancer **42**:2781-2793, 1978.

87 Williams RA, Whitehead R: Non-carcinoid epithelial tumours of the appendix — a proposed classification. Pathology **18**:50-53, 1986.

88 Wolff M, Ahmed N: Epithelial neoplasms of the vermiform appendix (exclusive of carcinoid). I. Adenocarcinoma of the appendix. Cancer **37**:2493-2510, 1976.

89 Wolff M, Ahmed N: Epithelial neoplasms of the vermiform appendix (exclusive of carcinoid). II. Cystadenomas, papillary adenomas, and adenomatous polyps of the appendix. Cancer **37**:2511-2522, 1976.

90 Woodruff R, McDonald JR: Benign and malignant cystic tumors of appendix. Surg Gynecol Obstet **71**:750-755, 1940.

OTHER LESIONS

91 Bolker H, Shapiro AL: Appendiceal metastasis in carcinoma of the breast. NY State J Med **40**:219-220, 1940.

92 Clark DE, Stocks JF, Wilkis JL: Mesoappendiceal paraganglioma. Am J Gastroenterol **80**:340-342, 1985.

93 Deschenes L, Couture J, Garneau R: Diverticulitis of the appendix. Report of sixty-one cases. Am J Surg **121**:706-709, 1971.

94 Droga BW, Levine S, Baker JJ: Heterotopic gastric and esophageal tissue in the vermiform appendix. Am J Clin Pathol **40**:190-193, 1963.

95 George, DH: Diverticulosis of the vermiform appendix in patients with cystic fibrosis. Hum Pathol **18**:75-79, 1987.

96 Hausman R: Granular cells in musculature of appendix. Arch Pathol **75**:360-372, 1963.

97 Johnston J, Helwig EB: Granular cell tumors of the gastrointestinal tract and perianal region. A study of 74 cases. Dig Dis Sci **26**:807-816, 1981.

98 Masson P: Carcinoids (argentaffin-cell tumors) and nerve hyperplasia of the appendicular mucosa. Am J Pathol **4**:181-211, 1928.

99 Michalany J, Galindo W: Classification of neuromas of the appendix. Beitr Pathol Bd **150**:213-228, 1973.

100 Nielsen M, Lykke J, Thomsen JL: Endometriosis of the vermiform appendix. Acta Pathol Microbiol Immunol Scand [A] **91**:253-256, 1983.

101 Olsen BS: Giant appendicular neurofibroma. A light and immunohistochemical study. Histopathology **11**:851-855, 1987.

102 Olsen BS, Holck S: Neurogenous hyperplasia leading to appendiceal obliteration. An immunohistochemical study of 237 cases. Histopathology **11**:843-849, 1987.

103 Rabinovitch J: Diverticulosis and diverticulitis of the vermiform appendix. Ann Surg **155**:434-440, 1962.

104 Sin IC, Ling E-T, Prentice RSA: Burkitt's lymphoma of the appendix. Report of two cases. Hum Pathol **11**:465-470, 1980.

105 Sobel HJ, Marquet E, Schwarz R: Granular degeneration of appendiceal smooth muscle. Arch Pathol **92**:427-432, 1971.

106 Stanley MW, Cherwitz D, Hagen K, Snover DC: Neuromas of the appendix. A light-microscopic, immunohistochemical and electron-microscopic study of 20 cases. Am J Surg Pathol **10**:801-815, 1986.

Large bowel

HIRSCHSPRUNG'S DISEASE AND RELATED DISORDERS

Hirschsprung's disease results from lack of function and coordinated propulsive movement of the distal portion of the large bowel. This is caused by the absence of parasympathetic ganglion cells in the intramural and submucosal plexuses, which in turn is due to either failure of migration from the neural crest or to focal neuronal necrosis[17,18,26,30,36] (Fig. 11-98). Eighty percent of the patients are male; 10%

have Down's syndrome, and another 5% have other serious neurologic abnormalities.[23] The symptoms usually begin shortly after birth, with gaseous distension and sometimes acute intestinal obstruction. With passage of time, the large bowel proximal to the lesion undergoes dilatation of the lumen and hypertrophy of the muscular wall, whereas the diseased segment appears grossly normal (Figs. 11-99 and 11-100).

Microscopically, there is absence of ganglion cells in *both* plexuses in the distal colorectum and in a variable length of the adjoining dilated bowel.[18,35] Hypertrophied, disorganized, nonmyelinated nerve fibers are found instead. In 70% to 80% of the cases, known as *short-segment Hirschsprung's disease,* the aganglionic segment involves only the rectum and rectosigmoid colon for a distance of several centimeters. In a rare variant of this form, known as *ultrashort,* the aganglionic segment is so narrow that the diagnosis can be missed if the biopsy is taken too high.[31] In *long-segment disease,* the abnormality is more extensive, involving most or all of the large bowel, and occasionally extending even to the small bowel[12,20,33]; these patients present with symptoms of intestinal obstruction without megacolon. In another variant, designated as *zonal colonic aganglionosis,* only a short segment of bowel is involved, with presence of ganglion cells above and *below* the aganglionic segment.[14,16]

The traditional approach to morphologic documentation of Hirschsprung's disease is the biopsy procedure described by Swenson et al.,[25] in which a full-thickness segment of the muscular wall of the rectum is excised and examined for the presence of ganglion cells in the myenteric plexus. Since ganglion cells are normally scanty near the internal anal sphincter, the standard guideline is that the biopsy should be taken at a point 2 cm above the anal valve in infants and 3 cm in older children.[1,34] Some authors believe

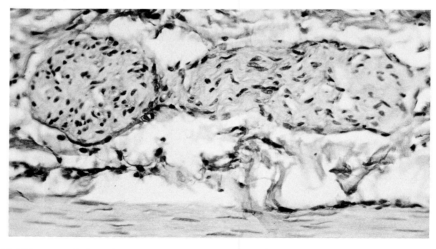

Fig. 11-98 Intramural plexus in narrow segment in patient with Hirschsprung's disease showing absence of ganglion cells and hypertrophy of nerve fibers.

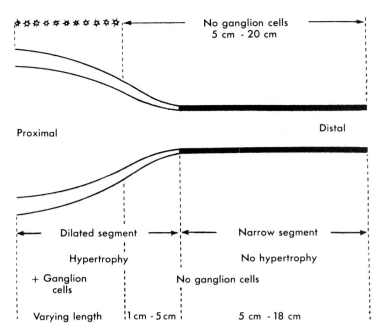

Fig. 11-99 Schematic diagram of gross and microscopic changes in fifteen cases of Hirschsprung's disease. (From Bodian M, Stephens FD, Ward BCH: Hirschsprung's disease and idiopathic megacolon. Lancet **1**:6-11, 1949.)

that biopsies taken at 1 to 1.5 cm from the anal valves may also be adequate.[31] Presence of squamous or transitional epithelium in a specimen indicates that the site of the biopsy is too low. This procedure is highly accurate, but it requires technical skill and general anesthesia, and it may lead to complications. For these reasons, the alternative of diagnosing Hirschsprung's disease with a rectal suction biopsy is now frequently employed.[2,8] This is based on the premise that the limit of aganglionosis in Hirschsprung's disease coincides closely in the submucosal and myenteric plexus, as shown by the careful microscopic mapping studies of Gherardi.[9] The ganglion cells of the submucosal plexus are smaller and more irregularly distributed than are those located intermuscularly, and their identification requires expertise, patience, and the performance of serial sections in the biopsy obtained. Yunis et al.[37] studied forty-seven patients with this technique and found that in experienced hands it is a simple and effective method for the exclusion of Hirschsprung's disease. These biopsies also can be evaluated for acetylcholinesterase activity, which is markedly increased throughout the lamina propria and muscularis mucosae in patients with this disorder.[3,13,15,19] The increase can be detected both by histochemical stains and biochemical analysis, the former being the more practical of the two.[6,21] In problematic cases, determination of the acethylcholinesterase-butyrylcholinesterase ratio may be helpful.[5a] Recently, two immunohistochemical techniques have been proposed as additional tools to the diagnosis of this disorder: neuron-specific enolase (which highlights the presence of hypertrophied nerve fibers and the absence of ganglion cells) and S-100 protein (which shows absence of the normal periganglionic satellite cells and accentuates the enlarged nerve bundles).[10,28,32] These changes are accompanied by a

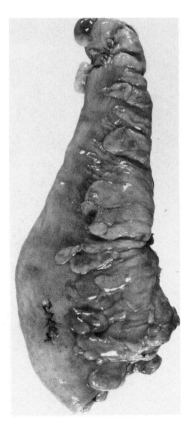

Fig. 11-100 Gross specimen of Hirschsprung's disease. Proximally dilated segment of bowel has been resected. Sutures correspond to biopsies taken to ascertain the presence of ganglion cells. (Courtesy Dr. J. Costa, Lausanne, Switzerland.)

marked decrease in the mucosal endocrine cells that secrete regulatory peptides, such as VIP, enteroglucagon, and somatostatin.[4,29] Another recently described abnormality is the frequent occurrence of fibromuscular dysplasia in the arteries located in the transitional zone.[27]

Frozen section is a practical method of documenting the absence of ganglion cells and is often used to determine the level of transection of the bowel at surgery. This procedure is facilitated if the surgeon gives the pathologist a rectangular piece of the entire muscular wall, so that the tissue can be properly oriented. In order for frozen section to be reliable, the piece examined should be at least 4 mm long, and multiple serial sections should be taken.

Hirschsprung's disease was uniformly fatal only 50 years ago; presently, the mortality rate has decreased to 5% to 10%.[5] The most common operations for the treatment of this disease are Swenson's proctectomy with pull-through of ganglionic bowel to the anus, the Duhamel side-to-side anastomosis of ganglionic bowel with the aganglionic rectal stump, and the Soave endorectal pull-through, in which the rectal mucosa is stripped away and the ganglionic bowel brought down to the anus.[11,23]

Hypoganglionosis is a disputed entity in which there is a deficiency rather than absence of ganglion cells.[35] It should be remembered that hypoganglionosis is usually present at the junction between normal and aganglionic bowel in Hirschsprung's disease. Another controversial entity is *colonic mucosal dysplasia*, in which hyperplasia of the myenteric nerves is accompanied by giant ganglia, isolated ganglion cells in the submucosa, and increase in acetylcholinesterase staining[22]; it has been described in association with Recklinghausen's disease and multiple endocrine adenomatosis.[5,24]

Megacolon can also result from *cytomegalovirus infec-tion* and *Chagas' disease*, as the result of acquired abnormalities of the neural plexus.[7]

DIVERTICULOSIS

Most cases of diverticulosis are acquired and occur in patients over the age of 40. Clinical evidence of diverticulosis is seen in slightly over 10% of the individuals in this age group, but surgical complications develop in only 10% of them. Naturally, the incidence of diverticulosis at autopsy is higher; in a study from Australia, 45% of 200 examined large bowels had diverticuli.[47] It is estimated that by the age of 80, about half the population is affected. There have been scattered reports of diverticula occurring in children, in young patients with Marfan's or Ehlers-Danlos syndrome, and in association with polycystic kidney disease.[38]

Diverticulosis shows a remarkable geographic difference in its frequency. It is common in North America, Europe, and Australia, but unusual in Asia, Africa, and parts of South America. The main protective factor seems to be a high residue diet, although the evidence is not conclusive.[42,57] This type of diet is thought to act by diminishing the degree of colonic segmentation, which is the mechanism responsible for mucosal herniation.[53] The disease is characteristically multiple and involves preferentially the left side of the colon. In the autopsy study from Australia previously mentioned,[47] the sigmoid colon was affected in 99% of the specimens. This was the only area of involvement in 41% of the cases; in 30%, the disease spread to the descending colon, in 4% to the transverse colon, and in 16% to the entire colon. The rectum is rarely affected. The distribution of the disease is different in Japanese patients, in whom there is a greater frequency of right-sided involvement.[56]

Grossly, the diverticuli are located on the mesenteric and

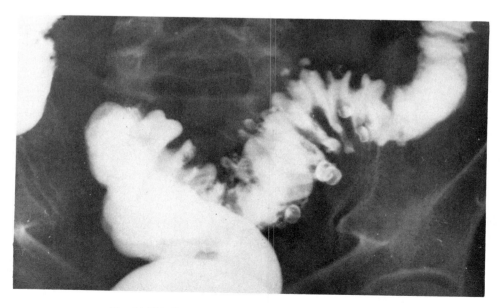

Fig. 11-101 Classic radiographic picture of diverticulosis.

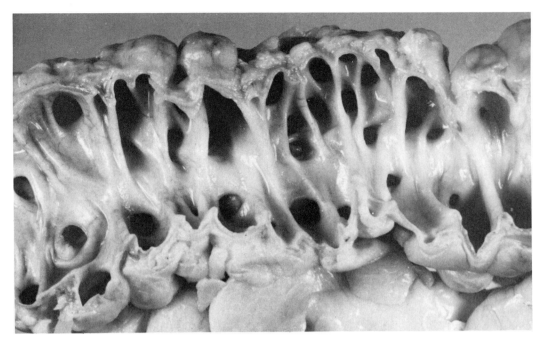

Fig. 11-102 Extensive diverticulosis of sigmoid colon with segmentation and shortening of bowel. Openings of diverticula can be seen clearly. Circular muscle is thick and corrugated.

lateral aspects of the bowel (Figs. 11-101 and 11-102). They have a flask-like shape and may be filled with feces or mucin. Some extend into the appendices epiploicae and bulge over the serosa, but they may still be difficult to recognize at the time of surgery in obese persons. The muscular wall of the bowel always appears abnormal in the area of diverticulosis. The teniae are prominent, with an almost cartilaginous look. The circular layer is also thickened, with a corrugated appearance corresponding to interdigitating processes of the muscle.[47,50] Microscopically, the diverticulum lacks a muscle layer except for residual bundles of muscularis mucosae. The adjacent bowel, including the myenteric plexus, shows no appreciable abnormalities.

Cecal diverticula may be of two types.[39] One, usually multiple, is similar in all aspects to diverticula of the left colon and is often associated with them. The other, thought to be congenital, is solitary and unassociated with diverticular disease elsewhere; it is usually located on the medial wall of the cecum near the ileocecal valve and contains an external muscle layer.[48]

The main complications of diverticulosis are hemorrhage, perforation, and diverticulitis.[52,55] The bleeding, which may be massive, results from rupture of one of the colonic nutrient vessels that run on the side of the diverticulum (Figs. 11-103 and 11-104). Arteriographic and microangiographic techniques have shown a characteristic asymmetric rupture of the vessel toward the lumen of the diverticulum precisely at its dome or antimesenteric margin.[49]

Perforation of the diverticulum may lead to a pericolic or pericecal abscess, which in later stages evolves into an indurated mass that may be confused with cancer clinically and radiographically[40,51] (Fig. 11-105). The abscess may drain into bladder or adjacent bowel and result in a fistulous formation ("dissecting diverticulitis"), resulting in double tracking on x-ray studies. Rarely, this fistulous track may extend into the perineum, scrotum, buttocks, hip, or even lower extremities.[54] Acute free perforation into the abdominal cavity is rare. Sometimes, release of mucin contained within the diverticula results in a pericolic mucocele-like formation.

Diverticulitis manifests radiographically with saw-tooth serrations and a narrowed lumen. It may resemble carcinoma, but the segment involved is usually longer and the mucosa is intact. Microscopically, there is acute or chronic inflammation in—but mainly around—the base of diverticulum. Pain, a common symptom of diverticular disease, may be secondary to these inflammatory changes; however, it may also be present in the absence of diverticulitis and is probably induced by the muscle abnormalities. Parenthetically, chronic corticosteroid therapy may lead to free perforation of the colon and closely simulate the picture of diverticulosis with diverticulitis.[58]

Surgical resection is being performed more frequently in patients with complications of diverticulitis such as perforation, obstruction, and hemorrhage.[44,45] The wisdom of prompt resection for patients with free diverticular perforation and spreading peritonitis has been repeatedly shown.[41,46] Naturally, morbidity and mortality rates are higher in these instances than when resections are performed for uncomplicated acute diverticulitis.[43] Other indications for surgery are repeated attacks of diverticulitis while on a good medical regimen and the development of urinary symptoms. The latter may imply impending sigmoid-vesical fistula. Welch et al.[59] reported an operative mortality of 2.6% among 114 patients treated by resection.

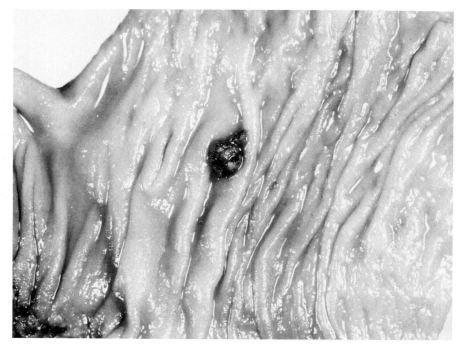

Fig. 11-103 Clot overlying orifice of uninflamed cecal diverticulum. Massively bleeding artery was open at neck of diverticulum.

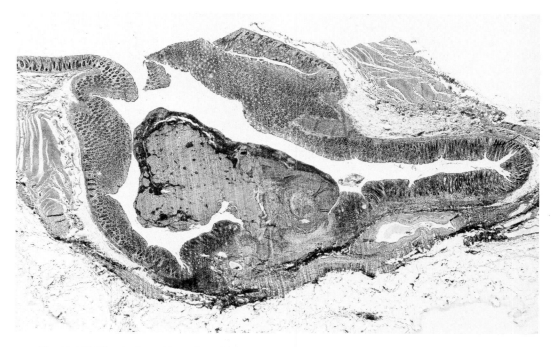

Fig. 11-104 Diverticulum of large bowel from which massive hemorrhage occurred. There is thrombus overlying vessels. Inflammation is absent.

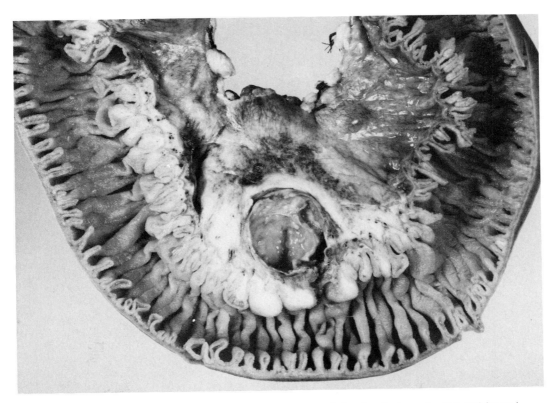

Fig. 11-105 In this colon with extensive diverticulosis, one of the diverticula perforated and formed large inflammatory mass in mesentery.

COLITIS
Ulcerative colitis

Ulcerative colitis occurs with equal frequency in both sexes. It appears most often in patients between 20 and 30 years of age, with a second peak between 70 and 80 years; however, it can occur at any age.[67,82] The etiology remains unknown. The duration is usually prolonged, with many remissions and exacerbations; nutritional deficiencies and anemia are common accompanying features.

Ulcerative colitis is characteristically a left-sided disease, which usually begins in the rectosigmoid area. In some cases, it remains localized to the rectum (ulcerative proctitis[65]), but in most instances it spreads proximally, sometimes to involve the entire colon (pancolitis).

The gross appearance of the lesions varies with the stage of the disease.[80] In the acute form, the mucosal surface of the bowel is wet and glaring from blood and mucus, and petechial hemorrhages are often seen. Various sized ulcers then appear. They have an irregular, somewhat geographic, configuration (Fig. 11-106). Some of these ulcers undermine the mucosa, so that mucosal bridges with an underlying inflammatory infiltrate develop. Extensive longitudinal ulcers, especially if connected by transverse ulcers, are *not* a feature of ulcerative colitis but rather of granulomatous colitis. Elevated sessile reddish nodules, known as *pseudopolyps*, are often seen in an otherwise flat surface (Fig. 11-107, *A*). They are typically small and multiple. Rarely, they may have a filiform configuration (Fig. 11-107, *B*);

sometimes they attain a giant size, thus raising the clinical and roentgenographic suspicion of carcinoma.[70,74]

In the more advanced stages of the process, the entire bowel becomes fibrotic, narrowed, and shortened. The cicatricial stenosis associated with an inflammatory mass may result in an erroneous clinical and roentgenographic diagnosis of carcinoma. If the colon has become defunctionalized with an ileostomy or colostomy before the colectomy, it may show extreme narrowing of the lumen, great atrophy of all the components of the wall, and marked increase in pericolic fat.[81] However, in the quiescent stage the ulceration is absent, the mucosa is atrophic, and there may be extensive submucosal fat deposition. In some of these cases, the mucosa may appear grossly normal.

Microscopically, ulcerative colitis is primarily a mucosal and submucosal disease.[93] In the acute phase, there is an increase in the number of inflammatory cells in the lamina propria.[67a] Crypt abscesses may also appear, preceded by collections of neutrophils at the base of the crypts (Fig. 11-108). This is accompanied by destruction of the glands, which show a marked decrease in cytoplasmic mucus and irregular shapes, resulting from a combination of atrophic and regenerative changes.[69] These regenerative changes are also manifested by nuclear enlargement and increased mitotic activity; the latter is no longer limited to the lower portion of the crypts, as in the normal mucosa, a feature also apparent by other techniques.[66,72] The decrease in total mucin is accompanied by an alteration in a particular species of mucin, a feature that has led some authors to postulate a specific mucin defect.[76] Paneth cells, usually absent beyond the cecum in normal individuals, appear as an expression of metaplasia.[92] Parenthetically, Paneth cells can also be encountered in other inflammatory and neoplastic disorders of the large bowel.[91] The stromal inflammatory infiltrate is composed of neutrophils, lymphocytes, plasma cells, a few histiocytes, and mast cells, but it does not contain epithelioid cells or giant cells.[83] The plasma cells represent a polyclonal population of IgG-, IgM-, and IgA-producing cells.[75] The infiltrate may be accompanied by numerous lymphoid follicles, particularly in the rectum, and may lead to marked distortion of the crypts.[87] The inflammation may remain above the muscularis mucosae or extend into the submucosa (Fig. 11-109). The ulcers are covered by nonspecific granulation tissue. The pseudopolyps are also largely composed of granulation tissue, mixed with inflamed and hyperemic mucosa. Occasionally, prominent reactive stromal cells are present in these pseu-

dopolyps, a feature that should not be confused with malignancy.[71] In some instances, the mucosal regeneration acquires a villous configuration reminiscent of small bowel mucosa.[79] Depending on the stage of the disease, the submucosa may appear normal or inflamed, hyperemic, infiltrated by fat, or fibrosed; sometimes, it contains glands that have herniated through gaps in the muscularis mucosae, which often appears hypertrophic.[61,64,89] In about 10% of the cases, the submucosal arteries show features of endarteritis obliterans, with or without thrombosis. The muscularis externa is usually normal or slightly hypertrophic, and there may be minor subserosal fibrosis.

In the quiescent or resolving stage of the disease, the mucosa may appear grossly normal, with nearly total restoration of the mucin content. This is especially true if steroid enemas have been administered; however, subtle microscopic abnormalities will be detected in the form of branching and irregular glands (rather than parallel, evenly

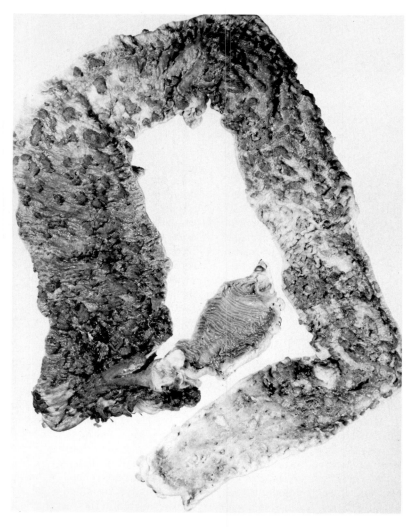

Fig. 11-106 Typical case of ulcerative colitis. Irregular ulcerations of geographic configuration surround small islands of residual mucosa, which are hyperemic and covered by inflammatory exudate.

spaced glands), a gap between the base of the crypts and the muscularis mucosae, appearance of Paneth's cells, hyperplasia of endocrine cells, presence of more than occasional neutrophils, and islands of lipocytes in the lamina propria.[62,87] If the rectal biopsy of a patient with colitis is *microscopically* normal, the diagnosis of ulcerative colitis is very unlikely.[85] In known instances of ulcerative colitis, the biopsy may demonstrate an active process before clinical relapse.

Ulcerative colitis can spread to other portions of the gastrointestinal tract. The ileum is involved in about one third of the cases. This involvement is superficial, of little clinical importance, always in continuity with the colonic disease, and rarely spread more than 10 cm from the ileocecal valve. The ileum is dilated, in striking contrast to the typical stenosis of Crohn's disease. The appendix is diseased in 20% to 60% of the cases, and anal lesions are seen in 10%. The latter may consist of midline dorsal fissures, skin excoriations, acute perianal and ischiorectal abscesses, or rectovaginal fistulas.

Some patients with ulcerative colitis have associated liver disease. This may consist of fatty infiltration, abscess, cirrhosis, sclerosing cholangitis, pericholangitis, and—rarely—carcinoma of the biliary tract.[63,84] Patients in whom the latter complication occurs are younger than those developing cancer *de novo*.[88] In the series reported by Akwari et al.[60] the mean duration of colitis before the onset of biliary symptoms from cancer was 19 years.

Other distant manifestations of ulcerative colitis include arthritis, uveitis, pyoderma gangrenosum, and limited forms of Wegener's granulomatosis.[73] These are usually limited to patients with extensive colonic involvement and appear only exceptionally in those with disease limited to the rectum.

Local complications of ulcerative colitis are perforation with peritonitis and abscess, toxic megacolon, venous thrombosis (most often in the iliac vein), and cancer. The latter complication is discussed in the next section.

The main differential diagnosis of ulcerative colitis is with Crohn's disease of the colon (granulomatous colitis) (see p. 583). For many years, the presence of a chronic inflammatory disease of the large bowel not attributed to a specific organism was equivalent to a diagnosis of ulcerative colitis. It is now apparent that many of these cases actually represent examples of Crohn's disease involving the colon. The clinical, roentgenographic, and morphologic differences between these two diseases have now been clearly delineated (Table 11-2). It also has become apparent that in about 15% of the cases features of both conditions are present and the

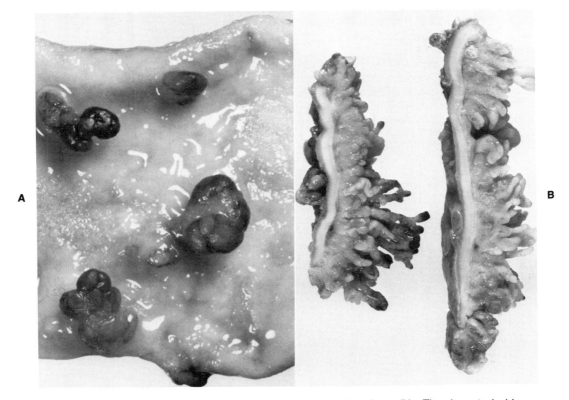

Fig. 11-107 A, Pseudopolyps associated with long-standing ulcerative colitis. They have typical hyperemic appearance and sessile configuration. **B,** Pseudopolyps of so-called filiform type. These lesions can be confused radiographically with carcinoma. (Courtesy Dr. J. Costa, Lausanne, Switzerland.)

Fig. 11-108 Typical crypt abscess with perforation. This occurs in ulcerative colitis but is not a pathognomonic finding.

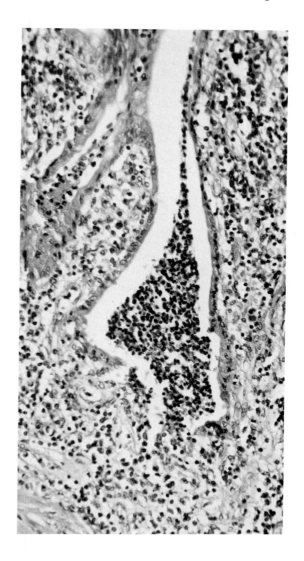

differential diagnosis becomes impossible. The term *indeterminate colitis* has been proposed under these circumstances.[78] The occurrence of such cases, the occasional co-existence of typical Crohn's disease of the small bowel and ulcerative colitis of the large bowel in the same patient, and the occurrence of both diseases in the same family[77] suggest that perhaps the distinction between these two entities has been too rigidly drawn.[68,90] In any event, there are enough clinical and pathologic differences in the majority of the cases to justify a separation that has prognostic and therapeutic implications.[85,86,94]

Carcinoma and dysplasia in ulcerative colitis

The incidence of carcinoma of the large bowel is markedly increased in patients with ulcerative colitis.

The overall incidence of this complication in older series ranged between 5% to 10%,[102,109,116] but the current rate is closer to 2%.[124] This represents only 1% of all cases of colorectal carcinoma in the general population.[124] The risk of carcinoma is higher when the entire colon is involved, when the disease is continuous, unremitting and long-standing (over 10 years),[102] and when the disease begins in childhood.[103,104] In a series of 396 cases of ulcerative colitis in children reported by Devroede et al.,[101] cancer developed in 3% by 10 years, in 23% by 20 years, and in 43% by 35 years after the onset of ulcerative colitis.

Early workers emphasized the atypical gross appearance of the cancer developing in ulcerative colitis, its more even distribution in the large bowel, its frequent multiplicity, the fact that it tends to occur in younger persons and that the site of origin is almost always a flat rather than a polypoid

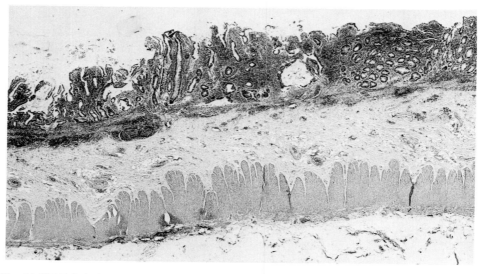

Fig. 11-109 Relatively quiescent area in chronic ulcerative colitis. Note that changes are restricted to mucosa and submucosa.

Table 11-2 Differences between ulcerative colitis and Crohn's disease (granulomatous colitis)

Features	Ulcerative colitis	Crohn's disease
Clinical		
Rectal bleeding	Common	Inconspicuous
Abdominal mass	Practically never	10%-15%
Abdominal pain	Usually left-sided	Usually right-sided
Sigmoidoscopy	Abnormal in 95%	Abnormal in less than 50%
Free perforation	12%	4%
Colon carcinoma	5%-10%	Very rare
Anal complications	Rare; minor	75%; fissures, fistulas, ulceration
Response to steroid therapy	75%	25%
Results of surgery	Very good	Fair
Ileostomy dysfunction	Rare	Common
Roentgenographic		
Sparing of rectum	Exceptional	90%
Involvement of ileum	Rare; dilated ("backwash ileitis")	Common; constricted
Strictures	Absent	Often present
Skip areas	Absent	Common
Internal fistulas	Absent	May be present
Longitudinal and transverse ulcers	Exceptional	Common
Fissuring	Absent	Common
Thumbprinting	Absent	Common
Morphologic		
Distribution of involvement	Diffuse; predominantly left-sided; mucosal and submucosal	Focal; predominantly right-sided; transmural
Mucosal atrophy and regeneration	Marked	Minimal
Cytoplasmic mucin	Diminished	Preserved
Lymphoid aggregates	Rare	Common
Edema	Minimal	Marked
Hyperemia	May be extreme	Minimal
Granulomas	Absent	Present in 60%
Fissuring	Absent	Present
Crypt abscesses	Common	Rare
Rectal involvement	Practically always	50%
Ileal involvement	Minimal; dilated not more than 10 cm	50%; constricted; transmural inflammation
Lymph nodes	Reactive hyperplasia	May contain granulomas

mucosa (Fig. 11-110).[100,109] Multiple tumors are present in 10% to 20% of the cases.[122] Carcinoma may also develop in the rectal stump following ileorectal anastomosis.[107,110] Morson[123] described the earliest gross change as a thick mucosa with a finely nodular or velvety surface configuration.

Microscopically, most of these tumors are adenocarcinomas of varying degrees of differentiation; however, the proportion of poorly differentiated and mucinous carcinomas is higher than for the tumors arising in an uninflamed mucosa.[122] It has been generally assumed that carcinomas developing on the basis of ulcerative colitis carry an ominous prognosis; however, in several recent series with control subjects from a population without colitis matched by stage and microscopic grade, no difference in survival between the two groups has been found.[111,114,117,129] The apparent discrepancy may be due to the fact that in the ulcerative colitis group there tends to be a higher proportion of inoperable and high-grade tumors.[129]

The development of adenocarcinoma is always accompanied—and probably always preceded—by dysplastic changes of the colorectal mucosa, as first described by Morson and Pang.[125] These dysplastic changes, which tend to occur in flat atrophic mucosa, should be distinguished from the more common ones resulting from regeneration atypia. As a rule, the diagnosis of dysplasia should not be made in areas of active inflammation. The evaluation of these changes is difficult and somewhat subjective, but, when properly done, has been successful in identifying a population at high risk for developing colorectal carcinoma.[132] The presence of dysplastic changes does not necessarily indicate that the patient harbors an invasive cancer elsewhere in the bowel[99] as the original report had claimed. Furthermore, the absence of such changes does not guarantee that the patient does not have cancer proximally, although it makes this possibility unlikely.[96,118] Multiple rectal biopsies are recommended for the detection of the dysplasia[128] (Figs. 11-111 and 11-112).

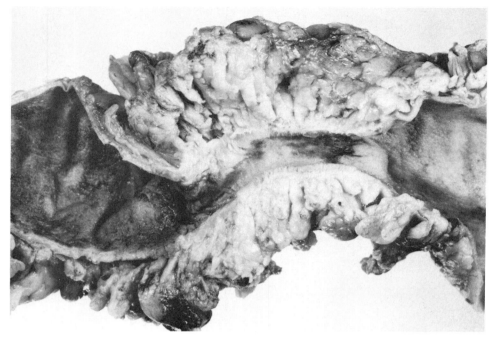

Fig. 11-110 Chronic ulcerative colitis with superimposed carcinoma in region of constriction.

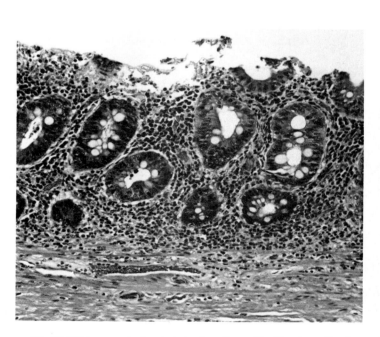

Fig. 11-111 Low-grade dysplasia in ulcerative colitis. Glands are lined by pseudostratified epithelium with mild hyperchromasia of nuclei.

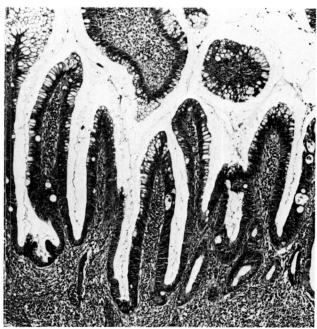

Fig. 11-112 High-grade dysplasia in ulcerative colitis. Mucosa has acquired papillary configuration. There is prominent pseudostratification by cells with markedly hyperchromatic nuclei.

A standardized classification of dysplasia has recently been recommended,[127] using the following terminology:

1 Negative for dysplasia
2 Indefinite for dysplasia, probably negative
3 Indefinite for dysplasia, unknown
4 Indefinite for dysplasia, probably positive
5 Positive for dysplasia, low grade
6 Positive for dysplasia, high grade

The reader is referred to the original publication for a detailed definition of these categories.[127] Whether morphometric analysis will improve the accuracy remains to be determined.[96a]

The implications for patient management are to continue regular follow-up in categories 1 and 2, to institute short-term follow-up in categories 3 and 4, and to consider colectomy for category 6 following confirmation of the diagnosis. For category 5, the recommendation is to either institute short-term follow-up or to consider colectomy following confirmation of the diagnosis, especially if a gross lesion is present. The importance of the detection of gross lesions endoscopically was emphasized by this and other studies for the detection of dysplasia or frank cancer; these lesions may be in the form of polypoid, elevated, nodular or villous formations, ulcers, or strictures.[97,126] The dysplastic changes are associated with a relative excess of sialomucin production,[105,106,108] higher reactivity for CEA,[95] decreased staining for the secretory component of immunoglobulin,[95] structural alterations as seen by scanning electron microscopy,[131] and abnormalities of DNA content as detected by flow cytometry.[112,113] Some of these special techniques may be helpful in confirming the presence of dysplasia, but at the present time this determination is largely based on the appearance of the epithelium in routinely stained sections. The surveillance protocols that have been devised for patients with ulcerative colitis, recommended to be started after 8 to 10 years of extensive colitis and after 15 years of left-sided colitis, depend on skill and experience with endoscopic and microscopic features on the part of the gastroenterologist and pathologist, respectively.[115,119,122,124,130] Whether this close surveillance will prove beneficial remains to be seen.[98]

Other colorectal malignancies that have occurred in association with ulcerative colitis are *carcinoid tumor* (usually atypical)[120,121] and *malignant lymphoma*.[126a]

Crohn's disease (granulomatous colitis)

Crohn's disease, originally described as a small bowel process, is now known to involve the large bowel in approximately 40% of all cases, with or without a concomitant ileal component.

The etiology remains undetermined. The possibility of a bacterial infection—mycobacterial or otherwise—is brought up periodically,[134] but definite proof of an infectious agent has not been forthcoming. Another possibility to consider is that Crohn's disease of the large bowel may not be a distinct entity but rather a pattern of reaction resulting from a variety of causes, including vascular disorders. It has been suggested that at least some of the cases of Crohn's disease in the elderly have a vascular pathogenesis.[141,157,160]

Grossly, segmental distribution of the lesions (with "skip" areas that can be demonstrated roentgenographically) and preference for the right side of the colon are two important diagnostic features.[144] Other gross findings of significance include stricture formation, fissuring, cobblestone appearance, and transmural involvement (Fig. 11-113). The ulcers are linear, serpiginous, and discontinuous, with an intervening normal or edematous (but not markedly abnormal) mucosa. Often, they run longitudinally for long distances and are connected by short transversal ulcers. Healing of this process leads to long rail-track scars. Sometimes, pseudopolyps of the usual filiform or giant type may develop, similar to those seen in ulcerative colitis.[133,143,149] The microscopic appearance of Crohn's disease in the large bowel is not qualitatively different from that seen in the

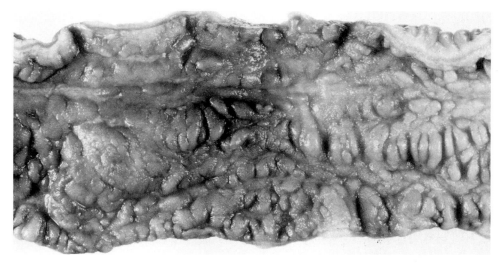

Fig. 11-113 Crohn's disease of large bowel. Extensive longitudinal ulcers joined by transverse ulcers separate edematous mucosa in patches, resulting in typical "cobblestone" appearance.

small bowel. Fissures, noncaseating sarcoid-like granulomas (present in 40% to 60% of the cases), and transmural involvement are typical (Fig. 11-114). The mucosa has a relatively normal appearance and retains a significant amount of mucus, even in areas immediately adjacent to ulcerations. Immunoglobulin-producing plasma cells are distinctly less common than in ulcerative colitis.[155] Presence of a well-defined focus of inflammatory cells surrounded by noninflamed and histologically normal mucosa is particularly suggestive of Crohn's disease, as is the predominance of inflammatory infiltrate deep into the mucosa and extending into the submucosa ("disproportionate inflammation").

The main features to look for in an endoscopic biopsy are granulomas, preservation of the goblet cell population, and maintenance of the architecture of the glands.[151] Serial sections may be necessary to demonstrate the granulomas, which are associated with the severity of the inflammation.[146,153,154,159] A rectal biopsy may be normal or show minor nonspecific changes.[148,152] As a matter of fact, a normal rectal biopsy in a definite case of colitis strongly favors Crohn's disease over ulcerative colitis.[148] If a colon involved by Crohn's disease contains diverticula, the inflammatory process often spreads to them.[145]

The ileum is involved in approximately 50% of the cases of Crohn's disease of the large bowel.[148] Anal lesions are seen in 75% of the cases and may present as chronic fissures, fistulas, and ulceration. They can be the first clinical manifestation of Crohn's disease and are recognized microscopically by the presence of granulomas.[138] These should not be confused with the foreign-body granulomas often seen in nonspecific anal fistulas. The regional lymph nodes are often enlarged. They do not differ significantly from those in patients with ulcerative colitis, except for the occasional presence of granulomas.[158]

One of the most common complications of Crohn's disease is the formation of fistulas, arising on the basis of fissuring. Although perianal fistulas can be seen in both Crohn's disease and ulcerative colitis, internal fistulas are virtually pathognomonic of the former.

Other complications of Crohn's disease include skin ulceration (of perianal skin, around colostomies and ileostomies, and elsewhere) and toxic megacolon.[139] In a series of 615 patients with Crohn's disease studied at the Cleveland Clinic,[137] the overall incidence of toxic megacolon was 4%. No cases were found when the disease was limited to the small bowel, but megacolon developed in 2% of the patients with ileocolic disease and in 11% when the disease was limited to the colon. It should be pointed out that if the bowel is removed at the time that a toxic megacolon has developed, it may be impossible to distinguish the nature of the underlying disease.[147] Specifically, the criterion of transmural inflammation as a differential diagnostic point loses its significance. Examination of biopsies taken during the quiescent phase may resolve the difficulty.[147]

The other important complication of Crohn's disease is the development of large bowel carcinoma. Although the incidence is much less than for ulcerative colitis, there is no doubt that the risk is substantially higher than for the normal population.[136,140,142] As in ulcerative colitis, the ma-

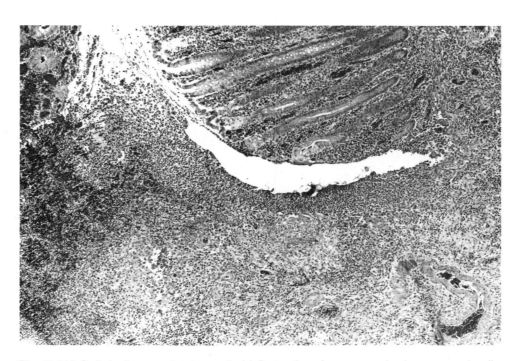

Fig. 11-114 Crohn's disease, showing marked inflammation of mucosa and submucosa and well-developed fissure ulcer.

lignancy can be difficult to identify grossly,[161] and it can also be accompanied and preceded by dysplastic changes of the colonic mucosa.[135,156,162] The criteria for the recognition and nomenclature of the dysplasia are the same in both conditions.[150]

Ischemic colitis

Ischemic colitis has been often confused in the past with Crohn's disease and ulcerative colitis. Most of the cases occur in patients past 50 years of age and the usual associations are arteriosclerosis, diabetes, and status postvascular surgery.[165] It has also been seen in younger patients in association with collagen-vascular disease (i.e. scleroderma and rheumatoid arthritis), Wegener's granulomatosis[166] and as a complication of birth control pills.[167] The process usually manifests itself by sudden onset of bleeding and abdominal pain. It is a segmental disease, the splenic flexure being the classic site of involvement due to its relative paucity of blood supply; however, other sites, including the rectum, can be involved. Morson[168] has described three morphologic variants: infarct, transient ischemia, and ischemic stricture. The last is more likely to be seen as a surgical specimen (Fig. 11-115). Roentgenographic, endoscopic, and intraoperative confusion with carcinoma may occur.[164] Grossly, pseudopolyps may be present in addition to the ulcerations and the fibrosis.[164] Microscopically, there is ulceration covered by granulation tissue, which extends into the submucosa and surrounds individual smooth muscle fibers of the muscularis mucosae. Hemosiderin is abundant. Hyaline thrombi can be seen in the lumen of small vessels. Fissures, lymphoid follicles, and granulomas are absent, but crypt abscesses may be seen.[163] Microscopic features suggestive of ischemia are the presence of a well-formed surface exudate of neutrophils and fibrin or mucosal necrosis in the acute stage, and of an increase of fibrous tissue in the lamina propria in the healed phase.

The main differential diagnosis is with Crohn's disease. Although the latter may be seen in any age group, it should be remembered that ischemic colitis is the most common form of colitis in the elderly.[163]

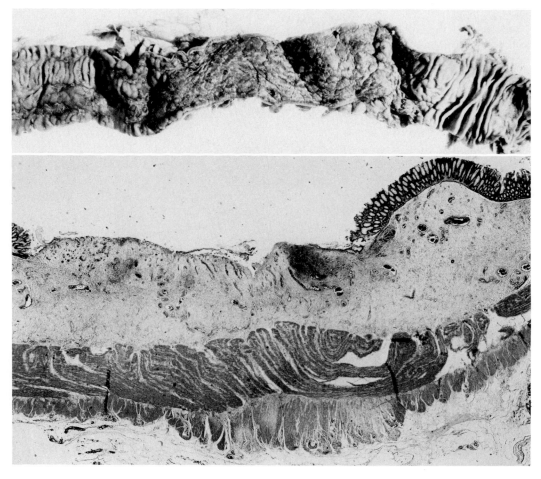

Fig. 11-115 Ischemic colitis involving portion of left colon in 70-year-old woman. **A,** Gross appearance of lesion. Note segmental nature and sharply circumscribed margins. **B,** Panoramic view of lesion, showing ulceration and marked vascularity of submucosa. (**A** and **B,** courtesy Dr. B. Morson, London, England.)

Other types of colitis

Nonspecific bacterial colitis (acute self-limited colitis; acute infectious-type colitis) is a self-limited diarrheal illness thought to be caused by infectious agents, particularly *Campylobacter, Salmonella,* and *Shigella;* however, in over half of the cases the etiology remains undetermined.[205] Microscopically, there is inflammatory infiltration of the lamina propria, edema, hyperemia, and hemorrhage; the changes may be indistinguishable from those of an early stage of ulcerative colitis,[172,220,221] so that a follow-up biopsy may be necessary to separate the two.[173] *Salmonella* and *Shigella* organisms are particularly well known for their capacity to simulate ulcerative colitis clinically and roentgenographically.[169] The microscopic appearance varies from nonspecific edematous and inflammatory changes to severe cases exhibiting crypt abscesses, extensive necrosis and hemorrhage, and microthrombi.[202] *Escherichia coli* has a tendency to cause acute hemorrhagic colitis,[171] with microscopic changes in the biopsy ranging from normal to those of an infectious-type colitis.[191] Acute inflammation out of proportion to chronic inflammation should suggest an infective etiology. Conversely, crypt distortion and plasma cell infiltration in the basal portion of the mucosa favor a diagnosis of ulcerative colitis.[198,217] The distinction between the two conditions is easier if the biopsy is taken within the first 4 days from the onset of symptoms.[183,205]

Allergic colitis and *proctitis* are related to foods (particularly cows' milk) and are seen more commonly in infants and children.[224] They present with rectal bleeding, sometimes accompanied by diarrhea. Biopsy shows a diffuse infiltration of the lamina propria and epithelium by eosinophils.[184]

Collagenous colitis presents clinically with chronic watery diarrhea and is characterized microscopically by collagen deposition beneath the surface epithelium, which shows evidence of focal or diffuse injury and infiltration by lymphocytes and other inflammatory cells.[187,222] Lymphocytes and neutrophils may be present in the crypts, and there is an increased number of inflammatory cells in the lamina propria. The basal lamina located over the thickened collagen is normal.[176] An immune pathogenesis has been postulated.[187] The clinical course is rather benign.[177,192] One case has been reported in association with colonic carcinoma.[181]

Pseudomembranous colitis is thought to be due in most cases to a toxin produced by *Clostridium difficile.*[182] A substantial number of cases have been associated with the use of the antibiotics lincomycin and clindamycin.[211] Florid cases of this condition are difficult to distinguish from ulcerative colitis and Crohn's disease on clinical and roentgenographic grounds.[203] Grossly, discrete yellow-white mucosal plaques are seen. The microscopic distinguishing feature is a "focal explosive mucosal lesion," characterized by the presence of a mushroom-like mass

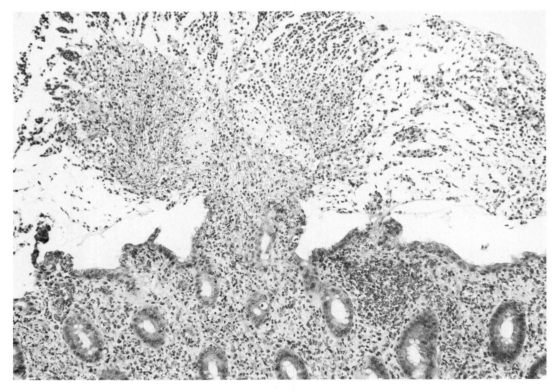

Fig. 11-116 Mucosal biopsy in pseudomembranous colitis due to clindamycin. Mushroomlike mass of mucus and neutrophils may be seen attached to mucosa, which is only slightly inflamed. (From Sumner HW, Tedesco FJ: Rectal biopsy in clindamycin-associated colitis. An analysis of 23 cases. Arch Pathol **99:**237-241, copyright 1975, American Medical Association.)

of mucus and neutrophils attached to the surface of the mucosal glands.[185,216] The mucosa immediately adjacent to these changes is remarkably normal (Fig. 11-116). The wall may show massive edema, probably due to vascular injury.[214]

Neonatal necrotizing enterocolitis is a condition primarily affecting infants who are either premature or who have had exchange transfusions.[193] A few cases have followed thrombosis of the abdominal aorta,[188,196] suggesting that ischemia is an important risk factor. The condition may also be seen as a complication of Hirschsprung's disease. Most cases begin in the first week of life and are manifested by abdominal distention, disappearance of bowel sounds, and passage of small amounts of blood-stained stool.[213,215]

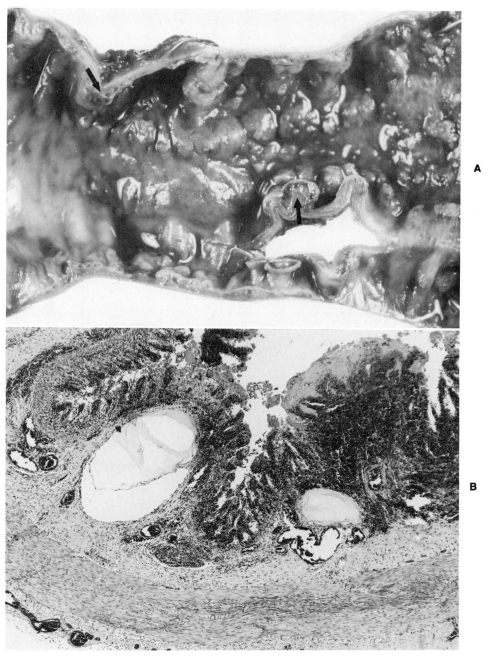

Fig. 11-117 Neonatal necrotizing enterocolitis. **A,** Gross appearance. Mucosa is necrotic and hemorrhagic. Numerous small gas-filled cysts are present (arrows). **B,** Microscopic appearance. There is extensive hemorrhagic infiltration of mucosa and loss of glandular epithelium. Two submucosal cysts can be seen.

The area of maximal involvement is the terminal ileum and ascending colon. The mucosa becomes necrotic and may partially slough off. Small submucosal gas-filled cysts are often present (Fig. 11-117); these can be seen roentgenographically, an important diagnostic sign.[209] Bowel perforation may occur. In these cases, resection of the perforated and necrotic bowel is indicated.[225]

Amebic colitis should always be considered in the differential diagnosis of inflammatory bowel disease. Clinically, it can closely simulate ulcerative colitis or Crohn's disease.[207] The classic sigmoidoscopic appearance is that of discrete areas of ulceration covered by exudate, with normal intervening mucosa; however, many cases depart from this description. Amebiasis may involve any part of the bowel, but it has a predilection for the cecum and ascending colon. In many cases the entire large bowel is involved, and there may even be extension into the terminal ileum.[170] Perforation occurs in 5% to 10% of the cases. The microscopic appearance of a rectal biopsy is rather nonspecific, although the relative paucity of inflammatory cells beneath the ulcer and the flask shape of the ulcer itself should alert the pathologist to the diagnosis. The confirmation rests on the identification of trophozoites of *Entamoeba histolytica*. They can be seen in hematoxylin-eosin slides, although the inexperienced observer may confuse them with macrophages (and vice versa). The PAS stain shows them particularly well.[201,208,210] They can also be demonstrated with immunoperoxidase techniques, both in sections and in smears.[194]

Tuberculosis may involve the gastrointestinal tract in the presence of minimal pulmonary disease.[174,190,206] The usual location is the ileocecal area, and a mass can be palpated in about half of the cases ("tuberculoma").[186] Grossly, there is ulceration with diffuse fibrosis extending through the wall, causing stenosis and obstruction (Fig. 11-118). Coexistent tuberculous peritonitis is seen in only a few of the cases. Microscopically, typical granulomas are usually present, accompanied by ulceration and extensive desmoplasia. The granulomas can be caseating, noncaseating, suppurative, or fibrous (healed).[179] In some instances, a nonspecific, diffuse, chronic inflammation with fibrosis without granulomas is seen focally or—very rarely—as the sole pattern.[179] Demonstration of acid-fast bacilli, either by stain of the sections or culture, is needed in order to establish a diagnosis. It

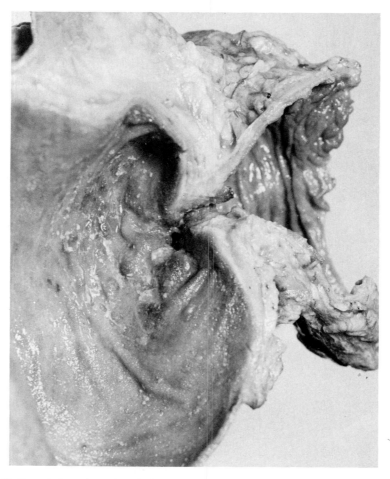

Fig. 11-118 Constricting tuberculous lesion at ileocecal valve occurring in young man. There was almost complete intestinal obstruction. Note extreme dilatation of small bowel on left with areas of tuberculous ulceration. After resection, patient completely recovered.

should be remembered that the large majority of cases of granulomatous disease of the ileocecal area seen in the United States and western Europe represent examples of Crohn's disease[199]; features favoring tuberculosis over Crohn's disease are caseation and coalescence of the granulomas.[219] Most patients with secondary ulcerating tuber-

culosis of the colon can be treated medically; surgery, sometimes in the form of ileocolectomy, is reserved for the large cecal tuberculomas.

Cytomegalovirus colitis is seen with increased frequency in immunocompromised patients, such as transplant recipients and individuals affected by AIDS.[195,204,218] The disease

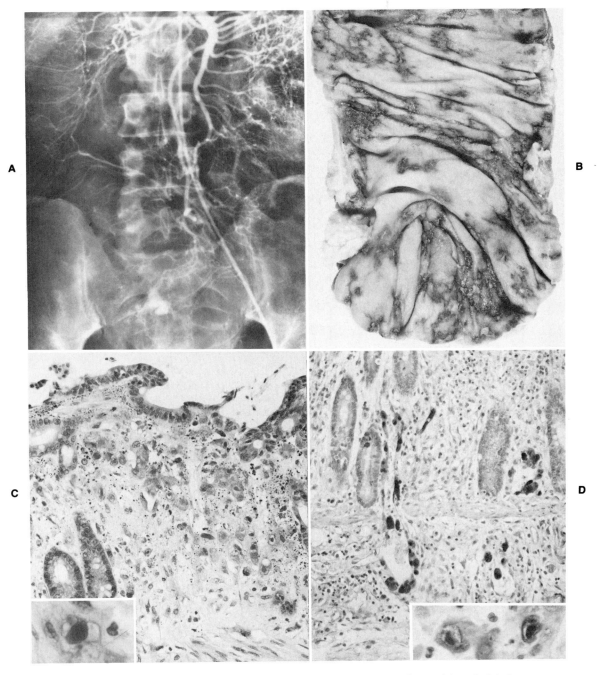

Fig. 11-119 Case of cytomegalovirus infection of large bowel in renal transplant recipient. **A,** Arteriogram showing site of bleeding in cecum. **B,** Gross appearance of resected specimen showing numerous superficial ulcerations. **C,** Microscopic section showing inflammation and erosions. **Inset** shows intranuclear inclusions. **D,** Immunoperoxidase stain for cytomegalovirus. Intranuclear and cytoplasmic stain may be seen in endothelial and epithelial cells. This is better appreciated in the high-power inset.

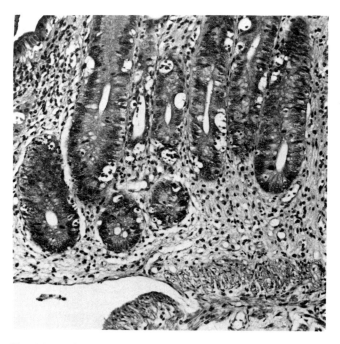

Fig. 11-120 Graft-versus-host disease. Rectal biopsy was taken at day 40 post-transplant. There is inflammation of stroma accompanied by proliferation of glands and individual cell necrosis at bottom of crypts. (Courtesy Dr. D. Snover, Minneapolis, MN.)

has a predilection for the ileocecal area and may be accompanied by extensive ulceration. Inclusion bodies are found mainly in cells located in the wall or lining the lumen of submucosal vessels showing features of vasculitis, but they may also be seen in fibroblasts and epithelial cells.[178] The diagnosis can be confirmed immunohistochemically[178] (Fig. 11-119 and Color plate 2, *D*). Surgical resection may be necessary in cases resulting in massive hemorrhage.

The colitis of *Behçet's syndrome* is characterized by multiple ulcers of various sizes, shapes, and depths involving any portion of the large bowel and is accompanied by lymphocytic vasculitis of the submucosal veins; it may resemble closely the appearance of Crohn's disease.[200]

Graft-versus-host disease, occurring in patients who have received bone marrow allografts, manifests in the gastrointestinal tract primarily as colitis. Microscopically, there is focal crypt epithelial cell degeneration ("apoptosis"), a feature that is thought to signify cell-mediated cytolysis[175,180,212] (Fig. 11-120). Crypt abscesses may also be present. Interestingly, similar changes are often seen in patients with AIDS, the pathogenesis being presumably related to immune rather than infectious factors.[197,223]

Several of the previously mentioned types of colitis may result in *toxic megacolon*, although the incidence of this complication is much less than in ulcerative colitis.[189]

OTHER NON-NEOPLASTIC LESIONS

Colonic atresia is much less common than in the small bowel; it is treated surgically with segmental resection and anastomosis.[252]

Heterotopic gastric epithelium may be rarely found in the rectum.[266]

Neuronal storage diseases of various types are accompanied by changes in the ganglion cells of the submucosal and myenteric plexuses, so that the condition may be diagnosed by rectal biopsy.[229,240,251]

Endometriosis may involve the wall of the large bowel, produce secondary smooth muscle hypertrophy, and result in almost complete obstruction[241,260] (Fig. 11-121). Microscopically, endometrial glands and stroma are seen surrounded by proliferated smooth muscle and clusters of hemosiderin-laden macrophages (Fig. 11-122). Occasionally, a carcinoma develops in these foci.[227]

Amyloidosis can be diagnosed in a rectal biopsy. In one series, a definitive diagnosis was possible in twenty-six of thirty patients.[236] These results are comparable to those obtained by renal biopsy and better than those from liver biopsy. It is important for the biopsy to include the submucosa, for this can be the only place of amyloid deposition.[242]

Volvulus of the large bowel is a rare cause of acute abdominal obstruction.[238] About 25% to 40% of the cases occur in the cecum.[247] Prompt surgical intervention is imperative. Gangrene will be found in approximately 25% of the cases at the time of exploration and is a definite indication for resection.

Malakoplakia can involve the colon diffusely[250,262] (Fig. 11-123). Most of the patients are adults, but cases in infants have been described.[257] Malakoplakia can occur as a complication of ulcerative colitis[244] and as a focal change in the stroma of adenomatous polyps (see p. 597).

Barium granulomas of the rectum and perirectal tissues can occur following barium enema. Barium escapes through a break in the mucosa produced by infection, tumor, foreign body, or trauma and provokes a granulomatous reaction. The crystals are easily visible under polarized light.[228]

Radiation changes in the colon and rectum can be accompanied by bizarre cellular changes in the epithelium of the crypts. Inflammation is also present, even with the formation of crypt abscesses; eosinophils may be numerous.[237,264] These acute changes usually subside within 1 to 2 months. Severe radiation changes include ulceration, necrosis, and hemorrhage.[253] In rare instances, glandular atypia develops, from which a postradiation adenocarcinoma may arise.[255]

Solitary cecal ulcers have an unknown etiology, and their microscopic appearance is nonspecific.[230,245]

Pneumatosis cystoides intestinalis occurring in infants is usually seen as a component of necrotizing enterocolitis and often has a fatal outcome.[265] A case in a child with cystic fibrosis has been reported.[267] In adults (mean age, 56 years), it may present as an idiopathic finding, or in association with mechanical intestinal obstruction or chronic lung disease.[258] When unassociated with other abnormalities, it follows a chronic and indolent clinical course, although in instances it may produce signs of intestinal obstruction and lead to an incorrect radiographic diagnosis of cancer. Grossly, polypoid grapelike masses formed by submucosal gas-filled cysts protrude through the mucosa (Fig. 11-124). Microscopically, the cysts are lined by multinucleated giant cells.[249] The overlying mucosa may show cryp-

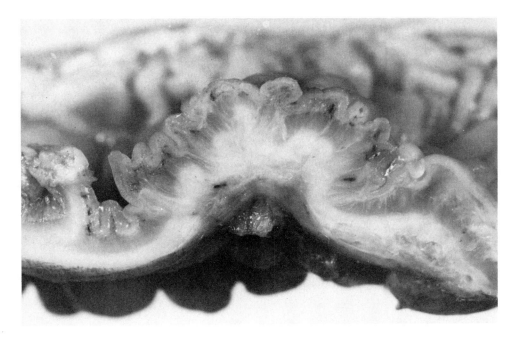

Fig. 11-121 Localized endometriosis of sigmoid producing partial obstruction.

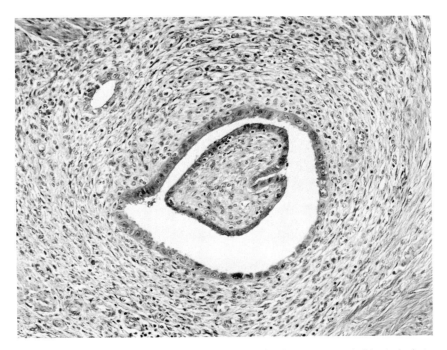

Fig. 11-122 Endometriosis of large bowel. Endometrial glands are surrounded by typical stroma.

titis, crypt abscesses, chronic inflammation, and granulomas.[248] It is believed that the gas is generated in the lumen or within inflamed crypts, from where it penetrates through the muscularis mucosa to accumulate in the form of submucosal cysts.[248] Some have suggested a lymphatic origin for the cysts, but this seems unlikely.[239]

It is possible that the peculiar condition described as *mucosal pseudolipomatosis* represents a lesion related to pneumatosis in which the gas-filled cysts are extremely small and limited to the lamina propria of the mucosa, resulting in an endoscopic appearance that simulates lipomatosis.[259]

Colitis cystica profunda is a non-neoplastic condition characterized by the presence of intramural mucus-containing cysts in the colon and rectum. It may present as a single polypoid mass or involve extensive areas of the bowel.[226,232] The localized form, also known as *hamartomatous inverted polyp*,[226] is typically located in the rectum, 5 to 12 cm from the anal margin. It presents as a plaque, nodule, or polyp and is associated with chronic proctitis.[263]

The diffuse form is in most cases the result of inflammation and ulceration of the bowel, as seen in ulcerative colitis, Crohn's disease, or irradiation change[246]; the ulcer-

ation provides the means by which mucosa can extend along granulation tracts and thus form lakes of mucus in the submucosa. This disease may be mistaken for a mucinous carcinoma of the rectum or rectosigmoid[256]; however, the mucin production in colitis cystica profunda is not accompanied by epithelial atypia and only rarely extends beyond the submucosa.

Solitary rectal ulcer (sometimes referred to as "solitary

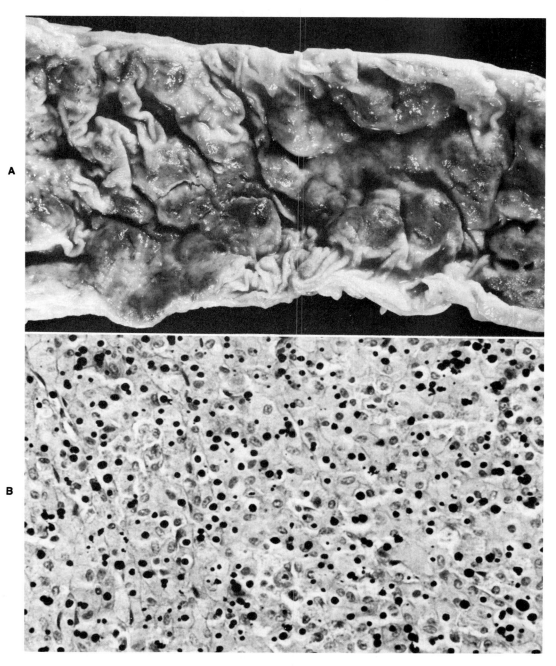

Fig. 11-123 Malakoplakia of colon. **A,** Gross photograph showing diffuse mucosal involvement and submucosal thickening. **B,** von Kossa's stain demonstrating innumerable Michaelis-Gutmann bodies among massive histiocytic infiltrate. (Courtesy Dr. J. Albores-Saavedra, Mexico City, Mexico.)

ulcer syndrome'' or benign idiopathic recurrent rectal ulceration [BIRRU]) presents as a solitary ulcerated or polypoid lesion located 4 to 18 cm from the anal margin, often in association with mucosal prolapse.[233,254] The usual symptoms are passage of blood and mucus per rectum, alteration in bowel habits, and pain.[233] Microscopically, there is a very superficial and irregular mucosal ulceration, hyperplasia of the crypts, a tendency towards villous configuration, obli-

teration of the lamina propria by fibroblasts and smooth muscle cells from the muscularis mucosae, reduction in the number of lymphocytes and plasma cells, and thickening of the muscularis mucosae with splaying of its fibers[234,254] (Fig. 11-125). In chronic cases, changes analogous to those of colitis cystica profunda may occur.[261] It is likely that the so-called *inflammatory cloacogenic polyp* is a further variation in the theme.[243] It has been proposed that solitary rectal

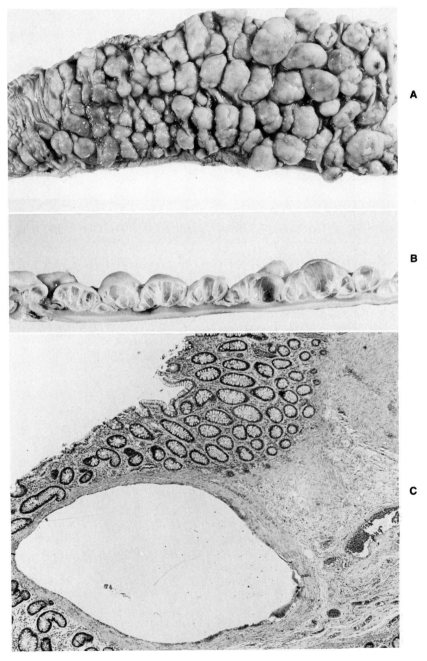

Fig. 11-124 A and **B,** Polypoid grapelike masses in pneumatosis cystoides intestinalis formed by submucosal gas-filled cysts. **C,** Biopsy showing one of these small cysts surrounded by granulomatous changes in stroma. (**A** to **C,** from Ramos AJ, Powers WE: Pneumatosis cystoides intestinalis. Report of a case. Am J Roentgenol Radium Ther Nucl Med **77**:678-683, 1957.)

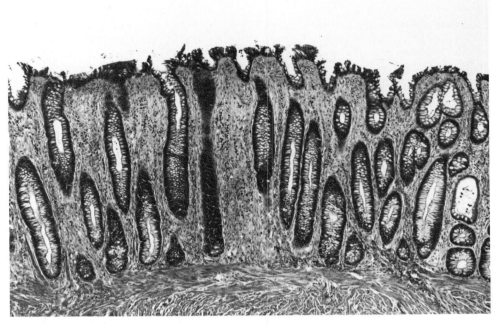

Fig. 11-125 So-called solitary rectal ulcer. There is lengthening of crypts, which are irregularly separated by inflamed and fibrous lamina propria. Surface epithelium has microvillous configuration. There is also mucin hypersecretion, with focal dilatation of glands.

ulcer is the result of the descending perineal syndrome in most cases, and the term *mucosal prolapse syndrome* has been suggested as a unifying concept for this and related disorders[231]; however, in some cases, there is no evidence of rectal prolapse.[235,254]

TUMORS
Epithelial polyps

The colorectal polyps included in this discussion are those of epithelial origin, which represent the large majority. They can be divided into five rather distinct categories, acknowledging the existence of transitional forms.[277]

Adenomatous polyps (tubular adenomas) are distributed rather regularly throughout the large bowel, with 40% found in the right colon, 40% in the left colon, and 20% in the rectum.[269,313] They are found at autopsy in about 30% to 35% of adult individuals, their frequency rising with age.[352] A familial predisposition has been detected and attributed to an inherited autosomal dominant gene for susceptibility.[276] Most are asymptomatic, but they may result in bleeding from twisting or vascular obstruction.[341] If large enough, they may cause changes in bowel habits or intussusception. Grossly, most measure under 1 cm in diameter. They may be sessile or pedunculated, have a short or a long stalk attached by a rather narrow base, and be single or multiple (Figs. 11-126 and 11-127). When multiple, they have a tendency to cluster.[287] Knob-like projections are frequently seen on the surface. Microscopically, there is an increase in the number of glands and cells per unit area as compared to the normal mucosa. The cells are crowded, contain enlarged hyperchromatic nuclei, and have an in-

creased number of mitoses.[301] Mucin production is highly variable but usually decreased. The basement membrane is not thickened. The changes first affect the superficial portion of the glands, a fact substantiated by in vivo incorporation of tritiated thymidine.[281] Obvious nuclear and cytoplasmic alterations, such as presence of abnormal secretory droplets, are evident at an electron microscopic level.[323] Immunohistochemically, CEA localization is seen, particularly in the highly atypical areas.[304]

Focal areas of villous configuration are not infrequent in adenomatous polyps.[293,344] Fung and Goldman[293] found them in 35% of sixty-seven polyps by careful examination of multiple sections taken with the guidance of a dissecting microscope. The incidence appeared to be related to the size of the polyp, reaching 76% in lesions larger than 1 cm in diameter. Polyps in which the adenomatous and villous components are present in approximately equal amounts are referred to as *villoglandular polyps, tubulovillous adenomas,* or *papillary adenomas;* the latter term should be avoided because of its possible confusion with villous adenoma.

The degree of atypia seen in adenomatous polyps is related to increasing age, number of polyps per patient, size of the polyps, and presence of villous changes.[313] It can be graded into mild, moderate, and severe; the latter is equivalent to carcinoma in situ.

Sometimes, clusters of atypical glands in an adenomatous or villoglandular polyp are seen beneath the muscularis mucosae and may lead to a mistaken diagnosis of malignant transformation.[295] This is not an uncommon event; as a matter of fact, it may be more prevalent than true malignant transformation of a polyp. The features that allow its rec-

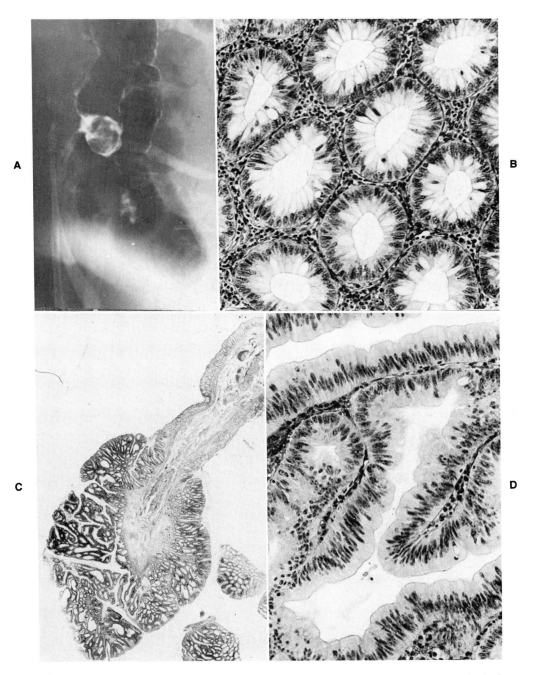

Fig. 11-126 A, Evacuation roentgenogram to demonstrate well-defined adenomatous polyp of splenic flexure. **B,** Cross section of glands in polyp shown in **A. C,** Adenomatous polyp shown in **A** demonstrating well-defined pedicle. There is no evidence of carcinoma. **D,** This section demonstrates deviation from normal glands with stratification of nuclei and beginning loss of nuclear polarity.

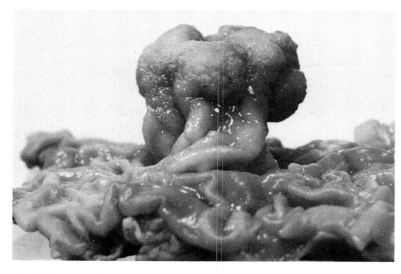

Fig. 11-127 Segmental resection of colon showing adenomatous polyp 2 cm in diameter.

ognition are the following[324]: (1) the cytologic features of the misplaced glands are similar to those in the surface; (2) the glands are surrounded by inflamed loose stroma and scattered bundles of muscularis mucosae, instead of the desmoplastic reaction associated with carcinoma; and (3) there are abundant hemosiderin granules around the neoplastic glands. Some of the glands may become cystic, rupture, and result in the formation of mucin lakes (Fig.

11-128). The overall appearance is reminiscent of, and probably pathogenetically analogous to, the localized form of colitis cystica profunda. Muto et al.[324] believe that this pseudocarcinomatous invasion is the result of repeated twisting of the stalk of the polyp.

Rarely, adenomatous polyps exhibit morular formation,[270,336] focal squamous metaplasia,[268] or a small component of Paneth cells and endocrine (Grimelius-positive)

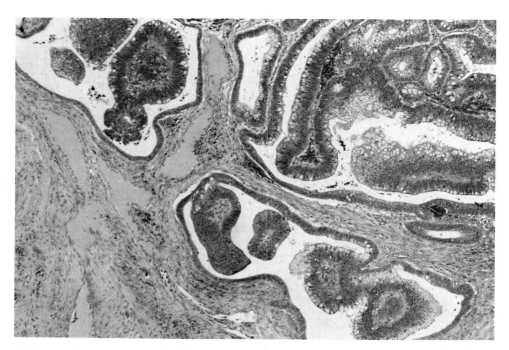

Fig. 11-128 Pseudoinvasion in adenomatous polyp. Irregular clusters of glands are seen, surrounded by hypertrophic bundles of muscularis mucosae. Clumps of hemosiderin-laden macrophages are present in stroma. These glands did not differ cytologically from those present in more superficial portion of polyp.

cells.[271] Even less frequent phenomena are the occurrence of focal malakoplakia in the stroma of the polyp[331] or the presence of metastases from another site within the polyp.[354]

The standard treatment for adenomatous and villoglandular polyps is polypectomy, followed by a repeated endoscopy 1 year later[314]; the incidence of development of new polyps in a group with a mean follow-up of 26 months was 30%.[326]

Familial polyposis of the large bowel (polyposis coli) must be segregated from the sporadic adenomatous polyps, despite the fact that the microscopic appearance of the individual lesions is indistinguishable by either light or electron microscopic criteria[285,299] (Figs. 11-129 to 11-132). This inherited defect is an autosomal mendelian dominant characteristic with a high degree of penetrance.[278,335] The responsible gene has been localized on chromosome 5.[273,315a] The tumors in familial polyposis become manifest much earlier than the usual adenomatous polyp, usually in the second decade of life.

Grossly, the bowel is studded with polyps ranging anywhere from very slight elevations of the normal mucosa to relatively large masses (Fig. 11-130). The presence of several adenomatous polyps in a patient does not necessarily indicate the presence of familial polyposis. A minimum of 100 polyps need to be present before such a diagnosis can be justified on morphologic grounds. Actually, in most examples of this condition the number of polyps is in the thousands. Microautoradiographic studies in patients with familial polyposis have shown persistence of DNA synthesis (as evidenced by the incorporation of tritiated thymidine) in the epithelial cells lining the polyps and also in the surface cells of the intervening flat mucosa.[286,317] Similarly, ornithine decarboxylase, an enzyme essential for intestinal mucosal proliferation, has been found to be elevated both in the polyps and intervening flat mucosa.[319]

Familial polyposis can involve other portions of the gastrointestinal tract, such as stomach (see earlier section on stomach) and small bowel.[330,355] It should be remembered, however, that most polypoid lesions of the ileum seen in patients with this disorder represent foci of lymphoid hyperplasia.[302,335]

If familial polyposis is left untreated, one or more carcinomas of the large bowel will develop in nearly every instance.[305] Malignant change is suggested by fixation or ulceration of the surface (Figs. 11-130 and 11-131). Carcinomas arising in a background of familial polyposis occur, on the average, some 20 years earlier than the ordinary colorectal cancers, most of them becoming manifest in the early thirties; therefore, prophylactic colectomy must be performed at 20 to 25 years of age, at the latest.[306] If the surgery performed is an abdominal colectomy with ileoproctostomy in order to preserve the anal function, a close monitoring of the rectal stump is indicated because of the possibility of development of polyps and carcinoma in it. Actually, the incidence of this complication is so high in some series (up to 59% of patients followed for 23 years after surgery) that some surgeons favor the initial performance of a proctocolectomy, if acceptable to the patient.[347]

Carcinomas developing in other organs, such as the gallbladder and adrenal gland, have also been reported in this disorder.[275,327]

Gardner's syndrome is a related familial condition in

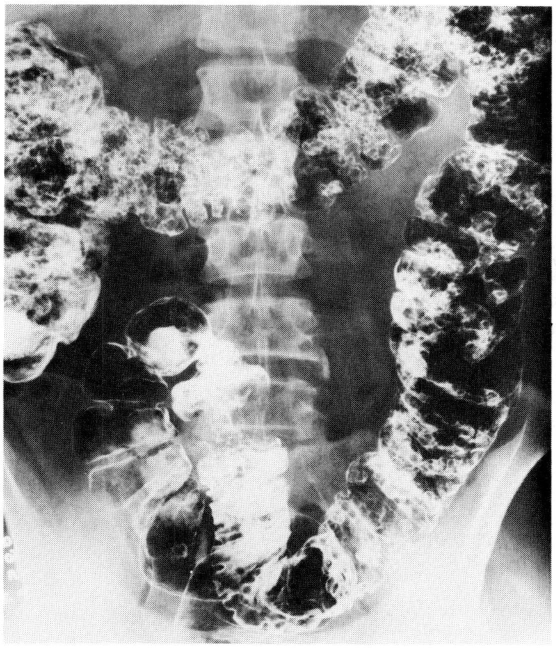

Fig. 11-129 Familial polyposis involving entire bowel.

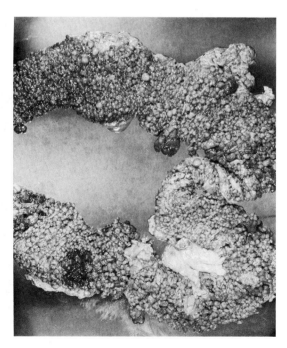

Fig. 11-130 Gross appearance of familial polyposis. There were four separate carcinomas present, but fortunately all 265 regional lymph nodes were negative.

which adenomatous polyps of the large bowel are seen associated with multiple osteomas of the skull and mandible, multiple keratinous cysts of the skin, and soft tissue neoplasms, especially fibromatosis.[294,339] Most of the fibromatoses are intra-abdominal and develop following surgical intervention. Because of the variable degree of penetrance, only one of the extracolonic manifestations may be present, such as fibromatosis.[308] Adenomatous polyps may also be present in the small bowel and stomach. The potential for development of large bowel cancer appears to be as high as for familial polyposis. In addition, patients with this syndrome can develop carcinomas of the small bowel, particularly in the periampullary area.[320] The recommended treatment for the colorectal component of Gardner's syndrome is similar to that of familial polyposis.[348]

Turcot's syndrome is the name given to the odd combination of colonic adenomatous polyps and brain tumors, usually of glioblastoma type.[288,316,338]

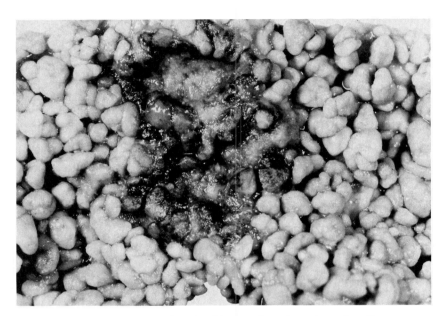

Fig. 11-131 Familial polyposis with area of carcinomatous ulceration.

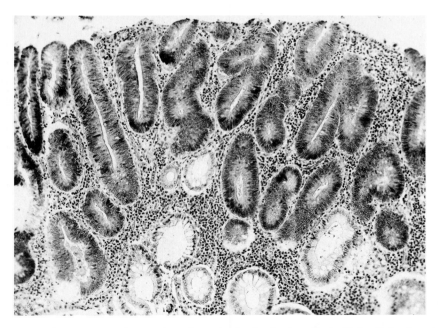

Fig. 11-132 Adenomatous changes in surface glands of polyp in patient with familial polyposis.

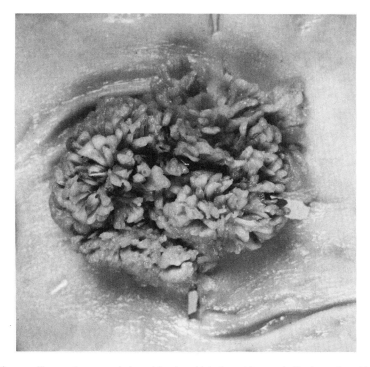

Fig. 11-133 Large villous adenoma of sigmoid colon. Note broad base of attachment and innumerable thin papillary projections.

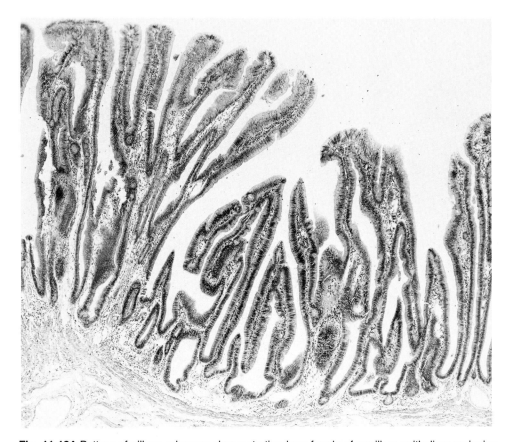

Fig. 11-134 Pattern of villous adenoma demonstrating long fronds of papillary epithelium springing directly from mucosal surface.

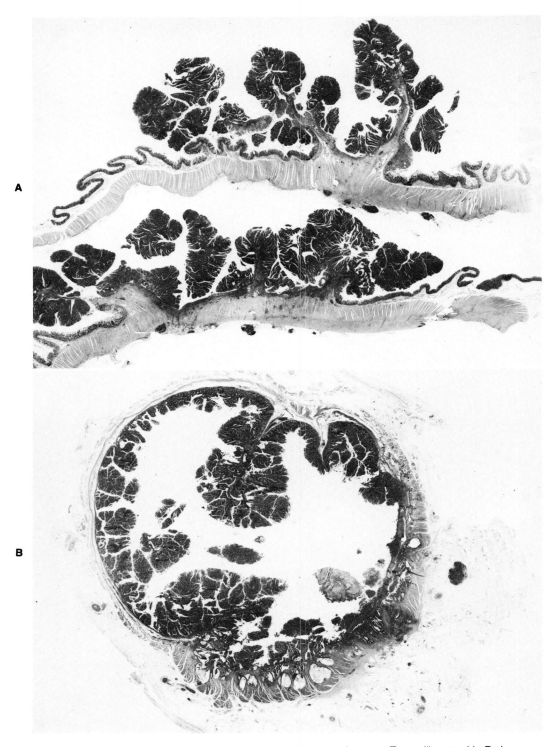

Fig. 11-135 Whole mount of two extensive villous adenomas of rectum. Tumor illustrated in **B** shows circumferential involvement of the mucosa and is associated with invasive mucinous carcinoma, see at lower part of specimen. (Courtesy Dr. C. Perez-Mesa, Columbia, MO.)

Other described associations are with hepatoblastoma[312] and multiple endocrine neoplasia.[328,337]

Villous adenoma (villous papilloma) is a distinctive, relatively infrequent type of polyp that in most cases presents as a single mass in the rectum or rectosigmoid of older patients, sometimes associated with fluid and electrolyte depletion.[342] With continuous growth the tumor may completely encircle the bowel. The consistency is so soft that the lesion can be missed completely on digital examination.[329] It has papillary villous projections and is usually attached by a wide base (Fig. 11-133), less than 10% of the cases being pedunculated; therefore, if a biopsy of a polypoid lesion having a definite stalk shows villous areas, the most likely diagnosis is that of villoglandular polyp. Microscopically, the villous projections ramify through a long, papillary, crown-like growth (Fig. 11-134). The pattern of mucin and CEA reactivity is similar to that seen in adenomatous polyps.[304] In time, a high percentage of these lesions become malignant (Fig. 11-135). The recorded incidence ranges from 29% to 70%.[270,349,350] On rectal palpation, the area of carcinoma has a firmer consistency than the surrounding adenoma; therefore, it is important to biopsy any indurated areas in villous adenomas. Local excision is the treatment of choice in the absence of cancer, but sometimes an abdominoperineal resection is needed because of the huge size of the lesion.[349]

Hyperplastic (metaplastic) polyps have often been misdiagnosed in the past as either normal mucosa or adenomatous polyps.[315] They are characteristically sessile and of small size, rarely exceeding 5 mm in diameter; however, they may be pedunculated and/or large, up to several centimeters.[289,353] If a careful gross examination of the colonic mucosa is made, hyperplastic polyps will be found in 30% to 50% of adult individuals.[280] Microscopically, elongated glands with intraluminal infoldings are seen, resulting in a sawtooth configuration (Fig. 11-136). The mitotic activity is increased only at the base, paralleling the pattern of the normal mucosa and in striking contrast with the behavior

of adenomatous polyps and villous adenomas.[351] Elsewhere, the epithelial cells have an inconspicuous basal nucleus and abundant cytoplasm filled with mucin. The basement membrane beneath the surface epithelium is thickened, a change that can be easily appreciated on hematoxylin-eosin-stained sections. The surface epithelium has a micropapillary appearance and is often infiltrated by "nuclear dust." Paneth's cells are present in about 8% of the cases. With increasing size, alterations in architecture and differentiation appear, accompanied by increased secretion of CEA, changes in blood group antigens expression,[282] reduced secretion of sialomucins,[307] and the appearance of focal adenomatous changes.[289,291] A variant of hyperplastic polyp, known as *inverted*, which is more frequent in the right colon, is characterized by an endophytic pattern of growth and penetration of the muscularis mucosae.[340]

Pure hyperplastic polyps do not become malignant; however, cancers have been found containing residual adenomatous and hyperplastic epithelium.[282a,345] Furthermore, in patients with the *multiple hyperplastic polyposis syndrome*, these polyps tend to be large and sometimes accompanied by adenocarcinoma.[272,353]

Juvenile (retention) polyp is the most frequent colonic polyp seen in children, but about one third of the cases occur in adults.[332] Traditionally, it has been described as single and located in the rectosigmoid area[300]; however, increased use of endoscopy has shown that in many cases there is more than one polyp present and that a high proportion of them occur proximal to the sigmoid colon.[283,321] The lesion usually presents with rectal bleeding; autoamputation is common, the polyp being sloughed off and passed per rectum.

Grossly, juvenile polyp has a granular, red surface, and a cystic, lattice-like appearance on cross section (Fig. 11-137, *A*). Microscopically, ulceration covered by granulation tissue is often seen at the surface. Beneath, there are cystically dilated glands filled with mucus, devoid of atypical features and separated by an inflamed and edematous stroma (Fig.

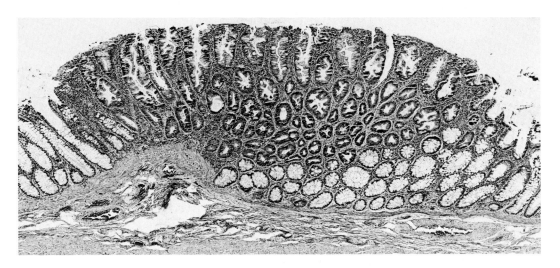

Fig. 11-136 Hyperplastic polyp of large bowel. Note maturation toward surface and serrated configuration of glands.

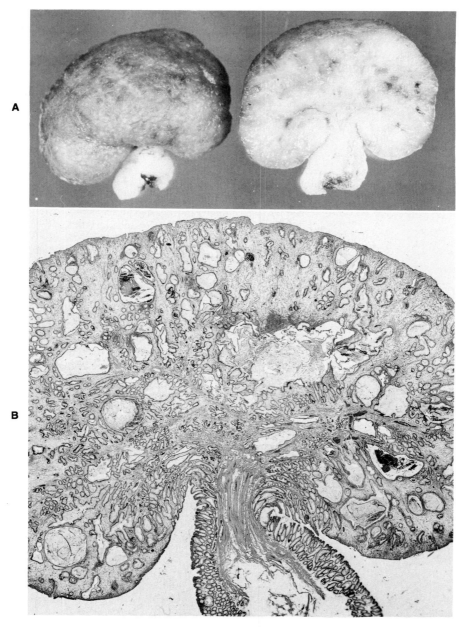

Fig. 11-137 Single juvenile polyp in child. **A,** Note cystic spaces. **B,** Same polyp with overproduction of mucus and surface ulceration. This type of polyp does not become malignant.

11-137, *B*). Hyperplastic mucosal changes are present in about 20% of the cases. It is unlikely that these lesions are true neoplasms,[290,303] although occasionally foci of severe atypia (carcinoma in situ) may be found in them.[309]

Rarely, multiple polyps of this type are seen throughout the bowel. This condition, known as *multiple juvenile polyposis,* can be life-threatening[298,346] and associated with the development of adenomatous polyps and adenocarcinoma of the large bowel, duodenum, stomach, or pancreas.* Some

of the polyps in this disorder have combined juvenile and adenomatous features.[292,322]

In *Cronkhite-Canada syndrome,* a nonhereditary disorder, multiple colorectal polyps of the juvenile type are associated with ectodermal changes (alopecia, nail atrophy, and hyperpigmentation).[284,311,334] In this condition, also, adenomatous changes and colorectal carcinoma may develop.[310] Another lesion with some morphologic resemblance to retention polyp (but mixed with elements of adenomatous polyp) is the *polypoid change* sometimes developing at the site of a ureterosigmoidostomy.

*See references 296, 297, 305, 318, 333, 343.

Peutz-Jeghers polyps are of hamartomatous type and have similar microscopic features to those seen in the small bowel. Lack of atypia, disorganization of glands, occurrence of several cell types (including Paneth cells), and the presence of smooth muscle fibers from the muscularis mucosae are the most important features. This pattern of glandular disorganization and epithelial misplacement simulating invasion should not be confused with malignancy[274,339a]; however, it should also be recognized that patients with this syndrome may also have adenomatous polyps with a marked degree of atypia and that some of these patients may develop colorectal adenocarcinoma.[325]

Cowden's syndrome (multiple hamartoma syndrome) is an autosomal dominant illness characterized by mucocutaneous stigmata (facial trichilemomas, acral keratoses, and oral mucosal papillomas), colorectal polyps, and an increased incidence of malignancy in various sites. The polyps have hamartomatous features, with disorganization and proliferation of the muscularis mucosae, but they differ microscopically from the polyps of Peutz-Jeghers syndrome.[279,299]

Transitional polyp is the name recently proposed for a small polypoid colorectal lesion characterized by elongated and widened crypts and enlarged goblet cells with increased mucin production[299a]; the appearance is similar to that often seen in the mucosa adjacent to carcinomas and other tumors.

Relationship with carcinoma and treatment

One can hardly think of a subject in tumor pathology that has been more controversial over the years than that of the precancerous nature of colorectal epithelial polyps.* Needless to say, the issue is a complex one. Yet, some basic and almost incontrovertible facts are known that provide us with guidelines to tackle the problem:

1 Solitary hyperplastic polyps (which represent the large majority of epithelial colonic polyps), retention polyps, and hamartomatous polyps do not become malignant or, if they do, the rate is negligible.

2 Patients with any type of polyposis syndrome are at an increased risk for the development of large bowel carcinoma. This incidence is extremely high (nearly 100%) in familial polyposis and Gardner's syndrome; it is lower, but still increased, in patients with Peutz-Jeghers' syndrome, juvenile polyposis, and hyperplastic polyposis. This is probably related to the fact that any of these polyposis syndromes can be accompanied by the development of adenomatous changes in some of the polyps.

3 Villous adenomas can become malignant, and they do so in a *high* proportion of cases (29% to 70%).

4 Adenomatous polyps *can* undergo malignant transformation. Every pathologist with experience has seen adenomatous polyps with focal cancer in them. This statement also applies to villoglandular polyps, which, for the purposes of this discussion, will be included with the adenomatous polyps.

5 *Not all* adenomatous polyps become malignant, at least not during the normal life span of an individual. If that were the case, and knowing the frequency of adeno-

matous polyps in the general population, the incidence of carcinoma should be at least twenty times higher than it actually is. Similarly, patients with familial colonic polyps (who have literally thousands of adenomatous polyps) who carry the disease in the large bowel for 20 or more years should develop not one or even several colorectal cancers but hundreds of them. The most important issue from a practical standpoint is trying to determine the likelihood of an adenomatous polyp becoming malignant during a reasonable life span. If we were to assume that all colorectal carcinomas arise on the basis of polyps (an assumption that has yet to be proved) and if we compare the rate of adenomatous polyps to carcinoma in the general population, we come up with a figure around 5%. Percentages lower than this are usually given in series that list the number of cases in which a focal carcinoma was found in an adenomatous polyp on pathologic examination, but this is understandable because these polyps are examined at only one point in time in their natural history. It also seems well established that the larger and more villous a polyp is, the greater the likelihood it will contain focal carcinoma.[375]

6 There is overwhelming evidence for a parallelism between adenomatous polyps and colonic cancer. Epidemiologic studies have shown that populations that have high incidence of polyps also have a high incidence of cancers and vice versa.[358,361,366] Large bowels with carcinomas have a higher incidence of polyps elsewhere in the specimen than those without carcinoma.[368] Adenomatous polyps are a good epidemiologic indicator of colon cancer risk. The morphologic, histochemical, immunochemical (CEA, blood group substances), flow cytometric, and ultrastructural features of adenocarcinomas and the most atypical areas of adenomatous polyps are extremely similar.* Furthermore, the adenoma-carcinoma sequence has also been shown with chemically induced colorectal tumors in animals.[377,382]

7 There is evidence suggesting that some colorectal cancers arise *de novo* rather than on the basis of preexisting polyps. Contrary to others,[369,385] it has been rare in our experience to find residual adenomatous epithelium at the edge of a carcinoma.[391] This has been the case even for extremely minute cancers (as small as 3 mm in diameter[390]) for which the interpretation that the malignant growth has totally overrun the polyp is hardly tenable. If anything, the existence of these cases seems to indicate that colonic cancers can arise from flat mucosa.[367,387] Furthermore, the distribution of polyps and carcinomas in the colon differ.[378] Finally, the incidence of carcinoma of the large bowel appears to be not significantly higher among patients with isolated small polyps when compared to those without polyps, although there seems to be a slightly increased incidence when the polyp is larger than 1 cm.[381]

8 It may be *impossible* grossly to distinguish an adenomatous polyp with or without focal carcinoma; there-

*See references 356, 360, 371, 383, 385, and 392.

*See references 357, 359, 364, 365, 389, 395, 399.

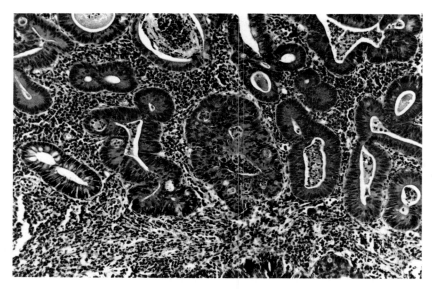

Fig. 11-138 Changes in tip of adenomatous polyp with morphologic features of carcinoma in situ. By convention, these changes are designated as severe dysplasia as long as they are restricted to lamina propria, as they are in this case.

fore, studies in which rectal polypoid lesions are cauterized under the assumption that they are adenomatous polyps may show that in so doing there is a decrease in the incidence of cancer in that population of patients, but such studies do not prove that such a goal is achieved by removing polyps; some of those lesions might have been small carcinomas.

These are the facts as we see them. Using this information, we can begin to address the main practical questions that arise in the management of patients with colonic polyps. First of all, there is no difficulty in the treatment of solitary juvenile polyps. Simple removal is sufficient. At the other extreme, since all untreated patients with familial polyposis eventually develop carcinoma of the colon, total colectomy is indicated even though the patient is young.[393]

Villous adenomas should be removed in toto, preferably in one piece. This allows a proper orientation of the specimen, so that in the presence of focal carcinoma the extent of the tumor can be assessed. This determination is of great importance in deciding whether further surgery is indicated.

The main difficulty resides in treating the patient with an isolated adenomatous polyp, although advent of the fiberoptic scope has revolutionized the approach to these lesions.[396-398] Since this technique has become available, the indication is that any polypoid lesion anywhere in the large bowel be removed as soon as it is detected, unless obvious contraindications exist.[375] This avoids the periodic roentgenographic examinations needed if the polyp is left in situ and the laparotomy that was once necessary to excise the proximally located lesions; however, it has not made things easier for the pathologist. The specimens obtained with this method are often fragmented and difficult to orient. When a focal cancer is present in a polyp, it may be impossible to decide whether invasion of the stalk has occurred. We have seen cases in which a small biopsy taken from the tip of a polypoid colonic lesion was correctly diagnosed microscopically as carcinoma, but examination of the subsequent colectomy specimen showed only an adenomatous polyp with focal carcinoma with a noninvolved stalk.

When several polyps are present, the patient can be safely managed by removing these polyps individually rather than performing a partial or total colectomy.

If a proximally located lesion is of large size, a small endoscopic biopsy may fail to detect the area of malignant transformation if present; therefore, such a lesion is best treated by anterior resection of a segment of bowel.

What should be the treatment for a patient in whom an area of carcinoma is found in an otherwise typical adenomatous polyp? In order to answer this question, one needs to realize that there are three distinct stages of the process that can be recognized pathologically and that bear a direct relationship to the therapeutic approach:

1 The cancerous glands may be present only in the mucosa and lamina propria above the muscularis mucosae ("carcinoma in situ") (Fig. 11-138)

2 They may extend beyond the muscularis mucosae but not invade the stalk of the polyp ("focal carcinoma") (Fig. 11-139, *A*)

3 They may extend to the base of the stalk or beyond ("focal carcinoma with stalk invasion"); in some of these cases, the tumor is seen to extend to the margin of resection, which is identified in a properly oriented specimen by the typical diathermy effect

The first situation, which is recognized by an architectural pattern of back-to-back glands with total loss of polarity and lack of intervening stroma, has *never* been found associated with lymph node metastases. This may be because

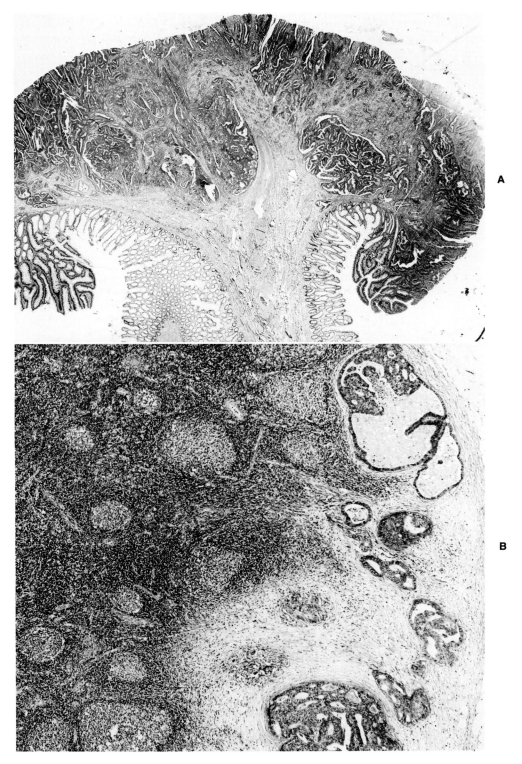

Fig. 11-139 Adenomatous polyp with focal invasive carcinoma. There is no tumor in stalk, yet regional lymph node in immediate vicinity of stalk showed partial replacement by tumor. This is an exceptionally rare occurrence. (**A** and **B,** courtesy Dr. F.T. Kraus, St. Louis, MO.)

the lamina propria of the large bowel—in contrast to that of the small bowel—seems to lack lymphatic vessels, although it has a rich capillary plexus.[370] It is obvious that under these circumstances, nothing other than a simple polypectomy needs to be done.[374] It is even questionable whether the diagnosis of carcinoma should be given at all under these circumstances. We prefer not to make such a diagnosis and simply designate these lesions as polyps with "severe atypia." Since every adenomatous polyp, by definition, shows some degree of atypia, we use the foregoing description *only* for those polyps that fulfill the morphologic criteria for carcinoma in situ.

The second situation ("focal carcinoma" with free stalk) can result in lymph node metastases[379,394] (Fig. 11-139, *B*), but the incidence is so low (less than 1%) that a simple polypectomy seems again the logical therapy for this lesion.[372,384] A possible exception to this approach is the rare lesion that is undifferentiated or is accompanied by obvious vascular invasion.[363,373,388]

Once invasion of the stalk has occurred (the third situation), the possibility of lymph node metastases, although still relatively low, is probably high enough to justify a formal bowel resection. This indication becomes more definite when the carcinoma is found in the submucosa of the underlying colonic wall and/or when it is present at the surgical margin.[376,380,386]

It is unlikely that total agreement in this field will be achieved in the near future. Indeed, articles appear periodically advocating a more aggressive surgical intervention, based on rather questionable figures.[362] In the meantime, we believe that following the rather conservative recommendations presented herein will help avoid subjecting patients with colorectal polyps to unnecessarily radical, costly, and potentially dangerous procedures.

Carcinoma
General features

Carcinoma of the large bowel is common in Northwest Europe, North America, and other Anglo-Saxon areas and low in Africa, Asia, and some parts of South America.[401,403] In the United States, it is by far the most common and most curable carcinoma of the gastrointestinal tract. There is some evidence of a further increase in its occurrence, particularly in young blacks.[410] Epidemiologic studies indicate that the incidence of colorectal cancer is closely related to environmental factors.[409] These factors are largely dietary, particularly in terms of fats and animal proteins and related to their influence on the intestinal microflora and ultimately on the chemical composition of the intraluminal content.[405] Specifically, there is a close association between beef consumption and the ingestion of large amounts of animal fat, and the incidence of bowel cancer; however, the issue is complex and the precise nature of the relationship is far from established.[416] The etiology of colorectal cancer may be multifactorial and not associated in a simple manner with dietary habits. For instance, it has recently been shown that about 20% of patients with sporadic colorectal carcinoma exhibit an allele loss in chromosome 5, a finding that correlates with the detection of the gene for familial polyposis in the same chromosome.[415] Furthermore, some cases of colorectal carcinoma not occurring in conjunction with familial polyposis show a definite hereditary pattern (Lynch syndrome).[407] This includes Torre-Muir syndrome, in which the colorectal tumor, often multiple, is associated with multiple sebaceous tumors and keratoacanthomas.[400]

The debated issue of the relationship between epithelial polyps and colorectal cancer has been already discussed. Patients with familial polyposis and with inflammatory bowel disease (particularly ulcerative colitis) have a definite predisposition to colorectal cancer, but they make up only a small percentage of the patients with bowel cancer in the general population. This is even truer for the other polyposis syndromes. A few cases of colorectal carcinomas have been reported as a late complication of pelvic irradiation, usually for carcinoma of the cervix.[402,412] Several cases of adenocarcinoma have been reported as arising at ureteral implantation sites.[413,414] Transitional cell carcinomas, undifferentiated carcinomas, and polyps of juvenile and/or adenomatous type can also occur at this juncture.[404,406,411] Interestingly, these changes are preceded by abnormal patterns of colonic mucin secretion.[408]

Diagnosis

Carcinomas of the large bowel may present with rectal bleeding, changes in bowel habits (such as diarrhea alternating with constipation), anemia resulting from chronic blood loss, and vague abdominal pain. Intestinal obstruction is common when the tumor is situated in the left colon and rare for tumors in the cecum or ascending colon. One out of four cecal carcinomas will present with signs suggestive of appendicitis (Fig. 11-140). Perforation may rarely occur, either at the site of the cancer or in the cecum as a result of distention caused by an obstructing rectosigmoid carcinoma. The endoscopic appearance is usually characteristic, but some inflammatory lesions may simulate cancer, and some undifferentiated carcinomas may have an innocent appearance.

Unfortunately, the previously mentioned symptoms are often indicative of advanced disease; therefore, many attempts have been made over the years to detect tumors at an earlier stage.[424] One such procedure is the performance of appropriately timed proctosigmoidoscopic examinations of both men and women over 40 years of age; such examinations should detect about 50% of the cases.[417,419] Whether routine examination of the entire large bowel with the fiberscope will prove rewarding as a screening method remains to be seen. Routine barium enemas are too expensive and not entirely without risk, although they are certainly indicated (preferably with air contrast) in any patient with symptoms. Guaiac stool examination for occult blood also has proved to be an efficient and inexpensive way of detecting cases of early, asymptomatic cancer.[418]

Another important advance has been the discovery of carcinoembryonic antigen (CEA), a glycocalix-related antigen that has been detected in the serum of 72% to 97% of patients with colorectal cancer.[422,426] It disappears after resection of the tumor and reappears in the event of recurrence or metastases. Higher values are found in tumors that have spread beyond the bowel wall, in poorly differentiated neoplasms, and in tumors associated with blood vessel,

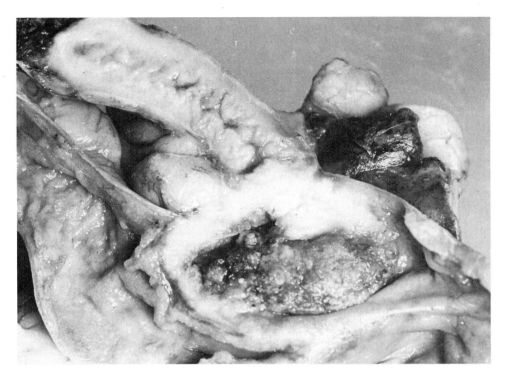

Fig. 11-140 Carcinoma blocking lumen of appendix, which caused symptoms and signs of obstructive appendicitis. At operation, large tumor mass was felt in region of cecum and ileocolectomy was done.

lymphatic, and perineural invasion.[425] Elevated circulating levels of CEA also have been described in carcinomas of the stomach, pancreas, breast, and prostate gland. Serum CEA is practically never elevated in normal individuals, but high values can be found in patients with chronic liver or renal disease.[425] Unfortunately, the test is often negative during the early stages of colorectal cancer and is therefore not a good screening procedure. Its main utility has been in the monitoring of therapy, in the early detection of metastases, and as an indicator for second-look surgery.[420]

CEA can also be detected in the tumor tissue by immunocytochemistry, radioimmunometric assay, or enzyme immunometric assay; its ability to discriminate between normal and carcinomatous tissue is higher than that of CA 19-9 and CA 125, two other recently described tumor-associated antigens.[421]

Biopsy. A positive biopsy should be obtained before radical surgery for colorectal carcinoma is undertaken. It is imperative that sufficient representative material be taken; small wisps of tissue are hardly adequate. In large lesions, it is advisable to perform several biopsies from diverse areas; those from the center may show only granulation tissue, and those from the very periphery may contain only hyperplastic colonic epithelium. Lesions below the peritoneal reflection should be removed *in toto* wherever possible to facilitate their orientation for section by the pathologist. Most adenocarcinomas are diagnosed easily, the main problems being presented by the better differentiated tumors and—paradoxically—the highly malignant signet ring car-

cinomas in which only a few tumor cells may be present. A sometimes more difficult (but just as critical) determination once the carcinoma has been recognized is to ascertain its position and extent. Obviously, the significance of the finding is markedly different if the fragment of tissue with adenocarcinoma was taken from the tip of a pedunculated polyp or from the side of a large ulcerated mass. Close communication with the endoscopist and surgeon, intact biopsy of an adequate size and depth, and proper orientation of the specimen are essential requisites for this determination.

Cytology. Cytology is unquestionably an effective way of diagnosing colorectal carcinoma but until now has proved of little practical value. Raskin and Pleticka[421a] studied eighty-seven patients with carcinoma and correctly identified the malignancy in seventy (80%); the incidence of false positives in 438 patients was 0.45%; however, the technique employed to obtain the specimen—which involves extensive cleansing of the colon followed by a diagnostic enema with manipulation of the patient—has led to an unenthusiastic response from clinicians.

Brush cytology can also be performed via the fiberopticscope, but whether this will improve the diagnostic yield over the conventional biopsy technique remains to be seen.[423]

Site and gross features

About 50% of all carcinomas occur in the rectosigmoid area, although their relative incidence seems to be decreasing.[431] Older patients have a relatively higher incidence of right-sided tumors.[433] Multicentric carcinomas are found in 3% to 6% of the cases.[429,430] Grossly, the typical tumor presents as a bulky mass with well-defined, rolled margins about an area of central ulceration. There is a sharp dividing line between the carcinoma and the normal bowel wall. In general, there is good correspondence between the gross and the microscopic margins. Retrograde intramural spread occurs in less than 5% of the cases.[427,432] On cross section, grayish white tissue is seen replacing the bowel wall. The edges may be well-demarcated or with finger-like projections extending from the main mass. Highly mucinous tumors have a gelatinous, glaring appearance, and layers of mucus may separate the layers of bowel wall.

Important features to evaluate at the time of gross inspection are whether the tumor is confined to the wall or whether it has extended to the pericolic tissues, whether gross invasion of veins is present,[428] and whether the remainder of the colon shows other carcinomas or polyps of any type.

Microscopic features

The usual carcinoma of the large bowel is a well to moderately differentiated adenocarcinoma secreting variable amounts of mucin. The cells represent a combination of columnar and goblet cells, with occasional participation of endocrine cells (see p. 611) and the exceptional occurrence of Paneth cells.[480] The carcinoma consistently elicits an inflammatory and desmoplastic reaction, which is particularly prominent at the edge of the tumor. Most of the inflammatory cells are T lymphocytes.[463] The tumor may be seen invading all the layers of the bowel and extending into the pericolic fat, permeating perineurial spaces, and invading veins. The latter feature, which is of prognostic significance, can be better appreciated with stains for elastic fibers (Verhoeff–van Giesen) or for smooth muscle actin (with immunohistochemical techniques). Rarely, the tumor stroma may exhibit metaplastic bone formation.[449]

The edge of the tumor may show foci of a residual polyp, but this has been an unusual finding in our experience. It is more common to see at this site a hyperplastic change

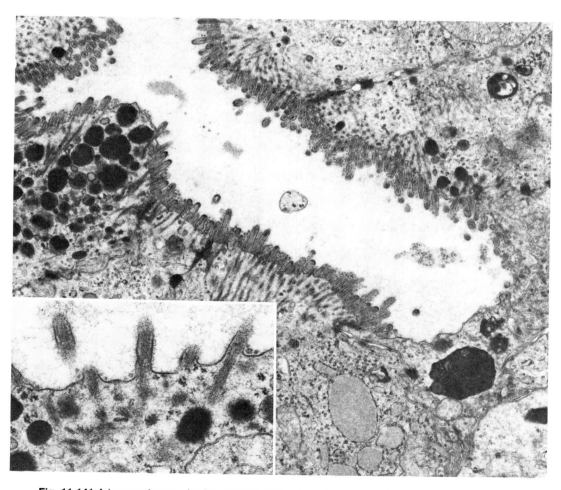

Fig. 11-141 Adenocarcinoma of colon with true lumen formation and mucin secretory product. Prominent collections of microfilaments that are related to brush border are characteristic of adenocarcinoma of colon and intestinal-type cancers of other organs. **Inset,** Microfilaments entering border and mucin secretory product. (×11,230; **inset** ×25,270.)

in the glands, which appear taller, more tortuous, and with more goblet cells than the normal mucosa.[476] This change, which is accompanied by histochemically detectable alterations in mucin secretion, has been referred to as *transitional mucosa*.[447,467] This is probably a reactive change, inasmuch as it can also occur at the edge of other tumors and non-neoplastic lesions, including anastomotic sites.[451,464,468,483]

Histochemically, the large majority of colorectal carcinomas are positive for mucin stains. Culling et al.[446] have devised a modification of the PAS technique that preferentially stains mucin of the lower intestinal tract. The stain is usually negative in adenocarcinomas of other sites, but unfortunately it will also stain tumors of intestinal type in those locations, thus diminishing its diagnostic utility.

Immunohistochemically, colorectal adenocarcinomas al-

ways show positivity for keratin.[448] Reactivity for CEA is also the rule; as a matter of fact, failure to demonstrate CEA in an adenocarcinoma makes it unlikely that the tumor is primary in the large bowel.[472] The positivity is equally distributed throughout the cell surface, as opposed to the polar distribution seen in normal mucosa and in the better differentiated tumors.[434,457] There is good correlation of the immunohistologic pattern with the serum levels but not with tumor staging or degree of differentiation.[453,469,475] A high percentage of colorectal carcinomas have shown immunohistochemical reactivity for HCG[440,455]; this seems particularly common in mucinous and poorly differentiated tumors.[440] Carcinomas of the large bowel often show loss of blood group isoantigens and of HLA-A, B, and C expression, particularly if poorly differentiated.[450,471] Correspondingly, these tumors acquire reactivity for blood group sub-

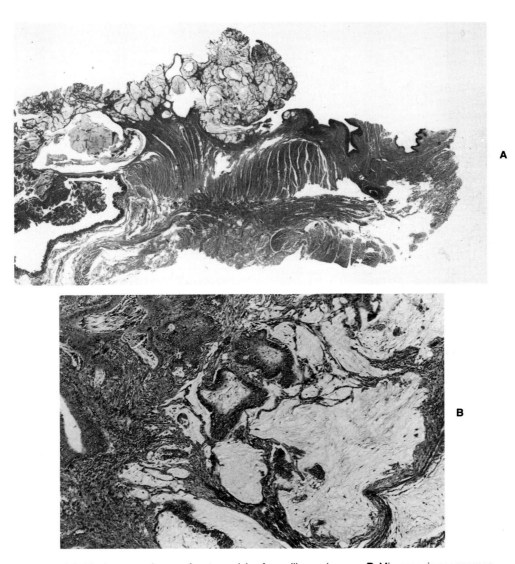

Fig. 11-142 A, Mucinous carcinoma of rectum arising from villous adenoma. **B,** Microscopic appearance of mucinous carcinoma. Well-differentiated neoplastic glands are seen associated with formation of large lakes of mucin surrounded by reactive fibrous tissue. (Courtesy Dr. C. Perez-Mesa, Columbia, MO.)

stance H.[443,478] Immunoreactivity for the secretory component of immunoglobulin is seen in about half of the cases and is particularly strong in the well-differentiated tumors.[437] Another tumor-associated antigen, designated as LEA (large external antigen), has been identified in the tumor tissue and sera of colorectal cancer cases; this may prove to be as useful as CEA for the monitoring of this malignancy.[439] Yet

another marker has been recently described in colorectal carcinoma. This is *ras* oncogene p21, as detected immunocytochemically in cytologic preparations.[446a]

Ultrastructurally, a constant feature of colorectal carcinoma is the presence of prominent collections of microfilaments running perpendicular to the cell membrane and entering the brush border[461] (Fig. 11-141).[461] This feature,

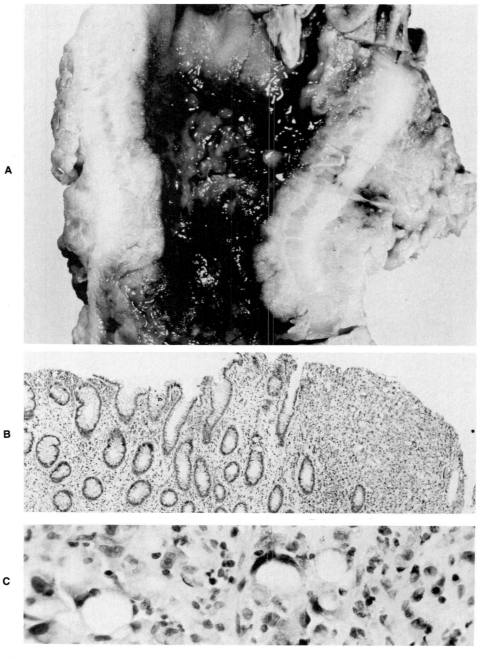

Fig. 11-143 Signet-ring carcinoma. **A,** This type is highly malignant, narrows lumen, and has pebbly mucosal surface and thickened muscular wall. **B,** Biopsy of carcinoma in **A** showing small area effacing glands. **C,** Area of biopsy showing signet-ring tumor cells. There were many lymph nodes involved in surgical specimen.

although helpful, is not diagnostic. We have also seen it in intestinal-type carcinomas of the stomach, small bowel, gallbladder, and pancreas.

Other microscopic types

Mucinous carcinoma is a special type of colorectal carcinoma in which large lakes of extracellular mucin are formed, mixed with collections of tumor cells[477] (Fig. 11-142). Some intracellular mucin may also be present. These tumors comprise 15% of colorectal carcinomas and occur most commonly in the rectum. In a series of 132 cases reported by Symonds and Vickery,[484] 31% were associated with villous adenomas, 7% with ulcerative colitis, 8% with colitis, and 5% with prior pelvic irradiation. Mucinous carcinomas are also more frequently associated with adenomas elsewhere in the colorectum than are conventional adenocarcinomas.[482] Their prognosis is somewhat worse than for the conventional type of adenocarcinoma, at least when located in the rectum.[470a,484]

Signet ring carcinoma (linitis plastica–type carcinoma) is a rare form of colorectal malignancy that usually affects young patients. Like its more common gastric counterpart, it usually presents grossly as a diffuse infiltration of the wall,[452,466] although it has also been described arising in an adenomatous polyp.[457a] Microscopically, the tumor grows in a diffuse fashion, with little if any glandular formation[435] (Fig. 11-143). Most or all of the mucin is intracellular, in contrast to the pattern seen in mucinous carcinoma. This intracellular accumulation of mucin results in displacement of the nucleus and a typical signet ring configuration of the cells. Metastases tend to develop in lymph nodes, the peritoneal surface, and the ovary rather than the liver. The prognosis is extremely poor.[436] The possibility of the colorectal lesion representing a metastasis from a gastric primary lesion should always be investigated before making a diagnosis of primary signet ring carcinoma.[438]

Squamous differentiation may be present in colorectal carcinoma; this is more common in cecal neoplasms but may be seen in any other area of the large bowel[445,462] (Fig. 11-144). In most instances, the squamous component is associated with glandular elements (adenosquamous carcinoma), but occasionally it is seen in a pure form (squamous cell carcinoma). One such case developed in a duplication of the colon,[460] and another led to hypercalcemia through the production of a parathyroid-like substance.[441] An association has been noted between squamous changes in colorectal carcinoma and ulcerative colitis.[446] It has been postulated that some of these squamous tumors may arise from areas of squamous differentiation in pre-existing adenomatous polyps.[487] For the squamous tumors located in the low rectum, the alternative possibility of upward extension or submucosal metastasis from a carcinoma of the anal canal should be considered.

Clear cell change can occur in the neoplastic epithelium as a result of glycogen accumulation.[464a]

Basaloid (cloacogenic) carcinoma, similar to its anal counterpart, has been reported on a few occasions in the colorectum, presumably developing on a metaplastic basis.[456]

Choriocarcinomatous differentiation can occur focally in colorectal adenocarcinoma, as it does in tumors of stom-

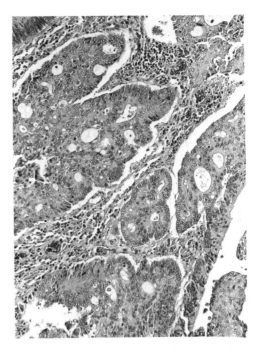

Fig. 11-144 Adenosquamous carcinoma of large bowel. Tumors with this appearance are more common in cecum than in other portions of colon.

ach and gallbladder.[465] HCG can be demonstrated immunohistochemically in the tumor cells.[474] Occasionally, the entire tumor has the appearance of a choriocarcinoma.[473] This phenomenon should be distinguished from the more common finding of HCG positivity in morphologically conventional adenocarcinomas (see p. 609).

Endocrine differentiation may manifest itself in a variety of ways, as it does elsewhere in the gastrointestinal tract. One manifestation is the presence of scattered endocrine cells in otherwise typical adenocarcinomas (particularly of the mucinous type), a feature that does not influence the prognosis or natural history of these tumors.[481,485] Another is in the form of tumors with a mixed composition, in which typical adenocarcinoma intermingles with a component exhibiting clearcut endocrine differentiation.[458,459] The existence of these tumors is explained by postulating an origin from endodermally derived multipotential cells located at the base of the crypts, which during the course of neoplastic transformation undergo differentiation along several different pathways.[444] Still another manifestation of endocrine differentiation is in the form of *small cell carcinoma,* a tumor having a microscopic appearance similar to that of its pulmonary homonym.[442] Electron microscopy usually reveals a few dense-core secretory granules in the cytoplasm, and immunohistochemical techniques may show positivity for neuron-specific enolase and other endocrine markers.[486] The entire tumor may have this appearance, or there may be foci of glandular differentiation, with or without mucin production.[454] Some of these small cell carcinomas arise on the basis of an adenoma, usually of villous type.[470] The prognosis is poor, with early metastases to lymph nodes and liver.[479]

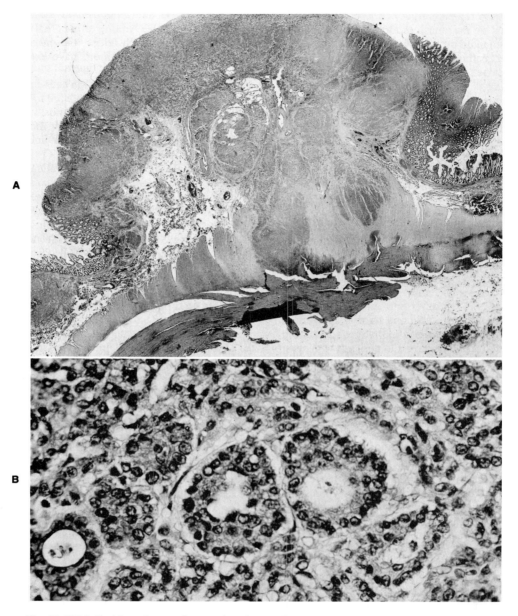

Fig. 11-145 A, Small carcinoma of rectum found on routine rectal examination. There were mestastases to many nodes, with blood vessel and nerve sheath invasion. **B,** Same lesion demonstrating poorly differentiated adenocarcinoma.

with colorectal carcinoma, whether one uses the original scheme or any of the modifications that have been subsequently proposed.[539] The 5-year survival rates are 90% or higher for Dukes' A, 50% to 65% for Dukes' B, and 15% to 25% for Dukes' C.[531,544]

15 *Pattern of lymph node reaction.* It has been shown that patients with colorectal cancer in whom the regional lymph nodes show morphologic evidence of a cell-mediated immune response (manifested by an increased number of paracortical immunoblasts and/or sinus histiocytosis) survive longer than those patients whose nodes do not show these changes.[527]

16 *DNA ploidy.* Flow cytometric determinations have been found to relate to the Dukes' stage and microscopic grade of differentiation.[514,534,541] The tumors are rather homogeneous in their DNA pattern; therefore, this technique is likely to prove of prognostic utility. Determination of S-phase fractions has shown a relation with survival rate in one study[509] but not in another.[521]

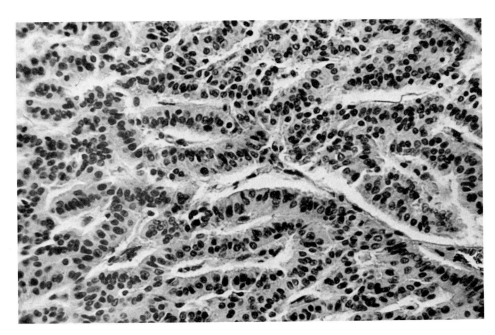

Fig. 11-146 Carcinoid tumor of rectum. Note typical pattern of festoons and ribbons.

17 *Oncogene expression.* Preliminary studies suggest that the expression of the c-myc oncogene is related to the degree of differentiation of the tumor[536]; therefore, the potential exists for this technique to be useful in determining prognosis.

Carcinoid tumor

Carcinoid tumors can occur in any portion of the large bowel but are more common in the rectum.[551] Those located in the colon tend to be large, to extend deeply through the wall of the bowel, and to involve the regional lymph nodes. In the rectum, they are often located in the anterior or lateral wall. Their shape is rounded, and ulceration is usually lacking. Of the 147 cases of rectal carcinoid examined by Caldarola et al.,[548] 105 measured less than 0.5 cm in diameter. Only three were associated with lymph node metastases, and all of these were larger than 2 cm in diameter. Multicentricity, a common finding in small bowel carcinoid tumors, is seen only exceptionally in rectal carcinoids.[553a] Rectal carcinoids have been reported in bowels affected by ulcerative colitis[550] and in association with ovarian carcinoid.[564] These tumors are practically never associated with the carcinoid syndrome. Grossly, their most distinctive feature is the yellow color that they acquire after formalin fixation. Microscopically, invasion of the stroma by small uniform cells growing in a ribbon or festoon fashion is seen[560] (Fig. 11-146). Argentaffin and argyrophil reactions are said to be usually negative,[547] but consistently positive results with the use of the Grimelius stain have been reported by several authors[552,558]; in addition, several examples of argentaffin rectal carcinoid tumors are on record.[565] Immunocytochemically, they stain for the pan-endocrine markers (neuron-specific enolase, chromogranin, synaptophysin), and for a variety of peptide hormones. Somatostatin, glucagon, substance P, and peptide YY are the ones most commonly represented, but gastrin/colecystokinin, calcitonin, and pancreatic polypeptide have also been demonstrated in some cases.[555,557,558,562,563] Many of the tumors are polyhormonal.[555] The presence of peptide YY is of particular interest because of its usual absence in carcinoid tumors of other sites.[553,557] Rectal carcinoid tumors have also been found often to exhibit immunoreactivity for human chorionic gonadotropin[549] and prostatic acid phosphatase.[559] The latter, whether real or the result of a cross-reaction, is of practical importance because metastatic prostatic carcinoma may enter in the differential diagnosis with carcinoid tumor; the distinction is made because the latter is consistently negative for prostatic specific antigen.[559]

Rectal carcinoid tumors smaller than 2 cm and limited to the mucosa or submucosa are best treated by local excision; those of larger size and/or exhibiting invasion of the muscularis externa need radical surgery, in view of their propensity for lymph node involvement.[548,554,556]

Malignant lymphoma and other lymphoid lesions

Malignant lymphomas are less frequently found in the large bowel or stomach, but they can occur at any level of the colorectum.[573] They may produce prominent mucosal folds, prominent ulceration, a large mass, or multiple small polyps distributed throughout the colorectum that also extend to the small bowel ("lymphomatous polyposis"[569]). The regional lymph nodes are involved in about half of the cases. These tumors are nearly always of non-Hodgkin's type, the large cell and small cleaved types being the predominant varieties. A few of these cases have been seen in renal transplant recipients and in patients with ulcerative colitis.[570,572] Some tumors show widespread plasmacytic differentiation with abundant immunoglobulin production and may be accompanied by amyloid deposition; these have been designated as *plasmacytomas*.[567,572a]

Lymphoid polyps of benign (reactive) nature are sometimes found in the rectal area.[571] They have also been designated as *lymphoid hyperplasia, pseudolymphoma,* and *rectal tonsil*. They appear as soft, superficial polyps usually covered by an intact, gray, smooth mucosa. The patient may complain of a mass, bleeding, or prolapse. In Helwig and Hanson's series,[568] forty were single and twenty-five were multiple. Microscopically, these lesions are located in the submucosa and are made up of lymphoid tissue with follicle formation, a lobular pattern, and germinal centers. They may distort the muscularis mucosae and even involve the muscularis externa.[566] At superficial or small biopsy they can be incorrectly diagnosed as malignant lymphoma. Local excision is curative.

Other tumors and tumorlike conditions

Vascular ectasias of the right colon are being increasingly recognized as an important cause of lower intestinal bleeding in the elderly. They have also been designated as angiomas, angiodysplasias, and arteriovenous malformations, these various names reflecting the uncertainty about their nature.[584] An acquired pathogenesis seems likely for most cases. They have been reported in association with aortic stenosis[593] and von Willebrand disease[578] and are sometimes found to contain cholesterol emboli. The lesions are often small, multiple, and easily demonstrated by arteriography but may be difficult to identify in a colonic biopsy or after they have collapsed following colectomy[591]; injection with a silicone rubber compound followed by clearing of the specimen shows them dramatically[575,586] (Fig. 11-147). These lesions should be distinguished from the *colonic varices* that may be seen as a complication of portal hypertension.[592]

Lipomas of the large bowel are rare; they are invariably submucosal and therefore may intussuscept[581] (Figs. 11-148 and 11-149). Some may exhibit atypical stomal cells and simulate malignancy. *Lipomatosis* (Fig. 11-150) of the ileocecal valve or other portions of the colon may be mistaken radiographically for a tumor.[576,597]

Smooth muscle tumors are usually located in the rectum, where they tend to be small and benign. Those situated higher up in the colon have a higher incidence of malignancy.[574,582,587,588]

Diffuse ganglioneuromatosis can occur in association with Recklinghausen's disease, multiple endocrine adenomatosis type IIB (III), or in the absence of either condition.[577] Most of these cases appear to arise from the neural plexuses in the bowel wall, but others with a predominantly mucosal distribution have been reported, sometimes in association with retention polyps, adenomatous polyps, and/or adenocarcinoma.[583,590,595]

Kaposi's sarcoma can involve the colon; occasionally, the disease may initially present with intestinal symptoms

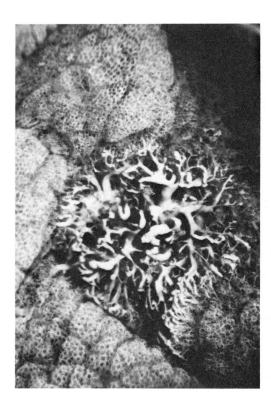

Fig. 11-147 Angiodysplasia of colonic mucosa demonstrated by silicone rubber injection and clearing of specimen. (Reprinted, by permission, from Case Records of the Massachusetts General Hospital—Weekly Clinicopathological Exercises: Case 36-1974. N Engl J Med **291**:569-575, 1974.)

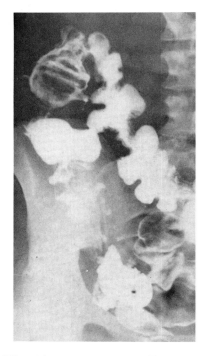

Fig. 11-148 Filling defect caused by lipoma. The appearance is highly characteristic.

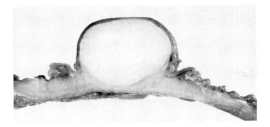

Fig. 11-149 Submucosal lipoma of sigmoid colon. Tumor is soft, yellow, and sharply circumscribed.

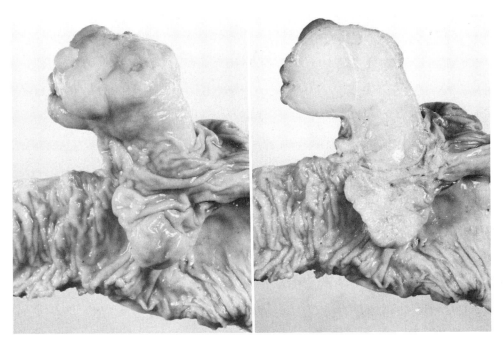

Fig. 11-150 External and cut surface of lipomatosis of ileocecal valve. Tumorlike mass of mature fat forms polypoid mass covered by normal mucosa. Ileum is on left side.

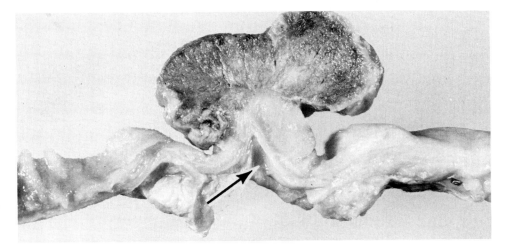

Fig. 11-151 Polypoid lesion of ileocecal area. Surface of lesion represents metastatic renal cell carcinoma, and base (arrow) represents primary carcinoid tumor.

and simulate the appearance of ulcerative colitis, particularly in AIDS patients.[589,594]

Other unusual types of reported primary tumors of the large bowel include *xanthogranuloma*,[585] *carcinosarcoma*,[596] and a neoplasm morphologically identical to *giant cell tumor* of bone or soft tissues.[579]

Metastatic malignant tumors occur as a part of a disseminated process. These tumors form disk-like areas in which there is a central area of ulceration; the normal mucosa extends to the ulcer, giving indirect evidence that the metastatic focus began in the submucosa. This phenomenon is particularly common in malignant melanoma and primary carcinoma of the lung. Our most exotic case was the metastasis of a renal cell carcinoma to an intestinal carcinoid tumor, simulating grossly an adenomatous polyp (Fig. 11-151). Prostatic carcinoma can extend into the rectum and simulate a primary rectal neoplasm.[580]

REFERENCES
HIRSCHSPRUNG'S DISEASE AND RELATED DISORDERS

1. Aldridge RT, Campbell PE: Ganglion cell distribution in the normal rectum and anal canal. A basis for the diagnosis of Hirschsprung's disease by anorectal biopsy. J Pediatr Surg 3:475-490, 1968.
2. Ariel I, Vinograd I, Lernau OZ, Nissan S, Rosenmann E: Rectal mucosal biopsy in aganglionosis and allied conditions. Hum Pathol 14:991-995, 1983.
3. Barr LC, Booth J, Filipe MI, Lawson JON: Clinical evaluation of the histochemical diagnosis of Hirschsprung's disease. Gut 26:393-399, 1985.
4. Bishop AE, Polak JM, Lake BD, Bryant MG, Bloom SR: Abnormalities of the colonic regulatory peptides in Hirschsprung's disease. Histopathology 5:679-688, 1981.
5. Blisard KS, Kleinman R: Hirschsprung's disease. A clinical and pathologic overview. Hum Pathol 17:1189-1191, 1986.
5a. Causse E, Vaysse P, Fabre J, Valdiguie P, Thouvenot J-P: The diagnostic value of acetylcholinesterase/butyrylcholinesterase ratio in Hirschsprung's disease. Am J Clin Pathol 88:477-480, 1987.
6. Challa VR, Moran JR, Turner CS, Lyerly AD: Histologic diagnosis of Hirschsprung's disease. The value of concurrent hematoxylin and eosin and cholinesterase staining of rectal biopsies. Am J Clin Pathol 88:324-328, 1987.
7. Dimmick JE, Bove KE: Cytomegalovirus infection of the bowel in infancy. Pathogenetic and diagnostic significance. Pediatr Pathol 2:95-102, 1984.
8. Dobbins WO III, Bill AH Jr: Diagnosis of Hirschsprung's disease excluded by rectal suction biopsy. N Engl J Med 272:990-993, 1965.
9. Gherardi GJ: Pathology of the ganglionic-aganglionic junction in congenital megacolon. Arch Pathol 69:520-523, 1960.
10. Hall CL, Lampert PW: Immunohistochemistry as an aid in the diagnosis of Hirschsprung's disease. Am J Clin Pathol 83:177-181, 1985.
11. Ikeda K, Goto S: Diagnosis and treatment of Hirschsprung's disease in Japan. An analysis of 1628 patients. Ann Surg 199:400-405, 1984.
12. Ikeda K, Goto S: Total colonic aganglionosis with or without small bowel involvement. An analysis of 137 patients. J Pediatr Surg 21:319-322, 1986.
13. Ito Y, Tatekawa I, Nishiyama F, Hirano H: Ultrastructural localization of acetylcholinesterase activity in Hirschsprung's disease. Arch Pathol Lab Med 111:161-165, 1987.
14. Kadair RG, Sims JE, Critchfield CF: Zonal colonic hypoganglionosis. JAMA 238:1838-1840, 1977.
15. Lake BD, Puri P, Nixon HH, Claireaux AE: Hirschsprung's disease. An appraisal of histochemically demonstrated acetylcholinesterase activity in suction rectal biopsy specimens as an aid to diagnosis. Arch Pathol Lab Med 102:244-247, 1978.
16. MacMahon RA, Moore CCM, Cussen LJ: Hirschsprung-like syndromes in patients with normal ganglion cells on suction rectal biopsy. J Pediatr Surg 16:835-839, 1981.
17. Madsen CM: Hirschsprung's disease. Springfield, Ill., 1964, Charles C Thomas, Publisher.
18. Meier-Ruge W: Hirschsprung's disease. Its aetiology, pathogenesis and differential diagnosis. In Grundmann E, Kirsten WH (eds): Current topics in pathology, vol. 59. New York, 1974, Springer-Verlag, New York, Inc., pp. 131-179.
19. Meier-Ruge W, Lutterbeck PM, Herzog B, Morger R, Moser R, Schärli A: Acetylcholinesterase activity in suction biopsies of the rectum in the diagnosis of Hirschsprung's disease. J Pediatr Surg 7:11-17, 1972.
20. N-Fékété C, Ricour C, Martelli H, Lortat Jacob S, Pellerin D: Total colonic aganglionosis (with or without ileal involvement). A review of 27 cases. J Pediatr Surg 21:251-254, 1986.
21. Patrick WJA, Besley GTN, Smith II: Histochemical diagnosis of Hirschsprung's disease and a comparison of the histochemical and biochemical activity of acetylcholinesterase in rectal mucosal biopsies. J Clin Pathol 33:336-343, 1980.
22. Scharli AF, Meier-Ruge W: Localized and disseminated forms of neuronal intestinal dysplasia mimicking Hirschsprung's disease. J Pediatr Surg 16:164-170, 1981.
23. Sieber WK: Hirschsprung's disease. In Welch KJ, Randolph JG, Ravitch MM (eds): Pediatric surgery, ed. 4. Chicago, 1986, Year Book Medical Publishers, pp. 995-1020.
24. Staple TW, McAlister WH, Anderson MS: Plexiform neurofibromatosis of the colon simulating Hirschsprung's disease. Am J Roentgenol Radium Ther Nucl Med 91:840-845, 1964.
25. Swenson O, Fisher JH, MacMahon HE: Rectal biopsy as an aid in the diagnosis of Hirschsprung's disease. N Engl J Med 253:632-635, 1955.
26. Swenson O, Rheinlander HG, Diamond I: Hirschsprung's disease. A new concept of the etiology. N Engl J Med 241:551-556, 1949.
27. Taguchi T, Tanaka K, Ikeda K: Fibromuscular dysplasia of arteries in Hirschsprung's disease. Gastroenterology 88:1099-1103, 1985.
28. Taguchi T, Tanaka K, Ikeda K: Immunohistochemical study of neuron specific enolase and S-100 protein in Hirschsprung's disease. Virchows Arch [Pathol Anat] 405:399-409, 1985.
29. Taguchi T, Tanaka K, Ikeda K, Matsubayashi S, Yanaihara N: Peptidergic innervation irregularities in Hirschsprung's disease. Immunohistochemistry-radioimmunoassay. Virchows Arch [Pathol Anat] 401:223-235, 1983.
30. Tam PKH, Lister J: Development profile of neuron-specific enolase in human gut and its implications in Hirschsprung's disease. Gastroenterology 90:1901-1906, 1986.
31. Venugopal S, Mancer K, Shandling B: The validity of rectal biopsy in relation to morphology and distribution of ganglion cells. J Pediatr Surg 16:433-437, 1981.
32. Vinores SA, May E: Neuron-specific enolase as an immunohistochemical tool for the diagnosis of Hirschsprung's disease. Am J Surg Pathol 9:281-285, 1985.
33. Walker AW, Kempson RL, Ternberg JL: Aganglionosis of the small intestine. Surgery 60:449-457, 1966.
34. Weinberg AG: The anorectal myenteric plexus. Its relation to hypoganglionosis of the colon. Am J Clin Pathol 54:637-642, 1970.
35. Weinberg AG: Hirschsprung's disease. A pathologist's view. In Rosenberg HS, Bolande RP (eds): Perspectives in pediatric pathology, vol. 2. Chicago, 1975, Year Book Medical Publishers, Inc., pp. 207-239.
36. Whitehouse FR, Kernohan JW: Myenteric plexus in congenital megacolon. Study of eleven cases. Arch Intern Med 82:75-111, 1948.
37. Yunis EJ, Dibbins AW, Sherman FE: Rectal suction biopsy in the diagnosis of Hirschsprung's disease in infants. Arch Pathol Lab Med 100:329-333, 1976.

DIVERTICULOSIS

38. Almy TP, Howell DA: Diverticular disease of the colon. N Engl J Med 302:324-331, 1980.
39. Bova JG, Hopens TA, Goldstein HM: Diverticulitis of the right colon. Dig Dis Sci 29:150-156, 1984.
40. Butler DB, Miller GV: Solitary diverticulitis of the cecum. Report of case. Arch Surg 68:355-358, 1954.
41. Eng K, Ranson JHC, Localio SA: Resection of the perforated segment. A significant advance in treatment of diverticulitis with free perforation or abscess. Am J Surg 133:67-72, 1977.
42. Fisher N, Berry CS, Fearn T, Gregory JA, Hardy J: Cereal dietary fiber consumption and diverticular disease. A lifespan study in rats. Am J Clin Nutr 42:788-804, 1985.
43. Giffin JM, Butcher HR Jr, Ackerman LV: The surgical management of colonic diverticulitis. Arch Surg 94:619-626, 1967.
44. Gouge TH, Coppa GF, Eng K, Ranson JHC, Localio SA: Management of diverticulitis of the ascending colon. Ten years' experience. Am J Surg 145:387-391, 1983.
45. Hackford AW, Veidenheimer MC: Diverticular disease of the colon. Current concepts and management. Surg Clin North Am 65:347-363, 1985.
46. Himal HS, Ashby DB, Duignan JP, Richardson DM, Miller SL, MacLean LD: Management of perforating diverticulitis of the colon. Surg Gynecol Obstet 144:225-226, 1977.
47. Hughes LE: Postmortem survey of diverticular disease of the colon. Part I. Diverticulosis and diverticulitis. II. The muscular abnormality in the sigmoid colon. Gut 10:336-351, 1969.

48 Magness LJ, Sanfelippo PM, van Heerden JA, Judd ES: Diverticular disease of the right colon. Surg Gynecol Obstet **140:**30-32, 1975.

49 Meyers MA, Alonso DR, Gray GF, Baier JW: Pathogenesis of bleeding colonic diverticulosis. Gastroenterology **71:**577-583, 1976.

50 Morson BC: The muscle abnormality in diverticular disease of the colon. Proc R Soc Med **56:**798-800, 1963.

51 Nicholas ER, Frymark WB, Raffensperger JR: Acute cecal diverticulitis. Report of 25 cases. JAMA **182:**157-160, 1962.

52 Noer RJ: Hemorrhage as a complication of diverticulitis. Ann Surg. **141:**674-485, 1955.

53 Painter NS, Burkitt DP: Diverticular disease of the colon. A deficiency disease of western civilization. Br Med J **2:**450-454, 1971.

54 Ravo B, Khan SA, Ger R, Mishrick A, Soroff HS: Unusual extraperitoneal presentations of diverticulitis. Am J Gastroenterol **80:**346-351, 1985.

55 Sorger K, Wacks MR: Exsanguinating arterial bleeding associated with diverticulating disease of the colon. Arch Surg **102:**9-14, 1971.

56 Sugihara K, Muto T, Morioka T, Asano A, Yamamoto T: Diverticular disease of the colon in Japan. A review of 615 cases. Dis Colon Rectum **27:**531-537, 1984.

57 Talbot JM: Role of dietary fiber in diverticular disease and colon cancer. Fed Proc **40:**2337-2342, 1981.

58 Warshaw AL, Welch JP, Ottinger LW: Acute perforation of the colon associated with chronic corticosteroid therapy. Am J Surg **131:**442-446, 1976.

59 Welch CE, Allen AW, Donaldson GA: An appraisal of resection of the colon for diverticulitis of the sigmoid. Ann Surg **138:**332-343, 1953.

COLITIS

Ulcerative colitis

60 Akwari OE, Van Heerden JA, Foulk WT, Baggenstoss AH: Cancer of the bile ducts associated with ulcerative colitis. Ann Surg **181:**303-309, 1975.

61 Allen DC, Biggart JD: Misplaced epithelium in ulcerative colitis and Crohn's disease of the colon and its relationship to malignant mucosal changes. Histopathology **10:**37-52, 1986.

62 Chambers TJ, Morson BC: Large bowel biopsy in the differential diagnosis of inflammatory bowel disease. Invest Cell Pathol **3:**159-173, 1980.

63 DeDombal FT, Goldie W, Watts JMcK, Goligher JC: Hepatic histologic changes in ulcerative colitis. Scand J Gastroenterol **1:**220-227, 1966.

64 Dyson JL: Herniation of mucosal epithelium into the submucosa in chronic ulcerative colitis. J Clin Pathol **38:**189-194, 1975.

65 Folley JH: Ulcerative proctitis. N Engl J Med **282:**1362-1364, 1970.

66 Franklin WA, McDonald GB, Stein HO, Gatter KC, Jewell DP, Clarke LC, Mason DY: Immunohistologic demonstration of abnormal colonic crypt cell kinetics in ulcerative colitis. Hum Pathol **16:**1129-1132, 1985.

67 Garland CF, Lilienfeld AM, Mendeloff AI, Markowitz JA, Terrell KB, Garland FC: Incidence rates of ulcerative colitis and Crohn's disease in fifteen areas of the United States. Gastroenterology **81:**1115-1124, 1981.

67a Goldman H, Antonioli DA: Mucosal biopsy of the rectum, colon, and distal ileum. Hum Pathol **13:**981-1012, 1982.

68 Goldman J, Hinrichs R, Glotzer DJ, Gardner RC, Zeitzel L: Ulcerative versus granulomatous colitis. Lab Invest **22:**497-498, 1970.

69 Hellstrom HR, Fisher ER: Estimation of mucosal mucin as an aid in the differentiation of Crohn's disease of the colon and chronic ulcerative colitis. Am J Clin Pathol **48:**259-268, 1967.

70 Hinrichs HR, Goldman J: Localized giant pseudopolyps of the colon. JAMA **205:**248-249, 1968.

71 Jessurun J, Paplanus SH, Nagle RB, Hamilton SR, Yardley JH, Tripp M: Pseudosarcomatous changes in inflammatory pseudopolyps of the colon. Arch Pathol Lab Med **110:**833-836, 1986.

72 Kanemitsu T, Koike A, Yamamoto S: Study of the cell proliferation kinetics in ulcerative colitis, adenomatous polyps, and cancer. Cancer **56:**1094-1098, 1985.

73 Kedziora JA, Wolff M, Chang J: Limited form of Wegener's granulomatosis in ulcerative colitis. Am J Roentgenol Radium Ther Nucl Med **125:**127-133, 1975.

74 Kelly JK, Langevin JM, Price LM, Hershfield NB, Share S, Blustein P: Giant and symptomatic inflammatory polyps of the colon in idiopathic inflammatory bowel disease. Am J Surg Pathol **10:**420-428, 1986.

75 Keren DF, Appelman HD, Dobbins WO III, Wells JJ, Whisenant B, Foley J, Dieterle R, Geisinger K: Correlation of histopathologic evidence of disease activity with the presence of immunoglobulin-containing cells in the colons of patients with inflammatory bowel disease. Hum Pathol **15:**757-763, 1984.

76 Kim YS, Byrd JC: Ulcerative colitis. A specific mucin defect? Gastroenterology **87:**1193-1195, 1984.

77 Kirsner JB: Ulcerative colitis; mysterious, multiplex, and menacing. J Chronic Dis **23:**681-684, 1971.

78 Lee KS, Medline A, Shockey S: Indeterminate colitis in the spectrum of inflammatory bowel disease. Arch Pathol Lab Med **103:**173-176, 1979.

79 Lee RG: Villous regeneration in ulcerative colitis. Arch Pathol Lab Med **111:**276-278, 1987.

80 Lennard-Jones JE, Ritchie JK, Hilde W, Spicer CC: Assessment of severity in colitis. Gut **16:**579-584, 1975.

81 Lumb GD, Protheroe RHB: Ulcerative colitis. A pathologic study of 152 surgical specimens. Gastroenterology **34:**381-407, 1958.

82 Mayberry JS: Some aspects of the epidemiology of ulcerative colitis. Gut **26:**968-974, 1985.

83 McAuley RL, Sommers SC: Mast cells in nonspecific ulcerative colitis. Am J Dig Dis **6:**233-236, 1961.

84 Morowitz DA, Glagov S, Dordal E, Kirsner JB: Carcinoma of the biliary tract complicating chronic ulcerative colitis. Cancer **27:**356-361, 1971.

85 Morson B: Current concepts of colitis. Lecture 1. Trans Med Soc Lond **86:**159-176, 1970.

86 Morson B: Crohn's disease. Lecture 2. Trans Med Soc Lond **86:**177-192, 1970.

87 Riddell RH, Goldman H, Ransohoff DF, Appelman HD, Fenoglio CM, Haggitt RC, Ahren C, Correa P, Hamilton SR, Morson BC, Sommers SC, Yardley JH: Dysplasia in inflammatory bowel disease. Standardized classification with provisional clinical applications. Hum Pathol **14:**931-968, 1983.

88 Ritchie JK, Allan RM, Macartney J, Thompson H, Hawley PR, Cooke WT: Biliary tract carcinoma associated with ulcerative colitis. Q J Med **43:**263-279, 1974.

89 Rubio CA: Ectopic colonic mucosa in ulcerative colitis and in Crohn's disease of the colon. Dis Colon Rectum **27:**182-186, 1984.

90 Schachter H, Goldstein MJ, Rappaport H, Fennessy JJ, Kirsner JB: Ulcerative and "granulomatous" colitis—validity of differential diagnostic criteria. A study of 100 patients treated by total colectomy. Ann Intern Med **72:**841-851, 1970.

91 Symonds DA: Paneth cell metaplasia in diseases of the colon and rectum. Arch Pathol **97:**343-347, 1974.

92 Watson AJ, Roy AD: Paneth cells in the large intestine in ulcerative colitis. J Pathol Bacteriol **80:**309-316, 1960.

93 Whitehead R: Mucosal biopsy of the gastrointestinal tract. In Bennington JL (consulting ed): Major problems in pathology, vol. 3, ed. 3. Philadelphia, 1985, W.B. Saunders Co.

94 Wright R: Ulcerative colitis. Gastroenterology **58:**875-897, 1970.

Carcinoma and dysplasia in ulcerative colitis

95 Allen DC, Biggart JD, Orchin JC, Foster H: An immunoperoxidase study of epithelial marker antigens in ulcerative colitis with dysplasia and carcinoma. J Clin Pathol **38:**18-29, 1985.

96 Allen DC, Biggart JD, Pyper PC: Large bowel mucosal dysplasia and carcinoma in ulcerative colitis. J Clin Pathol **38:**30-43, 1985.

96a Allen DC, Hamilton PW, Watt PCH, Biggart JD: Morphometrical analysis in ulcerative colitis with dysplasia and carcinoma. Histopathology **11:**913-926, 1987.

97 Butt JH, Konishi F, Morson BC, Lennard-Jones JE, Ritchie JK: Macroscopic lesions and dysplasia and carcinoma complicating ulcerative colitis. Dig Dis Sci **28:**18-26, 1983.

98 Collins RH Jr, Feldman N, Fordtran JS: Colon cancer, dysplasia, and surveillance in patients with ulcerative colitis. A critical review. N Engl J Med **316:**1654-1658, 1987.

99 Cook MG, Goligher JC: Carcinoma and epithelial dysplasia complicating ulcerative colitis. Gastroenterology **68:**1127-1136, 1975.

100 Counsell PB, Dukes CE: The association of chronic ulcerative colitis and carcinoma of the rectum and colon. Br J Surg **39:**485-495, 1952.

101 Devroede GJ, Taylor WF, Sauer WG, Jackman RJ, Stickler GB: Cancer risk and life expectancy of children with ulcerative colitis. N Engl J Med **285:**17-52, 1971.

102 Dukes CE, Lockhart-Mummery HE: Practical points in the pathology and surgical treatment of ulcerative colitis. A critical review. Br J Surg **45:**25-36, 1957.

103 Edwards FC, Truelove SC: The course and prognosis of ulcerative colitis. Gut **4:**299-315, 1963.

104 Edwards FC, Truelove SC: The course and prognosis of ulcerative colitis. III. Complications. Gut **5:**1-22, 1964.

105 Ehsannulah M, Filipe MI, Gazzard B: Mucin secretion in inflammatory bowel disease. Correlation with disease activity and dysplasia. Gut **23:**485-489, 1982.

106 Ehsannulah M, Morgan MN, Filipe MI, Gazzard B: Sialomucins in the assessment of dysplasia and cancer-risk patients with ulcerative colitis treated with colectomy and ileo-rectal anastomosis. Histopathology **9:**223-235, 1985.

107 Filipe MI, Edwards MR, Ehsannulah M: A prospective study of dysplasia and carcinoma in the rectal biopsies and rectal stump of eight patients following ileorectal anastomosis in ulcerative colitis. Histopathology **9:**1139-1153, 1985.

108 Fozard JBJ, Dixon MF, Axon ATR, Giles GR: Lectin and mucin histochemistry as an aid to cancer surveillance in ulcerative colitis. Histopathology **11:**385-394, 1987.

109 Goldgraber MB, Humphreys EM, Kirsner JB, Palmer WL: Carcinoma and ulcerative colitis. Gastroenterology **34:**809-839, 1958.

110 Grundfest AF, Fazio V, Weiss RA, Jagelman D, Lavery I, Weakley FL, Turnbull RB Jr: The risk of cancer following colectomy and ileorectal anastomosis for extensive mucosal ulcerative colitis. Ann Surg **193:**9-14, 1981.

111 Gyde SN, Prior P, Thompson H, Waterhouse JAH, Allan RN: Survival of patients with colorectal cancer complicating ulcerative colitis. Gut **25:**228-231, 1984.

112 Hammarberg C, Rubio C, Slezak P, Tribukait B, Ohman U: Flow-cytometric DNA analysis as a means for early detection of malignancy in patients with chronic ulcerative colitis. Gut **25:**905-908, 1984.

113 Hammarberg C, Slezak P, Tribukait B: Early detection of malignancy in ulcerative colitis. A flow-cytometric DNA study. Cancer **53:**291-295, 1984.

114 Hughes RG, Hall TJ, Block GE, Levin B, Moossa AR: The prognosis of carcinoma of the colon and rectum complicating ulcerative colitis. Surg Gynecol Obstet **146:**46-48, 1978.

115 Kewenter J, Hultén L, Ahrén C: The occurrence of severe epithelial dysplasia and its bearing on treatment of longstanding ulcerative colitis. Ann Surg **195:**209-213, 1982.

116 Kiefer ED, Eytinge DJ, Johnson AC: Malignant degeneration in chronic ulcerative colitis. Gastroenterology **19:**51-57, 1951.

117 Lavery IC, Chiulli RA, Jagelman DG, Fazio VW, Weakley FL: Survival with carcinoma arising in mucosal ulcerative colitis. Ann Surg **195:**508-512, 1982.

118 Lennard-Jones JE, Morson BC, Ritchie JK, Shove DC, Williams CB: Cancer in colitis. Assessment of the individual risk by clinical and histological criteria. Gastroenterology **73:**1280-1289, 1977.

119 Lennard-Jones JE, Ritchie JK, Morson BC, Williams CB: Cancer surveillance in ulcerative colitis. Experience over 15 years. Lancet **2:**149-152, 1983.

120 Lyss AP, Thompson JJ, Glick JH: Adenocarcinoid tumor of the colon arising in preexisting ulcerative colitis. Cancer **48:**833-839, 1981.

121 Miller RR, Sumner HW: Argyrophilic cell hyperplasia and an atypical carcinoid tumor in chronic ulcerative colitis. Cancer **50:**2920-2925, 1982.

122 Mir-Madjlessi SH, Farmer RG, Easley KA, Beck GJ: Colorectal and extracolonic malignancy in ulcerative colitis. Cancer **58:**1569-1574, 1986.

123 Morson BC: Current concepts of colitis. Lecture 1. Trans Med Soc Lond **86:**159-176, 1970.

124 Morson BC: Precancer and cancer in inflammatory bowel disease. Pathology **17:**173-180, 1985.

125 Morson BC, Pang LSC: Rectal biopsy as an aid to cancer control in ulcerative colitis. Gut **8:**423-434, 1967.

126 Ransohoff DF, Riddell RH, Levin B: Ulcerative colitis and colonic cancer. Problems in assessing the diagnostic usefulness of mucosal dysplasia. Dis Colon Rectum **28:**383-388, 1985.

126a Renton P, Blackshaw AJ: Colonic lymphoma complicating ulcerative colitis. Br J Surg **63:**542-545, 1976.

127 Riddell RH, Goldman H, Ransohoff DF, Appelman HD, Fenoglio CM, Haggitt RC, Ahren C, Correa P, Hamilton SR, Morson BC, Sommers SC, Yardley JH: Dysplasia in inflammatory bowel disease. Standardized classification with provisional clinical applications. Hum Pathol **14:**931-968, 1983.

128 Riddell RH, Morson BC: Value of sigmoidoscopy and biopsy in detection of carcinoma and premalignant change in ulcerative colitis. Gut **20:**575-580, 1979.

129 Ritchie JK, Hawley PR, Lennard-Jones JE: Prognosis of carcinoma in ulcerative colitis. Gut **22:**752-755, 1981.

130 Rosenstock E, Farmer RG, Petras R, Sivak MV Jr, Rankin GB, Sullivan BH: Surveillance for colonic carcinoma in ulcerative colitis. Gastroenterology **89:**1342-1346, 1985.

131 Shields HM, Bates ML, Goldman H, Zuckerman GR, Mills BA, Best CJ, Bair FA, Goran DA, DeSchryver-Kecskemeti K: Scanning electron microscopic appearance of chronic ulcerative colitis with and without dysplasia. Gastroenterology **89:**62-72, 1985.

132 Yardley JH, Keren DF: "Precancer" lesions in ulcerative colitis. A retrospective study of rectal biopsy and colectomy specimens. Cancer **34:**835-844, 1974.

Crohn's disease (granulomatous colitis)

133 Buchanan WM, Fyfe AHB: Giant pseudopolyposis in granulomatous colitis. J Pathol **127:**51-54, 1979.

134 Chiodini RJ, Van Kruiningen HT, Thayer WR, Merkal RS, Coutu JA: Possible role of mycobacteria in inflammatory bowel disease. I. An unclassified *Mycobacterium* species isolated from patients with Crohn's disease. Dig Dis Sci **29:**1073-1079, 1984.

135 Craft CF, Mendelsohn G, Cooper HS, Yardley JH: Colonic "precancer" in Crohn's disease. Gastroenterology **80:**578-584, 1981.

136 Farmer RG, Hawk WA, Turnbull RB Jr: Carcinoma associated with mucosal ulcerative colitis and with transmural colitis and enteritis (Crohn's disease). Cancer **28:**289-292, 1971.

137 Farmer RG, Hawk WA, Turnbull RB Jr: Clinical patterns in Crohn's disease. A statistical study of 1615 cases. Gastroenterology **68:**627-635, 1975.

138 Gray BK, Lockhart-Mummery HE, Morson BC: Crohn's disease of the anal region. Gut **6:**515-524, 1965.

139 Greenstein AJ, Janowitz HD, Sachar DB: The extraintestinal complications of Crohn's disease and ulcerative colitis. A study of 700 patients. Medicine [Baltimore] **55:**401-412, 1976.

140 Hamilton SR: Colorectal carcinoma in patients with Crohn's disease. Gastroenterology **89:**398-407, 1985.

141 Hoffman WA, Rosenberg MA: Granulomatous colitis in the elderly. Am J Gastroenterol **58:**508-518, 1972.

142 Jones JH: Colonic cancer and Crohn's disease. Gut **10:**651-654, 1969.

143 Kelly JK, Langevin J, Price LM, Hershfield NB, Share S, Blustein P: Giant and symptomatic inflammatory polyps of the colon in idiopathic inflammatory bowel disease. Am J Surg Pathol **10:**420-428, 1986.

144 Lockhart-Mummery HE, Morson BC: Crohn's disease of the large intestine. Gut **5:**493-509, 1964.

145 Meyers MA, Alonso DR, Morson BC, Bartram C: Pathogenesis of diverticulitis complicating granulomatous colitis. Gastroenterology **74:**24-31, 1978.

146 Petri M, Poulsen SS, Christensen K, Jarnum S: The incidence of granulomas in serial sections of rectal biopsies from patients with Crohn's disease. Acta Pathol Microbiol Immunol Scand [A] **90:**145-147, 1982.

147 Price AB: Overlap in the spectrum of non-specific inflammatory bowel disease— "colitis indeterminate." J Clin Pathol **31:**567-577, 1978.

148 Price AB, Morson BC: Inflammatory bowel disease. The surgical pathology of Crohn's disease and ulcerative colitis. Hum Pathol **6:**7-29, 1975.

149 Renison DM, Forouhar FA, Levine JB, Breiter JR: Filiform polyposis of the colon presenting as massive hemorrhage. An uncommon complication of Crohn's disease. Am J Gastroenterol **78:**413-416, 1983.

150 Riddell RH, Goldman H, Ransohoff DF, Appelman HD, Fenoglio CM, Haggitt RC, Ahren C, Correa P, Hamilton SR, Morson BC, Sommers SC, Yardley JH: Dysplasia in inflammatory bowel disease. Standardized classification with provisional clinical applications. Hum Pathol **14:**931-968, 1983.

151 Rotterdam H, Korelitz BI, Sommers SC: Microgranulomas in grossly normal rectal mucosa in Crohn's disease. Am J Clin Pathol **67:**550-554, 1977.

152 Schmitz-Moormann P, Himmelmann G-W, Brandes J-W: Relationships between clinical data and histology of the large bowel in Crohn's disease and ulcerative colitis. Pathol Annu **20**(Pt1)**:**281-301, 1985.

153 Schmitz-Moormann P, Pittner PM, Malchow H, Brandes JW: The granuloma in Crohn's disease. A bioptical study. Pathol Res Pract **178:**467-476, 1984.

154 Schmitz-Moormann P, Pittner PM, Sangmeister M: Probability of detecting a granuloma in a colorectal biopsy of Crohn's disease. Pathol Res Pract **178:**227-229, 1984.

155 Schneider H-M, Loos M, Storkel S, Gross M: Immunohistological differential diagnosis of inflammatory colonic diseases. Histopathology **8:**583-588, 1984.

156 Shamsuddin AKM, Phillips RM: Preneoplastic and neoplastic changes in colonic mucosa in Crohn's disease. Arch Pathol Lab Med **105:**283-286, 1981.

157 Shapiro PA, Peppercorn MA, Antonioli DA, Joffe N, Goldman H: Crohn's disease in the elderly. Am J Gastroenterol **76:**132-137, 1981.

158 Skinner JM, Whitehead R: A morphological assessment of immunoreactivity in colonic Crohn's disease and ulcerative colitis by a study of the lymph nodes. J Clin Pathol **27:**202-206, 1974.

159 Surawicz CM, Meisel JL, Ylvisaker T, Saunders DR, Rubin CE: Rectal biopsy in the diagnosis of Crohn's disease. Value of multiple biopsies and serial sectioning. Gastroenterology **81:**66-71, 1981.

160 Tchirkow G, Lavery IC, Fazio VW: Crohn's disease in the elderly. Dis Colon Rectum **26:**177-181, 1983.

161 Thompson EM, Clayden G, Price AB: Cancer in Crohn's disease. An "occult" malignancy. Histopathology **7:**365-376, 1983.

162 Warren R, Barwick KW: Crohn's colitis with carcinoma and dysplasia. Report of a case and review of 100 small and large bowel resections for Crohn's disease to detect incidence of dysplasia. Am J Surg Pathol **7:**151-159, 1983.

Ischemic colitis

163 Brandt L, Boley S, Goldberg L, Mitsudo S, Berman A: Colitis in the elderly. A reappraisal. Am J Gastroenterol **76:**239-245, 1981.

164 Brandt LJ, Katz HJ, Wolf EL, Mitsudo S, Boley SJ: Simulation of colonic carcinoma by ischemia. Gastroenterology **88:**1137-1142, 1985.

165 Gillespie IE: Intestinal ischaemia. Gut **26**:653-655, 1985.

166 Haworth SJ, Pusey CD: Severe intestinal involvement in Wegener's granulomatosis. Gut **25**:1296-1300, 1984.

167 Kilpatrick ZM, Silverman JF, Betancourt E, Farman J, Lawson JP: Vascular occlusion of the colon and oral contraceptives. Possible relation. N Engl J Med **278**:438-440, 1968.

168 Morson BC: Ischaemic colitis. Postgrad Med J **44**:665-666, 1968.

Other types of colitis

169 Anand BS, Malhotra V, Bhattacharya SK, Datta P, Datta D, Sen D, Bhattacharya MK, Mukherjee PP, Pal SC: Rectal histology in acute bacillary dysentery. Gastroenterology **90**:654-660, 1986.

170 Brandt H, Perez-Tamayo R: Pathology of human amebiasis. Hum Pathol **1**:351-385, 1970.

171 Cantey JR: Infectious diarrhea. Pathogenesis and risk factors. Am J Med **78**:65-75, 1985.

172 Choudari CP, Mathan M, Rajah DP, Raghavan R, Mathan VI: A correlative study of etiology, clinical features and rectal mucosal pathology in adults with acute infectious diarrhea in southern India. Pathology **37**:443-450, 1985.

173 Dickinson RJ, Gilmour HM, McClelland DBL: Rectal biopsy in patients presenting to an infectious disease unit with diarrhoeal disease. Gut **20**:141-148, 1979.

174 Ehsannulah M, Isaacs A, Filipe MI, Gazzard BG: Tuberculosis presenting as inflammatory bowel disease. Report of two cases. Dis Colon Rectum **27**:134-136, 1984.

175 Epstein RJ, McDonald GB, Sale GE, Shulman HM, Thomas ED: The diagnostic accuracy of the rectal biopsy in acute graft-versus-host disease. A prospective study of thirteen patients. Gastroenterology **78**:764-771, 1980.

176 Flejou JF, Grimaud JA, Molas G, Baviera E, Patet F: Collagenous colitis. Ultrastructural study and collagen immunotyping of four cases. Arch Pathol Lab Med **108**:977-982, 1984.

177 Foerster A, Fausa O: Collagenous colitis. Pathol Res Pract **180**:99-104, 1985.

178 Foucar E, Mukai K, Foucar K, Sutherland DER, Van Buren CT: Colon ulceration in lethal cytomegalovirus infection. Am J Clin Pathol **76**:788-801, 1981.

179 Gaffney EF, Condell D, Majmudar B, Nolan N, McDonald GSA, Griffin M, Sweeney EC: Modification of caecal lymphoid tissue and relationship to granuloma formation in sporadic ileocaecal tuberculosis. Histopathology **11**:691-704, 1987.

180 Gallucci BB, Sale GE, McDonald GB, Epstein R, Shulman HM, Thomas ED: The fine structure of human rectal epithelium in acute graft-versus-host disease. Am J Surg Pathol **6**:293-305, 1982.

181 Gardiner GW, Goldberg R, Currie D, Murray D: Colonic carcinoma associated with an abnormal collagen table. Collagenous colitis. Cancer **54**:2973-2977, 1984.

182 George RH, Symonds JM, Dimock F, Brown JD, Arabi Y, Shinagawa N, Keighley MRB, Alexander-Williams J, Burden DW: Identification of *Clostridium difficile* as a cause of pseudomembranous colitis. Br Med J **1**:695, 1978.

183 Goldman H: Acute versus chronic colitis. How and when to distinguish by biopsy. Gastroenterology **86**:199-201, 1984.

184 Goldman H, Proujansky R: Allergic proctitis and gastroenteritis in children. Clinical and mucosal biopsy features in 53 cases. Am J Surg Pathol **10**:75-86, 1986.

185 Goulston SJM, McGovern VJ: Pseudomembranous colitis. Gut **6**:207-212, 1965.

186 Howell JS, Knapton PJ: Ileo-caecal tuberculosis. Gut **5**:524-529, 1964.

187 Jessurun J, Yardley JH, Giardiello FM, Hamilton SR, Bayless TM: Chronic colitis with thickening of the subepithelial collagen layer (collagenous colitis). Histopathologic findings in 15 patients. Hum Pathol **18**:839-848, 1987.

188 Joshi VV, Draper DA, Bates RD III: Neonatal necrotizing enterocolitis. Occurrence secondary to thrombosis of abdominal aorta following umbilical arterial catheterization. Arch Pathol **99**:540-543, 1975.

189 Kalkay MN, Ayanian ZS, Lehaf EA, Baldi A: Campylobacter-induced toxic megacolon. Am J Gastroenterol **78**:557-559, 1983.

190 Kasulke RJ, Anderson WJ, Gupta SK, Gliedman ML: Primary tuberculous enterocolitis. Report of three cases and review of the literature. Arch Surg **116**:110-113, 1981.

191 Kelly JK, Pai CH, Jadusingh IH, Macinnis ML, Shaffer EA, Hershfield NB: The histopathology of rectosigmoid biopsies from adults with bloody diarrhea due to verotoxin-producing *Escherichia coli*. Am J Clin Pathol **88**:78-82, 1987.

192 Kingham JGC, Levison DA, Morson BC, Dawson Am: Collagenous colitis. Gut **27**:570-577, 1986.

193 Kliegman RM, Fanaroff AA: Necrotizing enterocolitis. N Engl J Med **310**:1093-1103, 1984.

194 Kobayashi TK, Koretoh O, Kamachi M, Watanabe S, Ishigooka S, Matsushita I, Sawaragi I: Cytologic demonstration of *Entamoeba histolytica* using immunoperoxidase techniques. Report of two cases. Acta Cytol [Baltimore] **29**:414-418, 1985.

195 Komorowski RA, Cohen EB, Kauffman HM, Adams MB: Gastrointestinal complications in renal transplant recipients. Am J Clin Pathol **86**:161-167, 1986.

196 Kosloske AM: Necrotizing enterocolitis in the neonate. Surg Gynecol Obstet **148**:259-269, 1979.

197 Kotler DP, Weaver SC, Terzakis JA: Ultrastructural features of epithelial cell degeneration in rectal crypts of patients with AIDS. Am J Surg Pathol **10**:531-538, 1986.

198 Kumar NB, Nostrant TT, Appelman HD: The histopathologic spectrum of acute self-limited colitis (acute infectious-type colitis). Am J Surg Pathol **6**:523-529, 1982.

199 Lee FD, Roy AD: Ileo-caecal granulomata. Gut **5**:517-523, 1964.

200 Lee RG: The colitis of Behçet's syndrome. Am J Surg Pathol **10**:888-893, 1986.

201 McAllister TA: Diagnosis of amoebic colitis on routine biopsies from rectum and sigmoid colon. Br Med J **1**:362-364, 1962.

202 McGovern VJ, Savutin LJ: Pathology of salmonella colitis. Am J Surg Pathol **3**:483-490, 1979.

203 Medline A, Shin DH, Medline NM: Pseudomembranous colitis associated with antibiotics. Hum Pathol **7**:693-703, 1976.

204 Meiselman MS, Cello JP, Margaretten W: Cytomegalovirus colitis. Report of the clinical, endoscopic, and pathologic findings in two patients with the acquired immune deficiency syndrome. Gastroenterology **88**:171-175, 1985.

205 Nostrant TT, Kumar NB, Appelman HD: Histopathology differentiates acute self-limited colitis from ulcerative colitis. Gastroenterology **92**:318-328, 1987.

206 Palmer KR, Patil DH, Basran GS, Riordan JF, Silk DBA: Abdominal tuberculosis in urban Britain. A common disease. Gut **26**:1296-1305, 1985.

207 Pittman FE, Hashimi WK, Pittman JC: Studies of human amebiasis. 1. Clinical and laboratory findings in eight cases of acute amebic colitis. Gastroenterology **65**:581-587, 1973.

208 Pittman FE, Hennigar GR: Sigmoidoscopic and colonic mucosal biopsy findings in amebic colitis. Arch Pathol **97**:155-158, 1974.

209 Pochaczevsky R, Kassner EG: Necrotizing enterocolitis in infancy. Am J Roentgenol Radium Ther Nucl Med **113**:283-296, 1971.

210 Prathap K, Gilman R: The histopathology of acute intestinal amebiasis. Am J Pathol **60**:229-245, 1970.

211 Price AB, Davies DR: Pseudomembranous colitis. J Clin Pathol **30**:1-12, 1977.

212 Sale GE, Shulman HM, McDonald GB, Thomas ED: Gastrointestinal graft-versus-host disease in man. A clinicopathologic study of the rectal biopsy. Am J Surg Pathol **3**:291-299, 1979.

213 Santulli TV, Schullinger JN, Heird WC, Gongaware RD, Wigger J, Barlow B, Blanc WA, Berdon WE: Acute necrotizing enterocolitis in infancy. A review of 64 cases. Pediatrics **55**:376-387, 1975.

214 Schnitt SJ, Antonioli DA, Goldman H: Massive mural edema in severe pseudomembranous colitis. Arch Pathol Lab Med **107**:211-213, 1983.

215 Stevenson JK, Graham CB, Oliver TK Jr, Goldenberg VE: Neonatal necrotizing enterocolitis. A report of twenty-one cases with fourteen survivors. Am J Surg **118**:260-272, 1969.

216 Sumner HW, Tedesco FJ: Rectal biopsy in clindamycin-associated colitis. An analysis of 23 cases. Arch Pathol **99**:237-241, 1975.

217 Surawicz CM, Belic L: Rectal biopsy helps to distinguish acute self-limited colitis from idiopathic inflammatory bowel disease. Gastroenterology **86**:104-113, 1984.

218 Sutherland DER, Chan FY, Foucar E, Simmons PL, Howard RJ, Najarian JS: The bleeding cecal ulcer in transplant patients. Surgery **86**:386-398, 1979.

219 Tandon HD, Prakash A: Pathology of intestinal tuberculosis and its distinction from Crohn's disease. Gut **13**:260-269, 1972.

220 Van Spreeuwel JP, Duursma GC, Meijer CJLM, Bax R, Rosekrans PCM, Lindeman J: Campylobacter colitis. Histological immunohistochemical and ultrastructural findings. Gut **26**:945-951, 1985.

221 Vesterby A, Baandrup U, Jacobsen NO, Albertsen K: Campylobacter enterocolitis. An important differential diagnosis in ulcerative colitis. Acta Pathol Microbiol Immunol Scand [A] **91**:31-33, 1983.

222 Wang KK, Perrault J, Carpenter HA, Schroeder KW, Tremaine WJ: Collagenous colitis. A clinicopathologic correlation. Mayo Clin Proc **62**:665-671, 1987.

223 Weber JR Jr, Dobbins WO III: The intestinal and rectal epithelial lymphocyte in AIDS. An electron-microscope study. Am J Surg Pathol **10**:627-639, 1986.

224 Whitehead R: Forms of colitis. A review of recent developments. Pathology **17**:204-208, 1985.

225 Wilson SE, Woolley MM: Primary necrotizing enterocolitis in infants. Arch Surg **99**:563-566, 1969.

OTHER NON-NEOPLASTIC LESIONS

226 Allen MS Jr: Hamartomatous inverted polyps of the rectum. Cancer **19:**257-265, 1966.

227 Amano S, Yamada N: Endometrioid carcinoma arising from endometriosis of the sigmoid colon. A case report. Hum Pathol **12:**845-848, 1981.

228 Beddoe H, Kaye S, Kaye S: Barium granuloma of the rectum. Report of case. JAMA **154:**747-748, 1954.

229 Brett EM, Berry CL: Value of rectal biopsy in pediatric neurology. Report of 165 biopsies. Br Med J **3:**400-403, 1967.

230 Brodey PA, Hill RP, Baron S: Benign ulceration of the cecum. Radiology **122:**323-327, 1977.

231 Du Boulay CE, Fairbrother J, Isaacson PG: Mucosal prolapse syndrome. A unifying concept for solitary ulcer syndrome and related disorders. J Clin Pathol **36:**1264-1268, 1983.

232 Epstein SE, Ascari WQ, Albow RC, Seaman WB, Lattes R: Colitis cystica profunda. Am J Clin Pathol **45:**186-201, 1966.

233 Ford MJ, Anderson JR, Gilmour HM, Holt S, Sircus W, Heading RC: Clinical spectrum of "solitary ulcer" of the rectum. Gastroenterology **84:**1533-1540, 1983.

234 Franzin G, Scarpa A, Dina R, Novelli P: "Transitional" and hyperplastic-metaplastic mucosa occurring in solitary ulcer of the rectum. Histopathology **5:**527-533, 1981.

235 Gad A: Benign idiopathic recurrent rectal ulceration (BIRRU). Scand J Gastroenterol **54**[Suppl]:111-113, 1979.

236 Gafni J, Sohar E: Rectal biopsy for the diagnosis of amyloidosis. Am J Med Sci **240:**332-336, 1960.

237 Gelfand MD, Tepper M, Katz LA, Binder HJ, Vesner R, Flock MH: Acute irradiation proctitis in man. Development of eosinophilic crypt abscesses. Gastroenterology **54:**401-411, 1968.

238 Grodsinsky C, Ponka JL: Volvulus of the colon. Dis Colon Rectum **20:**314-324, 1977.

239 Haboubi NY, Honan RP, Hasleton PS, Ali HH, Anfield C, Hobbiss J, Schofield PF: Pneumatosis coli. A case report with ultrastructural study. Histopathology **8:**145-155, 1984.

240 Kamoshita S, Landing BH: Distribution of lesions in myenteric plexus and gastrointestinal mucosa in lipidoses and other neurologic disorders of children. Am J Clin Pathol **49:**312-318, 1968.

241 Kratzer GL, Salvati EP: Collective review of endometriosis of the colon. Am J Surg **90:**866-869, 1955.

242 Kyle RA, Spencer RJ, Dahlin DC: Value of rectal biopsy in the diagnosis of primary systemic amyloidosis. Am J Med Sci **251:**501-506, 1966.

243 Lobert PF, Appelman HD: Inflammatory cloacogenic polyp. A unique inflammatory lesion of the anal transition zone. Am J Surg Pathol **5:**761-766, 1981.

244 MacKay EH: Malakoplakia in ulcerative colitis. Arch Pathol Lab Med **102:**140-145, 1978.

245 Madigan R, Morson BC: Solitary ulcer of the rectum. Gut **10:**871-881, 1969.

246 Magidson JG, Lewin KJ: Diffuse colitis cystica profunda. Report of a case. Am J Surg Pathol **5:**393-399, 1981.

247 O'Mara CS, Wilson TH Jr, Stonesifer GL, Cameron JL: Cecal volvulus. Analysis of 50 patients with long-term follow-up. Ann Surg **189:**724-731, 1979.

248 Pieterse AS, Leong AS-Y, Rowland R: The mucosal changes and pathogenesis of pneumatosis cystoides intestinalis. Hum Pathol **16:**683-688, 1985.

249 Ramos AJ, Powers WE: Pneumatosis cystoides intestinalis. Report of a case. Am J Roentgenol Radium Ther Nucl Med **77:**678-683, 1957.

250 Ranchod M, Kahn LB: Malakoplakia of the gastrointestinal tract. Arch Pathol **94:**90-97, 1972.

251 Rapola J, Santavuori P, Savilahti E: Suction biopsy of rectal mucosa in the diagnosis of infantile and juvenile types of neuronal ceroid lipofuscinoses. Hum Pathol **15:**352-360, 1984.

252 Rescorla FJ, Grosfeld JL: Intestinal atresia and stenosis. Analysis of survival in 120 cases. Surgery **98:**668-676, 1985.

253 Roswit B, Malsky SJ, Reid CB: Severe radiation injuries of the stomach, small intestine, colon, and rectum. Am J Roentgenol Radium Ther Nucl Med **114:**460-475, 1972.

254 Saul SH: Inflammatory cloacogenic polyp. Relationship to solitary rectal ulcer syndrome/mucosal prolapse and other bowel disorders. Hum Pathol **18:**1120-1125, 1987.

255 Shamsuddin AKM, Elias EG: Rectal mucosa. Malignant and premalignant changes after radiation therapy. Arch Pathol Lab Med **105:**150-151, 1981.

256 Silver H, Stolar J: Distinguishing features of well-differentiated mucinous adenocarcinoma of the rectum and colitis cystica profunda. Am J Clin Pathol **51:**493-500, 1969.

257 Sinclair-Smith C, Kahn LB, Cywes S: Malacoplakia in childhood. Case report

258 Smith BH, Welter LH: Pneumatosis intestinalis. Am J Clin Pathol **48:**455-465, 1967.

259 Snover DC, Sandstad J, Hutton S: Mucosal pseudolipomatosis of the colon. Am J Clin Pathol **84:**575-580, 1985.

260 Spjut HJ, Perkins DE: Endometriosis of the sigmoid colon and rectum. Am J Roentgenol Radium Ther Nucl Med **82:**1070-1075, 1959.

261 Stuart M: Proctitis cystica profunda. Incidence, etiology, and treatment. Dis Colon Rectum **27:**153-156, 1984.

262 Terner JY, Lattes R: Malakoplakia of colon and retroperitoneum. Am J Clin Pathol **44:**20-31, 1965.

263 Wayte DM, Helwig EB: Colitis cystica profunda. Am J Clin Pathol **48:**159-169, 1967.

264 Weisbrot IM, Liber AF, Gordon BS: The effects of therapeutic radiation on colonic mucosa. Cancer **36:**931-940, 1975.

265 Wilson SE, Woolley MM: Primary necrotizing enterocolitis in infants. Arch Surg **99:**563-566, 1969.

266 Wolff M: Heterotopic gastric epithelium in the rectum. A report of three new cases with a review of 87 cases of gastric heterotopia in the alimentary canal. Am J Clin Pathol **55:**604-616, 1971.

267 Wood RE, Herman CJ, Johnson KW, di Sant'Agnese PA: Pneumatosis coli in cystic fibrosis. Clinical, radiological, and pathological features. Am J Dis Child **129:**246-248, 1975.

TUMORS
Epithelial polyps

268 Almagro UA, Pintar K, Zellmer RB: Squamous metaplasia in colorectal polyps. Cancer **53:**2679-2682, 1984.

269 Arminski TC, McLean DW: Incidence and distribution of adenomatous polyps of the colon and rectum based on 1,000 autopsy examinations. Dis Colon Rectum **7:**249-261, 1964.

270 Bacon HE, Eisenberg SW: Papillary adenoma or villous tumor of the rectum and colon. Ann Surg **174:**1002-1008, 1971.

271 Bansal M, Fenoglio CM, Robboy SJ, West King D: Are metaplasias in colorectal adenomas truly metaplasias? Am J Pathol **115:**253-265, 1984.

272 Bengoechea O, Martínez-Peñuela JM, Larrínaga B, Valerdi J, Borda F: Hyperplastic polyposis of the colorectum and adenocarcinoma in a 24-year-old man. Am J Surg Pathol **11:**323-327, 1987.

273 Bodmer WF, Bailey CJ, Bodmer J, Bussey HJR, Ellis A, Gorman P, Lucibello FC, Murday VA, Rider SH, Scambler P, Sheer D, Solomon E, Spurr NK: Localization of the gene for familial adenomatous polyposis on chromosome 5. Nature **328:**614-616, 1987.

274 Bolwell JS, James PD: Peutz-Jeghers syndrome with pseudoinvasion of hamartomatous polyps and multiple epithelial neoplasms. Histopathology **3:**39-50, 1979.

275 Bombi JA, Rives A, Astudillo E, Pera C, Cardesa A: Polyposis coli associated with adenocarcinoma of the gallbladder. Report of a case. Cancer **53:**2561-2563, 1984.

276 Burt RW, Bishop DT, Cannon LA, Dowdle MA, Lee RG, Skolnick MH: Dominant inheritance of adenomatous colonic polyps and colorectal cancer. N Engl J Med **312:**1540-1544, 1985.

277 Bussey HJR: Gastrointestinal polyposis. Gut **11:**970-978, 1970.

278 Bussey HJR: Familial polyposis coli. Baltimore, 1975, Johns Hopkins University Press.

279 Carlson GJ, Nivatvongs S, Snover DC: Colorectal polyps in Cowden's disease (multiple hamartoma syndrome). Am J Surg Pathol **8:**763-770, 1984.

280 Chapman I: Adenomatous polypi of large intestine. Incidence and distribution. Ann Surg **157:**223-226, 1963.

281 Cole JW, McKalen A: Studies on the morphogenesis of adenomatous polyps in the human colon. Cancer **16:**998-1002, 1963.

282 Cooper HS, Marshall C, Ruggerio F, Steplewski Z: Hyperplastic polyps of the colon and rectum. An immunohistochemical study with monoclonal antibodies against blood groups antigens (sialosyl = Le^a^, Le^b^, Le^x^, Le^y^, A, B, H). Lab Invest **57:**421-428, 1987.

282a Cooper HS, Patchefsky AS, Marks G: Adenomatous and carcinomatous changes within hyperplastic colon epithelium. Dis Colon Rectum **22:**152-156, 1979.

283 Dajani YF, Kamal MF: Colorectal juvenile polyps. An epidemiological and histopathological study of 144 cases in Jordanians. Histopathology **8:**765-779, 1984.

284 Daniel ES, Ludwig SL, Lewin KJ, Ruprecht RM, Rajacich GM, Schwabe AD: The Cronkhite-Canada syndrome. An analysis of clinical and pathologic features and therapy in 55 patients. Medicine [Baltimore] **61:**293-309, 1982.

285 Dawson PA, Filipe MI, Bussey HJR: Ultrastructural features of the colonic epithelium in familial polyposis coli. Histopathology 1:105-113, 1977.

286 Deschner EE, Lipkin M: Proliferative patterns in colonic mucosa in familial polyposis. Cancer 35:413-418, 1975.

287 Eide TJ, Schweder T: Clustering of adenomas in the large intestine. Gut 25:1262-1267, 1984.

288 Erbe RW: Current concepts in genetics. Inherited gastrointestinal-polyposis syndromes. N Engl J Med 394:1101-1104, 1976.

289 Estrada RG, Spjut HJ: Hyperplastic polyps of the large bowel. Am J Surg Pathol 4:127-133, 1980.

290 Franzin G, Zamboni G, Dina R, Scarpa A, Fratton A: Juvenile and inflammatory polyps of the colon. A histological and histochemical study. Histopathology 7:719-728, 1983.

291 Franzin G, Zamboni G, Scarpa A, Dina R, Iannuci A, Novelli P: Hyperplastic (metaplastic) polyps of the colon. A histologic and histochemical study. Am J Surg Pathol 8:687-698, 1984.

292 Friedman CJ, Fechner RE: A solitary juvenile polyp with hyperplastic and adenomatous glands. Dig Dis Sci 27:946-948, 1982.

293 Fung CH, Goldman H: The incidence and significance of villous change in adenomatous polyps. Am J Clin Pathol 53:21-25, 1970.

294 Gardner EJ: Follow-up study of a family group exhibiting dominant inheritance for a syndrome including intestinal polyps, osteomas, fibromas, and epidermal cysts. Am J Hum Genet 14:375-389, 1962.

295 Greene FL: Epithelial misplacement in adenomatous polyps of the colon and rectum. Cancer 33:206-217, 1974.

296 Grigioni WF, Alampi G, Martinelli G, Piccaluga A: Atypical juvenile polyposis. Histopathology 5:361-376, 1981.

297 Grotsky HW, Rickert RR, Smith WD, Newsome JF: Familial juvenile polyposis coli. A clinical and pathologic study of a large kindred. Gastroenterology 82:494-501, 1982.

298 Haggitt RC, Pitcock JA: Familial juvenile polyposis of the colon. Cancer 26:1232-1238, 1970.

299 Haggitt RC, Reid BJ: Hereditary gastrointestinal polyposis syndromes. Am J Surg Pathol 10:871-887, 1986.

299a Heillmann KL, Schmidbauer G, Schyma G: The transitional polyp of the colorectal mucosa. Pathol Res Pract 182:690-693, 1987.

300 Helwig EB: Adenomas of the large intestine in children. Am J Dis Child 72:289-295, 1946.

301 Helwig EB: The evolution of adenomas of the large intestine and their relation to carcinoma. Surg Gynecol Obstet 84:36-49, 1947.

302 Helwig EB, Hanson J: Lymphoid polyps (benign lymphoma) and malignant lymphoma of the rectum and anus. Surg Gynecol Obstet 92:233-243, 1951.

303 Horrilleno EG, Eckert C, Ackerman LV: Polyps of the rectum and colon in children. Cancer 10:1210-1220, 1957.

304 Isaacson P, LeVann HP: The demonstration of carcinoembryonic antigen in colorectal carcinoma and colonic polyps using an immunoperoxidase technique. Cancer 38:1348-1356, 1976.

305 Järvinen H, Franssila KO: Familial juvenile polyposis coli. Increased risk of colorectal cancer. Gut 25:792-800, 1984.

306 Järvinen HJ: Time and type of prophylactic surgery for familial adenomatosis coli. Ann Surg 202:93-97, 1985.

307 Jass JR, Filipe MI, Abbas S, Falcon CAJ, Wilson Y, Lovell D: A morphologic and histochemical study of metaplastic polyps of the colorectum. Cancer 53:510-515, 1984.

308 Jones IT, Jagelman DG, Fazio VW, Lavery IC, Weakley FL, McGannon E: Desmoid tumors in familial polyposis coli. Ann Surg 204:94-97, 1986.

309 Jones MA, Hebert JC, Trainer TD: Juvenile polyp with intramucosal carcinoma. Arch Pathol Lab Med 111:200-201, 1987.

310 Katayama Y, Kimura M, Konn M: Cronkhite-Canada syndrome associated with a rectal cancer and adenomatous changes in colonic polyps. Am J Surg Pathol 9:65-71, 1985.

311 Kindblom L-G, Angervall L, Santesson B, Selander S: Cronkhite-Canada syndrome. Case report. Cancer 39:2651-2657, 1977.

312 Kingston JE, Herbert A, Draper GJ, Mann JR: Association between hepatoblastoma and polyposis coli. Arch Dis Child 58:959-962, 1983.

313 Konishi F, Morson BC: Pathology of colorectal adenomas. A colonoscopic survey. J Clin Pathol 35:830-841, 1982.

314 Lambert R, Sobin LH, Waye JD, Stalder GA: The management of patients with colorectal adenomas. CA 34:167-176, 1984.

315 Lane N, Kaplan H, Pascal RR: Minute adenomatous and hyperplastic polyps of the colon. Divergent patterns of epithelial growth with specific associated mesenchymal changes; contrasting roles in the pathogenesis of carcinoma. Gastroenterology 60:537-551, 1971.

315a Leppert M, Dobbs M, Scambler P, O'Connell P, Nakamura Y, Stauffer D, Woodward S, Burt R, Hughes J, Gardner E, Lathrop M, Wasmuth J, Lalouel J-M, White R: The gene for familial polyposis coli maps to the long arm of chromosome 5. Science 238:1411-1413, 1987.

316 Lewis JH, Ginsberg AL, Toomey KE: Turcot's syndrome. Evidence for autosomal dominant inheritance. Cancer 51:524-528, 1983.

317 Lipkin M, Blattner WA, Gardner EJ, Burt RW, Lynch H, Deschner E, Winawer S, Fraumeni JF Jr: Classification and risk assessment of individuals with familial polyposis, Gardner's syndrome, and familial non-polyposis colon cancer from [³H]thymidine labeling patterns in colonic epithelial cells. Cancer Res 44:4201-4207, 1984.

318 Lipper S, Kahn LB, Sandler RS, Varma V: Multiple juvenile polyposis. A study of the pathogenesis of juvenile polyps and their relationship to colonic adenomas. Hum Pathol 12:804-813, 1981.

319 Luk GD, Baylin SB: Ornithine decarboxylase as a biologic marker in familial colonic polyposis. N Engl J Med 311:80-83, 1984.

320 MacDonald JM, David WC, Crago HR, Berk AD: Gardner's syndrome and periampullary malignancy. Am J Surg 113:425-430, 1967.

321 Mestre JR: The changing pattern of juvenile polyps. Am J Gastroenterol 81:312-314, 1986.

322 Mills SE, Fechner RE: Unusual adenomatous polyps in juvenile polyposis coli. Am J Surg Pathol 6:177-183, 1982.

323 Mughal S, Filipe MI, Jass JR: A comparative ultrastructural study of hyperplastic and adenomatous polyps, incidental and in association with colorectal cancer. Cancer 48:2746-2755, 1981.

324 Muto T, Bussey HJR, Morson BC: Pseudo-carcinomatous invasion in adenomatous polyps of the colon and rectum. J Clin Pathol 26:25-31, 1973.

325 Narita T, Eto T, Ito T: Peutz-Jeghers syndrome with adenomas and adenocarcinomas in colonic polyps. Am J Surg Pathol 11:76-81, 1987.

326 Neugut AI, Johnsen CM, Forde KA, Treat MR: Recurrence rates for colorectal polyps. Cancer 55:1586-1589, 1985.

327 Painter TA, Jagelman DG: Adrenal adenomas and adrenal carcinomas in association with hereditary adenomatosis of the colon and rectum. Cancer 55:2001-2004, 1985.

328 Perkins JT, Blackstone MO, Riddell RH: Adenomatous polyposis coli and multiple endocrine neoplasia type 2b. A pathogenetic relationship. Cancer 55:375-381, 1985.

329 Ramirez RF, Culp CE, Jackman RJ, Dockerty MB: Villous tumors of the lower part of the large bowel. JAMA 194:121-125, 1965.

330 Ranzi T, Castagnone D, Velio P, Bianchi P, Polli EE: Gastric and duodenal polyps in familial polyposis coli. Gut 22:363-367, 1981.

331 Robert J, Lagace R, Delage C: Malakoplakia of the colon associated with a villous adenoma. Report of a case. Dis Colon Rectum 17:668-671, 1974.

332 Roth SI, Helwig EB: Juvenile polyps of the colon and rectum. Cancer 16:468-479, 1963.

333 Rozen P, Baratz M: Familial juvenile colonic polyposis with associated colon cancer. Cancer 49:1500-1503, 1982.

334 Ruymann FB: Juvenile polyps with cachexia. Report of an infant and comparison with Cronkhite-Canada syndrome in adults. Gastroenterology 57:431-438, 1969.

335 Sachatello CR: Familial polyposis of the colon. A four-decade follow-up. Cancer 28:581-587, 1971.

336 Sarlin JG, Mori K: Morules in epithelial tumors of the colon and rectum. Am J Surg Pathol 8:281-285, 1984.

337 Schneider NR, Cubilla AL, Chaganti RSK: Association of endocrine neoplasia with multiple polyposis of the colon. Cancer 51:1171-1175, 1983.

338 Schröder S, Moehrs D, von Weltzien J, Winkler R, Otto HF: The Turcot syndrome. Report of an additional case and review of the literature. Dis Colon Rectum 26:533-538, 1983.

339 Schuchardt WA Jr, Ponsky JL: Familial polyposis and Gardner's syndrome. Surg Gynecol Obstet 148:97-103, 1979.

339a Shepherd NA, Bussey HJR, Jass JR: Epithelial misplacement in Peutz-Jeghers polyps. A diagnostic pitfall. Am J Surg Pathol 11:743-749, 1987.

340 Sobin LH: Inverted hyperplastic polyps of the colon. Am J Surg Pathol 9:265-272, 1985.

341 Sobin LH: The histopathology of bleeding from polyps and carcinomas of the large intestine. Cancer 55:577-581, 1985.

342 Solomon SS, Moran JM, Nabseth DC: Villous adenoma of rectosigmoid accompanied by electrolyte depletion. JAMA 194:117-122, 1965.

343 Stemper TJ, Kent TH, Sommers RW: Juvenile polyposis and gastrointestinal carcinoma. A study of a kindred. Ann Int Med 83:639-646, 1975.

344 Thompson JJ, Enterline HT: The macroscopic appearance of colorectal polyps. Cancer 48:151-160, 1981.

345 Urbanski SJ, Kossakowska AE, Marcon N, Bruce WR: Mixed hyperplastic

adenomatous polyps. An underdiagnosed entity. Report of a case of adenocarcinoma arising within a mixed hyperplastic adenomatous polyp. Am J Surg Pathol **8**:551-556, 1984.

346 Veale AMO, McColl I, Bussey HJR, Morson BC: Juvenile polyposis coli. J Med Genet **3**:1-76, 1969.

347 Watne AL, Carrier JM, Durham JP, Hrabovsky EE, Chang W: The occurrence of carcinoma of the rectum following ileoproctostomy for familial polyposis. Ann Surg **197**:550-554, 1983.

348 Watne AL, Lai H-Y, Carrier J, Coppula W: The diagnosis and surgical treatment of patients with Gardner's syndrome. Surgery **82**:327-333, 1977.

349 Welch JP, Welch CE: Villous adenomas of the colorectum. Am J Surg **131**:185-191, 1976.

350 Wheat MW Jr, Ackerman LV: Villous adenomas of the large intestine. Clinicopathologic evaluation of 50 cases of villous adenomas with emphasis on treatment. Ann Surg **147**:476-487, 1958.

351 Wiebecke B, Brandts A, Eder M: Epithelial proliferation and morphogenesis of hyperplastic adenomatous and villous polyps of the human colon. Virchow Arch [Pathol Anat] **364**:35-49, 1974.

352 Williams AR, Balasooriya BAW, Day DW: Polyps and cancer of the large bowel. A necropsy study in Liverpool. Gut **23**:835-842, 1982.

353 Williams GT, Arthur JF, Bussey HJR, Morson BC: Metaplastic polyps and polyposis of the colorectum. Histopathology **4**:155-170, 1980.

354 Wiltz O, O'Toole K, Fenoglio CM: Breast carcinoma metastatic to a solitary adenomatous polyp in the colon. Arch Pathol Lab Med **108**:318-320, 1984.

355 Yonemoto RH, Slayback JB, Byron RL Jr, Rosen RB: Familial polyposis of the entire gastrointestinal tract. Arch Surg **99**:427-434, 1969.

Relationship with carcinoma and treatment

356 Ackerman LV: Malignant potential of polypoid lesions of the large intestine. Trans Stud Coll Physicians Phila **32**:5-14, 1964.

357 Banner BF, Chacho MS, Roseman DL, Coon JS: Multiparameter flow cytometric analysis of colon polyps. Am J Clin Pathol **87**:313-318, 1987.

358 Bat L, Pines A, Ron E, Rosenblum Y, Niv Y, Shemesh E: Colorectal adenomatous polyps and carcinoma in Ashkenazi and non-Ashkenazi Jews in Israel. Cancer **58**:1167-1171, 1986.

359 Boland CR, Montgomery CK, Kim YS: A cancer-associated mucin alteration in benign colonic polyps. Gastroenterology **82**:664-672, 1982.

360 Castleman B, Krikstein HI: Do adenomatous polyps of the colon become malignant? N Engl J Med **267**:469-475, 1962.

361 Clark JC, Collan Y, Eide TJ, Estève J, Ewen S, Gibbs NM, Jensen OM, Koskela E, MacLennan R, Simpson JG, Stalsberg H, Zaridze DG: Prevalence of polyps in an autopsy series from areas with varying incidence of large-bowel cancer. Int J Cancer **36**:179-186, 1985.

362 Colaccio TA, Forde KA, Scantlebury VP: Endoscopic polypectomy. Inadequate treatment for invasive colorectal carcinoma. Ann Surg **194**:704-707, 1981.

363 Cooper HS: Surgical pathology of endoscopically removed malignant polyps of the colon and rectum. Am J Surg Pathol **7**:613-623, 1983.

364 Cooper HS, Cox J, Patchevsky AS: Immunohistologic study of blood group substances in polyps of the distal colon. Expression of a fetal antigen. Am J Clin Pathol **73**:345-350, 1980.

365 Cooper HS, Reuter VE: Peanut lectin–binding sites in polyps of the colon and rectum. Lab Invest **49**:655-661, 1983.

366 Correa P, Strong JP, Reif A, Johnson WD: The epidemiology of colorectal polyps. Prevalence in New Orleans and international comparisons. Cancer **39**:2258-2264, 1977.

367 Crawford BE, Stromeyer FW: Small nonpolypoid carcinomas of the large intestine. Cancer **51**:1760-1763, 1983.

368 Eide TJ: Prevalence and morphological features of adenomas of the large intestine in individuals with and without colorectal carcinoma. Histopathology **10**:111-118, 1986.

369 Eide TJ: Remnants of adenomas in colorectal carcinomas. Cancer **51**:1866-1872, 1983.

370 Fenoglio CM, Kaye GI, Lane N: Distribution of human colonic lymphatics in normal, hyperplastic, and adenomatous tissue. Its relationship to metastasis from small carcinomas in pedunculated adenomas, with two case reports. Gastroenterology **64**:51-66, 1973.

371 Fenoglio CM, Lane N: The anatomical precursor of colorectal carcinoma. Cancer **34**:819-823, 1974.

372 Frei JV: Endoscopic large bowel polypectomy. Adequate treatment of some completely removed, minimally invasive lesions. Am J Surg Pathol **9**:355-359, 1985.

373 Fried GM, Hreno A, Duguid WP, Hampson LG: Rational management of malignant colon polyps based on long-term follow-up. Surgery **96**:815-822, 1984.

374 Fucini C, Wolff BG, Spencer RJ: An appraisal of endoscopic removal of malignant colonic polyps. Mayo Clin Proc **61**:123-126, 1986.

375 Gillespie PE, Chambers TJ, Chan KW, Doronzo F, Morson BC, Williams CB: Colonic adenomas. A colonoscopic survey. Gut **20**:240-245, 1979.

376 Haggitt RC, Glotzbach RE, Soffer EE, Wruble LD: Prognostic factors in colorectal carcinomas arising in adenomas. Implications for lesions removed by endoscopic polypectomy. Gastroenterology **89**:328-336, 1985.

377 Hermanek PJ Jr, Giedl J: The adenoma-carcinoma sequence in AMMN-induced colonic tumors of the rat. Pathol Res Pract **178**:548-554, 1984.

378 Hultborn KA: The causal relationship between benign epithelial tumors and adenocarcinoma of the colon and rectum. Acta Radiol **113**:1-71, 1954.

379 Kraus FT: Pedunculated adenomatous polyp with carcinoma in the tip and metastasis to lymph nodes. Dis Colon Rectum **8**:283-286, 1965.

380 Lipper S, Kahn LB, Ackerman LV: The significance of microscopic invasive cancer in endoscopically removed polyps of the large bowel. A clinicopathologic study of 51 cases. Cancer **52**:1691-1699, 1983.

381 Lotfi AM, Spencer RJ, Ilstrup DM, Melton LJ III: Colorectal polyps and the risk of subsequent carcinoma. Mayo Clin Proc **61**:337-343, 1986.

382 Madara JL, Harte P, Deasy J, Ross D, Lahey S, Steele G Jr: Evidence for an adenoma-carcinoma sequence in dimethylhydrazine-induced neoplasms of rat intestinal epithelium. Am J Pathol **110**:230-235, 1983.

383 Morson BC: The pathogenesis of colorectal cancer. In Bennington JL (consulting ed): Major problems in pathology, vol. 10. Philadelphia, 1978, W.B. Saunders Co.

384 Morson BC, Whiteway JE, Jones EA, Macrae FA, Williams CB: Histopathology and prognosis of malignant colorectal polyps treated by endoscopic polypectomy. Gut **25**:437-444, 1984.

385 Muto T, Bussey HJR, Morson BC: The evolution of cancer of the colon and rectum. Cancer **36**:2251-2270, 1975.

386 Riddell RH: Hands off "cancerous" large bowel polyps. Gastroenterology **89**:432-441, 1985.

387 Shamsuddin AM, Kato Y, Kunishima N, Sugano H, Trump BF: Carcinoma *in situ* in nonpolypoid mucosa of the large intestine. Report of a case with significance in strategies for early detection. Cancer **56**:2849-2854, 1985.

388 Shatney CH, Lober PH, Gilbertsen VA, Sosin H: The treatment of pedunculated adenomatous colorectal polyps with focal cancer. Surg Gynecol Obstet **139**:845-850, 1974.

389 Skinner JM, Whitehead R: Tumor-associated antigens in polyps and carcinoma of the human large bowel. Cancer **47**:1241-1245, 1981.

390 Spjut HJ, Frankel NB, Appel MF: The small carcinoma of the large bowel. Am J Surg Pathol **3**:39-46, 1979.

391 Spratt JS Jr, Ackerman LV: Small primary adenocarcinomas of the colon and rectum. JAMA **179**:337-346, 1962.

392 Spratt JS Jr, Moyer C, Ackerman LV: Relationship of polyps of the colon to colonic cancer. Ann Surg **148**:682-698, 1958.

393 Spratt JS Jr, Watson FR: The rationale of practice for polypoid lesions of the colon. Cancer **28**:153-159, 1971.

394 Stamm B, Ristivojevic B: Small pedunculated tubular adenoma of the colon with carcinoma restricted to the head, invasion of lymphatics and widespread metastases. Case report and review of the literature. Virchows Arch [Pathol Anat] **402**:83-89, 1983.

395 van den Ingh HF, Bara J, Cornelisse CJ, Nap M: Aneuploidy and expression of gastric-associated mucus antigens M_1 and CEA in colorectal adenomas. Am J Clin Pathol **87**:174-179, 1987.

396 Williams C, Muto T, Rutter KRP: Removal of polyps with fibreoptic colonoscope. A new approach to colonic polypectomy. Br Med J **1**:451-452, 1973.

397 Wolff WI, Shinya H: Endoscopic polypectomy. Therapeutic and clinicopathologic aspects. Cancer **36**:683-690, 1975.

398 Wolff WI, Shinya H: Polypectomy via the fiberoptic colonoscope. Removal of neoplasms beyond reach of the sigmoidoscope. N Engl J Med **288**:329-332, 1973.

399 Zotter S, Lossnitzer A, Hageman PC, Delemarre JFM, Hilkens J, Hilgers J: Immunohistochemical localization of the epithelial marker MAM-6 in invasive malignancies and highly dysplastic adenomas of the large intestine. Lab Invest **57**:193-199, 1987.

Carcinoma
General features

400 Alessi E, Brambilla L, Luporini G, Mosca L, Bevilacqua G: Multiple sebaceous tumors and carcinomas of the colon. Torre syndrome. Cancer **55**:2566-2574, 1985.

401 Berg JW, Howell MA: The geographic pathology of bowel cancer. Cancer **34**:807-814, 1974.

402 Black WC, Ackerman LV: Carcinoma of the large intestine as a late complication of pelvic radiotherapy. Clin Radiol **16**:278-281, 1965.

403 Boyle P, Zaridze DG, Smans M: Descriptive epidemiology of colorectal cancer. Int J Cancer **36**:9-18, 1985.

404 Cipolla R, Garcia RL: Colonic polyps and adenocarcinoma complicating ureterosigmoidostomy. Report of a case. Am J Gastroenterol **79**:453-457, 1984.

405 Hill MJ: Bacteria and the etiology of colonic cancer. Cancer **34**:815-818, 1974.

406 Lasser A, Acosta AE: Colonic neoplasms complicating ureterosigmoidostomy. Cancer **35**:1218-1222, 1975.

407 Lynch HT, Kimberling W, Albano WA, Lynch JF, Biscone K, Schuelke GS, Sandberg AA, Lipkin M, Deschner EE, Mikol YB, Elston RC, Bailey-Wilson JE, Danes BS: Hereditary nonpolyposis colorectal cancer (Lynch syndromes I and II). I. Clinical description of resource. Cancer **56**:934-938, 1985.

408 Marcheggiano A, Iannoni C, Pallone F, Frieri G, Gallucci M, Caprilli R: Abnormal patterns of colonic mucin secretion after ureterosigmoidostomy. Hum Pathol **15**:647-650, 1984.

409 Mendeloff AI: Dietary fiber and the gastrointestinal tract. Critical assessment. In Beek JE (ed): Developments in digestive diseases, Philadelphia, 1979. Lea & Febiger, pp. 43-56.

410 Mills SE, Allen MS Jr: Colorectal carcinoma in the first decades of life. Am J Surg Pathol **3**:443-448, 1979.

411 O'Higgins N, Digney J, Duff FA, Kelly DG: Three polypoid colorectal tumours associated with different types of ureterocolic implantation. Br J Urol **53**:278-279, 1981.

412 Qizilbash AH: Radiation-induced carcinoma of the rectum. A late complication of pelvic irradiation. Arch Pathol **98**:118-121, 1974.

413 Rivard J-Y, Bedard A, Dionne L: Colonic neoplasm following ureterosigmoidostomy. J Urol **113**:781-786, 1975.

414 Schipper H, Decter A: Carcinoma of the colon arising at ureteral implant sites despite early external diversion. Pathogenetic and clinical implications. Cancer **47**:2062-2065, 1981.

415 Solomon E, Voss R, Hall V, Bodmer WF, Jass JR, Jeffreys AJ, Lucibello FC, Patel I, Rider SH: Chromosome 5 allele loss in human colorectal carcinomas. Nature **328**:616-619, 1987.

416 Stemmermann GN, Nomura AMY, Heilbrun LK: Dietary fat and the risk of colorectal cancer. Cancer Res **44**:4633-4637, 1984.

Diagnosis

417 Gilbertsen VA: Proctosigmoidoscopy and polypectomy in reducing the incidence of rectal cancer. Cancer **34**:936-939, 1974.

418 Gilbertsen VA, McHugh R, Schuman L, Williams SE: The earlier detection of colorectal cancers. A preliminary report of the results of the occult blood study. Cancer **45**:2889-2901, 1980.

419 Gilbertsen VA, Nelms JM: The prevention of invasive cancer of the rectum. Cancer **41**:1137-1139, 1978.

420 Minton JP, Hoehn JL, Gerber DM, Horsley JS, Connolly DP, Salwan F, Fletcher WS, Cruz AB Jr, Gatchell FG, Oviedo M, Meyer KK, Leffall LD Jr, Berk RS, Stewart PA, Kurucz SE: Results of a 400-patient carcinoembryonic antigen second-look colorectal cancer study. Cancer **55**:1284-1290, 1985.

421 Quentmeier A, Möller P, Schwarz V, Abel U, Schlag P: Carcinoembryonic antigen, CA 19-9, and CA 125 in normal and carcinomatous human colorectal tissue. Cancer **60**:2261-2266, 1987.

421a Raskin HF, Pleticka S: The cytologic diagnosis of cancer of the colon. Acta Cytol [Baltimore] **8**:131-140, 1964.

422 Thompson DMP, Krupey J, Freedman SO, Gold P: The radioimmunoassay of circulating carcinoembryonic antigen of the human digestive system. Proc Natl Acad Sci USA **64**:161-167, 1969.

423 Winawer SJ, Leidner SD, Hajdu SI, Sherlock P: Colonoscopic biopsy and cytology in the diagnosis of colon cancer. Cancer **42**:2849-2853, 1978.

424 Winawer S, Schottenfeld D, Sherlock P: Screening for colorectal cancer. The issues. Gastroenterology **88**:841-844, 1985.

425 Zamcheck N, Doos WG, Prudente R, Lurie BB, Gottlieb LS: Prognostic factors in colon carcinoma. Correlation of serum carcinoembryonic antigen level and tumor histopathology. Hum Pathol **6**:31-45, 1975.

426 Zamcheck N, Moore TL, Dhar P, Kupchik H: Immunologic diagnosis and prognosis of human digestive-tract cancer. Carcinoembryonic antigens. N Engl J Med **286**:83-86, 1972.

Site and gross features

427 Black WA, Waugh JM: The intramural extension of carcinoma of the descending colon, sigmoid, and recto-sigmoid. Surg Gynecol Obstet **87**:457-464, 1948.

428 Dukes CE: Cancer of the rectum. An analysis of 1,000 cases. J Pathol Bacteriol **50**:527-539, 1940.

429 Ekelund GR: Multiple carcinomas of the colon and rectum. Cancer **33**:1630-1634, 1974.

430 Greenstein AJ, Slater G, Heimann TM, Sachar DB, Aufses AH Jr: A comparison of multiple synchronous colorectal cancer in ulcerative colitis, familial polyposis coli, and de novo cancer. Ann Surg **203**:123-128, 1986.

431 Netscher DT, Larson GM: Colon cancer. The left to right shift and its implications. Surg Oncol **2**:13-18, 1983.

432 Quer RE, Dahlin DC, Mayo CW: Retrograde intramural spread of carcinoma of the rectum and rectosigmoid. A microscopic study. Surg Gynecol Obstet **96**:24-30, 1953.

433 Slater G, Papatestas AE, Tartter PI, Mulvihill M, Aufses AH Jr: Age distribution of right- and left-sided colorectal cancers. Am J Gastroenterol **77**:63-66, 1982.

Microscopic features; other microscopic types

434 Ahnen DJ, Nakane PK, Brown WR: Ultrastructural localization of carcinoembryonic antigen in normal intestine and colon cancer. Abnormal distribution of CEA on the surfaces of colon cancer cells. Cancer **49**:2077-2090, 1982.

435 Almagro UA: Primary signet-ring carcinoma of the colon. Cancer **52**:1453-1457, 1983.

436 Amorn Y, Knight WA Jr: Primary linitis plastica of the colon. Report of two cases and review of the literature. Cancer **41**:2420-2425, 1978.

437 Arends JW, Wiggers T, Thijs CT, Verstijnen C, Swaen GJV, Bosman FT: The value of secretory component (SC) immunoreactivity in diagnosis and prognosis of colorectal carcinomas. Am J Clin Pathol **82**:267-274, 1984.

438 Balthazar EJ, Rosenberg HD, Davidian MM: Primary and metastatic scirrhous carcinoma of the rectum. AJR **132**:711-715, 1979.

439 Bleday R, Song J, Walker ES, Salcedo BF, Thomas P, Wilson RE, Chen LB, Steele G Jr: Characterization of a new monoclonal antibody to a cell surface antigen on colorectal cancer and fetal gut tissues. Cancer **57**:433-440, 1986.

440 Campo E, Palacin A, Benasco C, Quesada E, Cardesa A: Human chorionic gonadotropin in colorectal carcinoma. An immunohistochemical study. Cancer **59**:1611-1616, 1987.

441 Chevinsky AH, Berelowitz M, Hoover HC Jr: Adenosquamous carcinoma of the colon presenting with hypercalcemia. Cancer **60**:1111-1116, 1987.

442 Clery AP, Dockerty MB, Waugh JM: Small-cell carcinoma of the colon and rectum. A clinicopathologic study. Arch Surg **83**:164-172, 1961.

443 Compton C, Wyatt R, Konugres A, Ehrenthal D, Durda P: Immunohistochemical studies of blood group substance H in colorectal tumors using a monoclonal antibody. Cancer **59**:118-127, 1987.

444 Cox WF Jr, Pierce GB: The endodermal origin of the endocrine cells of an adenocarcinoma of the colon of the rat. Cancer **50**:1530-1538, 1982.

445 Crissman JD: Adenosquamous and squamous cell carcinoma of the colon. Am J Surg Pathol **2**:47-54, 1978.

446 Culling CFA, Reid PE, Burton JD, Dunn WL: A histochemical method of differentiating lower gastrointestinal tract mucin from other mucins in primary or metastatic tumours. J Clin Pathol **28**:656-658, 1975.

446a Czerniak B, Herz F, Koss LG, Schlom J: ras oncogene p 21 as a tumor marker in the cytodiagnosis of gastric and colonic carcinomas. Cancer **60**:2432-2436, 1987.

447 Dawson PA, Filipe MI: An ultrastructural and histochemical study of the mucous membrane adjacent to and remote from carcinoma of the colon. Cancer **37**:2388-2398, 1976.

448 Garin Chesa P, Rettig WJ, Melamed MR: Expression of cytokeratins in normal and neoplastic colonic epithelial cells. Implications for cellular differentiation and carcinogenesis. Am J Surg Pathol **10**:829-835, 1986.

449 Dukes CE: Ossification in rectal cancer. Proc R Soc Med **32**:1489-1494, 1939.

450 Ernst C, Thurin J, Atkinson B, Wurzel H, Herlyn M, Stromberg N, Civin C, Koprowski H: Monoclonal antibody localization of A and B isoantigens in normal and malignant fixed human tissues. Am J Pathol **117**:451-461, 1984.

451 Franzin G, Grigioni WF, Dina R, Scarpa A, Zamboni G: Mucin secretion and morphological changes of the mucosa in non-neoplastic diseases of the colon. Histopathology **7**:707-718, 1983.

452 Giacchero A, Aste H, Baracchini P, Conio M, Fulcheri E, Lapertosa G, Tanzi R: Primary signet-ring carcinoma of the large bowel. Report of nine cases. Cancer **56**:2723-2726, 1985.

453 Goslin R, O'Brien MJ, Steele G, Mayer R, Wilson R, Corson JM, Zamcheck N: Correlation of plasma CEA and CEA tissue staining in poorly differentiated colorectal cancer. Am J Med **71**:246-253, 1981.

454 Gould VE, Chejfec G: Neuroendocrine carcinomas of the colon. Ultrastructural and biochemical evidence of their secretory function. Am J Surg Pathol **2**:31-38, 1978.

455 Hainsworth JD, Greco FA: Human chorionic gonadotropin production by colon carcinoma. Biochemical heterogeneity and identification of a chemotherapy-sensitive cell subpopulation. Cancer **56**:1337-1340, 1985.

456 Hall-Craggs M, Toker C: Basaloid tumor of the sigmoid colon. Hum Pathol 13:497-500, 1982.

457 Hamada Y, Yamamura M, Hioki K, Yamamoto M, Nagura H, Watanabe K: Immunohistochemical study of carcinoembryonic antigen in patients with colorectal cancer. Correlation with plasma carcinoembryonic antigen levels. Cancer 55:136-141, 1985.

457a Hamazaki M, Kono S, Mimaya J, Ishihara A: Signet ring cell carcinoma in a polyp of the colon. A case report of a six-year old boy. Acta Pathol Jpn 37:1679-1684, 1987.

458 Hernandez FJ, Fernandez BB: Mucus-secreting colonic carcinoid tumors: light- and electron-microscopic study of three cases. Dis Colon Rectum 17:387-396, 1974.

459 Hernandez FJ, Reid JD: Mixed carcinoid and mucus-secreting intestinal tumors. Arch Pathol 88:489-496, 1969.

460 Hickey WF, Corson, JM: Squamous cell carcinoma arising in a duplication of the colon. Case report and literature review of squamous cell carcinoma of the colon and of malignancy complicating colonic duplication. Cancer 47:602-609, 1981.

461 Hickey WF, Seiler MW: Ultrastructural markers of colonic adenocarcinoma. Cancer 47:140-145, 1981.

462 Horne BD, McCulloch CF: Squamous cell carcinoma of the cecum. A case report. Cancer 42:1879-1882, 1978.

463 Horny H-P, Horst H-A: Lymphoreticular infiltrates in adenocarcinoma of the large intestine. Pathol Res Pract 182:222-227, 1987.

464 Isaacson P, Atwood PRA: Failure to demonstrate specificity of the morphological and histochemical changes in mucosa adjacent to colonic carcinoma (transitional mucosa). J Clin Pathol 32:214-218, 1979.

464a Jewell LD, Barr JR, McCaughey WTE, Nguyen G-K, Owen DA: Clear-cell epithelial neoplasms of the large intestine. Arch Pathol Lab Med 112:197-199, 1988.

465 Kubosawa H, Nagao K, Kondo Y, Ishige H, Inaba N: Coexistence of adenocarcinoma and choriocarcinoma in the sigmoid colon. Cancer 54:866-868, 1984.

466 Laufman H, Saphir O: Primary linitis plastica type of carcinoma of the colon. Arch Surg 62:79-91, 1951.

467 Lev R, Lance P, Camara P: Histochemical and morphologic studies of mucosa bordering rectosigmoid carcinomas. Comparisons with normal, diseased, and malignant colonic epithelium. Hum Pathol 16:151-161, 1985.

468 Listinsky CM, Riddell RH: Patterns of mucin secretion in neoplastic and non-neoplastic diseases of the colon. Hum Pathol 12:923-929, 1981.

469 Midiri G, Amanti C, Benedetti M, Campisi C, Santeusanio G, Castagna G, Peronace L, Di Tondo U, Di Paola M, Pascal RR: CEA tissue staining in colorectal cancer patients. A way to improve the usefulness of serial serum CEA evaluation. Cancer 55:2624-2629, 1985.

470 Mills SE, Allen MS Jr, Cohen AR: Small-cell undifferentiated carcinoma of the colon. A clinicopathological study of five cases and their association with colonic adenomas. Am J Surg Pathol 7:643-651, 1983.

470a Minsky BD, Mies C, Rich TA, Recht A, Chaffey JT: Colloid carcinoma of the colon and rectum. Cancer 60:3103-3112, 1987.

471 Momburg F, Degener T, Bacchus E, Moldenhauer G, Hämmerling GJ, Möller P: Loss of HLA-A, B, C and de novo expression of HLA-D in colorectal cancer. Int J Cancer 37:179-184, 1986.

472 O'Brien MJ, Zamsheck N, Burke B, Kirkham S, Saravis C, Gottlieb LS: Immunocytochemical localization of carcinoembryonic antigen in benign and malignant colo-rectal tissues. Assessment of diagnostic value. Am J Clin Pathol 75:283-290, 1981.

473 Ordóñez NG, Luna MA: Choriocarcinoma of the colon. Am J Gastroenterol 79:39-42, 1984.

474 Park CH, Reid JR: Adenocarcinoma of the colon with choriocarcinoma in its metastases. Cancer 46:570-575, 1980.

475 Pihl E, McNaughton J, Ma J, Ward HA, Nairn RC: Immunohistological patterns of carcinoembryonic antigen in colorectal carcinoma. Correlation with staging and blood levels. Pathology 12:7-13, 1980.

476 Saffos RO, Rhatigan RM: Benign (nonpolypoid) mucosal changes adjacent to carcinomas of the colon. A light microscopic study of 20 cases. Hum Pathol 8:441-449, 1977.

477 Sasaki O, Atkin WS, Jass JR: Mucinous carcinoma of the rectum. Histopathology 11:259-272, 1987.

478 Schoentag R, Williams V, Kuhns W: The distribution of blood group substance H and CEA in colorectal carcinoma. Cancer 53:503-509, 1984.

479 Schwartz AM, Orenstein JM: Small-cell undifferentiated carcinoma of the rectosigmoid colon. Arch Pathol Lab Med 109:629-632, 1985.

480 Shousha S: Paneth cell–rich papillary adenocarcinoma and a mucoid adenocarcinoma occurring synchronously in colon. A light and electron microscopic study. Histopathology 3:489-501, 1979.

481 Smith DM Jr, Haggitt RC: The prevalence and prognostic significance of argyrophil cells in colorectal carcinomas. Am J Surg Pathol 8:123-128, 1984.

482 Sunblad AS, Paz RA: Mucinous carcinomas of the colon and rectum and their relation to polyps. Cancer 50:2504-2509, 1982.

483 Sunter JP, Higgs MJ, Cowan WK: Mucosal abnormalities at the anastomosis site in patients who have had intestinal resection for colonic cancer. J Clin Pathol 38:385-389, 1985.

484 Symonds DA, Vickery AL Jr: Mucinous carcinoma of the colon and rectum. Cancer 37:1891-1900, 1976.

485 Ulich TR, Cheng L, Glover H, Yang K, Lewin KJ: A colonic adenocarcinoma with argentaffin cells. An immunoperoxidose study demonstrating the presence of numerous neuroendocrine products. Cancer 51:1483-1489, 1983.

486 Wick MR, Weatherby RP, Weiland LH: Small cell neuroendocrine carcinoma of the colon and rectum. Clinical, histologic, and ultrastructural study and immunohistochemical comparison with cloacogenic carcinoma. Hum Pathol 18:9-21, 1987.

487 Williams GT, Blackshaw AJ, Morson BC: Squamous carcinoma of the colorectum and its genesis. J Pathol 129:139-147, 1979.

Staging and grading

488 Astler VB, Coller FA: The prognostic significance of direct extension of carcinoma of the colon and rectum. Ann Surg 139:846-851, 1954.

489 Dukes CE: Histologic grading of rectal carcinoma. Proc R Soc Med 30:371-376, 1937.

490 Dukes CE: Peculiarities in the pathology of cancer of the anorectal region. Proc R Soc Med 39:763-765, 1946.

491 Hutter RVP, Sobin LH: A universal staging system for cancer of the colon and rectum. Let there be light. Arch Pathol Lab Med 110:367-368, 1986.

492 Jass JR, Atkin WS, Cuzick J, Bussey HJR, Morson BC, Northover JMA, Todd IP: The grading of rectal cancer. Historical perspectives and a multivariate analysis of 447 cases. Histopathology 10:437-459, 1986.

493 Kirklin JW, Dockerty MB, Waugh JM: The role of the peritoneal reflection in the prognosis of carcinoma of the rectum and sigmoid colon. Surg Gynecol Obstet 88:326-331, 1949.

494 Kyriakos M: The President's cancer, the Dukes classification, and confusion. Arch Pathol Lab Med 109:1063-1066, 1985.

495 Thomas GDH, Dixon MF, Smeeton NC, Williams NS: Observer variation in the histological grading of rectal carcinoma. J Clin Pathol 36:385-391, 1983.

Spread and metastases

496 Goldstein J, Mazor M, Leiberman JR: Primary carcinoma of the cecum with uterine metastases. Hum Pathol 12:1139-1140, 1981.

497 Moore JB, Law DK, Moore EE, Dean CM: Testicular mass. An initial sign of colon carcinoma. Cancer 49:411-412, 1982.

498 Rusthoven JJ, Fine S, Thomas G: Adenocarcinoma of the rectum metastatic to the oral cavity. Two cases and a review of the literature. Cancer 54:1110-1112, 1984.

Treatment

499 Balslev IB, Pedersen M, Teglbjaerg PS, Hanberg-Soerensen F, Bone J, Jacobsen NO, Overgaard J, Sell A, Bertelsen K, Hage E, Fenger C, Kronborg O, Hansen L, Hoestrup H, Noergaard-Pedersen, B: Postoperative radiotherapy in Dukes' B and C carcinoma of the rectum and rectosigmoid. A randomized multicenter study. Cancer 58:22-28, 1986.

500 Bühler H, Seefeld U, Deyhle P, Buchmann P, Metzger U, Ammann R: Endoscopic follow-up after colorectal cancer surgery. Early detection of local recurrence? Cancer 54:791-793, 1984.

501 Cole WH, McDonald GO, Roberts SS, Southwick HW: Dissemination of cancer. Prevention and therapy. New York, 1961, Appleton-Century-Croft, Inc.

502 Falterman KW, Hill CB, Markey JC, Fox JW, Cohn I Jr: Cancer of the colon, rectum, and anus. A review of 2313 cases. Cancer 34:951-959, 1974.

503 Foswit B, Higgins GA, Humphrey EW, Robinette CD: Preoperative irradiation of operable adenocarcinoma of the rectum and rectosigmoid colon. Report of a randomized study. Radiology 108:389-395, 1973.

504 Goligher JC, Dukes CE, Bussey HJR: Local recurrences after sphincter-saving excisions for carcinoma of the rectum and rectosigmoid. Br J Surg 39:199-211, 1951.

505 Higgins GA, Humphrey EW, Dwight RW, Roswit B, Lee LE Jr, Keehn RJ: Preoperative radiation and surgery for cancer of the rectum. Veterans Administration Surgical Oncology Group Trial II. Cancer 58:352-359, 1986.

506 Ottery FD, Bruskewitz RC, Weese JL: Endoscopic transrectal resection of rectal tumors. Cancer 57:563-566, 1986.

507 Stearns MW Jr, Sternberg SS, DeCosse JJ: Treatment alternatives. Localized rectal cancer. Cancer 54:2691-2694, 1984.

508 Withers HR, Romsdahl MM. Post-operative radiotherapy for adenocarcinoma of the rectum and rectosigmoid. Int J Radiat Oncol Biol Phys **2:**1069-1074, 1977.

Prognosis

509 Bauer KD, Lincoln ST, Vera-Roman JM, Wallemark CB, Chmiel JS, Madurski ML, Murad T, Scarpelli DG: Prognostic implications of proliferative activity and DNA aneuploidy in colonic adenocarcinomas. Lab Invest **57:**329-335, 1987.

510 Cass AW, Million RR, Pfaff WW: Patterns of recurrence following surgery alone for adenocarcinoma of the colon and rectum. Cancer **37:**2861-2865, 1976.

511 Dukes CE: The significance of the unusual in the pathology of intestinal tumor. Ann R Coll Surg Engl **4:**90-103, 1949.

512 Dukes CE: The surgical pathology of rectal cancer. J Clin Pathol **2:**95-98, 1949.

513 Eisenberg B, DeCosse JJ, Harford F, Michalek J: Carcinoma of the colon and rectum. The natural history reviewed in 1704 patients. Cancer **49:**1131-1134, 1982.

514 Enblad P, Glimelius B, Bengtsson A, Pontén J, Påhlman L: DNA content in carcinoma of the rectum and rectosigmoid. Acta Pathol Microbiol Immunol Scand [A] **93:**277-284, 1985.

515 Glenn F, McSherry CK: Carcinoma of the distal large bowel—32-year review of 1026 cases. Ann Surg **163:**838-849, 1966.

515a Griffin MP, Bergstralh EJ, Coffey RJ, Beart RW Jr, Melton LJ III: Predictors of survival after curative resection of carcinoma of the colon and rectum. Cancer **60:**2318-2324, 1987.

516 Gunderson LL, Sosin H: Areas of failure found at reoperation (second or symptomatic look) following "curative surgery" for adenocarcinoma of the rectum. Clinicopathologic correlation and implications for adjuvant therapy. Cancer **34:**1278-1292, 1974.

517 Hermanek P, Altendorf A: Classification of colorectal carcinomas with regional lymphatic metastases. Pathol Res Pract **173:**1-11, 1981.

518 Kaibara N, Koga S, Jinnai D: Synchronous and metachronous malignancies of the colon and rectum in Japan with special reference to a coexisting early cancer. Cancer **54:**1870-1874, 1984.

518a Krasna MJ, Flancbaum L, Cody RP, Shneibaum S, Ari GB: Vascular and neural invasion in colorectal carcinoma. Incidence and prognostic significance. Cancer **61:**1018-1023, 1988.

519 Lockhart-Mummery HE, Ritchie JK, Hawley PR: The results of surgical treatment for carcinoma of the rectum at St. Mark's Hospital from 1948 to 1972. Br J Surg **63:**673-677, 1976.

520 Lui IOL, Kung ITM, Lee JMH, Boey JH: Primary colorectal signet-ring cell carcinoma in young patients. Report of 3 cases. Pathology **17:**31-35, 1985.

521 Meyer JS, Prioleau PG: S-phase fractions of colorectal carcinomas related to pathologic and clinical features. Cancer **48:**1221-1228, 1981.

521a Minsky BD, Mies C, Recht A, Rich TA, Chaffey JT: Resectable adenocarcinoma of the rectosigmoid and rectum. II. The influence of blood vessel invasion. Cancer **61:**1417-1424, 1988.

522 Nacopoulou L, Azaris P, Papacharalampous N, Davaris P: Prognostic significance of histologic host response in cancer of the large bowel. Cancer **47:**930-936, 1981.

523 Newland RC, Chapuis PH, Pheils MT, MacPherson JG: The relationship of survival to staging and grading of colorectal carcinoma. A prospective study of 503 cases. Cancer **47:**1424-1429, 1981.

524 Newland RC, Chapuis PH, Smyth EJ: The prognostic value of substaging colorectal carcinoma. A prospective study of 1117 cases with standardized pathology. Cancer **60:**852-857, 1987.

525 Odone V, Chang L, Caces J, George SL, Pratt CB: The natural history of colorectal carcinoma in adolescents. Cancer **49:**1716-1720, 1982.

526 Patel SC, Tovee EB, Langer B: Twenty-five years of experience with radical surgical treatment of carcinoma of the extraperitoneal rectum. Surgery **82:**460-465, 1977.

527 Patt DJ, Brynes RK, Vardiman JW, Coppleson LW: Mesocolic lymph node histology is an important prognostic indicator for patients with carcinoma of the sigmoid colon. An immunomorphologic study. Cancer **35:**1388-1397, 1975.

528 Pilipshen SJ, Heilweil M, Quan SHQ, Sternberg SS, Enker WE: Patterns of pelvic recurrence following definitive resections of rectal cancer. Cancer **53:**1354-1362, 1984.

529 Pretlow TP, Keith EF, Cryar AK, Bartolucci AA, Pitts AM, Pretlow TG II, Kimball PM, Boohaker EA: Eosinophil infiltration of human colonic carcinomas as a prognostic indicator. Cancer Res **43:**2997-3000, 1983.

530 Rao BN, Pratt CB, Fleming ID, Dilawari RA, Green AA, Austin BA: Colon carcinoma in children and adolescents. A review of 30 cases. Cancer **55:**1322-1326, 1985.

531 Rich T, Gunderson LL, Lew R, Galdibini JJ, Cohen AM, Donaldson G: Patterns of recurrence of rectal cancer after potentially curative surgery. Cancer **52:**1317-1329, 1983.

532 Russell AH, Pelton J, Reheis CE, Wisbeck WM, Tong DY, Dawson LE: Adenocarcinoma of the colon. An autopsy study with implications for new therapeutic strategies. Cancer **56:**1446-1451, 1985.

533 Russell AH, Tong D, Dawson LE, Wisbeck W: Adenocarcinoma of the proximal colon. Sites of initial dissemination and patterns of recurrence following surgery alone. Cancer **53:**360-367, 1984.

534 Scott NA, Grande JP, Weiland LH, Pemberton JH, Beart RW Jr, Lieber MM: Flow cytometric DNA patterns from colorectal cancers. How reproducible are they? Mayo Clin Proc **62:**331-337, 1987.

535 Sessions RT, Reiddell DJ: Cancer of the large bowel in the young adult. Am J Surg **102:**66-69, 1961.

536 Sikora K, Chan S, Evan G, Gabra H, Markham N, Stewart J, Watson J: c-myc Oncogene expression in colorectal cancer. Cancer **59:**1289-1295, 1987.

537 Spratt JS Jr, Spjut HJ: Prevalence and prognosis of individual clinical and pathologic variables associated with colorectal carcinoma. Cancer **20:**1976-1985, 1967.

538 Steinberg SM, Barkin JS, Kaplan RS, Stablein DM: Prognostic indicators of colon tumors. The Gastrointestinal Tumor Study Group experience. Cancer **57:**1866-1870, 1986.

539 Steinberg SM, Barwick KW, Stablein DM: Importance of tumor pathology and morphology in patients with surgically resected colon cancer. Findings from the Gastrointestinal Tumor Study Group. Cancer **58:**1340-1345, 1986.

540 Talbot IC, Ritchie S, Leighton M, Hughes AO, Bussey HJR, Morson BC: Invasion of veins by carcinoma of rectum. Method of detection, histological features and significance. Histopathology **5:**141-163, 1981.

541 Tribukait B, Hammarberg C, Rubio C: Ploidy and proliferation patterns in colorectal adenocarcinomas related to Dukes' classification and to histopathological differentiation. A flow-cytometric DNA study. Pathol Microbiol Immunol Scand [A] **91:**89-95, 1983.

542 Welch JP, Donaldson GA: Perforative carcinoma of the colon and rectum. Ann Surg **180:**734-740, 1974.

543 Wolmark N, Cruz I, Redmond CK, Fisher B, Fisher ER and contributing NSABP investigators: Tumor size and regional lymph node metastasis in colorectal cancer. A preliminary analysis from the NSABP clinical trials. Cancer **51:**1315-1322, 1983.

544 Wolmark N, Fisher B, Wieand HS: The prognostic value of the modifications of the Dukes' C class of colorectal cancer. An analysis of the NSABP clinical trials. Ann Surg **203:**115-122, 1986.

545 Wolmark N, Fisher ER, Wieand HS, Fisher B and contributing NSABP investigators: The relationship of depth of penetration and tumor size to the number of positive nodes in Dukes C colorectal cancer. Cancer **53:**2707-2712, 1984.

546 Wolmark N, Wieand HS, Rockette HE, Fisher B, Glass A, Lawrence W, Lerner H, Cruz AB, Volk H, Shibata H, Evans J, Prager D and other NSABP investigators: The prognostic significance of tumor location and bowel obstruction in Dukes B and C colorectal cancer. Findings from the NSABP clinical trials. Ann Surg **198:**743-752, 1987.

Carcinoid tumor

547 Black WC: Enterochromaffin cell types and corresponding carcinoid tumors. Lab Invest **19:**473-486, 1968.

548 Caldarola VT, Jackman RJ, Moertel CG, Dockerty MB: Carcinoid tumors of the rectum. Am J Surg **107:**844-849, 1964.

549 Fukayama M, Hayashi Y, Koike M: Human chorionic gonadotropin in the rectosigmoid colon. Immunohistochemical study on unbalanced distribution of subunits. Am J Pathol **127:**83-89, 1987.

550 Gledhill A, Hall PA, Cruse JP, Pollock DJ: Enteroendocrine cell hyperplasia, carcinoid tumours and adenocarcinoma in long-standing ulcerative colitis. Histopathology **10:**501-508, 1986.

551 Horn RC Jr: Carcinoid tumors of the colon and rectum. Cancer **2:**819-837, 1949.

552 Hosoda J, Kito N, Nogaki M: Is rectal carcinoid argyrophilic? An application of Grimelius silver nitrate stain in four cases. Dis Colon Rectum **18:**386-390, 1975.

553 Iwafuchi M, Watanabe H, Ishihara N, Shimoda T, Iwashita A, Ito S: Peptide YY immunoreactive cells in gastrointestinal carcinoids. Immunohistochemical and ultrastructural studies of 60 tumors. Hum Pathol **17:**291-296, 1986.

553a Maruyama M, Fukayama M, Koike M: A case of multiple carcinoid tumors of the rectum with extraglandular endocrine cell proliferation. Cancer **60:**131-136, 1988.

554 Naunheim KS, Zeitels J, Kaplan EL, Sugimoto J, Shen K-L, Lee C-H, Straus FH II: Rectal carcinoid tumors. Treatment and prognosis. Surgery **94:**670-676, 1983.

555 O'Briain DS, Dayal Y, DeLellis RA, Tischler AS, Bendon R, Wolfe HJ: Rectal carcinoids as tumors of the hindgut endocrine cells. A morphological and immunohistochemical analysis. Am J Surg Pathol 6:131-142, 1982.

556 Peskin G, Orloff M: A clinical study of 25 patients with carcinoid tumors of the rectum. Surg Gynecol Obstet 109:673-682, 1959.

557 Ratzenhofer R, Gamse R, Höfler H, Auböck L, Popper H, Pohl P, Lembeck F: Substance P in an argentaffin carcinoid of the caecum. Biochemical and biological characterization. Virchows Arch [Pathol Anat] 392:21-31, 1981.

558 Shimoda T, Ishikawa E, Sano T, Watanabe K, Ikegami M: Histopathological and immunohistochemical study of neuroendocrine tumors of the rectum. Acta Pathol Jpn 34:1059-1077, 1984.

559 Sobin LH, Hjermstad BM, Sesterhenn IA, Helwig EB: Prostatic acid phosphatase activity in carcinoid tumors. Cancer 58:136-138, 1986.

560 Stout AP: Carcinoid tumors of the rectum derived from Erspamer's pre-enterochrome cells. Am J Pathol 18:993-1009, 1942.

561 Takatoh H, Iwamoto H, Ikezu M, Katoh N, Ito S, Kaneko H: Immunohistochemical demonstration of peptide YY in gastrointestinal endocrine tumors. Acta Pathol Jpn 37:737-746, 1987.

562 Wilander E, El-Salhy M, Lundqvist M, Grimelius L, Terenius L, Lundberg JM, Tatemoto K, Schwartz TW: Polypeptide YY (PYY) and pancreatic polypeptide (PP) in rectal carcinoids. An immunocytochemical study. Virchows Arch [Pathol Anat] 401:67-72, 1983.

563 Wilander E, Portela-Gomes G, Grimelius L, Lundqvist G, Skoog V: Enteroglucagon and substance P-like immunoreactivity in argentaffin and argyrophil rectal carcinoids. Virchows Arch [Cell Pathol] 25:117-124, 1977.

564 Williams RM: A light and electron microscopic study of an ovarian and rectal carcinoid. Histopathology 3:19-30, 1979.

565 Yoshida A, Yano M, Fujinaga Y, Sano C, Mori H, Yoshida H, Fukunishi R: Argentaffin carcinoid tumor of the rectum. Cancer 48:2103-2106, 1981.

Malignant lymphoma and other lymphoid lesions

566 Cornes JS, Wallace MH, Morson BC: Benign lymphomas of the rectum and anal canal. A study of 100 cases. J Pathol Bacteriol 82:371-382, 1961.

567 Gleason TH, Hammar SP: Plasmacytoma of the colon. Case report with lambda light chain, demonstrated by immunoperoxidase studies. Cancer 50:130-133, 1982.

568 Helwig EB, Hanson J: Lymphoid polyp (benign lymphoma) and malignant lymphoma of the rectum and anus. Surg Gynecol Obstet 92:233-243, 1951.

569 Isaacson PG, Maclennan KA, Subbuswamy SG: Multiple lymphomatous polyposis of the gastrointestinal tract. Histopathology 8:641-656, 1984.

570 Pinkus GS, Wilson RE, Corson JM: Reticulum cell sarcoma of the colon following renal transplantation. Cancer 34:2103-2108, 1974.

571 Ranchod M, Lewin KJ, Dorfman RF: Lymphoid hyperplasia of the gastrointestinal tract. A study of 26 cases and review of the literature. Am J Surg Pathol 2:383-400, 1978.

572 Renton P, Blackshaw AJ: Colonic lymphoma complicating ulcerative colitis. Br J Surg 63:542-545, 1976.

572a Schweers CA, Shaw MT, Nordquist RE, Rose D, Kell T: Solitary cecal plasmacytoma. Electron microscopic, immunologic, and cytochemical studies. Cancer 37:2220-2223, 1976.

573 Van der Henle B, Taylor CR, Terry R, Lukes RJ: Presentation of malignant lymphoma in the rectum. Cancer 49:2602-2607, 1982.

Other tumors and tumorlike conditions

574 Akwari OE, Dozois RR, Weiland LH, Beahrs OH: Leiomyosarcoma of the small and large bowel. Cancer 42:1375-1384, 1978.

575 Boley SJ, Sammartano R, Adams A, DiBiase A, Kleinhaus S, Sprayregen S: On the nature and etiology of vascular ectasias of the colon. Degenerative lesions of aging. Gastroenterology 72:650-660, 1977.

576 Cabaud PG, Harris LT: Lipomatosis of the ileocecal valve. Ann Surg 150:1092-1098, 1959.

577 DeSchryver-Kecskemeti K, Clouse RE, Goldstein MN, Gersell D, O'Neal L: Intestinal ganglioneuromatosis. A manifestation of overproduction of nerve growth factor? N Engl J Med 308:635-640, 1983.

578 Duray PH, Marcal JM, LiVolsi VA, Fisher R, Scholhamer C, Brand MH: Gastrointestinal angiodysplasia. A possible component of von Willebrand's disease. Hum Pathol 15:539-544, 1984.

579 Eshun-Wilson K: Malignant giant-cell tumor of the colon. Acta Pathol Microbiol Scand [A] 81:137-144, 1973.

580 Fry DE, Amin M, Harbrecht PJ: Rectal obstruction secondary to carcinoma of the prostate. Ann Surg 189:488-492, 1979.

581 Haller JD, Roberts TW: Lipomas of the colon. Clincopathologic study of 20 cases. Surgery 55:773-781, 1964.

582 MacKenzie DA, McDonald JR, Waugh JM: Leiomyoma and leiomyosarcoma of the colon. Ann Surg 139:67-75, 1954.

583 Mendelsohn G, Diamond MP: Familial ganglioneuromatous polyposis of the large bowel. Report of a family with associated juvenile polyposis. Am J Surg Pathol 8:515-520, 1984.

584 Meyer CT, Troncale FJ, Galloway S, Sheahan DG: Arteriovenous malformations of the bowel. An analysis of 22 cases and a review of the literature. Medicine [Baltimore] 60:36-48, 1981.

585 Morimatsu M, Shirozu K, Nakashima T, Fujimi T, Isomoto H: Xanthogranuloma of the rectum. Acta Pathol Jpn 35:165-171, 1985.

586 Pounder DJ, Rowland R, Pieterse AS, Freeman R, Hunter R: Angiodysplasias of the colon. J Clin Pathol 35:824-829, 1982.

587 Quan SHQ, Berg JW: Leiomyoma and leiomyosarcoma of the rectum. Dis Colon Rectum 5:418-425, 1962.

588 Ranchod M, Kempson RL: Smooth muscle tumors of the gastrointestinal tract and retroperitoneum. A pathologic analysis of 100 cases. Cancer 39:255-262, 1977.

589 Roth JA, Schell S, Panzarino S, Coronato A: Visceral Kaposi's sarcoma presenting as colitis. Am J Surg Pathol 2:209-214, 1978.

589a Snover DC: Atypical lipomas of the colon. Report of two cases with pseudomalignant features. Dis Colon Rectum 27:485-488, 1984.

590 Snover DC, Weigent CE, Sumner HW: Diffuse mucosal ganglioneuromatosis of the colon associated with adenocarcinoma. Am J Clin Pathol 75:225-229, 1981.

591 Stamm B, Heer M, Bühler H, Ammann R: Mucosal biopsy of vascular ectasia (angiodysplasia) of the large bowel detected during routine colonoscopic examination. Histopathology 9:639-646, 1985.

592 Vella-Camilleri FC, Friedrich R, Vento AO: Diffuse colonic varices. An uncommon cause of intestinal bleeding. Am J Gastroenterol 81:492-494, 1986.

593 Weaver GA, Alpern HD, Davis JS, et al.: Gastrointestinal angiodysplasia associated with aortic valve disease. Part of a spectrum of angiodysplasia of the gut. Gastroenterology 77:1-11, 1979.

594 Weber JN, Carmichael DJ, Boylston A, Munro A, Whitear WP, Pinching AJ: Kaposi's sarcoma of the bowel presenting as apparent ulcerative colitis. Gut 26:295-300, 1985.

595 Weidner N, Flanders DJ, Mitros FA: Mucosal ganglioneuromatosis associated with multiple colonic polyps. Am J Surg Pathol 8:779-786, 1984.

596 Weidner N, Zekan P: Carcinosarcoma of the colon. Report of a unique case with light and immunohistochemical studies. Cancer 58:1126-1130, 1986.

597 Yatto RP: Colonic lipomatosis. Am J Gastroenterol 77:436-437, 1982.

Anus

ANATOMY

The anal canal is a tubular structure 3 to 4 cm in length extending from the perineal skin to the lower end of the rectum and is demarcated by the proximal and distal margins of the internal sphincter (Fig. 11-152). The junction between the anal canal and the perineal skin is known as the *anal verge*, or Hilton's line, identified microscopically by the appearance of cutaneous adnexae. The pectinate (dentate) line is located at the very center of the anal canal. The segment of anal canal located immediately below this line exhibits a number of longitudinal folds known as *anal columns (of Morgagni)*. Homologous structures in the lower rectum are designated *rectal columns (of Morgagni)* and the depressions between them as *rectal sinuses (of Morgagni)*. The anal columns are connected at the dentate line by the *anal* or *semilunar valves (transverse plicae)*. The latter form the inner boundary of minute pockets designated as *anal crypts (of Morgagni)*.

The anal canal is lined by columnar epithelium in its upper portion and by keratinized or nonkeratinized squamous epithelium in its lower portion, which is known as *pecten*. At the interphase between the two, roughly corresponding to the pectinate line, there is a circular zone, 0.3 to 1.1 cm in width, with a glistening, wrinkled appearance made discontinuous by the presence of anal papillae.[1a] This zone is lined by epithelium known as *transitional, intermediate,* or *cloacogenic*, which resembles bladder epithelium; however, its ultrastructural appearance is different from that of urothelium.[2] Scattered endocrine cells are sometimes identified in the basilar portion of this epithelium.[3]

Anal papillae are toothlike, raised projections located on top of the anal columns, extending upward onto the rectum and representing ridges of squamous mucosa directly joining the rectal mucosa. Both anal crypts and papillae show marked individual variations and are occasionally absent. The anal glands discharge into the anal crypts through anal ducts, which can extend upward or, more commonly, downward. They penetrate the sphincters and sometimes extend into the perianal fat.[4,5] The epithelium that lines these ducts is similar to that of the overlying "transitional" epithelium and also exhibits sparse mucin production characterized by scarcity or absence of O-acylated sialic acids.[2]

It has been proposed that the strip of "transitional" epithelium represents a vestige of the cloacal membrane; although this is true, it should be pointed out that the entire anal canal, not just the transitional zone, is a cloacal deriv-

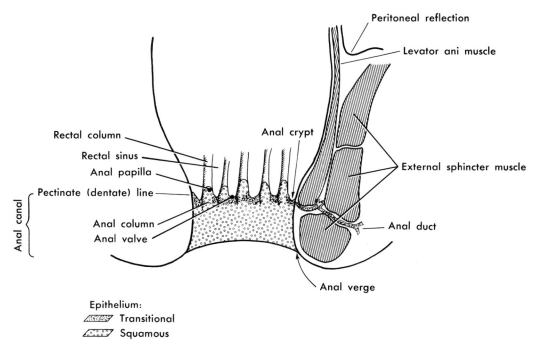

Fig. 11-152 Diagrammatic representation of normal anal structures. Most cases of anal carcinoma arise from small area of transitional epithelium.

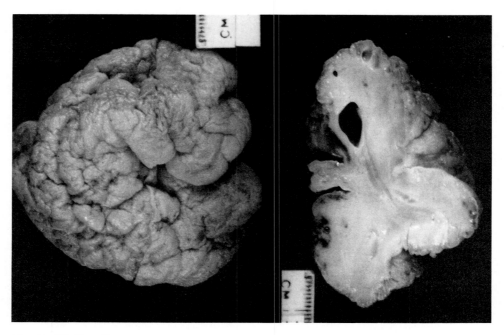

Fig. 11-153 Giant fibrous polyp of anus. This large lesion can be viewed as extremely exuberant form of hypertrophic anal papilla.

ative. A method for the gross demonstration of this anal transitional zone using whole-mount staining with Alcian dyes has been described.[1]

EMBRYOLOGIC DEFECTS

Anorectal anomalies occur in approximately 1 of every 1800 births.[6] They are divided into three major types depending on the relationship of the lower bowel to the puborectalis component of the levator ani muscle.[7] *High* or *supralevator anomalies* (40%) have a serious prognosis because of severe obstruction, common association with other congenital anomalies (in vertebrae and urinary tract), and defective innervation of the pelvic muscles. A fistulous tract to the bladder, urethra, or vagina is often present. A complicated sacroabdominoperineal approach is needed for reconstruction. In *low* or *translevator anomalies* (40%), obstruction is rarely severe. The pelvic innervation is normal, and associated anomalies are rare. Fistulas may or may not be present. A simple perineal operation will cure most of these patients. *Intermediate anomalies* are rare (15%). An abdominoperineal approach is usually needed for reconstruction. The remaining varieties, which are quite rare, include *perineal groove* and *persistent anal membrane*.

Familiarity with the anatomic variants of anorectal anomalies and a thorough radiologic investigation (plain x-ray films, cystograms, and fistulograms) are essential for accurate diagnosis and, therefore, proper treatment. Unsuccessful surgery leads to stricture and colonic obstruction, which may eventually necessitate a permanent colostomy.

FISSURE, ULCER, AND FISTULA

An anal *fissure* is a single linear separation of the tissues of the anal canal extending through the mucous membrane. About 90% of anal fissures are found at the posterior commissure overlying the bifurcation of the sphincter as it divides to circle the rectum.

An anal *ulcer* is a chronic process, usually oval in shape, that extends into the muscular layer. Above it is a hypertrophied papilla, and behind this papilla is an infected crypt. External to the ulcer is a skin tag, the result of chronic edema and fibrosis surrounding the ulcer.

An anal *fistula* is an abnormal track having an internal opening within the anal canal, usually at the dentate line.[10] The fistulous track may lead to the skin, or it may end blindly in the perianal soft tissues. A classification of anal fistulas into five categories on the basis of their anatomic relationships has been proposed.[14] The lining of the fistula is made of granulation tissue, although epithelium may eventually grow at either end of the track. Most cases of anal fistulas are caused by an intersphincteric abscess originating in an anal duct[12,15] and have a non-specific microscopic appearance. On the other hand, anal fistulas may be a manifestation of tuberculosis,[13] Crohn's disease,[9] ulcerative colitis,[11] and actinomycosis.[8] It is important therefore that tissue obtained from an anal fistula be examined microscopically in every case. The incidence of tuberculosis as a cause of anal fistulas dropped from 16% to less than 1% at St. Mark's Hospital (London) in a 50-year period.[13] The patients almost invariably show radiologic evidence of pulmonary tuberculosis. Fistulas caused by Crohn's disease are often complex and painless, with irregular edges and with little induration.[9] The diagnosis may be suggested by the presence of noncaseating granulomas, but it is important not to confuse them with the foci of foreign-body reaction sometimes seen in nonspecific fistulas.

HYPERTROPHIED PAPILLA

Anal papillae can enlarge as a result of edema, inflammation, and fibrosis, and protrude into the anal canal in polypoid fashion. They are often seen immediately above anal ulcers (Fig. 11-153). Microscopically, they are lined by squamous epithelium and contain a central core of edematous and inflamed fibrovascular stroma. Their appearance is similar to that of cutaneous "fibroepithelial polyps" or "skin tags." Occasionally, atypical stromal cells with large nuclei and stellate cytoplasmic outlines occur in them.[16]

HEMORRHOIDS

Stasis of blood in the veins of the hemorrhoidal plexus is usually caused simply by dependency. However, pathologic processes in the drainage path of those veins may cause secondary engorgement. Therefore the presence of hemorrhoids may be an indication of some other process such as cirrhosis of the liver with portal hypertension, carcinoma of the rectum, leiomyoma of the uterus, or pregnancy.

Hemorrhoids can be present either within or outside the anus. Thrombosis of these dilated veins is frequent. If the cause of venous obstruction is removed, the hemorrhoids may disappear, although in many instances resection is necessary. Inflammatory changes are secondary to surface ulceration rather than thrombosis.[18]

Microscopic examination of tissue submitted as hemorrhoids rarely may show nonspecific granulomas, tuberculosis, malignant lymphoma, koilocytotic atypia, Bowen's disease, epidermoid carcinoma, or even malignant melanoma.[16a,17]

TUMORS
Carcinoma

Anal carcinoma presents clinically with bleeding (50%), pain (40%; much higher than in colonic cancer), mass (25%), and pruritus (15%). About 25% of the patients are asymptomatic. The female/male ratio ranges from 2:1 to 4:1. In some instances, the tumor developed in association with Crohn's disease,[48] lymphogranuloma venereum,[46] condyloma acuminatum,[20] or independent carcinomas of the lower genital tract (particularly cervix) in females.[22] A strong association has also been found between anal carcinoma and receptive anal intercourse related to homosexual behavior.[24a] Grossly, it appears near the mucocutaneous junction and grows either upward into the rectum and surrounding tissues or outward to the perianal tissues[27a,35] (Fig. 11-154). At times, its gross appearance almost exactly simulates that of an adenocarcinoma of the rectum, and the correct diagnosis is made only with biopsy. Involvement of the perianal skin may be superficial, with only surface ulceration and slightly elevated margins. Such lesions can be mistaken for an inflammatory process. In other instances,

a typical deeply ulcerated neoplasm with rolled edges is seen (Fig. 11-155). Upward local extension may burrow beneath the overlying epithelium to ulcerate at a higher level. Because of the dual lymphatic supply of the pectinate line, lymph nodes along the rectum as well as those in the inguinal areas may contain metastases.

The interpretation of the microscopic pathology of carcinoma of the anal canal has changed considerably in the course of the years. Classically, these tumors were regarded and classified as epidermoid carcinomas.[25] Some years ago, it was proposed that there were two distinct types of carcinoma in this area: *epidermoid* carcinoma, analogous to its counterpart elsewhere in the skin; and *cloacogenic* (transitional, basaloid) carcinoma, supposedly originating from the transitional zone, a fact supported by ultrastructural examination.[31,33,42] The latter tumor, which was said to comprise about 20% of all anal cancers, was identified by the presence of solid tumor nests exhibiting peripheral palisading somewhat resembling that seen in cutaneous basal cell carcinoma (hence the term *basaloid*) (see Fig. 11-154, *D*), sometimes accompanied by foci of mucin secretion and areas of squamous differentiation.[40,43] With increased experience, it became obvious that distinguishing these two tumor types is not only difficult in practice but also histogenetically unwarranted. It seems likely that we are dealing with a carcinoma that is basically *epidermoid* in nature, but which manifests in various degrees a tendency toward glandular (adnexal) differentiation in a manner analogous to that sometimes seen in epidermoid carcinoma of oral cavity, larynx, or esophagus. Along these lines, Dougherty and Evans[26] have suggested classifying all these tumors as squamous cell carcinomas and subdividing them into five types: keratinizing, nonkeratinizing, basaloid, with mucous cysts, and pseudoadenoid cystic. We find this approach very sensible, although perhaps the number of subtypes is excessive.

Some anal carcinomas are accompanied by a massive infiltration by mature eosinophils.[41] Others have a spindle-cell (sarcomatoid) appearance.[39] Foci of dysplasia or carcinoma in situ are not uncommon in the epithelium adjacent to invasive anal carcinomas.[28]

Immunohistochemically, anal carcinomas exhibit reactivity for all cytokeratin classes, epithelial membrane antigen, CEA, and blood group isoantigens.[50]

Tumors described in the past as mucoepidermoid carcinomas of the anal canal are presently incorporated into this general scheme, although whether this is justified remains to be determined. Several of the cases that we have seen were located *proximal* to the pectinate line without encroaching upon it.

Some anal carcinomas are highly undifferentiated, formed by large solid nests of small hyperchromatic cells with central necrosis, with an appearance reminiscent of pulmonary *small cell carcinoma*. These tumors have been found to have signs of endocrine differentiation ultrastructurally and immunohistochemically.[50] Their behavior is extremely aggressive.

The standard therapy for anal carcinomas is abdominoperineal resection,[25,30] sometimes combined with hypogas-

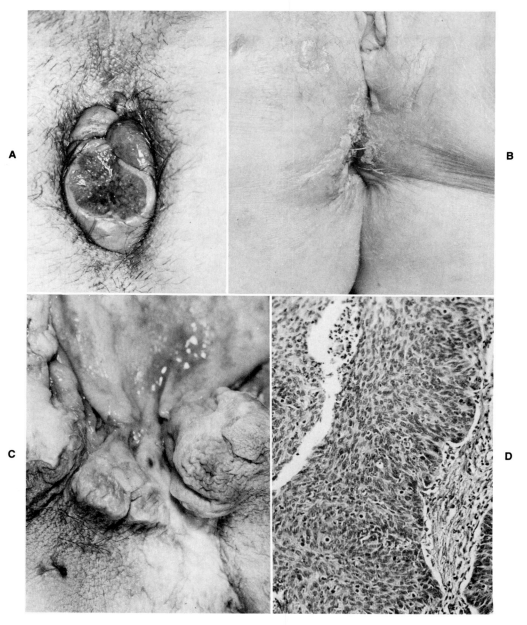

Fig. 11-154 A, Anal carcinoma extending into perianal skin. **B,** Same tumor showing excellent temporary results following irradiation. **C,** Tumor recurred locally, and abdominoperineal resection was done. Note irradiation effect in skin and narrowed anal canal. **D,** Microscopic appearance of persistent tumor. Note plexiform pattern and palisading of cells around border, resulting in a basaloid appearance. Regional lymph nodes were negative. Patient died of disseminated disease 4 years following microscopic diagnosis.

tric lymph node dissection and with posterior vaginectomy in women.[24,47] Alternative methods using radiation therapy and chemotherapy have been advocated.[29,44] Local excision is adequate for small tumors.[21,47] The overall 5-year survival rate ranges from 50% to 70% in the various series.[21,40]

The prognosis depends largely on the stage of the disease as determined by depth of invasion and regional nodal involvement.[21,26] Tumor size is related to stage and inversely related to prognosis. Involvement of inguinal lymph nodes

is an extremely grave prognostic sign.[38,47] Tumor recurrence in the pelvic or perineal regions following abdominoperineal resection carries an ominous prognosis; instead, subsequent development of inguinal lymph node metastases is compatible with long-term survival following the performance of an inguinal lymphadenectomy.[25,32] There is not much prognostic difference between the various microscopic *types*,[26,30,47] but an excellent correlation exists with the microscopic *grade* of the tumor.[21,43] In the series by Pang and

Fig. 11-155 Large excavated carcinoma involving dentate line and extending into rectal mucosa. Microscopically, it had basaloid features. All twenty-six lymph nodes were free of tumor. Patient, 56-year-old woman, is alive 7 years after surgery without evidence of tumor recurrence.

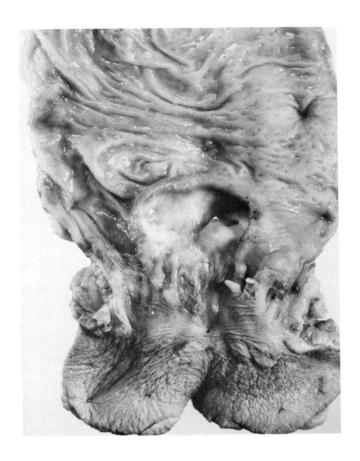

Morson,[43] the 5-year survival rate was 90%, 60%, and 0% for well-differentiated, moderately differentiated, and poorly differentiated tumors, respectively.

Verrucous carcinoma presents as a polypoid neoplasm that is microscopically composed of extremely well-differentiated squamous epithelium but which invades the underlying stroma in a pushing fashion. This lesion is closely related if not identical to the so-called giant condyloma acuminatum of Buschke-Loewenstein. Actually, a continuum seems to exist between the human papilloma virus–induced condyloma acuminatum, the "giant" form of this process, and verrucous carcinoma.[20] These lesions are morphologically identical to those seen in the lower female genital tract (Fig. 11-156) (see Chapter 19).

Mucinous adenocarcinomas are sometimes found in the anal region, often presenting with multiple fistulous tracts, and, on rare occasions, as vaginal cysts.[19] They are thought to arise from the epithelium of anal ducts, either *de novo* or on the basis of pre-existing anal fistulas.[27,51] Jones and Morson[37] have suggested that some of these carcinomas associated with fistulas arise in congenital duplications of

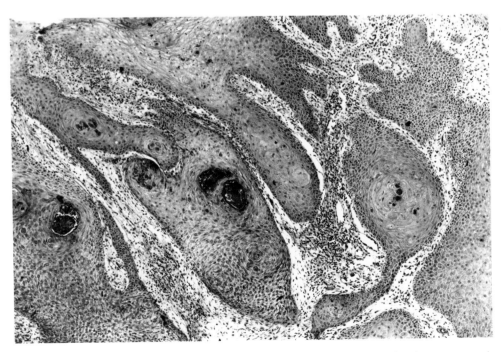

Fig. 11-156 Verrucous carcinoma of anus. Tongues of extremely well-differentiated squamous epithelium of bulbous shape are seen infiltrating inflamed stroma. Degree of cytologic atypia is minimal.

the distal end of the hindgut. These tumors need to be distinguished from low rectal, mucin-producing adenocarcinomas.[45] Cases have been reported of anorectal adenocarcinomas containing abundant melanin pigment in the cytoplasm of the tumor cells.[23]

True **basal cell carcinomas** can occur in the skin at the anal margin and can be cured either by local excision or by irradiation.[52]

Bowen's disease can involve the perianal skin in a diffuse or multicentric fashion and spread into the anal canal.[49] Some cases of Bowen's disease, as well as of superficially invasive anal carcinomas, are sometimes unexpectedly found in specimens obtained after minor anorectal surgery.[34] A routine microscopic examination of all these specimens is therefore mandatory.

Paget's disease of the anus presents as an erythematous, ulcerated lesion of eczematoid appearance. It is a malignant neoplasm of the intraepidermal portion of apocrine glands, with or without associated dermal involvement. The latter was found in thirteen of thirty-eight cases studied by Helwig and Graham.[36] Eleven patients had lymph node metastases, and all of them died of their disease. The cells of anogenital Paget's disease invariably contain acid mucosubstances, an important feature in the differential diagnosis with melanoma and Bowen's disease.[53]

Malignant melanoma

Approximately one melanoma is seen for every eight epidermoid carcinomas and one for every 250 adenocarcinomas

of the anorectal region.[58] Rectal bleeding is the most common complaint. The tumor usually begins at the pectinate line and tends to grow towards the rectal ampulla. The typical gross appearance is that of single or multiple polypoid masses covered by a smooth surface (Fig. 11-157). In the early stages, it can simulate clinically thrombosed hemorrhoids. Microscopically, the appearance is similar to that of other mucosal melanomas; a peripheral lentiginous appearance is often prominent. Sometimes melanoma extends proximally a long way along the submucosa and emerges through the mucosa at a high point, thus simulating a primary rectal tumor.[56] Rectal bleeding, palpable mass, and pain are the most common complaints.[55] Microscopically, the tumors are usually melanotic, and two thirds show a "junctional" component in the adjacent mucosa.[59] One reported case was of the desmoplastic variety.[54] The prognosis is extremely poor[57,59] and is directly related to tumor size and depth of invasion.

OTHER LESIONS

Granuloma inguinale may be confused clinically with epidermoid carcinoma (Fig. 11-158). Biopsy in such cases will allow a definite diagnosis if Donovan bodies are found.

Lymphogranuloma venereum is a sexually transmitted disease caused by *Chlamydia trachomatis*, the incidence of which is rising. It may cause a granulomatous proctitis very similar to Crohn's disease. Microscopically, the main changes are follicular lymphohistiocytic and plasmacellular infiltrate in the wall, associated with neuromatous hyper-

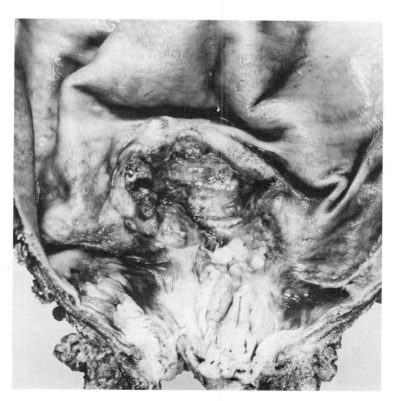

Fig. 11-157 Malignant melanoma growing into rectum to form polypoid mass. There were innumerable metastases.

plasia and extensive fibrosis.[62] Long-standing cases lead to rectal stricture and rectal squamous metaplasia. Occasionally, epidermoid carcinoma develops on the basis of these lesions (Fig. 11-159). *Pseudotumors* may be produced by sclerosing agents used to obliterate hemorrhoids. *Eosinophilic granuloma* (histiocytosis X) can involve the perianal skin.[64]

Inflammatory cloacogenic polyp is discussed in the bowel section.

The anus also can be the site of *keratinous cysts* of epidermal type,[61] as well as a variety of *sweat gland tumors* arising from the apocrine sweat glands of the perianal skin. Hydradenomas,[67] fibroadenomas,[60] and apocrine mixed tumors containing abundant cartilage have been described.

The only benign non-epithelial tumor that occurs with any frequency is *granular cell tumor;* it may grow to a relatively large size and ulcerate, thus simulating clinically the appearance of a malignant tumor.[63] Benign mesenchymal tumors are rare, especially if one avoids labeling hypertrophied anal papillae as "fibromas." A case of perianal spindle-cell lipoma has been reported.[65]

Embryonal rhabdomyosarcoma can occur in the perianal region of infants and children.[66] Some of these tumors are of the botryoid variety. Electron microscopy and immunohistochemistry are very useful in its recognition (Fig. 11-160).

Malignant lymphoma of the anorectal region has been observed in AIDS patients.[62a] *Metastases* to the anal region

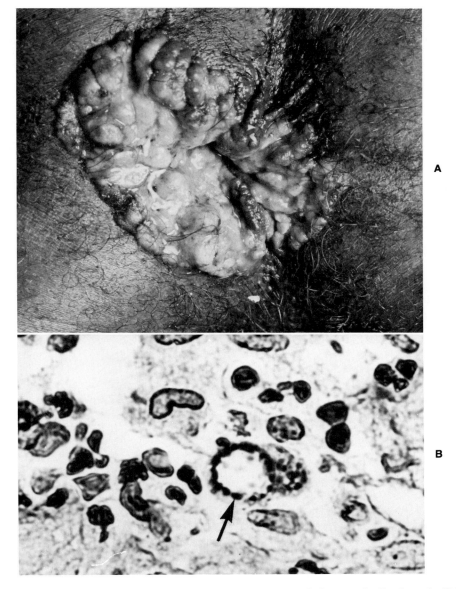

Fig. 11-158 A, Granuloma inguinale clinically simulating carcinoma. **B,** Donovan bodies (arrow) within cyst in cytoplasm of macrophage in patient with granuloma inguinale. (**B,** Warthin-Starry stain.)

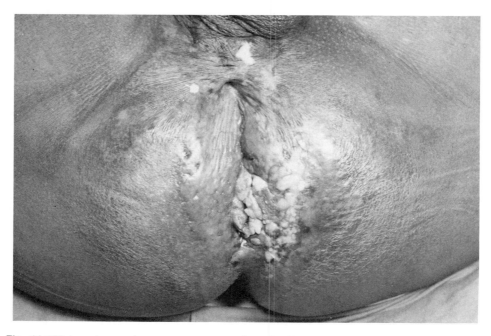

Fig. 11-159 Lymphogranuloma venereum complicated with epidermoid carcinoma. Frei test was positive.

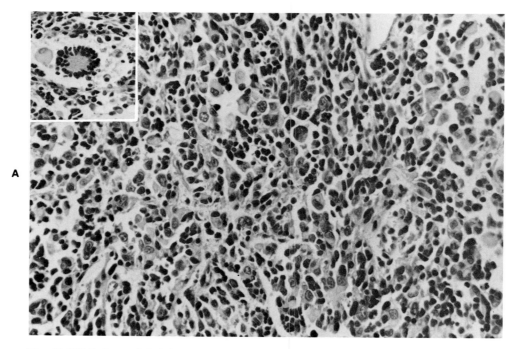

Fig. 11-160 Embryonal rhabdomyosarcoma arising from perianal region of 3-year-old boy. **A,** Light microscopic appearance is that of undifferentiated small cell tumor with occasional larger cells with acidophilic cytoplasm. **Inset** shows multinucleated tumor cell.

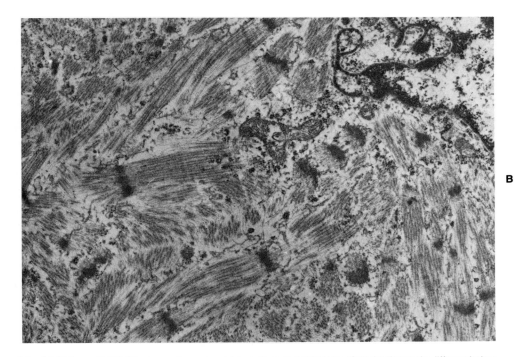

Fig. 11-160, cont'd B, Electron microscopy shows clear-cut evidence of skeletal muscle differentiation. Patient was treated by surgery followed by chemotherapy and is well 3 years later. (**B,** ×18,000; **A** and **B,** courtesy Dr. J. Magidson, Brookhaven, NY.)

often arise from rectal carcinomas. Sometimes, these metastases develop at the site of a recently performed hemorrhoidectomy.

REFERENCES
ANATOMY

1 Fenger C: The anal transitional zone. Acta Pathol Microbiol Scand [A] **86:**225-230, 1978.

1a Fenger C: Histology of the anal canal. Am J Surg Pathol **12:**41-55, 1988.

2 Fenger C, Knoth M: The anal transitional zone. A scanning and transmission electron microscopic investigation of the surface epithelium. Ultrastruct Pathol **2:**163-173, 1981.

3 Fetissof F, Dubois MP, Assan R, Arbeille-Brassart B, Baroudi A, Tharanne MJ, Jobard P: Endocrine cells in the anal canal. Virchows Arch [Pathol Anat] **404:**39-47, 1984.

4 Grinvalsky HT, Helwig EB: Carcinoma of the anorectal junction. I. Histological considerations. Cancer **9:**480-488, 1956.

5 Klotz RG, Pamukcoglu T, Souillard DH: Transitional cloacogenic carcinoma of the anal canal. Cancer **20:**1727-1745, 1967.

EMBRYOLOGIC DEFECTS

6 Louw JH, Cywes S, Cremin BJ: Anorectal malformations. Classification and clinical features. S Afr J Surg **9:**11-20, 1971.

7 Santulli TV, Kiesewetter WB, Bill AH Jr: Anorectal anomalies. A suggested international classification. J Pediatr Surg **5:**281-287, 1970.

FISSURE, ULCER, AND FISTULA

8 Fry GA, Martin WJ, Dearing WH, Culp CE: Primary actinomycosis of the rectum with multiple perianal and perineal fistulae. Mayo Clin Proc **40:**296-299, 1965.

9 Gray BK, Lockhart-Mummery HE, Morson BC: Crohn's disease of the anal region. Gut **6:**515-525, 1965.

10 Hanley PH: Anorectal abscess fistula. Surg Clin North Am **58:**487-503, 1978.

11 Lennard-Jones JE, Lockhart-Mummery HE, Chir M, Morson BC: Clinical and pathological differentiation of Crohn's disease and proctocolitis. Gastroenterology **54:**1162-1170, 1968.

12 Lilius HG: Fistula-in-ano. An investigation of human foetal anal ducts and intramuscular glands and a clinical study of 150 patients. Acta Chir Scand **383**[Suppl]:1-88, 1968.

13 Logan VS: Anorectal tuberculosis. Proc R Soc Med **62:**1227-1230, 1969.

14 Marks CG, Ritchie JK: Anal fistulas at St. Mark's Hospital. Br J Surg **64:**84-91, 1977.

15 Parks AG, Morson BC: The pathogenesis of fistula-in-ano. Proc R Soc Med **55:**751-754, 1962.

HYPERTROPHIED PAPILLA

16 Schinella RA: Stromal atypia in anal papillae. Dis Colon Rectum **19:**611-613, 1976.

HEMORRHOIDS

16a Foust R, Dean P, Moinuddin S, Stoler M: Squamous dysplasia and carcinoma arising in hemorrhoidal tissue. A study of 19 cases (abstract). Lab Invest **58:**31A, 1988.

17 Gordsky L: Unsuspected anal cancer discovered after minor anorectal surgery. Dis Colon Rectum **10:**471-478, 1967.

18 Laurence AE, Murray AJ: Histopathology of prolapsed and thrombosed hemorrhoids. Dis Colon Rectum **5:**56-61, 1962.

TUMORS
Carcinoma

19 Askin FB, Muhlendorf K, Walz BJ: Mucinous carcinoma of anal duct origin presenting clinically as a vaginal cyst. Cancer **42:**566-569, 1978.

20 Bogomoletz WV, Potet F, Molas G: Condylomata acuminata, giant condyloma acuminatum (Buschke-Loewenstein tumour) and verrucous squamous carcinoma of the perianal and anorectal region. A continuous precancerous spectrum? Histopathology **9:**1155-1169, 1985.

21 Boman BM, Moertel CG, O'Connell MJ, Scott M, Weiland LH, Beart RW, Gunderson LL, Spencer RJ: Carcinoma of the anal canal. A clinical and pathologic study of 188 cases. Cancer **54:**114-125, 1984.

22 Cabrera A, Tsukada Y, Pickren JW, Moore R, Bross IDJ: Development of lower genital carcinomas in patients with anal carcinomas. A more than casual relationship. Cancer **19:**470-480, 1966.

23 Chumas JC, Lorelle CA: Melanotic adenocarcinoma of the anorectum. Am J Surg Pathol 5:711-717, 1981.
24 Clark J, Petrelli N, Herrera L, Mittelman A: Epidermoid carcinoma of the anal canal. Cancer 57:400-406, 1986.
24a Daling JR, Weiss NS, Hislop TG, Maden C, Coates RJ, Sherman KJ, Ashley RL, Beagrie M, Ryan JA, Coney L: Sexual practices, sexually transmitted diseases, and the incidence of anal cancer. N Engl J Med 317:973-977, 1987.
25 Dillard BM, Spratt JS Jr, Ackerman LV, Butcher HR Jr: Epidermoid cancer of anal margin and canal. Review of 79 cases. Arch Surg 16:772-776, 1963.
26 Dougherty BG, Evans HL: Carcinoma of the anal canal. A study of 79 cases. Am J Clin Pathol 83:159-164, 1985.
27 Dukes CE, Galvin C: Colloid carcinoma arising within fistulae in the anorectal region. Ann R Coll Surg Engl 18:246-261, 1956.
27a Fenger C: Anal canal tumors and their precursors. Pathol Annu 23(Pt 1):45-46, 1988.
28 Fenger C, Nielsen VT: Precancerous changes in the anal canal epithelium in resection specimens. Acta Pathol Microbiol Immunol Scand [A] 94:63-69, 1986.
29 Flam MS, John M, Lovalvo LJ, Mills RJ, Ramalho LD, Prather C, Mowry PA, Morgan DR, Lau BP: Definitive nonsurgical therapy of epithelial malignancies of the anal canal. A report of 12 cases. Cancer 51:1378-1387, 1983.
30 Frost DB, Richards PC, Montague ED, Giacco GG, Martin RG: Epidermoid cancer of the anorectum. Cancer 53:1285-1293, 1984.
31 Gillespie JJ, MacKay B: Histogenesis of cloacogenic carcinoma. Fine structure of anal transitional epithelium and cloacogenic carcinoma. Hum Pathol 9:579-587, 1978.
32 Greenall MJ, Magill GB, Quan SHQ, DeCosse JJ: Recurrent epidermoid cancer of the anus. Cancer 57:1437-1441, 1986.
33 Grinvalsky HT, Helwig EB: Carcinoma of the anorectal junction. I. Histological consideration. Cancer 8:480-488, 1956.
34 Grodsky, L: Unsuspected anal cancer discovered after minor anorectal surgery. Dis Colon Rectum 10:471-478, 1967.
35 Grodsky L: Current concepts on cloacogenic transitional cell anorectal cancers. JAMA 207:2057-2061, 1969.
36 Helwig EB, Graham JH: Anogenital (extramammary) Paget's disease. A clinicopathological study. Cancer 16:387-403, 1963.
37 Jones EA, Morson BC: Mucinous adenocarcinoma in anorectal fistulae. Histopathology 8:279-292, 1984.
38 Judd ES Jr, Burleigh E DeT Jr: Squamous-cell carcinoma of the anus. Results of treatment. Surgery 37:220-228, 1955.
39 Kalogeropoulos NK, Antonakopoulos GN, Agapitos MB, Papacharalampous NX: Spindle cell carcinoma (pseudosarcoma) of the anus. A light, electron microscopic and immunocytochemical study of a case. Histopathology 9:987-994, 1985.
40 Klotz RG Jr, Pamukcoglu T, Souillard DH: Transitional cloacogenic carcinoma of the anal canal. Clinicopathologic study of three hundred and seventy-three cases. Cancer 20:1727-1745, 1967.
41 Lowe D, Fletcher CDM: Eosinophilia in squamous cell carcinoma of the oral cavity, external genitalia, and anus. Clinical correlations. Histopathology 8:627-632, 1984.
42 Morson BC, Pang LSC: Pathology of anal cancer. Proc R Soc Med 61:623-626, 1968.
43 Pang LSC, Morson BC: Basaloid carcinoma of the anal canal. J Clin Pathol 20:128-135, 1967.
44 Papillon J, Mayer M, Montbarbon JF, Gerard JP, Chassard JL, Bailly C: A new approach to the management of epidermoid carcinoma of the anal canal. Cancer 51:1830-1837, 1983.

45 Prioleau PG, Allen MS Jr, Roberts T: Perianal mucinous adenocarcinoma. Cancer 39:1295-1299, 1977.
46 Rainey R: The association of lymphogranuloma inguinale and cancer. Surgery 35:221-235, 1954.
47 Schraut WH, Wang C-H, Dawson PJ, Block GE: Depth of invasion, location, and size of cancer of the anus dictate operative treatment. Cancer 51:1291-1296, 1983.
48 Slater G, Greenstein A, Aufses AH Jr: Anal carcinoma in patients with Crohn's disease. Ann Surg 199:348-350, 1984.
49 Strauss RJ, Fazio VW: Bowen's disease of the anal and perianal area. Am J Surg 137:231-234, 1979.
50 Wick MR, Weatherby RP, Weiland LH: Small cell neuroendocrine carcinoma of the colon and rectum. Clinical, histologic, and ultrastructural study and immunohistochemical comparison with cloacogenic carcinoma. Hum Pathol 18:9-21, 1987.
51 Winkelman J, Grosfeld J, Bigelow B: Colloid carcinoma of anal-gland origin. Am J Clin Pathol 42:395-401, 1964.
52 Wittoesch JH, Woolner LB, Jackman RJ: Basal cell epithelioma and basaloid lesions of the anus. Surg Gynecol Obstet 104:75-80, 1957.
53 Wood WS, Culling CFA: Perianal Paget disease. Histochemical differentiation utilizing the borohydride-KOH-PAS reaction. Arch Pathol 99:442-445, 1975.

Malignant melanoma

54 Ackermann DM, Polk HC Jr, Schrodt GR: Desmoplastic melanoma of the anus. Hum Pathol 16:1277-1279, 1985.
55 Angeras U, Jönsson N, Jönsson P-E. Primary anorectal malignant melanoma. J Surg Oncol 22:261-264, 1983.
56 Mason JK, Helwig EB: Ano-rectal melanoma. Cancer 19:39-50, 1966.
57 Mills SE, Cooper PH: Malignant melanoma of the digestive system. Pathol Annu 18(Pt 2):1-26, 1983.
58 Morson BC, Volkstädt H: Malignant melanoma of the anal canal. J Clin Pathol 16:126-132, 1963.
59 Wanebo HJ, Woodruff JM, Farr GH, Quan SH: Anorectal melanoma. Cancer 47:1891-1900, 1981.

OTHER LESIONS

60 Assor D, Davis JB: Multiple apocrine fibroadenomas of the anal skin. Am J Clin Pathol 68:397-398, 1977.
61 Bonser GM, Raper FP, Shuchsmith HS: Epidermoid cysts in the region of the rectum and anus. A report of four cases. Br J Surg 37:303-306, 1950.
62 de la Monte SM, Hutchins GM: Follicular proctocolitis and neuromatous hyperplasia with lymphogranuloma venereum. Hum Pathol 16:1025-1032, 1985.
62a Joachim HL, Weinstein MA, Robbins RD, Sohn N, Lugo PN: Primary anorectal lymphoma. A new manifestation of the acquired immune deficiency syndrome (AIDS). Cancer 60:1449-1453, 1987.
63 Johnston J, Helwig EB: Granular cell tumors of the gastrointestinal tract and perianal region. A study of 74 cases. Dig Dis Sci 26:807-816, 1981.
64 Morales AR, Fine G, Horn RC Jr, Watson JHL: Langerhans cells in a localized lesion of the eosinophilic granuloma type. Lab Invest 20:412-423, 1969.
65 Robb JA, Jones RA: Spindle cell lipoma in a perianal location. Hum Pathol 13:1052, 1982.
66 Srouji MN, Donaldson MH, Chatten J, Koblenzer CS: Perianal rhabdomyosarcoma in childhood. Cancer 38:1008-1012, 1976.
67 Teloh HA: Apocrine adenoma of the anus. Cancer 7:367-372, 1954.

12 Major and minor salivary glands

NORMAL ANATOMY

Salivary gland tissue is distributed widely. The major salivary glands are the parotid, submaxillary, and sublingual glands. The parotid gland is the largest, the submaxillary gland is about one fourth its size, and the sublingual gland is about one third the size of the submaxillary gland. The main duct of the parotid gland (Stensen's duct) empties into the oral cavity, opposite the crown of the second maxillary molar. The ducts of both the submaxillary and sublingual glands open in the floor of the mouth.

Salivary gland tissue is present in many other locations, where it may give rise to inflammatory conditions, benign tumors, and malignant tumors. Its location influences, to some extent, the clinical signs and symptoms, the morphologic features, the pathology, and the treatment. It can be found in the lips (more often in the upper than the lower lip) and is present throughout the oropharynx, gingiva, floor of the mouth, cheek, hard and soft palates, tonsillar areas, and tongue.

Microscopically, salivary glands are composed of a ductal and an acinar portion, of either serous or mucinous type. The intercalated ducts and acini represent the terminal portion of the system (ducto-acinar unit). The reserve cells of the intercalated ducts are the source of regeneration of the acinar tissue and the terminal duct system and are probably the progenitors (together with the closely apposed myoepithelial cells) of most salivary gland tumors.[2]

HETEROTOPIA

Heterotopic salivary gland tissue is often found in lymph nodes within or near the parotid gland in both newborn infants and in adults.[1] It can also occur in other areas of the neck, including the supraclavicular area.[3,5] Youngs and Scofield[6] have described eleven such cases, the most common location being along the medial border of the right sternocleidomastoid muscle near the sternoclavicular joint. The majority of the cases were associated with cysts or sinus tracts, suggesting an embryologic relationship with the branchial apparatus. A variety of neoplasms can develop from heterotopic salivary gland tissue. Warthin's tumor is by far the most frequent (see p. 649), but several other benign and malignant types have been described.[4,4a]

SIALOLITHIASIS

Calculi may form in the major ducts of the submaxillary, sublingual, and parotid glands, sometimes in a multicentric and bilateral fashion. They are more common in the submaxillary gland than in the parotid gland, presumably because in the former the saliva is more saturated with calcium salts[8] (Fig. 12-1). Some of the stones have a foreign body or bacterial nidus. Others do not have an identifiable nidus, are laminated, and are composed of the crystalline compound carbonate apatite.[7] The formation of calculi blocks secretion and produces swelling of the distal salivary gland tissue. If ductal obstruction persists, the gland becomes inflamed and indurated as acinar tissue is destroyed. With obstructed ducts of the submaxillary and sublingual glands, marked induration can occur in the floor of the mouth that may be mistaken for neoplasm by palpation. The duct orifices become erythematous and swollen. Roentgenologic examination may demonstrate a radiopaque mass, and sialography will show partial or total blockage of the duct. Microscopic examination of glands that have been affected by stones shows dilatation of ducts, at times squamous metaplasia of the epithelium, moderate-to-prominent chronic inflammation, and a variable destruction of acinar tissue (Fig. 12-2).

CHRONIC SIALADENITIS

Mild lymphocytic infiltrations of the major salivary gland unaccompanied by clinical symptoms are relatively common. Some are of focal obstructive nature and are accompanied by various degrees of parenchymal atrophy and fibrosis; others, more common in females, are age-related, have a high statistical association with rheumatoid arthritis, and are probably immune-mediated.[9] In the clinically apparent cases, sialolithiasis is the most common cause.

Granulomatous sialadenitis can result from tuberculosis, mycosis, sarcoidosis, or because of duct obstruction from calculi or malignant tumors. In the latter instance, the granulomas result from rupture of ducts and may contain small pools of mucin.[10]

SALIVARY GLAND CYSTS

Most cystic lesions involving the major salivary gland are cystic neoplasms, usually Warthin's tumor but sometimes mucoepidermoid carcinoma, benign mixed tumor, or sebaceous lymphadenoma. The rare *non-neoplastic cysts* may be lined by squamous or glandular epithelium. Some have been interpreted as acquired and of retention type, but most are probably developmental and related to the so-called benign lymphoepithelial cysts[11,12] (see p. 652). In rare cases, a bilateral polycystic change may occur, presumably as the result of a developmental malformation of the ductal system.[11a,13]

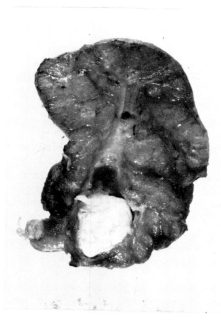

Fig. 12-1 Submaxillary gland with large calculus, blocking major duct, with dilatation of proximal portion.

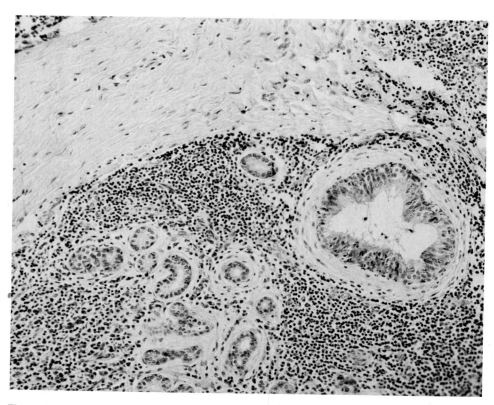

Fig. 12-2 Submaxillary gland demonstrating dilatation of ducts, acinar atrophy, and chronic inflammation. There were small stones in one of ducts leading to this area.

MIKULICZ'S DISEASE

Mikulicz's disease (benign lymphoepithelial lesion) is by far the most common cause of the Mikulicz's syndrome, defined as a diffuse and bilateral enlargement of salivary and lacrimal glands.[28] Some cases of the syndrome are said to result from malignant lymphoma, sarcoidosis, tuberculosis, and even syphilis, but this is very rare.

In Mikulicz's disease, the swelling of the salivary glands slowly increases and can become quite striking. It is usually bilateral and symmetric; however, we have seen several cases in which the parotid involvement was unilateral, at least when judged by clinical criteria. If the patient develops an infection, the process subsides only to recur.

Mikulicz's disease is one manifestation of a generalized symptom complex known as Sjögren's syndrome, the other components of which are keratoconjunctivitis, xerostomia, rheumatoid arthritis, and hypergammaglobulinemia.[15,21,23] Cases of this syndrome have been recently reported in AIDS patients.[27a]

Microscopically, the changes are similar in the salivary and lacrimal glands. The two main changes are lymphoid infiltration and epimyoepithelial islands.[24] The lymphoid tissue contains numerous well-formed germinal centers and is composed of a mixed population of B and T lymphocytes, accompanied by scattered histiocytes and dendritic reticulum cells. Immunohistochemically, the B lymphocytes may be polyclonal or exhibit light chain restriction.[19a,25a] The epimyoepithelial islands appear as solid nests surrounded and infiltrated by lymphoid cells[19] (Fig. 12-3). They represent collapsed acini in the process of involution and are largely composed of basal epithelial cells and modified myoepithelial cells, with very little participation from ductal epithelial cells.[16,17,20] A hyaline material is deposited between the cells, which is shown ultrastructurally to represent basal lamina material, including type IV collagen.[20,25]

The changes are similar in minor salivary glands of the oral cavity, except for the usual lack of epimyoepithelial islands; therefore, biopsy of the labial glands is often used to document the diagnosis of Mikulicz's disease.

In some patients with Sjögren's syndrome, the lymphoid proliferation involves other organs, such as lymph nodes, lung, kidney, bone marrow, skeletal muscle, skin, or liver. The appearance in the lung is usually that of a lymphoid interstitial pneumonitis, but it may be that of lymphomatoid granulomatosis.[29] Systemic vasculitis may occur.[27] Amyloid deposits can also be present. We have seen a case in which the skin infiltrates contained myoepithelial islands formed by the sweat glands. The term *pseudolymphoma* is sometimes applied to these benign extraglandular tumorlike aggregates.

Occasionally, true malignant lymphomas develop in these patients, either in the salivary gland or in extraglandular locations.[14,22,26] Most of these tumors are large cell lymphomas of B-cell type, many of them having an appearance

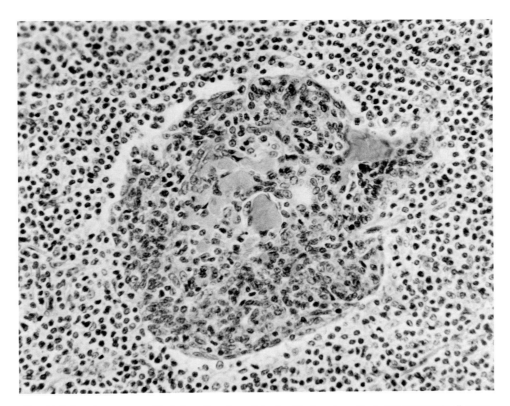

Fig. 12-3 Prominent myoepithelial proliferation of duct epithelium in patient with Mikulicz's disease.

consistent with immunoblastic and plasmacytoid differentiation. Others have the appearance of poorly differentiated lymphocytic (follicular center cell) lymphomas. Zulman et al.[30] have demonstrated monoclonal intracellular immunoglobulin (always of IgM kappa type) within their cytoplasm, whereas in the "pseudolymphomas" the immunoglobulin population is polyclonal. It is interesting that two patients with cytologically benign proliferations showed a predominance of cells containing IgM kappa; both patients developed a malignant lymphoma. These studies suggest that immunocytochemical determinations may be of prognostic significance and that there is a wide spectrum of lymphoid proliferation in Sjögren's syndrome, from the benign polyclonal lymphoplasmacytic infiltrates to the highly malignant large cell lymphomas. This is also suggested by the recent demonstration of immunoglobulin-gene rearrangement in several cases with benign histology, indicating the existence of a B-cell clonal expansion that may result from an immunoregulatory defect and that is obviously related to the increased incidence of lymphoma in this population.[18]

The development of lymphoma in these patients should not be confused with the entity known as *malignant lymphoepithelial lesion*. This represents a poorly differentiated carcinoma with prominent lymphoid stroma. This process, which we view as unrelated to Mikulicz's disease, is discussed on p. 663.

IRRADIATION EFFECT

The submaxillary glands, which are often included in the field of irradiation for tumors of the oral cavity, swell and become firm as a result of the therapy (Fig. 12-4). These changes may be mistaken clinically for metastatic carcinoma in submaxillary lymph nodes and sometimes have led to unnecessary radical surgery.[31] Microscopic examination shows atrophy of acinar elements and chronic inflammatory cells in the stroma (Fig. 12-5). The lining of the duct epithelium may show prominent squamous metaplasia.

OTHER NON-NEOPLASTIC LESIONS

Lymphoid disorders of reactive nature can involve the intraparotid lymph nodes and be confused clinically with a primary salivary gland tumor. These include nonspecific follicular hyperplasia, healed abscesses, and granulomatous inflammations, such as those produced by cat scratch disease.

Keratinous cysts of epidermal type can involve the parotid region (Fig. 12-6).

Amyloidosis may involve the salivary gland as part of a generalized process or as a localized pseudotumoral mass ("amyloid tumor") (Fig. 12-7).

Nodular fasciitis can present as a primary intraparotid lesion; its microscopic appearance is identical to that of its more common soft tissue counterpart.

EPITHELIAL TUMORS
Tumors with stromal differentiation
Benign mixed tumor (pleomorphic adenoma)

Benign mixed tumor is the most common neoplasm of the salivary glands. It is most frequent in women in the fourth decade of life, but it can be seen in children and in elderly persons of either sex.[33,48] It is about ten times more common in the parotid than in the submaxillary gland, and it is very rare in the sublingual gland. In the parotid gland, most tumors arise within the superficial lobe, from either the tail (50%) or the anterior portion (25%). The remaining 25% arise from the deep lobe and often present as a pharyngeal mass without external evidence of tumor.[36,42]

Grossly, the tumor forms a rubbery, resilient mass with a bosselated surface and may grow to a large size (Figs. 12-8 and 12-9). The consistency depends on the relative

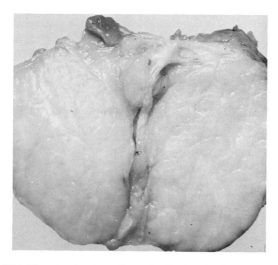

Fig. 12-4 Fibrosis of submaxillary gland related to irradiation. Note obliteration of normal pattern of salivary gland.

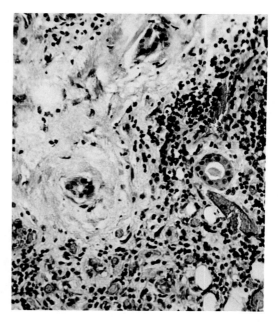

Fig. 12-5 Effect of irradiation on submaxillary gland. Note persistence of ducts, absence of acinar tissue, and presence of chronic inflammatory cells.

amount of epithelial cells and stroma and the type of the latter. Although the tumor tends to be well circumscribed, small extensions can be seen protruding into the adjacent normal tissue. The appearance of the cut surface again depends on the relative proportion of epithelium and stroma. Islands of cartilage can be recognized by their glistening, translucent appearance. In rare cases, foci of mature bone are identified.

Microscopically, benign mixed tumor is frequently misdiagnosed as carcinoma by the neophyte in pathology.[60] Its bewildering pattern, extreme cellularity, and the occasional penetration of the capsule by the neoplasm all make it most confusing. The typical tumor has a biphasic appearance resulting from the intimate admixture of epithelium and stroma (Fig. 12-10). Most of the epithelial component is of a glandular nature, but foci of squamous metaplasia are common, sometimes accompanied by keratinized epithelial plugs in the lumen. The neoplastic glands have a lining composed of two cell types, the basally located cells displaying morphologic features of myoepithelial cells.[38] They may be cuboidal, flattened, clear, spindle shaped, or "hyaline"[50] (Figs. 12-11 and 12-12). The stroma may have a

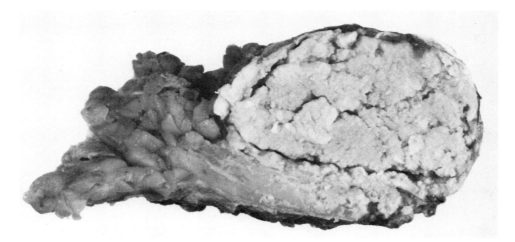

Fig. 12-6 Keratinous cyst of epidermal type located wtihin superficial lobe of parotid gland. It was clinically thought to represent a primary salivary gland tumor.

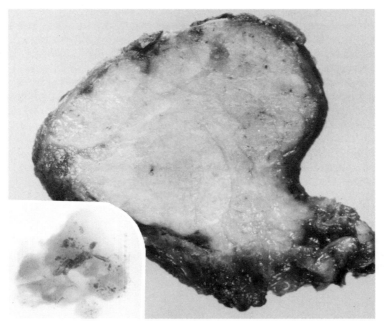

Fig. 12-7 Amyloid "tumor" of submaxillary gland. Lesion was bilateral. Note homogeneous, waxy appearance. **Inset,** X-ray appearance of surgical specimen, showing coarse foci of calcification.

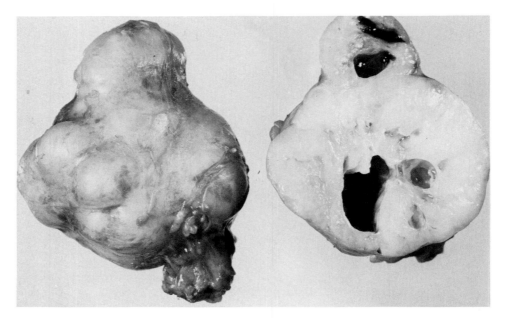

Fig. 12-8 External and cut surfaces of large benign mixed tumor of parotid gland. Cut surface shows areas of cystic change, and external surface has typical bosselated appearance.

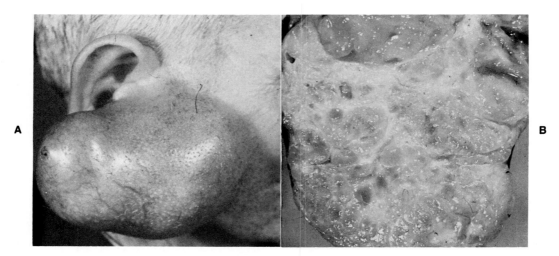

Fig. 12-9 A, Benign mixed tumor of parotid gland of long duration. There was no ulceration or facial nerve paralysis. **B,** Same tumor shown in **A.** Note variegated appearance with areas of mucoid change and cartilage-like material.

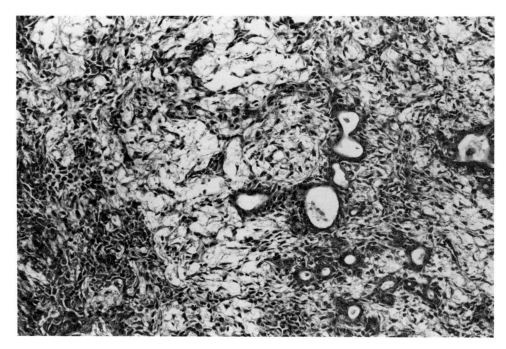

Fig. 12-10 Benign mixed tumor of parotid gland. Biphasic pattern resulting from well-differentiated ducts and myxochondroid stroma is characteristic.

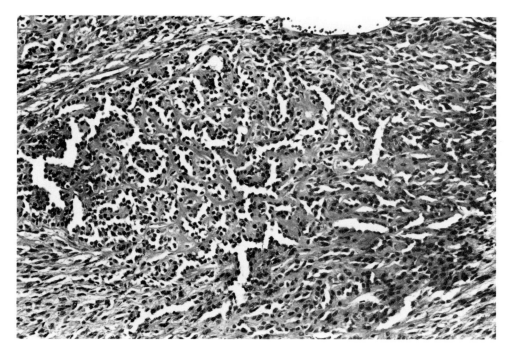

Fig. 12-11 Benign mixed tumor of parotid gland. In this area, branching appearance of neoplastic ducts results in pseudovascular configuration.

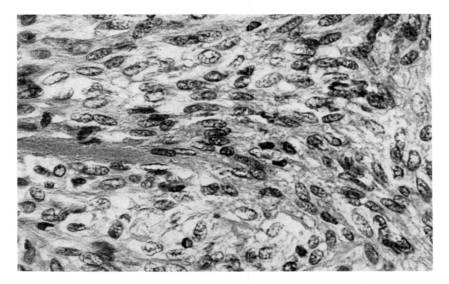

Fig. 12-12 Area of prominent cellularity and spindle-cell appearance in benign mixed tumor. These cells are probably of myoepithelial nature. In other areas, this tumor had well-defined glandular components.

nonspecific fibromyxoid appearance, sometimes containing abundant elastic tissue;[39] however, areas of clearcut cartilaginous differentiation are usually found.[64]

This phenomenon is more common and prominent in parotid and submaxillary tumors than in those arising from minor salivary glands. There is convincing morphologic, ultrastructural, and immunohistochemical evidence to suggest that these mesenchymal elements are derived from modified myoepithelial cells.[32,40] Actually, transitions between basally located myoepithelial cells and the myxochondroid cells of the stroma are often found. Ultrastructurally, a continuum of cytoplasmic features from epithelial to mesenchymal cells is present.[37,49,53]

Two types of mucin are formed by pleomorphic adenomas, one of epithelial and the other of connective tissue type.[32,59] The former is characterized by its high content of neutral glycoprotein, and the latter contains highly sulfated glycosaminoglycans. Both of these mucin types are probably secreted by cells of epithelial derivation, as shown by tissue culture and inoculation studies.[61] Occasionally, crystals containing tyrosine and other amino acids are found in the myxomatous areas.[34,45] Other extracellular substances sometimes found in this tumor are calcium oxalate crystals and amyloid.[62]

Some pleomorphic adenomas are extremely cellular, the tumor cells being either round or spindle shaped (Fig. 12-12). These may be confused with malignant tumors; however, follow-up studies have indicated that these tumors do not behave differently from the ordinary variety. The rarity of mitotic figures and absence of necrosis are of help in the differential diagnosis with true malignant neoplasms. Something similar can be said of pleomorphic adenomas having foci that superficially resemble the adenoid cystic pattern. The presence of these foci does not influence the prognosis and therefore should be disregarded.

Immunohistochemically, the ductal epithelial component is positive for keratin, epithelial membrane antigen,

secretory component, CEA, lysozyme, alpha-1-antitrypsin, alpha-1-antichymotrypsin, lactoferrin, and steroid C-21 hydroxylase.[41,44,47,54,55,60a] Conversely, amylase is usually absent.[47] The myoepithelial component is immunoreactive for keratin, actin, myosin, fibronectin, laminin, and S-100 protein.[57,63] The latter marker is also strongly expressed in the cartilaginous areas and in a subtype of the epithelial ductal cells. The immunohistochemical profile of the epithelial component is similar to that of the normal intercalated duct cells, particularly regarding the expression of lactoferrin and secretory component.[47] The demonstration in some of the tumors of glial fibrillary acidic protein and astroprotein, two glial markers, is more difficult to explain.[56,60b]

The *recurrence rate* of pleomorphic adenoma depends almost entirely on the adequacy of the primary excision.[58] Recurrence is very high if the tumor is removed by a simple enucleation (Fig. 12-13). This is because small inconspicuous nodules attached by threadlike filaments of neoplastic tissue may be present surrounding the main mass. They may have the shape and appearance of lymph nodes and be mistaken for nodal metastases by both the surgeon and the pathologist. If the tumor is enucleated these small remnants will be left behind and will provide the nidus for recurrence.[51] Most of these recurrences will appear during the first 18 months following surgery, but others supervene over an exceedingly long period (50 years or more). Because of this, long-term follow-up is essential. Usually the microscopic pattern of the recurrent tumor exactly mimics that of the original neoplasm. Surgery for recurrent tumor often fails. In about one fourth of the cases, further recurrences develop, often in the form of multiple foci.[42,52] The proper therapy for pleomorphic adenoma is its total surgical removal, along with a margin of normal salivary tissue that surrounds it. For the tumors located in the superficial lobe of the parotid gland, which represent the majority, the standard surgery is a superficial parotidectomy with preservation

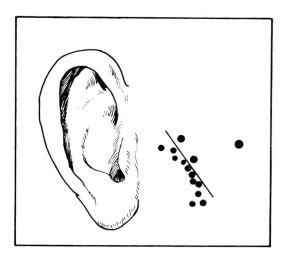

Fig. 12-13 Distribution of recurrent tumor nodules (shown as black dots) as demonstrated by careful histologic study of re-excision of benign mixed tumor which, at time of first operation, had apparently been enucleated. Surgical scar measured 3.5 cm. (Courtesy Dr. F. Leidler, Houston, TX.)

of the facial nerve. The incidence of recurrence following this procedure is almost zero, and the long-term prognosis for properly treated pleomorphic adenoma is excellent.[46] Under exceptionally rare circumstances, a pleomorphic adenoma of ordinary benign microscopic appearance will metastasize to the lungs or other organs, with the metastases appearing as benign as the original tumor.[35,43]

Malignant mixed tumor

Two major categories of malignant mixed tumor exist.[68,74] The first and most common can be viewed as a malignant transformation of a pre-existing benign mixed tumor. This complication takes place in about 5% to 10% of these neoplasms.[69,70] Clinical features that suggest this event in a longstanding tumor are sudden increase in growth, pain, and facial paralysis.[67,71] A history of previous surgery and/or radiation therapy is often obtained.[66] Documentation that a malignant salivary gland tumor arose from a pre-existent benign mixed tumor may be difficult to obtain. The above history, although suggestive of the process, is not by itself diagnostic. It is necessary to have microscopic evidence of a previously existing benign tumor or to have benign and malignant tumor in the same neoplasm.[65] This may require a thorough sampling of the tumor. Sometimes the pre-existing benign lesion is represented only by a totally hyalinized round nodule surrounded by carcinoma. The malignancy is limited to the epithelial component (Fig. 12-14). It has been stated that these malignant areas often assume the appearance of one of the well-recognized variants of salivary gland carcinoma (such as mucoepidermoid carcinoma or adenoid cystic carcinoma),[69] but this has rarely been the case in our experience. In the series of Tortoledo et al.,[74] the malignant component was classified as ductal carcinoma in thirteen cases, undifferentiated carcinoma in ten, terminal duct carcinoma in nine, myoepithelial carcinoma in three, and unclassified in two.

LiVolsi and Perzin[68] have pointed out that if the cytologically malignant foci are found entirely within a benign mixed tumor (i.e., in the form of carcinoma in situ), they are not associated with clinical malignancy. Only when invasion occurs beyond the capsule of the original neoplasm will the lesion behave clinically in a malignant fashion. For invasive tumors, the extent of invasion beyond the capsule is of importance. In one series, all patients whose malignant neoplasms extended for more than 8 mm beyond the capsule died of tumor.[74] Therefore the importance of thorough sampling cannot be overemphasized. Clinical malignancy also depends on the histologic type of carcinoma; the prognosis is substantially better if this component is of terminal duct type than any of the others.[74]

The most common sites of metastases are regional lymph nodes, lungs, bone (especially the vertebral column), and abdominal organs.[73]

The second type of malignant mixed tumor has a biphasic composition similar to that of benign mixed tumor, but both the epithelial and the mesenchyme-like elements have a malignant appearance, the former often in the form of a ductal carcinoma, and the latter in the form of chondrosarcoma (Fig. 12-15). Since no pre-existing benign tumor is found, the designation of *carcinoma ex pleomorphic adenoma* which has been suggested as an alternative term for malignant mixed tumor, is inappropriate.[71] Names such as *true malignant mixed tumor* and *carcinosarcoma* have been proposed instead.[72] This is an aggressive, often rapidly lethal neoplasm.

Tumors with oxyphilic (oncocytic) change

Oncocytes or oxyphilic cells are large ductal epithelial cells with a granular, deeply eosinophilic cytoplasm crowded with mitochondria. Their number in the normal salivary gland increases with age and their secretory activity is minimal, suggesting that they are the expression of a degenerative change. In some instances, they form well-defined clusters scattered throughout the gland. It is not clear whether these clusters represent an exaggeration of the age-related hyperplastic process or the emergence of a neoplasm, an uncertainty reflected by the terms that have been used to designate this process: *oncocytosis*,[81] *multinodular oncocytoma*,[77] and *multifocal adenomatous oncocytic hyperplasia*.[82]

Oxyphilic adenoma

Oxyphilic adenoma (oncocytoma; mitochondrioma) is defined as a benign tumor exclusively composed of oxyphilic cells.[79,80] The large majority occur in the parotid. Grossly, it presents as a solid, well-circumscribed mass, usually small and with a characteristic tan color. Microscopically, it is composed of large cells with round nuclei and abundant granular acidophilic cytoplasm (Fig. 12-16). Ultrastructurally, the cytoplasm is packed with mitochondria (Fig. 12-17). Some of these mitochondria contain large amounts of glycogen, and others are partitioned, suggesting division.[83] Mitotic figures are absent, and cellular transition from normal lining cells of the ducts may be seen. Occasionally, the cells undergo a clear change as a result of cystic dilatation of mitochondria. A case has been described

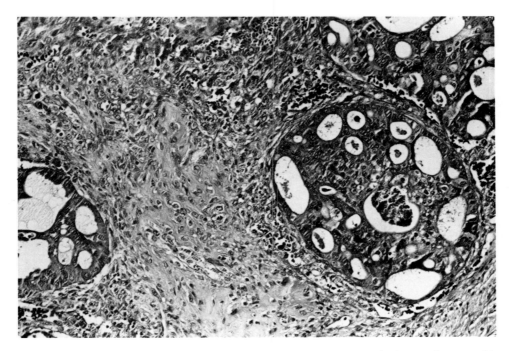

Fig. 12-14 Malignant mixed tumor. Epithelial component has appearance of adenocarcinoma and is surrounded by somewhat fibrous myxochondroid stroma.

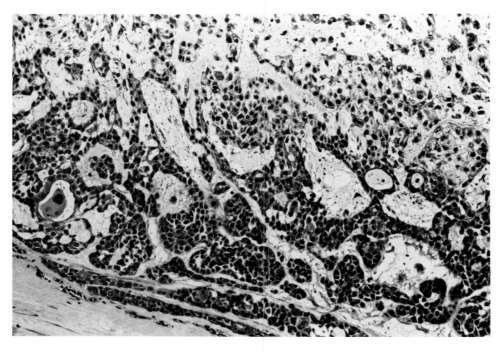

Fig. 12-15 Malignant mixed tumor in which both epithelial and cartilaginous-like elements have malignant appearance. There was no morphologic evidence of pre-existing benign mixed tumor.

containing psammoma bodies.[76] Focal collections of oncocytes may be present in the adjacent normal gland. Local excision is usually curative.[78]

Oxyphilic carcinoma (malignant oncocytoma) represents the malignant counterpart of oxyphilic adenoma, a tumor type so rare that it is a pathologic curiosity.[75,78]

Warthin's tumor

Warthin's tumor differs from other salivary gland tumors in several respects: it is more common in males, it is often multicentric, and it is bilateral in 10% to 15% of the cases. It comprises 70% of all bilateral salivary gland neoplasms.[107] This tumor is found almost exclusively in the parotid gland.[90,97] It often becomes cystic and occasionally is fixed to the overlying skin and mistaken for a malignant neoplasm. On cross section, it appears as a multicystic mass (Figs. 12-18 and 12-19). Between the fluid-filled cystic spaces, grayish lymphoid tissue can be seen. Occasionally the entire tumor undergoes necrotic changes consistent with hemorrhagic infarct.[90,102]

Microscopically, lymphoid tissue is prominent, often with germinal centers; this has led to the suggestion that this tumor originates from excretory ducts located within intraparotid lymph nodes.[106] This lymphoid stroma is predominantly composed of B lymphocytes,[88] but it also contains T lymphocytes, mast cells, and S-100 protein-positive dendritic cells.[87,103-105,110] The lymphocytic population is polyclonal,[96] with a predominance of IgA-producing cells.[94]

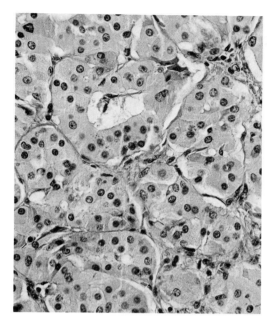

Fig. 12-16 Oxyphilic adenoma of parotid gland with large cells, granular cytoplasm, and uniform nuclei. This benign tumor arises from duct epithelium.

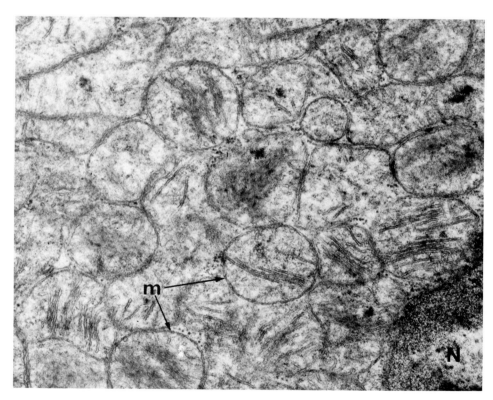

Fig. 12-17 Electron photomicrograph of oxyphilic adenoma showing cytoplasm packed with mitochondria, *m.* Portion of nucleus, *N,* is at right. ($\times$31,000.)

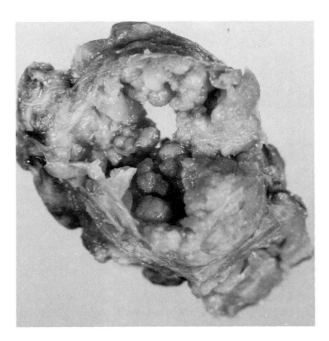

Fig. 12-18 Papillary cystadenoma lymphomatosum of parotid gland. Tumor had brownish gray color in fresh state. There are large cystic spaces present.

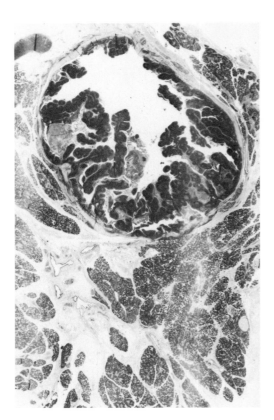

Fig. 12-19 Whole-mount view of Warthin's tumor of parotid gland. Good circumscription and cystic degeneration are particularly noticeable. (Courtesy Dr. C. Perez-Mesa, Columbia, MO.)

Covering the surface of this lymphoid tissue are large epithelial cells with granular cytoplasm, similar in most respects to those seen in oxyphilic adenoma (Fig. 12-20). These cells are arranged in two layers, with some morphologic and immunohistochemical differences between them.[95] Some of the apical cells may be ciliated.[90] These oncocytic cells are immunoreactive for keratin and secretory component, focally positive for ribonuclease, lactoferrin, CEA, and lysozyme, and negative for amylase, vimentin, and desmin;[96,100] there is no evidence for a myoepithelial cell component.[92] Interestingly, somatostatin has also been detected in some of these tumors.[93] Mucin-secreting cells and groups of sebaceous cells may also be present.[91] Occasionally, the lymphoid component is scanty or absent.[90] By electron microscopy, the cytoplasm of the granular cells is packed with mitochondria[98] (Fig. 12-21). Interestingly, the mitochondrial partitions commonly seen in oxyphilic adenoma are usually absent in Warthin's tumor.

The neoplasms associated with infarct-like necrosis may exhibit focal squamous metaplasia, sometimes with features analogous to those of necrotizing sialometaplasia as seen in the oral cavity.[109]

There have been cases of Warthin's tumor reported in the submaxillary gland, but it is probable that at least some of these represent tumors arising from the mandibular extension of the parotid gland. Similar lesions, but usually lacking

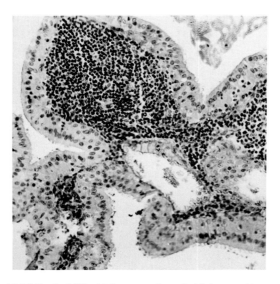

Fig. 12-20 Typical Warthin's tumor. Lymphoid tissue with germinal centers occurs beneath lining of large oxyphil cells.

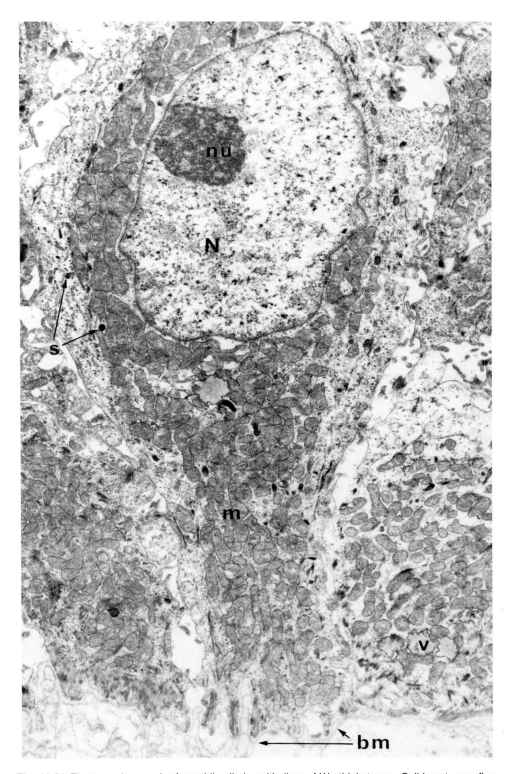

Fig. 12-21 Electron micrograph of oxyphil cells in epithelium of Warthin's tumor. Cell is set upon fine basement membrane, *bm*. Cytoplasm is packed with mitochondria, *m,* almost to exclusion of other organelles. Few vacuoles, *v,* containing lipid are present. Unidentified dense rods and spheres, *s,* are scattered through cytoplasm. Nucleolus, *nu,* is prominent. (×9,000.)

the granular acidophilia in the epithelial ductal cells, are sometimes found in the parotid or in upper cervical lymph nodes independent of the parotid gland.[108] Bernier and Bhaskar[85] called them *benign lymphoepithelial cysts*.

Simple excision of Warthin's tumor is curative.[98,106]

Malignant transformation of Warthin's tumor is an exceptional event, but has been documented both in terms of the lymphoid component evolving into malignant lymphoma[84,99] and the epithelial component evolving into adenocarcinoma or epidermoid carcinoma.[86,89,101]

Monomorphic adenoma

The term *monomorphic adenoma* was originally proposed for any benign epithelial salivary gland tumor other than benign mixed tumor (pleomorphic adenoma). It therefore includes tumors as disparate as oxyphilic adenoma, Warthin's tumor, sebaceous lymphadenoma, and basal cell adenoma.[112,113] The very inclusiveness of the term when so defined, and the fact that some people have used it instead as a synonym for only one member of the group, (i.e., for basal cell adenoma) has resulted in confusion. Therefore it is probably advisable to regard monomorphic adenoma not as a specific pathologic diagnosis but rather as the expression of a nosologic grouping and to name the tumors in this category according to their composition and appearance.[111]

Basal cell adenoma

Basal cell adenomas are grossly encapsulated and often cystic; as a group, they tend to be smaller than benign mixed tumors. Most cases occur in the parotid glands of adult patients; basal cell adenomas affect women slightly more often than they do men.[116] Microscopically, an important distinguishing feature is the palisading at the periphery of the epithelial nests, giving the tumor a "basaloid" appearance (Fig. 12-22). The pattern of growth may be predominantly tubular, trabecular, or solid.[119,122] In a variant of the latter designated by some as *membranous* or *dermal analogue tumor*, there is deposition of abundant basal lamina material around and within the epithelial nests, in a pattern nearly identical to that of the cutaneous sweat gland tumor known as eccrine dermal cylindroma[114,115] (Fig. 12-23). Actually, there have been cases of multiple dermal cylindromas co-existing with multiple parotid tumors with the same microscopic appearance.[123,129] Others have been seen to arise within periparotid lymph nodes.[126]

Another variant of basal cell carcinoma is characterized by the presence of bilayered strands or ribbons of columnar cells separated by a loose, well-vascularized stroma. This has been referred to as *canalicular adenoma* and is regarded by some authors as a separate entity from basal cell adenoma[120,122] (Fig. 12-24). However, the frequent occurrence in this tumor of foci of basaloid cells and the equally frequent merging of canalicular and trabecular structures suggest to us that a sharp separation between these entities is unwarranted. Foci of acinar differentiation have been observed in one case of basal cell adenoma, suggesting that the presence of acinar cells in a salivary gland tumor is not always indicative of acinic cell carcinoma.[128]

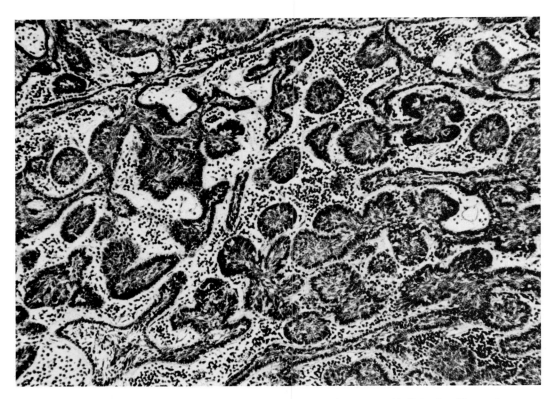

Fig. 12-22 Basal cell adenoma of salivary gland. Solid nests of uniform epithelial cells with prominent peripheral palisading can be seen.

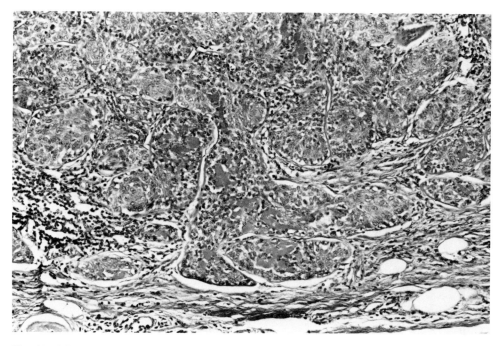

Fig. 12-23 Basal cell adenoma with appearance analogous to that of so-called dermal eccrine cylindroma. Note thick hyaline bands around tumor nests and round hyaline clusters within nests.

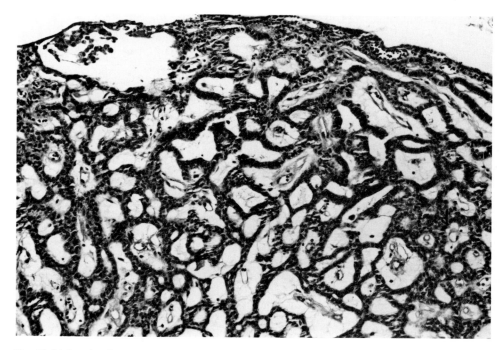

Fig. 12-24 Basal cell adenoma with canalicular pattern of growth. Some authors regard this tumor as a distinctive tumor entity.

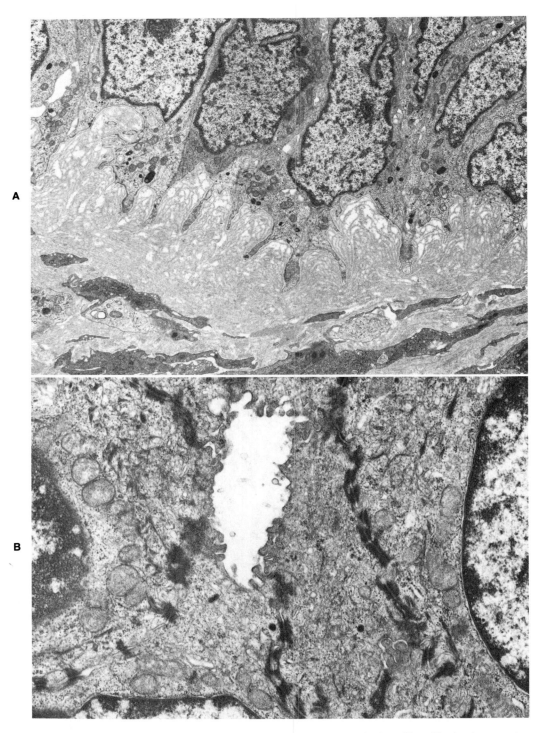

Fig. 12-25 Basal cell adenoma of parotid gland. **A,** Prominent reduplication of basal lamina is present. Cells are nondescript and are attached by numerous desmosomes. **B,** These epithelial cells contain numerous tonofilaments that are attached by desmosomes and form a true lumen. (**A,** ×5,065; **B,** ×16,850.)

The main differential diagnosis of basal cell adenoma is with benign mixed tumor and adenoid cystic carcinoma.[127] Basal cell carcinoma lacks the mesenchyme-like component of benign mixed tumor. In contrast to adenoid cystic carcinoma, it is encapsulated and devoid of stromal and perineurial invasion. Ultrastructural studies suggest that basal cell adenoma, like most other salivary gland tumors, derives from the intercalated portion of the duct, with little if any participation of myoepithelial cells[117,118,121,124] (Fig. 12-25, *A* and *B*). It behaves in a benign fashion, analogous to that of benign mixed tumor, and excision is curative.

Malignant transformation of basal cell adenomas rarely occurs; in six cases reported by Luna et al.,[125] the malignancy was diagnosed as adenoid cystic carcinoma in three and as basaloid carcinoma in the other three.

Tumors with sebaceous differentiation

Cells with a sebaceous appearance are rarely found within an otherwise normal parotid gland (Fig. 12-26). They are found with a higher frequency in a variety of salivary gland tumors. They are particularly common in Warthin's tumor but may also appear in benign mixed tumor, mucoepidermoid carcinoma, and adenoid cystic carcinoma.[130,131,135] The morphologic similarities of these tumor cells to normal cutaneous sebaceous glands are also evident on electron microscopic examination and thin-layer chromatography of the lipid material.[136]

Benign tumors with a predominant sebaceous component have been designated as *sebaceous adenoma* when pure and *sebaceous lymphadenoma* when accompanied by a prominent lymphoid stroma.[132,133] The latter tumor may present as a unilocular cystic mass on gross inspection.[134] Rare malignant counterparts of these tumors exist; these have been called *sebaceous carcinoma* and *sebaceous lymphadenocarcinoma*, respectively.[132]

Tumors with myoepithelial differentiation

Myoepithelial cells are a component of several types of benign and malignant salivary gland tumors, particularly benign mixed tumors, adenoid cystic carcinoma, and terminal duct carcinoma.[142,143,146] Tumors thought to be composed exclusively of myoepithelial cells are generically referred to as *myoepitheliomas*. Three major morphologic types exist: spindle cell, hyaline (plasmacytoid), and clear cell, acknowledging the existence of combined and intermediate forms.[148,158] The *spindle-cell type* tumors have a stromal-like appearance and can be confused with lesions of fibroblasts, Schwann cells, or smooth muscle derivation.[138] Collagen stroma is scanty, microcystic formations may be present, and various degrees of secondary myxoid change may be seen.[156] The *hyaline (plasmacytoid) cell type* tumors are composed of cells with eccentric nuclei degree of pleomorphism and hyperchromasia, but scanty or no mitotic activity. The cytoplasm is abundant, with a *diffuse* type of eosinophilia that is very different from the fine granular quality that one sees in oncocytes. The cell margins are polygonal and sharply outlined (Fig. 12-27). The appearance of hyaline cells may simulate that of neoplastic plasma cells or even skeletal muscle cells. Ultrastructurally, their main feature is the presence of abundant, uniformly dispersed microfilaments measuring 50 to 100 Å in diam-

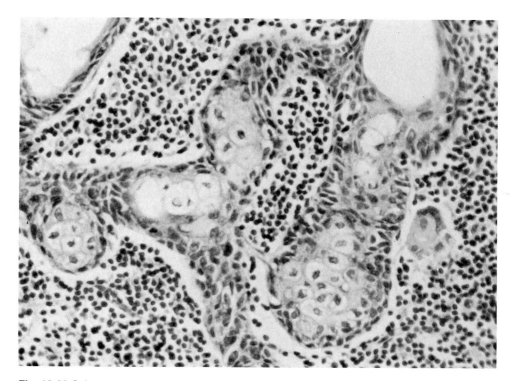

Fig. 12-26 Sebaceous gland hyperplasia associated with lymphocytic infiltration within parotid gland.

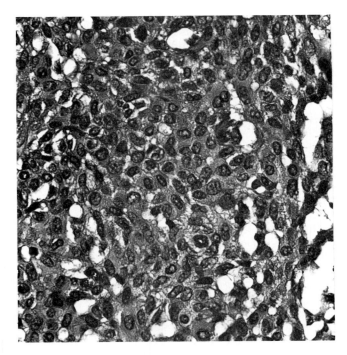

Fig. 12-27 Myoepithelioma composed of hyaline cells. Tumor cells have cuboidal appearance and homogeneous deeply acidophilic cytoplasm. This tumor type is more common in the palate than in major salivary glands.

eter.[157] The *clear cell type* tumors are composed of small tubules lined by a single layer of small cuboidal cells surrounded by one or more layers of prominent clear cells, with a prominent hyaline-like material in between (Fig. 12-28). These clear cells contain variable amounts of glycogen but no fat or mucin. In some areas, ductal formations are scanty, the lesion appearing as a sheet of clear cells. This type has also been described as clear cell adenoma, glycogen-rich adenoma, glycogen-rich adenocarcinoma, tubular carcinoma, and epithelial-myoepithelial carcinoma.[139,141,144,152,155]

Most of the reported cases of spindle cell and clear cell myoepitheliomas have occurred in the parotid gland, whereas most pure examples of hyaline myoepitheliomas have been described in minor salivary glands, particularly the palate.[149]

There seems to be a range of differentiation among these tumors, with both benign and malignant variants represented. The large majority of cases with a hyaline cell morphology have behaved in a benign fashion,[137] but malignant examples of the spindle-cell and particularly of the clear cell types have been described.[140] In general, these have been characterized by invasive properties and cytologic atypia.[137] According to some authors, all the myoepitheliomas of the clear cell type should be regarded as potentially malignant.[150] In one series there were local recurrences in 37%, lymph node metastases in 17%, distant metastases in 9%, and tumor-related deaths in 9%.[151]

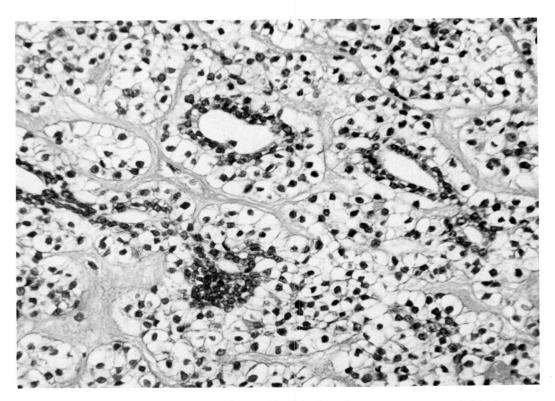

Fig. 12-28 Myoepithelioma of clear cell type. Glandular formations are seen surrounded by large collections of clear cells.

Immunohistochemically, the neoplastic myoepithelial cells may show reactivity for keratin and both forms of S-100 protein, and in some cases for vimentin, actin, and myosin.*

Tumors with clear cell change

Clear cell–containing neoplasms of the salivary gland do not constitute a specific type. In the presence of such neoplasms, the differential diagnosis should include clear cell myoepithelioma (positive for glycogen), sebaceous neoplasms (positive for fat), mucoepidermoid carcinoma (positive for mucin), acinic cell carcinoma (usually negative for all stains), and clear cell change in oncocytic tumors.

Mucoepidermoid carcinoma

Most cases of mucoepidermoid carcinoma are located in the parotid gland.[163,167,168] This lesion represents the most common malignant salivary gland tumor in children.[166] Microscopically, four cell types can be identified: mucin-producing, squamous, intermediate, and clear.[169] This tumor has been divided into low-grade and high-grade types.[164] The former presents grossly as a relatively well-circumscribed mass with cystic areas containing mucinous material. Microscopically, well-differentiated mucinous cells predominate (Fig. 12-29). The high-grade variety is more solid and has a more infiltrative pattern of growth. Squamous intermediate and clear cells predominate over the mucin-producing cells. It should be pointed out that marked nuclear atypia, frequent mitoses, and extensive necrosis are not

---

*See references 145, 147, 151, 152a, 153, and 154.

typical of mucoepidermoid carcinoma of any grade. When these features are present, the alternative possibilities of poorly differentiated adenocarcinoma and adenosquamous carcinoma should be considered.[162] Some authors divide mucoepidermoid carcinomas into three rather than two categories, but this seems unnecessary.[159]

When the mucin or keratin formed by mucoepidermoid carcinoma escapes into the interstitial tissue, it causes an inflammatory reaction. In the presence of mucin-filled cystic spaces in the parotid region, the possibility of a well-differentiated mucoepidermoid carcinoma should be ruled out by taking additional sections. We have seen several of these lesions that were originally underdiagnosed as "mucoceles." Sometimes, extensive fibrosis accompanies the spillage of mucin.[160]

Ultrastructural studies of mucoepidermoid carcinoma have shown a mixed population of luminal epithelial cells and a component identified as of myoepithelial nature.[161]

There is a marked difference in prognosis depending on the grade of the tumor. In the series reported by Jakobsson et al.[165] the determinate 5-year survival rate was 98% for the low-grade variety and 56% for the high-grade variety. Most of the latter showed their malignant behavior within the first 5 years following surgery, in contrast with the continuous fall in survival rate over a 20-year period seen with adenoid cystic carcinoma and acinic cell carcinoma. In another series involving 69 cases, all but two of the fourteen deaths and all six instances of distant metastases occurred in high-grade tumors, which were also associated with an increased incidence of local recurrence and regional lymph node metastases.[162]

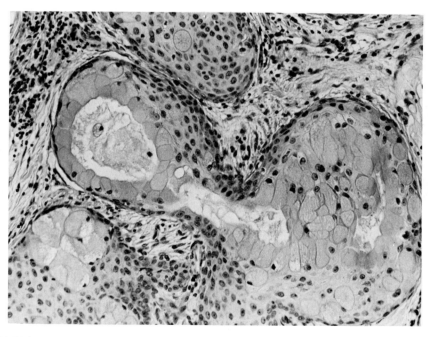

Fig. 12-29 Low-grade mucoepidermoid carcinoma. Well-differentiated squamous cells, together with mucin-producing cells, are present.

Acinic cell carcinoma

Acinic cell carcinoma comprises 1% to 3% of all salivary gland tumors. There is a male predominance and a peak incidence in the third decade of life.[175] The large majority are located in the parotid gland, but many examples in the minor salivary glands have been recorded.[171,172,174] Grossly, it presents as an encapsulated round mass with a solid, friable, grayish white cut surface, usually measuring less than 3 cm in diameter.[175] Occasionally it undergoes marked cystic degeneration.

The microscopic appearance shows considerable variations from case to case. The pattern of growth may be predominantly solid, microcystic, papillary-cystic, or follicular.[170] There is also marked variability in the appearance of the tumor cells. The most characteristic cell, known as acinic, has a basophilic granularity of the cytoplasm, an ultrastructural morphology, and a secretory behavior pattern analogous to those of acinic cells of normal salivary glands[176,178] (Fig. 12-30). Other cell types have been designated as intercalated duct, clear, vacuolated, and nonspecific glandular.[170] When the clear cell component predominates, the tumor acquires an "hypernephroid" appearance reminiscent of renal cell carcinoma (Fig. 12-31). These clear cells do not contain fat or mucin, but may have variable amounts of glycogen. However, focal mucin positivity can be encountered in the papillary-cystic or follicular areas.[181] The occurrence of these cytologic and architectural varia-

tions indicates that this neoplasm differentiates in the direction of the terminal ductular-acinar unit of the salivary gland, which includes secretory acinar cells, intercalated duct cells, pluripotential reserve cells, and myoepithelial cells.[173] Lymphoid follicles with germinal centers may be prominent at the periphery of the tumor, and laminated concretions with the appearance of psammoma bodies may be seen within the lumina.[170] Immunohistochemically, there is positivity for keratin and also focal reactivity for amylase, lactoferrin, secretory component, and proline-rich protein.[182] An endocrine component may also be present, identified by its argyrophilia and immunoreactivity for vasoactive intestinal peptide.[179]

In a series of thirty-seven cases examined by Eneroth and Jakobsson,[176] there was local recurrence in eleven and metastases in seven, four of them in regional lymph nodes. The determinate survival rate at 5 years was 89%, but it fell to 56% after 20 years. In a larger series reported by Ellis and Corio,[175] there was a recurrence rate of 12%, a metastatic rate of 7.8%, and a death rate of 6.1%. The regional lymph nodes are the most common site of metastases.[175]

Adequacy of surgical excision is of paramount importance. In the series of Perzin and LiVolsi,[180] recurrent tumor was found in fourteen of fifteen patients treated with limited local excisions but only in three of twenty-eight patients who had wide local excisions. This local recurrence was associated with an increased incidence of locally uncon-

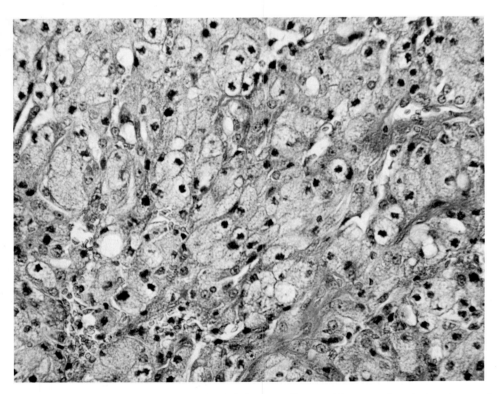

Fig. 12-30 Acinic cell tumor of parotid gland. Cells are uniform and have small central nucleus and abundant basophilic cytoplasm which, in some places, appears granular and in others vacuolated. Mucin stain was negative.

trollable and metastatic disease. Neck dissection does not appear warranted unless the nodes are clinically involved.[177] Radiation therapy has not proved effective for this neoplasm.[180]

Adenoid cystic carcinoma

Adenoid cystic carcinoma (formerly known as *cylindroma*) is a generally slow-growing but highly malignant neoplasm with a remarkable capacity for recurrence. In the parotid gland it is less common than mucoepidermoid carcinoma and acinic cell carcinoma, but in the minor salivary glands it is the most common malignant tumor.

Grossly, it usually has a solid appearance and an infiltrative pattern of growth, although some examples can be well-circumscribed. Microscopically, the typical adenoid cystic carcinoma has a pattern described as *cribriform:* nests and columns of cells of rather bland appearance are arranged concentrically around glandlike spaces ("pseudocysts") filled with PAS-positive material (Fig. 12-32). Most of these are not true glandular spaces; they represent instead cavities containing reduplicated basal lamina material produced by the tumor cells[198] (Fig. 12-33). Small true glandular lumina are also formed. Indeed, identification of *both* pseudocysts and true glandular lumina is required in order to make a diagnosis of adenoid cystic carcinoma. This tumor has a remarkable tendency for invasion of perineurial spaces, to the degree that the diagnosis of adenoid cystic carcinoma should be questioned if an adequate sample taken from the periphery of the tumor does not exhibit this feature (Fig. 12-34). The differential diagnosis with benign mixed tumor

can be difficult. Unfortunately, histochemical reactions are of no help in this regard, inasmuch as they are very similar in the two neoplasms.[185] Important points to remember are that adenoid cystic carcinoma is usually invasive and often associated with perineurial invasion and that mesenchyme-like areas and foci of squamous metaplasia are consistently absent. Some adenoid cystic carcinomas have a predominantly *tubular* pattern of growth, whereas others are mainly *solid.*[194,196] Combined patterns of growth are common. The main ultrastructural features are pseudocysts, intercellular spaces, abundant basal lamina, and true glandular lumens.[190] The cell types present combine features of intercalated ducts, myoepithelial cells, secretory cells, and pluripotential reserve cells.[188] Thus the composition of this tumor is not substantially different from that of benign mixed tumor, suggesting a similar histogenesis.[193]

Immunohistochemically, the tumor cells located in recognizable duct structures express a phenotype similar to that of the intercalated duct (positive for keratin, CEA, and S-100 protein), and those around pseudocysts have a phenotype suggestive of myoepithelial cell differentiation (positive for S-100 protein and actin and variably positive for keratin).[184,186,187] There is also strong reactivity for laminin, particularly along the inner luminal surface of the pseudocysts.[199]

Since the prognosis of adenoid cystic carcinoma is greatly influenced by its pattern of growth, this pattern has been used as a grading system.[191,192,194,197] In one series, the recurrence rate was 59% for the tubular tumors, 89% for the classic cribriform lesions, and 100% for the solid variety.[194]

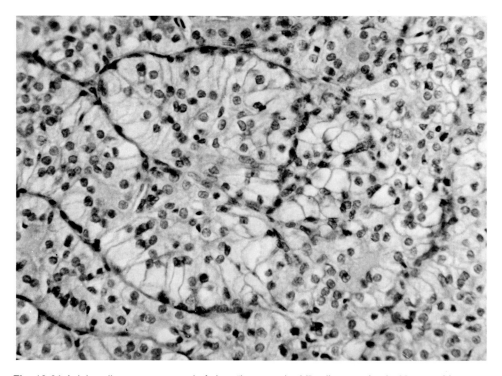

Fig. 12-31 Acinic cell tumor composed of clear "hypernephroid" cells occurring in 60-year-old woman. (Slide contributed by Dr. W. Drake, St. Louis, MO.)

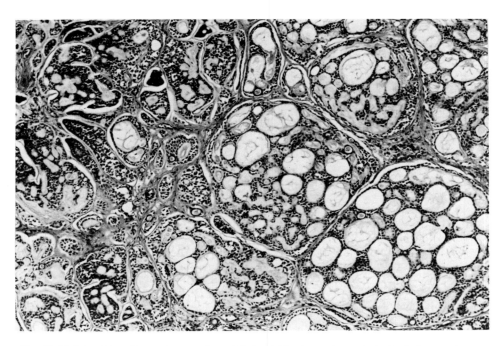

Fig. 12-32 Adenoid cystic carcinoma of parotid gland. The tumor has a typical cribriform pattern.

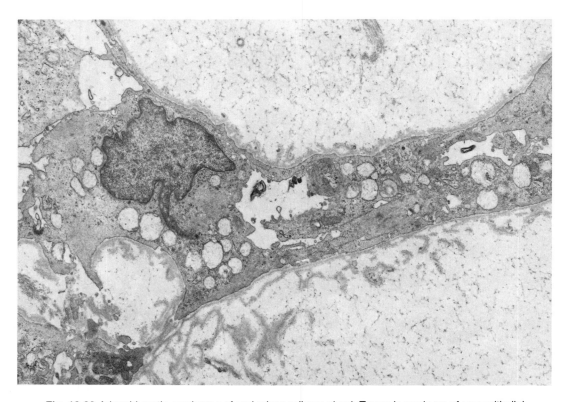

Fig. 12-33 Adenoid cystic carcinoma of oral minor salivary gland. Tumor is made up of myoepithelial cells covered by reduplicated basal lamina. False lumina are thus formed. (×7,450.)

In another series in which a somewhat similar grading system was used, the cumulative survival rates at 15 years were 39%, 26%, and 5% respectively.[197] The solid or anaplastic type of adenoid cystic carcinoma is also associated with a higher incidence of metastases and a rapid clinical course.[189,191] Other factors that influence the prognosis of adenoid cystic carcinoma are presence of tumor at the margins, anatomic site, size of the primary lesion, degree of atypia, and lymph node metastases[194,195,197] (Fig. 12-35).

Adenoid cystic carcinomas frequently metastasize to the lungs. These metastases are usually silent, and it is not unusual to find multiple nodules in the chest x-ray of a totally asymptomatic individual. Lymph node metastases are rare, at least at the time of the initial presentation; many of them seem to represent direct extension from the perinodal soft tissues rather than true embolic deposits.[183]

In the treatment of adenoid cystic carcinoma, a radical surgical approach should be used no matter how well differentiated the tumor appears under the microscope. Cures following tumor recurrence are very difficult to achieve. Radiation therapy is rarely curative, but it may improve results when combined with surgery,[191] and it may produce excellent temporary regression of inoperable recurrences.[192]

Salivary duct carcinoma

This type of carcinoma is usually seen in elderly males, most commonly in the parotid gland but also in the submaxillary gland.[202] Microscopically, it resembles ductal carcinoma of the breast, whether comedo, solid, papillary, or the usual invasive variety[200,201] (Fig. 12-36). This

is a highly aggressive tumor, with frequent metastases to both regional nodes and distant organs, and a mortality rate of 70%.[202]

Terminal duct carcinoma

This newly described type of salivary gland malignancy, also known as *lobular carcinoma* and *polymorphous low-grade adenocarcinoma*, is usually restricted to the minor salivary glands of the oral cavity and is therefore discussed in Chapter 5. Those occurring in the major salivary glands nearly always arise in a background of benign mixed tumor.

Papillary adenocarcinoma

Papillary adenocarcinoma comprises less than 3% of all parotid tumors.[203] It may grow large and be accompanied by hemorrhage and necrosis (Fig. 12-37). Microscopically, the presence of well-defined papillary structures is the most important distinguishing feature. Mucin production is usually present, but there are no squamous or intermediate components (Fig. 12-38). The differential diagnosis includes mucoepidermoid carcinoma, acinic cell carcinoma, and metastatic carcinoma, particularly from the thyroid. Blanck et al.[203] divided their cases into a high-grade and a low-grade variety on the basis of presence or absence of stromal invasion. The former had a poor prognosis, comparable to that of adenoid cystic carcinoma, whereas the latter did not differ prognostically from low-grade mucoepidermoid carcinoma.

Epidermoid carcinoma

Most epidermoid carcinomas in the parotid region represent metastases in the intraparotid lymph nodes of tumors located in the oral cavity, some other region in the upper aerodigestive tract, or the skin.

True pure epidermoid carcinomas of the salivary gland are rare. Some represent the malignant component of a mixed tumor, and others are predominantly epidermoid types of high-grade mucoepidermoid tumors, as shown by their focal positivity for mucin stains. An in situ malignant ductal component has been occasionally encountered.[204] These tumors grow rapidly and infiltrate surrounding structures. The treatment of choice is radical surgery, but radiation therapy is also effective.

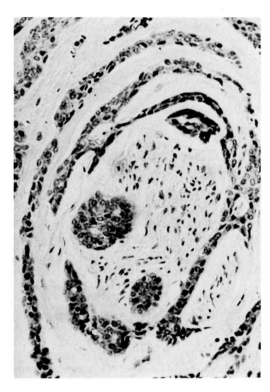

Fig. 12-34 Perineurial invasion in adenoid cystic carcinoma of salivary gland.

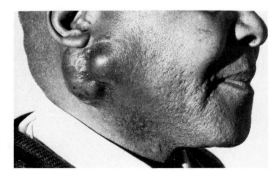

Fig. 12-35 Recurrent adenoid cystic carcinoma following conservative surgical therapy. Short time after reexcision, patient died as result of metastatic involvement to brain.

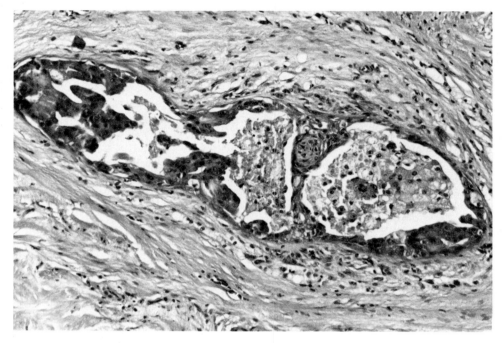

Fig. 12-36 Salivary duct carcinoma. Appearance of tumor is reminiscent of ductal carcinoma of breast.

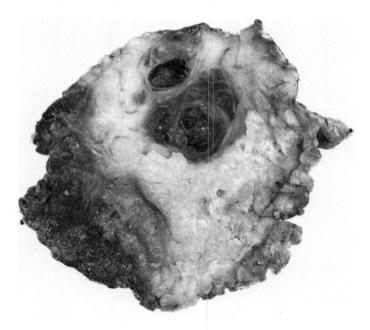

Fig. 12-37 Gross appearance of papillary adenocarcinoma of parotid gland. Tumor is hemorrhagic, partially cystic, and nonencapsulated.

Small cell carcinoma

Malignant tumors of the salivary gland exist that are entirely composed of a solid population of small cells with a darkly staining nucleus, high mitotic activity, and scanty cytoplasm[207,210] (Fig. 12-39). Some of these tumors are indistinguishable from small cell carcinomas of the lung. They may be pure or associated with areas of glandular or squamous differentiation.[205,206,209] Ultrastructurally, dense-core granules suggestive of endocrine differentiation are found in some but not all of the cases.[206a,208,210] In a few instances, these tumors have been found to have features analogous to those of Merkel cell carcinoma of skin.

Lymphoepithelioma-like carcinoma

Lymphoepithelioma-like carcinoma is the term we prefer for a type of salivary gland carcinoma that has been reported as malignant lymphoepithelial lesion and lymphoepithelial carcinoma.[214,216,217] This tumor is particularly frequent among Eskimos and Chinese, in whom it may show evidence of familial clustering.[211-213,215,217] It presents as a unilateral mass, either in the parotid or submaxillary glands in adult patients without any of the peripheral manifestations of Sjögren's syndrome. Its low-power appearance is reminiscent of Mikulicz's disease because of the mixture of epithelial solid islands and lymphoid tissue. However, high-power examination shows that the islands have malignant cytologic features throughout. The appearance is that of a nonkeratinizing large cell carcinoma, with occasional spin-dle-shaped areas, analogous by light and electron microscopy to the nasopharyngeal tumor classically known as lymphoepithelioma.[216,218] That the analogy may be more than morphologic is suggested by the fact that many of these patients have serologic evidence of Epstein-Barr virus infection.[217] Perineurial invasion may be present.[217] Immunohistochemically, there is strong positivity for keratin.[217] The reactive lymphoid tissue forms germinal centers and may exhibit focally a starry sky pattern. Regional lymph node metastases are very common, and distant metastases (particularly to lung, liver, and bone) also occur.[213] Wide variations in mortality rates have been reported, but the overall outcome in the better documented cases seems to be relatively good.[217]

Other primary carcinomas

Some *adenocarcinomas* of salivary gland do not fit into any of the above described patterns; these are usually high-grade neoplasms, the malignancy of which is already obvious at the clinical level.[220] Other large cell tumors grow in a *solid* or *undifferentiated* pattern throughout.[221,222] Some of these have been reported in children.[219]

MALIGNANT LYMPHOMA

Malignant lymphoma in the parotid region may arise from an intraparotid lymph node or in the gland itself. In the former instance, the histologic features and natural history of the disease are those of nodal lymphoma in general. When

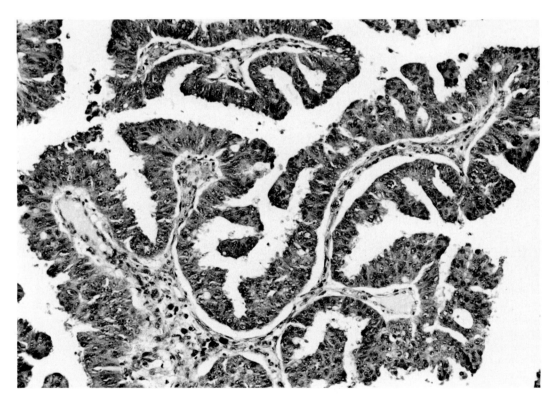

Fig. 12-38 Papillary adenocarcinoma of salivary gland. It was located in parotid gland of 65-year-old man. Note layering of cells and atypicality.

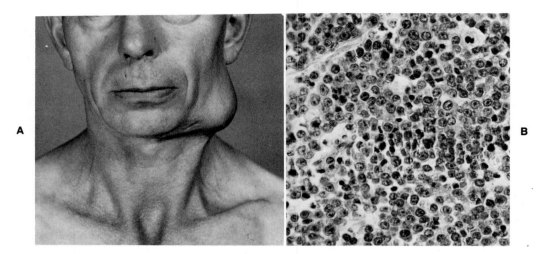

Fig. 12-39 Clinical appearance **(A)** and microscopic appearance **(B)** of small cell carcinoma of parotid gland.

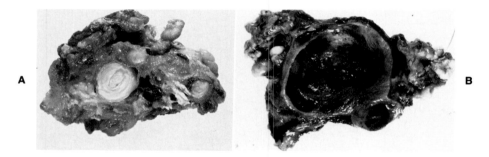

Fig. 12-40 A, Gross appearance of cavernous hemangioma of parotid gland. Note thrombi with laminated calcification. **B,** Gross appearance of cystic lymphangioma of parotid gland in infant. (Courtesy Dr. J. Costa, Lausanne, Switzerland.)

the involvement is within the salivary gland tissue, this may represent the expression of disseminated involvement or a primary process of this organ. The large majority of primary lymphomas of salivary gland involve the parotid, but several cases of submaxillary gland disease are on record.[224] In a series of thirty-three cases of lymphomas with initial involvement of major salivary gland, eighteen were classified as of large cell type, eight as lymphocytic, six as mixed, and one as Hodgkin's disease; twenty-one had a nodular pattern and twelve were diffuse.[225] Most of these tumors are of follicular center cell origin, nearly all of these exhibiting some degree of sclerosis.[229]

Primary parotid lymphoma may arise *de novo* or on a background of Mikulicz's syndrome. The former are usually of follicular center cell type and characterized by a very slow evolution and a good long-term prognosis.[229] Most of the latter are of immunoblastic type and run a rapidly progressive clinical course.[227] Clinically, most parotid lymphomas present as unilateral masses. In the cases associated with Mikulicz's disease, the differential diagnosis between a florid but still reactive immunoblastic process and malig-

nant lymphoma can be very difficult (see p. 641).

A few cases have also been observed of malignant lymphoma arising in Warthin's tumor.[223,226]

Isolated cases of *plasmacytoma* of the salivary gland have been reported, some later developing typical radiographic bone changes of multiple myeloma.[228]

OTHER PRIMARY NEOPLASMS

Vascular tumors of blood vessel and lymphatic vessel type occur in the parotid gland (Fig. 12-40, *A* and *B*).

Capillary hemangioma of the benign hemangioendothelioma type is the most common salivary gland tumor in infants and children. It is often congenital and usually involves the parotid gland. It forms a diffuse soft mass without fixation to the overlying skin. Microscopically, it is made up of anastomosing thin-walled capillaries growing between salivary ducts and acini. The solid proliferation of endothelial cells and the presence of mitotic figures may lead to a mistaken diagnosis of malignant tumor (Fig. 12-41). These lesions do not become malignant and can regress spontaneously.[234,238]

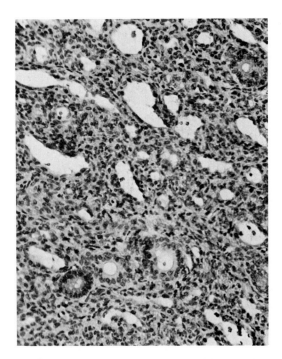

Fig. 12-41 Cellular capillary hemangioma involving parotid gland in child. Tumor replaces salivary gland, but ducts can still be seen.

Lipoma rarely involves the region of the parotid salivary gland.[231] It should be distinguished from *lipomatosis,* which is a diffuse nontumoral deposition of adipose tissue throughout the gland accompanied by enlargement of the organ. The latter has been seen in association with diabetes, cirrhosis, chronic alcoholism, malnutrition, and hormonal disturbances.[235] In some cases, this has been found to be preceded by hypertrophy of the serous acinar cells, interstitial edema, and ductal atrophy, a process known as *sialosis.*

Neurilemoma can arise from one of the fine radicals of the facial nerve and present clinically as a primary salivary gland tumor.[237] It is grossly encapsulated and its microscopic appearance is similar to that of neurilemomas elsewhere (see Chapter 25). Failure to recognize this neoplasm as benign may result in needless sacrifice of the facial nerve.[239]

Pilomatrixoma can present as an intraparotid or periparotid tumor and can be clinically confused with benign mixed tumor.

Embryoma is a term employed by Vawter and Tefft[241] for a highly cellular epithelial parotid tumor of infancy with an embryonal or blastomatous appearance. This tumor is probably of epithelial type and should be distinguished from the even rarer *teratoma* of salivary gland.[240]

Sarcomas are very rare and need to be distinguished from epithelial, myoepithelial, and melanocytic tumors with a spindle-cell pattern.[230] Malignant schwannoma and fibrosarcoma are the two most common types.[230] Malignant fibrous histiocytoma has also been observed.[233]

Giant cell tumors similar to those of bone or soft tissue can occasionally develop in the salivary gland.[232,236] The multinucleated giant cells resemble osteoclasts in all re-

spects. In two of the reported cases, the giant cell component was associated with foci of carcinoma, a phenomenon similar to that observed with giant cell tumors of other organs, such as pancreas, thyroid, or breast.[232,236]

METASTATIC TUMORS

Most metastatic tumors to this region begin in intraparotid or submandibular lymph nodes.[243] As the tumor grows, it closely mimics a primary neoplasm of the salivary gland. It should be remembered that the most common tumor in the submaxillary region is a metastatic carcinoma in the submaxillary nodes rather than a primary salivary gland neoplasm. The most common types are epidermoid carcinoma (from upper aerodigestive tract or skin) and malignant melanoma. Of the distant tumors metastasizing to this area, lung, kidney and breast are the most common.[242,243]

GENERAL FEATURES OF SALIVARY GLAND TUMORS
Relative incidence and malignancy

Salivary gland tumors are twelve times more frequent in the parotid than in the submaxillary gland, a difference that cannot be explained on the basis of gland size alone. The majority are benign, largely represented by the benign mixed tumor.[249,256]

In a series of 2,632 salivary gland tumors reported by Eneroth,[248] the incidence of malignancy was 17% for the parotid gland, 38% for the submaxillary gland, and 44% for the palate. The incidence of malignancy is highest for tumors of the sublingual gland.[249] The most common malignant tumor of the parotid gland is mucoepidermoid carcinoma, followed by undifferentiated carcinoma and acinic cell carcinoma. Adenoid cystic carcinoma comprises most submaxillary and palatal malignant salivary gland neoplasms.[246]

Tumors of minor salivary glands can be found anywhere in the oral cavity, including hard and soft palate, cheek, gingiva, tonsillar area, and tongue.[250] Their frequency seems to be roughly proportional to the amount of normal glandular tissue in this area, which may explain their marked predilection for the hard palate. They can also occur in the lip (particularly upper lip), nose and paranasal sinuses, ear, jaw, pharynx, larynx, trachea, and bronchi.[245] Furthermore, tumors of the salivary gland type may arise from a variety of glandular structures, particularly breasts and sweat glands. These neoplasms are discussed in the respective chapters.

Finally, salivary gland tumors of various types have been described as arising from lymph nodes located in or around the major salivary gland, presumably on the basis of ectopic salivary tissue. Warthin's tumor is by far the most common type, but examples of sebaceous lymphadenoma, benign mixed tumor, basal cell adenoma, acinic cell carcinoma, and mucoepidermoid carcinoma have also been reported.[253,255]

Little is known about the etiology of salivary gland tumors, and high-grade populations have not been identified except for the rare lymphoepithelioma-like carcinoma (see p. 663). An increased incidence of benign mixed tumors and other neoplasms has been observed following childhood irradiation.[254,257]

In children, the most common salivary gland tumor is benign mixed tumor, but the proportion of malignant tumors is higher than in adults. Among the malignant neoplasms, mucoepidermoid carcinoma, adenoid cystic carcinoma, and acinic cell carcinoma are the most common.[244,247,251]

Clinical diagnosis

Benign tumors of the minor salivary glands usually can be distinguished from the high-grade malignant varieties on the basis of their clinical and gross characteristics (Fig. 12-42; Table 12-1). Presence of facial nerve paralysis is almost diagnostic of malignancy. Unfortunately, this does not hold for the low-grade acinic cell carcinomas and mucoepidermoid carcinomas. In these, the clinical presentation is indistinguishable from that of benign neoplasms. The reverse also may be true, although only in rare cases. Warthin's tumor, for instance, may be clinically thought to be malignant because of its adherence to the skin.

Staging

A clinical staging system using the TNM classification scheme for salivary gland tumors has been proposed, which is based on five parameters: size of the primary tumor, local extension, palpability of the regional lymph nodes, degree of suspicion of the regional lymph nodes, and the presence or absence of distant metastases (Table 12-1).[252]

Table 12-1 Proposed staging system for major salivary gland cancer (parotid and submandibular)

Stage	Description
T0	No clinical evidence of primary tumor
T1	Tumor 0.1-2 cm in diameter without significant local extension
T2	Tumor 2.1-4 cm in diameter without significant local extension
T3	Tumor 4.1-6.0 cm in diameter without significant local extension
T4a	Tumor >6 cm in diameter without significant local extension
T4b	Tumor of any size with significant local extension
N0	No evidence of regional lymph node involvement (including palpable but not suspicious regional lymph nodes)
N1	Evidence of regional lymph node involvement (including palpable and suspicious regional lymph nodes)
NX	Regional lymph nodes not assessed
M0	No distant metastases
M1	Distant metastases such as to bone, lung, etc.

Stage I	T1N0M0
	T2N0M0
Stage II	T3N0M0
Stage III	T1N1M0
	T2N1M0
	T4aN0M0
	T4bN0M0
Stage IV	T3N1M0
	T4aN1M0
	T4bN1M0
	Any T Any N and M1

From Spitz MR, Batsakis JG: Major salivary gland carcinoma. Descriptive epidemiology and survival of 498 patients. Arch Otolaryngol **110:**45-49, copyright 1984, American Medical Association.

Biopsy and cytology

Tumors of the submaxillary gland are usually treated by removal of the gland without previous biopsy. For tumors of the parotid glands, several choices are available depending on the size and location of the tumor, clinical features, and expertise of the pathologist. Tumors involving the superficial parotid lobe lacking clinical features of malignancy can be properly handled by a superficial lobectomy with frozen section, any subsequent therapy depending on the diagnosis of the frozen section. Obviously malignant tumors with skin invasion can usually be diagnosed with a small incisional biopsy and treated accordingly. Other options are core-needle biopsy and fine-needle aspiration. Although the former usually provides diagnostic material, the possibility of implantation along the needle tract and the difficulty sometimes encountered in the differential diagnosis (particularly between adenoid cystic carcinoma, monomorphic adenoma, and benign mixed tumor) have resulted in a less than enthusiastic response from clinicians and pathologists. Instead, fine-needle aspiration has been used successfully by several European institutions (particularly the Karolinska Institute in Sweden), and has now become widespread in this country.[261,265,267] The overall accuracy rate has been over 90% in most reported series.[258,262,264]

Frozen section

Intraoperative examination of salivary gland tumors is an accurate procedure that can be of help to the surgeon in determining the extent of the surgery needed, particularly for parotid neoplasms.[259] Obviously, the usefulness of this

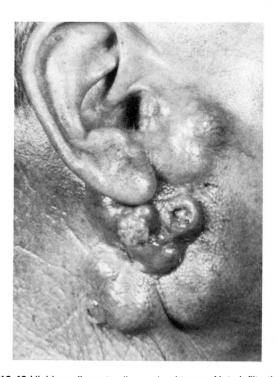

Fig. 12-42 Highly malignant salivary gland tumor. Note infiltration of skin with secondary ulceration.

procedure depends on the expertise of the pathologist in providing accurate diagnoses and the wisdom of the surgeon in applying this information.[266] The most common error when using this technique is to misdiagnose a mucoepidermoid carcinoma as a benign neoplasm.[260,263]

Treatment

The extent of surgical treatment of parotid tumors is determined by their microscopic type and the anatomic peculiarities of the parotid gland, particularly its intimate relationship with the facial nerve.[270] The normal parotid gland is composed of a broad superficial lobe and a smaller deep lobe, with the facial nerve running in between. Variations of this anatomy and the distribution of the facial nerve may occur.[268] Fortunately, most parotid tumors arise from the superficial lobe, so that a superficial parotidectomy with preservation of the nerve can be carried out; actually, the nerve can be preserved in selected cases even if the entire gland is removed.

Most low-grade malignant tumors of mucoepidermoid or acinic cell type can be treated in a similar fashion. If the carcinoma is advanced and/or high grade, total parotidectomy with sacrifice of the facial nerve is usually necessary. If there is clinical evidence of nodal involvement, this procedure needs to be coupled with radical neck dissection.

The surgical treatment of submaxillary tumors, whether benign or malignant, is total removal of the gland. The recurrence rate of carcinomas of this particular gland is relatively high because of the close relation of the gland to the mandible.

Patients who develop post-operative recurrence of high-grade malignant salivary gland tumors do poorly; most have a relatively short survival, and subsequent treatment is effective in only one out of four cases.

Radiation therapy has been used as the primary form of therapy in inoperable tumors and as a post-operative modality in cases selected on the basis of the microscopic type and surgical procedure. There is some evidence that this may result in a decrease in the incidence of local recurrence.[269,271]

Prognosis

The prognosis of salivary gland tumors is influenced by the location, clinical staging, and microscopic type[273,274] (Fig. 12-43). Malignant tumors of the submaxillary gland have a worse prognosis than parotid tumors of the same type.[272] For adenoid cystic carcinoma, the prognosis is best when located in the palate, intermediate when in the parotid, and worst in the submaxillary gland. For parotid malignant tumors, the presence of facial nerve paralysis is an ominous prognostic sign. In regard to microscopic types, the prognosis is best for the low-grade variants of mucoepidermoid and acinic cell carcinoma, and worst for the high-grade variants of these tumors and for adenoid cystic carcinoma, malignant mixed tumor, poorly differentiated adenocarcinoma, and epidermoid carcinoma.

Some preliminary data suggest that determination of DNA ploidy by flow cytometry may provide important prognostic information in adenoid cystic carcinoma and other malignancies of salivary glands.[275]

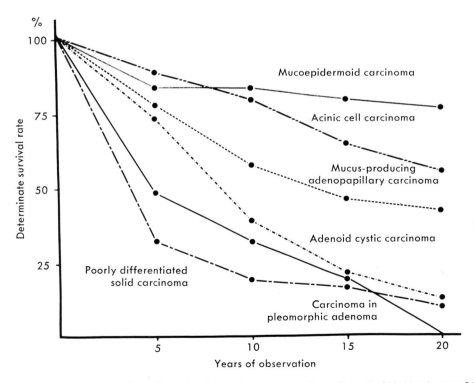

Fig. 12-43 Survival rates in malignant salivary gland tumors. (From Eneroth CM, Hamberger CA: Principles of treatment of different types of parotid tumors. Laryngoscope **84:**1732-1740, 1974.)

REFERENCES
NORMAL ANATOMY; HETEROTOPIA

1 Brown RB, Gaillard RA, Turner JA: Significance of aberrant or heterotopic parotid gland tissue in lymph nodes. Ann Surg **138:**850-856, 1953.
2 Dardick I, van Nostrand AWP: Morphogenesis of salivary gland tumors. A prerequisite to improving classification. Pathol Annu **22**(Pt 1):1-53, 1987.
3 Jernstrom P, Prietto CA: Accessory parotid gland tissue at base of neck. Arch Pathol **73:**473-480, 1962.
4 Ludmer B, Joachims HZ, Ben-Arie J, Eliachar I: Adenocarcinoma in heterotopic salivary tissue. Arch Otolaryngol **107:**547-548, 1981.
4a Luna M, Monheit J: Salivary gland neoplasms arising in lymph nodes. A clinicopathologic analysis of 13 cases (abstract). Lab Invest **58:**58A, 1988.
5 Singer MI, Applebaum EL, Loy KD: Heterotopic salivary gland tissue in the neck. Laryngoscope **89:**1772-1777, 1979.
6 Youngs LA, Scoffield HH: Heterotopic salivary gland tissue in the lower neck. Arch Pathol **83:**550-556, 1967.

SIALOLITHIASIS

7 Blatt IM, Denning RM, Zumberge JH, Maxwell JH: Studies in sialolithiasis. Ann Otol Rhinol Laryngol **67:**595-617, 1958.
8 Husted E: Sialolithiasis. Acta Chir Scand **105:**161-171, 1953.

CHRONIC SIALADENITIS

9 Kurashima C, Hirokawa K: Age-related increase of focal lymphocytic infiltration in the human submandibular glands. J Oral Pathol **15:**172-178, 1986.
10 Van der Walt JD, Leake J: Granulomatous sialadenitis of the major salivary glands. A clinicopathological study of 57 cases. Histopathology **11:**131-144, 1987.

SALIVARY GLAND CYSTS

11 Cohen MN, Rao U, Shedd DP: Benign cysts of the parotid gland. J Surg Oncol **27:**85-88, 1984.
11a Dobson CM, Ellis HA: Polycystic disease of the parotid glands. Case report of a rare entity and review of the literature. Histopathology **11:**953-961, 1987.
12 Pieterse AS, Seymour AE: Parotid cysts. An analysis of 16 cases and suggested classification. Pathology **13:**225-234, 1981.
13 Seifert G, Thomsen St, Donath K: Bilateral dysgenetic polycystic parotid glands. Morphological analysis and differential diagnosis of a rare disease of the salivary glands. Virchows Arch [Pathol Anat] **390:**273-288, 1981.

MIKULICZ'S DISEASE

14 Anderson LG, Talal N: The spectrum of benign to malignant lymphoproliferation in Sjögren's syndrome. Clin Exp Immunol **9:**199-221, 1971.
15 Bloch KJ, Buchanan WW, Wohl MJ, Bunim JJ: Sjögren's syndrome. A clinical, pathological and serological study of sixty-two cases. Medicine (Baltimore) **44:**187-231, 1965.
16 Caselitz J, Osborn M, Wustrow J, Seifert G, Weber K: Immunohistochemical investigations on the epimyoepithelial islands in lymphoepithelial lesions. Use of monoclonal keratin antibodies. Lab Invest **55:**427-432, 1986.
17 Chaudhry AP, Cutler LS, Yamane GM, Satchidanand S, Labay G, Sunder Raj M: Light and ultrastructural features of lymphoepithelial lesions of the salivary glands in Mikulicz's disease. J Pathol **146:**239-250, 1986.
18 Fishleder A, Tubbs R, Hesse B, Levine H: Uniform detection of immunoglobulin-gene rearrangement in benign lymphoepithelial lesions. N Engl J Med **316:**1118-1121, 1987.
19 Hamperl H: The myothelia (myoepithelial cells). Normal state; regressive changes; hyperplasia; tumors. Curr Top Pathol **53:**161-220, 1970.
19a Hyjek E, Smith WJ, Isaacson PG: Primary B-cell lymphoma of salivary gland and its relationship to myoepithelial sialadenitis. Hum Pathol (In press).
20 Kahn LB: Benign lymphoepithelial lesion (Mikulicz's disease) of the salivary gland. An ultrastructural study. Hum Pathol **10:**99-104, 1979.
21 Kassan SS, Gardy M: Sjögren's syndrome. An update and overview. Am J Med **64:**1037-1046, 1978.
22 Miller DG: The association of immune disease and malignant lymphoma. Ann Intern Med **66:**507-521, 1967.
23 Molina R, Provost TT, Arnett FC, Bias WB, Hochberg MC, Wilson RW, Alexander EL: Primary Sjögren's syndrome in men. Clinical, serologic, and immunogenetic features. Am J Med **80:**23-31, 1986.
24 Morgan WS, Castleman B: A clinicopathologic study of "Mikulicz's disease." Am J Pathol **29:**471-503, 1953.
25 Palmer RM, Eveson JW, Gusterson BA: "Epimyoepithelial" islands in lymphoepithelial lesions. Virchows Arch [Pathol Anat] **408:**603-609, 1986.

25a Schmid U, Helbron D, Lennert K: Development of malignant lymphoma in myoepithelial sialadenitis (Sjögren's syndrome). Virchows Arch [Pathol Anat] **395:**11-43, 1982.
26 Talal N, Sokoloff L, Barth WF: Extrasalivary lymphoid abnormalities in Sjögren's syndrome (reticulum cell sarcoma, "pseudolymphoma," macroglobulinemia). Am J Med **43:**50-64, 1967.
27 Tsokos M, Lazarou SA, Moutsopoulos HM: Vasculitis in primary Sjögren's syndrome. Histologic classification and clinical presentation. Am J Clin Pathol **88:**26-31, 1987.
27a Ulirsch RC, Jaffe ES: Sjögren's syndrome-like illness associated with the acquired immunodeficiency syndrome-related complex. Hum Pathol **18:**1063-1068, 1987.
28 von Mikulicz J: Concerning a peculiar symmetrical disease of the lacrimal and salivary glands. Med Classics **2:**165-186, 1937.
29 Weisbrot IM: Lymphomatoid granulomatosis of the lung, associated with a long history of benign lymphoepithelial lesions of the salivary glands and lymphoid interstitial pneumonitis. Report of a case. Am J Clin Pathol **66:**792-801, 1976.
30 Zulman J, Jaffe R, Talal N: Evidence that the malignant lymphoma of Sjögren's syndrome is a monoclonal B-cell neoplasm. N Engl J Med **299:**1215-1220, 1978.

IRRADIATION EFFECT

31 Evans JC, Ackerman LV: Irradiated and obstructed submaxillary salivary glands simulating cervical lymph node metastasis. Radiology **62:**550-555, 1954.

EPITHELIAL TUMORS
Tumors with stromal differentiation
Benign mixed tumor (pleomorphic adenoma)

32 Azzopardi JG, Smith OD: Salivary gland tumours and their mucins. J Pathol Bacteriol **77:**131-140, 1959.
33 Byars LT, Ackerman LV, Peacock E: Tumors of salivary gland origin in children. A clinical pathologic appraisal of 24 cases. Ann Surg **146:**40-52, 1957.
34 Chaplin AJ, Darke P, Patel S: Tyrosine-rich crystals in pleomorphic adenomas of parotid glands. J Oral Pathol **12:**342-346, 1983.
35 Chen KTK: Metastasizing pleomorphic adenoma of the salivary gland. Cancer **42:**2407-2411, 1978.
36 Chu W, Strawitz JG: Parapharyngeal growth of parotid tumors. Report of two cases. Arch Surg **112:**709-711, 1977.
37 Dardick I, van Nostrand AWP, Jeans MTD, Rippstein P, Edwards V: Pleomorphic adenoma. II. Ultrastructural organization of "stromal" regions. Hum Pathol **14:**798-809, 1983.
38 Dardick I, van Nostrand AWP, Phillips MJ: Histogenesis of salivary gland pleomorphic adenoma (mixed tumor) with an evaluation of the role of the myoepithelial cell. Hum Pathol **13:**62-75, 1982.
39 David R, Buchner A: Elastosis in benign and malignant salivary gland tumors. Cancer **45:**2301-2310, 1980.
40 Erlandson RA, Cardon-Cardo C, Higgins PJ: Histogenesis of benign pleomorphic adenoma (mixed tumor) of the major salivary glands. An ultrastructural and immunohistochemical study. Am J Surg Pathol **8:**803-820, 1984.
41 Fantasia JE, Lally ET: Localization of free secretory component in pleomorphic adenomas of minor salivary gland origin. Cancer **53:**1786-1789, 1984.
42 Frazell EL: Clinical aspects of tumors of the major salivary glands. Cancer **7:**637-659, 1954.
43 Gerughty RM, Scofield HH, Brown FM, Hennigar GR: Malignant mixed tumors of salivary gland origin. Cancer **24:**471-486, 1969.
44 Gusterson BA, Lucas RB, Ormerod MG: Distribution of epithelial membrane antigen in benign and malignant lesions of the salivary glands. Virchows Arch [Pathol Anat] **397:**227-233, 1982.
45 Harris BR, Shipkey F: Tyrosine-rich crystalloids in neoplasms and tissues of the head and neck. Arch Pathol Lab Med **110:**709-712, 1986.
46 Kirklin JW, McDonald JR, Harrington SW, New GB: Parotid tumors. Histopathology, clinical behavior, and end results. Surg Gynecol Obstet **92:**721-733, 1951.
47 Korsrud FR, Brandtzaeg P: Immunofluorescence study of secretory epithelial markers in pleomorphic adenomas. Virchows Arch [Pathol Anat] **403:**291-300, 1984.
48 Krolls SO, Trodahl JN, Boyers RC: Salivary gland lesions in children. A survey of 430 cases. Cancer **30:**459-469, 1972.
49 Lam RMY: An electron microscopic histochemical study of the histogenesis of major salivary gland pleomorphic adenoma. Ultrastruct Pathol **8:**207-223, 1985.
50 Lomax-Smith JD, Azzopardi JG: The hyaline cell. A distinctive feature of "mixed" salivary tumours. Histopathology **2:**77-92, 1978.

51 Malett KJ, Harrison MS: The recurrence of salivary gland tumours. J Laryngol Otol **85:**439-448, 1971.
52 Maran AGD, Mackenzie IJ, Stanley RE: Recurrent pleomorphic adenomas of the parotid gland. Arch Otolaryngol **110:**167-171, 1984.
53 Mills SE, Cooper PH: An ultrastructural study of cartilaginous zones and surrounding epithelium in mixed tumors of salivary glands and skin. Lab Invest **44:**6-12, 1981.
54 Mori M, Sumitomo S, Iwai Y, Meenagham MA: Immunolocalization of keratins in salivary gland pleomorphic adenoma using monoclonal antibodies. Oral Surg Oral Med Oral Pathol **61:**611-616, 1986.
55 Murase N, Kobayashi K, Mitani H, Mori M: Immunohistochemical localization of α1-antitrypsin and α1-antichymotrypsin in salivary pleomorphic adenomas. Virchows Arch [Pathol Anat] **408:**107-116, 1985.
56 Nakazato Y, Ishizeki J, Takahashi K, Yamaguchi H, Kamei T, Mori T: Localization of S-100 protein and glial fibrillary acidic protein-related antigen in pleomorphic adenoma of the salivary glands. Lab Invest **46:**621-626, 1982.
57 Palmer RM, Lucas RB, Knight J, Gusterson B: Immunocytochemical identification of cell types in pleomorphic adenoma, with particular reference to myoepithelial cells. J Pathol **146:**213-220, 1985.
58 Patey DH, Thackray AC: The treatment of parotid tumours in the light of a pathological study of parotidectomy material. Br J Surg **45:**477-487, 1958.
59 Quintarelli G, Robinson L: The glycosaminoglycans of salivary gland tumors. Am J Pathol **511:**19-37, 1967.
60 Ryan RE Jr, DeSanto LW, Weiland LH, Devine KD, Beahrs OH: Cellular mixed tumors of the salivary glands. Arch Otolaryngol **104:**451-453, 1978.
60a Sasano H, Ohkubo T, Sasano N: Immunohistochemical demonstration of steroid C-21 hydroxylase in normal and neoplastic salivary glands. Cancer **61:**750-753, 1988.
60b Stead RH, Qizilbash AH, Kontozoglou T, Daya AD, Riddell RH: An immunohistochemical study of pleomorphic adenomas of the salivary gland. Glial fibrillary acidic protein-like immunoreactivity identifies a major myoepithelial component. Hum Pathol **19:**32-40, 1988.
61 Takeuchi J, Sobue M, Yoshida M, Esaki T, Katok Y: Pleomorphic adenoma of the salivary gland. With special reference to histochemical and electron microscopic studies and biochemical analysis of glycosaminoglycans in vivo and in vitro. Cancer **36:**1771-1789, 1975.
62 Tandler B: Amyloid in a pleomorphic adenoma of the parotid gland. Electron microscopic observations. J Oral Pathol **10:**158-163, 1981.
63 Toto PD, Hsu DJ: Product definition of pleomorphic adenoma of minor salivary glands. J Oral Pathol **14:**818-832, 1985.
64 Welsh RA, Meyer AT: Mixed tumors of human salivary gland, histogenesis. Arch Pathol **85:**433-447, 1968.

Malignant mixed tumor

65 Beahrs OH, Woolner LB, Kirklin JW, Devine KD: Carcinomatous transformation of mixed tumors of the parotid gland. Arch Surg **75:**605-614, 1957.
66 Buxton RW, Maxwell JH, Cooper DR: Tumors of the parotid gland. Laryngoscope **59:**565-594, 1949.
67 Eneroth C-M: Histological and clinical aspects of parotid tumours. Acta Otolarynol (Stockh) **191**[Suppl]:1-99, 1964.
68 LiVolsi VA, Perzin KH: Malignant mixed tumors arising in salivary glands. I. Carcinomas arising in benign mixed tumors. A clinicopathologic study. Cancer **39:**2209-2230, 1977.
69 Moberger JG, Eneroth C-M: Malignant mixed tumors of the major salivary glands. Special reference to the histologic structure in metastases. Cancer **21:**1198-1211, 1968.
70 Nagao K, Matsuzaki O, Saiga H, Sugano I, Shigematsu H, Kaneko T, Katoh T, Kitamura T: Histopathologic studies on carcinoma in pleomorphic adenoma of the parotid gland. Cancer **48:**113-121, 1981.
71 Spiro RH, Huvos AG, Strong EW: Malignant mixed tumor of salivary origin. A clinicopathologic study of 146 cases. Cancer **39:**388-396, 1977.
72 Stephen J, Batsakis JG, Luna MA, von der Heyden U, Byers RM: True malignant mixed tumors (carcinosarcoma) of salivary glands. Oral Surg Oral Med Oral Pathol **61:**597-602, 1986.
73 Thomas WH, Coppola ED: Distant metastasis from mixed tumors of the salivary glands. Am J Surg **109:**724-730, 1965.
74 Tortoledo ME, Luna MA, Batsakis JG: Carcinomas ex pleomorphic adenoma and malignant mixed tumors. Histomorphologic indexes. Arch Otolaryngol **110:**172-176, 1984.

Tumors with oxyphilic (oncocytic) change
Oxyphilic adenoma

75 Bazaz-Malik G, Gupta DN: Metastasizing (malignant) oncocytoma of the parotid gland. Z Krebsforsch **70:**193-197, 1968.

76 Feiner HD, Goldstein S, Ittman M, Pelton K, Jacobs J: Oncocytic adenoma of the parotid gland with psammoma bodies. Arch Pathol Lab Med **110:**640-644, 1986.
77 Ghandur-Mnaymneh L: Multinodular oncocytoma of the parotid gland. A benign lesion simulating malignancy. Hum Pathol **15:**485-486, 1984.
78 Gray SR, Cornog JL Jr, Seo IS: Oncocytic neoplasms of salivary glands. A report of fifteen cases including two malignant oncocytomas. Cancer **38:**1306-1317, 1976.
79 Hamperl H: Benign and malignant oncocytoma. Cancer **15:**1019-1027, 1962.
80 Meza-Chavez L: Oxyphilic granular cell adenoma of the parotid gland (oncocytoma). Report of five cases and study of oxyphilic granular cells (oncocytes) in normal parotid glands. Am J Pathol **25:**523-547, 1949.
81 Schwartz IS, Feldman M: Diffuse multinodular oncocytoma ("oncocytosis") of the parotid gland. Cancer **23:**636-640, 1969.
82 Sørensen M, Baunsgaard P, Frederiksen P, Haahr PA: Multifocal adenomatous oncocytic hyperplasia of the parotid gland. (Unusual clear cell variant in two female siblings.) Pathol Res Pract **181:**254-257, 1986.
83 Tandler B, Hutter RVP, Erlandson RA: Ultrastructure of oncocytoma of the parotid gland. Lab Invest **23:**567-580, 1970.

Warthin's tumor

84 Banik S, Howell JS, Wright DH: Non-Hodgkin's lymphoma arising in adenolymphoma. A report of two cases. J Pathol **146:**167-177, 1985.
85 Bernier JL, Bhaskar SN: Lymphoepithelial lesions of salivary glands. Histogenesis and classification based on 186 cases. Cancer **11:**1156-1179, 1958.
86 Brown LJR, Aparicio SR: Malignant Warthin's tumour. An ultrastructural study. J Clin Pathol **37:**170-175, 1984.
87 Caselitz J, Salfelder A, Seifert G: Adenolymphoma. An immunohistochemical study with monoclonal antibodies against lymphocyte antigens. J Oral Pathol **13:**438-447, 1984.
88 Cossman J, Deegan MJ, Batsakis JG: Warthin tumor. B-lymphocytes within the lymphoid infiltrate. Arch Pathol Lab Med **101:**354-356, 1977.
89 Damjanov I, Sneff EM, Delerme AN: Squamous cell carcinoma arising in Warthin's tumor of the parotid gland. A light, electron microscopic, and immunohistochemical study. Oral Surg Oral Med Oral Pathol **55:**286-290, 1983.
90 Eveson JW, Cawson RA: Warthin's tumor (cystadenolymphoma) of salivary glands. A clinicopathologic investigation of 278 cases. Oral Surg Oral Med Oral Pathol **61:**256-262, 1986.
91 Gnepp DR: Warthin tumor exhibiting sebaceous differentiation and necrotizing sialometaplasia. Virchows Arch [Pathol Anat] **391:**267-273, 1981.
92 Gustafsson H, Kjörell U, Carlsöö B: Cytoskeletal proteins in oncocytic tumors of the parotid gland. Arch Otolaryngol **111:**99-105, 1985.
93 Hayashi Y, Saito H, Saito S, Yanagawa T, Yoshida H, Yura Y, Sato M: Immunoreactive somatostatin in Warthin's tumor. Am J Pathol **123:**250-255, 1986.
94 Hsu S-M, Hsu P-L, Nayak RN: Warthin's tumor. An immunohistochemical study of its lymphoid stroma. Hum Pathol **12:**251-257, 1981.
95 Hsu S-M, Raine L: Warthin's tumor. Epithelial cell differences. Am J Clin Pathol **77:**78-81, 1982.
96 Korsrud FR, Brandtzaeg P: Immunohistochemical characterization of cellular immunoglobulins and epithelial marker antigens in Warthin's tumor. Hum Pathol **15:**361-367, 1984.
97 Martin H, Ehrlich HE: Papillary cystadenoma lymphomatosum (Warthin's tumor) of the parotid gland. Surg Gynecol Obstet **79:**611-623, 1944.
98 McGavran MH: The ultrastructure of papillary cystadenoma lymphomatosum of the parotid gland. Virchows Arch [Pathol Anat] **338:**195-202, 1965.
99 Miller R, Yanagihara ET, Dubrow AA, Lukes RJ: Malignant lymphoma in a Warthin's tumor. Report of a case. Cancer **50:**2948-2950, 1982.
100 Morley DJ, Hodes JE, Calland J, Hodes ME: Immunohistochemical demonstration of ribonuclease and amylase in normal and neoplastic parotid glands. Hum Pathol **14:**969-973, 1983.
101 Nakashima N, Goto K, Takeuchi J: Malignant papillary cystadenoma lymphomatosum. Light and electron microscopic study. Virchows Arch [Pathol Anat] **399:**207-219, 1983.
102 Patey DH, Thackray AC: Infected adenolymphomas. A new parotid syndrome. Br J Surg **57:**569-572, 1970.
103 Ruco LP, Rosati S, Remotti D, Modesti A, Vitolo D, Baroni CD: Immunohistology of adenolymphoma (Warthin's tumour). Evidence for a role of vascularization in the organization of the lympho-epithelial structure. Histopathology **11:**557-565, 1987.
104 Scevola A: Studio istomorfologico della quota linfatica nel tumore di Warthin. Otorinolaringol Ital **37:**85-98, 1968.
105 Takahashi H, Tsuda N, Tezuka F, Okabe H: An immunoperoxidase investigation

of S-100 protein in the epithelial component of Warthin's tumor. Oral Surg Oral Med Oral Pathol **62:**57-62, 1986.

106 Thompson AS, Bryant HC Jr: Histogenesis of papillary cystadenoma lymphomatosum (Warthin's tumor) of the parotid salivary gland. Am J Pathol **26:**807-849, 1950.

107 Turnbull AD, Frazell EL: Multiple tumors of the major salivary glands. Am J Surg **118:**787-789, 1969.

108 Weidner N, Geisinger KR, Sterling RT, Miller TR, Yen TSB: Benign lymphoepithelial cysts of the parotid gland. A histologic, cytologic, and ultrastructural study. Am J Clin Pathol **85:**395-401, 1986.

109 Weiss LM, Brodsky GL: Adenolymphoma with massive necrosis and squamous metaplasia. Acta Pathol Jpn **34:**1469-1474, 1984.

110 Yamamoto H, Caselitz J, Seifert G: Cystadenolymphoma. An immunohistochemical study with special reference to Ig E and mast cells. Pathol Res Pract **180:**364-368, 1985.

Monomorphic adenoma

111 Gardner DG, Daley TD: The use of the terms *monomorphic adenoma, basal cell adenoma,* and *canalicular adenoma* as applied to salivary gland tumors. Oral Surg Oral Med Oral Pathol **56:**608-615, 1983.

112 Mintz GA, Abrams AM, Melrose RJ: Monomorphic adenomas of the major and minor salivary glands. Report of twenty-one cases and review of the literature. Oral Surg Oral Med Oral Pathol **53:**375-386, 1982.

113 Thawley SE, Ward SP, Ogura JH: Basal cell adenoma of the salivary glands. Laryngoscope **84:**1756-1766, 1974.

Basal cell adenoma

114 Batsakis JB: Basal cell adenoma of the parotid gland. Cancer **29:**226-230, 1972.

115 Batsakis JG, Brannon RB: Dermal analogue tumours of major salivary glands. J Laryngol Otol **95:**155-164, 1981.

116 Batsakis JG, Brannon RB, Sciubba JJ: Monomorphic adenomas of major salivary glands. A histologic study of 96 tumours. Clin Otolaryngol **6:**129-143, 1981.

117 Chaudhry AP, Cutler LS, Satchidanand S, Labay G, Sunder Raj M: Ultrastructure of monomorphic adenoma (ductal type) of the minor salivary glands. Arch Otolaryngol **109:**118-122, 1983.

118 Chaudhry AP, Cutler LS, Satchidanand S, Labay G, Sunder Raj M, Lin C-C: Monomorphic adenomas of the parotid glands. Their ultrastructure and histogenesis. Cancer **52:**112-120, 1983.

119 Crumpler C, Scharfenberg JC, Reed RJ: Monomorphic adenomas of salivary glands. Trabecular, tubular, canalicular, and basaloid variants. Cancer **38:**193-200, 1976.

120 Daley TD, Gardner DG, Smout MS: Canalicular adenoma. Not a basal cell adenoma. Oral Surg Oral Med Oral Pathol **57:**181-188, 1984.

121 Dardick I, Kahn HJ, van Nostrand AWP, Baumal R: Salivary gland monomorphic adenoma. Ultrastructural, immunoperoxidase, and histogenetic aspects. Am J Pathol **115:**334-348, 1984.

122 Gardner DG, Daley TD: The use of the terms *monomorphic adenoma, basal cell adenoma,* and *canalicular adenoma* as applied to salivary gland tumors. Oral Surg Oral Med Oral Pathol **56:**608-615, 1983.

123 Herbst EW, Utz W: Multifocal dermal-type basal cell adenomas of parotid glands with co-existing dermal cylindromas. Virchows Arch [Pathol Anat] **403:**95-102, 1984.

124 Jao W, Keh PC, Swerdlow MA: Ultrastructure of the basal cell adenoma of parotid gland. Cancer **37:**1322-1333, 1976.

125 Luna MA, Batsakis JG, Tortoledo ME, del Junco G: Carcinoma ex monomorphic adenoma of salivary glands. Lab Invest (In press.)

126 Luna MA, Tortoledo ME, Allen M: Salivary dermal analogue tumors arising in lymph nodes. Cancer **59:**1165-1169, 1987.

127 Nagao K, Matsuzaki O, Saiga H, Sugano I, Shigematsu H, Kaneko T, Katoh T, Kitamura T: Histopathologic studies of basal cell adenoma of the parotid gland. Cancer **50:**736-745, 1982.

128 Pulitzer DR, Reed RJ, Megehee JA: Tubuloalveolar adenoma of salivary gland. Hum Pathol **16:**641-644, 1985.

129 Reingold IM, Keasbey LE, Graham JH: Multicentric dermal-type cylindromas of the parotid glands in a patient with florid turban tumor. Cancer **40:**1702-1710, 1977.

Tumors with sebaceous differentiation

130 Cramer SF, Gnepp DR, Kiehn CL, Levitan J: Sebaceous differentiation in adenoid cystic carcinoma of the parotid gland. Cancer **46:**1405-1410, 1980.

131 Gnepp DR: Sebaceous neoplasms of salivary gland origin. A review. Pathol Annu **18**(Pt 1):71-102, 1983.

132 Gnepp DR, Brannon R: Sebaceous neoplasms of salivary gland origin. Report of 21 cases. Cancer **53:**2155-2170, 1984.

133 McGavran MH, Bauer WC, Ackerman LV: Sebaceous lymphadenoma of the parotid salivary gland. Cancer **13:**1185-1187, 1960.

134 Merwin WH Jr, Barnes L, Myers EN: Unilocular cystic sebaceous lymphadenoma of the parotid gland. Arch Otolaryngol **111:**273-275, 1985.

135 Rawson AJ, Horn RC Jr: Sebaceous glands and sebaceous gland–containing tumors of parotid salivary gland, with consideration of histogenesis of papillary cystadenoma lymphomatosum. Surgery **27:**93-101, 1950.

136 Tschen JA, McGavran MH: Sebaceous lymphadenoma. Ultrastructural observations and lipid analysis. Cancer **44:**1388-1392, 1979.

Tumors with myoepithelial differentiation

137 Barnes L, Appel BN, Perez H, El-Attar AM: Myoepitheliomas of the head and neck. Case report and review. J Surg Oncol **28:**21-28, 1985.

138 Chaudhry AP, Satchidanand S, Peer R, Cutler LS: Myoepithelial cell adenoma of the parotid gland. A light and ultrastructural study. Cancer **49:**288-293, 1982.

139 Corio RL, Sciubba JJ, Brannon RB, Batsakis JG: Epithelial-myoepithelial carcinoma of intercalated duct origin. A clinicopathologic and ultrastructural assessment of sixteen cases. Oral Surg Oral Med Oral Pathol **53:**280-287, 1982.

140 Crissman JD, Wirman JA, Harris A: Malignant myoepithelioma of the parotid gland. Cancer **40:**3042-3049, 1977.

141 Daley TD, Wysocki GP, Smout MS, Slinger RP: Epithelial-myoepithelial carcinoma of salivary glands. Oral Surg Oral Med Oral Pathol **57:**512-519, 1984.

142 Dardick I, van Nostrand AWP: Myoepithelial cells in salivary gland tumors—revisited. Head Neck Surg **7:**395-408, 1985.

143 Dardick I, van Nostrand AWP, Jeans MTD, Rippstein P, Edwards V: Pleomorphic adenoma. I. Ultrastructural organization of "epithelial" regions. Hum Pathol **14:**780-797, 1983.

144 Goldman RL, Klein HZ: Glycogen-rich adenoma of the parotid gland. An uncommon benign clear-cell tumor resembling certain clear-cell carcinomas of salivary origin. Cancer **30:**749-754, 1972.

145 Hara K, Ito M, Takeuchi J, Iijima S, Endo T, Hidaka H: Distribution of S-100b protein in normal salivary glands and salivary gland tumors. Virchows Arch [Pathol Anat] **401:**237-249, 1983.

146 Hubner G, Klein HJ, Kleinsasser O, Schieffer HG: Role of myoepithelial cells in the development of salivary gland tumors. Cancer **27:**1255-1261, 1971.

147 Kahn HJ, Baumal R, Marks A, Dardick I, van Nostrand AWP: Myoepithelial cells in salivary gland tumors. An immunohistochemical study. Arch Pathol Lab Med **109:**190-195, 1985.

148 Kahn LB, Schoub L: Myoepithelioma of the palate. Histochemical and ultrastructural observations. Arch Pathol **95:**209-212, 1973.

149 Lomax-Smith JD, Azzopardi JG: The hyaline cell. A distinctive feature of "mixed" salivary tumors. Histopathology **2:**77-92, 1978.

150 Luna MA, Batsakis JG, Ordóñez NG, Mackay B, Tortoledo ME: Salivary gland adenocarcinomas. A clinicopathologic analysis of three distinctive types. Semin Diagn Pathol **4:**117-135, 1987.

151 Luna MA, Ordóñez NG, Mackay B, Batsakis JG, Guillamondegui O: Salivary epithelial-myoepithelial carcinomas of intercalated ducts. A clinical, electron microscopic, and immunocytochemical study. Oral Surg Oral Med Oral Pathol **59:**482-490, 1985.

152 Mohamed AH, Cherrick HM: Glycogen-rich adenocarcinoma of minor salivary glands. A light and electron microscopic study. Cancer **36:**1057-1066, 1975.

152a Morinaga S, Nakajima T, Shimosato Y: Normal and neoplastic myoepithelial cells in salivary glands. An immunohistochemical study. Hum Pathol **18:**1218-1226, 1987.

153 Nilsen R, Donath K: Actin containing cells in normal human salivary glands. An immunohistochemical study. Virchows Arch [Pathol Anat] **391:**315-322, 1981.

154 Palmer RM: The identification of myoepithelial cells in human salivary glands. A review and comparison of light microscopical methods. J Oral Pathol **15:**221-229, 1986.

155 Saksela E, Tarkkanen J, Wartiovaara J: Parotid clear-cell adenoma of possible myoepithelial origin. Cancer **30:**742-748, 1972.

156 Sciubba JJ, Brannon RB: Myoepithelioma of salivary glands. Report of 23 cases. Cancer **49:**562-572, 1982.

157 Stromeyer FW, Haggitt RC, Nelson JF, Hardman JM: Myoepithelioma of minor salivary gland origin. Light and electron microscopical study. Arch Pathol **99:**242-245, 1975.

158 Tanimura A, Nakamura Y, Nagayama K, Tanaka S, Hachisuka H: Myoepithelioma of the parotid gland. Report of two cases with immunohistochemical technique for S-100 protein and electron microscopic observation. Acta Pathol Jpn **35:**409-417, 1985.

Mucoepidermoid carcinoma

159 Accetta PA, Gray GF Jr, Hunter RM, Rosenfeld L: Mucoepidermoid carcinoma of salivary glands. Arch Pathol Lab Med 108:321-325, 1984.

160 Chan JKC, Saw D: Sclerosing mucoepidermoid tumour of the parotid gland. Report of a case. Histopathology 11:203-207, 1987.

161 Dardick I, Daya D, Hardie J, van Nostrand AWP: Mucoepidermoid carcinoma. Ultrastructural and histogenetic aspects. J Oral Pathol 13:342-358, 1984.

162 Evans HL: Mucoepidermoid carcinoma of salivary glands. A study of 69 cases with special attention to histologic grading. Am J Clin Pathol 81:696-701, 1984.

163 Foote FW, Becker WF: Mucoepidermoid tumors of the salivary glands. Ann Surg 122:820-844, 1945.

164 Healey WV, Perzin KH, Smith L: Mucoepidermoid carcinoma of salivary gland origin. Classification, clinical-pathologic correlation, and results of treatment. Cancer 26:368-388, 1970.

165 Jakobsson PA, Blanck C, Eneroth C-M: Mucoepidermoid carcinoma of the parotid gland. Cancer 22:111-124, 1968.

166 Krolls SO, Trodahl JN, Boyers RC: Salivary gland lesions in children. A survey of 430 cases. Cancer 30:459-469, 1972.

167 Nascimento AG, Amaral ALP, Prado LAF, Kligerman J, Silveira TRP: Mucoepidermoid carcinoma of salivary glands. A clinicopathologic study of 46 cases. Head Neck Surg 8:409-417, 1986.

168 Spiro RH, Huvos AG, Berk R, Strong EW: Mucoepidermoid carcinoma of salivary gland origin. Am J Surg 136:461-468, 1978.

169 Woolner LB, Pettet JR, Kirklin JW: Mucoepidermoid tumors of major salivary glands. Am J Clin Pathol 24:1350-1362, 1954.

Acinic cell carcinoma

170 Abrams AM, Cornyn J, Scofield HH, Hansen LS: Acinic cell adenocarcinoma of the major salivary glands. A clinicopathologic study of 77 cases. Cancer 18:1145-1162, 1965.

171 Abrams AM, Melrose RJ: Acinic cell tumors of minor salivary gland origin. Oral Surg 46:220-233, 1978.

172 Batsakis JG, Chinn EK, Weimert TA, Work WP, Krause CJ: Acinic cell carcinoma. A clinicopathologic study of thirty-five cases. J Laryngol Otol 93:325-340, 1979.

173 Chaudhry AP, Cutler LS, Leifer C, Satchidanand S, Labay G, Yamane G: Histogenesis of acinic cell carcinoma of the major and minor salivary glands. An ultrastructural study. J Oral Pathol 148:307-320, 1986.

174 Chen SY, Brannon RB, Miller AS, White DK, Hooker SP: Acinic cell adenocarcinoma of minor salivary glands. Cancer 42:678-685, 1978.

175 Ellis GL, Corio RL: Acinic cell adenocarcinoma. A clinicopathologic analysis of 294 cases. Cancer 52:542-549, 1983.

176 Eneroth C-M, Jakobsson PA: Acinic cell carcinoma of the parotid gland. Cancer 19:1761-1772, 1966.

177 Godwin JT, Foote FW Jr, Frazell EL: Acinic cell adenocarcinoma of the parotid gland. Report of 27 cases. Am J Pathol 30:465-477, 1954.

178 Gustafsson H, Carlsöö B, Henriksson R: Ultrastructural morphometry and secretory behavior of acinic cell carcinoma. Cancer 55:1706-1710, 1985.

179 Hayashi Y, Nishida T, Yoshida H, Yanagawa T, Yura Y, Sato M: Immunoreactive vasoactive intestinal polypeptide in acinic cell carcinoma of the parotid gland. Cancer 60:962-968, 1987.

180 Perzin KH, LiVolsi VA: Acinic cell carcinomas arising in salivary glands. A clinicopathologic study. Cancer 44:1434-1457, 1979.

181 Spiro RH, Huvos AG, Strong EW: Acinic cell carcinoma of salivary origin. A clinicopathologic study of 67 cases. Cancer 41:924-935, 1978.

182 Warner TFCS, Seo IS, Azen EA, Hafez GR, Zarling TA: Immunocytochemistry of acinic cell carcinomas and mixed tumors of salivary glands. Cancer 56:2221-2227, 1985.

Adenoid cystic carcinoma

183 Allen MS Jr, Marsh WL Jr: Lymph node involvement by direct extension in adenoid cystic carcinoma. Absence of classic embolic lymph node metastasis. Cancer 38:2017-2021, 1976.

184 Azumi N, Battifora H: The cellular composition of adenoid cystic carcinoma. An immunohistochemical study. Cancer 60:1589-1598, 1987.

185 Bloom GD, Carlsöö B, Gustafsson H, Henriksson R: Distribution of mucosubstances in adenoid cystic carcinoma. A light and electron microscopic study. Virchows Arch [Pathol Anat] 375:1-12, 1977.

186 Caselitz J, Becker J, Seifert G, Weber K, Osborn M: Coexpression of keratin ad vimentin filaments in adenoid cystic carcinomas of salivary glands. Virchows Arch [Pathol Anat] 403:337-344, 1984.

187 Caselitz J, Jaup T, Seifert G: Immunohistochemical detection of carcinoembryonic antigen (CEA) in parotid gland carcinomas. Analysis of 52 cases. Virchows Arch [Pathol Anat] 394:49-60, 1981.

188 Chaudhry AP, Leifer C, Cutler LS, Satchidanand S, Labay GR, Yamane GM: Histogenesis of adenoid cystic carcinoma of the salivary glands. Light and electronmicroscopic study. Cancer 58:72-82, 1986.

189 Eby LS, Johnson DC, Baker HW: Adenoid cystic carcinoma of the head and neck. Cancer 29:1160-1168, 1972.

190 Lawrence JB, Mazur MT: Adenoid cystic carcinoma. A comparative pathologic study of tumors in salivary gland, breast, lung, and cervix. Hum Pathol 13:916-924, 1982.

191 Matsuba HM, Spector GJ, Thawley SE, Simpson JR, Mauney M, Pikul FJ: Adenoid cystic salivary gland carcinoma. A histopathologic review of treatment failure patterns. Cancer 57:519-524, 1986.

192 Nascimento AG, Amaral ALP, Prado LAF, Kligerman J, Silveira TRP: Adenoid cystic carcinoma of salivary glands. A study of 61 cases with clinicopathologic correlation. Cancer 57:312-319, 1986.

193 Orenstein JM, Dardick I, van Nostrand AWP: Ultrastructural similarities of adenoid cystic carcinoma and pleomorphic adenoma. Histopathology 9:623-638, 1985.

194 Perzin KH, Gullane P, Clairmont AC: Adenoid cystic carcinomas arising in salivary glands. A correlation of histologic features and clinical course. Cancer 42:265-282, 1978.

195 Smith LC, Lane N, Rankow RM: Cylindroma (adenoid cystic carcinoma). Am J Surg 110:519-526, 1965.

196 Spiro RH, Huvos AG, Strong EW: Adenoid cystic carcinoma of salivary origin. A clinicopathologic study of 242 cases. Am J Surg 128:512-520, 1974.

197 Szanto PA, Luna MA, Tortoledo ME, White RA: Histologic grading of adenoid cystic carcinoma of the salivary glands. Cancer 54:1062-1069, 1984.

198 Tandler B: Ultrastructure of adenoid cystic carcinoma of salivary gland origin. Lab Invest 24:504-512, 1971.

199 Toida M, Takeuchi J, Hara K, Sobue M, Tsukidate K, Goto K, Nakashima N: Histochemical studies of intercellular components of salivary gland tumors with special reference to glycosaminoglycan, laminin and vascular elements. Virchows Arch [Pathol Anat] 403:15-26, 1984.

Salivary duct carcinoma

200 Chen KTK, Hafez GR: Infiltrating salivary duct carcinoma. A clinicopathologic study of five cases. Arch Otolaryngol 107:37-39, 1981.

201 Garland TA, Innes DJ, Fechner RE: Salivary duct carcinoma. An analysis of four cases with review of literature. Am J Clin Pathol 81:436-441, 1984.

202 Luna MA, Batsakis JG, Ordonez NG, Mackay B, Tortoledo ME: Salivary gland adenocarcinomas. A clinicopathologic analysis of three distinctive types. Semin Diagn Pathol 4:117-135, 1987.

Papillary adenocarcinoma

203 Blanck C, Eneroth C-M, Jakobsson PÅ: Mucus-producing adenopapillary (nonepidermoid) carcinoma of the parotid gland. Cancer 28:676-685, 1971.

Epidermoid carcinoma

204 Leader M, Jass JR: In situ neoplasia in squamous cell carcinoma of the parotid. A case report. Histopathology 9:325-329, 1985.

Small cell carcinoma

205 Gnepp DR, Corio RL, Brannon RB: Small cell carcinoma of the major salivary glands. Cancer 58:705-714, 1986.

206 Hayashi Y, Nagamine S, Yanagawa T, Yoshida H, Yura Y, Azuma M, Sato M: Small cell undifferentiated carcinoma of the minor salivary gland containing exocrine, neuroendocrine, and squamous cells. Cancer 60:1583-1588, 1987.

206a Huntrakoon M: Neuroendocrine carcinoma of the parotid gland. A report of two cases with ultrastructural and immunohistochemical studies. Hum Pathol 18:1212-1217, 1987.

207 Koss LG, Spiro RH, Hajdu S: Small cell (oat cell) carcinoma of minor salivary gland origin. Cancer 30:737-741, 1972.

208 Kraemer BB, Mackay B, Batsakis JG: Small cell carcinomas of the parotid gland. A clinicopathologic study of three cases. Cancer 52:2115-2121, 1983.

209 Leipzig B, Gonzales-Vitale JC: Small cell epidermoid carcinoma of salivary glands. "Pseudo" oat cell carcinoma. Arch Otolaryngol 108:511-514, 1982.

210 Wirman JA, Battifora HA: Small cell undifferentiated carcinoma of salivary gland origin. An ultrastructural study. Cancer 37:1840-1848, 1976.

Lymphoepithelioma-like carcinoma

211 Arthaud JB: Anaplastic parotid carcinoma ("malignant lymphoepithelial lesion") in seven Alaskan natives. Am J Clin Pathol 57:275-289, 1972.

liver.[4a,13] Therefore the surgeon should perform not only an incisional biopsy but also a deeper needle biopsy.

Liver biopsy is indicated for several reasons: (1) to diagnose cases in which clinical and laboratory studies are equivocal, (2) to assess the cause of hepatomegaly (both positive and negative features of the biopsy are important in this regard), (3) to distinguish between medical and surgical jaundice, (4) to evaluate the degree of injury present in a particular disease, (5) to monitor the evolution of a disease and its response to therapy, and (6) to determine hepatic involvement in systemic, neoplastic, and familial disorders. Generally speaking, in patients with acute jaundice, the clinical and laboratory findings often provide a definitive diagnosis. It is in patients with chronic jaundice or hepatomegaly that needle biopsy is most often required for the diagnosis.[4]

The clinical value of liver biopsy was assessed in a series of biopsies from 1,324 patients over a 14-year period.[17] The biopsy was a significant aid in establishing the diagnosis in approximately 75% of the cases. In about 50% of patients the biopsy confirmed the clinical impression, whereas in approximately 25% it altered the clinical impression.

The needle biopsy represents about 1/50,000 of the hepatic parenchyma.[16] Therefore the possibility of sampling error should always be borne in mind. Fortunately, many hepatic diseases affect the organ quite homogeneously. The pathologist should not attempt diagnosis of a needle biopsy without having the clinical and laboratory data. This information is necessary if one is to render an interpretation rather than merely a description of the biopsy.

There is reasonably good correlation between the clinical state of the patient and the liver function tests, but at times there may be very little correlation between either of these two parameters and the microscopic appearance of the liver.[15] It is not uncommon to encounter prominent structural derangement of the liver parenchyma in a patient with only minimal clinical evidence of liver disease. As Popper et al.[14] emphasized, the morphologic changes in the liver persist long after there has been pronounced clinical and laboratory improvement.

VIRAL HEPATITIS

The outcomes of exposure to the agents of viral hepatitis are quite variable. They range from anicteric flulike syndromes to fulminant hepatic failure to various chronic liver diseases. The reasons for this are multifactorial and incompletely understood. Characteristics of both the host and the infectious agent play a role.[30,62] The variables include (1) characteristics of the infectious agent (hepatitis A; B; non-A, non-B; and delta hepatitis), (2) regenerative capacity of the host, (3) character of the immune response, and (4) magnitude of the initial hepatocellular insult.

Most instances of *hepatitis A* infection are anicteric and undiagnosed. Although patients with clinical hepatitis can have significant symptoms and laboratory abnormalities, type A hepatitis is essentially a self-limited illness. Fatalities occur in less than 0.5% of the patients in whom the diagnosis is made. The chronic carrier state has not been shown to exist.[22]

The implications of infection by *hepatitis B* virus are somewhat more serious. As is the case with hepatitis A, most persons exposed to hepatitis B have a subclinical illness. However, over 10% of the patients developing symptomatic B hepatitis have something other than a "typical" bout of viral hepatitis.[30] These atypical forms include both acute fulminant illness and a variety of chronic disease states.

Non-A, non-B hepatitis is responsible for most cases of post-transfusion hepatitis (80% to 90%) and is also a common type of hepatitis among IV drug abusers.* Similar to hepatitis B infection, chronic hepatitis may complicate acute non-A, non-B infection and has been reported in 21% to 67% of acutely infected patients.[24,47,53,57] Chronic persistent hepatitis, chronic active hepatitis, and cirrhosis may complicate the course of chronic non-A, non-B hepatitis. In addition these patients are also at risk for developing hepatocellular dysplasia and hepatocellular carcinoma.[41,52,55,60]

Characteristics of the host also play a role in determining the outcome of exposure to hepatitis virus. Genetic factors may explain the vastly differing incidence of the hepatitis B chronic carrier state in different populations.[48] Elderly individuals more often have serious sequelae to viral hepatitis.[35,62] This might be a reflection of impaired regenerative capacity.[62] The character of the immune response determines the ability of patients to rid themselves of the virus and is a factor in determining the amount of hepatocellular injury.[29]

The morphologic features of acute viral hepatitis have been well described.[25-27,49,62,63] In evaluating biopsies, one should assess the degree of hepatocellular damage, the presence of regenerative activity, and the characteristics of the inflammatory and stromal response.

Typical *acute viral hepatitis* is a panlobular disease. Lobular disarray, as evidenced by irregularity of hepatic cell plates caused by variability in hepatocyte size and intrusion of inflammatory and reticuloendothelial cells, is prominent. Hepatocellular injury is manifested by ballooning degeneration and shrunken acidophilic bodies (Fig. 13-1). Ultrastructural changes and aspects of the pathophysiology have been detailed.[70,75] Typically, the extent of hepatocellular loss or "drop out" is focal (unicellular) or limited to small groups of several hepatocytes. Both lobular disarray and areas of "drop out" are well visualized with a reticulin stain. The inflammatory infiltrate expands the portal tracts and involves the lobules. Mononuclear cells predominate, although neutrophils and eosinophils also may be seen. Kupffer cells are prominent. Their cytoplasm may contain impressive amounts of both lipofuscin and iron, especially in the subsiding phase of hepatitis.[74]

The histologic appearances of acute infection by hepatitis A virus, hepatitis B virus, and hepatitis non-A, non-B virus(es) are similar and some have maintained that they can not be distinguished by biopsy.[58] Others, however, have described different patterns of inflammation and cell injury with infection by different infectious agents.[23,33,71,77] Non-A, non-B viral infection induces a cytopathic injury pattern rather than the immune lymphocytic infiltration characteristic of hepatitis B infection.[33] Accordingly alterations of the hepatocytes including microvesicular steatosis and eo-

---

*See references 34, 39, 40, 47, 53, and 57.

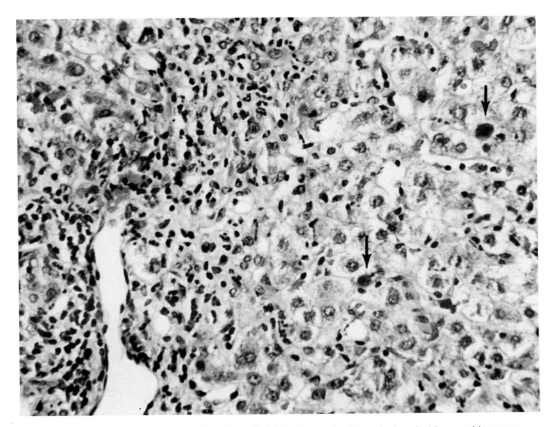

Fig. 13-1 Viral hepatitis 6 months following administration of blood transfusions in 36-year-old woman. Australia antigen was present. Liver shows marked inflammatory portal inflammation and panlobular disease, evidenced by hyperplasia of Kupffer cells, swollen hepatocytes, and scattered acidophilic bodies (arrows).

sinophilic alteration of hepatocyte cytoplasm characterize non-A, non-B infection[33] (Fig. 13-2). Sinusoidal cell proliferation is also more intense in non-A, non-B infection. Acute hepatitis A infection demonstrates inflammation and cell injury that is more limited to portal and periportal areas in contrast to the uniform lobular involvement that is characteristic of acute infection by hepatitis B virus of non-A, non-B virus(es).[23,33]

Cholestatic viral hepatitis, with biochemical features simulating mechanical obstruction, has been observed in both sporadic and epidemic form.[36] The observation of a hepatitis *independent* of cholestasis can enable one to distinguish this from mechanical obstruction.

In 1977 Rizzetto et al.[67] discovered a new viral agent while investigating the distribution of hepatitis B virus antigen in chronic HB_sA_g carriers. This new antigen was called the delta agent (later the delta virus) and was soon discovered to be a defective RNA virus that requires concurrent hepatitis B virus infection for its own replication. Nonetheless the delta virus has been found to be highly virulent and infectious and has been responsible for several epidemics of lethal hepatitis all over the world.* *Delta hepatitis* can occur in three clinical situations: (1) simultaneous acute

delta and acute type B hepatitis, (2) acute delta infection superimposed upon chronic hepatitis B, and (3) chronic delta hepatitis superimposed upon chronic hepatitis B. The histologic picture of delta hepatitis is similar to other forms of viral hepatitis, and although it tends to be more severe, it can not be reliably distinguished from hepatitis B or non-A, non-B hepatitis.[32,56,76] Verme et al. found the most characteristic microscopic features to be a marked intralobular infiltration by mononuclear cells and a degenerative eosinophilic change of the cytoplasm of infected hepatocytes.[76] In a study of HB_sA_g with or without delta infection, Lok et al. found delta hepatitis patients to have more inflammation on biopsy, more severe symptoms, and to be younger.[56] Overall, however, the same range of changes from mild to moderate acute hepatitis to hepatitis with bridging or confluent necrosis to cirrhosis has been observed. Serologic tests for delta antibody and immunohistochemical analysis for delta antigens in tissue are more reliable methods of documenting infection.[32,43,45,76]

A small number of biopsies in acute viral hepatitis show unusual patterns of necrosis that are predictive of atypical clinical outcomes. In 1970, Boyer and Klatskin[28] called attention to a variant of acute viral hepatitis termed subacute hepatic necrosis. The pattern of necrosis in this lesion differed from the focal necrosis of "typical" viral hepatitis. It

---

*See references 31, 32, 45, 46, 64, 67, 72, and 73.

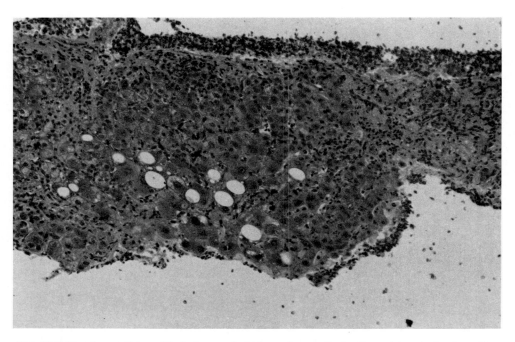

Fig. 13-2 Non-A, non-B hepatitis in fragmented biopsy from patient with post-transfusion hepatitis, which has evolved to chronic hepatitis and cirrhosis. Characteristic features of non-A, non-B etiology include steatosis and cytotoxic degenerative injury to hepatocytes, sinusoidal cell proliferation, and dense eosinophilic alteration of cytoplasm of many of hepatocytes.

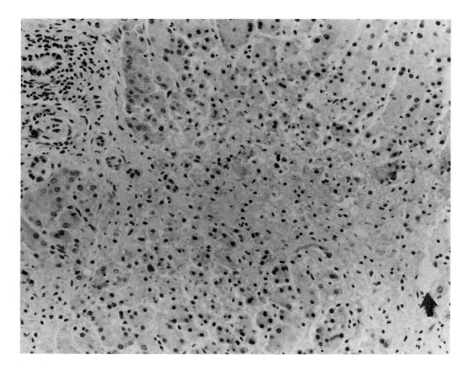

Fig. 13-3 Confluent area of hepatocellular necrosis extends from portal triad to adjacent central vein (arrow) in patient with acute hepatitis with bridging necrosis. Relatively intact hepatocytes may be seen above and below this area of bridging necrosis.

was characterized by areas of confluent hepatocellular necrosis that *bridged* adjacent portal triads and central veins (Fig. 13-3). Currently, the term *acute viral hepatitis with bridging necrosis* is preferred to that of subacute hepatic necrosis. The outcome in Boyer and Klatskin's group of fifty-two patients[28] was drastically different from that in patients with conventional viral hepatitis, with 19% of the group dying in progressive hepatic failure, the course being either fulminant (days) or subacute (months). Cirrhosis developed in 37% of the fifty-two patients.[28] In another study of the significance of hepatitis with bridging necrosis, Ware et al.[78] found that about 30% of their patients had a poor outcome. Boyer[29] recommends that at least two, and preferably three, definite bridges be present in an adequately sized (at least 2 cm) biopsy. More unusual still are cases of viral hepatitis with *multilobular* (areas confluent between adjacent lobules) or *massive* (entire lobules) necrosis. The patients typically show fulminant hepatic failure.[51,68] Mortality is high (50% to 90%), especially in patients over 40 years old. Survivors usually do not develop chronic liver disease.[51]

The *acquired immune deficiency syndrome (AIDS)* is a condition frequently complicated by hepatitis, and a variety of types and patterns have been observed both in biopsy and autopsy series.* The liver is frequently involved by *Mycobacterium avium intracellulare* as a component of systemic infection, and the organisms may be seen either within granulomas or within nonaggravated Kupffer cells or other macrophages. Infection by hepatitis B virus and cytomegalovirus (CMV) are also frequent. Cytomegalovirus infection is often widespread in this syndrome and liver involvement is usually asymptomatic.[52a] Liver biopsy may also show Kaposi's sarcoma or malignant lymphoma in AIDS victims but this is more frequently seen at autopsy.[42,65] The entire histologic range of chronic hepatitis (see the following discussion) may be encountered in AIDS patients and this may be caused by hepatotrophic viruses and/or nonhepatotrophic viruses. Liver biopsy for histology and culture should be considered in any AIDS patient with unexplained fever, hepatomegaly, or abnormal liver function tests because of the high yield of diagnosis of potentially treatable infections.[50,54,59] The changes present, however, in hepatic biopsies in this patient population are within the overall range of hepatitis and histologic alterations that occur are not specific for AIDS.[38,42,54]

CHRONIC HEPATITIS

For two decades the classification of chronic hepatitis has followed what the International Group first proposed in 1968 and then revised in 1977.[92,93] Two morphologic categories were recognized and later expanded to three: (1) chronic persistent hepatitis, (2) chronic active hepatitis, and (3) chronic lobular hepatitis. In the intervening time since the initial proposal of this classification, several clinical pathologic studies have underscored its usefulness. In general, it is recognized that patients with chronic persistent hepatitis have low risk of it evolving into end stage liver disease or cirrhosis, whereas this risk is much higher for patients with

*See references 37, 38, 42, 44, 50, 53a, 59, 61, 65, 69, and 79.

chronic active hepatitis.[81,88,105] Individuals with chronic lobular hepatitis appear to have a clinical outcome similar to chronic persistent hepatitis, although this conclusion deserves further study.[83,85,104,111] Chronic hepatitis occurring in childhood is an increasing problem especially in areas of the world where hepatitis B virus is endemic. The same histologic patterns of chronic hepatitis have been observed in children as occur in adults.[82a,91a]

Chronic persistent hepatitis is defined histologically by restriction of the inflammatory infiltrate to the portal tracts without piecemeal necrosis and is the most common long-term sequela to viral hepatitis. Piecemeal necrosis has been defined as "the destruction of liver cells at an interface between parenchyma and connective tissue, together with predominantly lymphocytic or plasma cell infiltrate."[92] No significant lobular inflammation is present, and liver cell injury is mild or absent. Minimal erosion of the limiting plate without cell necrosis is not evidence of chronic active hepatitis. Chronic persistent hepatitis may follow either B or non-A, non-B viral hepatitis. The disease may wax and-wane both clinically and pathologically.[82]

Chronic active hepatitis (formally also called chronic aggressive hepatitis) is histologically defined by the presence of piecemeal necrosis (Fig. 13-4). Chronic active hepatitis is a disorder with both varied etiology and variable histologic features.[81,87,109] Mild forms consist of an inflammatory infiltrate that erodes minimally into adjacent parenchyma with necrosis of periportal hepatocyte. Severe cases include those characterized by bridging necrosis and by the deposition of fibrous tissue in the periportal region or bridging portal to portal or portal to central regions (Fig. 13-5). Confluent necrosis or multilobular necrosis may also be seen in severe examples.

Chronic lobular hepatitis is characterized by spotty or patchy inflammation within the lobules with minimal portal tract inflammation. This form of hepatitis can mimic acute viral hepatitis, and it is important to apply the generally accepted definition of chronic hepatitis, which requires the presence of clinical or laboratory evidence of disease for at least 6 months.

One variant of chronic active hepatitis has been called *"lupoid"* or *autoimmune chronic hepatitis.* It is important to be aware that this is more a clinical and laboratory characterization than a histological one. The definition of autoimmune chronic liver disease includes striking hypergammaglobulinemia, circulating autoantibodies, lymphoid infiltration within portal tracts of the liver, therapeutic response to steroids, and association with other autoimmune disorders.[107] This variant cannot be reliably identified by histologic changes. In fact even in laboratory evaluation there is a confusing overlap with various types of chronic liver disease, including primary biliary cirrhosis.[95,102]

Careful histologic documentation of the activity of inflammation on biopsies from patients with chronic hepatitis is important in predicting clinical outcome. The presence of chronic active hepatitis has been shown in several studies to place individuals at high risk for evolution to cirrhosis if followed for a significant interval of time.[80,85,101] The severity of inflammation in the spectrum of chronic active hepatitis is also important for predicting outcome in patients

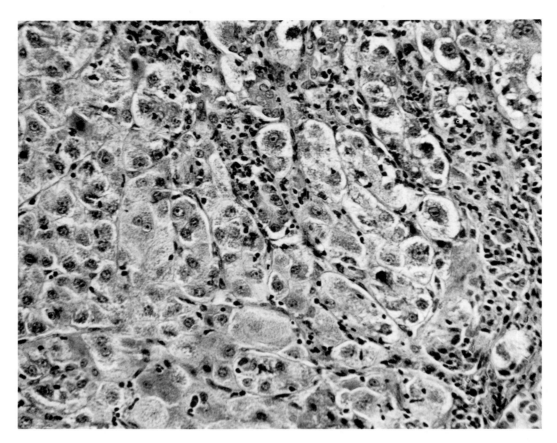

Fig. 13-4 Chronic active hepatitis in 28-year-old man. Portal inflammatory infiltrate disrupts limiting plate and surrounds individual hepatocytes, some of which exhibit degenerative changes.

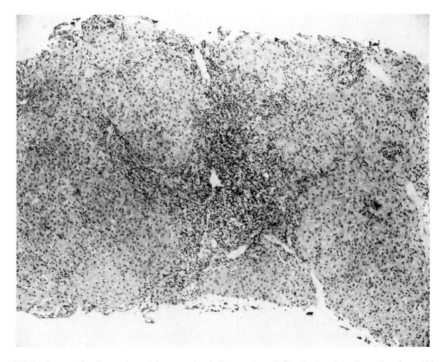

Fig. 13-5 Linkage of adjacent portal areas by inflammatory infiltrate in chronic active hepatitis with piecemeal necrosis. Limiting plate is indistinct because of extension of infiltrate into lobule.

who show bridging necrosis or confluent necrosis because they are at greater risk than those showing only mild piecemeal necrosis.[80] A biopsy report of chronic active hepatitis should document the degree of inflammation and the type of necrosis, whether piecemeal, bridging, confluent, or submassive. There appears to be a low risk that chronic persistent hepatitis will evolve into cirrhosis or chronic liver failure, although this has largely been based on studies with limited follow-up, and some recent studies have demonstrated that follow-up biopsies upon patients with chronic persistent hepatitis may often show chronic active hepatitis.[83,85,89] The assumption can be made that continued follow-up would ultimately demonstrate evolution into fibrosis or cirrhosis. Furthermore, in a recent commentary on classifications of chronic hepatitis, Scheuer has commented that there is a need to re-examine the implication of severe lobular necrosis that may be found independent of portal inflammation.[111] Although this is uncommon, he proposes that chronic hepatitis should be subdivided not only according to the severity and extent of piecemeal necrosis but also according to the presence or absence of lobular necrosis. A grading scale for histologic activity both in lobular areas and in the portal area has recently been defined and applied for chronic hepatitis B with superimposed delta virus infection.[98] A similar study using a scoring system for chronic hepatitis B found numeric scoring of histologic activity to be more predictive of clinical and histologic outcome than the use of routine chronic hepatitis diagnostic terminology.[97a] Additional studies are needed to fully explore the implication of lobular inflammation independent of portal and periportal activity.

Also of importance is whether or not the disease is associated with hepatitis B.[108] The prognosis in HB_sA_g-positive chronic active hepatitis was formerly considered to be somewhat better than in the "autoimmune" or idiopathic variety. However, in the study by De Groote et al.,[87] cirrhosis developed in 71% of the HB_sA_g-positive patients versus 31% of the HB_sA_g-negative patients. The series from the Mayo Clinic also showed that treatment failure and death were significantly more frequent in HB_sA_g-positive than in HB_sA_g-negative patients.

Three controlled studies have shown that corticosteroids can benefit both patients with chronic active hepatitis and patients with cirrhosis combined with chronic active hepatitis.[84,100,114,116] However, further studies are necessary to more precisely characterize the prognostic and therapeutic implications of *piecemeal* versus *bridging* necrosis in chronic active hepatitis. In addition, the role of corticosteroids in HB_sA_g-positive disease has not been adequately defined.

Asymptomatic carriers have been discovered with increasing frequency in blood bank screening for HB_sA_g. This state is usually defined as persistent antigenemia (longer than 6 months) with normal transaminases and no clinical symptoms. In the 167 reported cases reviewed by Shrago et al.,[113] only one patient had cirrhosis. The common findings in this group were normal liver (20%), mild nonspecific inflammatory changes (36%), chronic persistent hepatitis (7%), and ground-glass hepatocytes only (15%).

Ground-glass cytoplasm in hepatocytes is a reflection of marked proliferation of the smooth endoplasmic reticulum. It was observed by Klinge and Bannasch[96] in 1968 as an adaptive phenomenon with a variety of drugs (barbiturates, chlorpromazine). Subsequently, the ground-glass change was described in biopsies from HB_sA_g carriers.[91] Ultrastructurally, this showed proliferated smooth endoplasmic reticulum containing tubular profiles of HB_sA_g.[115] Shikata et al.[112] showed that the HB_sA_g-associated, ground-glass hepatocytes could be stained with orcein or aldehyde fuchsin. This staining was thought to depend on disulfide bonds present in the viral antigen. The drug-induced ground-glass hepatocytes do not show these staining characteristics.[94] A positive orcein or aldehyde-fuchsin reaction for HB_sA_g shows *diffuse* staining of the cytoplasm of isolated hepatocytes.[97] It should be noted that orcein and aldehyde-fuchsin also react with copper-protein complexes in the liver. This results in *coarse granular* staining of the hepatocyte cytoplasm that is easily distinguished from that seen with HB_sA_g (Fig. 13-6).

Antibody probes are available for immunohistochemical characterization of hepatitis A, hepatitis B, and delta hepatitis.[90] Hepatitis A viral antigen may be detected in liver tissue for several weeks following onset of infection.[99] However, serum determination of IgM anti-HAV is more reliable, rendering immunohistochemistry for hepatitis A of limited clinical value.[90]

Several hepatitis B viral antigens may be detected immunohistochemically including surface antigen (HB_sA_g), core antigen (HB_cA_g), and e antigen (HB_eA_g). Again because of the availability of reliable, sensitive serologic markers, immune staining of tissue for diagnosis of acute hepatitis B infection is of limited use. Immunostaining may be very helpful, however, in the characterization of chronic HBV infection.[86,90] Acute exacerbation of clinical disease in a chronic HBV carrier may be caused by superinfection by HAV or delta virus or may be secondary to reactivation of HBV replication. Characterization of HB_eA_g and HB_cA_g versus HAV antigen or delta virus antigen can assist in this differential. However, the greatest use for this tissue marker at the current time may be in clinical trials for the treatment of hepatitis B to monitor response to therapy.[90]

A newer and increasingly important tool in diagnosing hepatitis B infection is molecular hybridization techniques for HBV-DNA in serum and liver tissue.[103,106] The presence of HBV-DNA can sometimes be detected in the absence of all other markers of active disease. DNA hybridization techniques can be accomplished retrospectively in formalin-fixed liver biopsies.[106] Another potentially important area of investigation in understanding the pathogenesis of chronic hepatitis following HBV infection is the characterization of antigen-specific immune responses. Recent data suggest the HBV nucleoprotein may be a major target antigen for both helper and cytotoxic T lymphocytes.[99a]

Hepatitis D viral antigen can be detected in the nuclei or, less commonly, in the cytoplasm of hepatocytes infected by HDV.[90] It can be of particular clinical value in that serum IgM anti HD may not always be detectable in the presence of active infection.

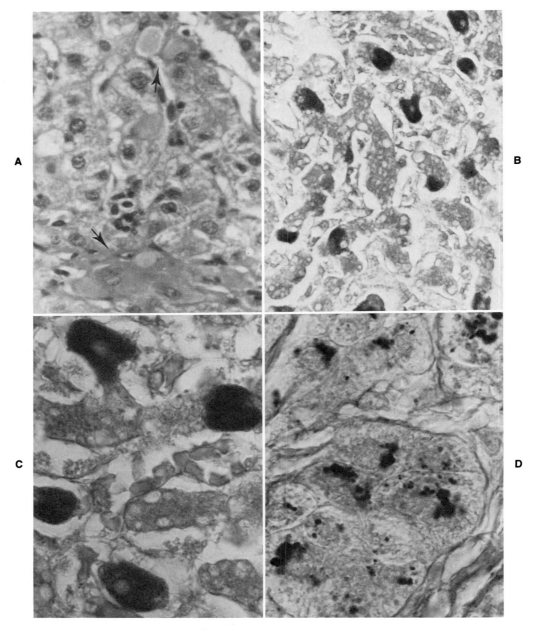

Fig. 13-6 A, Two clusters of ground-glass hepatocytes (arrows) are evident. Patient had HB$_s$A$_g$-positive chronic active hepatitis. **B,** With orcein stain, ground-glass hepatocytes are readily apparent. Patient was asymptomatic HB$_s$A$_g$ carrier. **C,** Orcein stain of HB$_s$A$_g$ ground-glass hepatocytes shows diffuse staining of cytoplasm; note negatively stained nucleus. **D,** Orcein stain also can demonstrate excess copper. Coarse granular staining of copper-protein complexes is quite distinct from that seen with HB$_s$A$_g$. Patient had primary biliary cirrhosis.

DRUG-INDUCED LIVER DISEASE

Drug-induced liver disease is a heterogenous and complex set of disorders that can mimic essentially any form of acute or chronic liver disease both clinically and pathologically.[127] An overview of the general principles will be provided here and the reader is referred to recent reviews for more in depth discussion.* The different categories of lesions may be outlined as follows:

Hepatocellular
  Acute
    Panlobular hepatitis (viral hepatitis-like)
    Zonal hepatitis
    Fatty change
  Chronic
    Chronic persistent hepatitis
    Chronic active hepatitis
Cholestatic
  Bland cholestasis
  Cholestatic hepatitis
Granulomatous hepatitis
Vascular
  Occlusive
    Budd-Chiari syndrome
    Veno-occlusive disease
  Ectatic
    Sinusoidal dilatation
    Peliosis hepatitis
Neoplastic
  Hepatocellular
  Vascular

*See references 121, 127, 129, 131, 146, and 147.

It is helpful to attempt to categorize the disease process in this way. Unfortunately, some overlap occurs, and certain drugs can cause a variety of reactions.[135] The injury may be either dose-related and predictable or idiosyncratic. These latter unpredictable instances are considered hypersensitivity reactions.[118]

Several types of predominantly hepatocellular lesions have been described. *Panlobular hepatitis,* a lesion histologically indistinguishable from viral hepatitis, has been seen with a number of drugs. These include methyldopa, halothane, monoamine oxidase inhibitors, and antituberculous agents.[128,135] Both direct toxicity and hypersensitivity reactions can result in this viral hepatitis–like picture. The severity of these reactions range from mild spotty hepatocellular necrosis to "typical" panlobular hepatitis to hepatitis with bridging necrosis.[141]

Zonal hepatic necrosis is an expression of a direct toxic injury. The centrilobular (Rappaport's zone 3)[130] lesion of carbon tetrachloride and the periportal (Rappaport's zone 1) necrosis seen with yellow phosphorus are well known.[128] Some therapeutic agents also cause a zonal injury pattern. The lesion seen with acetaminophen is an example, with necrosis being most evident in the centrilobular area[126,138] (Fig. 13-7). Tetracycline is one example of a drug causing *fatty change* in the liver. The fat here is microvesicular in appearance. The lesion ranges from mild to fatal hepatic steatosis, the latter seen most often in pregnancy.[136]

A chronic liver disease that fulfills the clinical pathologic criteria of *chronic active hepatitis* has been seen with several drugs.[132] Chief among these are oxyphenisatin, isoni-

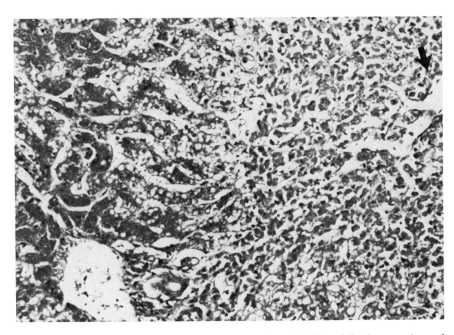

Fig. 13-7 Patient, a chronic alcoholic, died in fulminant hepatic failure following overdose of acetaminophen. Drug was being taken for abdominal pain caused by pancreatitis. Zonal nature of acetaminophen lesion is apparent. Necrosis is most evident in centrilobular area (arrow on central vein); there is relative sparing of periportal region. Chronic alcoholics appear particularly susceptible to hepatotoxic effects of acetaminophen.

azid, and methyldopa. In addition, some cases of *chronic persistent hepatitis* appear drug induced.

The most common types of drug-induced liver lesions are those that are predominantly or exclusively cholestatic.[142] *Bland cholestasis*, unaccompanied by inflammation or cellular degeneration, has been seen with both contraceptive and anabolic steroids.[136] *Cholestatic hepatitis* describes a lesion that is predominantly cholestatic, though accompanied by some degree of inflammation and hepatocellular degeneration. The ability of phenothiazines to cause such a lesion is well recognized. The clinical and pathologic features of phenothiazine-induced liver disease have been well described.[124] Over 20% of the patients reported by Ishak and Irey[124] underwent surgical exploration, an indication of how this can mimic mechanical obstruction. Eosinophilia and clinical symptoms of a hypersensitivity reaction are frequent in these patients.

The list of drugs causing a *granulomatous hepatitis* is ever expanding. Examples include phenylbutazone, oxyphenbutazone, the sulfonamides, and sulfonylurea derivatives.[125] An extensive discussion of specific drugs and their effects on the liver is presented by Klatskin.[128] More recent reviews are provided by Kaplowitz et al.[127] and by Ludwig and Axelsen.[131]

Both occlusive and ectatic vascular lesions have been ascribed to drugs. Cases of the *Budd-Chiari syndrome*, occlusion of the vena cava or major hepatic vein, have been attributed to oral contraceptives.[145] *Veno-occlusive disease* is characterized by sclerotic occlusive lesions of the terminal hepatic veins (central veins); there is associated sinusoidal congestion. The lesion is caused by pyrrolozidine alkaloids (bush tea poisoning).[143] It has more recently been attributed to certain therapeutic agents. Azathioprine and 6-thioguanine have been implicated, as has radiation of the liver.[123,133,140]

Sinusoidal dilatation, most pronounced in the periportal area, has been attributed to oral contraceptives.[144] *Peliosis hepatis* is a more pronounced vascular ectatic lesion characterized by grossly visible blood-filled cysts. It has been seen in patients treated with androgenic anabolic steroids and, less commonly, with contraceptive steroids.[117,134] While the majority of reported cases of this unusual condition have followed drug administration, peliosis hepatis has also occurred in renal transplant recipients,[123a] in hematologic disorders,[119a] and as a complication of exposure to vinyl chloride.[143a] Characteristically, the blood-filled spaces of peliosis hepatis lack an endothelial lining histologically. The pathogenesis of this lesion is not fully elucidated, but it may be that subcellular changes on the sinusoidal endothelial cells are the initial event.[145a]

Drugs have been implicated as a cause of both benign and malignant tumors. These include focal nodular hyperplasia, hepatocellular adenoma, and hepatocellular carcinoma.[120,122] Angiosarcomas of the liver have been described with exposure to Fowler's solution (potassium arsenite) and thorium dioxide (Thorotrast) in addition to polyvinyl chloride and "Bordeaux mixture" (a fungicide containing copper sulfate and lime).[119,130,137] These neoplsms are discussed in more detail later in this chapter.

Table 13-1 Liver biopsy in the chronic alcoholic

Major histologic feature	%
Normal	15
Simple fatty change	40
Alcoholic hepatitis	15
Cirrhosis	10
Other (viral hepatitis, drug hepatitis, chronic active hepatitis, mechanical biliary obstruction)	20

ALCOHOL-INDUCED LIVER DISEASE

Experiments, both in human volunteers and animal models, have established the hepatotoxicity of ethanol.[147a,173,174] A wide spectrum of pathologic changes can be seen with alcohol abuse. Several variables, including amount and duration of ethanol exposure, nutritional status, and immunologic factors may determine the type of lesion a particular patient develops.[153,163,164]

The true incidence of the various histologic changes in chronic alcoholism is difficult, if not impossible, to determine. A large series of liver biopsies in a truly unselected group of alcoholics is not available. Using several series of biopsies in somewhat selected groups of alcoholics, a rough approximation may be reached[152,155,161] (Table 13-1).

Fatty change is the most common pathologic change on liver biopsy in alcoholics. The lipid, predominantly triglyceride, tends to accumulate first in the centrilobular area (Rappaport's zone 3). In severe cases the entire lobule is involved. The significance of the fatty liver is not clear. The prevalent opinion is that simple fatty liver is not a precirrhotic lesion and that significant fibrosis occurs only after the stage of alcoholic hepatitis is reached.[153]

An important although poorly understood lesion that occurs in alcohol-induced liver disease is progressive fibrosis of the central vein and pericentral parenchymal.* This begins as subtle thickening of the wall of the central vein (Fig. 13-8) and progresses to involve the adjacent parenchyma often in a spider-like pattern that isolates individual or some clusters of hepatocytes (Fig. 13-9). Whether these changes result as a complication of circulatory alterations in alcohol-induced liver disease or are responsible for such alterations is disputed, but it is likely that central fibrosis plays an important role in the evolution of cirrhosis in alcohol-induced liver disease.[154,177]

Alcoholic hepatitis shows both inflammation and hepatocellular degeneration; the changes are most evident in the centrilobular area.[156] They may be superimposed on a fatty, fibrotic, or cirrhotic liver. The inflammatory infiltrate is characteristically neutrophilic. An important feature is the presence of Mallory bodies in the cytoplasm of hepatocytes. These bodies appear as irregular refractile cytoplasmic structures that often have a beaded appearance and frequently assume a C-shaped configuration about the nucleus. The structures have been shown both by electron microscopy

---

*See references 154, 157, 160, 167, 168, 177, and 179.

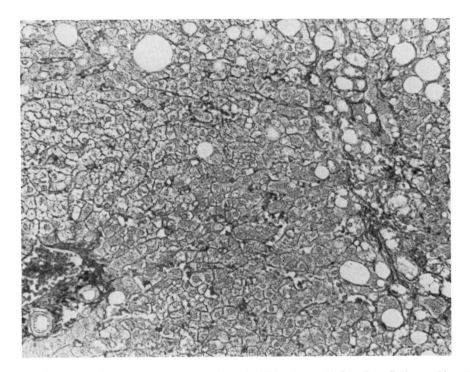

Fig. 13-8 Early sclerosis in region about central vein (right) is apparent in fatty liver. Patients with such a lesion are probably at greater risk of developing more serious alcoholic liver disease.

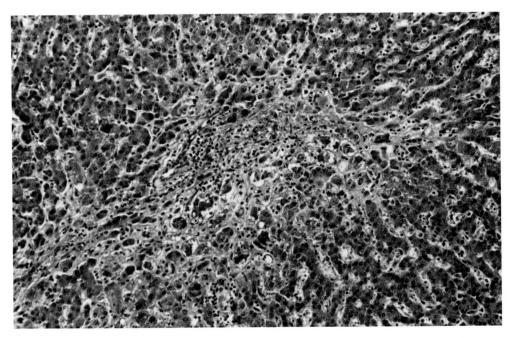

Fig. 13-9 More advanced example of central sclerosis in alcohol-induced liver disease. At this stage central vein is no longer readily apparent, making recognition of lobular architecture difficult on small biopsies.

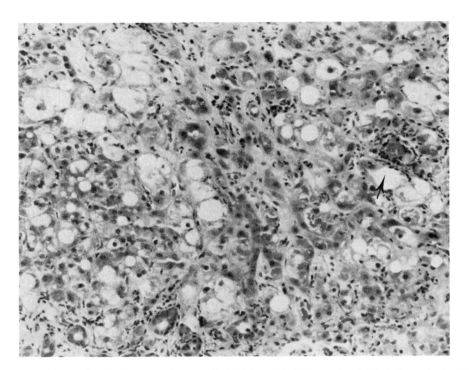

Fig. 13-10 Biopsy showing features of severe alcoholic hepatitis. Inflammatory infiltrate is predominantly neutrophilic. There is sclerosis of centrilobular area. Hepatocytes show fatty change; many contain alcoholic hyaline. Some hyaline-containing hepatocytes are surrounded by rim of neutrophils, the "unit lesion" of alcoholic hepatitis (arrow).

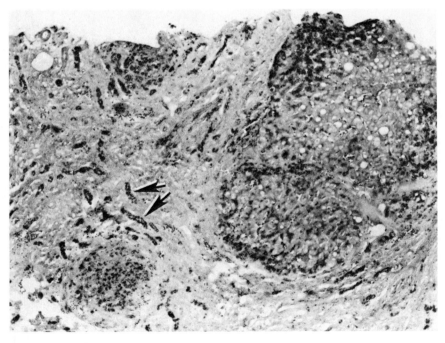

Fig. 13-11 Massive iron deposition is evident in biopsy from alcoholic with cirrhosis. Iron may be seen in parenchymal nodules, fibrous septa, and bile duct epithelium (arrows).

and immunohistochemistry to be aggregated keratin proteins.

This peculiar form of hepatocellular degeneration is characteristic, though not pathognomonic, of alcohol-induced liver disease. Mallory bodies can be seen in other conditions, including primary biliary cirrhosis, Wilson's disease, Indian childhood cirrhosis, nonalcoholic steatohepatitis, and extrahepatic biliary obstruction. Interestingly, some of these other conditions are associated with an excess of hepatic copper.[176] Seen in the proper clinical setting (history of alcohol abuse), a fatty liver with centrilobular sclerosis, neutrophilic infiltration, and Mallory bodies is strongly suggestive of alcoholic liver disease (Fig. 13-10). It must be remembered, however, that the exact histologic appearance is also seen in nonalcoholic steatohepatitis (see discussion following) and in some forms of drug-induced liver disease, notably amiodarone-associated hepatotoxicity.[171,175] At times, alcoholic hepatitis may present with striking cholestatic features, including an acute cholangitis on liver biopsy.[148,149,158,169] In such cases it can be exceedingly difficult to distinguish between *cholestatic alcoholic hepatitis* and mechanical obstruction in an alcoholic.

Alcoholics are not immune to other liver diseases. Levin et al.[165] found clinically unsuspected *nonalcoholic* liver disease in over 20% of liver biopsies performed on alcoholics. These diseases include viral hepatitis, drug (e.g., acetaminophen) hepatitis, chronic active hepatitis, and portal fibrosis secondary to chronic pancreatitis.[159,166] In addition, massive iron deposition can be seen in the liver of chronic alcoholics (Fig. 13-11). Iron may be seen in bile ducts in addition to hepatocytes and Kupffer's cells. It can be difficult or impossible to distinguish this from genetic hemochromatosis (see p. 696).

Mitochondrial abnormalities are frequent ultrastructural findings in alcoholic liver disease.[172] *Giant mitochondria* also can be seen light microscopically (Fig. 13-12). They are distinguishable from alcoholic Mallory bodies and are PAS-negative. Giant mitochondria have been observed in all types of alcohol-induced liver disease from fatty liver to cirrhosis.[151,178] Although not specific for alcohol, they are suggestive of that etiology and can serve as a diagnostic clue.

NONALCOHOLIC STEATOHEPATITIS

A condition that closely mimics alcoholic liver disease pathologically and clinically is nonalcoholic steatohepatitis. It has been recognized for many years that obesity and glucose intolerance contribute to fatty liver,[191,197] but the clinicopathologic disorder that Ludwig et al. named nonalcoholic steatohepatitis in 1980[192] has only been well characterized in the last few years.[181-186,188,189,195,196] The condition occurs in children as well as adults[190,193] and is similar histologically and probably pathogenetically to liver disease that complicates jejunoileal bypass.[187,195] However, the precise mechanisms of injury for these lesions remains unknown. The incidence of abnormal liver histology and function in large biopsy series in individuals with glucose intolerance or obesity has ranged from 60% to 90% with a 3:1 female predominance.[195] Prevalence in the general population is unknown. Histologic features are identical to al-

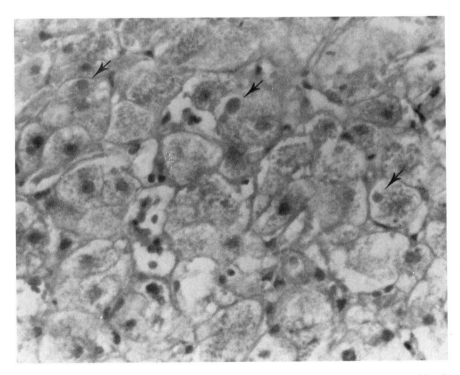

Fig. 13-12 Biopsy in which several giant mitochondria are evident. They resemble red blood cells; however, they are within cytoplasm of hepatocytes (arrows).

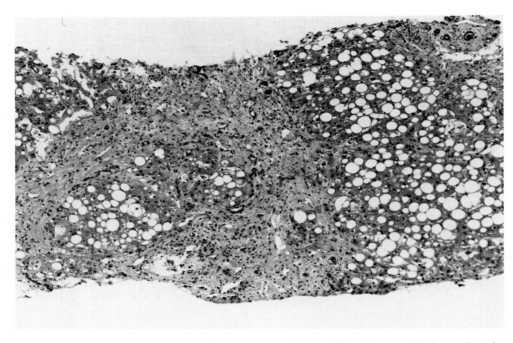

Fig. 13-13 Nonalcoholic steatohepatitis as demonstrated in liver biopsy from a diabetic, moderately obese 68-year-old woman. Changes of steatosis, Mallory bodies, and cirrhosis are identical to those that may be present in advanced alcohol-induced liver disease.

coholic liver disease, ranging from fatty liver to steatohepatitis with hepatocellular degeneration, Mallory bodies, and neutrophilic infiltration to central sclerosis to fibrosis and cirrhosis (Fig.13-13). Ultrastructural features are also identical to those found in alcohol-induced liver disease.[194] The recognition of this disease complex has rendered the designation alcoholic hepatitis solely as a histologic diagnosis inappropriate. Differentiation of alcoholic versus nonalcoholic forms of steatohepatitis is very difficult and cannot be accomplished by biopsy.

EXTRAHEPATIC BILIARY OBSTRUCTION

Needle biopsy is frequently used to distinguish between intrahepatic and extrahepatic causes of cholestasis. Primary hepatocellular diseases, including viral and alcoholic hepatitis, can present with predominantly cholestatic features. These can be difficult to distinguish from mechanical biliary obstruction. It is often helpful to separate the parenchymal from the portal changes in analyzing such biopsies.

The initial parenchymal change is centrolobular cholestasis. Bile stasis is evident both in hepatocytes and canaliculi. This stage of bland cholestasis is followed by a variety of parenchymal and portal alterations. In mechanical biliary obstruction, the parenchymal changes observed should be *attributable to* cholestasis. Hepatocellular alteration, predominantly ballooning or feathery degeneration, should be related to areas of cholestasis. In cholestatic variants of primary hepatocellular diseases (e.g., cholestatic viral hepatitis), one should be able to discern a hepatitis *independent of* cholestasis. Acidophilic bodies, few in number, can be

seen in extrahepatic obstruction.[198,199] More than an occasional acidophilic body, unrelated to areas of cholestasis, points against an obstructive disease.

The portal changes commonly seen in extrahepatic obstruction are ductular proliferation, periductal edema, and portal inflammation.[200,201] Periductal edema is most apparent about the larger interlobular ducts (Fig. 13-14). The ductular proliferation characteristically occurs along the margins of the portal triad[198] (Fig. 13-15). The inflammatory infiltrate is predominantly neutrophilic with some mononuclear cells. Neutrophils are often most evident at the periphery of a triad among the proliferating ductules.[198] These portal changes, though characteristic, are not specific for mechanical obstruction.[201a]

The presence of bile plugs in interlobular ducts and bile infarcts are strong evidence for obstruction. Unfortunately, these rather specific indicators are rarely present.[203] While fibrosis occurs with protracted obstruction, true cirrhosis is rare.[202,204]

PRIMARY BILIARY CIRRHOSIS (CHRONIC NONSUPPURATIVE DESTRUCTIVE CHOLANGITIS)

Primary biliary cirrhosis, once considered to be a rare disease, has undergone an apparent increase in incidence in the last several years.[218] In addition to a possible true increase in the occurrence of the disease, at least two other factors may contribute to this apparent increase: (1) increased clinical awareness of the disease and (2) frequent early diagnosis in an asymptomatic state. Study of asymp-

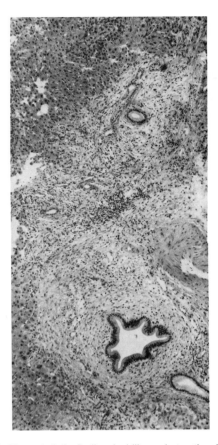

Fig. 13-14 Characteristic finding in biliary obstruction is pallor or edema of portal triads.

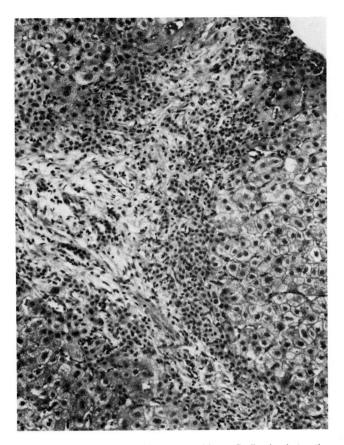

Fig. 13-15 Another reasonably common biopsy finding in obstruction is ductular (cholangiolar) proliferation at periphery of portal triads. Neutrophils are present between ductules.

tomatic patients with primary biliary cirrhosis has altered our understanding of the disorder in that a number of reports have concluded that these patients have a normal life expectancy compared with age-matched controls.[206,207,209,212,219] This is sharply in contrast to the prevalent earlier belief that, although insidious, this was always fatal disorder.

Antimitochrondrial antibodies are found in about 90% to 95% of patients but are also present in as many as one fifth of patients with severe chronic active hepatitis.[210,224] Subdivision of antimitochondrial antibodies into subtypes may aid in this distinction and may provide prognostic information for patients with primary biliary cirrhosis.[9a,226] There is also emerging evidence that determination of class II antigens of the major histocompatibility complex may provide information relative to the etiology and prognosis of primary biliary cirrhosis.[226] A number of recent reviews discuss these issues as well as the pathogenesis and therapy of primary biliary cirrhosis.[210,217,217a,218,223]

Several stages in the histologic evolution of the disease have been recognized.[213,220,222,224] Four stages are commonly proposed: (1) florid duct lesion, (2) ductular proliferation, (3) scarring, and (4) cirrhosis. The first, or so-called "florid duct" stage, is pathognomonic.[224] A lymphocytic and plasma-cellular infiltrate is *centered* about interlobular bile

ducts (Fig. 13-16). The ductal epithelium may show degeneration or necrosis. Granulomas, often poorly defined, are occasionally seen adjacent to involved ducts. Extension of the inflammatory infiltrate into the surrounding parenchyma is characteristically minimal. At times, however, the limiting plate is eroded.

With subsequent inflammation and destruction, there is a diminution in the number of ducts and a proliferation of ductules. To reliably assess whether the number of ducts is diminished, a wedge biopsy and a standardized method of counting may be necessary.[205] The histometric method described by Nakanuma and Ohta[216] can be used. Later in the disease, there is fibrosis and eventually cirrhosis. Biopsy in these later stages of the disease may be "suggestive" or "consistent with" the diagnosis but is rarely diagnostic. It is important to recognize that more than one histologic stage may be represented on a single biopsy and that many patients may not advance though these proposed histologic stages in an orderly fashion.[215,218]

The distinction between primary biliary cirrhosis and chronic active hepatitis is occasionally difficult to make.[208,211] Some cases of the former show piecemeal necrosis; conversely, in chronic active hepatitis one occasionally sees evidence of bile duct injury. Special stains for

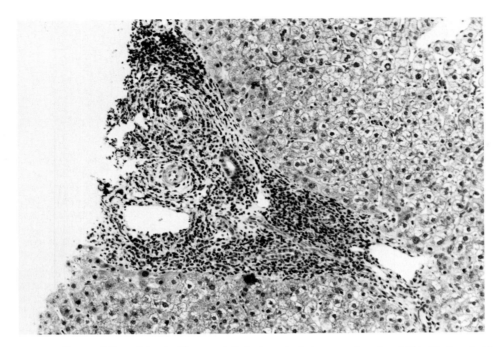

Fig. 13-16 Primary biliary cirrhosis. Characteristic features include expansion of portal triad by lymphoid aggregates and histocytes, degenerative changes of bile ductule epithelium, and infiltration of ductule in lower portion of field by lymphocytes.

copper can help in these difficult cases.[221,225] Copper is normally excreted in the bile. In chronic cholestatic conditions, such as chronic nonsuppurative destructive cholangitis, there is marked accumulation of copper in the liver. The copper is bound to a carrier protein.[227] Excess copper can be demonstrated by either the rhodanine method (a histochemical stain for copper) or Shikata's orcein stain (which reacts with the copper-protein complex).[213,214] In the difficult case, the presence of excess coppper is a point in favor of primary biliary cirrhosis.

At least two studies have demonstrated that the presence of granulomas on liver biopsy is a favorable prognostic feature for both symptomatic and asymptomatic cases of primary biliary cirrhosis.[206,215] In contrast, associated autoimmune disorders noted clinically or serologically carry an unfavorable implication.[206] Liver transplantation is now a means of therapy for end-stage patients with primary biliary cirrhosis. This is the most frequent or one of the most frequent indications for transplantation in several medical centers.[206a,398,400]

NONSPECIFIC REACTIVE HEPATITIS

As the name indicates, nonspecific reactive hepatitis is a nonspecific hepatic reaction to a variety of infectious and toxic agents.[228] Microscopically, the main change is a mild intralobular and/or portal inflammation, sometimes accompanied by mild proliferation of bile ducts and Kupffer's cells and very rare necrotic hepatocytes. Usually not all portal tracts are involved by inflammation.[4a] A subsiding viral hepatitis may exhibit a microscopic appearance indis-

tinguishable from that of nonspecific reactive hepatitis. Nonspecific reactive hepatitis is often the histologic picture documented by liver biopsy in an AIDS patient.[4a] Liaw and colleagues studied sixty-two Taiwanese patients with histologic features of nonspecific reactive hepatitis and found that in this population (endemic for hepatitis B virus infection), most patients were HB_sA_g positive and many evolved either to chronic lobular hepatitis (43%) or to chronic active hepatitis (7%).[229] They suggest that nonspecific reactive hepatitis may be a variant of chronic lobular hepatitis at least in the spectrum of HVB infection.

GRANULOMATOUS HEPATITIS

Granulomas are present in 3% to 10% of liver biopsies performed in general hospitals.[235] Lists of the possible etiologies can be quite lengthy.[230,233-236] Causes include systemic granulomatous disorders, numerous infectious agents, intrinsic hepatic diseases, a variety of drugs, and neoplasms. The granulomas are found predominantly in the portal areas in most of the diseases. It is unusual to be able to arrive at a specific etiologic diagnosis solely on histologic grounds. In 10% to 37% of the patients, the etiology of the granulomas remains obscure despite thorough investigation.[234,235,237] Also, the presence of granulomas in a liver biopsy does not necessarily imply an underlying systemic granulomatous disease.[237]

The commonest causes of a granulomatous hepatitis are sarcoidosis, intrinsic liver disease (especially primary biliary cirrhosis), and tuberculosis.[237-241] In endemic areas, histoplasmosis may account for a significant percentage of cases.[240] Acid-fast bacilli are demonstrable in only about 10% of cases of hepatic granulomas thought to be tuberculous in nature.[237]

Hepatic granulomas are demonstrable on biopsy in 60% to 90% of the patients with sarcoidosis.[235] The majority of these patients have no evidence of liver disease. However, in a small percentage of patients, portal hypertension and evidence of hepatocellular dysfunction can dominate the clinical picture.[239] Another rare manifestation is a cholestatic liver disease that is something of a hybrid between sarcoidosis and primary biliary cirrhosis.[242]

A distinction should be made between epithelioid granulomas and lipogranulomas. The latter are frequently found in liver biopsies if carefully sought after and may form in response to both endogenous and dietary lipid.[231,232] Their importance lies chiefly in their distinction from epithelioid granulomas and generally they require no additional evaluation.

NEONATAL HEPATITIS AND BILIARY ATRESIA

There are numerous causes of hyperbilirubinemia in early life. Some are self-limited disorders; others are life threatening. Some require prompt surgical intervention; others are made worse by the surgical and anesthetic insult. Separating these disorders in a timely fashion is both crucial and difficult.[244]

An initial laboratory distinction is made between unconjugated and conjugated hyperbilirubinemia. The commonest cause of unconjugated hyperbilirubinemia is, of course, "physiologic" jaundice. Breast milk jaundice also occurs with some frequency, affecting about 1% of breast-fed infants. Obstruction of the proximal small intestine also can cause unconjugated hyperbilirubinemia. A rare cause is hereditary glucuronide transferase deficiency; both autosomal dominant and recessive (Crigler-Najjar) forms exist.[250]

The list of causes of conjugated hyperbilirubinemia in infancy is lengthy.[246,250,255] Some causes are primarily hepatocellular (the neonatal hepatitis syndrome); others are secondary to mechanical obstruction. Liver biopsy can play an important role in making this distinction.

Neonatal hepatitis is a broad clinical *syndrome*. Typically, jaundice is first noted between 1 week and 2 months of age. In the majority of cases a particular etiology is not discovered. Over the years, however, several specific infectious and metabolic diseases have been split off from the large inhomogeneous neonatal hepatitis syndrome. The list of recognized infections includes bacterial sepsis, *Listeria monocytogenes*, toxoplasmosis, hepatitis B, cytomegalovirus, and herpes simplex. Metabolic causes include alpha₁-antitrypsin deficiency, galactosemia, cystic fibrosis, hereditary tyrosinemia, hereditary fructose intolerance, and parenteral hyperalimentation.[250,255]

The large prospective series of Danks et al.[247] included 105 infants who fit into the broad neonatal hepatitis syndrome. Of these, 20% had identifiable infectious causes, 5% had galactosemia, and about 7% had alpha₁-antitrypsin deficiency. In an additional 10%, the disease appeared familial. The remainder had "idiopathic" neonatal hepatitis.

The long-term prognosis for infants who fit into the neonatal hepatitis syndrome is related to the etiology but in general is not good. Death in the first few months or evolution to cirrhosis has occurred in over 30% of patients in some series.[248] Subjecting the infants to surgery, in order to rule out extrahepatic biliary atresia, can further increase morbidity and mortality. This is particularly true if surgery is performed prior to 4 months of age.[254]

Mechanical biliary obstruction in the neonatal period may be caused by extrahepatic biliary atresia, the bile plug syndrome, and choledochal cyst.[246] The large majority of these cases are secondary to extrahepatic biliary atresia. This is defined as a partial or total absence of permeable bile ducts between porta hepatis and the duodenum.[243] The intrahepatic component of this disease evolves through progressive histologic changes manifested by biliary ductular proliferation in the earlier stages followed by fibrosis with regression and ultimate disappearance of bile ductules.[245,251,256] Landing et al. studied the time course of these intrahepatic changes and observed that there is an early phase of rapid bile ductular proliferation that peaks at 205 days followed by rapid duct regression at approximately 400 days with slower duct loss thereafter.[252] Biopsy of the extrahepatic biliary tree usually shows evolving inflammation and bile duct injury (Fig. 13-17).

Kasai[251] has shown that hepatic porto-enterostomy performed early in life, preferably before 10 weeks of age, can restore bile flow in an appreciable number of these infants. On the contrary, surgery after 4 months of age is rarely, if ever, successful. Pathologic examination of the resected porta hepatis yields important prognostic information. If one or more bile ducts are found that measure more than 200 μm in diameter, there is a reasonable chance of success (ten of twenty-two patients cured). Of seventeen patients who had bile ducts with a maximum diameter less than 200 μm, only one was cured.[251]

The therapeutic goal is prompt surgical intervention in biliary atresia, while not subjecting infants with the neonatal hepatitis syndrome to harmful, unnecessary surgery. Liver biopsy is an important and accurate diagnostic tool in making that distinction. In Brough and Bernstein's series of 158 patients, biopsy yielded the correct diagnosis in 94%.[246]

The degree of hepatocellular giant cell transformation and the character of the inflammatory infiltrate are of little importance in distinguishing between the neonatal hepatitis syndrome and biliary atresia. A very important diagnostic finding is bile duct proliferation. In extrahepatic biliary atresia, all or almost all of the portal areas show duct and ductular proliferation. Using *diffuse bile duct proliferation* as their single most important diagnostic criterion, Brough and Bernstein[246] were able to achieve their impressive accuracy rates.

The most common diagnostic error (seven cases in Brough and Bernstein's series of 158) was interpreting neonatal hepatitis as biliary atresia. A small proportion of cases of neonatal hepatitis will, unfortunately, have diffuse bile duct proliferation histologically indistinguishable from biliary atresia. Another source of error (two cases) was interpreting alpha₁-antitrypsin deficiency as obstruction.[246]

In addition to distinguishing between biliary atresia and neonatal hepatitis, biopsy can, at times, help split specific entities off the latter syndrome. In some cases, a particular

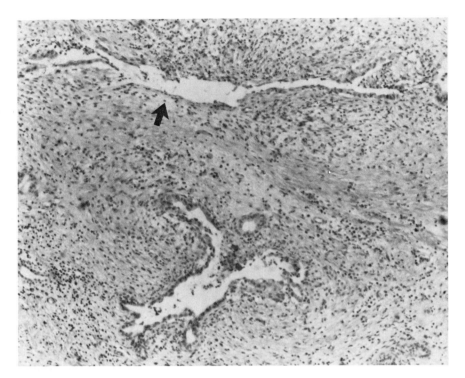

Fig. 13-17 Specimen from resected porta hepatitis of infant with extrahepatic biliary "atresia" showing evolving character of lesion. There are ongoing inflammation and sloughing of ductal epithelium (arrow).

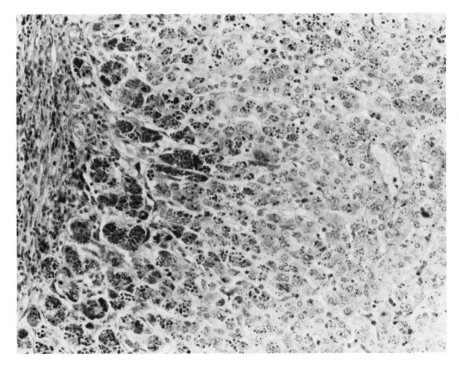

Fig. 13-18 Diastase-resistant, PAS-positive globules of alpha-1-antitrypsin deficiency show definite zonal distribution. In noncirrhotic liver, they are most evident in periportal resion (Rappaport's zone 1), while in the cirrhotic liver illustrated here, they are most abundant at periphery of parenchymal nodules. (PAS with diastase.)

infectious etiology might be apparent. Alpha-1-antitrypsin deficiency can be diagnosed if looked for. In an inflamed liver it is extremely difficult to see the periportal cytoplasmic globules characteristic of alpha-1-antitrypsin deficiency on sections stained with hematoxylin-eosin, a point in favor of routinely doing PAS-diastase stains on liver biopsies in this setting (Fig. 13-18). A paucity of inflammatory cell infiltrate in a case of neonatal hepatitis might point toward a metabolic etiology.[246] In addition, marked fatty change is not a usual feature of "idiopathic" neonatal hepatitis but is regularly seen with certain metabolic disorders, such as galactosemia and hereditary fructose intolerance.[255]

A current problem once the diagnosis of extrahepatic biliary atresia is established is deciding the best mode of therapy. Only 10% to 15% of individuals undergoing the Kasai procedure (hepatic porto-enterostomy) are long-term cures.[253] Liver transplantation is becoming an attractive alternative but the shortage of organs does not allow this for many patients.[253] Liver histology has proved useful to predict those patients who will do well after the Kasai operation. Increase in inflammation and fibrosis identify patients who will have short-term functional failure following surgery.[249] These patients may most benefit from consideration of transplantation.

TOTAL PARENTERAL NUTRITION–ASSOCIATED LIVER DISEASE

Total parenteral nutrition (TPN) has evolved into a major method of nutritional therapeutic support for a number of disorders including prematurity, malabsorption, surgical loss of bowel, severe inflammatory bowel disease, and various forms of congenital gastrointestinal disorders such as gastroschisis and intestinal atresia.[264] Unfortunately, hepatic complications of TPN are common at least in neonates and in certain adult groups such as those suffering major loss of bowel.[257,260,262,265-267] The pathogenesis of hepatic injury associated with TPN is incompletely understood but seems to include: (1) prematurity with functional immaturity of bile secretory mechanism, (2) toxic effect of infused amino acids, (3) increased hepatic lipoprotein synthesis and decreased secretion, (4) effects of fasting with a lack of luminal secretion of gut hormones involved in biliary secretion and intestinal motility, and (5) associated sepsis.[257,259,262] Hepatic histology evolves through a complex sequence of events that progresses through seatosis, cholestasis, fibrosis, and cirrhosis.[259-263] In infants laboratory evidence of hepatic dysfunction provided by elevated alkaline phosphatase, increased bilirubin, and increased transaminases may be seen within 5 days after initiating TPN. Steatosis followed by canalicular cholestasis may be present within 2 weeks.[260] Moderate to severe portal fibrosis may be present after 90 days.[260]

Ninety percent of infants will have histologic abnormalities after 4 months of TPN.[258,262] Liver histology may be variable and changes include steatosis, cholestasis, nonspecific triaditis, and lipofuscin bearing macrophages in early biopsies evolving to portal fibrosis, dramatic portal ductular proliferation, and micronodular cirrhosis in later biopsies

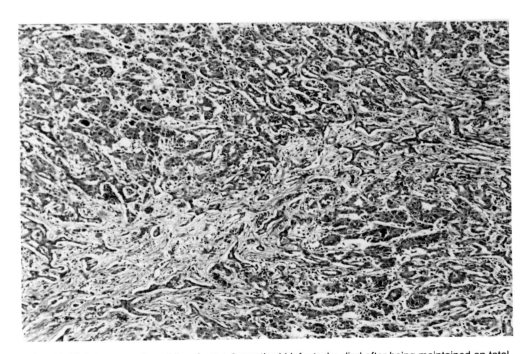

Fig. 13-19 Autopsy section of liver from a 3-month-old infant who died after being maintained on total parenteral nutrition from birth. Marked portal fibrosis and bile ductule proliferation are evident. Extreme lobular disarray and cholestasis are also present.

(Fig. 13-19).[257,259-262,266] The earlier histologic abnormalities are usually reversible after termination of TPN but mild cholestasis may persist for several months.[261]

LIVER DISEASE DURING PREGNANCY

Liver disease during pregnancy is uncommon but may present unusual difficulties in terms of diagnosis, monitoring, and therapy.[286] This is partly because some routine liver function tests may fall outside of the usual normal range as a consequence of the altered physiology of a normal pregnancy.[286] Mild increases in total and direct bilirubin may be observed in 20% of pregnant women. In spite of this, histologic changes are generally absent by light microscopy although minor subcellular changes, especially involving bile canaliculi, have been observed.[271] Disorders that affect the liver during pregnancy may be divided into three groups: (1) liver disease unique to pregnancy, (2) intercurrent liver disease occurring during pregnancy but etiologically unrelated to it, and (3) pre-existing liver disease.[280,286] As a general rule pre-existing and intercurrent liver disease is not significantly affected by gestation, with exceptions such as cirrhosis with portal hypertension, chronic active hepatitis, and the Dubin-Johnson syndrome.[280] Diseases that are unique to pregnancy include acute fatty liver of pregnancy, liver disease in toxemia of pregnancy, intrahepatic cholestasis of pregnancy, and liver disease in hyperemesis gravidarum.

Acute fatty liver of pregnancy is a disease of the third trimester usually occurring from the 30th to the 40th week of gestation and usually affecting primiparas.[272,275,277,279,280]

The apparent increase in prevalence of this uncommon disorder to one case per 13,328 in 1980[275] is probably because of greater awareness and recognition of the disease.[272] The cause of acute fatty liver of pregnancy is unknown although there is no evidence to support infectious or inherited metabolic disorders.[272] Grossly the affected liver is pale, yellow, and small, reflecting fat content and parenchymal loss. The most typical microscopic finding is microvesicular steatosis, which may be pan-acinar or zonal, affecting zones 2 and 3 or zone 3 alone (Fig. 13-20).[279,280] Marked ballooning of hepatocytes and macrovesicular fat is also encountered in acute fatty liver of pregnancy, creating a spectrum of histologic changes that may also include intrahepatic cholestasis, acute cholangiolitis, and liver cell necrosis. This array of histologic changes may complicate recognition of acute fatty liver of pregnancy and its differentiation from other disease processes. When acute fatty liver is in the differential diagnosis, a small piece of a biopsy should be frozen for fat staining by oil red 0.[269,272,280] The prognosis of this serious complication of pregnancy has improved considerably in recent years, with fetal and maternal mortality rates now as low as 23% and 18%.[281] In severe cases immediate delivery is indicated.[269,270,272]

Liver disease in toxemia of pregnancy (preeclampsia/eclampsia), like acute fatty liver, also occurs in the third trimester, usually affecting primigravida, and the two diseases exhibit considerable clinical overlap.[276] Hepatic involvement in preeclampsia/eclampsia is not primary, but secondary damage at least in mild forms is probably common.[276] Mildly affected patients may be mistaken as suf-

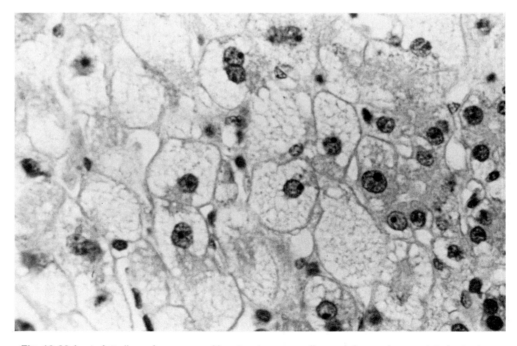

Fig. 13-20 Acute fatty liver of pregnancy. Hepatocytes are swollen and show pale vacuolated cytoplasm characteristic of microvesicular steatosis. This should be confirmed and differentiated from other forms of cell injury by fat stain. (Courtesy Dr. G. Klatskin.)

fering from acute viral hepatitis or other abdominal complications.[280] Macroscopic changes in severe cases include diffuse fine or confluent hemorrhage that may be parenchymal or capsular. Areas of infarction are frequent and may be massive.[281] Microscopically, changes are most typically found in the preportal regions and include hemorrhage, fibrin deposition, and hepatocellular necrosis. These changes are usually present at autopsy but may be seen in only about one fourth of needle biopsies from women with eclampsia, probably caused by sample artifact.[281] Periportal fibrin deposition may extend into the lobules to occlude sinusoids, and thrombi may also occur in portal tract capillaries. Less frequent changes include bile inspissation in canaliculi and ductules, macrovesicular or microvesicular steatosis, and a portal lymphoplasmacytic infiltrate.[281] Eclampsia and its complications continue to be a leading cause of maternal death; this is in large part secondary to a frequent delay in diagnosis with consequent lack of initiation of therapy.[268]

Intrahepatic cholestasis of pregnancy is second only to viral hepatitis as a cause of jaundice during pregnancy. It may occur at any time during gestation but is most frequent during late pregnancy. This disorder is presumably induced by the effects of pregnancy-associated steroids on the liver.[285] Patients usually experience pruritus, which persists with jaundice until delivery. Biopsy is usually not performed for this benign disorder, but when obtained it characteristically shows bland cholestasis predominantly within canaliculi in zone 3. Greater risk for the fetus exists in this disorder than for the mother; fetal distress, premature delivery, and fetal death have been observed.[273,284] Transplacental passage of maternal bile salts may partially underlie the observed four-fold increase in fetal perinatal mortality.[274]

Viral hepatitis occurring during pregnancy is the leading cause of gestational jaundice, a fact that must be tempered by the observation that it is also the most common cause of jaundice in nonpregnant women of childbearing age.[282] Although the clinical presentation, complications, and course of gestational viral hepatitis are similar to nongestational cases, it is important to recognize and accurately diagnose the disease during pregnancy to prevent risk to the fetus. Maternal infection with hepatitis B virus represents a risk to the fetus that is three-fold: (1) acute infection, (2) chronic carrier state, and (3) increased likelihood of hepatocellular carcinoma.[282,283] Fetal infection may result from transplacental transmission of the virus or from exposure to infectious maternal blood at delivery. Immunoprophylaxis of the newborn with hyperimmune serum and HBV vaccine will dramatically lessen risk of infection.[282]

ALPHA-1-ANTITRYPSIN DEFICIENCY AND CYSTIC FIBROSIS

Hereditary deficiency of alpha-1-antitrypsin (AAT) may present as liver disease, lung disease, or a combination of both.[291] ATT is the major alpha-I globulin of human plasma and is synthesized by the liver. It serves to inhibit several proteolytic enzymes, including trypsin. More than thirty variants of AAT have been identified by immunoelectrophoresis and each has been assigned a Pi (protease inhibitor) phenotypic designation. The normal phenotype of the Pi system is M. The most common deficiency state that exists

occurs when individuals have a Z allele instead of an M, and individuals homogeneous for the Z allele (Pi-ZZ) have AAT levels 10% to 15% of normal. Risk of liver disease in AAT deficiency has been best defined by Svenger in his prospective study of 200,000 newborn infants.[306] Of 120 Pi-ZZ infants encountered (incidence is 1 in 2,000 to 4,000 live births), 66% developed evidence of liver disease ranging from cholestasis to advanced cirrhosis, liver failure, and death. By age 4, 2.5% of these infants had died.

Although AAT deficiency is predominantly a cause of liver disease in children and young adults, it also can be a cause of cirrhosis and liver failure presenting later in adulthood.[296,303,307] An increased risk for hepatocellular carcinoma has been documented in patients with AAT deficiency, although this risk may be significant only in males.[292] The diagnosis of AAT deficiency is best accomplished by determination of the AAT phenotype by immunodiffusion of electrophoresis.[298] Diagnosis may also be accomplished prenatally.[288,289] Liver biopsy is confirmatory for the diagnosis of AAT deficiency and determines the extent of histologic damage.

The most characteristic histologic feature of AAT deficiency is the presence of diastase resistant, PAS-positive cytoplasmic globules (see Fig. 13-18). A wide range of changes may be seen, however, including hepatocellular degeneration, giant cell formation, cholestasis, portal fibrosis, cholangitis, and cirrhosis.[293a,296] This range of histological alterations and the lack of specificity for cytoplasmic globules makes further evaluation by phenotypic determination mandatory in suspected cases.[297] Immunohistochemistry may be performed to confirm the presence of AAT globules within the cytoplasm of hepatocytes but the significance of this is lessened by the finding of such globules in several forms of liver disease, including hepatic congestion.[296a,308]

Cystic fibrosis is one of the most common and most lethal hereditary diseases among whites.[290] The observation that it is rare among blacks and almost unreported in Orientals supports the hypothesis that this poorly understood disease complex has at least a partial genetic basis. The liver is usually unaffected at birth but becomes involved to some extent as the individual grows older.[299,301] Earlier autopsy studies upon the liver in patients dying from cystic fibrosis concentrated upon bile plugs within dilated ductules together with the accompanying inflammatory and proliferative changes, but it is evident that earlier, more subtle histologic alterations are common.[294,295,302]

The incidence of liver disease in cystic fibrosis varies with age and method of detection.[302] The range extends from 2.2% of patients who have clinical evidence of liver disease[305] to 40% who have abnormal liver scans[293] to one half of patients with abnormal liver function studies[287] or abnormalities documented at autopsy[300] to 100% of a small number of biopsies that were carefully studied by light and electron microscopy.[294]

Steatosis is the most common hepatic lesion in cystic fibrosis. This is usually macrovesicular and without a zonal pattern. The lesion that has been considered pathognomonic is termed focal biliary cirrhosis and is characterized by inspissated granular eosinophilic material within portal bile

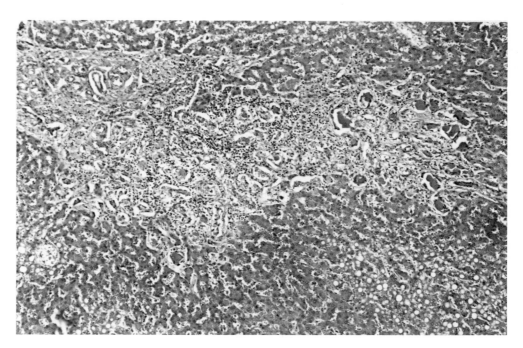

Fig. 13-21 Focal biliary cirhosis in liver of 7-year-old boy who died of pulmonary complications of cystic fibrosis. Changes of fibrosis, chronic inflammation, and bile duct proliferation were scattered randomly throughout the liver, which otherwise showed normal lobular architecture. Note presence of inssipated bile-like material in ductules in right side of field.

ductules, a chronic portal infiltrate, bile duct proliferation, and focal distribution within the liver[300] (Fig. 13-21). In a limited number of patients, reaching about 10% after age 25, cirrhosis may develop as a complication of cystic fibrosis.[302,304] Ultrastructural studies early in the disease process have documented an increase in the number of Ito cells and accompanying portal and periportal collagen deposition before these changes become evident by light microscopy.[294]

Therapy for both AAT deficiency and hepatic complications of cystic fibrosis has largely been ineffective and experimental. A selected group of patients with these disorders have undergone liver transplantation which, in the case of AAT deficiency, is theoretically curative.

REYE'S SYNDROME

In 1963 Reye and colleagues described the clinical and pathologic features of a usually lethal disease characterized by encephalopathy and fatty degeneration of the liver and other viscera.[317] Since that time Reye's syndrome has been well characterized both clinically and pathologically and earlier, usually nonlethal, stages of the disorder have been defined.[311] In spite of this, the etiology and pathogenesis remain poorly understood.[311] In recent years the incidence of Reye's syndrome in children has leveled off and even fallen, but the incidence in adults has risen.[309,313] The decline in children and consequent overall decline in incidence may be in part because of the recognition of the potentiating effect of aspirin in precipitating the disease when used to treat viral illnesses of children. Awareness of this has led

to a subsequent decline in use of salicylates for pediatric patients.[311] The characteristic hepatic lesion in Reye's syndrome is diffuse panlobular microvesicular steatosis, which may appear only as cytoplasmic pallor (Fig. 13-22, *A*). A fat stain may be a vital aid in recognizing this lesion (Fig. 13-22, *B*).[310] Inflammation is typically absent. As the hepatic lesion evolves, however, it can become more complex and may exhibit zonal or massive coagulative necrosis and accompanying inflammation, creating a differential diagnosis with infectious forms of hepatitis.[310,312] Ultrastructural features are characteristic, showing enlarged pleomorphic mitochondria with expanded matrix and fewer mitochondrial dense bodies.[310,315,316] Familiarity with these lesions and ensuring that cryostat sections for fat section and tissue for electron microscopy are taken is essential when the diagnosis of Reye's syndrome is considered. Recognition of early forms of Reye's syndrome and careful supportive therapy has greatly improved the clinical outcome for affected patients.[311,314]

HEMOCHROMATOSIS AND WILSON'S DISEASE

Genetic disorders of iron and copper metabolism have been considered to be rare causes of hepatic disease. However, hemochromatosis in particular may be more common than previously believed. The frequency of the hemochromatosis gene in North America and Western Europe is about 0.05.[323,328,341] This implies a heterozygote frequency of about 1 in 10 and a homozygote frequency of 2 to 3 persons per

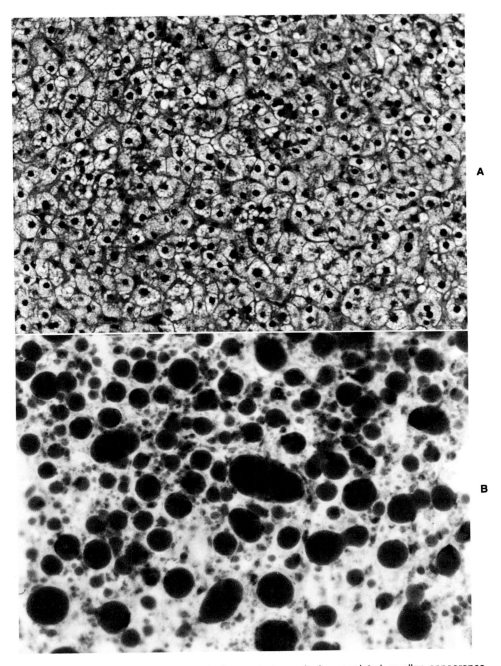

Fig. 13-22 Reye's syndrome. **A,** Microvesicular steatosis results in vacuolated, swollen appearance of hepatocytes with loss of definition of liver plates. **B,** Oil red O stains on cryostat section reveals striking degree of fat within liver.

1,000. A city of one million would contain 2,000 to 3,000 persons at high risk for hemochromatosis, almost epidemic levels.[331]

Early diagnosis of abnormalities of iron and copper metabolism is essential. Serious complications can be avoided by appropriate therapy, and a recent study has demonstrated that precirrhotic hemochromatosis individuals can have a normal life expectancy when treated by venesection.[340] In contrast, cirrhotic individuals have shortened life expectancy and increased risk of hepatocellular carcinoma. Screening for hemochromatosis can be accomplished by determining serum ferritin, transferritin saturation, serum iron concentration, and total iron-binding capacity. The best combination of these tests for screening continues to be debated. The discovery of a patient with idiopathic hemochromatosis mandates the screening of relatives. As mentioned, a number of screening schema have recently been advocated.* HLA-typing can also be of value, since hemochromatosis is associated with HLA-A3 and HLA-B14.[331,338,351] In a newly encountered patient with iron overload demonstrated on liver biopsy, the most sensitive way to differentiate primary hemachromatosis from secondary siderosis is by quantitative analysis of iron on desiccated liver tissue. Individuals with the former condition have much higher concentrations within the liver tissue.†

Familial (idiopathic) hemochromatosis is a genetic dis-

order characterized by excessive iron absorption.[345] In early cases, discovered incidentally or by screening affected families, the biopsy may show substantial iron deposition in the absence of fibrosis or other evidence of hepatocellular injury (Fig. 13-23). Rowe et al.[349] found no relationship between the degree of iron deposition and fibrosis. The iron is deposited more heavily in the periportal area. This zonal feature is of limited differential diagnostic value, because other causes of iron overload (e.g., multiple transfusions) also are characterized by predominantly periportal deposition. It will, however, tend to differentiate iron deposition secondary to circulatory disturbances, which has a predominantly centrilobular distribution.[337] Predominantly hepatocellular iron deposition favors familial hemochromatosis, whereas predominantly reticuloendothelial siderosis or mixed (roughly equal) parenchymal and reticuloendothelial siderosis favor iron deposition secondary to other disorders.[337] Except for the presence of excessive iron, the hepatocytes in familial hemochromatosis typically are fairly normal in appearance. Other alterations, such as ballooning degeneration or piecemeal necrosis, tend to favor another diagnosis.[345]

Another form of hemochromatosis that does not appear to be familial is neonatal hemochromatosis.[317a,322a,350a] This rare condition affects infants who are often born prematurely and usually die in the neonatal period with excessive iron deposition in the liver and multiple other organs. The relationship of this disorder and adult hemochromatosis is currently unclear.[317a]

---

*See references 320, 321, 331, 335, 340, and 357.
†See references 319, 320, 327, 330, 332, and 344.

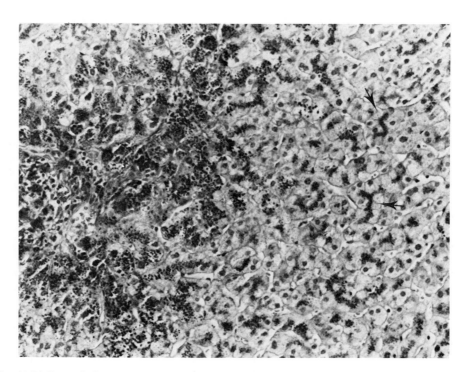

Fig. 13-23 Case of idiopathic hemochromatosis that was discovered incidentally. Biopsy shows heavy parenchymal iron deposition that is most marked in periportal area. In less involved central area, pericanalicular distribution of iron is better appreciated (arrows.) Hepatocytes appear unremarkable except for excess iron. Trichrome stain showed no increase in connective tissue.

As the disease progresses, fibrosis and eventually cirrhosis are seen. It would be helpful if liver biopsy could distinguish between advanced cases of familial hemochromatosis and secondary causes of iron overload (e.g., alcoholic cirrhosis with excess iron). Unfortunately, this is often impossible. There are, however, some features that may be of value in making such a distinction.

Powell and Kerr[345] observed a somewhat distinctive form of fibrosis in patients with familial hemochromatosis. The lesion was somewhat inhomogeneous: nodular cirrhotic areas *alternated* with areas of partially preserved parenchyma having normal central veins. The finding of normal central veins can be of value in distinguishing this from alcoholic liver disease in which one would typically observe fibrosis around the central veins. Needless to say, such differential architectural features are better appreciated in wedge biopsies than in Menghini needle specimens. In addition, the distinction between familial hemochromatosis and alcoholic liver disease with secondary iron overload is blurred by the fact that 30% of patients with familial hemochromatosis drink excessive amounts of alcohol.[342,343]

The risk of developing hepatocellular carcinomas as a complication of hemochromatosis is disputed, but there does appear to be an increased risk. Bradbear et al. followed 208 patients with genetic hemochromatosis from the time of diagnosis and observed sixteen new cases of hepatocellular carcinoma, representing a 200-fold increase in expected cases.[324] Individuals with liver disease from hemochromatosis appear to be at increased risk for HBV, and this may play a role in the observed incidence of liver cancer.[326]

Wilson's disease is a genetic defect in copper metabolism that is inherited as an autosomal recessive trait.[329] Characteristically, the patients present in late childhood or early adult life. The most common mode of presentation is as a neuropsychiatric disorder. Hepatic disease is second in frequency. Rarely, hemolytic anemia or bone disease may be the presenting feature.[325]

The hepatic manifestations of Wilson's disease are quite variable. The disorder may present as acute hepatitis, chronic active hepatitis, fulminant hepatic failure, or cirrhosis.* Typically, there is a picture of chronic active hepatitis with fibrosis or the patients already have cirrhosis. In addition to the features of chronic active hepatitis, the biopsy will often show fatty change and nuclear vacuolation.[350] Mallory bodies are frequently present.[356]

A small proportion (2% to 5%) of patients presenting with apparent chronic active hepatitis will, when properly studied, be shown to have Wilson's disease.[325,354] Screening procedures for Wilson's disease have been recommended in adults under 30 years of age with idopathic chronic hepatitis or cryptogenic cirrhosis.[325,354] Hepatic disease as the initial symptom has been observed in a patient 55 years of age.[333]

The screening procedures used are (1) slit-lamp examination for Kayser-Fleischer rings, (2) determination of serum ceruloplasmin (<20 mg/dl in 85% to 95% of patients with Wilson's disease); (3) measurement of urinary copper excretion (typically well in excess of the 30 to 50 µg/24

*See references 318, 322, 339, 346, 347, 350, and 354.

hr seen in normal subjects.).[334,347] Liver biopsy with hepatic copper determination (>250 µg/g dry weight in untreated Wilson's disease) is occasionally necessary. In screening families, hypoceruloplasminemia is found in 10% of heterozygotes. Biopsy with chemical copper determination is at times the only way to distinguish these healthy individuals from presymptomatic homozygotes. Heterozygotes will have copper concentration of <250 µg/g dry weight.[325]

Histochemical stains for copper should in no way be considered an adequate screening test for Wilson's disease. Rubeanic acid stain is used in many laboratories. This was positive in only three of the seventeen patients reported by Scott et al.[350] The rhodanine method is probably a better histochemical stain for copper. Shikata's orcein stain also can be used. Fetal liver serves as an adequate positive control.[336]

There are, on occasion, difficulties in making the diagnosis of Wilson's disease. Kayser-Fleischer rings can rarely be encountered in patients without the disorder.[334] Patients with chronic cholestasis (particularly primary biliary cirrhosis) may have increased hepatic copper concentration (>250 µg/g dry weight) and increased urinary copper excretion.[348] Hypoceruloplasminemia may occasionally be seen in patients with fulminant hepatic failure of any cause.[355] Nevertheless, the most common difficulty in establishing the diagnosis is failure to consider the entity. Liver transplantation has been used as a successful form of therapy for selected patients with Wilson's disease.[352,353]

FIBROPOLYCYSTIC LIVER DISEASES

The family of fibropolycystic diseases shows a variety of clinical and pathologic appearances. Hepatic lesions are frequently accompanied by renal lesions, and disease of either organ may dominate the clinical picture. The mode of inheritance in adult polycystic disease is an autosomal dominant one, while that of congenital hepatic fibrosis is autosomal recessive.[359]

Polycystic liver disease is characterized by multiple variably sized hepatic cysts. These range in size from a few millimeters to over 10 cm. The cysts do not communicate with the biliary tree. In Melnick's autopsy survey of seventy cases, the cysts were lined by cuboidal epithelium in 90%.[367] The remaining cases either had a flat epithelial lining or no epithelial lining. In 40% the liver also contained von Meyenburg's complexes. It is unusual for polycystic liver disease to become symptomatic. Often it is an incidental finding in patients who are symptomatic because of their accompanying adult polycystic renal disease. An occasional patient may become jaundiced secondary to compression of the biliary tree by a large cyst.[363] Rarely, massive hepatomegaly may occur presumably due to enlargement of cysts that arise from von Meyenberg complexes.[364a]

Congenital hepatic fibrosis was the term coined by Kerr et al.[364] to describe a fibrotic disease distinct from cirrhosis. It is characterized by fibrous septa that partially or completely surround islands of essentially normal parenchyma (Fig. 13-24). These septa contain numerous bile ducts. The configuration of the ducts may have a hamartomatous appearance. The diagnosis can sometimes be suggested by a biopsy showing ductal cholestasis in the absence of paren-

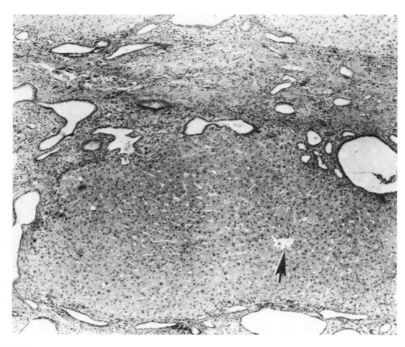

Fig. 13-24 Features of this case are admixture of congenital hepatic fibrosis and Caroli's disease. Biopsy shows typical appearance of congenital hepatic fibrosis. Fibrous septa containing numerous oddly shaped bile ducts surround normal parenchymal lobules. Central vein is evident (arrow). Several ducts are dilated. Patient's initial presentation (at 43 years of age) was with episode of cholangitis.

chymal cholestasis.[358] The major clinical manifestations are caused by portal hypertension.

Caroli's disease (communicating cavernous biliary ectasia) is characterized by multiple cystically dilated bile ducts.[369] These ectatic ducts *communicate* with the biliary tree, in contrast to the cysts of the polycystic liver. Patients may suffer repeated bouts of cholangitis.

The relationship of congenital hepatic fibrosis to Caroli's disease, and the relationship of these to infantile polycystic renal disease has been long debated.[358,359,362,368] These three entities show considerable clinical and pathologic overlap. They might be considered as a disease spectrum rather than separate or coincidental disorders.[358,362,368] Regarding the hepatic lesions, the ends of the spectrum do show fairly pure examples of congenital hepatic fibrosis on the one hand and Caroli's on the other. The remainder of cases, however, show a variable admixture of hepatic fibrosis and duct ectasia.[366,369] Symptomatology in these cases depends on whether the fibrosis (portal hypertension) or ectasia (cholangitis) predominates.

Renal anomalies frequently accompany these hepatic lesions. The essential feature of the renal lesion is ectasia of medullary collecting ducts.[360] The renal disease varies considerably in severity. In some cases there is renal failure in infancy. Conversely, clinically inapparent medullary ectasia is at times an incidental finding in a patient symptomatic because of congenital hepatic fibrosis.

There have been several instances of carcinoma arising in association with the fibropolycystic liver diseases. Carcinoma complicating polycystic liver disease is exception-

ally rare. In congenital hepatic fibrosis and Caroli's disease, where the ducts are in contact with bile, the incidence of adenocarcinoma is somewhat higher (1% to 7%).[361]

CIRRHOSIS

Cirrhosis may be defined as a diffuse scarring of the liver characterized by (1) loss of lobular architecture, (2) regeneration of hepatocytes with nodule formation, and (3) diffuse fibrosis. Localized scars, either subcapsular or parenchymal, do not constitute cirrhosis, although the surgeon who biopsies such a focal process may receive a mistaken diagnosis if its focality is not communicated. Because of the unreliability of clinical and laboratory features, liver biopsy constitutes an important aspect of the diagnosis of cirrhosis.

Many classifications of cirrhosis have been published, and the lack of consensus regarding concepts and terminology has generated much confusion. It has not always been appreciated that cirrhosis represents the final common pathway of a number of different diseases, only a few of which leave specific traces late in the course.[371] Well-meaning attempts to name cirrhosis according to presumed etiology (e.g., alcoholic cirrhosis) without supporting clinical or laboratory evidence have been misleading. In recent years morphologic classifications have been proposed, which have restored some order to the approach to cirrhosis.[370,373,377] A WHO-sponsored group recognized three categories: (1) micronodular, (2) macronodular, and (3) mixed.[370]

Micronodular cirrhosis is a lesion in which almost all the parenchymal nodules are less than 3 mm in diameter[370] (Fig. 13-25). The septa are thin (usually less than 2 mm)

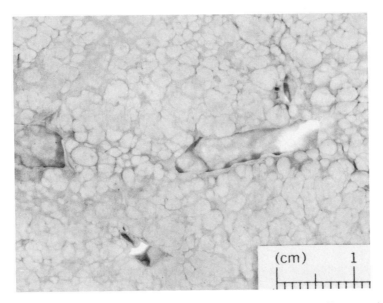

Fig. 13-25 This represents a reasonably "pure" case of micronodular cirrhosis. Regenerative nodules are smaller than 3 mm in size. Patient was a chronic alcoholic.

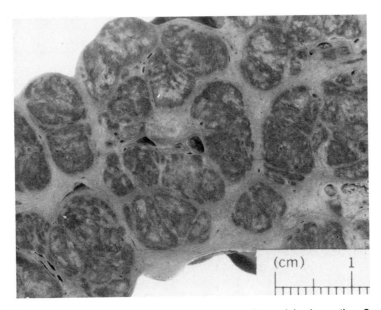

Fig. 13-26 This case of macronodular cirrhosis shows regenerative nodules larger than 3 mm. Fibrous bands are also quite thick, Patient was a chronic alcoholic.

and uniform.[377] Only rarely do the nodules contain portal tracts or hepatic veins. The regularity of the lesion suggests a uniform pathogenetic process. The cirrhosis associated with alcoholism and long-standing biliary obstruction, for instance, tends to be of this type.

Macronodular cirrhosis is characterized by variably sized nodules, many of which are over 3 mm in diameter[370] (Fig. 13-26). Nodule size ranges up to 2 to 3 cm. The septa are likewise variable; some are delicate, while others are broad scars. The parenchymal nodules may contain portal tracts and hepatic vein radicles. The variability of the lesion suggests irregularity of the preceding insult and parenchymal regeneration.[377] A subtype of macronodular cirrhosis, *incomplete septal fibrosis,* is characterized by macronodules separated by rather delicate septa. The septa tend to form portal-portal connections and at times end blindly.[370] The delicate pattern of fibrosis can make gross and microscopic recognition of this subtype difficult. The term *mixed cirrhosis* can be used when there is a fairly equal mixture of micronodules and macronodules.

Cirrhosis is usually not a static process but rather a dynamic combination of inflammation, cell injury and death, fibrosis, and regeneration. These changes frequently result in transistion of micronodular cirrhosis to macronodular cirrhosis.[372,374,376,379] The Copenhagen Study Group for Liver Diseases studied 156 cirrhotic patients and observed a conversion ratio of micro- to macrolobular cirrhosis of about 90% in 10 years.[372] Median time interval between the diagnosis of micro- and macronodular cirrhosis was 2.25 years. The association of late complications of cirrhosis (such as hepatocellular carcinoma) with macronodular cirrhosis more than with the micronodular pattern probably simply reflects their later occurrence in the disease process.

The diagnosis of cirrhosis is usually straightforward in wedge biopsies although subcapsular fibrosis can confuse interpretation of a superficial wedge biopsy. On needle biopsy, however, it can be quite difficult. The needle biopsy may not contain parenchymal nodules with surrounding fibrous septa. In such instances, other features may help to make or suggest the diagnosis. These features include (1) fragmentation of the biopsy into nodules that are partly surrounded by a thin layer of connective tissue, (2) altered architecture with abnormal numbers and spacing of hepatic veins, and (3) two-cell thick hepatic cell plates; these can sometimes be recognized by the position of the nuclei along the sinusoidal surfaces.[370,378]

Evaluation of the *activity* of the cirrhotic process is also extremely important.[376] The magnitude of the inflammatory infiltrate and the amount of ongoing hepatocellular necrosis should be assessed. The activity may be specific for the disease process (i.e., cirrhosis with ongoing acute alcoholic hepatitis) or independent of the original insult. The borders between the fibrous septa and parenchymal nodules deserve careful scrutiny. Necrosis at this interface (piecemeal necrosis) can be a significant indicator of progression of the lesion.[376] The activity of the cirrhosis can be expressed as mild, moderate, or severe.

The biopsy should be examined for histologic features indicative of an etiology. There are several morphologic markers, including Mallory bodies, ground-glass hepatocytes, excess iron or copper, or PAS-positive globules that may help to suggest an etiology. These should be specifically looked for. Depending on the etiology, patients may benefit from specific therapy, systemic steroids, or withdrawal of the causative agent.

Several questions should be answered in evaluating the liver biopsy in cirrhosis: (1) Does the patient, in fact, have cirrhosis? (2) What type? (3) Is the lesion active or quiescent? (4) Does the biopsy indicate a specific etiology?

Cirrhosis must be distinguished from *nodular regenerative hyperplasia,* also known as nodular transformation of the liver.[380a,380b] This entity can mimic micronodular cirrhosis both grossly and microscopically. The lesion consists of small nodules of regenerating hepatocytes distributed diffusely throughout the liver.[375] Nodular regenerative hyperplasia is distinct from cirrhosis in that these regenerative nodules are not surrounded by fibrous septa. One does, however, observe compressed reticulin fibers at the periphery of the nodules. It should also be distinguished from focal nodular hyperplasia (p. 705). The patients' symptoms are caused by portal hypertension.[380] Some cases have been seen in association with rheumatoid arthritis, Felty's syndrome, and neoplasms of other organs.

LIVER TRANSPLANTATION

Liver transplantation is now a recognized form of treatment for patients with advanced liver disease that is unresponsive to conventional therapy, where the prognosis is less than 1 year, or where the effects of the disease make life intolerable for the patient.[398] An increasing number of medical centers now practice liver transplantation in both adult and pediatric patients[383,391,392] and several reviews that discuss selection of patients and preoperative prognostic prediction are available.* More recently, experience with emergency liver transplantation for fulminant hepatitis (including delta virus hepatitis) has been described.[381a]

The major risk for orthotopic liver recipients is allograft rejection. At the University of Pittsburg approximately 16% of transplant patients underwent retransplantation following liver failure secondary to graft rejection.[386] At the University of Minnesota 77% of the patients experienced one or more episodes of rejection following transplantation.[401] The most effective method for diagnosing and monitoring rejection is percutaneous liver biopsy.[389,401,402,406] Most transplant centers, including our own, now monitor therapeutic response to immunosuppressive agents primarily with liver biopsy.

The pathology of liver allograft rejection has been described by several institutions.† Snover et al. recognized a triad of histologic changes that characterize acute rejection: a mixed lymphocytic-polymorphonuclear portal infiltrate, bile duct damage, and endothelialitis, or, in the absence of endothelialitis, a mixed infiltrate and more than 50% of bile ducts damaged[401,402] (Figs. 13-27 and 13-28). Nondiagnostic changes are common on post-transplant biopsies and include mild portal inflammatory infiltrate and minimal bile duct injury. Chronic rejection may be diagnosed by the presence of obliterative endarteritis, portal fibrosis with bridging, paucity of bile ducts in association with fibrosis, and cirrhosis.[387,389,401] The changes of arteritis indicating evolution to chronic rejection may be difficult to document by percutaneous biopsy and, unfortunately, are better seen at autopsy.[387] Histologic changes, which may predict chronic rejection or an adverse outcome, include arteritis, paucity of bile ducts, and hepatocellular ballooning together with hepatocellular dropout and necrosis.[401]

Several attempts at grading hepatic allograft rejection have been undertaken.[389,401,406] The grading system of the University of Minnesota was devised in an attempt to preduct clinical outcome and to allow more accurate therapeutic intervention.[401] Three grades of acute rejection were defined: (1) lymphocytic or mixed portal infiltrate, less than 50% damaged bile ducts, and endothelialitis; (2) lymphocytic or mixed portal infiltrate and greater than 50% damaged bile ducts with or without endothelialitis; and (3) acute rejection

---

*See references 381, 382, 385, 388, 393, 396a, 398, 400, and 404.
†See references 387, 389, 395, 401, 402, 405, and 406.

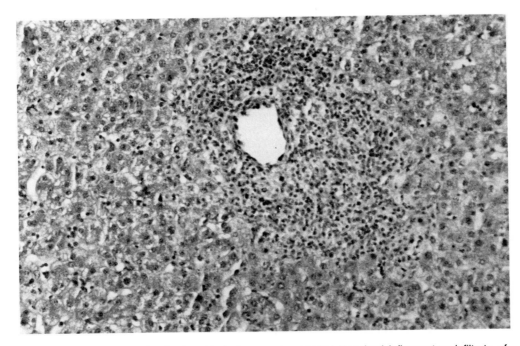

Fig. 13-27 Liver allograft rejection. Marked expansion of triad by mixed inflammatory infiltrate of lymphocytes, histiocytes, eosinophils, and neutrophils. No bile ductule is apparent and has presumably been eroded by inflammation. Endothelium of ectatic venule is swollen and disrupted.

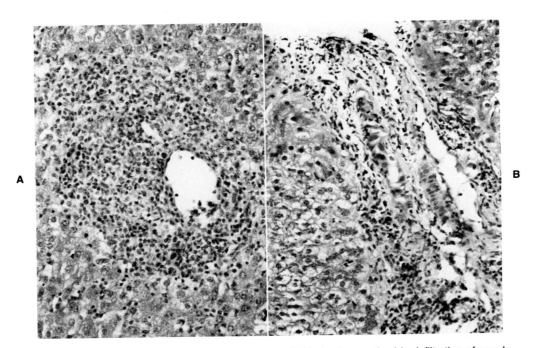

Fig. 13-28 Changes of allograft rejection. **A,** Endothelialitis is characterized by infiltration of venule wall and disruption of endothelial lining. Note lymphocytes adherent to endothelial cells. Bile ductule (above and to left of venule) shows extensive injury and inflammatory infiltration. **B,** Another biopsy shows bile duct injury characterized by lymphocyte infiltration into epithelial cells and accompanying cytoplasmic vacuolization.

plus arteritis, paucity of bile ducts, or central hepatocellular balloning with confluent dropout of hepatocytes.

Hyperacute graft rejection, which is relatively common in renal transplantation, appears to be unusual in liver transplantation, and most graft failures immediately post-operatively result from occlusive or nonocclusive ischemia or from infection.[384,407] At least two patients have been reported, however, who showed clinical and pathologic evidence of hyperacute rejection.[402] Another incompletely understood complication of the early post-operative period has been called the acute vanishing bile duct syndrome.[396,405] This is an irreversible condition that occurs within 100 days following transplantation and is characterized histologically by destructive cholangitis and loss of ducts.[396]

Liver allograft recipients are at risk for developing forms of disease other than rejection, including redevelopment of their original pathology.[387,397] They are also at significant risk of infection as a consequence of immunosuppression.[390,394,403] Masih et al. have recently described a method of rapid identification of cytomegalovirus in liver allograph biopsies using an in situ hybridization technique on formalin-fixed tissue.[397a] Other potential changes that the surgical pathologist must exclude are drug-induced injury, vascular thrombosis, and bile duct complications such as obstruction from post-operative scarring. Differentiating these processes from rejection can be problematic, but in general nonrejection alterations in allografts are identical to those occurring in native livers. As is the case in liver pathology in general, difficult biopsies should only be interpreted in view of the overall clinical, laboratory, and histologic picture of the patient.

HETEROTOPIA

Heterotopic liver tissue is a very uncommon finding. It has been described in the gallbladder, spleen, pancreas, umbilicus, adrenal glands, and lesser omentum; often, this tissue has some attachment to the liver. Exceptional instances of heterotopic liver in the lung have also been recorded.[408]

ABSCESS

The incidence of hepatic abscess has been fairly stable over the past 50 years.[410,411] However, the character of the disease has changed drastically during that time. In the past, hepatic abscesses often affected young adults; most were amebic or secondary to pylephlebitis. Today, the disease usually affects older patients, and enteric bacteria are the most common pathogens. The incidence of culture-negative abscesses diminished markedly when proper anaerobic cultures are obtained. Mortality remains considerable, ranging from 30% to 80%.[410,411]

Currently, the predisposing factors, in descending order of frequency, are (1) biliary tract obstruction/infection, (2) systemic bacteremia, (3) direct extension from a contiguous infection, (4) trauma (penetrating and nonpenetrating), and (5) pylephlebitis.[410] Secondary bacterial infection of metastatic tumor nodules is another cause.[412] Rarely, hepatic abscess may complicate inflammatory bowel disease.[412a] Hepatic abscesses vary tremendously in size. In two thirds of the patients reported by Rubin et al.[410] the lesions were

macroscopic; the remainder had microabscesses. Multiplicity of lesions is seen in about half of the pyogenic abscesses and a fourth of amebic abscesses.[409]

ECHINOCOCCUS CYST

Echinococcus or hydatid disease of the liver is rare in the United States but frequent in Iceland, Sicily, Australia, Turkey, South America, and New Zealand.[414-416] It is caused by the larval or cystic stage of the dog tapeworm. Four species of the parasite have been identified: *Echinococcus granulosus* (by far the commonest), *Echinococcus obligarthrus*, *Echinococcus patagonicus*, and *Echinococcus multilocularis*.[416] Its definitive hosts are dogs, wolves, cats, and other carnivora. The intermediate or cystic stage is present in sheep, hogs, and cows, but man or other mammals can become infected.

The most common sites of echinococcus cysts are the liver (60% to 70% of patients) and the lung, but they can occur in many other locations. We have seen them in the spleen, soft tissue, bone, breast, brain, and spinal extradural space. When the cyst is viable, the skin and complement fixation tests are often positive, and eosinophilia is frequent. Death of the parasite is accompanied by collapse of the wall and calcification. At this stage, the skin test is of little value, and eosinophilia is present in less than 5% of the cases. Communication with the biliary tract and superimposed infection are frequent.[413] Rupture of the cysts into the peritoneal cavity may result in a fatal anaphylactic reaction or in the formation of innumerable small granulomas closely resembling peritoneal tuberculosis. The diagnosis is made by identifying fragments of germinal membrane or scoleces in their center. Hepatic echinococcus cysts also can rupture inside the gallbladder or through the diaphragm into the pleural space and lung.

Grossly, hydatidosis of the liver is usually of the unilocular type. The cysts average 1 to 7 cm in diameter (Fig. 13-29). About 75% are in the right lobe, the majority on the inferior surface extending downward into the peritoneal cavity. Histologic examination of the cyst wall shows an outer *chitinous* (or fibrous laminar) layer and an inner *germinal layer* surrounded by granulation tissue or a fibrous capsule (so-called pericyst layer). Calcification in the latter layer signifies that the cyst is dead. The neighboring liver parenchyma often shows pressure atrophy and a moderately intense portal infiltrate in which eosinophils may be prominent. The viable cyst is filled with colorless fluid, which contains daughter cysts and brood capsules with scoleces. The latter can be easily identified after macerating a portion of the germinal layer in saline solution. They have characteristic hooklets, 20 μm to 40 μm in length. The best treatment for uncomplicated hydatic cyst is evacuation, scolicidal irrigation, and primary closure.[413]

SOLITARY NONPARASITIC CYST

Solitary nonparasitic cysts of the liver are not well discussed in the literature and, when mentioned, are touted to be unusual.[420] The unilocular cyst, which is usually encountered incidentally at autopsy is of uncertain pathogenesis but is presumed to be a retention cyst of bile ductule derivation. The presence of a simple columnar epithelial lining supports this hypothesis. Some of these solitary cysts, however, may be congenital.[416a,418] Although usually asymptomatic, rare complications such as rapid enlargement,[416a] torsion,[417,419a] rupture,[417,419a] or obstructive jaundice may occur.

Ciliated foregut cyst is a type of solitary unilocular cyst lined by ciliated pseudostratified columnar epithelium resting on a wall that contains abundant smooth muscle.[420a]

Epidermoid cyst has been reported a few times, both in children and adults.[419]

Endometrial cyst of the liver has been observed in a 21-year-old woman by Finkel et al.[417a]

TUMORS AND TUMORLIKE CONDITIONS
Liver cell tumors and tumorlike conditions
Focal nodular hyperplasia

Focal nodular hyperplasia can occur in any age group, including childhood; most cases, however, are seen during the third to fifth decades of life.[423] The female to male ratio is about 2:1 in adult cases, but as high as 4:1 in pediatric cases.[433] In about 80% of the cases, the lesion is asymptomatic.[430a] Hemoperitoneum is extremely rare. The lesion is usually solitary; the presence of several independent nodules has been described in 20% of the adult cases and in a higher percentage of the pediatric cases.[433] A possible relationship to oral contraceptives has been postulated in many reports,[421,428] but it is not as clearcut as for liver cell adenoma.[423a,425,426,427] There is no question that this disease occurred prior to the widespread use of oral contraceptives

and that it can occur in males, particularly in association with chronic alcohol abuse.[425a]

The arteriographic appearance, characterized by a centrifugal filling pattern, is distinctive.[424] Grossly, it usually presents as a gray-white, solid mass beneath the capsule, sometimes pedunculated. On cut section, a white depressed area of fibrosis is seen in the center, with broad strands radiating from it to the periphery in a stellate configuration (Fig. 13-30). Microscopically, *all the components of the normal liver lobule are present*. The cellular morphology and relationship between hepatocytes and bile ducts are essentially those of normal liver, both by light and electron microscopic criteria.

Some of the hepatocytes have increased amounts of glycogen and fat. In most of the cases, there is immunoreactivity for alpha-1-antitrypsin, a feature shared with liver cell adenoma and liver cell carcinoma.[429] Acute or chronic inflammatory cells are common. Fibrous septa containing eccentrically thickened vessels divide the lesion into lobules with a pattern resembling that of cirrhosis (Fig. 13-31).[422]

The differential diagnosis should be made with liver cell adenoma,[430] well-differentiated liver cell carcinoma, and *nodular regenerative hyperplasia* (nodular transformation) (see p. 700).[434,434a] In the latter condition, *the entire liver* shows nodulation, and central scars are absent in the nodules. It is not clear whether the rare cases described as *focal* or *partial* nodular transformation,[431,432] which may be associated with portal hypertension, are pathogenetically

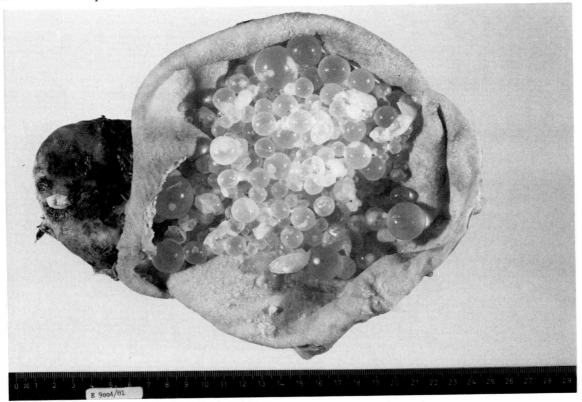

Fig. 13-29 Hydatidosis of liver. Innumerable daughter cysts are contained within huge cystic cavity. (Courtesy Dr. J. Costa, Lausanne, Switzerland.)

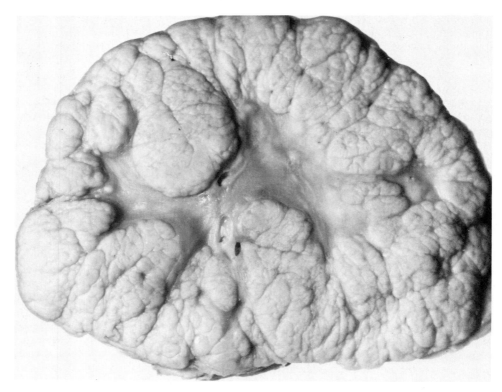

Fig. 13-30 Focal nodular hyperplasia removed from liver of 20-year-old woman. Mass measured 5 cm × 5 cm × 8.5 cm. Note typical central scar with stellate configuration.

related to focal nodular hyperplasia or to nodular regenerative hyperplasia, but the latter seems more likely.

Liver cell adenoma

True adenomas of the liver are very rare. They have a striking predilection for females and are statistically related to the use of oral contraceptives,[440,446] a fact further corroborated by the detection of cytoplasmic progesterone receptors in the tumor cells[437] and the occasional total regression of this tumor following discontinuation of the hormones.[436] These neoplasms have also been reported following anabolic androgenic steroid therapy[438,450] and in association with glycogen storage diseases.[439] When compared with focal nodular hyperplasia, the adenomas are more often symptomatic and can lead to severe and even fatal peritoneal hemorrhage.[435] Most of the patients are in the third to fifth decades of life, but cases have also been reported in children.[451] The majority of the lesions (70%) are solitary,[445] but on occasion there are ten or more tumors, a condition known as *liver cell adenomatosis*.[441] They are usually visualized as defects on ^{99m}technetium-sulfur colloid liver scans. Grossly, they have a well-defined capsule and a color different from the surrounding liver. The typical central scar of nodular hyperplasia is absent (Fig. 13-32). Microscopically, the tumor is composed of well-differentiated hepatocytes with abundant eosinophilic granular cytoplasm. *There are no portal triads or central veins*, and there is no connection with the biliary system. Kupffer cells are always present, in a pattern comparable to that seen in normal liver.[443] Unusual features

of adenoma include oncocytic changes,[449] presence of Mallory's alcoholic hyaline,[444] and secondary granulomatous reaction.[447]

Multiple sections should be carefully evaluated to rule out a well-differentiated liver cell carcinoma. Search for blood vessel invasion is particularly important. Not infrequently, the differential diagnosis between these two entities is impossible, and only the clinical course establishes the true nature of the lesion. Thus some of the androgen-induced tumor originally diagnosed as liver cell carcinoma have been reclassified as adenomas because of the benign long-term evolution.[448] Sometimes, an unequivocal focus of liver cell carcinoma is seen in a lesion having otherwise the features of adenoma.[446] Galloway et al.[442] have proposed the somewhat unsatisfactory term *minimal deviation hepatoma* for lesions that cannot be clearly categorized as benign or malignant.

The most important differences between focal nodular hyperplasia and liver cell adenoma are listed in Table 13-2.

Liver cell carcinoma

General features. Liver cell carcinoma (hepatocellular carcinoma, hepatoma) is relatively rare in this country, but very common in all African countries south of the Sahara and in Southeast Asia.[455] In the People's Republic of China, this tumor is responsible for over 100,000 deaths per year. Most cases are seen in patients over the age of 50 years, but this tumor can also occur in younger individuals and

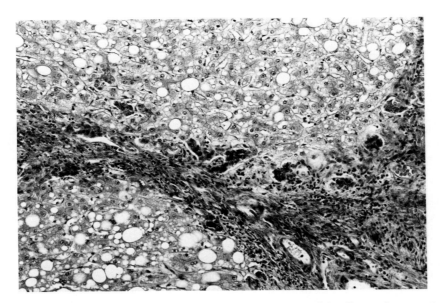

Fig. 13-31 Focal nodular hyperplasia. Nodules are separated by cellular fibrous tissue containing inflammatory cells. Hepatocytes within nodules show marked fatty metamorphosis. Note proliferating bile duct structures at interface between parenchyma and stroma.

even in children.[453,456] It is more common in males than in females, especially when associated with cirrhosis.

It usually presents with abdominal pain, ascites, and liver enlargement. Sometimes liver cell carcinoma is associated with systemic manifestations such as hypoglycemia, hypercholesterolemia, erythrocytosis, hypercalcemia, carcinoid syndrome, serum elevation of proline hydroxylase, ectopic production of chorionic gonadotropin and prostaglandin, dysfibrinogenemia, and several others.[455a,457,459]

Alpha-fetoprotein can be detected by immunodiffusion or radioimmunoassay in a large percentage of patients with liver cell carcinoma.[460] The incidence of positivity is higher in places in which the tumor is endemic (more than 75%) than in Europe or the United States (40% to 60%). The tests also may be positive with malignant germ cell tumors and, rarely, with metastatic carcinomas to the liver, hepatitis, and posttraumatic liver regeneration. However, increases over one hundred times normal levels are virtually diagnostic of liver cell carcinoma if a malignant germ cell tumor can be excluded[461]; therefore, serial determinations of serum alpha-fetoprotein levels offer a good clue to early detection in high-risk populations. CT scan or nuclear magnetic resonance imaging usually result in the accurate determination of the location of the tumor, the extent of its invasiveness, and the presence or absence of multicentricity.

The diagnosis is confirmed by core or fine needle biopsy.[452,458,463] The better differentiated the tumor, the more difficult the diagnosis. In fine needle material, the most useful diagnostic criteria are similarity of tumor cells to liver cells, prominence of nucleoli, and trabecular pattern.[454] Two rare but well-documented complications of needle biopsy are implantation along the tract and intra-abdominal hemorrhage.[462]

Predisposing and associated factors. A large propor-

tion of liver cell carcinomas have been found to be associated with one or another of the following items, strongly suggesting a pathogenetic relationship.

1 *Cirrhosis.* In the United States, 60%-80% of the cases develop in livers affected by cirrhosis. This is usually of the macronodular type, including that caused by hemochromatosis.[475] Cases of liver cell carcinoma have also been reported in association with biliary cirrhosis secondary to congenital bile duct atresia,[472] familial cholestatic cirrhosis of childhood[471,497] cirrhosis caused by alpha-1-antitrypsin deficiency[484] or tyrosinemia,[499] and congenital hepatic fibrosis associated with adult polycystic kidneys.[486]

The liver cell carcinomas associated with cirrhosis show widespread hepatic involvement more often than those arising in a previously normal liver.

2 *Hepatotropic viruses.* There is strong evidence of a pathogenetic role of hepatotropic viruses in the development of liver cell carcinoma, not only through the production of cirrhosis but also in noncirrhotic livers.[485,489] The incidence of hepatitis B surface antigenemia in patients with liver cell carcinoma is over 50%, both in the United States and overseas.[469,496,498] Both surface and core antigens can be detected by immunoperoxidase techniques in the cytoplasm of the tumor cells and the non-neoplastic hepatocytes in many of the cases[479,480,494,495] (Fig. 13-33). Integration of hepatitis B virus DNA into the genome of the tumor cells has also been documented.[468,481,491]

Presence of *liver cell dysplasia* (defined as cellular enlargement, nuclear pleomorphism, and multinucleation) in the non-neoplastic portion of an organ harboring a liver cell carcinoma has also been used as indirect evidence for viral participation in the pro-

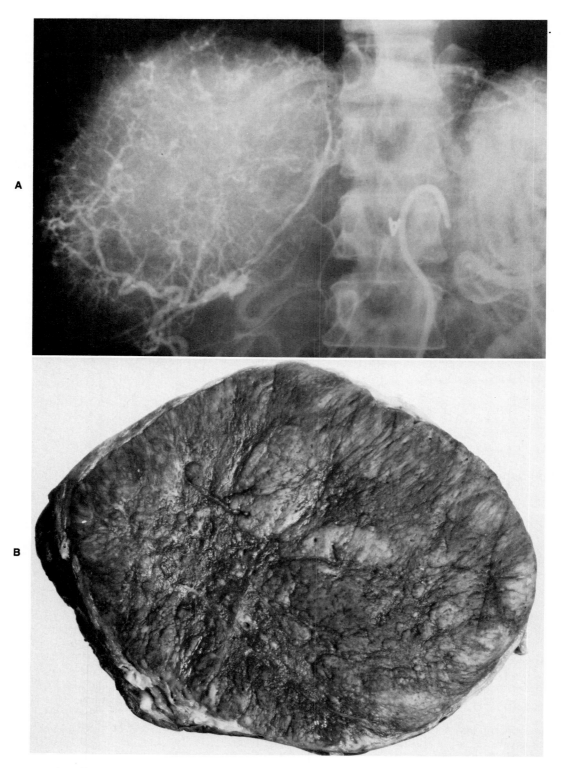

13-32 A, Arteriogram showing large well-vascularized mass in right lobe of liver in 43-year-old woman. **B,** Gross appearance of lesion. Tumor is well encapsulated and irregularly lobulated. Microscopically, it was composed throughout by well-differentiated hepatocytes. Diagnosis was liver cell adenoma. Patient is alive and well 3 years following partial hepatectomy.

Table 13-2 Comparison of clinical, radiologic, and pathologic characteristics of focal nodular hyperplasia and liver cell adenoma

Features	Focal nodular hyperplasia	Liver cell adenoma
Clinical		
Incidence	Uncommon	Rare
Age	All ages	Third, fourth decades
Sex	85% females	Nearly all females
Oral contraceptive use	Occasionally	Nearly always
Clinical presentation	Usually asymptomatic, 35% abdominal mass, abdominal discomfort	Often abdominal emergency 45% abdominal mass, acute abdominal pain
Hemoperitoneum	Less than 1%	25%
Liver function tests	Nearly always normal	Nearly always normal
Malignant potential	None	Probably none
Therapy	Resection if operative risk negligible	Resection
Angiography		
Vascularity	Hypervascular with dense capillary blush	Hypovascular
Hematoma formation	Rare	Common
Necrosis	Rare	Common
Septation	Present 50%	Absent
Liver scan		
Uptake	Normal or slightly decreased	None
Pathology		
Capsule	No capsule	Partial to ample encapsulation
Location	Usually subcapsular, 20% pedunculated Often multiple	Usually subcapsular, 7% pedunculated Usually solitary
Stellate scar	Present	Absent
Parenchyma	Nodular	Homogeneous
Hemorrhage, necrosis	Rare	Common
Bile stasis	Absent	Present
Hepatocytes	Cytologically normal	Glycogen rich, vacuolated
Bile ductules	Present	Absent
Kupffer cells	Present	Reduced or absent
Vascularity	Large thick-walled vessels	Thin-walled sinusoids
Ultrastructure	Normal	Simplified

From Knowles DM II, Casarella WJ, Johnson PM, Wolff M: The clinical, radiologic, and pathologic characterization of benign hepatic neoplasms. Alleged association with oral contraceptives. Medicine [Baltimore] **57**:223-237, 1978; © 1978 The Williams & Wilkins Co., Baltimore.

cess. Anthony et al.[466] studied the incidence of this change in a large group of patients from Uganda and found it in only 1% of patients with normal liver, in 6.9% of patients with liver cell carcinoma occurring in an otherwise normal liver, in 20.3% of patients with cirrhosis, and in 64.5% of patients with cirrhosis *and* liver cell carcinoma. They also documented a strong relationship between dysplasia and the presence of hepatitis B surface antigen, and concluded that the presence of liver cell dysplasia identifies a group of patients who are at high risk for developing liver cell carcinoma. The statistical relation of hepatocytic dysplasia with both hepatitis B virus infection and the development of liver cell carcinoma has been confirmed by several other groups.[464,477] These dysplastic changes can also be seen in other forms of viral hepatitis.[483]

3 *Thorium dioxide exposure.* Administration of thorium dioxide suspension (Thorotrast) as a radiographic contrast medium has resulted in the development of many liver cell carcinomas, the average latent period being 20 years.[493]

4 *Androgenic anabolic steroids.* Several cases of liver tumors have been reported in males in association with long-term administration of androgenic anabolic steroids.[467,474,482] Most of these have been diagnosed as liver cell carcinoma but their behavior has been generally benign, casting some doubts on the correctness of the diagnosis. Many of these are probably adenomas analogous to those seen in females in association with contraceptive pills.[476,488]

5 *Progestational agents.* Several cases of liver cell carcinomas, either alone or in association with liver cell adenomas, have been reported in women taking contraceptive pills.[478,490,492]

6 *Alpha-1-antitrypsin deficiency.* Cases of cirrhosis caused by this inborn error of metabolism complicated by liver cell carcinoma are on record, but there is still controversy as to whether this condition *per se* is a pre-neoplastic condition.[470,473]

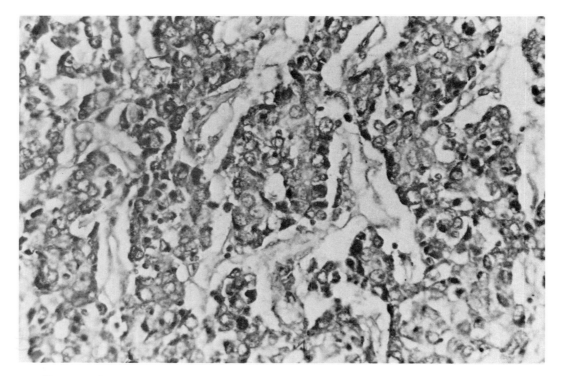

Fig. 13-33 Positive immunoperoxidase reaction for hepatitis B surface antigen in cytoplasm of liver cell carcinoma.

7 *Tyrosinemia.* The chronic form of this inborn error of metabolism is associated with a high incidence of liver cell carcinoma. In one series, 37% of 43 patients surviving beyond 2 years of age develop this malignancy.[499] All of the patients with tumor also have cirrhosis.

8 *Ataxia-telangiectasia.* A few cases of liver cell carcinomas have been observed in patients with this form of congenital immune deficiency.[500]

9 *Aflatoxins.* The peculiar geographic distribution of liver cell carcinoma has suggested to some a relationship with the ingestion of aflatoxins, metabolic products of the growth of the ubiquitous fungus *Aspergillus flavus.*[465] A good correlation exists between the level of contamination of foods with aflatoxins and the incidence of liver cancer; elimination of this contamination has resulted in a decrease in the number of tumors.

10 *Schistosomiasis.* There is no convicing evidence that schistosomiasis *per se* predisposes to liver cell carcinoma.[487]

Pathologic features. Grossly, liver cell carcinoma may present as a single large mass, as multiple nodules, or as diffuse liver involvement; these are sometimes referred to as massive, nodular, and diffuse forms, respectively.[527] Some lesions are surrounded by a grossly distinct capsule.[529] In rare cases, the tumor is pedunculated, presumably because it arises in an accessory lobe.[503,514] The tumor size varies a great deal from case to case. In recent years, prog-

ress in diagnostic procedures has led to the detection of an increased number of *small* or *minute* tumors, variously defined as measuring less than 3 cm, 3.5 cm, or 5 cm.[516,519,523]

Portal vein thrombosis is found in a high proportion of the advanced cases[501] (Fig. 13-34).

Microscopically, the pattern of growth may be trabecular, solid, or tubular.[511,521] The latter, which has also been referred to as pseudoglandular or acinar, may result in vaguely papilloid formations and can lead to diagnostic confusion with bile duct carcinoma[521,522] A network of sinusoidal vessels surrounds the tumor cells, an important diagnostic feature; some of these sinusoids seem to be lined by tumor cells.[528] The stroma is usually scanty, in contrast to bile duct carcinoma; however, a rare *sclerosing* form of liver cell carcinoma has been described, especially following therapy.[521] Invasion of veins in the portal tract is a frequent finding. Cytologically, there is a wide range of differentiation from tumor to tumor, which correlates closely with the DNA pattern.[509a] The lesser differentiated cases show great pleomorphism, bizarre mitotic figures, and tumor giant cells.[502,509] Nuclei and nucleoli are prominent, and the cytoplasm is scanty and basophilic (Fig. 13-35). It may be difficult or impossible to identify these tumors with certainty as liver cell carcinomas. Conversely, the better differentiated tumors may be difficult to categorize as malignant. An occasional cluster of enlarged hyperchromatic nuclei, an atypical mitotic figure, or a blood vessel with a thrombus may be the only clue to the malignant nature of the lesion.

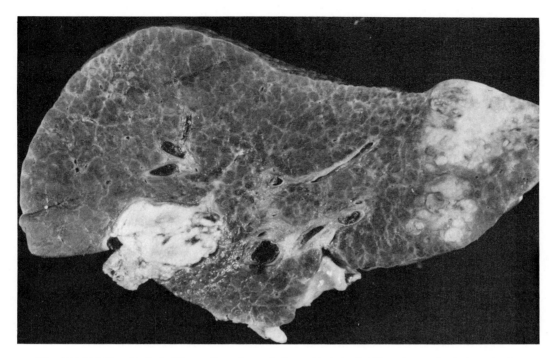

Fig. 13-34 Multicentric foci of liver cell carcinoma in liver with cirrhosis. There is portal vein thrombosis by tumor. As is usually the case, cirrhosis is of multilobular (postnecrotic) type. (Courtesy Dr. J. Murray, Johannesburg, South Africa.)

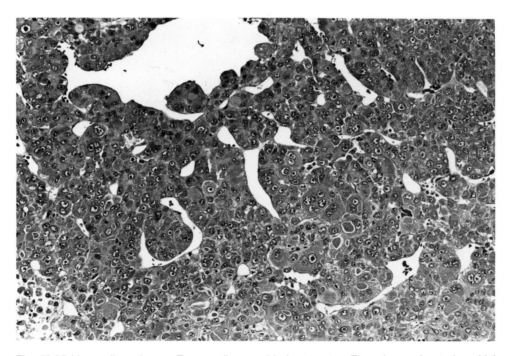

Fig. 13-35 Liver cell carcinoma. Tumor cells resemble hepatocytes. There is prominent sinusoidal pattern, an important clue to diagnosis.

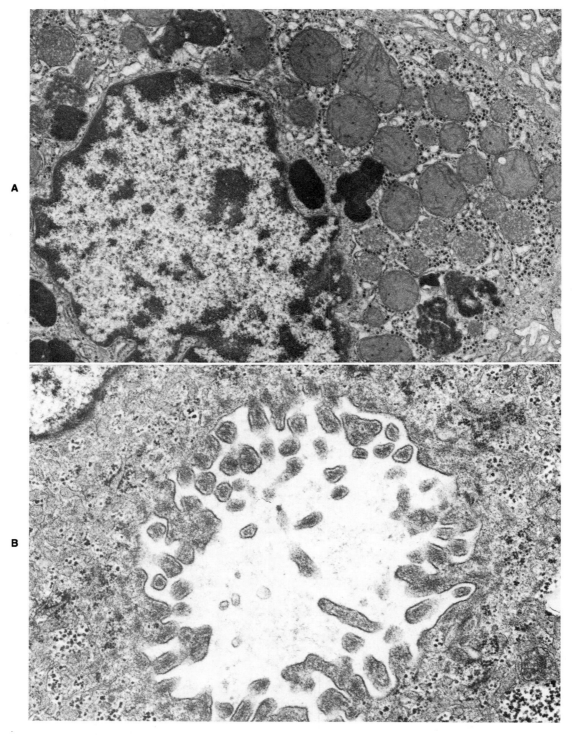

Fig. 13-36 Ultrastructural appearance of liver cell carcinoma. **A,** Malignant hepatocyte with numerous mitochondria, microbodies, and abundant glycogen. Cells also contain intracytoplasmic bile products. **B,** Intracytoplasmic canaliculus is present in this malignant cell. (**A,** ×11,200; **B,** ×25,270.)

The tumor cells often contain intranuclear pseudoinclusions caused by cytoplasmic invaginations. The cytoplasm may contain Mallory's hyaline similar to that seen in alcoholic liver disease, round hyaline globules (some containing alpha-fetoprotein and others alpha-1-antitrypsin),[506,530] copper,[512,513] or bile pigment; the latter is an important diagnostic feature. Both the copper and copper-binding proteins can be detected histochemically.[510a] In some tumors, the cytoplasm has a ground-glass appearance, presumably because of synthesis of fibrinogen.[532] In one remarkable case, the tumor was black due to the accumulation of a Dubin-Johnson–like pigment.[531]

In about 9% of the cases, the cytoplasm is clear because of the accumulation of glycogen and/or fat.[533] These tumors, known as *clear cell carcinomas*, closely resemble renal or adrenal cortical carcinomas.[505] Rarely, a combination of liver cell carcinoma and bile duct carcinoma is encountered (see p. 715). Another unusual event is the presence of sarcomatoid areas in the tumor, composed of spindle and/or multinucleated tumor cells [518] or osteoclast-like giant cells.[524] In rare cases, bone or cartilage formation is seen in them. Yet another exceptional occurrence is the presence of features of endocrine differentiation in some of the tumor cells.[504]

Kuppfer cells may be present in liver cell carcinoma, but they are usually scanty and irregularly distributed.

The ultrastructure of liver cell carcinoma recapitulates in some respects that of the normal adult hepatocyte and is different from that of hepatoblastoma[515] (Fig. 13-36).

Immunohistochemically, reactivity has been found for alpha-fetoprotein, alpha-1-antitrypsin, fibrinogen, IgG, fibronectin, transferrin receptor, and ferritin.* CEA and *cytoplasmic* keratin are usually negative or only focally positive, an important factor in the differential diagnosis with bile duct carcinoma and metastatic carcinoma.[510,520] In regard to the keratins, it has been shown that most liver cell carcinomas are immunoreactive for monoclonal antibody Cam 5.2 (which recognizes keratins 8, 18, and 19) but not for monoclonal antibody AE1 (which recognizes keratins 10, 14, 15, 16, and 19).[517a] Unfortunately, none of these reactions is useful in the differential diagnosis between benign and malignant hepatocytic tumors.[520] An important diagnostic feature is the production of bile canalicular structures between the tumor cells. These can be demonstrated in cytologic preparations or in plastic-embedded material with stains for alkaline phosphatase, biliary glycoprotein, or low molecular weight keratin.[520] The claim that this canalicular staining pattern as demonstrated by alkaline phosphatase staining is present in the benign but not in the malignant hepatocytic tumors[508] seems to us to be of doubtful validity.

The cells of liver cell carcinoma have also been found to possess both estrogen and androgen receptors.[525,526]

Fibrolamellar variant. Fibrolamellar carcinoma (also know as polygonal cell type hepatocellular carcinoma with fibrous stroma and oncocytic hepatocellular tumor) is a distinctive morphologic variant of liver cell carcinoma seen predominantly in young patients without cirrhosis and associated with a favorable prognosis.[534,535] Almost half of the

---

*See references 507, 509b, 510, 517, 520, and 531a.

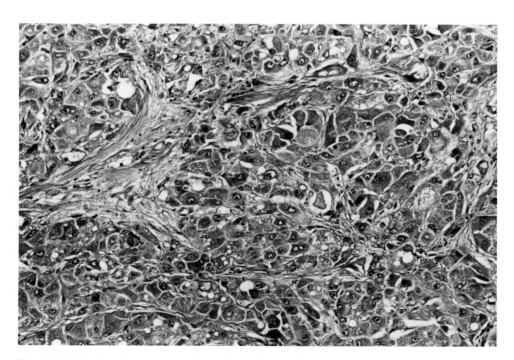

Fig. 13-37 Fibrolamellar variant of liver cell carcinoma. Tumor cells have abundant cytoplasm of polygonal shape and are separated in nests by prominent fibrohyaline stroma.

liver cell carcinomas seen in this country in patients younger than 35 years belong to this type.[536] The most characteristic microscopic feature is fibrosis arranged in a lamellar fashion around the neoplastic hepatocytes. The tumor cells are polygonal and deeply eosinophilic (Fig. 13-37). These features can also be appreciated in material from fine needle aspiration.[540]

Ultrastructurally, the tumor cells have numerous mitochondria, in keeping with their oncocytic appearance at the light microscopic level.[537] Dense-core granules of neurosecretory type have been reported in some cases.[538]

The architectural similarities between this tumor and focal nodular hyperplasia, and the occasional co-existence of the two entities suggest that they may be pathogenetically related.[539]

Over half of the fibrolamellar carcinomas are resectable, and the cure rate is about 50%.

Spread and metastasis. Liver cell carcinomas quickly permeate the liver through the portal venous system, spread to the lung, and grow into the pulmonary arterial tree. They may also grow into the hepatic vein and from there reach the inferior vena cava and the right atrium.[543] Gross tumor invasion of the biliary tree is less common but it does occur.[542] Local invasion of the diaphragm and metastases to regional lymph nodes also are common. In rare cases wide dissemination through the bloodstream takes place, with the development of adrenal and extensive bone metastases.[541,544,545] In some of the cases, a pathologic fracture or some other sign attributable to bone metastasis is the first sign of the disease.[545,546]

Treatment and prognosis. The overall median survival of liver cell carcinoma is about 4 months.[548,554] The major causes of death are hepatic failure and gastrointestinal bleeding.[558] Sometimes the terminal event is spontaneous rupture[547] or localized submassive liver cell necrosis.[556]

The only effective treatment of liver cell carcinoma is complete resection.[559] Encouraging reports from Japan indicate that if the tumor is diagnosed and excised at an early stage, good chances of cure exist.[557] The Japan Liver Cancer Study Group reported that, as of the end of 1974, twenty-five of 297 patients who had had hepatectomy had survived for more than 5 years, the longest survival being more than 17 years.[552]

Factors to be mentioned in relation to the prognosis of liver cell carcinoma include the following:

1 *Stage*. This constitutes the most important prognostic determinator.[558]
2 *Size*. Tumor size *per se* does not show a strong relationship with survival.[551]
3 *Encapsulation*. The rare liver cell carcinomas that are totally surrounded by a capsule behave in a less aggressive fashion.[551]
4 *Number of tumors*. As expected, single lesions are associated with a longer survival rate than multiple tumors.
5 *Microscopic type*. As already indicated, the fibrolamellar variant is associated with a definitely better prognosis. No consistent correlations have been found between prognosis and the many other morphologic variants of liver cell carcinoma.

6 *Presence of cirrhosis*. Carcinomas associated with cirrhosis have a worsened prognosis, probably because of the combination of a lesser functional defense and frequent widespread tumor involvement.[553,555]
7 *Viral antigenemia*. No significant prognostic differences exist between hepatitis B antigen positive and negative cases.[549,550]
8 *Use of progestational hormones*. It has been stated that tumors in patients who have taken contraceptive pills have a better prognosis than the others.
9 *Sex and age*. In most series, these parameters have not been found to correlate with tumor prognosis.

Hepatoblastoma

Hepatoblastoma occurs almost exclusively in infants, although isolated instances in older children and adults have been reported.[563,567] It has been reported in association with a variety of congenital abnormalities (particularly hemihypertrophy), coexistent Wilms' tumor of kidney, and glycogen storage disease.[567,569,571] In contrast with liver cell carcinoma, hepatoblastoma does not have a relationship with cirrhosis. Some patients present with virilization as a result of ectopic sex hormone production.[562,572] Serum levels of alpha-fetoprotein are often elevated. Hepatic angiography and CT scans provide the most valuable preoperative assessment of the tumor location and extent.[565] Grossly, hepatoblastoma is solid, well circumscribed, and more often solitary than multiple. Microscopically, most of the tumors are composed exclusively of immature hepatocytic elements and are referred to as *pure* or epithelial.[561] Some of these, known as *fetal,* consist of hepatocytes arranged in irregular two-cell thick laminae, recapitulating those of the fetal liver (Fig. 13-38, *A*). Others, designated as *embryonal,* have a more immature appearance, and a pattern of growth that is predominantly solid but which may also exhibit ribbons, rosettes, and papillary formations.[577,579] Some tumors are largely made up of anaplastic small cells.[571] The number of mitoses varies widely, but in general it is higher in the embryonal forms. Foci of extramedullary hematopoiesis are often seen, invariably associated with the fetal pattern.[564] Multinucleated giant cells may be present, particularly in the tumors associated with hormone production.[574,576] Transitions between the fetal and the embryonal patterns are common. Gonzalez-Crussi et al.[566] have further described a *macrotrabecular type,* resembling liver cell carcinoma. The main light microscopic differences between hepatoblastoma and liver cell carcinoma are listed in Table 13-3.

About a fourth of hepatoblastomas (referred to as *mixed*) contain, in addition to the epithelial cells, a stromal component that may be undifferentiated or develop into bone or cartilage, resulting in an appearance reminiscent of Wilms' tumor (Fig. 13-38, *B*). This feature supports the interpretation that these tumors arise from a multipotential blastema capable of both epithelial and mesenchymal differentiation.[573]

Ultrastructurally, the epithelial tumor cells have features of immature hepatocytes.[568,578] Immunohistochemically, reactivity has been found for epithelial membrane antigen, keratin (focally), vimentin, alpha-fetoprotein, and HCG.[560,575,577]

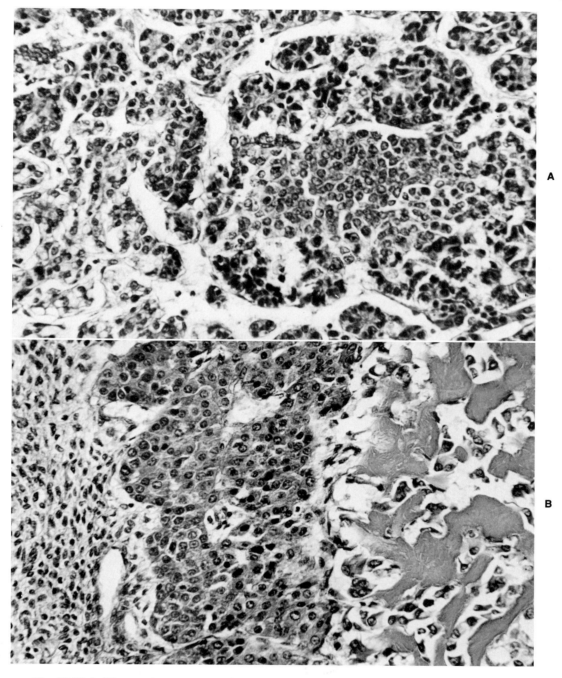

Fig. 13-38 A, Microscopic appearance of "pure" hepatoblastoma. Tumor cells resemble embryonal hepatocytes in different stages of development. **B,** Hepatoblastoma of mixed type. Tumor is composed of spindle cells of embryonal appearance (left), solid cords of hepatocytes (center), and malignant osteoid (right).

Hepatoblastoma invades locally and gives rise to metastases in regional nodes, lung, brain, and other organs. Some patients with hepatoblastoma have a peculiar adenomatoid transformation of the epithelium lining the Bowman's capsule of the renal glomeruli; the pathogenesis of this transformation is unknown.[570]

The treatment of choice is surgical excision with adjunctive chemotherapy. The survival rate is substantially better than for liver cell carcinoma and largely determined by the clinical stage.[566] Among the histologic subtypes, the fetal pattern is associated with a better prognosis than the embryonal variety.[579] The anaplastic subtype is a particularly

Table 13-3 Morphologic comparison between epithelial type of hepatoblastoma and liver cell carcinoma

Histologic findings	Hepatoblastoma	Liver cell carcinoma
Tumor mass	Single	Single or multiple
Pseudocapsule	Present	Usually absent
Trabeculae	Usually two cells thick	Usually many cells thick
Canaliculi	Present	Present
"Light and dark" pattern	Present	Usually absent
Size of cells compared to uninvolved hepatocytes	Smaller	Larger
Pleomorphism	Absent to minimal	Present
Tumor giant cells	Absent	Present
Multinucleated tumor cells	Absent	Present
Bile formation	Present	Present
Glycogen	Present	Present or absent
Fat	Present	Present or absent
Cytoplasmic globular and other inclusions	Absent	Present or absent
Extramedullary hematopoiesis	Present	Absent
Associated cirrhosis	Absent	Present or absent

From Ishak KG, Glunz PR: Hepatoblastoma and hepatocarcinoma in infancy and childhood. Cancer **20**:396-422, 1967.

aggressive form[571] According to Gonzalez-Crussi et al.[566] the macrotrabecular type is also associated with a poor prognosis.

Bile duct tumors and tumorlike conditions
Bile duct hamartoma

Bile duct hamartoma, also known as von Meyenburg or Moschcowitz complex and ductal plate anomaly, presents as multiple, small, whitish nodules scattered throughout the liver, which may be mistaken for metastatic carcinoma by the surgeon. Microscopically, these nodules appear as a focal disorderly collection of bile ducts and ductules surrounded by abundant fibrous stroma.[580,583] It has been suggested that at least some of these lesions are the result of hepatic ischemia.[582] Isolated instances of malignant transformation in the form of bile duct carcinomas have been reported.[581]

Bile duct adenoma

True bile duct adenomas are solitary in over 80% of the cases. Grossly, they appear as well-circumscribed wedge-like white masses, sometimes with a central depression, closely resembling metastatic carcinoma.[586] Most of the lesions are less than 1 cm in diameter and are located subcapsularly.[585] Microscopically, they are made up of small tubular structures with little or no lumen.[584] Inflammation and/or fibrosis are often present (Fig. 13-39). Immunohistochemically, there is reactivity for CEA, EMA, and keratin.[583a] The behavior is benign.

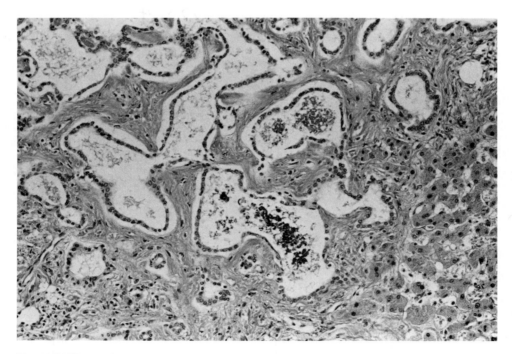

Fig. 13-39 Bile duct hamartoma. Bile ducts show abnormal arrangement but no cytologic abnormalities. They are surrounded by dense fibrous stroma and their dilated lumina contain inspissated bile.

Biliary cystadenoma and cystadenocarcinoma

Benign and malignant cystic tumors of biliary origin can arise in the liver or, less frequently, in the extrahepatic biliary system. In the series of Ishak et al.,[589] all the patients were adults. Grossly, the neoplasms are multilocular and contain a mucinous or clear fluid. The benign tumors are lined by a single layer of cuboidal to tall columnar mucin-producing cells, whereas the malignant varieties show pleomorphism, anaplasia, and stromal infiltration. Benign and malignant areas may coexist, emphasizing the need for thorough sampling. In some cases, occurring only in females, the underlying layer of connective tissue is quite cellular and closely resembles ovarian stroma.[591] In rare cases, the malignant epithelial cells of a cystadenocarcinoma acquire a spindle-shaped pseudosarcomatous appearance.[590]

Some of these cystic bile duct tumors are thought to be related to congenital abnormalities of the bile ducts, such as congenital cysts.[588] Other malignant tumors that have been reported in association with these anomalies include cholangiocarcinoma (see following discussion) and squamous cell carcinoma.[587]

Bile duct carcinoma (cholangiocarcinoma)

Malignant tumors of intrahepatic bile ducts are less common than those of hepatocytes and have no direct relationship with cirrhosis.[592] Some cases have arisen within congenitally dilated intrahepatic bile ducts (Caroli's disease),[593,598] on the basis of congenital hepatic fibrosis,[596]

following Thorotrast administration[604] or anabolic steroid therapy,[605] or in association with intrahepatic lithiasis.[600,601] Most cases of bile duct carcinoma are seen after the age of 60 years. Microscopically, the tumor is an adenocarcinoma, the duct-like structures being lined by cuboidal or columnar cells (Fig. 13-40). A common feature, and one of great diagnostic significance, is the heterogeneity of the neoplastic epithelial cells within the same gland.[606] The tumor has a tendency to spread between hepatocyte plates, along duct walls, and in relation to nerves. The stroma, usually abundant, is sometimes arranged circumferentially around the neoplastic glands. The prominent sinusoidal pattern of liver cell carcinoma is absent. Mucin stains are nearly always positive.[606] Sometimes this mucin production is very abundant and accompanied by the formation of signet ring cells.[595] Immunohistochemically there is consistent reactivity for keratin, EMA, and CEA, features of importance in the differential diagnosis with liver cell carcinoma.[594] The positivity for keratin is seen with monoclonal antibody Cam 5.2 *and also* with monoclonal antibody AE1.[599a] The tumor has also been shown to stain for tissue polypeptide antigen, in contrast to pure liver cell carcinomas.[603]

Although hepatic tumors composed of a mixture of liver cell carcinoma and cholangiocarcinoma do occur,[599] many tumors so designated are, in reality, liver cell carcinomas with focal ductular differentiation, perhaps recapitulating the structure of Herring ducts (so-called cholangiolocellular carcinoma). The ductular formations are lined by tumor cells

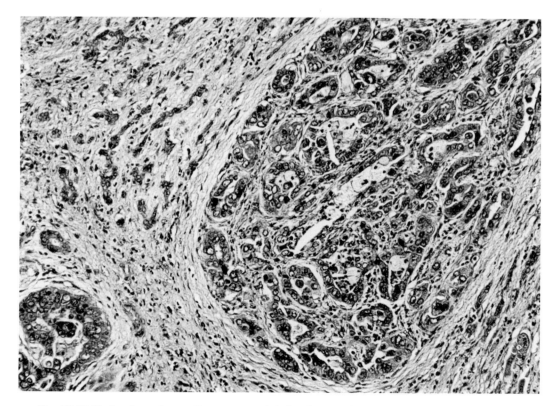

Fig. 13-40 Cholangiocarcinoma. Tumor was entirely intrahepatic. Glandular structures grow in cellular nests, separated by fibrous stroma containing strands of less differentiated tumor cells. Bile pigment is absent.

resembling hepatocytes rather than bile duct cells, both at the light and electron microscopic level,[602] and the luminal content is mucin-negative. The main clinical and pathologic differences between liver cell carcinoma and cholangiocarcinoma are listed in Table 13-4.

We have seen an example of an extremely well-differentiated cholangiocarcinoma, originally diagnosed as bile duct adenoma, which in the course of 15 years replaced almost the entire liver and metastasized to the lung.[597]

Mesenchymal tumors and tumorlike conditions
Vascular tumors

Hemangioma is the most common benign tumor of the liver. In most cases, it is found incidentally at laparotomy or autopsy. Occasionally, it grows large enough to form a clinically apparent mass. When this is the case, complications such as spontaneous bleeding with rupture and se-

questration of platelets resulting in thrombocytopenic purpura may develop. The mass usually projects only slightly above the cut surface, but it may be pedunculated. On section, the spongy appearance and dark red color are characteristic (Fig. 13-41). Microscopically, most liver hemangiomas are of the cavernous type, constituted by widely dilated nonanastomotic vascular spaces lined by flat endothelial cells and supported by fibrous tissue. Thrombi in different stages of organization are often encountered.

Lymphangioma is usually seen in infants or children; in most reported cases, the liver involvement is part of a multicentric process affecting other organs.[629]

Hemangioendothelioma is a highly cellular variant of hemangioma occurring almost exclusively in children (Fig. 13-42). In the series reported by Dehner and Ishak,[610] 87% of the cases were diagnosed prior to 6 months of age. The tumors can be solitary or multiple. The latter are not infre-

Table 13-4 Main clinical and pathologic differences between liver cell carcinoma and bile duct carcinoma

Features	Liver cell carcinoma	Bile duct carcinoma
Cell of origin	Hepatocyte	Bile duct cell
Geographic distribution	Marked variability	Worldwide
Age predilection	Young persons	Older persons
Sex predilection	Males	None
Presence of cirrhosis	Common	Exceptional
Liver cell dysplasia	May be present	Absent
Alpha-fetoprotein	Present	Absent
Bile production	May be present	Absent
Mucin secretion	Absent	Usually present
Gross appearance	Soft and hemorrhagic	Hard and whitish
Preferential spread	Through veins	Through lymphatics

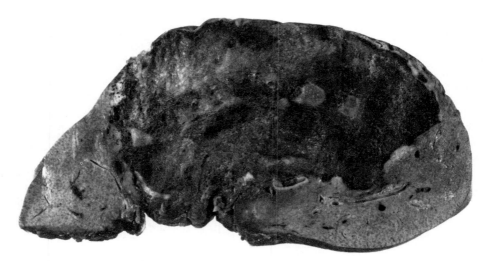

Fig. 13-41 Gross appearance of cavernous hemangioma of liver. Spongy hemorrhagic mass is seen sharply demarcated from liver parenchyma but not encapsulated. There are several nodular foci of degeneration, probably secondary to focal thrombosis. (Courtesy Dr. J. Costa, Lausanne, Switzerland.)

quently associated with hemangiomas in other sites, particularly the skin.[622] There may be a serum elevation of alphafetoprotein. These tumors are associated with a high mortality rate, largely as a result of hepatic failure or congestive heart failure.[610] Microscopically and ultrastructurally, the blood vessels of hemangioendothelioma are lined by one or more layers of plump endothelial cells.[613] The lumen is small or collapsed in most vessels, but cavernous foci can sometimes be identified. A lobular configuration is focally apparent, and anastomosing channels are not a feature.

Epithelioid (histiocytoid) hemangioendothelioma is a distinctive vascular tumor originally described as histiocytoid hemangioma.[625] Most patients are adult females, and there may be a relationship with oral contraceptive use.[609] Grossly, the tumors are often multiple and involve both hepatic lobes. Microscopically, the neoplastic endothelial cells infiltrate sinusoids and veins. These cells are plump, with an acidophilic cytoplasm that is often vacuolated. Immunohistochemically, they exhibit focally positive staining for factor VIII–related antigen, and Weibel-Palade bodies may be seen ultrastructurally.[626] The stroma, usually abundant, may have myxoid, sclerotic, or calcifying features. In retrospect, it is likely that the tumors described by Ludwig et al.[618] and Echevarria et al.[611] belong to the same category. The prognosis is much more favorable than for angiosarcoma, but extrahepatic metastases occurred in 28% of the thirty-two patients reported by Ishak et al.[614] The lung metastases closely simulate the appearance of intravenous bronchiolo-alveolar tumor, a fact that is not surprising in view of their common histogenesis.

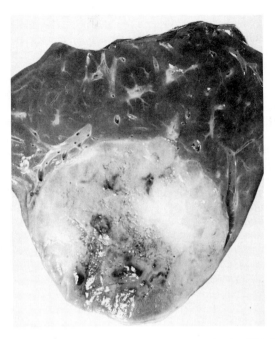

Fig. 13-42 Hemangioendothelioma of liver occurring in child. It was removed successfully.

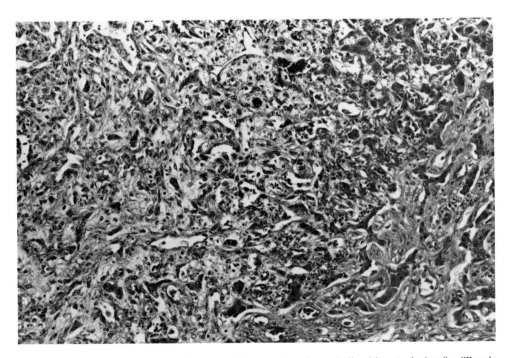

Fig. 13-43 Angiosarcoma of liver. Anastomosing vascular channels lined by atypical cells diffusely permeate liver parenchyma. There are numerous extravasated red blood cells.

Angiosarcoma (hemangiosarcoma; malignant hemangioendothelioma) is characterized by the formation of freely anastomosing vascular channels (Fig. 13-43). The degree of differentiation varies a great deal from case to case, with the better differentiated examples simulating peliosis hepatis or other benign conditions[619] and the poorly differentiated types being difficult to distinguish from primary or metastatic epithelial neoplasms. Factor VIII–related antigen can be detected immunohistochemically in all but the most undifferentiated neoplasms.[621] Most cases occur in adults, but well-documented cases in infants also are on record.[607,612,615,623]

An increased risk for the development of angiosarcoma of the liver in adults has been documented in the following conditions:

1 *Cirrhosis.* It is present in approximately one third of the adult cases and is usually of the macronodular (postnecrotic) type, including the variant that is caused by hemochromatosis.[627]

2 *Vinyl chloride exposure.* It has been shown that hepatic angiosarcoma occurs with undue frequency in workers of chemical plants that produce polyvinyl chloride (PVC), a component of most plastic products such as water pipes, wrapping materials, and building materials.[608] In the series of Makk et al.,[620] the average time of exposure was 16.9 years. Grossly, most tumors are multicentric, hemorrhagic, and necrotic, with areas of cystic degeneration and fibrosis. The non-neoplastic liver often exhibits subcapsular and portal fibrosis, sinusoidal dilatation, and endothelial hyperplasia.[628] The disease is invariably fatal; at autopsy, most of the cases are restricted to the liver or invade the local structures by direct extension; in contrast to the non-PVC-related hepatic angiosarcoma, distant metastases are rare.[620]

3 *Thorium dioxide exposure.* The administration of a suspension of thorium dioxide (Thorotrast) for radiographic purposes has been linked with the late development of hepatic angiosarcoma, the latent period ranging from 20 to 40 years.[617,624] As in the previous group, these tumors are often associated with sinusoidal dilatation and endothelial hyperplasia in the non-neoplastic areas.[617] In some of these patients, the angiosarcoma may be combined with liver cell carcinoma and/or cholangiocarcinoma.[616,630]

4 *Arsenic exposure.* Some cases of hepatic angiosarcomas have followed prolonged therapeutic administration of arsenic in the form of Fowler's solution.

Mesenchymal hamartoma

Mesenchymal hamartoma is a rare benign lesion with a predilection for infants, in whom it appears as a solitary, spherical, reddish nodule.[632] Some examples have a prominent cystic component.[633] Most are asymptomatic and present during the first 2 years of life with abdominal swelling and a palpable abdominal mass.[635] Microscopically, the main component is a well-vascularized mature connective tissue intermixed with elongated branching bile ducts. The low-power appearance is reminiscent of fibroadenoma of the breast[636] (Fig. 13-44). Ultrastructurally, the cells have a mesenchymal, fibroblast-like appearance.[631,634] It has been

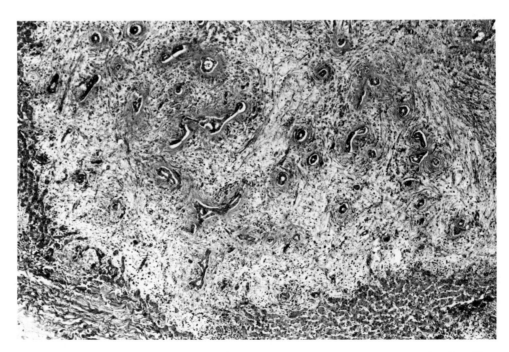

Fig. 13-44 Mesenchymal hamartoma of liver. Combination of collapsed ducts of abundant fibro-edematous stroma is reminiscent of fibroadenoma of breast.

postulated that this lesion arises from the connective tissue of the portal tracts.[631]

Malignant mesenchymoma

Malignant mesenchymoma, also known as undifferentiated or embryonal sarcoma, occurs predominantly in children and is composed of a mixture of highly atypical mesenchymal elements with ultrastructural features of fibroblast-like cells.[637-639] Near the periphery of the tumor, there are entrapped hyperplastic or degenerating bile duct-like structures. PAS-positive hyaline globules frequently are found. Grossly, these tumors are usually large, solitary, and well circumscribed, with multiple areas of necrosis, hemorrhage, and cystic degeneration. The prognosis is very poor; in the series by Stocker and Ishak,[640] the median survival was less than 1 year following diagnosis.

Other mesenchymal tumors

Angiomyolipoma of liver is similar to its more common renal counterpart, being composed of tortuous blood vessels, smooth muscle, and fat.[644] The tumor may have necrosis and pleomorphic epithelioid smooth muscle cells, which may result in a mistaken diagnosis of malignancy. Some lesions contain prominent hematopoietic elements (angiomyo-myelo-lipomas or myelolipomas).[653] In contrast to the renal tumors, hepatic angiomyolipomas are not associated with tuberous sclerosis.

Leiomyoma can present as a solitary hepatic nodule, the obvious differential diagnosis being a metastasis from a well-differentiated leiomyosarcoma.[645] *Lipoma* presents as a single round intraparenchymal mass[647]; it should be distinguished from so-called *hepatic pseudolipoma,* which is a round nodule of fat attached to Glisson's capsule, probably representing entrapped, detached appendix epiploica.[648]

Localized fibrous tumor (so-called localized fibrous mesothelioma) may arise from beneath the liver capsule and involve this organ.[649]

Sarcomas primary in the liver are exceptional. Their differential diagnosis includes metastases from sarcomas of other sites and sarcomatoid liver cell carcinomas. Types of reported primary sarcoma of liver in adults include *fibrosarcoma,*[641] *leiomyosarcoma,*[643,651] *malignant fibrous histiocytoma,*[642] *osteosarcoma,*[654,655] and *osteoclastoma-like giant cell tumor.*[646,650] In infants and children, there have been isolated reports of *embryonal rhabdomyosarcoma* and *rhabdoid tumor.*[652]

Other primary tumors and tumorlike conditions

Epidermoid carcinoma of the liver has been reported as arising from congenital cyst, as a component of teratoma, and in association with intrahepatic lithiasis.[662,670]

Carcinoid tumor in the liver, whether solitary or multiple, represents in the overwhelming majority of the cases the expression of metastatic involvement from a primary tumor usually located in the gastrointestinal tract; however, on some occasions, a typical carcinoid tumor has been seen in the liver in the absence of a neoplasm in any other site after prolonged clinical search or at autopsy.[667a,673] Primary carcinoid tumors of the small bowel can be extremely small,

and it is difficult to dismiss entirely the possibility of their having been missed during the dissection. Yet, under these circumstances it is appropriate to regard the carcinoid tumor as probably originating within the liver. Actually, this occurrence should be expected in view of the presence of Kultschitsky's cells in the normal bile tract and the well-documented occurrence of carcinoid tumors in the gallbladder and extrahepatic biliary system. Hepatic tumors having a lesser differentiated appearance than carcinoids but still exhibiting neuroendocrine features have also been described.[674] The occasional occurrence of neuroendocrine differentiation in liver cell carcinoma was discussed on p. 713.

Teratoma of the liver, an exceptionally rare neoplasm seen predominantly in children but also described in adults, should be distinguished from the mixed type of hepatoblastoma, which is a much more common occurrence.[661,667] Cases of apparently primary *yolk sac tumor* of the liver have been reported.[663,668] Heaton et al.[665] studies two cases of *malignant trophoblastic tumor* with the appearance of choriocarcinoma presenting as liver primaries with massive hemorrhage.

Malignant lymphoma confined to the liver is an exceptionally rare occurrence.[656,668a] Most of the reported cases have been of diffuse large cell type.[660,671,672] A few of the cases have occurred in children.[666] When confined to a single large mass, treatment by hepatic lobectomy may be compatible with long-term survival.[659] Secondary involvement of the liver by non-Hodgkin's lymphoma or Hodgkin's disease is common in stage IV disease.

Leukemic involvement of the liver is frequent in both chronic lymphocytic and chronic myelocytic leukemia. In the former, the infiltrate is predominantly periportal and in the latter predominantly sinusoidal, but many exceptions to this rule exist.

Tumorlike masses in the liver may result from abscesses, congenital hepatic fibrosis,[664] *inflammatory pseudotumors* accompanied by occlusive phlebitis,[658,669] or so-called *solitary necrotic nodules.*[657] It has been suggested that some of the latter may have their origin in sclerosing hemangiomas.[657]

Metastatic tumors

Primary malignant tumors of the gallbladder, extrahepatic bile ducts, pancreas, and stomach frequently involve the liver by direct extension. Carcinomas of the large bowel, lung, breast, pancreas, kidney, stomach, and other organs metastasize to the liver with appalling frequency. Sarcomas of soft tissues or internal organs and malignant melanomas also frequently metastasize to this organ. Within the highly receptive liver parenchyma, these metastases often grow to hugh dimensions.

In a series of 8,455 autopsies of adult patients with malignant tumors, 39% had liver metastases.[681] Only 6% of these were solitary. In eighty-one patients (2.5%), the metastases were confined to this organ; this phenomenon was seven times more frequent for tumors drained by the portal venous system than for the others.

Grossly, metastatic tumors in the liver form discrete masses that may locally elevate the capsule and appear as poorly defined yellow or gray masses. Central necrosis with umbilication occurs in the larger nodules. The absence of visible nodules on the external surface of the liver does not rule out the possibility of metastatic involvement. Sometimes large metastases are completely hidden within the parenchyma.[684]

A certain correlation exists between the site of the primary tumor and the gross appearance of the liver metastases. Metastases from carcinoma of the large bowel often result in a few large nodules with marked central umbilication; when mucin production is abundant, they tend to undergo marked calcification that may be apparent roentgenographically. Well-differentiated squamous cell carcinomas result in very soft nodules because of necrosis and keratinization. The nodules from lung or breast cancer are usually medium sized, without extensive necrosis or hemorrhage, and with early central umbilication. The metastases from gallbladder carcinoma cluster around the gallbladder bed and progressively diminish in size as they move farther into the hepatic parenchyma. Occasionally, extremely small, almost miliary metastatic lesions are seen spreading throughout the liver and even simulating cirrhosis[675]; they are usually the result of tumors from the breast, prostate, or stomach.

It is often said that liver metastases from cancers of the right colon tend to be located in the right lobe and those from the left colon and rectum in the left lobe, but the difference in frequency—if any—probably has no statistical validity.[683] Metastatic breast carcinoma treated with chemotherapy can result in the coarsely lobulated liver appearance known as *hepar lobatum*, traditionally associated with syphilis.[682]

Many benign lesions may have a gross appearance indistinguishable from metastatic carcinoma. This is true of fibrous scars, healed granulomas, bile duct hamartoma or adenoma, and nodular hyperplasia. Therefore *it is imperative that a microscopic confirmation be obtained in every patient in whom lesions suggestive of liver metastases are detected at laparotomy*, regardless of how typical grossly they might seem to the surgeon or the pathologist.

A percutaneous liver biopsy will be positive in about 75% of the cases with widespread metastatic liver disease. For laparoscopically directed biopsies, the incidence of positivity is much higher. Fine needle biopsy aspiration is being increasingly used for the diagnosis of liver metastases with excellent results.[676-678,685]

Naturally, the finding of multiple hepatic metastases at exploration makes all surgical attempts of only temporary palliative value. However, in carefully selected patients with a single bloodborne metastatic lesion or with direct extension into the liver by a neighboring malignant tumor, partial hepatectomy may result in long-term palliation and, exceptionally, in cure.[679,686] Resection of hepatic metastases is particularly worthwhile in patients with metastatic carcinoid because of the dramatic amelioration of the symptoms of the carcinoid syndrome often achieved.[680]

REFERENCES
BIOPSY

1 Bull HJM, Gilmore IT, Bradley RD, Marigold RD, Thompson RPH: Experience with transjugular liver biopsy. Gut 24:1057-1060, 1983.
2 Combes B: The initial morphologic lesion in chronic hepatitis, important or unimportant? Hepatology 6:518-522, 1986.
3 Czaja AJ, Wolf AM, Baggenstoss AH, Schoenfield LJ: Clinical assessment of cirrhosis in severe chronic active liver disease. Specificity and sensitivity of physical and laboratory findings. Mayo Clin Proc 55:360-364, 1980.
4 Edmonson HA, Peters RL: Diagnostic problems in liver biopsies. Pathol Annu 2:213-242, 1967.
4a Gerber MA, Thung SN: Histology of the liver. Am J Surg Pathol 11:709-722, 1987.
5 Hall-Craggs MA, Lees WR: Fine needle biopsy. Cytology, histology or both? Gut 28:233-236, 1987.
6 Hegarty JE, Williams R: Liver biopsy. Techniques, clinical applications and complications. Br Med J 288:1254-1256, 1984.
7 Limberg B, Hopker WW, Kommerell B: Histologic differential diagnosis of focal liver lesions by ultrasonically guided fine needle aspiration. Gut 28:237-241, 1987.
8 Lindner H: Grenzen und Gefahren der perkutanen Leberbiopsie mit der Menghini-Nadel. Erfahrungen bei 80,000 Leberbiopsien. Dtsch Med Wochenschr 92:1751-1757, 1967.
9 Maharaj B, Maharaj RJ, Leary WP, Coopan RM, Naran AD, Pirie D, Pudifin DJ: Sampling variability and its influence on the diagnostic yield of percutaneous needle biopsy of the liver. Lancet 1:523-525, 1986.
10 Menghini G: One-second needle biopsy of the liver. Gastroenterology 35:190-199, 1958.
11 Menghini G: One-second biopsy of the liver. Problems of its clinical application. N Engl J Med 283:582-585, 1970.
11a Miruk GY, Sutherland LR, Wiseman DA, MacDonald FR, Ding DL: Prospective study of the incidence of ultrasound-detected intrahepatic and subcapsular hematomas in patients randomized to 6 or 24 hours of bed rest after percutaneous liver biopsy. Gastroenterology 92:290-293, 1987.
12 Morris JS, Gallo GA, Scheuer PJ, Sherlock S: Percutaneous liver biopsy in patients with large bile duct obstruction. Gastroenterology 68:750-754, 1975.
13 Petrelli M, Scheuer PJ: Variation in subcapsular liver structure and its significance in the interpretation of wedge biopsies. J Clin Pathol 20:743-748, 1967.
14 Popper H, Steigman F, Meyer KA, Kozoll DD, Franklin M: Correlation of liver function and liver structure. Am J Med 6:278-291, 1949.
15 Post J, Rose JV: Clinical, functional, and histologic studies in Laennec's cirrhosis of the liver. Am J Med 8:300-313, 1950.
16 Scheur PJ: Liver biopsy interpretation. London, 1973, Baillière Tindall.
17 Schiff L, Gall E, Oikawa Y: In Proceedings of World Congress on Gastroenterology, Baltimore, 1958, The Williams & Wilkins Co.
18 Schlichting P, Holund B, Poulsen H: Liver biopsy in chronic aggressive hepatitis. Diagnostic reproducibility in relation to size of specimen. Scand J Gastroenterol 18:27-32, 1983.
19 Soloway RD, Baggenstoss AH, Schonfield LJ, Summerskill WHJ: Observer error and sampling variability in evaluation of hepatitis and cirrhosis by liver biopsy. Am J Dig Dis 16:1082-1086, 1971.
20 Thaler H: Uber Vorteil und Risiko der Leberbiopsiemethod nach Menghini. Wien Klin Wochenschr 76:533-538, 1964.
21 Whitmore LF, Galambos JT: Image guided percutaneous hepatic biopsy. Diagnostic accuracy and safety. J Clin Gastroenterol 7:511-515, 1985.

VIRAL HEPATITIS

22 Aach RD: Viral hepatitis. A to E. Med Clin North Am 62:59-69, 1978.
23 Abe H, Beninger PR, Ikejiri N, Setayama H, Sara M, Tarikawa K: Light microscopic findings of liver biopsy specimens from patients with hepatitis type A and comparison with type B. Gastroenterology 82:938-947, 1982.
24 Berman M, Alter HJ, Ishak KG, Purcell RH, Jones EA: The chronic sequelae of non-A, non-B hepatitis. Ann Intern Med 91:1-6, 1979.
25 Bianchi L: Liver biopsy interpretation in hepatitis. II. Histopathology and classification of acute and chronic hepatitis. Pathol Res Pract 178:170-213, 1983.
26 Bianchi L: Necroinflammatory liver diseases. Semin Liver Dis 6:185-198, 1986.
27 Bianchi L, De Groote J, Desmet VJ, Gedigk P, Korb G, Popper H, Poulsen H, Scheuer PJ, Schmid M, Thaler H, Wepler W: Morphological criteria in viral hepatitis. Lancet 1:333-337, 1971.
28 Boyer JL, Klatskin G: Pattern of necrosis in acute viral hepatitis. Prognostic value of bridging (subacute hepatic necrosis). N Engl J Med 283:1063-1071, 1970.

29 Boyer JL: Chronic hepatitis. A perspective on classification and determinants of prognosis. Gastroenterology **70**:1161-1171, 1976.

30 Boyer JL: The diagnosis and pathogenesis of clinical variants in viral hepatitis. Am J Clin Pathol **65**:898-908, 1976.

31 Buitrago B, Popper H, Hadler SC, Thung SN, Gerber MA, Purcell RH, Maynard JE: Specific histologic features of Santa Marta hepatitis. A severe form of hepatitis delta virus infection in northern South America. Hepatology **6**:1285-1291, 1986.

32 Craig JR, Govindarajan S, DeCock KM: Delta viral hepatitis. Histopathology and course. Pathol Annu **21**(Pt 2):1-21, 1986.

33 Dienes HP, Popper H, Arnold W, Lobeck H: Histologic observations in human hepatitis non-A, non-B. Hepatology **2**:562-571, 1982.

34 Dienstag JL: Non-A, non-B hepatitis. I. Recognition, epidemiology and clinical features. Gastroenterology **85**:439-462, 1983.

35 Dietrichson O, Zoffman H, Christoffersen P, Hilden M, Juhl E, Thomsen A: Chronic acute hepatitis. A prognostic study with observation time up to 37 years. Acta Med Scand **202**:271-276, 1977.

36 Dubin IN, Sullivan BH, LeGolvan PC, Murphy LC: The cholestatic form of viral hepatitis. Experiences with viral hepatitis at Brooke Army Hospital during the years 1951 to 1953. Am J Med **29**:55-72, 1960.

37 Duffy LF, Daum F, Kahn E, Teichberg S, Pahwa R, Fagin J, Kenigsberg K, Kaplan M, Fisher SE, Pahwa S: Hepatitis in children with acquired immunodeficiency syndrome. Histopathologic and immunocytologic features. Gastroenterology **90**:173-181, 1986.

38 Dworkin BM, Stahl RE, Giardina MA, Wormser GP, Weiss L, Jankowski R, Rosenthal WS: The liver in acquired immunodeficiency syndrome. Emphasis on patients with intravenous drug abuse. Am J Gastroenterol **82**:231-236, 1987.

39 Fagan EA, Williams R: Non-A, non-B hepatitis. Semin Liver Dis **4**:314-355, 1984.

40 Fagan EA, Williams R: Viral hepatitis (excluding hepatitis B). Practitioner **231**:380-385, 1987.

41 Gilliam JH, Geisinger KR, Richter JE: Primary hepatocellular carcinoma after chronic non-A, non-B posttransfusion hepatitis. Ann Intern Med **1001**:794-795, 1984.

42 Glasglow BJ, Anders K, Layfield LJ, Steinsaper KD, Gitnick GL, Lewin KJ: Clinical and pathologic findings of the liver in the acquired immune deficiency syndrome (AIDS). Am J Clin Pathol **83**:582-588, 1985.

43 Govindarajan S, DeCock KM, Peters RL: Morphologic and immunohistochemical features of fulminant delta hepatitis. Hum Pathol **16**:262-268, 1985.

44 Guarda LA, Luna MA, Smith JL Jr, Mansell PW, Gyorkey F, Roca AN: Acquired immunodeficiency syndrome. Postmortem findings. Am J Clin Pathol **81**:549-557, 1984.

45 Hadler SC, de Monzon M, Ponzetta A, Anzola E, Rivero D, Mondolfi A, Bracho A, Francis DP, Gerber MA, Thung S: Delta virus infection and severe hepatitis. An epidemic in the Yucpa Indians of Venezuela. Ann Intern Med **100**:223-229, 1983.

46 Hansson BG, Moestrup T, Widell A, Nordenfelt E: Infection with delta agent in Sweden. Introduction of a new hepatitis agent. J Infect Dis **146**:472-478, 1982.

47 Hay CRM, Triger DR, Preston FE, Underwood JCE: Progressive liver disease in haemophilia. An understated problem? Lancet **2**:1495-1498, 1985.

48 Hug G: Genetic factors and autoimmunity in viral hepatitis. Am J Clin Pathol **65**:870-875, 1976.

49 Ishak KG: Light microscopic morphology of viral hepatitis. Am J Clin Pathol **65**:787-827, 1976.

50 Kahn SA, Saltzman BR, Klein RS, Mahadevia PS, Friedland GH, Brandt LJ: Hepatic disorders in the acquired immune deficiency syndrome. A clinical and pathological study. Am J Gastroenterol **81**:1145-1148, 1986.

51 Karvountzis GG, Redeker AG, Peters RL: Long-term follow-up studies of patients surviving fulminant viral hepatitis. Gastroenterology **67**:870-877, 1974.

52 Kiyosawa K, Akahane Y, Nagata A, Furuta S: Hepatocellular carcinoma after non-A, non-B posttransfusion hepatitis. Am J Gastroenterol **79**:777-781, 1984.

52a Klatt EC, Shibata D: Cytomegalovirus infection in the acquired immunodeficiency syndrome. Arch Pathol Lab Med **112**:540-544, 1988.

53 Koretz RL, Stone O, Mousa M, Gitnick GL: Non-A, non-B posttransfusion hepatitis. A decade later. Gastroenterology **88**:125-1254, 1985.

53a Lebovics E, Dworkin BM, Heier SK, Rosenthal WS: The hepatobiliary manifestations of human immunodeficiency virus infection. Am J Gastroenterol **83**:1-7, 1988.

54 Lebovics E, Thung SN, Schaffner F, Radensky PW: The liver in the acquired immunodeficiency syndrome. A clinical and histologic study. Hepatology **5**:293-293, 1985.

55 Lefkowitch JH, Apfelbaum TF: Liver cell dysplasia and hepatocellular carcinoma in non-A, non-B hepatitis. Arch Pathol Lab Med **111**:170-173, 1987.

56 Lok ASF, Lindsay I, Scheuer PJ, Thomas HC: Clinical and histologic features of delta infection in chronic hepatitis B virus carriers. J Clin Pathol **38**:530-533, 1985.

57 Mathieson RD, Sampliner RE, Latham PS, Rogers EL, Alter MJ: Chronic liver disease following community acquired non-A, non-B hepatitis. Am J Clin Pathol **85**:353-356, 1986

58 Mck Thorne CH, Higgans GR, Ulich TR, Gitnick GL, Klaus I, Lewin J: A histologic comparison of hepatitis B with non-A, non-B chronic active hepatitis. Arch Pathol Lab Med **106**:433-436, 1982.

59 Nakanuma Y, Liew CT, Peters RL, Govindarajan S: Pathologic features of the liver in acquired immunodeficiency syndrome (AIDS). Liver **6**:158-166, 1986.

60 Okuda K: Primary liver cancer. Quadrennial review lecture. Dig Dis Sci **31**(Suppl):133S-146S, 1985.

61 Orenstein MS, Tavitian A, Yonk B, Dincsoy HP, Zerega J, Iyer SK, Straus EW: Granulomatous involvement of the liver in patients with AIDS. Gut **26**:1220-1226, 1985.

62 Peters RL: Viral hepatitis. A pathologic spectrum. Am J Med Sci **270**:17-31, 1975.

63 Popper H: General pathology of the liver. Light microscopic aspects serving diagnosis and interpretation. Semin Liver Dis **6**:175-184, 1986.

64 Popper H, Thung SN, Gerber MA, Hadler SC, de Monzon M, Ponzetto A, Anzola E, Rivera D, Mondolfi A, Brachos A, Francis DP, Gerin JL, Maynard JE, Purcell RH: Histologic studies of severe delta agent infection in Venezuelan Indians. Hepatology **3**:906-912, 1983.

65 Reichert CM, O'Leary TJ, Levens DL, Simrell CR, Macher AM: Autopsy pathology in the acquired immunodeficiency syndrome. Am J Pathol **112**:357-382, 1983.

66 Rizzetto M: The delta agent. Hepatology **3**:729-737, 1983.

67 Rizzetto M, Canese MG, Arico S, Crivelli O, Trepo C, Bonino F, Verme G: Immunofluoresence detection of new antigen-antibody system associated with hepatitis B virus in liver and serum of HB$_s$A$_g$ carriers. Gut **18**:997-1003, 1977.

68 Rueff B, Benhanion JP: Acute hepatic necrosis and fulminant hepatic failure. Gut **14**:805-815, 1973.

69 Rustgi VK, Hoofnagle JH, Gerin JL, Gelmann EP, Reichert CM, Cooper JN, Macher AM: Hepatitis B virus infection in the acquired immunodeficiency syndrome. Ann Intern Med **101**:795-797, 1984.

70 Schaffner F: The structural basis of altered hepatic function in viral hepatitis. Am J Med **49**:659-667, 1970.

71 Schmid M, Pirovino M, Altorfer J, Gudat F, Bianchi L: Acute hepatitis non-A, non-B. Are there specific light microscopic features? Liver **2**:61-67, 1982.

72 Shiels MT, Czaja AJ, Taswell HF, Gerin JL, Purcell RH, Ludwig J, Rakela J, Nelson CA: Frequency and significance of delta antibody in acute and chronic hepatitis B. A United States experience. Gastroenterology **89**:1230-1234, 1985.

73 Smedile A, Lavarini C, Farci P, Arico S, Marinucci G, Dentico P, Guiliani G, Cargnel A, Del Vecchio Blanco C, Rizzetto M: Epidemiologic patterns of infection with the hepatitis B virus associated delta agent in Italy. Am J Epidemiol **117**:223-229, 1983.

74 Teixeira MR, Weller IVD, Murray A, Bamber M, Thomas HC, Sherlock S, Scheurer PJ: The pathology of hepatitis A in man. Liver **2**:53-60, 1982.

75 Trump BF, Kim KM, Iseri OA: Cellular pathophysiology of hepatitis. Am J Clin Pathol **65**:828-847, 1976.

76 Verme G, Amoroso P, Lettieri G, Pierri P, David E, Sessa F, Rizzi R, Bonino F, Recchia S, Rizzetto M: A histologic study of hepatitis delta virus liver disease. Hepatology **6**:1303-1307, 1986.

77 Volmer J, Lüders CJ, Henning H: Semiquantitative and morphometric investigations on the histopathology of chronic hepatitis non-A, non-B. Z Gastroenterol **23**:632-642, 1985.

78 Ware A, Eigenbradt EH, Combes B: Prognostic significance of subacute hepatic necrosis in acute hepatitis. Gastroenterology **68**:519-524, 1975.

79 Welch K, Finkbeiner W, Alpers CE, Blumenfeld W, Davis RL, Smuckler EA, Beckstead JH: Autopsy findings in the acquired immunodeficiency syndrome. JAMA **252**:1152-1159, 1984.

CHRONIC HEPATITIS

80 Baggenstoss AH, Soloway RD, Summerskill WHJ, Schoenfield LJ: Chronic active liver disease. The range of histologic lesions, their response to treatment, and evaluation. Hum Pathol **3**:183-198, 1972.

81 Boyer JL: Chronic hepatitis. A perspective on classification and determinants of prognosis. Gastroenterology **70**:1161-1171, 1976.

82 Chadwick RG, Galizzi J Jr, Heathcote J, Lyssiotis T, Cohen BJ, Scheuer PJ, Sherlock S: Chronic persistent hepatitis. Hepatitis B virus markers and histological follow-up. Gut 20:372-377, 1979.

82a Chang M-H, Hwang L-Y, Hsu H-C, Lee C-Y, Beasley RP: Prospective study of asymptomatic HB$_x$A$_g$ carrier children infected in the perinatal period. Clinical and liver histologic studies. Hepatology 8:374-377, 1988.

83 Combes B: The initial morphologic lesion in chronic hepatitis, important or unimportant? Hepatology 6:518-522, 1986.

84 Cook GC, Mulligan R, Sherlock S: Controlled perspective trial of cortiosteroid therapy in active chronic hepatitis. Q J Med 40:159-185, 1971.

85 Cooksley WGE, Bradbear RA, Robinson W, Harrison M, Halliday JW, Powell LW, Ng HS, Seah CS, Okuda K, Scheur PJ, Sherlock S: The prognosis of chronic active hepatitis without cirrhosis in relation to bridging necrosis. Hepatology 6:345-348, 1986.

86 Cuccurullo L, Rambaldi M, Iaquinto G, Ferraraccio F, Ambrosone L, Giardullo N, Devita A: Importance of showing HB$_s$A$_g$ and HB$_c$A$_g$ positivity for better aetiologic definition of chronic liver disease. J Clin Pathol 40:167-171, 1987.

87 De Groote J, Fevery J, Lepoutre L: Long-term follow-up of chronic active hepatitis of moderate severity. Gut 19:510-513, 1978.

88 Dietrichson O: Chronic persistent hepatitis. A clinical, serological, and prognostic study. Scand J Gastroenterol 10:249-255, 1975.

89 Dietrichson O, Christoffersen P: The prognosis of chronic aggressive hepatitis. Scand J Gastroenterol 12:289-295, 1977.

90 Gerber MA, Thung SN: The diagnostic value of immunohistochemical demonstration of hepatitis viral antigens in the liver. Hum Pathol 18:771-774, 1987.

91 Hadziyannis S, Gerber MA, Vissoulis C, Popper H: Cytoplasmic hepatitis B antigen in "ground glass" hepatocytes of carriers. Arch Pathol 96:327-330, 1973.

91a Hsu H-C, Lin Y-H, Chang M-H, Su I-J, Chen D-S: Pathology of chronic hepatitis B virus infection in children. With special reference to the intrahepatic expression of hepatitis B virus antigens. Hepatology 8:378-382, 1988.

92 International Group: A classification of chronic hepatitis. Lancet 2:626-628, 1968.

93 International Group: Acute and chronic hepatitis revisited. Lancet 2:914-919, 1977.

94 Ishak KG: Light microscopic morphology of viral hepatitis. Am J Clin Pathol 65:787-827, 1976.

95 Kenny RP, Czaja AJ, Ludwig J, Dickson ER: Frequency and significance of antimitochondrial antibodies in severe chronic active hepatitis. Dig Dis Sci 31:705-711, 1986.

96 Klinge O, Bannasch P: Zur Vermehrung der glutten endoplasmatischen Retikulum in Hepatocyten menschlicher Leberpunktate. Verh Dtsch Ges Pathol 52:568-573, 1968.

97 Kostich ND, Ingham D: Detection of hepatitis B surface antigen by means of orcein staining of liver. Am J Clin Pathol 67:20-30, 1977.

97a Lindh G, Weiland O, Glaumann H: The application of a numerical scoring system for evaluating the histologic outcome in patients with chronic hepatitis B followed in long term. Hepatology 8:98-103, 1988.

98 Lok ASF, Lindsay I, Scheuer PJ, Thomas HC: Clinical and histologic features of delta infection in chronic hepatitis B virus carriers. J Clin Pathol 38:530-533, 1985.

99 Mathiesen JL, Fauerholdt L, Moller AM, Aldershule J, Dietrichson O, Hardt F, Nielsen JO, Skin Hoj P, The Copenhagen Hepatitis Acuta Programme: Immunofluoresence studies for hepatitis A virus and hepatitis B surface and core antigen in liver biopsies from patients with acute viral hepatitis. Gastroenterology 77:623-628, 1979.

99a Mondelli MU, Manas M, Ferrari C: Does the immune response play a role in the pathogenesis of chronic liver disease? Arch Pathol Lab Med 112:489-497, 1988.

100 Murray-Lyon IM, Stern RB, Williams R: Controlled trial of prednisone and azathioprine in active chronic hepatitis. Lancet 1:735-737, 1973.

101 Okuno T, Okanoue T, Takino T, Mori K: Prognostic significance of bridging necrosis in chronic active hepatitis. Gastroenterol Jpn 18:577-584, 1983.

102 Penner E: Nature of immune complexes in autoimmune chronic active hepatitis. Gastroenterology 92:304-308, 1987.

103 Pontisso P, Chemello L, Fattovich G: Relationship between HB$_c$A$_g$ in serum and liver and HBV replication in patients with HB$_s$A$_g$ positive chronic liver disease. J Med Virol 17:145-150, 1985.

104 Popper H: Changing concepts of the evolution of chronic hepatitis and the role of piecemeal necrosis. Hepatology 3:758-762, 1983.

105 Redeker AG: Viral hepatitis. Clinical aspects. Am J Med Sci 270:9-16, 1975.

106 Rijntjes PJ, van Ditzhuijsen TJ, Van Loon AM, Van Hoelst UJ, Bronkhorst FB, Yap SH: Hepatitis B virus DNA detected in formalin-fixed liver specimens and its relation with serologic markers and histopathologic features in chronic liver disease. Am J Pathol 120:411-418, 1985.

107 Schaffner F: Autoimmune chronic active hepatitis. Three decades of progress. Prog Liver Dis 8:486-503, 1986.

108 Sampliner R: Chronic active hepatitis in hepatitis B surface antigen (HBsAg) carriers. The need for liver biopsy. JAMA 237:50-51, 1977.

109 Schalm SW, Korman MG, Summerskill WHJ, Czaja AJ, Baggenstoss AH: Severe chronic active liver disease. Prognostic significance of initial morphological patterns. Am J Dig Dis 22:973-980, 1977.

110 Schalm SW, Summerskill WHJ, Gitnick GL, Elvebuck LR: Contrasting features and responses to treatment of severe chronic active liver disease with and without HB$_s$A$_g$. Gut 17:781-786, 1976.

111 Scheuer PJ: Changing views on chronic hepatitis. Histopathology 10:1-4, 1986.

112 Shikata T, Uzawa T, Yoshiwara N, Akatuska T, Yamazaki S: Staining methods of Australian antigen in paraffin section. Detection of cytoplasmic inclusion bodies. Jpn J Exp Med 44:25-35, 1974.

113 Shrago SS, Auslander MO, Gitnick GL: Hepatic pathologic condition in asymptomatic Australia antigen carriers. Arch Pathol Lab Med 101:648-651, 1977.

114 Soloway RD, Summerskill WHJ, Baggenstoss AH, Geall MG, Gitnick GL, Elveback LR, Schoenfield LJ: Clinical, biochemical, and histological remission of severe chronic active liver disease. A controlled study of treatement and early prognosis. Gastroenterology 63:820-833, 1972.

115 Trump BF, Kim KM, Iseri OA: Cellular pathophysiology of hepatitis. Am J Clin Pathol 65:828-847, 1976.

116 Wright EC, Seeff LB, Berk PD, Jones EA, Plotz PH: Clinical trends and topics. Treatment of chronic active hepatitis. An analysis of three controlled trials. Gastroenterology 73:1422-1430, 1977.

DRUG-INDUCED LIVER DISEASE

117 Bagheri SA, Boyer JL: Peliosis hepatis associated with androgenic-anabolic steroid therapy. Ann Intern Med 81:610-618, 1974.

118 Berthelot P: Mechanisms and prediction of drug-induced liver disease. Gut 14:332-339, 1973.

119 Brady J, Liberatore F, Harper P, Greenwald P, Burnett W, Davies JNP, Bishop M, Polan A, Vianna N: Angiosarcoma of the liver. An epidemiologic survey. J Natl Cancer Inst 59:1383-1385, 1977.

119a Chopra S, Edelstein A, Koff RS, Zimelman AP, Lacson A, Neiman RS: Peliosis hepatis in hematologic disease. JAMA 240:1153-1155, 1978.

120 Christopherson WM, Mays ET: Liver tumors and contraceptive steroids. Experience with the first one hundred registry patients. J Natl Cancer Inst 58:167-171, 1977.

121 Farrell GC: The hepatic side effects of drugs. Med J Aust 145:600-604, 1986.

122 Fechner RE: Benign hepatic lesions and orally administered contraceptives. A report of seven cases and a critical analysis of the literature. Hum Pathol 8:255-268, 1977.

123 Griner PF, Elbadawi A, Packman CH: Veno-occlusive disease of the liver after chemotherapy of acute leukemia. Ann Intern Med 85:578-582, 1976.

123a Hillian D, de View E, Bargue A, Bruet A, Dongrade G, Frendler JP: Peliosis hepatis in a chronic hemodialysis patient. Nephron 35:205-206, 1983.

124 Ishak KG, Irey NS: Hepatic injury associated with the phenothiazines. Arch Pathol 93:283-304, 1972.

125 Ishak KG, Kirchner JP, Dhar JK: Granulomas and cholestatic-hepatocellular injury associated with phenylbutazone. Report of two cases. Am J Dig Dis 22:611-617, 1977.

126 Johnson GK, Tolman KG: Chronic liver disease and acetaminophen. Ann Intern Med 87:302-304, 1977.

127 Kaplowitz N, Aw TY, Simon FR, Stolz A: Drug induced hepatotoxicity. Ann Intern Med 104:826-839, 1986.

128 Klatskin G: Toxic and drug-induced hepatitis. In Schiff L (ed): Disease of the liver, ed. 4. Philadelphia, 1975, J.B. Lippincott Co., pp. 604-710.

129 Koch HK, Gropp A, Oehlert W: Drug-induced liver injury in liver biopsies of the years 1981 and 1983. Their prevalence and type of presentation. Pathol Res Pract 179:469-480, 1985.

130 Lander JJ, Stanley RJ, Sumner HW, Boswell DC, Aach RD: Angiosarcoma of the liver associated with Fowler's solution (potassium arsenite). Gastroenterology 68:1582-1586, 1975.

131 Ludwig J, Axelsen R: Drug effects upon the liver. Dig Dis Sci 7:651-666, 1983.

132 Maddrey WC, Boitnott JK: Progress in hepatology. Drug-induced chronic liver disease. Gastroenterology 72:1348-1353, 1977.

133 Marubbio AT, Danielson B: Hepatic veno-occlusive disease in a renal transplant patient receiving azathioprine. Gastroenterology 69:739-743, 1975.

134 Nadell J, Kosek J: Peliosis hepatis. Twelve cases associated with oral androgen therapy. Arch Pathol Lab Med 101:405-410, 1977.

135 Paton A: Diseases of the alimentary system. Drug jaundice. Br Med J 2:1126-1127, 1976.

136 Perez V, Schaffner F, Popper H: Hepatic drug reactions. Prog Liv Dis 4:597-625, 1972.

137 Pimentel JC, Menezes AP: Liver disease in vineyard sprayers. Gastroenterology **72**:275-283, 1977.

138 Portmann B, Talbot IC, Day DW, Davidson AR, Murray-Lyon IM, Williams R: Histopathological changes in the liver following a paracetamol overdose. Correlation with clinical and biochemical parameters. J Pathol **117**:169-181, 1974.

139 Rappaport AM, Borowy ZJ, Lougheed WM, Lotto WN: Subdivision of hexagonal liver lobules into a structural and functional unit. Role in hepatic physiology and pathology. Anat Rec **119**:11-34, 1954.

140 Reed GB, Cox AJ: The human liver after radiation injury. A form of venoocclusive disease. Am J Pathol **48**:597-611, 1966.

141 Spitz RD, Keren DF, Boitnott JK, Maddrey WC: Bridging hepatic necrosis. Etiology and prognosis. Am J Dig Dis **23**:1076-1078, 1978.

142 Stenger RJ: Liver disease. Hum Pathol **8**:603-619, 1977.

143 Stuart KL, Bras G: Veno-occlusive disease of the liver. Q J Med **26**:291-320, 1957.

143a Thomas LB, Popper H, Berk PD, Selikoff I, Fank H: Vinyl chloride induced liver disease. N Engl J Med **292**:17-22, 1975.

144 Winkler K, Poulsen H: Liver disease with periportal sinusoidal dilatation. A possible complication to contraceptive steroids. Scand J Gastroenterol **10**:699-704, 1975.

145 Wu SM, Spurny OM, Klotz AP: Budd-Chiari syndrome after taking oral contraceptives. A case report and review of 14 reported cases. Am J Dig Dis **22**:623-628, 1977.

145a Zafrani ES, Grazier A, Brandelot AM, Feldman G: Ultrastructural lesions of the liver in human peliosis. A report of 12 cases. Am J Pathol **114**:329-359, 1984.

146 Zimmerman HJ: Drug-induced liver disease. An overview. Semin Liver Dis **1**:93-103, 1981.

147 Zimmerman HJ: Hepatotoxic effects of oncotherapeutic agents. Prog Liver Dis **8**:621-642, 1986.

ALCOHOL-INDUCED LIVER DISEASE

147a Achord JL: Nutrition, alcohol and the liver. Am J Gastroenterol **83**:244-248, 1988.

148 Afshani P, Littenberg GD, Wollman J, Kaplowitz N: Significance of microscopic cholangitis in alcoholic liver disease. Gastroenterology **75**:1045-1050, 1978.

149 Ballard H, Bernstein M, Farrar J: Fatty liver presenting as obstructive jaundice. Am J Med **30**:196-201, 1961.

150 Barbatis C, Morton J, Woods JC, Burns J, Bradley J, McGee JO: Disorganization of intermediate filament structure in alcoholic and other liver disorders. Gut **27**:765-770, 1986.

151 Bruguera M, Bertran A, Bombi J, Rodes J: Giant mitochondria in hepatocytes. A diagnostic hint for alcoholic liver disease. Gastroenterology **73**:1383-1387, 1977.

152 Bruguera M, Bordas J, Rodes J: Asymptomatic liver disease in alcoholics. Arch Pathol Lab Med **101**:644-647, 1977.

153 Brunt PW: Alcohol and the liver. Gut **12**:222-229, 1971.

154 Burt AD, MacSween RNM: Hepatic vein lesions in alcoholic liver disease. Retrospective biopsy and necropsy study. J Clin Pathol **29**:63-67, 1986.

155 Christoffersen P, Nielsen K: Histological changes in human liver biopsies from chronic alcoholics. Acta Pathol Microbiol Scand [A] **80**:557-565, 1972.

156 Edmondson H, Peters R, Reynolds T, Kuzma O: Sclerosing hyalin necrosis of the liver in the chronic alcoholic. Ann Intern Med **59**:646-673, 1963.

157 Fallon HJ: Alcohol and the terminal hepatic venule. Early lesion or late residual? Gastroenterology **83**:930-932, 1982.

158 Glover S, McPhie J, Brunt P: Cholestasis in acute alcoholic liver disease. Lancet **1**:1305-1307, 1977.

159 Goldberg S, Mendenhall C, Connell A, Chedid A: "Nonalcoholic" chronic hepatitis in the alcoholic. Gastroenterology **72**:598-604, 1977.

160 Goodman ZD, Ishak KG: Occlusive venous lesions in alcoholic liver disease. A study of 200 cases. Gastroenterology **83**:786-796, 1982.

161 Insunza I, Iturriaga H, Ugarte G, Altschiller H: Clinical and histological liver abnormalities in alcoholics. Acta Hepatosplenol (Stuttg) **18**:460-470, 1971.

162 Kimoff RJ, Huang S-N: Immunocytochemical and immunoelectron microscopic studies on Mallory bodies. Lab Invest **45**:491-503, 1981.

163 Leevy C, Chen T, Luisada-Opper A, Kanagasundaram N, Zetterman R: Liver disease of the alcoholic. Role of immunologic abnormalities in pathogenesis, recognition, and treatment. Prog Liver Dis **5**:516-530, 1976.

164 Lelbach W: Epidemiology of alcoholic liver disease. Prog Liver Dis **5**:494-515, 1976.

165 Levin DM, Baker AL, Riddell RH, Rochman H, Boyer JL: Nonalcoholic liver disease. Overlooked causes of liver injury in patients with heavy alcohol consumption. Am J Med **66**:429-434, 1979.

166 Morgan MY, Sherlock S, Scheuer PJ: Portal fibrosis in the livers of alcoholic patients. Gut **19**:1015-1021, 1978.

167 Nakano M, Wormer TM, Lieber CS: Perivenular fibrosis in alcoholic liver injury. Ultrastructural and histologic progression. Gastroenterology **83**:777-785, 1982.

168 Nasrallah SM, Nasser VH, Galambos JT: Importance of terminal hepatic venule thickening. Arch Pathol Lab Med **104**:84-86, 1980.

169 Perrillo RP, Griffin R, DeSchryver-Kecskemeti K, Lander JJ, Zuckerman GR: Alcoholic liver disease presenting with marked elevation of serum alkaline phosphatase. A combined clinical and pathological study. Am J Dig Dis **23**:1061-1066, 1978.

170 Ray MB: Distribution patterns of cytokeratin antigen determinants in alcoholic and nonalcoholic liver diseases. Hum Pathol **18**:61-66, 1987.

171 Rigas B, Rosenfeld L, Barwick KW, Enriquez R, Helzberg J, Batsford WP, Josephson ME, Riely CA: Amiodarone hepatotoxicity. A clinicopathologic study of five patients. Ann Intern Med **104**:348-351, 1986.

172 Rubin E, Lieber C: Early fine structural changes in the human liver induced by alcohol. Gastroenterology **52**:1-13, 1967.

173 Rubin E, Lieber C: Alcohol induced hepatic injury in nonalcoholic volunteers. N Engl J Med **278**:869-876, 1968.

174 Rubin E, Lieber C: Fatty liver, alcoholic hepatitis in cirrhosis produced by alcohol in primates. N Engl J Med **290**:128-135, 1974.

175 Simon JB, Manley PN, Brien JF, Armstrong PW: Amiodarone hepatotoxicity simulating alcoholic liver disease. N Engl J Med **311**:167-172, 1984.

176 Sternlieb I: Copper and the liver. Gastroenterology **78**:1615-1628, 1980.

177 Takada A, Nei J, Matsuda Y, Kanayama R: Clinicopathological study of alcoholic fibrosis. Am J Gastroenterol **77**:660-666, 1982.

178 Uchida T, Kronborg I, Peters RL: Giant mitochondria in the alcoholic liver diseases. Their identification, frequency and pathologic significance. Liver **4**:29-38, 1984.

179 Van Waes L, Lieber C: Early perivenular sclerosis in alcoholic fatty liver: an index of progressive liver injury. Gastroenterology **73**:646-650, 1977.

180 Yokoo H, Minick O, Batti F, Kent G: Morphologic variants of alcoholic hyalin. Am J Pathol **69**:25-32, 1972.

NONALCOHOLIC STEATOHEPATITIS

181 Adler M, Schaffner F: Fatty liver hepatitis and cirrhosis in obese patients. Am J Med **67**:811-816, 1979.

182 Anderson T, Gluud C: Liver morphology in morbid obesity. A literature study. Int J Obes **8**:97-106, 1984.

183 Braillon A, Capron JP, Hervema A, Degott C, Quenum C: Liver in obesity. Gut **26**:133-139, 1985.

184 Eriksson S, Eriksson KF, Bondesson L: Nonalcoholic steatohepatitis in obesity. A reversible condition. Acta Med Scand **220**:83-88, 1986.

185 Falchuk KR, Fiske SC, Haggitt RC, Federman M, Trey C: Pericentral hepatic fibrosis and intracellular hyalin in diabetes mellitus. Gastroenterology **78**:535-541, 1980.

186 Galambos JT, Wills CE: Relationship between 505 paired liver tests and biopsies in 242 obese patients. Gastroenterology **74**:1191-1195, 1978.

187 Haines N, Baker AL, Boyer JL, Glagov S, Schneir H, Jaspan J, Ferguson DJ: Prognostic indicators of hepatic injury following jejunoileal bypass performed for refractory obesity. A prospective study. Hepatology **1**:161-167, 1981.

188 Hornboll P, Olsen TS: Fatty changes in the liver. The relation to age, overweight, and diabetes mellitus. Acta Pathol Microbiol Scand [A] **90**:199-205, 1982.

189 Itoh S, Matsuo S, Ichinoe A, Yamaka Y, Miyazawa M: Nonalcoholic steatohepatitis and cirrhosis with Mallory's hyalin. With ultrastructural study of one case. Dig Dis Sci **27**:341-346, 1982.

190 Kingasa A, Tsunamoto K, Furukawa N, Sawada T, Kusunoki T, Shimada N: Fatty liver and its fibrous changes found in simple obesity of children. J Pediatr Gastroent Nutr **3**:408-414, 1984.

191 Leevy CM: Fatty liver. A study of 270 patients with biopsy proven fatty liver and review of the literature. Medicine [Baltimore] **41**:249-276, 1962.

192 Ludwig J, Viggiano TR, McGill DB, Oh BJ: Nonalcoholic steatohepatitis. Mayo Clinic experience with a hitherto unnamed disease. Mayo Clin Proc **55**:434-438, 1980.

193 Moran JR, Ghishan FK, Halter SA, Greene HL: Steatohepatitis in obese children. A cause of chronic liver dysfunction. Am J Gastroenterol **78**:374-377, 1983.

194 Rubin E, Lieber C: Early fine structural changes in the human liver induced by alcohol. Gastroenterology **52**:1-13, 1967.

195 Schaffner F, Thaler H: Nonalcoholic fatty liver disease. Prog Liver Dis **8**:283-298, 1986.

196 Van Theil DH: Diabetes mellitus and biliary disease. Curr Concepts Gastroenterol **10**:3-11, 1985.

197 Westwater JO, Fainter D: Liver impairment in the obese. Gastroenterology **34**:686-693, 1958.

EXTRAHEPATIC BILIARY OBSTRUCTION

198 Christofferson P, Poulsen H: Histological changes in human liver biopsies following extrahepatic biliary obstruction. Acta Pathol Microbiol Scand [A] (Suppl) 222:150-157, 1970.

199 Gall EA, Dobrogorski O: Hepatic alteration in obstructive jaundice. Am J Clin Pathol 41:120-139, 1964.

200 Poulsen H, Christoffersen P: Histological changes in liver biopsies from patients with surgical bile duct disorders. Acta Pathol Microbiol Scand [A] 78:571-579, 1970.

201 Scheuer PJ: Liver biopsy interpretation. London, 1973, Baillière Tindall.

201a Shimada H, Nihmoto S, Matsuba A, Nakagawara G: Acute cholangitis. A histopathologic study. J Clin Gastroenterol 10:197-200, 1988.

202 Shorter RG, Baggenstoss AH: Extrahepatic cholestasis. I. Histologic changes in hepatic interlobular bile ducts and ductules in extrahepatic cholestasis. Am J Clin Pathol 32:1-4, 1959.

203 Shorter RG, Baggenstoss AH: Extrahepatic cholestasis. II. Histologic features of diagnostic importance. Am J Clin Pathol 32:5-9, 1959.

204 Shorter RG, Baggenstoss AH: Extrahepatic cholestasis. III. Chronology of histologic changes in the liver. Am J Clin Pathol 32:10-17, 1959.

PRIMARY BILIARY CIRRHOSIS (CHRONIC NONSUPPURATIVE DESTRUCTIVE CHOLANGITIS)

205 Baggenstoss AH, Foulk WT, Butt HR, Bahn RC: The pathology of primary biliary cirrhosis with emphasis on histogenesis. Am J Clin Pathol 42:259-276, 1964.

206 Beswick DR, Klatskin G, Boyer JL: Asymptomatic primary cirrhosis. A progress report on long term follow-up and natural history. Gastroenterology 89:267-271, 1985.

206a Esquivel CO, Van Thiel DH, Demetris AJ, Bernardos A, Iwatsuki S, Markus B, Goidon RD, Marsh JW, Makowa L, Tzakis AG, Todo S, Gavaler JS, Starzl TE: Transplantation for primary biliary cirrhosis. Gastroenterology 94:1207-1216, 1988.

207 Fleming CR, Ludwig J, Dickson ER: Asymptomatic primary biliary cirrhosis. Mayo Clin Proc 53:587-593, 1978.

208 Geubel AP, Baggenstoss AH, Summerskill WHJ: Responses to treatment can differentiate chronic active liver disease with cholangitic features from the primary biliary cirrhosis syndrome. Gastroenterology 71:444-449, 1976.

209 James O, Mackton AF, Watson AJ: Primary biliary cirrhosis. A revised clinical spectrum. Lancet 1:1278-1281, 1981.

210 Kaplan MM: Primary biliary cirrhosis. N Engl J Med 316:521-528, 1987.

211 Kenny RP, Czaja AJ, Ludwig J, Dickson ER: Frequency and significance of antimitochrondrial antibodies in severe chronic active hepatitis. Dig Dis Sci 31:705-711, 1986.

212 Long RG, Scheuer PJ, Sherlock S: Presentation and course of asymptomatic primary biliary cirrhosis. Gastroenterology 72:1204-1207, 1977.

213 Ludwig J, Dickson ER, McDonald GSA: Staging of chronic nonsuppurative destructive cholangitis (syndrome of primary biliary cirrhosis). Virchows Arch [Pathol Anat] 379:103-112, 1978.

214 Ludwig J, McDonald GSA, Dickson ER, Elveback LR, McCall JT: Copper stains and the syndrome of primary biliary cirrhosis. Arch Pathol Lab Med 103:467-470, 1979.

215 MacSween RNM, Sumithran E: Histopathology of primary biliary cirrhosis. Semin Liver Dis 1:282-292, 1981.

216 Nakanuma Y, Ohta G: Histometric and serial section observations of the intrahepatic bile ducts in primary biliary cirrhosis. Gastroenterology 76:1326-1332, 1979.

217 Neuberger J: Primary biliary cirrhosis. Dig Dis 4:162-177, 1986.

217a Olomu AB, Vickers CR, Waring RH, Clements D, Babbs C, Warnes TW, Elias E: High incidence of poor sulfoxidation in patients with primary biliary cirrhosis. N Engl J Med 318:1089-1092, 1988.

218 Peters RL: Primary biliary cirrhosis. Gastroenterology 88:1998-2000, 1985.

219 Roll J, Boyer JL, Klatskin G: The prognostic importance of clinical and histologic features in asymptomatic and symptomatic primary biliary cirrhosis. N Engl J Med 308:1-7, 1983.

220 Rubin E, Schaffner F, Popper H: Primary biliary cirrhosis. Am J Pathol 46:387-407, 1965.

221 Salaspuro MP, Sipponen P, Ikkala E, Kolho L, Makkonen HM, Miettinen TA, Rasanen JA, Siurala M: Clinical correlations and significance of orcein positivity in chronic active hepatitis and primary biliary cirrhosis. Ann Clin Res 8:206-215, 1976.

222 Scheuer PJ: Primary biliary cirrhosis. Proc R Soc Med 60:1257-1260, 1967.

223 Sherlock S, Epstein O: Primary biliary cirrhosis. The present position. Ann NY Acad Sci 465:378-385, 1986.

224 Sherlock S, Scheuer PJ: The presentation and diagnosis of 100 patients with primary biliary cirrhosis. N Engl J Med 289:674-678, 1973.

225 Sipponen P, Salaspuro MP, Makkonen H: Histological characteristics of chronic hepatitis and primary biliary cirrhosis with special reference to orcein positive hepatocellular accumulations. Ann Clin Res 8:200-205, 1976.

226 Smith ND, Boyer JL: Are antimitochondrial antibodies of prognostic value in primary biliary cirrhosis? Hepatology 6:739-741, 1986.

227 Sternlieb I: Copper and the liver. Gastroenterology 78:1615-1628, 1980.

NONSPECIFIC REACTIVE HEPATITIS

228 Bianchi L: Liver biopsy interpretation in hepatitis. II. Histopathology and classification of acute and chronic hepatitis. Pathol Res Pract 178:170-213, 1983.

229 Liaw YN, Sheen IS, Chu CM, Chen TJ: Chronic hepatitis with nonspecific histologic changes. Is it a distinct variant of chronic hepatitis? Liver 4:55-60, 1984.

GRANULOMATOUS HEPATITIS

230 Cunningham D: Hepatic granulomas. Experience over a 10 year period in the west of Scotland. Q J Med 202:162-168, 1982.

231 Delladetsima JK, Horn T, Poulsen H: Portal tract lipogranulomas in liver biopsies. Liver 7:9-17, 1987.

232 Dincsoy HP, Weesner RE, MacGee J: Lipogranulomas in non-fatty liver. A mineral oil induced environmental disease. Am J Clin Pathol 78:35-41, 1982.

233 Fauci AS, Wolff SM: Granulomatous hepatitis. Prog Liver Dis 5:609-621, 1976.

234 Gilinsky NH, Campbell JH, Kirsch RE: The clinical spectrum of hepatic granuloma. S Afr Med J 60:691-698, 1981.

235 Guckian JG, Perry JE: Granulomatous hepatitis. Analysis of 63 cases and review of the literature. Ann Intern Med 65:1081-1100, 1966.

236 Ishak KG, Kirchner JP, Dhar JK: Granulomas and cholestatic-hepatocellular injury associated with phenylbutazone. Report of two cases. Am J Dig Dis 22:611-617, 1977.

237 Klatskin G: Hepatic granulomata. Problems in interpretation. Ann NY Acad Sci 278:427-432, 1976.

238 Lee RG, Epstein O, Jauregui H, Sherlock S, Scheuer PJ: Granulomas in primary biliary cirrhosis. A prognostic feature. Gastroenterology 81:983-986, 1981.

239 Maddrey WC, Johns CJ, Boitnott JK, Iber FL: Sarcoidosis and chronic hepatic disease. A clinical and pathologic study of 20 patients. Medicine [Baltimore] 49:375-395, 1970.

239a Mir-Madjlessi SH, Farmer Rg, Hawk WA: Granulomatous hepatitis. A review of 50 cases. Am J Gastroenterol 60:122-134, 1973.

240 Neville E, Piyasera KHG, James DG: Granulomas of the liver. Postgrad Med J 51:361-365, 1975.

241 Rudzki C, Ishak KG, Zimmerman HJ: Chronic intrahepatic cholestasis of sarcoidosis. Am J Med 59:373-387, 1975.

242 Fagan EA, Moore-Gillon JC, Turner-Warwick M: Multiorgan granulomas and mitochondrial antibodies. N Engl J Med 308:527-575, 1983.

NEONATAL HEPATITIS AND BILIARY ATRESIA

243 Alagille D: Extrahepatic biliary atresia. Hepatology 4(Suppl):7S-10S, 1984.

244 Altman RP, Abramson S: Potential errors in the diagnosis and surgical management of neonatal jaundice. J Pediatr Surg 20:529-534, 1985.

245 Bill AH, Hass JE, Foster GL: Biliary atresia. Histopathologic observations and reflections upon its natural history. J Pediatr Surg 12:977-982, 1977.

246 Brough AJ, Bernstein J: Conjugated hyperbilirubinemia in early infancy. A reassessment of liver biopsy. Hum Pathol 5:507-516, 1974.

247 Danks DM, Campbell PE, Jack I, Rogers J, Smith AL: Studies of the aetiology of neonatal hepatitis and biliary atresia. Arch Dis Child 52:360-367, 1977.

248 Danks DM, Campbell PE, Smith AL, Rogers J: Prognosis of babies with neonatal hepatitis. Arch Dis Child 52:368-372, 1977.

249 Dessanti AD, Ohi R, Hansmatsu M, Mochizuchi I, Chiba T, Kasai M: Short term histological liver changes in extrahepatic biliary atresia with good postoperative bile drainage. Arch Dis Child 60:739-742, 1985.

250 Johnson JD: Neonatal nonhemolytic jaundice. N Engl J Med 292:194-197, 1975.

251 Kasai M: Treatment of biliary atresia with special reference to hepatic portoenterostomy and its modifications. Prog Pediatr Surg 6:5-52, 1974.

252 Landing BH, Wells TR, Ramicone E: The course of the intrahepatic lesion of extrahepatic biliary atresia. A morphometric study. Pediatr Pathol 4:309-319, 1985.

253 Lilly JR, Hall RJ, Altman RP: Liver transplantation and Kasai operation in the first year of life. Therapeutic dilemma in biliary atresia. J Pediatr 110:561-562, 1987.

254 Thaler MM, Gellis SS: Studies in neonatal hepatitis and biliary atresia. Am J Dis Child 116:257-261, 1968.

255 Watkins JB, Katz AJ, Grand RJ: Neonatal hepatitis. A diagnostic approach. Adv Pediatr **24:**399-454, 1977.

256 Witzleben CL, Buck BE, Schnaufer L, Brzosko WJ: Studies on the pathogenesis of biliary atresia. Lab Invest **38:**525-532, 1978.

TOTAL PARENTERAL NUTRITION–ASSOCIATED LIVER DISEASE

257 Baker AL, Rosenberg IH: Hepatic complications of total parenteral nutrition. Am J Med **82:**489-497, 1987.

258 Beale EF, Nelson RM, Bucciarelli RL, Donnelly WH, Eitzman DV: Intrahepatic cholestasis associated with parenteral nutrition in premature infants. Pediatrics **64:**342-347, 1979.

259 Benjamin DR: Hepatobiliary dysfunction in infants and children associated with long-term total parenteral nutrition. A clinico-pathologic study. Am J Clin Pathol **76:**276-283, 1981.

260 Cohen C, Olsen MM: Pediatric total parenteral nutrition. Liver histopathology. Arch Pathol Lab Med **105:**152-156, 1981.

261 Dahms BB, Halpin TC: Serial liver biopsies in parenteral nutrition–associated cholestasis of early infancy. Gastroenterology **82:**136-144, 1981.

262 Gutcher G, Cutz E: Complications of parenteral nutrition. Semin Perinatol **10:**196-207, 1986.

263 Merritt RJ: Cholestasis associated with total parenteral nutrition. J Pedriatr Gastroenterol Nutr **5:**9-22, 1986.

264 Robin AP, Grieg PD: Basic principles of intravenous nutritional support. Clin Chest Med **7:**29-39, 1986.

265 Roy CC, Belli DC: Hepatobiliary complications associated with TPN. An enigma. J Am Coll Nutrit **4:**651-660, 1985.

266 Stanko RT, Nathan G, Mendelow H, Adibi SA: Development of hepatic cholestasis and fibrosis in patients with massive loss of intestine supported by prolonged parenteral nutrition. Gastroenterology **92:**197-202, 1987.

267 Whitington PB: Cholestasis associated with total parenteral nutrition. Hepatology **5:**693-696, 1985.

LIVER DISEASE DURING PREGNANCY

268 Alexander J, Cueller RE, Van Thiel DH: Toxemia of pregnancy and the liver. Semin Liver Dis **7:**55-58, 1987.

269 Ebert EC, Sun EA, Wright SH, Decker JP, Librizzi RJ, Bolognese RJ, Lipshutz WH: Does early diagnosis and delivery in acute fatty liver of pregnancy lead to improvement in maternal and infant survival? Dig Dis Sci **29:**453-455, 1984.

270 Hou UH, Levin S, Ahola S, Lister J, Omicioli V, Dandrow R, Papageorge W, Kaplan M: Acute fatty liver of pregnancy. Survival with early cesarean section. Dig Dis Sci **39:**449-452, 1984.

271 Ishak KG: Hepatic lesions caused by anabolic and contraceptive steroids. Semin Liver Dis **1:**116-128, 1981.

272 Kaplan MM: Acute fatty liver of pregnancy. N Engl J Med **313:**367-370, 1985.

273 Kregs GJ: Jaundice during pregnancy. Semin Liver Dis **3:**73-82, 1983.

274 Laatikainen T, Tulenheimo A: Maternal serum bile acid levels and fetal distress in cholestasis of pregnancy. Int J Gynaecol Obstet **22:**91-94, 1984.

275 Pockros PJ, Peters RL, Reynolds TB: Idiopathic fatty liver of pregnancy. Findings in ten cases. Medicine [Baltimore] **63:**1-11, 1984.

276 Riely CA: The liver in preeclampsia/eclampsia. The tip of the iceberg. Am J Gastroenterol **81:**1218-1219, 1986.

277 Riely CA: Acute fatty liver of pregnancy. Semin Liver Dis **7:**47-54, 1987.

278 Riely CA, Latham PS, Romero R, Duffy TP: Acute fatty liver of pregnancy. A reassessment based on observations in nine patients. Ann Intern Med **106:**703-706, 1987.

279 Rolfes DB, Ishak KG: Acute fatty liver of pregnancy. A clinicopathologic study of 35 cases. Hepatology **5:**1149-1158, 1985.

280 Rolfes DB, Ishak KG: Liver disease in pregnancy. Histopathology **10:**555-570, 1986.

281 Rolfes DB, Ishak KG: Liver disease in toxemia of pregnancy. Am J Gastroenterol **81:**1138-1144, 1986.

282 Rustgi VK, Hoofnagle JH: Viral hepatitis during pregnancy. Semin Liver Dis **7:**40-46, 1987.

283 Snydman DR: Hepatitis in pregnancy. N Engl J Med **313:**1398-1401, 1985.

284 Steven MM: Pregnancy and liver disease. Gut **22:**592-614, 1981.

285 Van Theil DH, Gavaler JS: Pregnancy-associated sex steroids and their effects on the liver. Semin Liver Dis **7:**1-7, 1987.

286 Varma RR: Course and prognosis of pregnancy in women with liver disease. Semin Liver Dis **7:**59-66, 1987.

ALPHA-1-ANTITRYPSIN DEFICIENCY AND CYSTIC FIBROSIS

287 Boat TF, Doershuk CF, Stern RC, Matthews LW: Serum alkaline phosphatase in cystic fibrosis. Clin Pediatr [Phila] **13:**505-512, 1974.

288 Corney G, Whitehouse DB, Hopkinson DA, et al.: Prenatal diagnosis of alpha-1-antitrypsin deficiency by fetal blood sampling. Prenat Diagn **7:**101-108, 1986.

289 Cox DW, Mansfield T: Prenatal diagnosis of alpha-1-antitrypsin deficiency and estimates of fetal risk for disease. J Med Genet **24:**52-59, 1987.

290 Di Sant Agnese PA, Talamo C: Cystic fibrosis of the pancreas. N Engl J Med **277:**1287-1294, 1967.

291 Eriksson SG: Liver disease in alpha-1-antitrypsin deficiency. Aspects of incidence and prognosis. Scand J Gastroenterol **20:**907-911, 1985.

292 Eriksson S, Carolson J, Velez R: Risk of cirrhosis and primary liver cancer in alpha-1-antitrypsin deficiency. N Engl J Med **314:**736-739, 1986.

293 Feigelson J, Pecau Y, Catheleau J: Additional data on hepatic function tests in cystic fibrosis. Acta Paediatr Scand **64:**337-344, 1975.

293a Ghishan FK, Greene HL: Liver disease in children with PiZZ alpha-1-antitrypsin deficiency. Hepatology **8:**307-310, 1988.

294 Hultcrantz R, Mengarelli S, Strandvik B: Morphologic findings in the liver of children with cystic fibrosis. A light and electron microscopical study. Hepatology **6:**881-889, 1986.

295 Isenberg JN: Cystic fibrosis. Its influence in the liver, biliary tree and bile salt metabolism. Semin Liver Dis **2:**302-313, 1982.

296 Kage M, Liew Ct, Xu Y, Peters RL: Alpha-1-antitrypsin deficiency in adults. Acta Pathol Jpn **36:**1139-1148, 1986.

296a Klatt EC, Koss MN, Young TS, Macauley L, Martin SE: Hepatic hyaline globules associated with passive congestion. Arch Pathol Lab Med **112:**510-513, 1988.

297 Larcher V: Chronic active hepatitis and related disorders. Clin Gastroenterol **15:**173-198, 1986.

298 Malfait R, Gorus F, Sevens C: Electrophoresis of serum protein to detect alpha-1-antitrypsin deficiency. Five illustrative cases. Clin Chem **31:**1379-1399, 1985.

299 Oppenheimer EH, Esterly JR: Hepatic changes in young infants with cystic fibrosis. Possible relation to focal biliary cirrhosis. J Pediatr **86:**683-689, 1975.

300 Oppenheimer EH, Esterly JR: Pathology of cystic fibrosis. Review of the literature and comparison with 146 autopsied cases. Perspect Pediatr Pathol **2:**241-278, 1975.

301 Psacharopoulos HT, Howard ER, Postman B, Mowat AP, Williams R: Hepatic complications of cystic fibrosis. Lancet **ii:**78-80, 1981.

302 Roy CC, Weber AM, Morin CL, Lepage G, Brisson G, Yousef I, LaSalle R: Hepatobiliary disease in cystic fibrosis. A survey of current issues and concepts. J Pediatr Gastroenterol Nutr **1:**469-478, 1982.

303 Sassaris MP, Trinkl W, Meka R, Gonzales P, Torres O, Leach R, Hunter FM: Alpha-1-antitrypsin deficiency and liver cirrhosis in adults. South Med J **78:**52-57, 1985.

304 Shwachman H, Kowalski M, Khaw KT: Cystic fibrosis. A new outlook: 70 patients about 25 years of age. Medicine [Baltimore] **56:**129-149, 1977.

305 Stern RC, Stevens DP, Boat TF, Doershuk CF, Izant RJ Jr, Matthews LW: Symptomatic hepatic disease in cystic fibrosis. Incidence, course and outcome of portal systemic shunting. Gastroenterology **70:**645-649, 1976.

306 Sveger T: Liver disease in alpha-1-antitrypsin deficiency detected by screening of 200,000 infants. N Engl J Med **294:**1316-1319, 1976.

307 Thatcher BS, Windelman EI, Tuthill RJ: Alpha-1-antitrypsin deficiency presenting as cryptogenic cirrhosis in adults over 50. J Clin Gastroenterol **7:**405-408, 1985.

308 Theaker JM, Fleming KA: Alpha-1-antitrypsin and the liver. A routine immunohistological screen. J Clin Pathol **39:**58-62, 1986.

REYE'S SYNDROME

309 Barrett MJ, Hurwitz ES, Schonberger LB, Rogers MF: Changing epidemiology of Reye's syndrome in the United States. Pediatrics **77:**598-602, 1986.

310 Bove KE, McAdams J, Partin JC, Partin JS, Hug G, Schubert WK: The hepatic lesion in Reye's syndrome. Gastroenterology **69:**685-697, 1975.

311 Heubi JE, Partin JC, Partin JS, Schubert WK: Reye's syndrome. Current concepts. Hepatology **7:**155-164, 1987.

312 Kimura A, Yoshida I, Yamashita F: Necessity of liver biopsy for accurate diagnosis of Reye's syndrome (letter). J Pediatr Gastroenterol Nutr **6:**153-154, 1987.

313 Meythaler JM, Varma RR: Reye's syndrome in adults. Diagnostic considerations. Arch Intern Med **147:**61-64, 1987.

314 Mortimer EA: Reye's syndrome, salicylates, epidemiology, and public health policy. JAMA **257:**1941, 1987.

315 Partin JC, Schubert WK, Partin JS: Mitochondrial ultrastructure in Reye's syndrome (encephalopathy and fatty degeneration of the viscera). N Engl J Med **185:**1339-1343, 1971.

316 Partin JS, Daugherty CE, McAdams AJ, Partin JC, Schubert WK: A comparison of liver ultrastructure in salicylate intoxication and Reye's syndrome. Hepatology **4:**687-690, 1984.

317 Reye RDK, Morgan G, Baral J: Encephalopathy and fatty degeneration of the viscera. A disease entity in childhood. Lancet **2:**749-752, 1963.

Hemochromatosis and Wilson's disease

317a Adams PC, Searle J: Neonatal hemochromatosis. A case and review of the literature. Am J Gastroenterol **83:**422-425, 1988.

318 Adler R, Mahnovski V, Heuser ET, Presser DH, Robinson RG: Fulminant hepatitis, a presentation of Wilson's disease. Am J Dis Child **131:**870-872, 1977.

319 Baldus WP, Fairbanks VF, Dickson ER, Baggenstoss AH: Deferoxamine-chelatable iron in hemochromatosis and other disorders of iron overload. Mayo Clin Proc **53:**157-165, 1978.

320 Bassett ML, Halliday JW: Value of hepatic iron measurement in early hemochromatosis and determination of the critical level associated with fibrosis. Hepatology **6:**24-29, 1986.

321 Bassett ML, Halliday JW, Ferris RA, Powell LW: Diagnosis of hemochromatosis in young subjects. Predictive accuracy of biochemical screening tests. Gastroenterology **87:**628-632, 1984.

322 Bernuau J, Rueff B, Benhamou JP: Fulminant and subfulminant liver failure. Definitions and causes. Semin Liver Dis **6:**97-106, 1986.

322a Blisard KS, Bartow SA: Neonatal hemochromatosis. Hum Pathol **17:**376-383, 1986.

323 Borwein ST, Ghent CN, Flanagan PR, Chamberlain MJ, Valberg LS: Genetic and phenotypic expression of hemochromatosis in Canadians. Clin Invest Med **6:**171-179, 1983.

324 Bradbear RA, Bain C, Siskind V, Schofield FD, Webb S, Axelsen EM, Halliday JW, Bassett ML, Powell LW: Cohort study of internal malignancy in genetic hemochromatosis and other chronic nonalcoholic liver diseases. J Natl Cancer Inst **75:**81-84, 1985.

325 Cartwright GE: Diagnosis of treatable Wilson's disease. N Engl J Med **298:**1347-1350, 1978.

326 Conte D, Piperno A, Mandelli C, Fargion S, Cesana M, Brunelli L, Ferrario L, Velio P, Zaramella G, Tiribelli C, Fiorella G, Bianchi PA: Clinical, biochemical and histologic features of primary hemochromatosis. A report of 67 cases. Liver **6:**310-315, 1986.

327 Crosby WH: Serum ferritin fails to indicate hemochromatosis. Nothing gold can stay. N Engl J Med **294:**333-334, 1976.

328 Dadone MM, Kushner JP, Edwards CQ, Bishop DT, Skolnick MH: Hereditary hemochromatosis. Analysis of laboratory expression of the disease by genotype in 18 pedigrees. Am J Clin Pathol **78:**196-207, 1982.

329 Danks DM: Of mice and men, metals and mutations. J Med Genet **32:**99-106, 1986.

330 Edwards CQ, Carroll M, Bray P, Cartwright GE: Hereditary hemochromatosis. N Engl J Med **297:**7-12, 1977.

331 Fairbanks VF, Baldus WP: Hemochromatosis. The neglected diagnosis. Mayo Clin Proc **61:**296-298, 1986.

332 Feller ER, Pont A, Wands JR, Carter EA, Foster G, Kourides IA, Isselbacher KJ: Familial hemochromatosis. Physiologic studies in the precirrhotic stage of the disease. N Engl J Med **296:**1422-1426, 1977.

333 Fitzgerald MA, Gross JB, Goldstein NP, Wahner HW, McCall JT: Wilson's disease (hepatolenticular degeneration) of late adult onset. Mayo Clin Proc **50:**438-442, 1975.

334 Frommer D, Morris J, Sherlock S, Abrams J, Newman S: Kayer-Fleischer–like rings in patients without Wilson's disease. Gastroenterology **72:**1331-1335, 1977.

335 Gollan JL: Diagnosis of hemochromatosis. Gastroenterology **84:**418-421, 1983.

336 Irons RD, Schenk EA, Lee JCK: Cytochemical methods for copper. Arch Pathol Lab Med **101:**298-301, 1977.

337 Kent G, Popper H: Liver biopsy in diagnosis of hemochromatosis. Am J Med **44:**837-841, 1968.

338 LeSage GD, Baldus WP, Fairbanks VF, Baggenstoss AH, McCall JT, Moore SB, Taswell HF, Gordon M: Hemochromatosis. Genetic or alcohol induced? Gastroenterology **84:**1471-1477, 1983.

339 McCullough AJ, Fleming CR, Thistle JL, Baldus WP, Ludwig J, McCall JT, Dickson ER: Diagnosis of Wilson's disease presenting as fulminant hepatic failure. Gastroenterology **84:**161-164, 1983.

340 Niederau C, Fischer R, Sonnenberg A, Stremmel W, Trampisch HJ, Strohmeyer G: Survival and causes of death in cirrhotic and noncirrhotic patients with primary hemochromatosis. N Engl J Med **313:**1256-1262, 1985.

341 Olsson KS, Ritter B, Rosen U, Heedman PA, Staugård F: Prevalence of iron overload in central Sweden. Acta Med Scand **213:**145-150, 1983.

342 Powell LW: The role of alcoholism in hepatic iron storage disease. Ann NY Acad Sci **252:**124-134, 1975.

343 Powell LW, Bassett ML, Halliday JW: Hemochromatosis. 1980 update. Gastroenterology **78:**374-381, 1980.

344 Powell LW, Halliday JW: The detection of early hemochromatosis. Am J Dig Dis **23:**377-379, 1978.

345 Powell LW, Kerr JFR: The pathology of the liver in hemochromatosis. Pathobiol Annu **5:**317-337, 1975.

346 Rector WG, Uchida T, Kanel GC, Redeker AG, Reynolds TB: Fulminant hepatic and renal failure complicating Wilson's disease. Liver **4:**341-347, 1984.

347 Riely CA: Wilson's disease. Pediatr Rev **5:**217-222, 1984.

348 Ritland S, Steinnes E, Skrede S: Hepatic copper content, urinary copper excretion, and serum ceruloplasmin in liver disease. Scand J Gastroenterol **12:**81-88, 1977.

349 Rowe JW, Wands JR, Mezey E, Waterbury LA, Wright JR, Tobin J, Andres R: Familial hemochromatosis. Characteristics of the precirrhotic stage in a large kindred. Medicine [Baltimore] **56:**197-211, 1977.

350 Scott J, Gollan JL, Samourian S, Sherlock S: Wilson's disease, presenting as chronic active hepatitis. Gastroenterology **74:**645-651, 1978.

350a Silver MM, Beverly DW, Valberg LS, Cutz E, Phillips J, Shaheed WA: Perinatal hemochromatosis. Clinical, morphologic and quantitative iron studies. Am J Pathol **128:**538-554, 1987.

351 Simon M, Bourel M, Genetet B, Fauchet R: Idiopathic hemochromatosis. Demonstration of recessive transmission and early detection by family HLA typing. N Engl J Med **297:**1017-1021, 1977.

352 Sokol RJ, Francis PD, Gold SH, Ford DM, Lum GM, Ambruso DR: Orthotopic liver transplantation for acute fulminant Wilson's disease. J Pediatr **107:**549-552, 1985.

353 Sternlieb I: Diagnosis of Wilson's disease. Gastroenterology **74:**787-793, 1978.

354 Sternlieb I: Wilson's disease. Indications for liver transplants. Hepatology **4**(Suppl):158-178, 1984.

355 Sternlieb I, Scheinberg IH: Chronic hepatitis as a first manifestation of Wilson's disease. Ann Intern Med **76:**59-64, 1972.

356 Stromeyer FW, Ishak KG: Histology of the liver in Wilson's disease. A study of 34 cases. Am J Clin Pathol **73:**12-24, 1980.

357 Valberg LS, Ghent CN: Diagnosis and management of hereditary hemochromatosis. Annu Rev Med **36:**27-37, 1985.

FIBROPOLYCYSTIC LIVER DISEASES

358 Baldus WP, Sherlock S, Carlson HC, Baggenstoss AH, Danadio JW, Adson MA: Fibropolycystic disease of the hepatobiliary system and kidneys. Am J Dig Dis **21:**1058-1069, 1976.

359 Bernstein J: What is Caroli's disease? Gastroenterology **68:**417-419, 1975.

360 Bernstein J: A classification of renal cysts. In Gardner KD Jr (ed): Cystic diseases of the kidney. New York, 1976, John Wiley & Sons, Inc.

361 Bloustein PA: Association of carcinoma with congenital cystic conditions of the liver and bile ducts. Am J Gastroenterol **67:**40-46, 1977.

362 Foulk WT: Congenital malformations of the intrahepatic biliary tree in the adult. Gastroenterology **58:**253-256, 1970.

363 Howard RJ, Hanson RF, Delaney JP: Jaundice associated with polycystic liver disease. Arch Surg **111:**816-817, 1976.

364 Kerr DNS, Harrison CV, Sherlock S, Walker RM: Congenital hepatic fibrosis. Q J Med **30:**91-117, 1961.

364a Kwok MK, Lewin KJ: Massive hepatomegaly in adult polycystic liver disease. Am J Surg Pathol **12:**321-324, 1988.

365 Longmire WP, Mandiola SA, Gordon HE: Congenital cystic disease of the liver and biliary system. Ann Surg **174:**711-726, 1971.

366 Mall JC, Ghahremani GG, Boyer JL: Caroli's disease associated with congenital hepatic fibrosis and renal tubular ectasia. Gastroenterology **66:**1029-1035, 1974.

367 Melnick PJ: Polycystic liver. Arch Pathol **59:**162, 1955.

367a Morin ME, Baker DN, Vanoganas T, Tass A, Sue HK: Solitary nonparasitic hepatic cyst causing obstructive jaundice. Am J Gastroenterol **73:**434-436, 1980.

368 Murray-Lyon IM, Ockenden BG, Williams R: Congenital hepatic fibrosis. Is it a single clinical entity? Gastroenterology **64:**653-656, 1973.

369 Murray-Lyon IM, Shilkin KB, Laws JW, Illing RC, Williams R: Non-obstructive dilatation of the intrahepatic biliary tree with cholangitis. Q J Med **41:**477-489, 1972.

CIRRHOSIS

370 Anthony PP, Ishak KG, Nayak NC, Poulsen HE, Scheuer PJ, Sobin LH: The morphology of cirrhosis. J Clin Pathol **31:**395-414, 1978.

371 Epstein O: Management aspects of cirrhosis. Practitioner **231:**395-401, 1987.

372 Fauerholdt L, Schlichting P, Christensen E, Poulsen H, Tygstrup N, Juhl E: Conversion of micronodular cirrhosis into macronodular cirrhosis. Hepatology **3:**928-931, 1983.

373 Galambos JT: Classification of cirrhosis. Am J Gastroenterol **64:**437-451, 1975.

374 Gluud C, Christoffersen P, Eriksen J, Wantzin P, Knudsen BB, Copenhagen Study Group for Liver Diseases: Influence of ethanol on development of hyperplastic nodules in alcoholic men with micronodular cirrhosis. Gastroenterology **93:**256-260, 1987.

375 Miyai K, Bonin ML: Nodular regenerative hyperplasia of the liver. Report of 3 cases and review of the literature. Am J Clin Pathol **73**:267-271, 1980.

376 Popper H: What are the major types of hepatic cirrhosis? In Ingelfinger FJ, Relman AS, Finland M (eds): Controversy in internal medicine. Philadelphia, 1966, W.B. Saunders Co., pp. 233-243.

377 Popper H: Pathologic aspects of cirrhosis. Am J Pathol **87**:228-258, 1977.

378 Popper H: General pathology of the liver. Light microscopic aspects serving diagnosis and interpretation. Semin Liver Dis **6**:175-184, 1986.

379 Saunders JB, Walters JRF, Davies P, Paton A: A 20-year prospective study of cirrhosis. Br Med J **282**:263-266, 1981.

380 Stromeyer FW, Ishak KG: Nodular transformation (nodular "regenerative" hyperplasia) of the liver. Hum Pathol **12**:60-71, 1981.

380a Waneless IR: The use of morphometry in the study of nodular and vascular lesions of the liver. Analyt Quant Cytol Histol **9**:39-41, 1987.

380b Waneless IR, Mawdsley C, Adams R: On the pathogenesis of focal nodular hyperplasia of the liver. Hepatology **5**:1194-1200, 1985.

LIVER TRANSPLANTATION

381 Bismuth H, Gugenheim S, Ciardualo M: Indicators for hepatic transplantation in alcoholic liver cirrhosis. Transplant Proc **18**:83-85, 1986.

381a Bismuth H, Samuel D, Gugenheim J, Costaing D, Brennau J, Rueff B, Benhamon J-P: Emergency liver transplantation for fulminant hepatitis. Ann Intern Med **107**:337-341, 1987.

382 Busuttil RW, Goldstein LI, Danovitch GM, Ament ME, Memsic LD: Liver transplantation today. Ann Intern Med **104**:377-389, 1986.

383 Calne RY, Williams R, Rolles K: Liver transplantation in the adult. World J Surg **10**:422-431, 1986.

384 Cuervas-Mons V, Julio Martinez AJ, Dekker A, Starzl TE, Van Thiel DH: Adult liver transplantation. An analysis of the early causes of death in 40 consecutive cases. Hepatology **6**:495-501, 1986.

385 Cuervas-Mons V, Millan I, Gavaler JS, Starzl TE, Van Thiel DH: Prognostic value of preoperatively obtained clinical and laboratory data transplantation. Hepatology **6**:922-927, 1986.

386 Demetris AJ, Jaffe R, Sheahan DG, Burnham J, Spero J, Iwatsuki S, Van Thiel DH, Starzl TE: Recurrent hepatitis B in liver allograft recipients. Differentiation between viral hepatitis B and rejection. Am J Pathol **125**:161-172, 1986.

387 Demetris AJ, Lasky S, Van Thiel DH, Starzl TE, Whiteside T: Pathology of hepatic transplantation. A review of 62 allograft recipients immunosuppressed with cyclosporin/steroid regimen. Am J Pathol **118**:151-161, 1985.

388 de Silva BG, Gore SM, White DJG, Bourgeon K, Rolles K, Calne RY: Analysis of risk factors in liver transplantation. Transplant Proc **18**:1210-1212, 1986.

389 Eggink HF, Hofstee N, Gips CH, Krom RA, Houthoff HJ: Histopathology of serial graft biopsies from liver transplant recipients. Am J Pathol **114**:18-31, 1984.

390 Esquivel O, Jaffe R, Gordon RD, Marsh WJ, Starzl TE: Liver rejection and its differentiation from other causes of graft dysfunction. Semin Liver Dis **5**:369-374, 1985.

391 Esquivel O, Koneru B, Karrer F, Todo S, Iwatsuki S, Gordon RD, Makowka L, Marsh WJ, Starzl TE: Liver transplantation before one year of age. J Pediatr **110**:545-548, 1987.

392 Flye MW, Jendrisak MD: Liver transplantation in the child. World J Surg **10**:432-441, 1986.

393 Gordon RD, Shaw BW, Iwatsuki S, Esquivel O, Starzl TE: Indications for liver transplantation in the cyclosporin era. Surg Clin North Am **66**:541-556, 1986.

394 Ho M, Miller G, Atchison RW, Breinig MK, Dummer JS, Andiman W, Starzl TE, Eastman R, Griffith BP, Hardesty RL: Epstein-Barr virus infections and DNA hybridization studies in post-transplantation lymphoma and lymphoproliferative lesions. The role of primary infection. J Infect Dis **152**:876-886, 1985.

395 Hubscher SG, Clements D, Elias E, McMaster P: Biopsy findings in cases of rejection of liver allograft. J Clin Pathol **38**:1366-1373, 1985.

396 Ludwig J, Weisner RH, Batts KP, Perkins JD, Krom RA: The acute vanishing bile duct syndrome (acute irreversible rejection) after orthotopic liver transplantation. Hepatology **7**:476-483, 1987.

396a Malatack JJ, Schoid DJ, Urbach AH, Gartner JC, Zitelli BJ, Rockette H, Fischer J, Starzl TE, Iwatsuki S, Shaw BW: Choosing a pediatric recipient for orthotopic liver transplantation. J Pediatr **111**:479-489, 1987.

397 Margreiter R: Indications for liver transplantation for primary and secondary tumors. Transplant Proc **18**:74-77, 1986.

397a Masih AS, Linder J, Shaw BW, Wood P, Donovan JP, White R, Markin RS: Rapid identification of cytomegalovirus in liver allograft biopsies by in situ hybridization. Am J Surg Pathol **12**:362-367, 1988.

398 Neuberger J: Liver transplantation. Indications and timing. Cur Opin Gastroenterol **3**:402-407, 1987.

399 Neuberger J, Portman B, MacDougall BRD, Caine RY, Williams R: Recurrence of primary biliary cirrhosis after liver transplantation. N Engl J Med **36**:1-4, 1982.

400 O'Grady J, Williams RW: Liver transplantation. Practitioner **231**:387-394, 1987.

400a Rizzetto M, Macagno S, Chiaberge E, Verme G, Negro F, Marinucci G, DiGiacoma C, Alfani D, Cortesini R, Milozzo F, Doglia M, Fassati LR, Galmarini D: Liver transplantation in heptitis delta virus disease. Lancet **2**:467-471, 1987.

401 Snover D, Freese DK, Sharp HL, Bloomer JR, Najarian JS, Ascher NL: Liver allograft rejection. An analysis of the use of biopsy in determining outcome of rejection. Am J Surg Pathol **11**:1-10, 1987.

402 Snover DC, Sibley RK, Freese DK, Sharp HL, Bloomer JR, Najarian JS, Ascher NL: Orthotopic liver transplantation. A pathologic study of 63 serial biopsies from 17 patients with specific reference to the diagnostic features and natural history of rejection. Hepatology **4**:1212-1222, 1984.

403 Tennapel CHH, Houthoff HJ, Van Thiel DH: Cytomegalovirus in normal and immune compromised hosts. Liver **4**:184-194, 1984.

404 van der Putten ABMM, Bijeveld CMA, Sloof MJH, Wesenhagen H, Gips CH: Selection criteria and decisions in 375 patients with liver disease, considered for liver transplantation during 1977-1985. Liver **7**:84-90, 1987.

405 Vierling JM, Fennell RH: Histopathology of early and late human hepatic allograft rejection. Evidence of progressive destruction of interlobular bile ducts. Hepatology **5**:2076-2082, 1985.

406 Williams JW, Peters TG, Vera SR, Britt LG, van Voorst SJ, Haggitt RC: Biopsy directed immunosuppression following hepatic transplantation in man. Transplantation **39**:589-596, 1985.

407 Wozney P, Zajko AB, Bron KM, Point S, Starzl TE: Vascular complications after liver transplantation. A 5 year experience. AJR **147**:657-664, 1986.

HETEROTOPIA

408 Mendoza A, Voland J, Wolf P, Benirschke K: Supradiaphragmatic liver in the lung. Arch Pathol Lab Med **110**:1085-1086, 1986.

ABSCESS

409 Greenstein AJ, Barth J, Dicker A, Bottone EJ, Aufses AH Jr: Amebic liver abscess. A study of 11 cases compared with a series of 38 patients with pyogenic liver abscess. Am J Gastroenterol **80**:472-478, 1985.

410 Rubin RH, Swartz MN, Malt R: Hepatic abscess. Changes in clinical, bacteriologic and therapeutic aspects. Am J Med **57**:601-610, 1974.

411 Satiani B, Davidson ED: Hepatic abscesses. Improvement in mortality with early diagnosis and treatment. Am J Surg **135**:647-650, 1978.

412 Trump DL, Fahnestock R, Cloutier CT, Dickman MD: Anaerobic liver abscess and intrahepatic metastases. A case report and review of the literature. Cancer **41**:682-686, 1978.

412a Weinberg RJ, Klish WJ, Brown MR, Smalley JR, Emmens RW: Hepatic abscess as a complication of Crohn's disease. J Pediatr Gastroenterol Nutr **2**:171-174, 1983.

ECHINOCOCCUS CYST

413 Langer JC, Rose DB, Keystone JS, Taylor BR, Langer B: Diagnosis and management of hydatid disease of the liver. A 15-year North American experience. Ann Surg **199**:412-417, 1984.

414 Kahn JB, Spruance S, Harbottle J, Connor P, Schultz MG: Echinococcosis in Utah. Am J Trop Med Hyg **21**:185-188, 1972.

415 Katz AM, Pan C-T: Echinococcus disease in the United States. Am J Med **25**:759-770, 1958.

416 Williams JF, Lopez AH, Trejos A: Current prevalence and distribution of hydatidosis with special reference to the Americas. Am J Trop Med Hyg **20**:224-236, 1971.

SOLITARY NONPARASITIC CYST

416a Byrne WJ, Fonkalsrud EW: Congenital solitary nonparasitic cyst of the liver. A rare cause of rapidly enlarging abdominal mass in infancy. J Pediatr Surg **17**:316-317, 1982.

417 Cousoftides, Herman RE: Nonparasitic cysts of the liver. Surg Gynecol Obstet **138**:906-910, 1974.

417a Finkel L, Marchensky A, Cohen B: Endometrial cyst of the liver. Am J Gastroenterol **81**:576-578, 1986.

418 Longmire WP, Mandiola SA, Gordon HE: Congenital cystic disease of the liver and biliary system. Ann Surg **174**:711-726, 1971.

419 Schullinger JN, Wigger HJ, Price JB, Benson M, Harris RC: Epidermoid cysts of the liver. J Pediatr Surg **18**:240-242, 1983.

419a Sood SC, Watson A: Solitary cyst of the liver presenting as an abdominal emergency. Postgraduate Med J **50**:48-50, 1974.

420 Wellwood JM, Madar JL, Cady B, Haggitt RC: Large intrahepatic cysts and pseudocysts. Am J Surg **135:**57-64, 1978.

420a Wheeler DA, Edmondson HA: Ciliated hepatic foregut cyst. Am J Surg Pathol **8:**467-470, 1984.

TUMORS AND TUMORLIKE CONDITIONS
Liver cell tumors and tumorlike conditions
Focal nodular hyperplasia

421 Baum JK, Bookstein JJ, Holtz F, Klein EW: Possible association between benign hepatomas and oral contraceptives. Lancet **2:**926-929, 1973.

422 Benz EJ, Baggenstoss AH: Focal cirrhosis of liver. Its relation to so-called hamartoma (adenoma, benign hepatoma). Cancer **6:**743-755, 1953.

423 Christopherson WM, Mays ET, Barrows G: A clinicopathologic study of steroid-related liver tumors. Am J Surg Pathol **1:**31-41, 1977.

423a Fechner RE: Benign hepatic lesions and orally administered contraceptives. A report of seven cases and a critical analysis of the literature. Hum Pathol **8:**255-268, 1977.

424 Fechner RE, Roehm JOF Jr: Angiographic and pathologic correlations of hepatic focal nodular hyperplasia. Am J Surg Pathol **1:**217-224, 1977.

425 Gold JH, Guzman IJ, Rosai J: Benign tumors of the liver. Pathologic examination of 45 cases. Am J Clin Pathol **70:**6-17, 1978.

425a Karhunen PJ, Penttilä A, Liesto K, Männikkö A, Möttönen MM: Occurrence of benign hepatocellular tumors in alcoholic men. Acta Pathol Microbiol Immunol Scand [A] **94:**141-147, 1986.

426 Knowles DM II, Casarella WJ, Johnson PM, Wolff M: The clinical, radiologic, and pathologic characterization of benign hepatic neoplasms. Alleged association with oral contraceptives. Medicine [Baltimore] **57:**223-237, 1978.

427 Knowles DM II, Wolff M: Focal nodular hyperplasia of the liver. A clinicopathologic study and review of the literature. Hum Pathol **7:**533-545, 1976.

428 Nissen ED, Kent DR, Nissen SE: Liver tumors and the pill. Analyzing the data. Contemp Obst/Gynecol **8:**103-111, 1976.

429 Palmer PE, Christopherson WM, Wolfe HJ: Alpha-1-antitrypsin. Protein marker in oral contraceptive-associated hepatic tumors. Am J Clin Pathol **68:**736-739, 1977.

430 Phillips MJ, Langer B, Stone R, Fisher MM, Ritchie S: Benign liver cell tumors. Classification and ultrastructural pathology. Cancer **32:**463-470, 1973.

430a Ramchand S, Suh HS, Gonzalez-Crussi F: Focal nodular hyperplasia of the liver. Can J Surg **13:**22-26, 1970.

431 Sherlock S, Feldman CA, Moran B, Scheuer PJ: Partial nodular transformation of liver with portal hypertension. Am J Med **40:**195-203, 1966.

432 Steiner PE: Nodular regenerative hyperplasia of the liver. Am J Pathol **35:**943-953, 1959.

433 Stocker JT, Ishak KG: Focal nodular hyperplasia of the liver. A study of 21 pediatric cases. Cancer **48:**336-345, 1981.

434 Stromeyer FW, Ishak KG: Nodular transformation (nodular "regenerative" hyperplasia) of the liver. A clinicopathologic study of 30 cases. Hum Pathol **12:**60-71, 1981.

434a Weinbren K, Mutum SS: Pathological aspects of diffuse nodular hyperplasia of the liver. J Pathol **143:**81-92, 1984.

Liver cell adenoma

435 Ameriks JA, Thompson NW, Frey CF, Appelman HD, Walter JF: Hepatic cell adenomas, spontaneous liver rupture, and oral contraceptives. Arch Surg **110:**548-557, 1975.

436 Bühler H, Pirovino M, Akovbiantz A, Altorfer J, Weitzel M, Maranta E, Schmid M: Regression of liver cell adenoma. A follow-up study of three consecutive patients after discontinuation of oral contraceptive use. Gastroenterology **82:**775-782, 1982.

437 Carbone A, Vecchio FM: Presence of cytoplasmic progesterone receptors in hepatic adenomas. A report of two cases. Am J Clin Pathol **85:**325-329, 1986.

438 Chandra RS, Kapur SP, Kelleher J, Luban N, Patterson K: Benign hepatocellular tumors in the young. A clinicopathologic spectrum. Arch Pathol Lab Med **108:**168-171, 1984.

439 Coire CI, Qizilbash AH, Castelli MF: Hepatic adenomata in type Ia glycogen storage disease. Arch Pathol Lab Med **111:**166-169, 1987.

440 Edmondson HA, Henderson B, Benton B: Liver-cell adenomas associated with use of oral contraceptives. N Engl J Med **294:**470-472, 1976.

441 Flejou JF, Barge J, Menu Y, Degott C, Bismuth H, Potet F, Benhamou JP: Liver adenomatosis. An entity distinct from liver adenoma? Gastroenterology **89:**1132-1138, 1985.

442 Galloway SJ, Casarella WJ, Lattes R, Seaman WB: Minimal deviation hepatoma. A new entity. Am J Roentgenol Radium Ther Nucl Med **125:**184-192, 1975.

443 Goodman ZD, Mikel UV, Lubbers PR, Ros PR, Langloss JM, Ishak KG: Kupffer cells in hepatocellular adenomas. Am J Surg Pathol **11:**191-196, 1987.

444 Heffelfinger S, Irani DR, Finegold MJ: "Alcoholic hepatitis" in a hepatic adenoma. Hum Pathol **18:**751-754, 1987.

445 Ishak KG, Rabin L: Benign tumors of the liver. Med Clin North Am **59:**995-1013, 1975.

446 Kerlin P, Davis GL, McGill DB, Weiland LH, Adson MA, Sheedy PF II: Hepatic adenoma and focal nodular hyperplasia. Clinical, pathologic, and radiologic features. Gastroenterology **84:**994-1002, 1983.

447 Malatjalian DA, Graham CH: Liver adenoma with granulomas. The appearance of granulomas in oral contraceptive-related hepatocellular adenoma and in the surrounding nontumorous liver. Arch Pathol Lab Med **106:**244-246, 1982.

448 McCaughan GW, Bilous MJ, Gallagher ND: Long-term survival with tumor regression in androgen-induced liver tumors. Cancer **56:**2622-2626, 1985.

449 Salisbury JR, Portmann BC: Oncocytic liver cell adenoma. Histopathology **11:**533-539, 1987.

450 Westaby D, Portmann B, Williams R: Androgen related primary hepatic tumors in non-Fanconi patients. Cancer **51:**1947-1952, 1983.

451 Wheeler DA, Edmondson HA, Reynolds TB: Spontaneous liver cell adenoma in children. Am J Clin Pathol **85:**6-12, 1986.

Liver cell carcinoma
General features

452 Chlebowski RT, Tong M, Weissman J, Block JB, Ramming KP, Weiner JM, Bateman JR, Chlebowski JS: Hepatocellular carcinoma. Diagnostic and prognostic features in North American patients. Cancer **53:**2701-2706, 1984.

453 Farhi DC, Shikes RH, Murari PJ, Silverberg SG: Hepatocellular carcinoma in young people. Cancer **52:**1516-1525, 1983.

454 Greene C-A, Suen KC: Some cytologic features of hepatocellular carcinoma as seen in fine needle aspirates. Acta Cytol [Baltimore] **28:**713-725, 1984.

455 Higginson J: The epidemiology of primary carcinoma of the liver. In Pack GT, Islami AH (eds): Tumors of the liver. Vol. 26 of Recent results in cancer research. Heidelberg, 1970, Springer-Verlag.

455a Ikeda T, Tozuka S, Hasumura Y, Takeuchi J: Prostaglandin E-producing hepatocellular carcinoma with hypercalcemia. Cancer **61:**1813-1814, 1988.

456 Lack EE, Neave C, Vawter GF: Hepatocellular carcinoma. Review of 32 cases in childhood and adolescence. Cancer **52:**1510-1515, 1983.

457 Margolis S, Homey C: Systemic manifestations of hepatoma. Medicine [Baltimore] **51:**381-391, 1972.

458 Noguchi S, Yamamoto R, Tatsuta M, Kasugai H, Okuda S, Wada A, Tamura H: Cell features and patterns in fine-needle aspirates of hepatocellular carcinoma. Cancer **58:**321-328, 1986.

459 Primack A, Wilson J, O'Conor GT, Engelman K, Canellos GP: Hepatocellular carcinoma with the carcinoid syndrome. Cancer **27:**1182-1189, 1971.

460 O'Conor GT, Tatarinov YS, Abelev GI, Uriel J: A collaborative study for the evaluation of a serologic test for primary liver cancer. Cancer **25:**1091-1098, 1970.

461 Ruoslahti E, Seppala M, Vuopio P, Saksela E, Peltokallio P: Radioimmunoassay of alpha-fetoprotein in primary and secondary cancer of the liver. J Natl Cancer Inst **49:**623-630, 1972.

462 Sakurai M, Okamura J, Seki K, Kuroda C: Needle tract implantation of hepatocellular carcinoma after percutaneous liver biopsy. Am J Surg Pathol **7:**191-195, 1983.

463 Tao LC, Ho CS, McLoughlin MJ, Evans WK, Donat EE: Cytologic diagnosis of hepatocellular carcinoma by fine-needle aspiration biopsy. Cancer **53:**547-552, 1984.

Predisposing and associated factors

464 Akagi G, Furuya K, Kanamura A, Chihara T, Otsuka H: Liver cell dysplasia and hepatitis B surface antigen in liver cirrhosis and hepatocellular carcinoma. Cancer **54:**315-318, 1984.

465 Alpert ME, Davidson CS: Mycotoxins. A possible cause of primary carcinoma of the liver. Am J Med **46:**325-327, 1969.

466 Anthony PP, Vogel CL, Barker LF: Liver cell dysplasia. A premalignant condition. J Clin Pathol **26:**217-223, 1973.

467 Boyd PR, Mark GJ: Multiple hepatic adenomas and a hepatocellular carcinoma in a man on oral methyl testosterone for eleven years. Cancer **40:**1765-1770, 1977.

468 Brambilla C, Tackney C, Hirschman SZ, Colombo M, Dioguardi ML, Donato MF, Paronetto F: Varying nuclear staining intensity of hepatitis B virus DNA in human hepatocellular carcinoma. Lab Invest **55:**475-481, 1986.

469 Chlebowski RT, Tong M, Weissman J, Block JB, Ramming KP, Weiner JM, Bateman JR, Chlebowski JS: Hepatocellular carcinoma. Diagnostic and prognostic features in North American patients. Cancer **53:**2701-2706, 1984.

470 Cohen C, Berson SD, Budgeon LR: Alpha-1-antitrypsin deficiency in southern African hepatocellular carcinoma patients. An immunoperoxidase and histochemical study. Cancer **49**:2537-2540, 1982.

471 Dahms BB: Hepatoma in familial cholestatic cirrhosis of childhood. Its occurrence in twin brothers. Arch Pathol Lab Med **103**:30-33, 1979.

472 Deoras MP, Dicus W: Hepatocarcinoma associated with biliary cirrhosis. A case due to congenital bile duct atresia. Arch Pathol **86**:338-341, 1968.

473 Eriksson S, Carlson J, Velez R: Risk of cirrhosis and primary liver cancer in α-1-antitrypsin deficiency. N Engl J Med **314**:736-739, 1986.

474 Farrell GC, Uren RF, Perkins KW, Joshua DE, Baird PJ, Kronenberg H: Androgen-induced hepatoma. Lancet **1**:430-432, 1975.

475 Gall EA: Primary and metastatic carcinoma of the liver. Relationship to hepatic cirrhosis. Arch Pathol **70**:226-232, 1960.

476 Hernandez-Nieto L, Bruguera M, Bombi JA, Camacho L, Rozman C: Benign liver-cell adenoma associated with long-term administration of an androgenic-anabolic steroid (methandienone). Cancer **40**:1761-1764, 1977.

477 Ho JCI, Wu P-C, Mak T-K: Liver cell dysplasia in association with hepatocellular carcinoma, cirrhosis and hepatitis B surface antigen in Hong Kong. Int J Cancer **28**:571-574, 1981.

478 Hromas RA, Srigley J, Murray JL: Clinical and pathological comparison of young adult women with hepatocellular carcinoma with and without exposure to oral contraceptives. Am J Gastroenterol **80**::479-485, 1985.

479 Hsu H-C, Lin W-S-J, Tsai M-J: Hepatitis-B surface antigen and hepatocellular carcinoma in Taiwan. With special reference to types and localization of HB$_s$A$_g$ in the tumor cells. Cancer **52**:1825-1832, 1983.

480 Ilardi CF, Ying YY, Ackerman LV, Elias JM: Hepatitis B surface antigen and hepatocellular carcinoma in the People's Republic of China. Cancer **46**:1612-1616, 1980.

481 Imazeki F, Omata M, Yokosuka O, Okuda K: Integration of hepatitis B virus DNA in hepatocellular carcinoma. Cancer **58**:1055-1060, 1986.

482 Johnson FL, Feagler JR, Lerner KG, Majerus PW, Siegel M, Hartman JR, Thomas ED: Association of androgenic-anabolic steroid therapy with development of hepatocellular carcinoma. Lancet **2**:1273-1276, 1972.

483 Lefkowitch JH, Apfelbaum TF: Liver cell dysplasia and hepatocellular carcinoma in non-A, non-B hepatitis. Arch Pathol Lab Med **111**:170-173, 1987.

484 Lieberman J, Silton RM, Agliozzo CM, McMahon J: Hepatocellular carcinoma and intermediate α-1-antitrypsin deficiency (MZ phenotype). Am J Clin Pathol **64**:304-310, 1975.

485 London WT: Primary hepatocellular carcinoma. Etiology, pathogenesis, and prevention. Hum Pathol **12**:1085-1097, 1981.

486 Manes JL, Kissane JM, Valdes AJ: Congenital hepatic fibrosis, liver cell carcinoma and adult polycystic kidneys. Cancer **39**:2619-2623, 1977.

487 Nakashima T, Okuda K, Kojiro M, Sakamoto K, Kubo Y, Shimokawa Y: Primary liver cancer coincident with schistosomiasis japonica. A study of 24 necropsies. Cancer **36**:1483-1489, 1975.

488 Neuberger J, Nunnerley HB, Davis M, Portmann B, Laws JW, Williams R: Oral-contraceptive–associated liver tumours. Occurrence of malignancy and difficulties in diagnosis. Lancet **1**:273-276, 1980.

489 Okuda K, Nakashima T, Sakamoto K, Ikari T, Hidaka H, Kubo Y, Sakuma K, Motoike Y, Okuda H, Obata H: Hepatocellular carcinoma arising in noncirrhotic and highly cirrhotic livers. A comparative study of histopathology and frequency of hepatitis B markers. Cancer **49**:450-455, 1982.

490 Pryor AC, Cohen RJ, Goldman RL: Hepatocellular carcinoma in a woman on long-term oral contraceptives. Cancer **40**:884-888, 1977.

491 Shafritz DA, Shouval D, Sherman HI, Hadziyannis SJ, Kew MC: Integration of hepatitis B virus DNA into the genome of liver cells in chronic liver disease and hepatocellular carcinoma. N Engl J Med **305**:1067-1073, 1981.

492 Shar SR, Kew MC: Oral contraceptives and hepatocellular carcinoma. Cancer **49**:407-410, 1982.

493 Smoron GL, Battifora HA: Thorotrast-induced hepatoma. Cancer **30**:1252-1259, 1972.

494 Suzuki K, Uchida T, Horiuchi R, Shikata T: Localization of hepatitis B surface and core antigens in human hepatocellular carcinoma by immunoperoxidase methods. Replication of complete virions of carcinoma cells. Cancer **56**:321-327, 1985.

495 Thung SN, Gerber MA, Sarno E, Popper H: Distribution of five antigens in hepatocellular carcinoma. Lab Invest **41**:101-105, 1979.

496 Tong MJ, Sun SC, Schaeffer BT, Chang NK, Lo KJ, Peters RL: Hepatitis-associated antigen and hepatocellular carcinoma in Taiwan. Ann Intern Med **75**:687-691, 1971.

497 Ugarte N, Gonzalez-Crussi F: Hepatoma in siblings with progressive familial cholestatic cirrhosis of childhood. Am J Clin Pathol **76**:172-177, 1981.

498 Vogel CL, Mody N, Anthony PP, Barker LF: Hepatitis-associated antigen in Ugandan patients with hepatocellular carcinoma. Lancet **2**:621-624, 1970.

499 Weinberg AG, Mize CE, Worthen HG: The occurrence of hepatoma in the chronic form of hereditary tyrosinemia. J Pediatr **88**:434-438, 1976.

500 Weinstein S, Scottolini AG, Loo SYT, Caldwell PC, Bhagavan NV: Ataxia telangiectasia with hepatocellular carcinoma in a 15-year-old girl and studies of her kindred. Arch Pathol Lab Med **109**:1000-1004, 1985.

Pathologic features

501 Albacete RA, Matthews MJ, Saini N: Portal vein thromboses in malignant hepatoma. Ann Intern Med **67**:337-348, 1967.

502 Anthony PP: Primary carcinoma of the liver. A study of 282 cases in Ugandian Africans. J Pathol **110**:37-48, 1973.

503 Anthony PP, James K: Pedunculated hepatocellular carcinoma. Is it an entity? Histopathology **11**:403-414, 1987.

504 Barsky SH, Linnoila I, Triche TJ, Costa J: Hepatocellular carcinoma with carcinoid features. Hum Pathol **15**:892-894, 1984.

505 Buchanan TF Jr, Huvos AG: Clear-cell carcinoma of the liver. A clinicopathologic study of 13 patients. Am J Clin Pathol **61**:529-539, 1974.

506 Cohen C: Intracytoplasmic hyaline globules in hepatocellular carcinomas. Cancer **37**:1754-1758, 1976.

507 Cohen C, Berson SD, Shulman G, Budgeon LR: Immunohistochemical ferritin in hepatocellular carcinoma. Cancer **53**:1931-1935, 1984.

508 Cohen MB, Beckstead JH, Ferrell LD, Yen TSB: Enzyme histochemistry of hepatocellular neoplasms. Am J Surg Pathol **10**:789-794, 1986.

509 Edmonson HA, Steiner PE: Primary carcinoma of the liver. A study of 100 cases among 48,900 necropsies. Cancer **7**:462-503, 1954.

509a Ezaki T, Kanematsu T, Okamura T, Sonoda T, Sugimachi K: DNA analysis of hepatocellular carcinoma and clinicopathologic implications. Cancer **61**:106-109, 1988.

509b Ferrandez-Izquierdo A, Llombart-Bosch A: Immunohistochemical characterization of 130 cases of primary hepatic carcinomas. Pathol Res Pract **182**:783-791, 1987.

510 Goodman ZD, Ishak KG, Langloss JM, Sesterhenn IA, Rabin L: Combined hepatocellular-cholangiocarcinoma. A histologic and immunohistochemical study. Cancer **55**:124-135, 1985.

510a Guigui B, Mavier P, Lescs M-C, Pinaudeau Y, Dhumeaux D, Zafrani ES: Copper and copper-binding protein in liver tumors. Cancer **61**:1155-1158, 1988.

511 Hamperl H: The classification of liver tumors. In Pack GT, Islami AH (eds): Tumors of the liver. Vol. 26 of Recent results in cancer research. Heidelberg, 1970, Springer-Verlag.

512 Haratake J, Horie A, Nakashima A, Takeda S, Mori A: Minute hepatoma with excessive copper accumulation. Report of two cases with resection. Arch Pathol Lab Med **110**:192-194, 1986.

513 Haratake J, Horie A, Takeda S, Kobori K, Sato H, Tokudome S: Tissue copper content in primary and metastatic liver cancers. Acta Pathol Jpn **37**:231-238, 1987.

514 Horie Y, Katoh S, Yoshida H, Imaoka T, Suou T, Hirayama C: Pedunculated hepatocellular carcinoma. Report of three cases and review of literature. Cancer **51**:746-751, 1983.

515 Horie A, Kotoo Y, Hayashi I: Ultrastructural comparison of hepatoblastoma and hepatocellular carcinoma. Cancer **44**:2184-2193, 1979.

516 Hsu H-C, Sheu J-C, Lin Y-H, Chen D-S, Lee C-S, Hwang L-Y, Beasley RP: Prognostic histologic features of resected small hepatocellular carcinoma (HCC) in Taiwan. A comparison with resected large HCC. Cancer **56**:672-680, 1985.

517 Jagirdar J, Ishak KG, Colombo M, Brambilla C, Paronetto F: Fibronectin patterns in hepatocellular carcinoma and its clinical significance. Cancer **56**:1643-1648, 1985.

517a Johnson DE, Herndier BG, Medeiros LJ, Warnke RA, Rouse RV: The diagnostic utility of the keratin profiles of hepatocellular carcinoma and cholangiocarcinoma. Am J Surg Pathol **12**:187-197, 1988.

518 Kakizoe S, Kojiro M, Nakashima T: Hepatocellular carcinoma with sarcomatous change. Clinicopathologic and immunohistochemical studies of 14 autopsy cases. Cancer **59**:310-316, 1987.

519 Kanai T, Hirohashi S, Upton MP, Noguchi M, Kishi K, Makuuchi M, Yamasaki S, Hasegawa H, Takayasu K, Moriyama N, Shimosato Y: Pathology of small hepatocellular carcinoma. A proposal for a new gross classification. Cancer **60**:810-819, 1987.

520 Koelma IA, Nap M, Huitema S, Krom RAF, Houthoff HJ: Hepatocellular carcinoma, adenoma, and focal nodular hyperplasia. Comparative histopathologic study with immunohistochemical parameters. Arch Pathol Lab Med **110**:1035-1040, 1986.

521 Kondo Y: Histologic features of hepatocellular carcinoma and allied disorders. Pathol Annu 20(Pt 2):405-430, 1985.

522 Kondo Y, Nakajima T: Pseudoglandular hepatocellular carcinoma. A morphogenetic study. Cancer 60:1032-1037, 1987.

523 Kondo Y, Niwa Y, Akikusa B, Takazawa H, Okabayashi A: A histopathologic study of early hepatocellular carcinoma. Cancer 52:687-692, 1983.

524 Kuwano H, Sonoda T, Hashimoto H, Enjoji M: Hepatocellular carcinoma with osteoclast-like giant cells. Cancer 54:837-842, 1984.

525 Nagusue N, Ito A, Yukaya H, Ogawa Y: Estrogen receptors in hepatocellular carcinoma. Cancer 57:87-91, 1986.

526 Nagasue N, Yukaya H, Chang Y-C, Ogawa Y, Kohno H, Ito A: Active uptake of testosterone by androgen receptors of hepatocellular carcinoma in humans. Cancer 57:2162-2167, 1986.

527 Nagasue N, Yukaya H, Hamada T, Hirose S, Kanashima R, Inokuchi K: The natural history of hepatocellular carcinoma. A study of 100 untreated cases. Cancer 54:1461-1465, 1984.

528 Nakashima T, Kojiro M, Kawano Y, Shirai F, Takemoto N, Tomimatsu H, Kawasaki H, Okuda K: Histologic growth pattern of hepatocellular carcinoma. Relationship to orcein (hepatitis B surface antigen)-positive cells in cancer tissue. Hum Pathol 13:563-568, 1982.

529 Okuda K, Musha H, Nakajima Y, Kubo Y, Shimokawa Y, Nagaski Y, Sawa Y, Junnouchi S, Kaneko T, Obata H, Hisamitsu T, Motoike S, Okazaki N, Kojiro M, Sakamoto K, Nakashima T: Clinicopathologic features of encapsulated hepatocellular carcinoma. A study of 26 cases. Cancer 40:1240-1245, 1977.

530 Palmer PE, Wolfe HJ: α-1-antitrypsin deposition in primary hepatic carcinomas. Arch Pathol Lab Med 100:232-236, 1976.

531 Roth JA, Berman E, Befeler D, Johnson FB: A black hepatocellular carcinoma with Dubin-Johnson–like pigment and Mallory bodies. A histochemical and ultrastructural study. Am J Surg Pathol 6:375-382, 1982.

531a Sciot R, Paterson AC, Van Eyken P, Callea F, Kew MC, Desmet VJ: Transferrin receptor expression in human hepatocellular carcinoma. An immunohistochemical study of 34 cases. Histopathology 12:53-63, 1988.

532 Stromeyer FW, Ishak KG, Gerber MA, Mathew T: Ground-glass cells in hepatocellular carcinoma. Am J Clin Pathol 74:254-258, 1980.

533 Wu PC, Lai CL, Lam KC, Lok ASF, Lin HJ: Clear cell carcinoma of liver. An ultrastructural study. Cancer 52:504-507, 1983.

Fibrolamellar variant

534 Berman MM, Libbey NP, Foster JH: Hepatocellular carcinoma. Polygonal cell type with fibrous stroma. An atypical variant with a favorable prognosis. Cancer 46:1448-1455, 1980.

535 Craig JR, Peters RL, Edmondson HA, Omata M: Fibrolamellar carcinoma of the liver. A tumor of adolescents and young adults with distinctive clinicopathologic features. Cancer 46:372-379, 1980.

536 Farhi DC, Shikes RH, Murari PJ, Silverberg SG: Hepatocellular carcinoma in young people. Cancer 52:1516-1525, 1983.

537 Farhi DC, Shikes RH, Silverberg SG: Ultrastructure of fibrolamellar oncocytic hepatoma. Cancer 50:702-709, 1982.

538 Payne CM, Nagle RB, Paplanus SH, Graham AR, Berman MM: Fibrolamellar carcinoma of liver. A primary malignant oncocytic carcinoid? Ultrastruct Pathol 10:539-552, 1986.

539 Saul SH, Titelbaum DS, Gansler TS, Varello M, Burke DR, Atkinson BF, Rosato EF: The fibrolamellar variant of hepatocellular carcinoma. Its association with focal nodular hyperplasia. Cancer 60:3049-3055, 1987.

540 Suen KC, Magee JF, Halparin LS, Chan NH, Greene C-A: Fine needle aspiration cytology of fibrolamellar hepatocellular carcinoma. Acta Cytol [Baltimore] 29:867-872, 1984.

Spread and metastasis

541 Becker FF: Hepatoma. Nature's model tumor. A review. Am J Pathol 74:179-200, 1974.

542 Kojiro M, Kawabata K, Kawano Y, Shirai F, Takemoto N, Nakashima T: Hepatocellular carcinoma presenting as intrabile duct tumor growth. A clinicopathologic study of 24 cases. Cancer 49:2144-2147, 1982.

543 Kojiro M, Nakahara H, Sugihara S, Murakami T, Nakashima T, Kawasaki H: Hepatocellular carcinoma with intra-atrial tumor growth. A clinicopathologic study of 18 autopsy cases. Arch Pathol Lab Med 108:989-992, 1984.

544 Linder GT, Crook JN, Cohn I Jr: Primary liver carcinoma. Cancer 33:1624-1629, 1974.

545 Okazaki N, Yoshino M, Yoshida T, Hirohashi S, Kishi K, Shimosato Y: Bone metastasis in hepatocellular carcinoma. Cancer 55:1991-1994, 1985.

546 Talerman A, Magyar E: Hepatocellular carcinoma presenting with pathologic fracture due to bone metastases. Cancer 32:1477-1481, 1973.

Treatment and prognosis

547 Chearanai O, Plengvanit U, Asavanich C, Damrongsak D, Sindhvananda K, Boonyapisit S: Spontaneous rupture of primary hepatoma. Report of 63 cases with particular reference to the pathogenesis and rationale treatment by hepatic artery ligation. Cancer 51:1532-1536, 1983.

548 Chlebowski RT, Tong M, Weissman J, Block JB, Ramming KP, Weiner JM, Bateman JR, Chlebowski JS: Hepatocellular carcinoma. Diagnostic and prognostic features in North American patients. Cancer 53:2701-2706, 1984.

549 Falkson G, Böhmer RH, Adam M, Coetzer BJ: Hepatitis-B as a prognostic discriminant in patients with primary liver cancer. Cancer 57:812-815, 1986.

550 Fisher RL, Scheuer PJ, Sherlock S: Primary liver cell carcinoma in the presence or absence of hepatitis B antigen. Cancer 38:901-905, 1976.

551 Hsu H-C, Sheu J-C, Lin Y-H, Chen D-S, Lee C-S, Hwang L-Y, Beasley RP: Prognostic histologic features of resected small hepatocellular carcinoma (HCC) in Taiwan. A comparison with resected large HCC. Cancer 56:672-680, 1985.

552 Ishikawa K, et al.: Statistics of liver surgery in Japan. III. A study by Japan Liver Cancer Study Group. Acta Hepatol Jpn 17:460-465, 1976.

553 Lin DY, Liaw Y-F, Chu CM, Chang-Chien CS, Wu CS, Chen PC, Sheen IS: Hepatocellular carcinoma in noncirrhotic patients. A laparoscopic study of 92 cases in Taiwan. Cancer 54:1466-1468, 1984.

554 Nagasue N, Yukaya H, Hamada T, Hirose S, Kanashima R, Inokuchi K: The natural history of hepatocellular carcinoma. A study of 100 untreated cases. Cancer 54:1461-1465, 1984.

555 Nagasue N, Yukaya H, Ogawa Y, Sasaki Y, Chang Y-C, Niimi K: Clinical experience with 118 hepatic resections for hepatocellular carcinoma. Surgery 99:694-702, 1986.

556 Okuda K, Musha H, Kanno H, Kojiro M, Sakamoto K, Nakashima T, Igarashi M, Nakano M, Shimokawa Y, Kubo Y, Arishima T, Hashimoto M, Nagata P: Localized submassive liver cell necrosis as a terminal event of liver carcinoma. Cancer 37:1965-1972, 1976.

557 Okuda K, Nakashima T, Obata H, Kubo Y: Clinicopathological studies of minute hepatocellular carcinoma. Analysis of 20 cases, including 4 with hepatic resection. Gastroenterology 73:109-115, 1977.

558 Okuda K, Ohtsuki T, Obata H, Tomimatsu M, Okazaki N, Hasegawa H, Nakajima Y, Ohnishi K: Natural history of hepatocellular carcinoma and prognosis in relation to treatment. Study of 850 patients. Cancer 56:918-928, 1985.

559 Patt YZ, Claghorn L, Charnsangavej C, Soski M, Cleary K, Mavligit GM: Hepatocellular carcinoma. A retrospective analysis of treatments to manage disease confined to the liver. Cancer 61:1884-1888, 1988.

Hepatoblastoma

560 Abenoza P, Manivel JC, Wick MR, Hagen K, Dehner LP: Hepatoblastoma. An immunohistochemical and ultrastructural study. Hum Pathol 18:1025-1035, 1987.

561 Baggenstoss AH: Pathology of tumors of liver in infancy and childhood. In Pack GT, Islami AH (eds): Tumors of the liver, Vol. 26 of Recent results in cancer research. Heidelberg, 1970, Springer-Verlag.

562 Behrle FC, Mantz FA Jr, Olson RL, Trombold JC: Virilization accompanying hepatoblastoma. Pediatrics 32:265-271, 1963.

563 Carter R: Hepatoblastoma in the adult. Cancer 23:191-197, 1969.

564 Emura I, Ohnishi Y, Yamashita Y, Iwafuchi M: Immunohistochemical and ultrastructural study on erythropoiesis in hepatoblastoma. Acta Pathol Jpn 35:79-86, 1985.

565 Giacomantonio M, Ein SH, Mancer K, Stephens CA: Thirty years of experience with pediatric primary malignant liver tumors. J Pediatr Surg 19:523-526, 1984.

566 Gonzalez-Crussi F, Upton MP, Maurer HS: Hepatoblastoma. Attempt at characterization of histologic subtypes. Am J Surg Pathol 6:599-612, 1982.

567 Ishak KG, Glunz PR: Hepatoblastoma and hepatocarcinoma in infancy and childhood. Cancer 20:396-422, 1967.

568 Ito J, Johnson WW: Hepatoblastoma and hepatoma in infancy and childhood, light and electron microscopic studies. Arch Pathol 87:259-266, 1969.

569 Ito E, Sato Y, Kawauchi K, Munakata H, Kamata Y, Yodono H, Yokoyama M: Type Ia glycogen storage disease with hepatoblastoma in siblings. Cancer 59:1776-1780, 1987.

570 Knowlson GTG, Cameron AH: Hepatoblastoma with adenomatoid renal epithelium. Histopathology 3:201-208, 1979.

571 Lack EE, Neave C, Vawter GF: Hepatoblastoma. A clinical and pathologic study of 54 cases. Am J Surg Pathol 6:693-705, 1982.

572 McArthur JW, Toll GD, Russfield AB, Reiss AM, Quinby WC, Baker WH: Sexual precocity attributable to ectopic gonadotropin secretion by hepatoblastoma. Am J Med 54:390-403, 1973.

573 Misugi K, Okajima H, Misugi N, Newton WA Jr: Classification of primary malignant tumors of liver in infancy and childhood. Cancer **20:**1760-1771, 1967.

574 Morinaga S, Yamaguchi M, Watanabe I, Kasai M, Ojima M, Sasano N: An immunohistochemical study of hepatoblastoma producing human chorionic gonadotropin. Cancer **51:**1647-1652, 1983.

575 Nakagawara A, Ikeda K, Hayashida Y, Tsuneyoshi M, Enjoji M, Kawaoi A: Immunocytochemical identification of human chorionic gonadotropin- and alpha-fetoprotein–producing cells of hepatoblastoma associated with precocious puberty. Virchows Arch [Pathol Anat] **398:**45-51, 1982.

576 Nakagawara A, Ikeda K, Tsuneyoshi M, Daimaru Y, Enjoji M, Watanabe I, Iwafuchi M, Sawada T: Hepatoblastoma producing both alpha-fetoprotein and human chorionic gonadotropin. Clinicopathologic analysis of four cases and a review of the literature. Cancer **56:**1636-1642, 1985.

577 Schmidt D, Harms D, Lang W: Primary malignant hepatic tumours in childhood. Virchows Arch [Pathol Anat] **407:**387-403, 1985.

578 Silverman JF, Fu Y-S, McWilliams NB, Kay S: An ultrastructural study of mixed hepatoblastoma with osteoid elements. Cancer **36:**1436-1443, 1975.

579 Weinberg AG, Finegold MJ: Primary hepatic tumors of childhood. Hum Pathol **14:**512-537, 1983.

Bile duct tumors and tumorlike conditions
Bile duct hamartoma

580 Chung EB: Multiple bile-duct hamartomas. Cancer **26:**287-296, 1970.

581 Honda N, Cobb C, Lechago J: Bile duct carcinoma associated with multiple von Meyenburg complexes in the liver. Hum Pathol **17:**1287-1290, 1986.

582 Popovsky MA, Costa JC, Doppman JL: Meyenburg complexes of the liver and bile cysts as a consequence of hepatic ischemia. Hum Pathol **10:**425-432, 1979.

583 Thommesen N: Biliary hamartomas (von Meyenburg complexes) in liver needle biopsies, Acta Pathol Microbiol Scand [A] **86:**93-99, 1978.

Bile duct adenoma

583a Allaire G, Rabin L, Ishak KG: Bile duct adenoma. A study of 152 cases. (abstract). Lab Invest **58:**3A, 1988.

584 Govindarajan S, Peters RL: The bile duct adenoma. A lesion distinct from Meyenburg complex. Arch Pathol Lab Med **108:**922-924, 1984.

585 Ishak KG, Rabin L: Benign tumors of the liver. Med Clin North Am **59:**995-1013, 1975.

586 Mixter CG, Mixter CG Jr: Liver nodules encountered at laparotomy. Significance and treatment. Ann Surg **138:**230-239, 1953.

Biliary cystadenoma and cystadenocarcinoma

587 Bloustein PA, Silverberg SG: Squamous cell carcinoma originating in an hepatic cyst. Case report with a review of the hepatic cyst-carcinoma association. Cancer **38:**2002-2005, 1976.

588 Devine P, Ucci AA: Biliary cystadenocarcinoma arising in a congenital cyst. Hum Pathol **16:**92-94, 1985.

589 Ishak KG, Willis GW, Cummins SD, Bullock AA: Biliary cystadenoma and cystadenocarcinoma. Report of 14 cases and review of the literature. Cancer **38:**322-338, 1977.

590 Unger PD, Thung SN, Kaneko M: Pseudosarcomatous cystadenocarcinoma of the liver. Hum Pathol **18:**521-523, 1987.

591 Wheeler DA, Edmondson HA: Cystadenoma with mesenchymal stroma (CMS) in the liver and bile ducts. A clinicopathologic study of 17 cases, 4 with malignant change. Cancer **56:**1434-1445, 1985.

Bile duct carcinoma (cholangiocarcinoma)

592 Anthony PP: Primary carcinoma of the liver. A study of 282 cases in Ugandan Africans. J Pathol **110:**37-48, 1973.

593 Azizah N, Paradinas FJ: Cholangiocarcinoma coexisting with developmental liver cysts. A distinct entity different from liver cystadenocarcinoma. Histopathology **4:**391-400, 1980.

594 Bonetti F, Chilosi M, Pisa R, Novelli P, Zamboni G, Menestrina F: Epithelial membrane antigen expression in cholangiocarcinoma. A useful immunohistochemical tool for differential diagnosis with hepatocarcinoma. Virchows Arch [Pathol Anat] **401:**307-313, 1983.

595 Chou ST, Chan CW, Ng WL: Mucin histochemistry of human cholangiocarcinoma. J Pathol **118:**165-170, 1976.

596 Daroca PJ Jr, Tuthill R, Reed RJ: Cholangiocarcinoma arising in congenital hepatic fibrosis. A case report. Arch Pathol **99:**592-595, 1975.

597 Foucar E, Kaplan LR, Gold JH, Kiang DT, Sibley RK, Bosl G: Well differentiated peripheral cholangiocarcinoma with an unusual clinical course. Gastroenterology **77:**347-353, 1979.

598 Gallagher PJ, Millis RR, Mitchinson MJ: Congenital dilatation of the intrahepatic bile ducts with cholangiocarcinoma. J Clin Pathol **25:**804-808, 1972.

599 Goodman ZK, Ishak KG, Langloss JM, Sesterhenn IA, Rabin L: Combined hepatocellular-cholangiocarcinoma. A histologic and immunohistochemical study. Cancer **55:**124-135, 1985.

599a Johnson DE, Herndier BG, Medeiros LJ, Warnke RA, Rouse RV: The diagnostic utility of the keratin profiles of hepatocellular carcinoma and cholangiocarcinoma. Am J Surg Pathol **12:**187-197, 1988.

600 Koga A, Ichimiya H, Yamaguchi K, Miyazaki K, Nakayama F: Hepatolithiasis associated with cholangiocarcinoma. Possible etiologic significance. Cancer **55:**2826-2829, 1985.

601 Nakanuma Y, Terada T, Tanaka Y, Ohta G: Are hepatolithiasis and cholangiocarcinoma aetiologically related? A morphological study of 12 cases of hepatolithiasis associated with cholangiocarcinoma. Virchows Arch [Pathol Anat] **406:**45-58, 1985.

602 Ordóñez NG, Mackay B: Ultrastructure of liver cell and bile duct carcinomas. Ultrastruct Pathol **5:**201-241, 1983.

603 Pastolero GC, Wakabayashi T, Oka T, Mori S: Tissue polypeptide antigen. A marker antigen differentiating cholangiolar tumors from other hepatic tumors. Am J Clin Pathol **87:**168-173, 1987.

604 Rubel LR, Ishak KG: Thorotrast-associated cholangiocarcinoma. An epidemiologic and clinicopathologic study. Cancer **50:**1408-1415, 1982.

605 Stromeyer FW, Smith DH, Ishak KG: Anabolic steroid therapy and intrahepatic cholangiocarcinoma. Cancer **43:**440-443, 1979.

606 Weinbren K, Mutum SS: Pathological aspects of cholangiocarcinoma. J Pathol **139:**217-238, 1983.

Mesenchymal tumors and tumorlike conditions
Vascular tumors

607 Baggenstoss AH: Pathology of tumors of liver in infancy and childhood. In Pack GT, Islami AH (eds): Tumors of the liver, Vol. 26 of Recent results in cancer research. Heidelberg, 1970, Springer-Verlag.

608 Dannaher CL, Tamburro CH, Yam LT: Occupational carcinogenesis. The Louisville experience with vinyl chloride–associated hepatic angiosarcoma. Am J Med **70:**279-287, 1981.

609 Dean PJ, Haggitt RC, O'Hara CJ: Malignant epithelioid hemangioendothelioma of the liver in young women. Relationship to oral contraceptive use. Am J Surg Pathol **10:**695-704, 1985.

610 Dehner LP, Ishak KG: Vascular tumors of the liver in infants and children. A study of 30 cases and review of the literature. Arch Pathol **92:**101-111, 1971.

611 Echevarria RA, Arean YM, Galindo L: Hepatic tumors of long duration with eventual metastases. Two cases of leiomyosarcomatosis possibly arising from hamartomas of liver. Am J Clin Pathol **69:**624-631, 1978.

612 Falk H, Herbert JT, Edmonds L, Heath CW Jr, Thomas LB, Popper H: Review of four cases of childhood hepatic angiosarcoma. Elevated environmental arsenic exposure in one case. Cancer **47:**382-391, 1981.

613 Feldman PS, Shneidman D, Kaplan C: Ultrastructure of infantile hemangioendothelioma of the liver. Cancer **42:**521-527, 1978.

614 Ishak KG, Sesterhenn IA, Goodman MZD, Rabin L, Stromeyer FW: Epithelioid hemangioendothelioma of the liver. A clinicopathologic and follow-up study of 32 cases. Hum Pathol **15:**839-852, 1984.

615 Kauffman SL, Stout AP: Malignant hemangioendothelioma in infants and children. Cancer **14:**1186-1196, 1961.

616 Kojiro M, Kawano Y, Kawasaki H, Nakashima T, Ikezaki H: Thorotrast-induced hepatic angiosarcoma, and combined hepatocellular and cholangiocarcinoma in a single patient. Cancer **49:**2161-2164, 1982.

617 Kojiro M, Nakashima T, Ito Y, Ikezaki H, Mori T, Kido C: Thorium dioxide-related angiosarcoma of the liver. Pathomorphologic study of 29 autopsy cases. Arch Pathol Lab Med **109:**853-857, 1985.

618 Ludwig J, Grier MW, Hoffman HN II, McGill DB: Calcified mixed malignant tumor of the liver. Arch Pathol **99:**162-166, 1975.

619 Ludwig J, Hoffman HN II: Hemangiosarcoma of the liver. Spectrum of morphologic changes and clinical findings. Mayo Clin Proc **50:**255-263, 1975.

620 Makk L, Delmore F, Creech JL Jr, Ogden LL, Fadell EH, Songster CL, Clanton J, Johnson MN, Christopherson WM: Clinical and morphologic features of hepatic angiosarcoma in vinyl chloride workers. Cancer **37:**149-163, 1976.

621 Manning JT Jr, Ordóñez NG, Barton JH: Endothelial cell origin of thorium oxide–induced angiosarcoma of liver. Arch Pathol Lab Med **107:**456-458, 1983.

622 McLean RH, Moller JH, Warwick WJ, Satran L, Lucas RV Jr: Multinodular hemangiomatosis of the liver in infancy. Pediatrics **49:**563-573, 1972.

623 Noronha R, Gonzalez-Crussi F: Hepatic angiosarcoma in childhood. A case report and review of the literature. Am J Surg Pathol **8:**863-871, 1984.

624 Rakov HL, Smalldon TR, Derman H: Hepatic hemangioendotheliosarcoma. Report of a case due to thorium. Arch Intern Med **112:**173-178, 1963.

625 Rosai J, Gold J, Landy R: The histiocytoid hemangiomas. A unifying concept embracing several previously described entities of skin, soft tissue, large vessels, bone, and heart. Hum Pathol 10:707-730, 1979.

626 Ruebner BH, Eggleston JC: What is new in epithelioid hemangioendothelioma of the liver? Pathol Res Pract 182:110-112, 1987.

627 Sussman EB, Nydick I, Gray GF: Hemangioendothelial sarcoma of the liver and hemochromatosis. Arch Pathol 97:39-42, 1974.

628 Thomas LB, Popper H, Berk PD, Selikoff I, Falk H: Vinyl-chloride–induced liver disease. From idiopathic portal hypertension (Banti's syndrome) to angiosarcomas. N Engl J Med 292:17-22, 1975.

629 Van Steenbergen W, Joosten E, Marchal G, Baert A, Vanstapel MJ, Desmet V, Wijnants P, DeGroote J: Hepatic lymphangiomatosis. Report of a case and review of the literature. Gastroenterology 88:1968-1972, 1985.

630 Winberg CD, Ranchod M: Thorotrast induced hepatic cholangiocarcinoma and angiosarcoma. Hum Pathol 10:108-112, 1979.

Mesenchymal hamartoma

631 Dehner LP, Ewing SL, Sumner HW: Infantile mesenchymal hamartoma of the liver. Histologic and ultrastructural observations. Arch Pathol 99:379-382, 1975.

632 Lack EE: Mesenchymal hamartoma of the liver. A clinical and pathologic study of nine cases. Am J Pediatr Hematol/Oncol 8:91-98, 1986.

633 Raffensperger JG, Gonzalez-Crussi F, Skeehan T: Mesenchymal hamartoma of the liver. J Pediatr Surg 18:585-587, 1983.

634 Rhodes RH, Marchildon MB, Luebke DC, Edmondson HA, Mikitz VG: A mixed hamartoma of the liver. Light and electron microscopy. Hum Pathol 9:211-221, 1978.

635 Srouji MN, Chatten J, Schulman WM, Ziegler MM, Koop CE: Mesenchymal hamartoma of the liver in infants. Cancer 42:2483-2489, 1978.

636 Sutton CA, Eller JL: Mesenchymal hamartoma of the liver. Cancer 22:29-34, 1968.

Malignant mesenchymoma

637 Dehner LP: Hepatic tumors in the pediatric age group. A distinctive clinico-pathologic spectrum. Perspect Pediatr Pathol 4:217-268, 1978.

638 Keating S, Taylor GP: Undifferentiated (embryonal) sarcoma of the liver. Ultrastructural and immunohistochemical similarities with malignant fibrous histiocytoma. Hum Pathol 16:693-699, 1985.

639 Stanley RJ, Dehner LP, Hesker AE: Primary malignant mesenchymal tumors (mesenchymoma) of the liver in childhood. An angiographic-pathologic study of three cases. Cancer 32:973-984, 1973.

640 Stocker JT, Ishak KG: Undifferentiated (embryonal) sarcoma of the liver. Report of 31 cases. Cancer 42:336-348, 1978.

Other mesenchymal tumors

641 Alrenga DP: Primary fibrosarcoma of the liver. Case report and review of the literature. Cancer 36:446-449, 1975.

642 Arends JW, Willebrand D, Blaauw AMM, Bosman FT: Primary malignant fibrous histiocytoma of the liver. A case report with immunocytochemical observations. Histopathology 11:427-431, 1987.

643 Bloustein PA: Hepatic leiomyosarcoma. Ultrastructural study and review of the differential diagnosis. Hum Pathol 9:713-715, 1978.

644 Goodman ZD, Ishak KG: Angiomyolipomas of the liver. Am J Surg Pathol 8:745-750, 1984.

645 Hawkins EP, Jordan GL, McGavran MH: Primary leiomyoma of the liver. Successful treatment by lobectomy and presentation of criteria for diagnosis. Am J Surg Pathol 4:301-304, 1980.

646 Horie Y, Hori T, Hirayama C, Hashimoto K, Yumoto T, Tanikawa K: Osteoclast-like giant cell tumor of the liver. Acta Pathol Jpn 37:1327-1335, 1987.

647 Ishak KG, Rabin L: Benign tumors of the liver. Med Clin North Am 59:995-1013, 1975.

648 Karhunen PJ: Hepatic pseudolipoma. J Clin Pathol 38:877-879, 1985.

649 Kim H, Damjanov I: Localized fibrous mesothelioma of the liver. Report of a giant tumor studied by light and electron microscopy. Cancer 52:1662-1665, 1983.

650 Munoz PA, Rao MS, Reddy JK: Osteoclastoma-like giant cell tumor of the liver. Cancer 46:771-779, 1980.

651 O'Leary MR, Hill RB, Levine RA: Peritoneoscopic diagnosis of primary leiomyosarcoma of liver. Hum Pathol 13:76-78, 1982.

652 Parham DM, Peiper SC, Robicheaux G, Ribeiro RC, Douglass EC: Malignant rhabdoid tumor of the liver. Evidence for epithelial differentiation. Arch Pathol Lab Med 112:61-64, 1988.

653 Rubin E, Russinovich NAE, Luna RF, Tishler JMA, Wilkerson JA: Myelolipoma of the liver. Cancer 54:2043-2046, 1984.

654 Sumiyoshi A, Niho Y: Primary osteogenic sarcoma of the liver. Report of an autopsy case. Acta Pathol Jpn 21:305-312, 1971.

655 von Hochstetter AR, Hättenschwiler J, Vogt M: Primary osteosarcoma of the liver. Cancer 60:2312-2317, 1987.

Other primary tumors and tumorlike conditions

656 Bagley CM Jr, Thomas LB, Johnson RE, Chretien PB, De Vita T Jr: Diagnosis of liver involvement by lymphoma. Results in 96 consecutive peritoneoscopies. Cancer 31:840-847, 1973.

657 Berry CL: Solitary "necrotic nodule" of the liver. A probable pathogenesis. J Clin Pathol 38:1278-1280, 1985.

658 Chen KTK: Inflammatory pseudotumor of the liver. Hum Pathol 15:694-696, 1984.

659 Daniel SJ, Attiyeh FF, Dire JJ, Pyun HJ, Carroll DS, Attia A: Primary lymphoma of the liver treated with extended left hepatic lobectomy. Cancer 55:206-209, 1985.

660 DeMent SH, Mann RB, Staal SP, Kuhajda FP, Boitnott JK: Primary lymphomas of the liver. Report of six cases and review of the literature. Am J Clin Pathol 88:255-263, 1987.

661 Edmondson HA: Tumors of the liver and intrahepatic bile ducts. In Atlas of human pathology, Sect. 4, Fasc. 25. Washington, D.C., 1958, Armed Forces Institute of Pathology.

662 Gresham GA, Rue LW III: Squamous cell carcinoma of the liver. Hum Pathol 16:413-416, 1985.

663 Hart WR: Primary endodermal sinus (yolk sac) tumor of the liver. First reported case. Cancer 35:1453-1458, 1975.

664 Hausner RJ, Alexander RW: Localized congenital hepatic fibrosis presenting as an abdominal mass. Hum Pathol 9:473-476, 1978.

665 Heaton GE, Matthews TH, Christopherson WM: Malignant trophoblastic tumors with massive hemorrhage presenting as liver primary. A report of two cases. Am J Surg Pathol 10:342-347, 1986.

666 Miller ST, Wollner N, Meyers PA, Exelby P, Jereb B, Miller DR: Primary hepatic or hepatosplenic non-Hodgkin's lymphoma in children. Cancer 52:2285-2288, 1983.

667 Misugi K, Reiner CB: A malignant true teratoma of liver in childhood. Arch Pathol 80:409-412, 1965.

667a Miura K, Shirasawa H: Primary carcinoid tumor of the liver. Am J Clin Pathol 89:561-564, 1988.

668 Robinson RA, Nelson L: Hepatic teratoma in an anencephalic fetus. Arch Pathol Lab Med 10:655-657, 1986.

668a Ryan J, Straus DJ, Lange C, Filippa DA, Botet JF, Sanders LM, Shiu MH, Fortner JG: Primary lymphoma of the liver. Cancer 61:370-375, 1988.

669 Someren A: "Inflammatory pseudotumor" of liver with occlusive phlebitis. Report of a case in a child and review of the literature. Am J Clin Pathol 69:176-181, 1978.

670 Song E, Kew MC, Grieve T, Isaacson C, Myburgh JA: Primary squamous cell carcinoma of the liver occurring in association with hepatolithiasis. Cancer 53:542-546, 1984.

671 Strayer DS, Reppun TS, Levin M, Deschryver-Kecskemetic K: Primary lymphoma of the liver. J Gastroenterol 78:1571-1576, 1980.

672 Torres A, Bollozos GD: Primary reticulum cell sarcoma of liver. Cancer 27:1489-1492, 1971.

673 Warner TFCS, Seo IS, Madura JA, Polak JM, Pearse AGE: Pancreatic-poly-peptide–producing apudoma of the liver. Cancer 46:1146-1151, 1980.

674 Yu-Ping X, Ji-yao Y: Primary neuroendocrine carcinoma of the liver. Ultrastruct Pathol 10:331-336, 1986.

Metastatic tumors

675 Borja ER, Hori JM, Pugh RP: Metastatic carcinomatosis of the liver mimicking cirrhosis. Case report and review of the literature. Cancer 35:445-449, 1975.

676 Hajdu SI, D'Ambrosio FG, Fields V, Lightdale CJ: Aspiration and brush cytology of the liver. Semin Diagn Pathol 3:227-238, 1986.

677 Johansen P, Svendsen KN: Scan-guided fine needle aspiration biopsy in malignant hepatic disease. Acta Cytol [Baltimore] 22:292-296, 1978.

678 Lundquist A: Fine needle aspiration biopsy for cytodiagnosis of malignant tumor in the liver. Acta Med Scand 188:465-470, 1970.

679 McKenzie AD, Wilson JW: Hepatic resection for blood borne metastases from large bowel carcinoma. Case report and review of literature. Can J Surg 13:159-162, 1970.

680 Mosenthal WT: Resection of massive liver metastases in the malignant carcinoid syndrome. Surg Clin North Am **43**:1253-1262, 1963.

681 Pikren JW, Tsukada Y, Lane WW: Liver metastases. Analysis of autopsy data. In Weiss L, Gilber HA (eds): Liver metastases. Boston, 1982, G.K. Hall & Co.

682 Qizilbash A, Kontozoglou T, Sianos J, Scully K: Hepar lobatum associated with chemotherapy and metastatic breast cancer. Arch Pathol Lab Med **111**:58-61, 1987.

683 Schulz W, Hagen CH, Hort W: The distribution of liver metastases from colonic cancer. A quantitative postmortem study. Virchows Arch [Pathol Anat] **406**:279-284, 1985.

684 Schulz W, Hort W: The distribution of metastases in the liver. A quantitative postmortem study. Virchows Arch [Pathol Anat] **394**:89-96, 1981.

685 Sherlock P, Kim YS, Koss IG: Cytology diagnosis of cancer from aspirated material obtained at liver biopsy. Am J Dig Dis **12**:396-402, 1967.

686 Wilson SM, Adson MA: Surgical treatment of hepatic metastases from colorectal cancers. Arch Surg **111**:330-334, 1976.

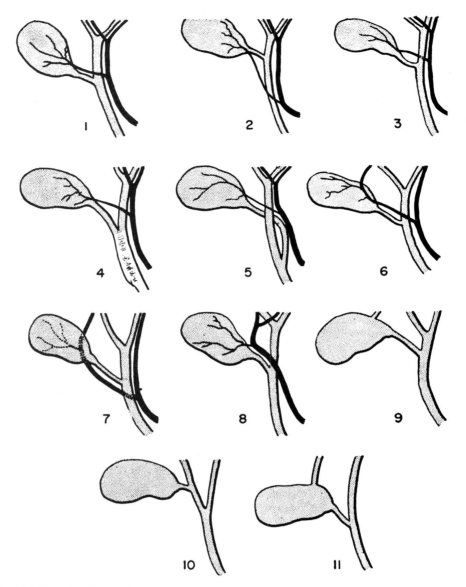

Fig. 14-1 Normal and anomalous arrangements of extrahepatic bile ducts and their adjoining arteries.

1, Normal arrangement.

2, Caudad origin of cystic artery (frequent variation).

3, Placement of cystic artery posterior to common hepatic duct.

4, Long cystic duct attached to common hepatic duct for some distance prior to confluence to form common bile duct.

5, Long cystic duct passing behind common hepatic duct and joining it medially at lower level.

6, Normal ductal system with anomalous right hepatic artery reaching gallbladder wall, where it gives off cystic artery and then turns into liver. In this anomaly, which is not rare, right hepatic artery is often ligated either with cystic duct or as separate structure erroneously identified as cystic artery.

7, Anomalous right hepatic artery in posterior position presenting same dangers as mentioned in 6.

8, Very dangerous anomaly of entire hepatic artery which follows cystic duct to gallbladder before turning into liver. Accidental ligation on entire hepatic artery was almost always fatal before advent of penicillin and chlortetracycline, and it is still hazardous.

9, Anomalous bile duct entering gallbladder through its bed in liver. Cholecystectomy in such instances is usually followed by profuse drainage of bile and is likely to result in fatal peritonitis unless external drainage is afforded.

10, Anomalous insertion of cystic duct into right hepatic duct. Section of right hepatic duct caudad to its junction with cystic duct can easily be mistaken for cystic duct and ligated, thus shutting off drainage of right lobe of liver into intestine.

11, Anomalous arrangement of right hepatic duct in which it enters gallbladder so that all of bile from right lobe of liver must drain through cystic duct.

(From Rhoads JE: Liver, gallbladder and bile passages. In Rhoads JE, Allen JG, Harkins HN, Moyer CA: Surgery: principles and practice, ed. 4. Philadelphia, 1970, J.B. Lippincott Co.)

by supersaturation with cholesterol and rapid in vitro nucleation of cholesterol crystals.[26]

Stones in the gallbladder are four times more frequent in women than in men. About 20% of the stones contain sufficient calcium to be radiopaque. Of the nonopaque stones about 50% are manifest only by nonvisualization of the gallbladder by cholecystography. The others show as a negative shadow when the gallbladder concentrates the dye. The technique of sonography has been successfully used for the identification of gallbladder stones and it has become the method of choice for their detection.

The incidence of stones in the general population of the United States is 11%, as determined by the Framingham study.[19] Torvik and Höivik[27] report a frequency of 19.5% in autopsy material from Scandinavia. The incidence increases with age until at 60 years about one out of every four women has stones.

Gallstones vary considerably in chemical composition, the basic constituents being cholesterol, calcium bilirubinate, and calcium carbonate, either alone or in combination.[25]

Pure gallstones (10%) are composed of only one of the substances mentioned. *Cholesterol stones* are single, spheroidal, coarsely nodular, and have a translucent bluish white color. On fracture, they show large, flat crystals (Fig. 14-2). Most cholesterol stones are found in multiparous women; this is probably related to the fact that cholesterol metabolism is altered during pregnancy and to the clinical observation that the first signs and symptoms of cholelithiasis often develop shortly after pregnancy.[20] However, no correlation exists between the presence of cholesterol stones in the gallbladder and the level of cholesterol in the blood.

Calcium bilirubinate stones are multiple, small, brown to jet black, faceted and measure 2 to 5 mm in diameter. They are associated with cirrhosis and with hemolytic disorders, such as sickle cell anemia, thalassemia, hereditary spherocytosis, and artificial cardiac valves.[24] *Calcium carbonate stones* are amorphous and grayish white.

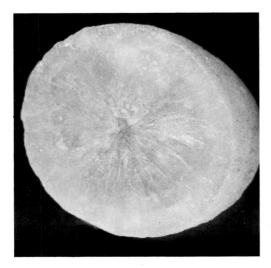

Fig. 14-2 Cross section of solitary, pure cholesterol stone showing typical crystalline structure.

The gallbladder containing pure gallstones shows little or no inflammatory reaction if the cystic duct is not obstructed.

Mixed gallstones (80%) consist of various combinations of cholesterol, calcium bilirubinate, and calcium carbonate. Their size and number vary. They are usually multiple, faceted, and laminated. Chronic cholecystitis is almost always present (Fig. 14-3). Several crops may be present, suggesting that the causes for their formation may operate at different times.

Combined gallstones (10%) are characteristically large and single. They may have a pure nucleus with a mixed shell or the reverse. *Barrel stones,* a type of combined stone, are usually two in number, large, and faceted on one surface, and the thick-walled gallbladder is closely wrapped around them (Fig. 14-4). Combined stones are always accompanied by chronic inflammation of the gallbladder and occasionally by biliary fistulas.

Sequential cholecystographic studies and C[14] dating suggest that gallbladder stones grow at a rate of approximately 1 to 2 mm per year and that they are usually present for 5 to 20 years before they are removed.[23]

Gallstones are formed in the gallbladder, from which they may escape into the cystic and other extrahepatic ducts. Their independent formation in the extrahepatic ducts is rare.[22] Choledocholithiasis, with or without obstruction, is nearly always secondary to cholelithiasis.[21] The appearance of symptoms of choledocholithiasis some time after cholecystectomy for stones is usually caused by stones that were overlooked at the time of surgery. However, the occasional finding of multiple small intrahepatic stones indicates that they can also be formed in the hepatic duct system outside the gallbladder.

Impaction of the stone in the cystic duct may lead to acute cholecystitis, and impaction in the terminal third of the common duct or ampulla of Vater will result in severe, colicky pain and obstructive jaundice.

CHOLESTEROSIS

Cholesterosis of the gallbladder occurs, for the most part, in multiparous women. The gross appearance is characteristic; linear yellow streaks are seen in the prominences of the ridges, surrounded by a congested mucosa ("strawberry gallbladder") (Fig. 14-5). The bile is usually dark, thick, and shows a high concentration of cholesterol by chemical analysis.

Microscopically, collections of lipid-filled foamy cells are present in the tips of the villi (Fig. 14-6). Inflammatory changes are usually insignificant, unless the cholesterosis is accompanied by stones in the cystic duct. The rarity of the coexistence of cholesterosis with advanced cholecystitis has suggested that the inflammatory process induces in some way the resorption of the lipid deposits.

Although cholesterosis of the gallbladder is in all likelihood a morphologic marker for a functional abnormality of bile metabolism, it is probably erroneous to ascribe the symptoms that these patients might have to the mere presence of the foamy histiocytes, especially in view of the fact that these changes are restricted to the gallbladder mucosa and do not ordinarily extend to the mucosa of the extrahepatic bile ducts.

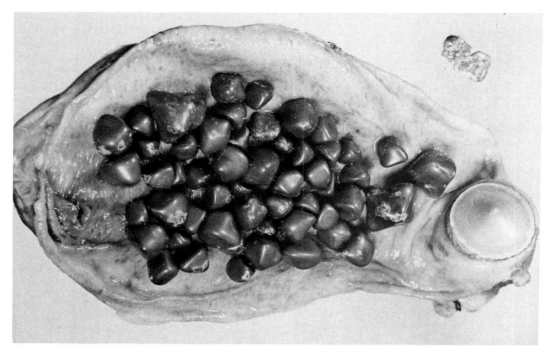

Fig. 14-3 Numerous stones of mixed type in chronically inflamed gallbladder. There is also a large combined stone totally occluding cystic duct.

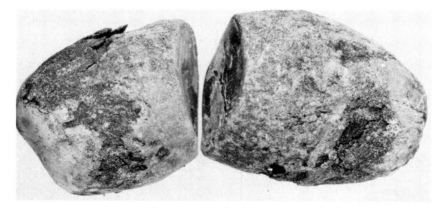

Fig. 14-4 Two typical barrel stones of combined type faceted on only one surface. These stones completely filled thick-walled gallbladder.

ACUTE CHOLECYSTITIS

The main clinical symptoms of acute cholecystitis are pain in the right upper quadrant, nausea and vomiting, and fever.[39] Grossly, the gallbladder wall is markedly edematous and the mucosa has an angry red color.[45] When stones are present (95% of the cases), the disease is known as *acute calculous cholecystitis*. The luminal content often has a yellow, grumous appearance; this may appear grossly as empyema, but in reality the material is not pus but an emulsion of calcium carbonate and/or cholesterol. Often, acute changes are seen superimposed on an organ with chronic

cholecystitis. Microscopically, the tissue response is characterized in most cases by edema, hyperemia, extravasation of red blood cells, and widespread fibroblastic proliferation rather than by the customary polymorphonuclear infiltrate. The mucosa may be intact or show focal or extensive areas of ulceration. Fresh thrombi are often found within small veins.[28]

The pathogenesis of acute calculous cholecystitis is thought to be in most cases chemical or ischemic rather than infectious and is nearly always related to a stone impacted in the cystic duct.[32,36,42] Such impaction may lead to changes

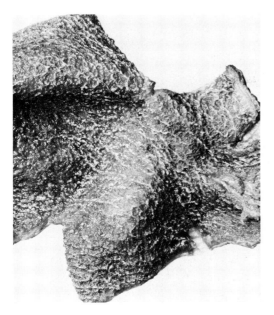

Fig. 14-5 Cholesterosis of gallbladder. Small yellow flecks are present along mucosal ridges.

in the concentration and composition of the bile and also to interference with the venous supply of the gallbladder by obstructing the tortuous venous channels surrounding the cystic duct. The hypothesis that most cases of acute cholecystitis have a chemical rather than an infectious pathogenesis is supported by the experimental production of acute cholecystitis by injecting concentrated bile into the gallbladder,[46] by the fact that 25% to 50% of bile cultures from acutely inflamed gallbladders are sterile, and by observation that free perforation of these gallbladders is only rarely followed by bacterial peritonitis.

The chemical agents that have been proposed as mediators of acute cholecystitis are trypsin from pancreatic juice, unconjugated bile salts, and the phospholipid lysolecithin.[43] In an acutely distended gallbladder, these agents may leak through the intact wall and cause *bile peritonitis,* a condition with an ominous prognosis.[38]

Free perforation into the peritoneal cavity has become a relatively rare occurrence because of the awareness by surgeons of the importance of an operation promptly after onset of symptoms of gallbladder disease. In a study reported by van der Linden and Sunzel,[44] one half of 140 patients with acute cholecystitis had early operation (within 24 hours), whereas the remaining had delayed operation (2 months later). The patients in the latter group had more protracted fever, longer hospital stay, and greater loss of time from work.

Bacterial invasion in acute calculous cholecystitis is usually a secondary event. If the organisms are of the gasforming type, the condition known as *emphysematous* or *acute gaseous cholecystitis* may result;[29] this complication is particularly common in diabetics.

Acute acalculous cholecystitis accounts for about 5% of all cases of acute cholecystitis and a higher proportion of cases in children.[33-35,37] It may follow systemic infections such as hemolytic streptococcal septicemia or typhoid fever.[35] Cases of chemical acalculous cholecystitis have also been seen following the administration of hepatic arterial chemotherapy.[41]

Occasionally, a gallbladder removed because of acute inflammation will show fibrinoid necrosis of the muscular arteries, indistinguishable from that seen in polyarteritis nodosa.[30,31] Later on some of these patients show evidence of

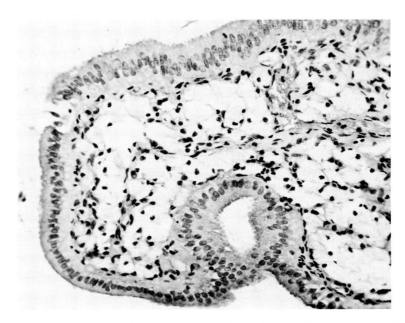

Fig. 14-6 Cholesterosis of gallbladder. Large foamy cells can be seen beneath normal epithelium of a villus.

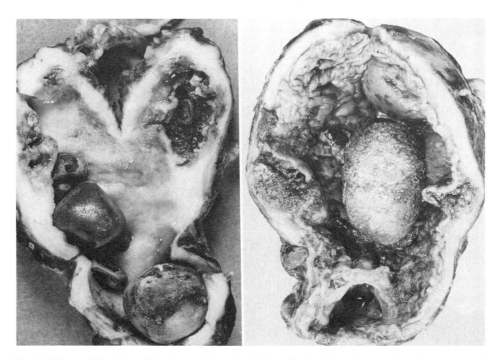

Fig. 14-7 Two gallbladders with advanced chronic cholecystitis. In both, subserosal portions are greatly thickened. In one, there is ulceration of mucosal surface. One gallbladder shows single large stone, and other shows multiple faceted stones.

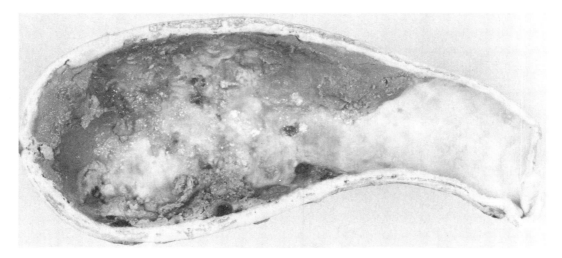

Fig. 14-8 Chronically inflamed gallbladder in which extensive calcification has occurred, resulting in condition known as "porcelain gallbladder." Epithelium was largely eroded. Stones were removed before photograph was taken.

a multisystem disorder,[40] but others remain asymptomatic thereafter, indicating that the vascular changes are not always part of a systemic disease.

CHRONIC CHOLECYSTITIS AND CHOLANGITIS

Chronic cholecystitis is rarely seen in the absence of lithiasis, although pure stones of the cholesterol and calcium bilirubinate types may be present without inflammation. Thickening of the wall is always present, sometimes to a striking degree (Fig. 14-7). Occasionally this is associated with diffuse calcification, a condition known as "porcelain gallbladder" (Fig. 14-8). In most instances, stones are of the mixed or combined type (see Figs. 14-3 and 14-8). Ulceration of the mucosa may result from pressure by the stones.

Microscopically, the mucosa of a chronically inflamed gallbladder shows varying degrees of mononuclear infiltration and fibrosis (Figs. 14-9 and 14-10). The epithelium may be relatively normal, atrophic, or show hyperplastic and metaplastic changes.[54] The metaplasia can be of goblet

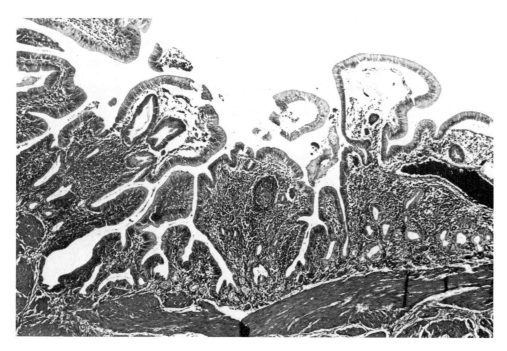

Fig. 14-9 Chronic cholecystitis with expansion of mucosa resulting from accumulation of chronic inflammatory cells. Fibrosis is absent.

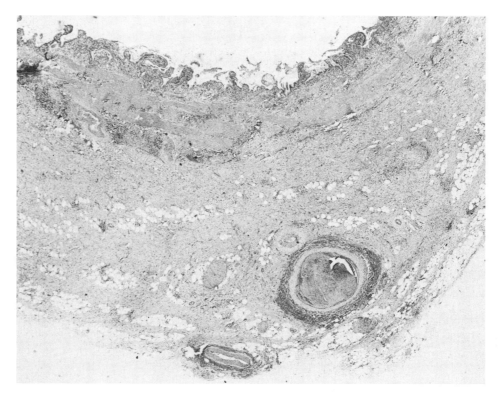

Fig. 14-10 Advanced chronic cholecystitis. There is extreme subserosal fibrosis and recent thrombus can be seen within a vessel.

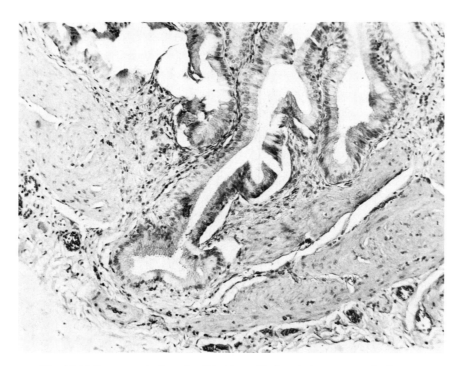

Fig. 14-11 Deep penetration of gallbladder epithelium between muscular layers.

cell type or pseudopyloric type, the former being accompanied by the appearance of Paneth cells and endocrine cells.[61,71] These endocrine cells can exhibit immunocytochemical reactivity for serotonin, somatostatin, cholecystokinin, gastrin, and pancreatic polypeptide.[47] The incidence of these metaplastic changes increases steadily with age.[59]

The gallbladder wall may show fibrosis, muscle hypertrophy, encrusted stones, or nodular collections of foamy macrophages. Irregularly shaped tubular structures are present within the wall in over half of the cases (Fig. 14-11). They are lined by columnar or cuboidal epithelium and may contain bile or stones. These tubular structures, traditionally known as Rokitansky-Aschoff sinuses, are thought to represent diverticula resulting from increased intraluminal pressure.[65] Similar but smaller tubular formations, sometimes found in the subserosal layer and known as Luschka's ducts, probably have a similar origin, but their communication with the lumen has been cut off so that they have become cysts with bud-like branches.[65]

Exaggerated examples of gallbladder diverticulosis associated with muscular hypertrophy have been dignified with the impressive but inaccurate names of *adenomyoma* (when focal), and *adenomyomatosis* (when diffuse).[58] The localized form may involve any segment of the organ but in most cases is located in the fundus, where it results in a sharply circumscribed lesion[49] (Fig. 14-12).

Several morphologic variants of chronic cholecystitis have been described. *Follicular cholecystitis* is characterized by widespread formation of lymphoid follicles in all layers of the gallbladder.[55] *Eosinophilic cholecystitis* shows a massive outpouring of mature eosinophils.[74] *Xanthogranulomatous cholecystitis*,[56] *cholecystic granuloma*,[57] and *ceroid gran-*

uloma[48] refer to the presence in the wall of diffuse or nodular collections of macrophages containing neutral fat and lipofuscin (ceroid) pigment. Some of these lesions are probably the result of rupture of Rokitansky-Aschoff sinuses. *Malakoplakia* may rarely involve the gallbladder; it is identified by the presence of calcium and iron-positive Michaelis-Guttman bodies in the cytoplasm of histiocytes.[52]

Other rare inflammatory gallbladder diseases include *schistosomiasis*,[64b] *amebiasis*,[74] and *Crohn's disease*.[64]

It has often been argued that all gallbladders that contain stones should be removed surgically because of the risk of cancer, this risk being greater than the operative mortality. This argument lacks validity since the incidence of carcinoma in gallbladders with lithiasis is less than 1%.[66] A more valid reason for removing gallbladders containing stones relates to the serious inflammatory and obstructive complications that may arise from them.[76] Lund[63] followed 526 nonoperated cases of cholelithiasis and found that one third to one half of the patients subsequently developed severe symptoms or complications from the disease; he therefore concluded that prophylactic removal of the gallbladder containing stones is indicated in all patients who are good surgical risks. Similar findings were obtained in the National Cooperative Gallstone Study involving 305 patients.[69]

Gallstones may lead to ***internal biliary fistulas.*** Over 90% of them are located between the gallbladder and the duodenum, the gallbladder and the colon, or the common bile duct and the duodenum.[72] These fistulas are created by the formation of inflammatory adhesions between the biliary tree and adjacent organs and the subsequent erosion of a stone through the gallbladder or the common duct into the gastrointestinal tract. Continuing choledochal obstruction contributes to the persistence of the fistula. Biliary fistulas may become evident by the patient vomiting or passing per rectum a large gallstone, by detecting air in the biliary tree in a plain abdominal roentgenogram, or by seeing the outline of the biliary tree in an upper gastrointestinal series or a barium enema. With cholecystocolic fistulas, infection often is severe. Repair of these fistulas requires cholecystectomy and closure or resection of the involved portion of bowel.

Strictures of the common duct are usually caused by surgical trauma in which the duct is injured or ligated inadvertently.[60] Anatomic variations of the ducts and blood vessels may cause such an error. Strictures may also be the result of infection following operation.[53]

The goal of therapy is to establish a wide, tension-free anastomosis between the normal portion of the bile duct and the bowel, with mucosa-to-mucosa apposition. This is usu-

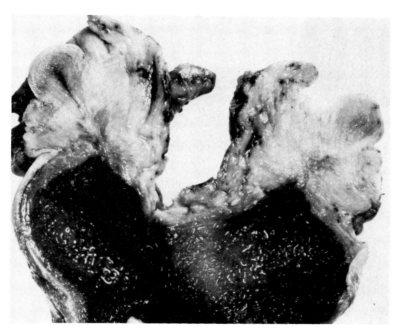

Fig. 14-12 Gallbladder with "adenomyoma" of fundus.

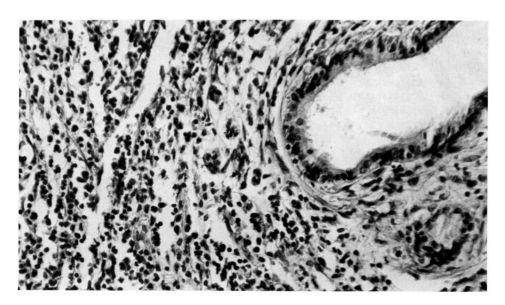

Fig. 14-13 Sclerosing cholangitis. Prominent chronic inflammatory change is seen surrounding cystic bile duct. Note intact mucosa. Continuous T-tube drainage will often relieve process. (Slide contributed by Dr. W.B. Sorrell, Montgomery, AL.)

ally accomplished by an end-to-end choledochoduodenostomy or a Roux-en-Y hepaticojejunostomy.[64a,73]

Sclerosing cholangitis is a relatively rare disorder of unknown etiology, characterized by diffuse thickening of the wall, which, if severe enough, will lead to obstruction of the lumen.[50,75] Microscopically there is dense fibrosis, a sparse mixed inflammatory infiltrate (sometimes containing eosinophils), and a relatively intact epithelium[62,67] (Fig. 14-13). The most typical microscopic changes are seen in the early stages of the disease not in the extrahepatic bile ducts but in the liver biopsy and are characterized by a fibrous obliterative cholangitis leading to replacement of duct segments by solid cords of connective tissue and eventually to complete loss of bile ducts.[62] Sclerosing cholangitis has been reported in association with Riedel's thyroiditis, retroperitoneal or mediastinal fibrosis, orbital pseudotumor, Crohn's disease, and, in particular, ulcerative colitis.[68,70] Patients with primary sclerosing cholangitis associated with ulcerative colitis have a marked increase in the frequency of serum anticolon antibodies.[51] The diagnosis of sclerosing, well-differentiated adenocarcinoma should always be considered before making a diagnosis of sclerosing cholangitis (see p. 752).

TUMORS
Benign tumors and tumorlike conditions

Cholesterol polyps are multilobular yellow formations composed of aggregates of foamy histiocytes covered by an intact mucosa; they represent a morphologic variation in the theme of cholesterosis. *Inflammatory polyps* are always associated with chronic cholecystitis.[78] *Adenomatous hyperplasia* and the already mentioned *adenomyomatous hyperplasia* are also reactive mucosal changes secondary to inflammation and/or lithiasis.[78] *Villous papillomas* of the gallbladder have been seen in infants with metachromatic leukodystrophy.[87] *Adenomas* resemble their homologues in the gastrointestinal tract; they may be sessile or pedunculated and can exhibit tubular, tubulovillous, or villous patterns of growth[86] (Fig. 14-14). Some degree of atypia is always present, and a few will show changes of carcinoma in situ or focal invasive carcinoma. As in the colorectum, the larger the adenoma, the more likely that an area of malignant change will be found.[81]

Paragangliomas arise from small paraganglia known to occur in the gallbladder serosa.[84] *Granular cell tumors* present as small nodules in the gallbladder wall, sometimes in association with similar lesions in the extrahepatic biliary tree.[88]

Benign tumors of the extrahepatic bile duct are exceptional.[79] Those of epithelial nature have been designated as *adenomas, cystadenomas,* and *papillomas,* depending on their configuration.[80] *Granular cell tumors* may occur anywhere along the intra- and extrahepatic biliary system.[77,83] *Traumatic neuromas* occur most often following operations in the area; their most common site is the stump of the cystic duct following a cholecystectomy. They

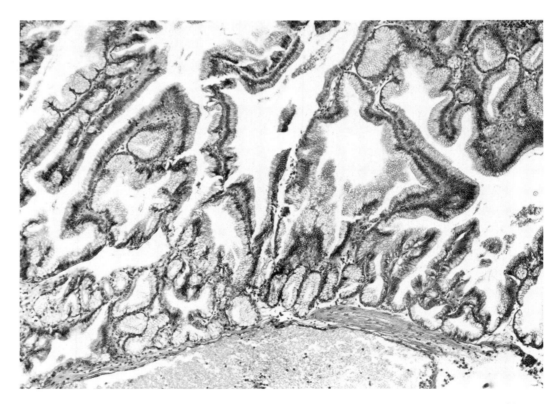

Fig. 14-14 Papillary adenoma of gallbladder. Tumor, which was seen in cholecystogram, measured 2 cm in diameter.

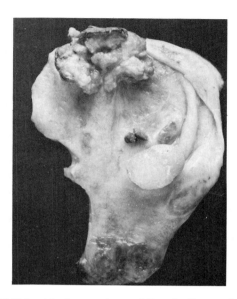

Fig. 14-15 Polypoid adenocarcinoma 2.5 cm in diameter in fundus. Stones are also present. Patient was well 8 years after cholecystectomy. (From Appleman RM, Morlock CG, Dahlin DC, Adson MA: Long term survival in carcinoma of the gallbladder. Surg Gynecol Obstet **117**:459-464, 1963; by permission of Surgery, Gynecology & Obstetrics.)

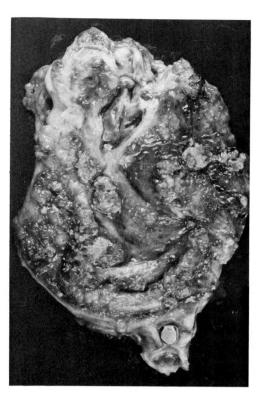

Fig. 14-16 Diffuse multicentric papillary carcinoma. Despite penetration of lesion through muscle in several areas, patient survived 5 years after cholecystectomy. Note stone in cystic duct. (From Appleman RM, Morlock CG, Dahlin DC, Adson MA: Long term survival in carcinoma of the gallbladder. Surg Gynecol Obstet **117**:459-464, 1963; by permission of Surgery, Gynecology & Obstetrics.)

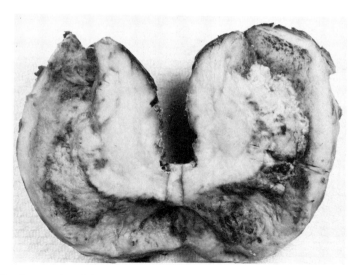

Fig. 14-17 Carcinoma of gallbladder with almost complete replacement of wall and infiltration of surrounding structures. Stones were present.

may cause postcholecystectomy pain or obstructive jaundice.[82] Some cases have occurred in the absence of previous surgery, perhaps as an expression of a hyperplastic reactive change.[85]

Carcinoma of gallbladder
General features

Carcinoma of the gallbladder is more frequent in females (3 to 4:1 ratio); over 90% of the patients are 50 years of age or older at the time of diagnosis. It is more common in some Latin American countries than in the United States. In this country, there is a concentration of cases in the Southwest, North central, and Appalachian regions.[100] The incidence is high in American Indians, relatively low in whites of European extraction, and very rare in blacks.

A definite epidemiologic parallel exists between gallbladder carcinoma and cholelithiasis, but it is not clear what is the pathogenetic relationship between them, if any. In the non-Indian, non-Hispanic population of the United States, the incidence of carcinoma in gallbladders with lithiasis is less than 1%.[118]

Other conditions associated with an increased risk of gallbladder carcinoma are cholecystoenteric fistula, porcelain gallbladder, ulcerative colitis, polyposis coli,[99] Gardner's syndrome,[123] and anomalous connection between the common bile duct and the pancreatic duct.[109]

Gross features

Grossly, the carcinoma may present as a diffusely growing (70%) or polypoid (30%) mass[120] (Figs. 14-15 and 14-16). When diffuse, the gross distinction from chronic cholecystitis may be difficult. Gallbladders with carcinomas usually also exhibit stones (80% to 90% of the cases) and marked fibrosis of the wall (Fig. 14-17). The latter may represent reaction to the tumor or the expression of a preexisting chronic cholecystitis. The fact that some gallbladder carcinomas are not obvious on gross examination indicates the need for microscopic examination of every excised gallbladder. We have seen several patients in whom an unexpected metastatic tumor was found in the liver sometime following the removal of a gallbladder thought to have only lithiasis and inflammation on gross examination by the surgeon and therefore discarded.

Microscopic features

Microscopically, most gallbladder cancers are adenocarcinomas showing varying degrees of differentiation (Fig. 14-18). Many have a papillary surface, but they may also be deeply invasive. Most tumors have a morphologic appearance that is common to adenocarcinomas of the pancreatobiliary region—well-formed glands with wide lumina lined by one or few rows of highly atypical cuboidal cells, surrounded by a cellular stroma often arranged in a concentric fashion. It is characteristic for these glands to seem well differentiated at an architectural level but poorly differentiated at a cytologic level. The mucin produced by these tumors is variable in amount and typically of the sialomucin type in contrast to the predominantly sulfomucin type secreted by the normal, inflamed, or obstructed gallbladder.[102,112] Keratin and CEA are strongly positive.[93]

Foci of intestinal differentiation are common, with appearance of goblet cells, endocrine cells, and even Paneth

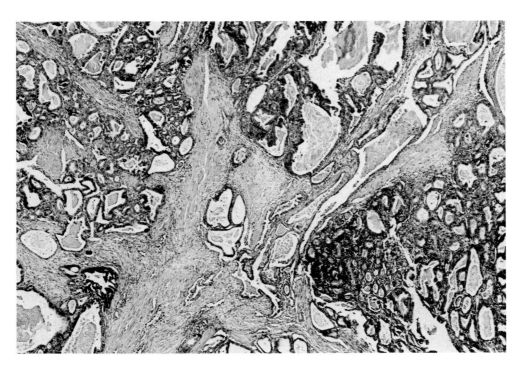

Fig. 14-18 Adenocarcinoma of gallbladder showing extensive infiltration of muscular wall.

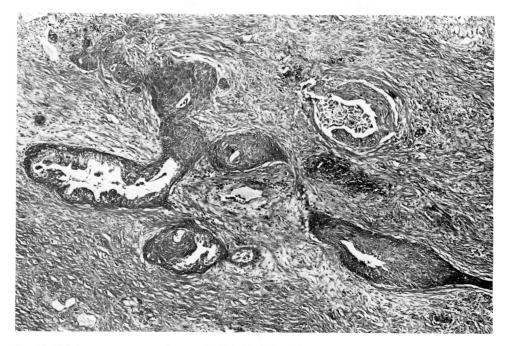

Fig. 14-19 Adenosquamous carcinoma of gallbladder. Well-differentiated neoplastic glandular structure merges with solid nests of squamous epithelium.

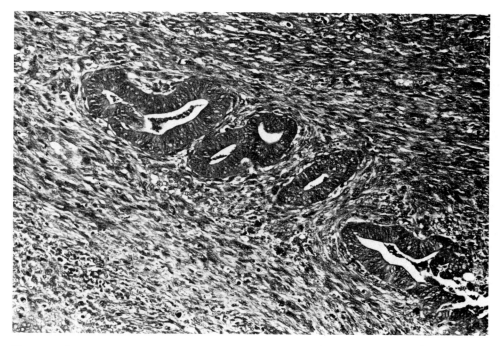

Fig. 14-20 Sarcomatoid carcinoma of gallbladder. Sharp interface between adenocarcinoma and spindle cell sarcoma−like elements has given rise to alternative term of carcinosarcoma for this tumor.

cells. Occasionally, the entire tumor is of intestinal type on morphologic, histochemical, and immunohistochemical grounds.[92,113] Some adenocarcinomas are combined with areas of carcinoid tumor ("adenocarcinoids"), in a fashion similar to that more often seen in the appendix.[114]

Other microscopic types

Adenocarcinomas of the gallbladder may exhibit varying degrees of squamous metaplasia; terms such as *adenoacanthoma* and *adenosquamous carcinoma* have been used for them, depending on whether the squamous component was, respectively, well or poorly differentiated[121] (Fig. 14-19). Pure *squamous cell carcinomas* are exceptional.[108]

Undifferentiated (anaplastic, pleomorphic, sarcomatoid) carcinomas occur in a variety of morphologic presentations (giant cell, spindle cell), many of them closely simulating sarcomas.[90,96,104a] The tumors in which the carcinomatous and sarcoma-like components segregate in a biphasic pattern have also been called malignant mixed tumor and carcinosarcoma[106,122] but current evidence suggests that the sarcoma-like component is also of epithelial derivation[95] (Fig. 14-20).

Some gallbladder adenocarcinomas have *choriocarcinoma-like areas*.[90] Others have a morphology equivalent to that of pulmonary *oat cell carcinoma;* these have also been referred as neuroendocrine carcinoma and may be seen in association with well-differentiated adenocarcinoma. Ultrastructurally, dense core secretory granules can be found. These are highly aggressive neoplasms, which metastasize early and cause death shortly after diagnosis.[94]

Precursor lesions

The precursor lesions of invasive adenocarcinoma of the gallbladder have not been studied in detail until recently.[89,91,98,111,116] Intestinal metaplasia is commonly seen in the mucosa adjacent to the carcinoma.[101,110] It is thought that in most cases the invasive tumor arises from a sequence of intestinal metaplasia, dysplasia, and carcinoma in situ[98] (Fig. 14-21). In a study done in Mexico City (a place with a very high incidence of gallbladder carcinoma), lesions interpreted as carcinoma in situ were found in the mucosa adjacent to invasive carcinoma in 79% of thirty-nine surgical cases.[89] Also, mucosal lesions interpreted as atypical hyperplasia and carcinoma in situ were observed in 13.5% and 3.5%, respectively, of 200 consecutive specimens of cholecystectomy performed for cholelithiasis or cholecystitis. In a subsequent study from the same group, eighteen cases of carcinoma in situ were reported.[91] Grossly, the lesions could not be distinguished from chronic cholecystitis. Two of the tumors had a papillary configuration, and four exhibited beginning invasion of the underlying lamina propria. One of these four patients died with liver metastases; all of the others were cured by cholecystectomy.

The pattern of CEA distribution in these lesions is similar to that of other mucosae in the digestive tract: in the normal epithelium it is limited to the apical surface, whereas in dysplasias and carcinomas it is abundantly present in the cytoplasm and lumen.[93]

Spread and metastases

Gallbladder carcinoma has a great propensity to invade the liver directly, as well as the stomach and duodenum; it

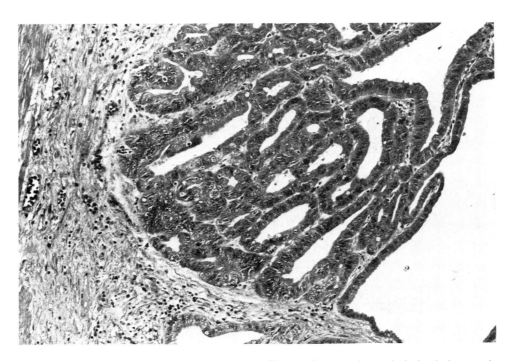

Fig. 14-21 Adenocarcinoma in situ of gallbladder. Cluster of extremely atypical glands is seen in mucosa, without stromal invasion. Packing of glands has resulted in obliteration of lamina propria.

also metastasizes frequently to the liver, to pericholedochal lymph nodes in the lesser omentum, and to lymph nodes behind the first portion of the duodenum.[103] Almost half of the patients already have metastatic disease at the time of surgery.[105]

Treatment and prognosis; staging and grading

By the time the diagnosis of carcinoma of the gallbladder can be made clinically, the tumor is advanced and usually inoperable.[117] Under such circumstances, the chances of cure—even following heroic surgical measures—are minimal.[107,119] Even when the carcinoma becomes apparent to the surgeon at the time of exploration of the gallbladder for stones, it is often incurable because of its tendency to spread through the wall of the gallbladder and its propensity to invade the liver, pericolic tissues, and lymph nodes, and even infiltrate the duodenum. In a series of eighty cases recently reported, there was only one long-term survivor.[105] The best possibility of cure is when the cancer is found incidentally by the pathologist on gross or microscopic examination.[104]

Nevin et al.[115] found a close correlation between staging and survival. Patients with stage I (intramucosal only) and stage II (mucosa and muscularis) disease were generally cured by cholecystectomy alone. Stage V disease (involvement of liver or other organs) was uniformly fatal and palliation alone was recommended. In patients with stage III (involvement of all three layers) and stage IV disease (involvement of all three layers plus cystic lymph node), the 5-year survival rate was approximately 11%. For these two latter groups, the authors suggested radical surgery, including right hepatic lobectomy and lymphadenectomy. Histologic grading was also related to prognosis in this and other series, with well-differentiated papillary tumors having the most favorable prognosis.[97] A combination of staging and microscopic grading seems to offer the best prognostic correlation.[115]

Carcinoma of extrahepatic bile ducts

Bile duct carcinoma (cholangiocarcinoma) occurs with equal frequency in males and females[141]; the average age of presentation is 60 years. About 90% of the patients present with jaundice. An increased incidence of this disease has been reported in patients with ulcerative colitis,[124,128,140] sclerosing cholangitis (see p. 746), *Clonorchis sinensis* infestation,[141] and in a variety of congenital abnormalities of the intrahepatic and extrahepatic bile ducts, such as congenital dilatation of the bile duct (including choledochal cyst), Caroli's disease, congenital hepatic fibrosis, polycystic disease, and abnormal pancreatico-choledochal junction.[130,140a,142]

These tumors can develop at any level of the biliary tree. They have been divided anatomically into upper third, including hilum (50% to 75%), middle third (10% to 25%), and lower third (10% to 20%).[125,138,146] Tumors arising from the intrahepatic bile ducts are discussed in Chapter 13 and

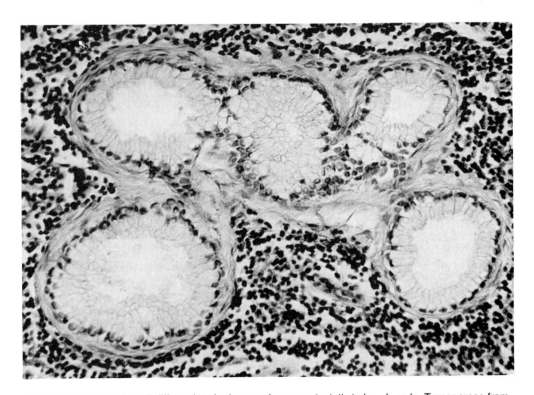

Fig. 14-22 Extremely well-differentiated adenocarcinoma metastatic to lymph node. Tumor arose from hepatic duct, but it was 6 years before patient died of this cancer. Concentric fibrosis seen around neoplastic glands is characteristic of tumors in this location. (Slide contributed by Dr. R.E. Johnson, Columbia, MO.)

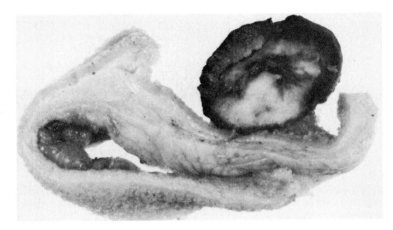

Fig. 14-23 Malignant melanoma metastatic to gallbladder, resulting in single polypoid mass. Primary lesion was in skin.

those located in the ampulla of Vater in Chapter 15. The presence and location of these tumors are best shown by retrograde endoscopic cholangiography or percutaneous transhepatic cholangiography. With the latter technique, Elias et al.[129] demonstrated the site of the extrahepatic obstruction in 95% of the cases.

Grossly, bile duct carcinomas can be polypoid and superficial, but most are nodular or sclerosing, with deep penetration into the wall.[145] Occasionally, they are multicentric and/or associated with carcinoma of the gallbladder.[133] Direct extension to the liver is common in upper third lesions.[127] Metastases to regional and peripancreatic nodes are also frequent.

Microscopically, the large majority of bile duct malignancies are well-differentiated mucin-secreting adenocarcinomas.[145] A papillary surface may be seen in the more distal lesions. The tumors can be so well differentiated— even in metastatic sites—that their identification as malignant is very difficult (Fig. 14-22). Heterogeneity of cells within the same gland, increased nucleocytoplasmic ratio, nucleolar prominence, stromal and *perineurial* invasion, and concentric layering of cellular stroma around the neoplastic glands are the most important identifying features. As Weinbren and Mutum have emphasized,[145] the juxtaposition of normal-appearing cells with cells having large nuclei with prominent nucleoli is a particularly important diagnostic clue. Clusters of small acini, normally present in the wall and known as periluminal sacculi of Beale, should not be misinterpreted as invasive carcinoma.

In addition to these morphologic features, bile duct carcinoma resembles gallbladder carcinoma in its expression of mucosubstances and CEA,[137,145] common detection of metaplastic and dysplastic changes in the adjacent epithelium,[134] and the occasional occurrence of variants with squamous metaplasia[132] or neuroendocrine features.[147]

A somewhat distinct variant of bile duct carcinoma is *sclerosing carcinoma* (Altemeier-Klatskin's tumor).[126,131] It begins at the hepatic duct junction and spreads from there to long segments of the biliary tree; it is characterized by a long clinical course and a well-differentiated microscopic

appearance, associated with extensive fibrosis. The main differential diagnosis, both roentgenographically and pathologically, is with sclerosing cholangitis.[139] It is possible that some cases of sclerosing carcinomas actually arise in a background of sclerosing cholangitis and that this is the reason for the striking similarities between the two entities.[136,144]

Surgical resection offers the only possibility of cure for bile duct carcinoma.[135] Proximal lesions are treated with resection (which may include hepatic lobectomy) and Roux-en-Y hepaticojejunostomy; distal lesions are treated by the Whipple procedure.[131a] The prognosis is poor. The overall survival rate is 10%; the survival for patients with tumors of the lower third is about 25%.[143]

Other malignant tumors

Carcinoid tumors can occur in the gallbladder and extrahepatic bile ducts.[153,160a] One such tumor, located in the cystic duct, had the immunohistochemical features of somatostatinoma.[152]

Primary malignant melanoma may present as a mass inside the gallbladder[149,159] or the common bile duct.[150] Most cases have already metastasized by the time of diagnosis. Before making the diagnosis of primary melanoma of this organ, the more likely possibility of a metastasis from a cutaneous or ocular source needs to be ruled out (Fig. 14-23).

Malignant lymphoma and *leukemia* can involve the gallbladder or extrahepatic bile ducts as part of a systemic disease; their initial presentation in these sites is exceptional but has been recorded.[154,158,161]

Botryoid rhabdomyosarcoma is the most common malignant tumor of extrahepatic bile ducts in children.[151] It can also involve the gallbladder,[156] and a few cases have been described in adults.[148] Obstructive jaundice is the usual presenting sign. Grossly, it has a deceptively soft polypoid appearance. Microscopically, small undifferentiated spindle cells concentrate beneath an intact epithelium ("cambium layer"). Cross striations may or may not be present in them (Fig. 14-24). The prognosis is poor, but the combination of surgery, radiation therapy, and chemotherapy has resulted

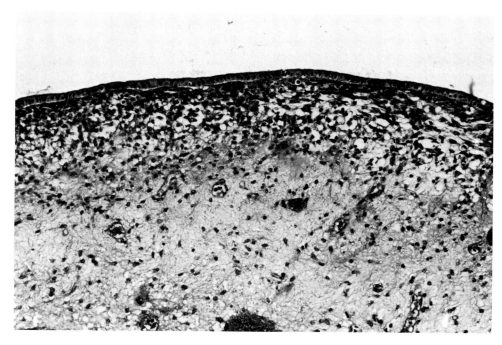

Fig. 14-24 Botryoid rhabdomyosarcoma of common bile duct. Beneath single layer of cuboidal epithelium, there is highly cellular layer of small tumor cells (Nicholson's cambium layer). Tumor beneath has deceptively benign-looking edematous appearance.

in long-term survivals.[160] Metastases occur in about 40% of the cases, but death is usually due to the local effects of the tumor.[155]

Other *sarcomas* of the gallbladder occur in adults, such as leiomyosarcoma,[157,162,163] but before making such a diagnosis, the alternative diagnosis of sarcomatoid carcinoma should always be considered.

REFERENCES

CONGENITAL ABNORMALITIES

1 Alonso-Lej F, Rever WB Jr, Pessagno DJ: Congenital choledocal cyst, with a report of 2 and an analysis of 94 cases. Int Abst Surg 108:1-30, 1959.

2 Altman RP: The portoenterostomy procedure for biliary atresia. A five-year experience. Ann Surg 188:351-362, 1978.

3 Bloustein PA: Association of carcinoma with congenital cystic conditions of the liver and bile ducts. Am J Gastroenterol 67:40-46, 1977.

4 Busuttil A: Ectopic adrenal within the gall-bladder wall. J Pathol 113:231-233, 1974

5 Christensen AH, Ishak KG: Benign tumors and pseudotumors of the gallbladder. Report of 180 cases. Arch Pathol 90:423-432, 1970.

6 Corcoran DB, Wallace KK: Congenital anomalies of the gallbladder. Am Surg 20:709-725, 1954.

7 Curtis LE, Shehan DG: Heterotopic tissues in the gallbladder. Arch Pathol 88:677-683, 1969.

8 Gautier M, Eliot N: Extrahepatic biliary atresia. Morphological study of 98 biliary remnants. Arch Pathol Lab Med 105:397-402, 1981.

9 Järvi O, Meurman L: Heterotopic gastric mucosa and pancreas in the gallbladder with reference to the question of heterotopias in general. Ann Acad Sci Fenn 106[Suppl 22]:1-42, 1964.

10 Komi N, Tamura T, Tsuge S, Miyoshi Y, Udaka H, Takehara H: Relation of patient age to premalignant alterations in choledochal cyst epithelium. Histochemical and immunohistochemical studies. J Pediatr Surg 21:430-433, 1986.

11 Landing B: Considerations on the pathogenesis of neonatal hepatitis, biliary atresia, and choledochal cyst—the concept of infantile obstructive cholangiopathy. In Bill AH, Kasai M (eds): Progress in pediatric surgery, vol. 6. Baltimore, 1974, University Park Press, p. 113.

12 Matsumoto Y, Uchida K, Nakase A, Houjo I: Clinicopathologic classification of congenital cystic dilatation of the common bile duct. Am J Surg 134:569-574, 1977.

13 Miyano T, Suruga K, Tsuchiya H, Suda K: A histopathological study of the remnant of extrahepatic bile duct in so-called uncorrectable biliary atresia. J Pediatr Surg 12:19-25, 1977.

14 Nagorney DM, McIlrath DC, Adson MA: Choledochal cysts in adults. Clinical management. Surgery 96:656-663, 1984.

15 Ober WB, Wharton RN: On the "phrygian cap." N Engl J Med 255:571-572, 1956.

16 Olbourne NA: Choledochal cysts. A review of the cystic anomalies of the biliary tree. Ann R Coll Surg Engl 56:26-32, 1975.

17 Trout HH III, Longmire WP Jr: Long-term follow-up study of patients with congenital cystic dilatation of the common bile duct. Am J Surg 121:68-86, 1971.

18 Witzleben CL, Buck BE, Schnaufer L, Brzosko WJ: Studies on the pathogenesis of biliary atresia. Lab Invest 38:525-532, 1978.

CHOLELITHIASIS

19 Friedman GD, Kannel WF, Dawber TR: The epidemiology of gallbladder diseases. Observations in the Framingham study. J Chronic Dis 19:273-292, 1966.

20 Gerwig WH, Thistlethwaite JR: Cholecystitis and cholelithiasis in young women following pregnancy. Surgery 28:983-996, 1950.

21 Jordan GL Jr: Choledocholithiasis. Curr Probl Surg 19:723-798, 1982.

22 Madden JL, Vanderheyden L, Kandalaft S: The nature and surgical significance of common duct stones. Surg Gynecol Obstet 126:2-8, 1968.

23 Mok HYI, Druffel ERM, Rampone WM: Chronology of cholelithiasis. Dating gallstones from atmospheric radiocarbon produced by nuclear bomb explosions. N Engl J Med 314:1075-1077, 1986.

24 Ostrow JD: The etiology of pigment gallstones. Hepatology 4:215S-222S, 1984.

25 Small DM: Gallstones. N Engl J Med 279:588-592, 1968.

26 Smith BF, LaMont JT: The sequence of events in gallstone formation. Lab Invest 56:125-126, 1987.

27 Torvik A, Höivik B: Gallstones in an autopsy series. Acta Chir Scand 120:168-174, 1960.

ACUTE CHOLECYSTITIS

28 Andrews E: Pathologic changes of diseased gallbladders. Arch Surg **31**:767-793, 1935.

29 Bigler FC: Acute gaseous cholecystitis. Am J Med **29**:181-186, 1960.

30 Bohrat MG, Bodon GR: Isolated polyarteritis nodosa of the gallbladder. Am Surg **36**:681-685, 1970.

31 Dillard BM, Black, WC: Polyarteritis nodosa of the gallbladder and bile ducts. Am Surg **36**:423-427, 1970.

32 Glenn F: Acute cholecystitis. Surg Gynecol Obstet **143**:56-60, 1976.

33 Glenn F: Acute acalculous cholecystitis. Ann Surg **189**:458-465, 1979.

34 Glenn F, Becker CG: Acute acalculous cholecystitis. An increasing entity. Ann Surg **195**:131-136, 1982.

35 Glenn F, Hill MR Jr: Primary gallbladder disease in children. Ann Surg **139**:302-311, 1954.

36 Hallendorf LC, Dockerty MB, Waugh JM: Gangrenous cholecystitis. A clinical and pathologic study of 100 cases. Surg Clin North Am **28**:979-998, 1948.

37 Hanson BA, Mahour GH, Woolley MM: Diseases of the gallbladder in infancy and childhood. J Pediatr Surg **6**:277-283, 1971.

38 Kent SJS, Menzies-Gow N: Biliary peritonitis without perforation of the gallbladder in acute cholecystitis. Br J Surg **61**:960-962, 1974.

39 Lahey FH: Acute cholecystitis. Surg Clin North Am **32**:837-845, 1952.

40 LiVolsi VA, Perzin KH, Porter M: Polyarteritis nodosa of the gallbladder, presenting as acute cholecystitis. Gastroenterology **65**:115-123, 1973.

41 Marymont JV, Dakhil SR, Travers H, Housholder DF: Chemical cholecystitis associated with hepatic arterial chemotherapy delivered by a permanently implanted pump. Hum Pathol **16**:986-990, 1985.

42 Mechling RS, Watson JR: The solitary gallstone. Surg Gynecol Obstet **91**:404-408, 1950.

43 Sjödahl R, Tagesson C, Wetterfors J: On the pathogenesis of acute cholecystitis. Surg Gynecol Obstet **146**:199-202, 1976.

44 van der Linden W, Sunzel H: Early versus delayed operation for acute cholecystitis. A controlled clinical trial. Am J Surg **120**:7-13, 1970.

45 Weedon D: Pathology of the gallbladder. New York, 1984, Masson Publishing USA, Inc.

46 Womack NA, Bricker EM: Pathogenesis of cholecystitis. Arch Surg **44**:658-676, 1942.

CHRONIC CHOLECYSTITIS AND CHOLANGITIS

47 Albores-Saavedra J, Nadji M, Henson DE, Ziegels-Weissman J, Mones JM: Intestinal metaplasia of the gallbladder. A morphologic and immunocytochemical study. Hum Pathol **17**:614-620, 1986.

48 Amazon F, Rywlin AM: Ceroid granulomas of the gallbladder. Am J Clin Pathol **73**:123-127, 1980.

49 Beilby JO: Diverticulosis of the gall bladder. The fundal adenoma. Br J Exp Pathol **48**:455-461, 1967.

50 Cameron JL, Gayler BW, Sanfey H, Milligan F, Kaufman S, Maddrey WC, Herlong HF: Sclerosing cholangitis. Anatomical distribution of obstructive lesions. Ann Surg **200**:54-60, 1984.

51 Chapman RW, Cottone M, Selby WS, Shepherd HA, Sherlock S, Jewell DP: Serum autoantibodies, ulcerative colitis and primary sclerosing cholangitis. Gut **27**:86-91, 1986.

52 Charpentier P, Prade M, Bognel C, Gadenne C, Duvillard P: Malacoplakia of the gallbladder. Hum Pathol **14**:827-828, 1983.

53 Cole WH, Ireneus C, Raynolds JT: Strictures of the common duct. Ann Surg **133**:684-695, 1951.

54 Elfving G, Silvonen E, Tier H: Mucosal hyperplasia of the gallbladder in cases of cholecystolithiasis. Acta Chir Scand **135**:519-522, 1969.

55 Estrada RL, Brown NM, James CE: Chronic follicular cholecystitis. Radiological, pathological, and surgical aspects. Br J Surg **48**:205-209, 1958.

56 Goodman ZD, Ishak KG: Xanthogranulomatous cholecystitis. Am J Surg Pathol **5**:653-659, 1981.

57 Hanada M, Tujimura T, Kimura M: Cholecystic granulomas in gallstone disease. A clinicopathologic study of 17 cases. Acta Pathol Jpn **31**:221-231, 1981.

58 Jutras JA, Levesque HP: Adenomyoma and adenomyomatosis of gallbladder. Radiologic and pathologic correlations. Radiol Clin North Am **4**:483-500, 1966.

59 Kozuka S, Hackisuka K: Incidence by age and sex of intestinal metaplasia in the gallbladder. Hum Pathol **15**:779-784, 1984.

60 Lahey RH, Pyrtek LJ: Experience with the operative management of 280 strictures of the bile ducts. Surg Gynecol Obstet **91**:25-56, 1950.

61 Laitio M, Nevalainen T: Ultrastructure of endocrine cells in metaplastic epithelium of human gall bladder. J Anat **120**:219-225, 1975.

62 LaRusso NF, Wiesner RH, Ludwig J, MacCarty RL: Primary sclerosing cholangitis. N Engl J Med **310**:899-903, 1984.

63 Lund J: Surgical indication in cholelithiasis. Prophylactic cholecystectomy elucidated on the basis of long-term follow up on 526 nonoperated cases. Ann Surg **151**:153-162, 1960.

64 McClure J, Banerjee SS, Schofield PS: Crohn's disease of the gall bladder. J Clin Pathol **37**:516-518, 1984.

64a Pitt HA, Miyamoto T, Parapatis SK, Tompkins RK, Longmire WP Jr: Factors influencing outcome in patients with postoperative biliary strictures. Am J Surg **144**:14-21, 1982.

64b Rappaport I, Albukerk J, Schneider IJ: Schistosomal cholecystitis. Arch Pathol **99**:227-228, 1975.

65 Robertson HE, Ferguson WJ: The diverticula (Luschka's crypts) of the gallbladder. Arch Pathol **40**:312-333, 1945.

66 Russell PW, Brown CH: Primary carcinoma of the gallbladder. Ann Surg **132::**121-128, 1950.

67 Schwartz SI, Dale WA: Primary sclerosing cholangitis. Review and report of six cases. Arch Surg **77**:439-451, 1958.

68 Sivak MV Jr, Farmer RG, Lalli AF: Sclerosing cholangitis. Its increasing frequency of recognition and association with inflammatory bowel disease. J Clin Gastroenterol **3**:261-266, 1981.

69 Thistle JL, Cleary PA, Lachin JM, Tyor MP, Hersh T: The natural history of cholelithiasis. The National Cooperative Gallstone Study. Ann Intern Med **101**:171-175, 1984.

70 Thompson HH, Pitt HA, Tompkins RK, Longmire WP Jr: Primary sclerosing cholangitis. A heterogenous disease. Ann Surg **196**:127-136, 1982.

71 Tsutsumi Y, Nagura H, Osamura RY, Watanabe K, Yanaihara N: Histochemical studies of metaplastic lesions in the human gallbladder. Arch Pathol Lab Med **108**:917-921, 1984.

72 Waggoner CM, LeMone DV: Clinical and roentgen aspects of internal biliary fistulas. Report of twelve cases. Radiology **53**:31-41, 1949.

73 Warren KW, Mountain JC, Midell AL: Management of strictures of the biliary tract. Surg Clin North Am **51**:711-731, 1971.

74 Weedon D: Pathology of the gallbladder. New York, 1984, Masson Publishing USA, Inc.

75 Wiesner RH, LaRusso NF: Clinicopathologic features of the syndrome of primary sclerosing cholangitis. Gastroenterology **79**:200-206, 1980.

76 Wenchert A, Robertson B: The natural course of gallstone disease. Eleven-year review of 781 nonoperated cases. Gastroenterology **50**:376-381, 1966.

TUMORS
Benign tumors and tumorlike conditions

77 Chandrasoma P, Fitzgibbons P: Granular cell tumor of the intrapancreatic common bile duct. Cancer **53**:2178-2182, 1984.

78 Christensen AH, Ishak KG: Benign tumors and pseudotumors of the gallbladder. Report of 180 cases. Arch Pathol **90**:423-432, 1970.

79 Chu PT: Benign neoplasms of the extrahepatic biliary ducts. Review of the literature and report of a case of fibroma. Arch Pathol **50**:87-97, 1950.

80 Ishak KG, Willis GW, Cummins SD, Bullock AA: Biliary cystadenoma and cystadenocarcinoma. Report of 14 cases and review of the literature. Cancer **39**:322-338, 1977.

81 Kozuka S, Tsubone M, Yasui A, Hachisuka K: Relation of adenoma to carcinoma in the gallbladder. Cancer **50**:2226-2234, 1982.

82 Larson DM, Storsteen KA: Traumatic neuroma of the bile ducts with intrahepatic extension causing obstructive jaundice. Hum Pathol **15**:287-290, 1984.

83 LiVolsi VA, Perzin KH, Badder EM, Price JB Jr, Porter M: Granular cell tumors of the biliary tract. Arch Pathol **95**:13-17, 1973.

84 Miller TA, Weber TR, Appelman HD: Paraganglioma of the gallbladder. Arch Surg **105**:637-639, 1972.

85 Peison B, Benisch B: Traumatic neuroma of the cystic duct in the absence of previous surgery. Hum Pathol **16**:1168-1169, 1985.

86 Sato H, Mizushima M, Ito J, Doi K: Sessile adenoma of the gallbladder. Reappraisal of its importance as a precancerous lesion. Arch Pathol Lab Med **109**:65-69, 1985.

87 Warfel KA, Hull MT: Villous papilloma of the gallbladder in association with leukodystrophy. Hum Pathol **15**:1192-1194, 1984.

88 Yamaguchi K, Kuroki S, Daimaru Y, Hashimoto H, Enjoji M: Granular cell tumor of the gallbladder: Report of a case. Acta Pathol Jpn **35**:687-691, 1985.

Carcinoma of gallbladder

89 Albores-Saavedra J, Alcantara-Vazquez A, Curz-Ortiz H, Herrera-Goepfert R: The precursor lesions of invasive gallbladder carcinoma. Hyperplasia, atypical hyperplasia and carcinoma in situ. Cancer **45**:919-927, 1980.

90 Albores-Saavedra J, Cruz-Ortiz H, Alcantara-Vazques A, Henson DE: Unusual types of gallbladder carcinoma. A report of 16 cases. Arch Pathol Lab Med **105**:287-293, 1981.

91 Albores-Saavedra J, de Jesus Manrique J, Angeles-Angeles A, Henson DE: Carcinoma in situ of the gallbladder. A clinicopathologic study of 18 cases. Am J Surg Pathol **8**:323-333, 1984.

92 Albores-Saavedra J, Nadji M, Henson DE: Intestinal-type adenocarcinoma of the gallbladder. A clinicopathologic and immunocytochemical study of seven cases. Am J Surg Pathol **10**:19-25, 1986.

93 Albores-Saavedra J, Nadji M, Morales AR, Henson DE: Carcinoembryonic antigen in normal, preneoplastic and neoplastic gallbladder epithelium. Cancer **52**:1069-1072, 1983.

94 Albores-Saavedra J, Soriano J, Larraza-Hernandez O, Aguirre J, Henson DE: Oat cell carcinoma of the gallbladder. Hum Pathol **15**:639-646, 1984.

95 Alpers CE, Smuckler EA: Pleomorphic carcinoma of the gallbladder. Case report and ultrastructural study. Ultrastruct Pathol **6**:29-38, 1984.

96 Appelman HD, Coopersmith N: Pleomorphic spindle-cell carcinoma of the gallbladder. Relation to sarcoma of the gallbladder. Cancer **25**:535-541, 1970.

97 Appelman RM, Morlock CG, Dahlin DC, Adson MA: Long term survival in carcinoma of the gallbladder. Surg Gynecol Obstet **117**:459-464, 1963.

98 Black WC: The morphogenesis of gallbladder carcinoma. Prog Surg Pathol **2**:207-223, 1980.

99 Bombi JA, Rives A, Astudillo E, Pera C, Cardesa A: Poliposis coli associated with adenocarcinoma of the gallbladder. Report of a case, Cancer **53**:2561-2563, 1984.

100 Diehl AK: Epidemiology of gallbladder cancer. A synthesis of recent data. J Natl Cancer Inst **65**:1209-1214, 1980.

101 Dowling GP, Kelly JK: The histogenesis of adenocarcinoma of the gallbladder. Cancer **58**:1702-1708, 1986.

102 Esterly JR, Spicer SS: Mucin histochemistry of human gallbladder. Changes in adenocarcinoma, cystic fibrosis, and cholecystitis. J Natl Cancer Inst **40**:1-10, 1968.

103 Fahim RB, McDonald JR, Richards JC, Ferris DO: Carcinoma of the gallbladder. A study of its modes of spread. Ann Surg **156**:114-124, 1962.

104 Frank SA, Spjut HJ: Inapparent carcinoma of the gallbladder. Am Surg **33**:367-372, 1967.

104a Guo K-J, Yamaguchi K, Enjoji M: Undifferentiated carcinoma of the gallbladder. A clinicopathologic, histochemical, and immunohistochemical study of 21 patients with a poor prognosis. Cancer **61**:1872-1879, 1988.

105 Hamrick RE Jr, Liner FJ, Hastings PR, Cohn I Jr: Primary carcinoma of the gallbladder. Ann Surg **195**:270-273, 1982.

106 Inoshita S, Iwashita A, Enjoji M: Carcinosarcoma of the gallbladder. Report of a case and review of the literature. Acta Pathol Jpn **36**:913-920, 1986.

107 Jones CJ: Carcinoma of the gallbladder. A clinical and pathologic analysis of 50 cases. Ann Surg **132**:110-120, 1950.

108 Karasawa T, Itoh K, Komukai M, Ozawa U, Sakurai I, Shikata T: Squamous cell carcinoma of gallbladder. Report of two cases and review of literatures. Acta Pathol Jpn **31**:299-308, 1981.

109 Kinoshita H, Nagata E, Hirohashi K, Sakai K, Kobayashi Y: Carcinoma of the gallbladder with an anomalous connection between the choledochus and the pancreatic duct. Report of 10 cases and review of the literature in Japan. Cancer **54**:762-769, 1984.

110 Kozuka S, Kurashina M, Tsubone M, Hachisuka K, Yasui A: Significance of intestinal metaplasia for the evolution of cancer in the biliary tract. Cancer **54**:2277-2285, 1984.

111 Laitio M: Histogenesis of epithelial neoplasms of human gallbladder. I. Dysplasia. Pathol Res Pract **178**:51-56, 1983.

112 Laitio M: Histogenesis of epithelial neoplasms of human gallbladder. II. Classification of carcinoma on the basis of morphological features. Pathol Res Pract **178**:57-66, 1983.

113 Laitio M, Käkkinen I: Intestinal-type carcinoma of gallbladder. A histochemical and immunologic study. Cancer **36**:1668-1674, 1975.

114 Muto Y, Okamato K, Mechimura M: Composite tumor (ordinary adenocarcinoma, typical carcinoid and goblet cell adenocarcinoid) of the gallbladder. A variety of composite tumor. Am J Gastroenterol **79**:645-649, 1984.

115 Nevin JE, Moran TJ, Ray S, King R: Carcinoma of the gallbladder. Staging, treatment and prognosis. Cancer **37**:141-148, 1976.

116 Ojeda VJ, Shilkin KB, Walters MNI: Premalignant epithelial lesions of the gallbladder. A prospective study of 120 cholecystectomy specimens. Pathology **17**:451-454, 1985.

117 Piehler JM, Crichlow RW: Primary carcinoma of the gallbladder. Surg Gynecol Obstet **147**:929-942, 1978.

118 Russell PW, Brown CH: Primary carcinoma of the gallbladder. Ann Surg **132**:121-128, 1950.

119 Solan MJ, Jackson BT: Carcinoma of the gall-bladder. A clinical appraisal and review of 57 cases. Br J Surg **58**:593-597, 1971.

120 Sons HU, Borchard F, Joel BS: Carcinoma of the gallbladder. Autopsy findings in 287 cases and review of the literature. J Surg Oncol **28**:199-206, 1985.

121 Suster S, Huszar M, Herczeg E, Bubis JJ: Adenosquamous carcinoma of the gallbladder with spindle cell features. A light microscopic and immunocytochemical study of a case. Histopathology **11**:209-214, 1987.

122 Von Kuster LC, Cohen C: Malignant mixed tumor of the gallbladder. Report of two cases and a review of the literature. Cancer **50**:1166-1170, 1982.

123 Walsh N, Qizilbash A, Banerjee R, Waugh GA: Biliary neoplasia in Gardner's syndrome. Arch Pathol Lab Med **111**:76-77, 1987.

Carcinoma of extrahepatic bile ducts

124 Akwari OE, Van Heerden JA, Foulk WT, Baggenstoss AH: Cancer of the bile ducts associated with ulcerative colitis. Ann Surg **181**:303-309, 1975.

125 Alexander F, Rossi RL, O'Bryan M, Khettry U, Braasch JW, Walkins E Jr: Biliary carcinoma. A review of 109 cases. Am J Surg **147**:503-509, 1984.

126 Altemeier WA, Gall EA, Zinninger MM, Hoxworth PI: Sclerosing carcinoma of the major intrahepatic bile ducts. Arch Surg **75**:450-461, 1957.

127 Beazley RM, Hadjis N, Benjamin IS, Blumgart LH: Clinicopathological aspects of high bile duct cancer. Experience with resection and bypass surgical treatments. Ann Surg **199**:623-636, 1984.

128 Converse CF, Reagan JW, DeCosse JJ: Ulcerative colitis and carcinoma of the bile ducts. Am J Surg **121**:39-45, 1971.

129 Elias E, Hamlyn AN, Jain S, Long RG, Summerfield JA, Sherlock S: A randomized trial of percutaneous transhepatic cholangiography with the Chiba needle versus endoscopic retrograde cholangiography for bile duct visualization in jaundice. Gastroenterology **71**:439-443, 1976.

130 Gallagher PJ, Millis RR, Mitchinson MJ: Congenital dilatation of the intrahepatic bile ducts with cholangiocarcinoma. J Clin Pathol **25**:804-808, 1972.

131 Klatskin G: Adenocarcinoma of the hepatic duct as its bifurcation within the porta hepatis. An unusual tumor with distinctive clinical and pathological features. Am J Med **38**:241-256, 1965.

131a Iida S, Tsuzuki T, Ogata Y, Yoneyama K, Iri H, Watanabe K: The long-term survival of patients with carcinoma of the main hepatic duct junction. Cancer **60**:1612-1619, 1987.

132 Koo J, Ho J, Wong J, Ong GB: Mucoepidermoid carcinoma of the bile duct. Ann Surg **196**:140-148, 1982.

133 Kozuka S, Tsubone M, Hachisuka K: Evolution of carcinoma in the extrahepatic bile ducts. Cancer **54**:65-72, 1984.

134 Laitio M: Carcinoma of extrahepatic bile ducts. A histopathologic study. Pathol Res Pract **178**:67-72, 1983.

135 Langer, JC, Langer B, Taylor BR, Zeldin R, Cummings B: Carcinoma of the extrahepatic bile ducts. Results of an aggressive surgical approach. Surgery **98**:752-759, 1985.

136 MacCarty RL, LaRusso NF, May GR, Bender, CE, Wiesner RH, King JE, Coffey RJ: Cholangiocarcinoma complicating primary sclerosing cholangitis. Cholangiographic appearances. Radiology **156**:43-46, 1985.

137 Nagura H, Tsutsumi Y, Watanabe K, Hasegawa H, Fujimoto T, Sugita T, Mitomi T: Immunohistochemistry of carcinoembryonic antigen, secretory component and lysozyme in benign and malignant common bile duct tissues. Virchows Arch [Pathol Anat] **403**:271-280, 1984.

138 Okuda K, Kubo Y, Okazaki N, Arishima T, Hashimoto M, Jinnouchi S, Sawa Y, Shimokawa Y, Nakajima Y, Noguchi T, Nakano M, Kojiro M, Nakashima T: Clinical aspects of intrahepatic bile duct carcinoma including hilar carcinoma. A study of 57 autopsy-proven cases. Cancer **39**:232-246, 1977.

139 Qualman SJ, Haupt HM, Bauer TW, Taxy JB: Adenocarcinoma of the hepatic duct junction. A reappraisal of the histologic criteria of malignancy. Cancer **53**:1545-1551, 1984.

140 Richtie JK, Allan RM, Macartney J, Thompson H, Hawley PR, Cooke WT: Biliary tract carcinoma associated with ulcerative colitis. Q J Med **43**:263-279, 1974.

140a Sameshima Y, Uchimura M, Muto Y, Maeda J, Tsuchiyama H: Coexistent carcinoma in congenital dilatation of the bile duct and anomalous arrangement of the pancreatico-bile duct. Carcinogenesis of coexistent gallbladder carcinoma. Cancer **60**:1883-1890, 1987.

141 Strom BL, Hibberd PL, Soper KA, Stolley PD, Nelson WL: International variations in epidemiology of cancers of the extrahepatic biliary tract. Cancer Res **45**:5165-5168, 1985.

142 Suda K, Matsumoto Y, Miyano T: An extended common channel in patients with biliary tract carcinoma and congenital biliary dilatation. Surg Pathol **1**:65-69, 1988.

143 Tompkins RK, Thomas D, Wile A, Longmire WP Jr: Prognostic factors in bile duct carcinoma. Analysis of 96 cases. Ann Surg **194**:447-457, 1981.

144 Wee A, Ludwig J, Coffey RJ, LaRusso NF, Wiesner RH: Hepatobiliary carcinoma associated with primary sclerosing cholangitis and chronic ulcerative colitis. Hum Pathol **16**:719-726, 1985.

145 Weinbren K, Mutum SS: Pathological aspects of cholangiocarcinoma. J Pathol **139**:217-238, 1983.

146 Whelton MJ, Petrelli M, George P, Young WB, Sherlock S: Carcinoma of the junction of the main hepatic ducts. Q J Med **38**:211-230, 1969.

147 Yamamoto M, Nakajo S, Tahara E, Miyoshi N: Endocrine cell carcinoma of extrahepatic bile duct. Acta Pathol Jpn **36**:587-593, 1986.

Other malignant tumors

148 Aldabagh SM, Shibata CS, Taxy JB: Rhabdomyosarcoma of the common bile duct in an adult. Arch Pathol Lab Med **110**:547-550, 1986.

149 Borja SR, Meyer WR, Cahill JP: Malignant melanoma of the gallbladder. Report of a case. Cancer **54**:929-931, 1984.

150 Carstens PHB, Ghazi C, Carnighan RH, Brewer MS: Primary malignant melanoma of the common bile duct. Hum Pathol **17**:1282-1285, 1986.

151 Davis GL, Kissane JM, Ishak KG: Embryonal rhabdomyosarcoma (sarcoma botryoides) of the biliary tree. Report of five cases and review of the literature. Cancer **24**:333-342, 1969.

152 Goodman ZD, Albores-Saavedra J, Lundblad DM: Somatostatinoma of the cystic duct. Cancer **53**:498-502, 1984.

153 Judge DM, Dickman PS, Trapukdi BS: Nonfunctioning argyrophilic tumor (APUDoma) of the hepatic duct. Simplified methods of detecting biogenic amines arising in tissue. Am J Clin Pathol **66**:40-45, 1976.

154 King DK, Ewen SWB, Sewell HF, Dawson AA: Obstructive jaundice. An unusual presentation of granulocytic sarcoma. Cancer **60**:114-117, 1987.

155 Lack EE, Perez-Atayde AR, Schuster SR: Botryoid rhabdomyosarcoma of the biliary tract. Report of five cases with ultrastructural observations and literature review. Am J Surg Pathol **5**:643-652, 1981.

156 Mihara S, Matsumoto H, Tokunaga F, Yano H, Ota M, Yamashita S: Botryoid rhabdomyosarcoma of the gallbladder in a child. Cancer **49**:812-818, 1982.

157 Newmark H III, Kliewer K, Curtis A, DenBesten L, Enenstein W: Primary leiomyosarcoma of gallbladder seen on computed tomography and ultrasound. Am J Gastroenterol **81**:202-204, 1986.

158 Nguyen G: Primary extranodal non-Hodgkin's lymphoma of the extrahepatic bile ducts. Report of a case. Cancer **50**:2218-2222, 1982.

159 Peison B, Rabin L: Malignant melanoma of the gallbladder. Report of three cases and review of the literature. Cancer **37**:2448-2454, 1976.

160 Ruymann FB, Raney B Jr, Crist WM, Lawrence W Jr, Lindberg RD, Soule EH: Rhabdomyosarcoma of the biliary tree in childhood. A report from the Intergroup Rhabdomyosarcoma Study. Cancer **56**:575-581, 1985.

160a Shiffman MA, Juler G: Carcinoid of the biliary tract. Arch Surg **89**:113-115, 1964.

161 Van Slick EJ, Schuman BM: Lymphocytic lymphosarcoma of the gallbladder. Cancer **30**:810-816, 1972.

162 Willen R, Willen H: Primary sarcoma of the gallbladder. A light and electron-microscopical study. Virchows Arch [Pathol Anat] **396**:91-102, 1982.

163 Yasuma T, Yanaka M: Primary sarcoma of the gallbladder. Report of three cases. Acta Pathol Jpn **21**:285-304, 1971.

15 Pancreas and periampullary region

Pancreas
ANNULAR PANCREAS

Annular pancreas is a rare embryologic abnormality in which the ventral anlage of the pancreas fails to rotate properly.[1,3] Encirclement of the duodenum by pancreatic parenchyma occurs and may lead to constriction of the lumen. The duct in the annular pancreas originates anteriorly, courses to the right over the duodenum and then posteriorly and to the left behind the duodenum, passing near the common duct. These anatomic variations have to be kept in mind when surgery is contemplated. Pancreatitis may develop in association with this anomaly.

Microscopically, the annular pancreas contains a large number of PP cells in its islet cell component, in keeping with its origin from the ventral primordium.[2]

HETEROTOPIC PANCREAS

Heterotopia of pancreatic tissue is a relatively frequent congenital anomaly.[4,5] It is most common in the duodenum (particularly the second portion), stomach, and jejunum, but also occurs in the ileum, Meckel's diverticulum, gastric and intestinal diverticula, gallbladder and bile ducts, large bowel, splenic capsule, omentum, and several other locations.

Grossly, the heterotopic tissue resembles normal pancreas. Firm, yellow, lobulated nodules measuring up to 4 cm are seen sharply circumscribed from the surrounding tissues. Central umbilication is often present in the cases located beneath a mucosa, corresponding to a central duct that opens into the lumen; both the umbilication and the duct can be demonstrated roentgenographically and constitute an important diagnostic sign.[6] Microscopically, acinar and ductal tissues are always present, whereas islet tissue is found in only one third of the cases. In some cases, there is also a component of pyloric-type mucous glands. The islet component contains all the major types of endocrine cells, but their relative number varies a great deal from case to case. In most instances, the islets are rich in alpha cells and poor in PP cells (dorsal type), although in others the reverse is true (ventral type).[7]

Every pathologic change that occurs in the pancreas can occur in its heterotopic counterpart, including acute pancreatitis and neoplasms. Heterotopic pancreas in the stomach may cause hemorrhage, ulceration, or pyloric obstruction. When located in the area of the ampulla of Vater, it may result in obstructive jaundice.

PANCREATITIS
Acute pancreatitis

The pathogenesis of acute pancreatitis still remains controversial.[18,20,25] Experimental work has been hampered by the fact that most laboratory animals do not suffer naturally from this illness. Opie[21] postulated an obstructive mechanism after demonstrating in his famous case of pancreatitis the presence of a small stone lodged in the ampulla. This stone had converted the common bile duct and the main pancreatic duct (duct of Wirsung) into a common channel so that bile might have passed into the pancreatic duct. This could have activated trypsinogen, thus beginning a series of events that included the digestion of the duct wall, adjacent parenchyma, and vessel walls by trypsin, as well as the splitting of fat and formation of calcium soaps by lipase. Theoretically, fibrosis of the sphincter of Oddi or a neoplasm in this region could induce a similar process. Indeed, cases of pancreatitis secondary to tumors of the periampullary area or in the head of the pancreas have been recorded.

The difficulty with this theory is that the formation of a common channel with a stone impacted in the ampulla occurs in less than 5% of patients with pancreatitis. As Dragstedt et al.[13] pointed out many years ago, the union of the pancreatic duct and the bile duct to form an ampulla must occur at a sufficient distance from the duodenal opening to permit obstruction of the orifice without obstruction of either duct. Furthermore, the stone must be just the right size. If it is too small, it will not block the ampullary opening; if it is too large, it will block either or both the common bile duct and the main pancreatic duct.

Some of these objections might be circumvented by postulating a transient blockage of the ampulla of Vater by a migrating gallstone or by a spasm of the sphincter of Oddi, which could produce a common channel in the absence of a stone. Acosta and Ledesma[8] recovered gallstones in the feces of thirty-four of thirty-six patients with pancreatitis, but in only three out of thirty-six control subjects (patients with lithiasis of the gallbladder but no pancreatitis). Sphincter spasm can be demonstrated in experimental animals and in human beings by chemical and roentgenographic studies performed under different conditions, including the administration of drugs resulting in sphincter spasm (such as morphine) and relaxation (such as nitrites). The pancreatic duct is visualized in about 25% of the patients having postoperative T-tube cholangiograms. If the common duct T tube is in place and pancreatic secretion is injected intravenously, almost pure pancreatic juice comes from the T tube.[12] If spasm of the sphincter of Oddi is produced by morphine and if radiopaque material is injected through the T tube into the common duct, the whole pancreatic system may be visualized. Bile taken from the common duct or gallbladder often contains pancreatic enzymes. Conversely, bile may be found in the peripancreatic tissues of patients operated on for pancreatitis, possibly because of rupture of a pancreatic duct.

All these experiments demonstrate that a common channel may indeed occur under physiologic circumstances and that the relative secretory pressures of the gallbladder, bile ducts, and pancreatic ducts (which fluctuate greatly under different conditions) and the status of the sphincter of Oddi will determine the type and direction of the flow.

Another approach to the problem is a careful anatomic examination of the system in an attempt to determine how often a common channel is possible on anatomic grounds alone. Several autopsy studies have shown that there are many anatomic variations in the ampullary area that preclude such an occurrence. These include separation of common and pancreatic ducts by a septum and independent emptying of the main pancreatic duct into the duodenum. The consensus reached from these anatomic studies is that a common channel is anatomically present in 50% to 60% of all individuals.[16]

The anatomic arrangement of the accessory (Santorini's) pancreatic duct is also important because this duct has no sphincter; therefore, if it communicates with the duct of Wirsung and the latter in turn communicates with the common bile duct, the biliary duct pressure will predominate. In the study of Howard and Jones,[16] the duct of Santorini communicated with the duct of Wirsung in fifty-four (36%)

of the 150 cases. Interestingly enough, this communication was present in almost 50% of the cases in which reflux could be demonstrated but in less than 15% of those in whom no reflux occurred.

A variation of the obstructive theory for the pathogenesis of pancreatitis postulates that partial or total obstruction of the pancreatic duct *alone* is enough to induce the production of pancreatitis—through a mechanism of increased secretion, rupture of ductules and acini, and liberation of pancreatic enzymes into the parenchyma. Rich and Duff[24] postulated that squamous metaplasia of the pancreatic duct might result in such an obstruction. Such type of metaplasia, however, can be found at autopsy in at least 6% of otherwise normal pancreases.[11] Interestingly, if a patient with heterotopic pancreas develops acute pancreatitis, the inflammatory process will also affect the heterotopic foci. Recently, it has been postulated that buthyl cholinesterase normally present in large amounts in the pancreatic acinar cells may be directly involved in the production of pancreatitis.[14,15] Regardless of what the precise pathogenetic mechanism will prove to be, it is a fact that the large majority of cases of acute pancreatitis are associated with biliary tract disease (63%), alcoholism (8%), and trauma.

The gross changes vary from a swollen and edematous but otherwise well-preserved organ (associated with a 10% to 15% mortality) to a hemorrhagic and necrotic mass of tissue (associated with a mortality of about 50%). Yellow plaques and nodules representing fat necrosis are seen within the pancreas as well as throughout the mesenteric and peritoneal fat (Fig. 15-1). Sometimes the process spreads to the neighboring colon, and it may result in localized ileus, stenosis, perforation, fistulous formations, and ischemic necrosis.[17]

Microscopically, the earlier changes in the pancreas are represented by acinar cell homogenization, ductal dilatation with epithelial degeneration, diffuse interstitial edema, leukocytic infiltration, and fibroblastic reaction.[23] Whether the pancreatitis is initiated in the acinar cell or in the interstitial space is controversial. If the disease progresses, extensive necrosis and hemorrhage of pancreatic tissue supervene. The foci of peritoneal fat necrosis become almost immediately surrounded and infiltrated by neutrophils; this population later changes to foamy histiocytes and lymphocytes. Calcification occurs early and extensively in these areas.

Acute pancreatitis is characteristically associated with serum elevation of amylase, an alteration that can also be found with duodenal ulcer, volvulus, gangrenous cholecystitis, ruptured aortic aneurysm, and mesenteric thrombosis.[9]

The mortality rate for acute pancreatitis is about 20%.[10] The current therapeutic approach is to treat medically suspected cases of acute pancreatitis vigorously for 4 to 6 hours; if the diagnosis is in doubt and the patient is deteriorating despite therapy, emergency laparotomy is indicated. The presence of an upper abdominal mass suspected of being a pseudocyst and persistent rising jaundice are also indications for surgical intervention.[19]

Postoperative pancreatitis is in most, but not all, cases the result of direct operative trauma to the pancreatic region.[22] Of seventy cases reported by White et al.,[26] the original operation had included exploration of the common

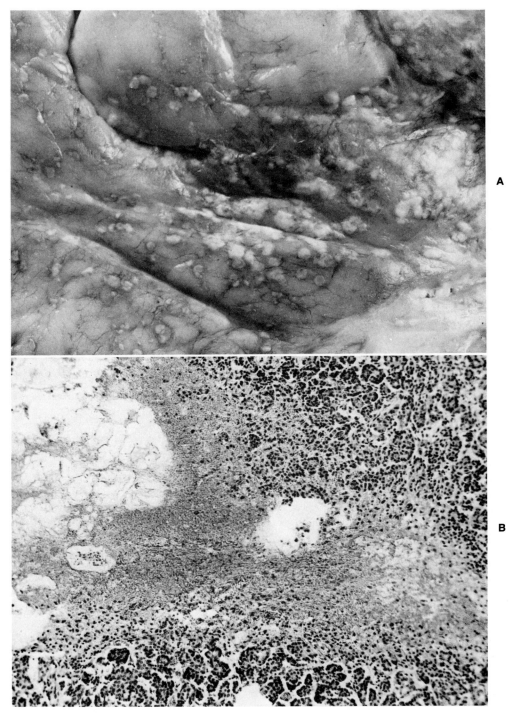

Fig. 15-1 A, Fat necrosis of pancreatic origin. Well-defined yellowish areas are scattered over mesentery. **B,** Fat necrosis in pancreas.

bile duct in twenty-eight and gastric resection in seventeen. In sixteen patients, the surgical procedure was such that the possibility of local trauma could be excluded.

Chronic pancreatitis

Chronic pancreatitis characteristically presents with abdominal pain, which can be very severe.[37] Two major anatomic forms have been described, one associated with obstruction of the major pancreatic ducts and the other accompanied by extensive parenchymal calcification.

Obstructive chronic pancreatitis is the result of narrowing or occlusion of the pancreatic ducts, the most common causes being carcinoma and stones. In the latter condition, known as chronic pancreatitis with lithiasis, most of the stones are found in the duct of Wirsung within 2 to 4 cm of the ampulla of Vater.[30] In the twenty-two cases reported by Stobbe et al.,[39] the calculi were restricted to a small portion of the gland. None of the patients had symptoms of pancreatic origin, none had hyperparathyroidism, and only one had a history of alcoholism.

Chronic calcifying pancreatitis is characterized grossly by a pancreas that is nodular, hard, and misshapen; it may be either enlarged or atrophic. Microscopically, the main features are dilatation of ducts and acini, squamous metaplasia, intraluminal eosinophilic mucoprotein plugs (which often calcify), acinar atrophy, and perilobular and intralobular sclerosis.[36] Proliferative changes in the ductal epithelium are frequent.[42] Interestingly, chronic pancreatitis is often accompanied by hyperplasia of Brunner's glands in the duodenum.[40]

In a series of twenty-three patients reported by Stobbe et al.[39] six patients had hyperparathyroidism, three had associated pancreatic carcinoma, and ten had a history of alcoholism. In other series, a history of alcoholism has been obtained in approximately 75% of the patients with chronic pancreatitis.[41] It is estimated that about 7% of hyperparathyroid patients develop chronic pancreatitis as a result of the hypercalcemia.[32]

Rare types of pancreatitis include a hereditary form manifested during childhood and inherited as an autosomal mendelian dominant trait,[29] a variety accompanying polyarteritis nodosa, a chronic form following mumps infection,[28] a "tropical" form seen in some third world countries,[35] and tuberculous infection.[38]

A rare complication of both acute and chronic pancreatitis is the occurrence of widespread metastatic fat necrosis, presumably as a consequence of the liberation of lipase by the damaged organ. Subcutaneous tissue (particularly in the legs), mediastinum, pleura, pericardium, bone marrow, periarticular fat, and liver can be involved.[34] Erythema nodosum–like lesions of the skin, polyarthropathy, and avascular bone necrosis are some of the diseases that may develop as a result.

Chronic pancreatitis can result in a marked proliferation of islet cells, which may grow in cords and small clusters.[31] Sometimes they even may simulate a malignant neoplasm. Immunohistochemical stains have shown that all major types of islet cells are represented[27] (Fig. 15-2).

The treatment of chronic pancreatitis includes pancreatic duct drainage, partial pancreatic resection, and near-total pancreatectomy with or without islet autotransplantation.[33]

Abscess

Pancreatic abscess is most often seen as a complication of acute pancreatitis. In contrast to pseudocysts, pancreatic abscesses are bonafide infections; pus is present in them, and bacteria are recovered in over 90% of the cases.[43]

Pseudocysts

Pseudocysts are related to pancreatitis, trauma, and, rarely, to neoplastic duct obstruction. Blockage of ducts leads to an accumulation of secretion and the formation of cysts. These pseudocysts often become large, spread beyond the substance of the pancreas into the lesser peritoneal cavity, and present through the gastrocolic or gastrohepatic ligament. They are multiple in about 15% of the cases.[44] They do not have an epithelial lining. The fluid within them has a high amylase content.

Complications of pancreatic pseudocyst include perforation and hemorrhage. The splenic artery is the most common source of intracystic hemorrhage, which can be massive and result in sudden death.[45]

Small pseudocysts located in the body or tail of the pancreas can be treated with excision. Most of the others are treated by external drainage (preferred for the infected cysts) or internal drainage, in the form of transgastric cystgastrostomy or cystojejunostomy to a Roux-en-Y loop of jejunum.

TRUE CYSTS

Cysts lined by non-neoplastic glandular epithelium are usually congenital and associated with similar cysts of other viscera such as liver or kidney.

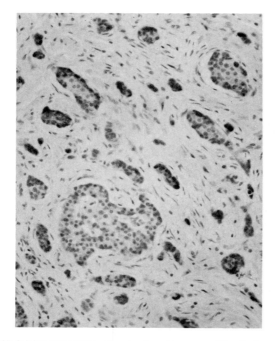

Fig. 15-2 Islet cell proliferation in chronic pancreatitis. By immunoperoxidase, all major cells were represented. Despite apparently invasive pattern, lesion is probably non-neoplastic.

A rare form of cyst has been described that is lined by squamous epithelium with a thick wall of lymphoid tissue beneath (lymphoepithelial cyst).[46]

TUMORS
Ductal adenocarcinoma
General features

Ductal adenocarcinoma of the exocrine pancreas comprises about 85% of all cases of pancreatic malignancy.[49,58] It constitutes the fourth most common cause of death from cancer in the United States, and its incidence is increasing.[55] Cases have been described in families,[52] in patients with Peutz-Jeghers syndrome,[47] and in workers exposed to beta-naphthylamine or benzidine.[56] Cigarette smoking has also been cited as a risk factor.[57] It has been suggested that the pancreaticobiliary ductal anatomy may be related to the incidence of carcinoma, in view of the fact that lack of a common channel has been found at autopsy to be associated with abnormalities of the ductal epithelium.[51] There is an increase in the incidence of diabetes in patients with pancreatic carcinoma, but this usually develops within a short time of the diagnosis of cancer, suggesting that it is a secondary event. Most patients with pancreatic carcinoma are elderly, and there is a slight male preponderance (1.6:1 ratio).[57]

Because of its strategic location in relation to the extrahepatic bile ducts, carcinoma of the head of the pancreas usually causes progressive jaundice that is associated with pain in at least one half of the patients; however, the diagnosis in most cases is made when the tumor is relatively large (about 5 cm) and has extended beyond the pancreas (85% of the cases). Carcinomas of the body and tail of the pancreas grow insidiously and often have already metastasized at the time of diagnosis. They are associated with peripheral venous thrombi in about 25% of the patients.[54]

Various techniques have been used with various degrees of success to detect pancreatic carcinoma at an early stage. These include CT scan, nuclear magnetic resonance, celiac angiography, sonography, endoscopic retrograde cholangiopancreatography (ERCP), selenomethionine scan, duodenal aspiration, and serum tests.[53] The latter use monoclonal antibodies against various cancer-related antigens. Of these, those measuring levels of S pan-1 and CA 19-9 antigen seem more effective than those measuring CEA or other markers.[48,50,53a,59]

Location and gross features

Pancreatic carcinoma is located in the head of the pancreas in two thirds of the patients and in the body or tail in the other third. Multiple tumors are found in about 20% of the cases. Most are poorly delineated and firm, with a yellowish gray cut surface. The duodenal wall is invaded by direct extension in one fourth of the tumors arising from the pancreatic head. The involved pancreatic ducts frequently become greatly dilated and plugged with necrotic tumor. This dilatation may extend for a considerable distance beyond the main mass of the tumor. Extrapancreatic extension is common; when extensive, it may be very difficult to determine whether or not a given tumor is of pancreatic origin. Cubilla and Fitzgerald [60] found that one third of the cases clinically regarded as pancreatic cancers were not of pancreatic origin but rather of duodenal, retroperitoneal, or metastatic origin. Of twenty-eight patients in whom the cancer was grossly located in the area of the head of the pancreas, an origin from the pancreatic ducts could be proved in only fourteen. In five, the site of origin could not

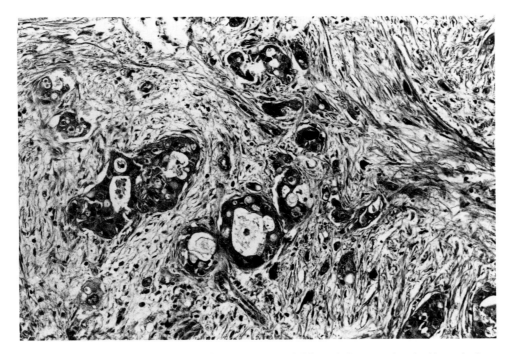

Fig. 15-3 Pancreatic adenocarcinoma. Good architectural differentiation associated with marked nuclear atypia is typical of tumors of this organ. Note extensive desmoplastic reaction.

be determined; in the others, the tumors originated in the duodenum, ampulla, or bile ducts.

The non-neoplastic pancreas distal to the tumor may show extensive atrophy, fibrosis, and ductal dilatation.

Microscopic features

Pancreatic duct adenocarcinomas can be well differentiated, moderately differentiated, or poorly differentiated (Fig. 15-3). Their pattern of growth may be papillary, but usually it is not.[63] In the well-differentiated tumors, the microscopic diagnosis can be extremely difficult.[71] Close attention must be given to cytologic details. At low-power examination, the glands are often well formed, have a large lumen, and are lined by one or a few layers of cylindrical epithelium. Their overall low-power appearance may not be particularly suggestive of carcinoma, except for the irregularities in the shape and distribution of the glands and the peculiar desmoplastic stroma that surrounds them; however, high-power examination of the lining epithelium will show one or more features which, in this location, are indicative of malignancy: marked nuclear pleomorphism, loss of polarity, prominent nucleoli, and mitotic activity. Perineurial invasion, which is present in 90% of the cases, constitutes an important diagnostic sign (Fig. 15-4). However, it is not pathognomonic of malignancy: benign epithelial inclusions have been observed in pancreatic nerves,[65] and perineurial extension of islet cells can occur in chronic pancreatitis.[61] Invasion of blood vessels, particularly veins, is seen in half of the cases.

Immunohistochemically, there is positivity for keratin, EMA, CEA, CA19-9 antigen, and laminin, a rough correlation existing between the expression of these markers and the degree of differentiation.[62,70,72,80] A high proportion of these tumors also contain a minor population of endocrine cells.[68,73] In rare instances, a mixture of ductal and insular patterns is seen in the same tumor.[77,78]

Carcinoma in situ is found in the duct epithelium adjacent to the carcinoma in about 20% to 30% of the cases, sometimes at a distance from the main tumor mass and even at the point of surgical transection.[67,79] Atypia and papillary hyperplasia of duct epithelium are present in one third of the cases with carcinoma, whereas the incidence of these abnormalities in the pancreases of control subjects is very low.[64,66,75,76] Conversely, the prevalence of squamous metaplasia, pyloric gland metaplasia, mucous hypertrophy, and focal epithelial hyperplasia is not significantly different among the two groups.[66,74]

Because of ductal occlusion by the carcinoma, the lobular tissue may be completely destroyed. The islet tissue is usually well preserved, resulting in an appearance designated as *insular pancreas;* however, both atrophic and hypertrophic changes can occur in the islets. Most commonly, destruction of a variable amount of islet tissue mass results in a subclinical or overt diabetic picture. Rarely, hypertrophy of the islets occurs distal to a ductal adenocarcinoma and produces hypoglycemia. Gambill[69] found significant pancreatitis in twenty-six (10%) of 255 patients with pancreatic or ampullary carcinoma. The presence of pancreatitis resulted in a considerable delay in the diagnosis of carcinoma.

Other microscopic types

Uncommon but reasonably distinctive variants of pancreatic adenocarcinoma include *adenosquamous carcinoma* (a term preferable to *mucoepidermoid carcinoma* or *adenoacanthoma*),[85] *oncocytic carcinoma, clear cell carcinoma,*[85a] *signet ring carcinoma,* and *mucinous carcinoma*[83] (Fig. 15-5). The latter can result in pseudomyxoma peritonei.[82] The few reported cases of pure *epidermoid car-*

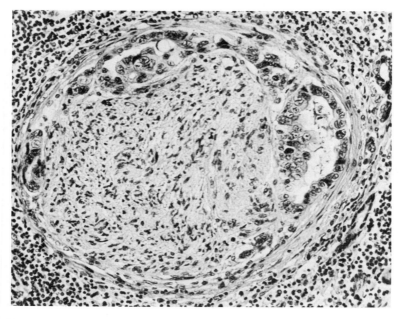

Fig. 15-4 Perineurial invasion in well-differentiated adenocarcinoma of pancreas.

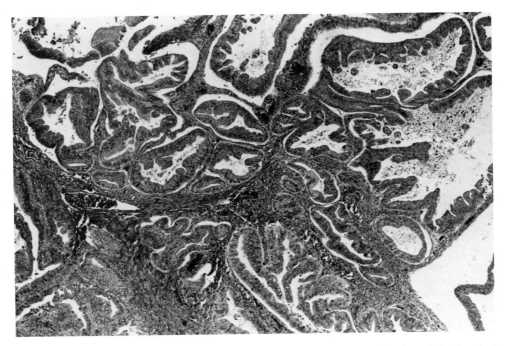

Fig. 15-5 Mucinous adenocarcinoma of pancreas. Large well-differentiated glands contain abundant mucin in their lumina.

cinoma of the pancreas probably represent a variant of adenosquamous carcinoma in which the squamous component has overrun the glandular elements; this tumor can be associated with hypercalcemia.[81]

Metastases

Pancreatic duct adenocarcinoma tends to metastasize to multiple lymph nodes of the superior head, superior body, and posterior pancreaticoduodenal groups (88%). Cubilla et al.[86] found that in 33% of patients with pancreatic cancer, nodal metastases were present in groups of nodes not usually removed with the standard Whipple's procedure. Some of these metastases occur very early in the course of the disease.[88,89]

The most common sites of distant metastases are liver, peritoneum, lung, adrenal, bone, distant lymph node groups, skin, and central nervous system.[87] Sometimes, a distant nodal metastasis (particularly in the supraclavicular region) is the first manifestation of pancreatic carcinoma.

Cytology

Cytologic material for the diagnosis of pancreatic periampullary carcinoma can be obtained from different sources, with various degrees of success.

1 Duodenal secretion, sometimes enriched with pancreatic secretion by the intravenous administration of secretin (Fig. 15-6). The reported success rate for identifying pancreatic cancer is 66% overall, 79% for tumors of the head, and 33% for those of the tail.[92,94]

2 Pancreatic juice obtained during the performance of an endoscopic retrograde cholangiopancreatography (ERCP). The yield rate has ranged from 50% to 85% in the reported series.[90,96]

3 Percutaneous fine needle aspiration with ultrasonic, angiographic, or CT guidance.[91,93,95,97,98] The accuracy of this method is over 90%.[91]

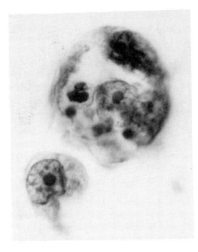

Fig. 15-6 Cluster of tumor cells obtained from duodenal lavage that led to diagnosis of adenocarcinoma. At operation, tumor was found to be primary in terminal third of common bile duct.

4 Intraoperative fine needle aspiration. The accuracy of this technique is well over 90% (see next section).

Exploration and frozen section

At the time of exploration for a presumptive diagnosis of carcinoma of pancreas or periampullary region, evidence of metastatic disease in the peripancreatic nodes, liver, and peritoneum should be searched for and a frozen section requested if a lesion in any of these sites is encountered. In the absence of detectable metastases, search for the primary tumor should then be undertaken. If a mass is palpated in the pancreas, this should be examined microscopically by either an incisional biopsy, core needle biopsy, or fine needle aspiration. The latter technique is becoming increasingly popular because it minimizes the possibilities of hemorrhage, pancreatitis, and tumor seeding that exist with the biopsy procedures.[99-101] When biopsying the pancreatic head, experience is required to avoid the common bile duct, the gastroduodenal artery, and the portal vein.

During exploration of the jaundiced patient in whom no obvious pancreatic tumor is detected, the head of the pancreas should be mobilized and carefully palpated, and the common bile duct should be exposed. If the latter is dilated, it should be explored. If no tumor or stones are found in it, duodenotomy should follow and the ampullary region should be inspected; in the presence of a mass in the area, a biopsy should be submitted for frozen section. In papillary lesions, the biopsy should be deep in order to detect the invasive component if present. One should remember that dilatation of the common duct and of the gallbladder in the presence of jaundice and in the absence of biliary tract stones is almost always caused by carcinoma.

Frozen section interpretation of pancreatic lesions can be very difficult because of the well-differentiated nature of many carcinomas on one hand and the architectural distortion resulting from chronic pancreatitis on the other.[104,105] One should search for perineurial invasion and also evaluate carefully the cytologic features of the glandular formations.[102] When examining sections from the terminal portion of the common bile duct or the ampullary region, one should be careful not to misinterpret accessory pancreatic ducts or Beale's periluminal sacculi as malignant.[103]

Treatment

The treatment of pancreatic carcinoma is primarily surgical, its extent depending on the site and size of the tumor. Neoplasms of body and tail are treated with a distal pancreatectomy. Neoplasms of the pancreatic head and periampullary region are generally treated with the Whipple operation, the alternative for this being total pancreatectomy.[106-108] These operations carry a 10% to 20% mortality rate.[110,112]

Unfortunately, most tumors have already extended outside the pancreas at the time of laparotomy and are therefore not amenable to curative surgery. These tumors are better treated with palliative bypass operations, which result in similar overall survival times with much less operative morbidity and mortality. Locally unresectable pancreatic carcinomas are also treated with radiation therapy (sometimes administered intraoperatively) and/or chemotherapy.[109,111]

Table 15-1 Staging of pancreatic carcinoma

Stage	Description
I	T1, T2, N0, M0—No (or unknown) direct extension, or limited direct extension of tumor to adjacent viscera, with no (or unknown) regional node extension and absence of distant metastases. Limited direct extension is defined as involvement of organs adjacent to the pancreas (duodenum, common bile duct, or stomach) that can be removed *en bloc* with the pancreas if a curative resection is attempted.
II	T3, N0, M0—Further direct extension of tumor into adjacent viscera, with no (or unknown) lymph node involvement and no distant metastases, which precludes surgical resection.
III	T1-3, N1, M0—Regional node metastases without clinical evidence of distant metastases.
IV	T1-3, N0-1, M1—Distant metastatic disease in liver or other sites.

Definitions of TNM categories for cancer of the pancreas

T	Primary tumor
	T1: No direct extension of the primary tumor beyond the pancreas
	T2: Limited direct extension (to duodenum, bile ducts, or stomach), still possibly permitting tumor resection
	T3: Further direct extension, incompatible with surgical resection
	Tx: Direct extension not assessed or not recorded
N	Regional lymph node involvement
	N0: Regional nodes not involved
	N1: Regional nodes involved
	Nx: Regional node involvement not assessed or not recorded
M	Distant metastases
	M0: No distant metastases
	M1: Distant metastatic involvement
	Mx: Distant metastatic involvement not assessed or not recorded

From Pollard HM, Anderson WAD, Brooks, FP, Cohn I Jr, Copeland MM, Connelly RR, Fortner JG, Kissane JM, Lemon HM, Palmer PES, Thomas LB, Webster PD III, Carter S: Staging of cancer of the pancreas. Cancer of the Pancreas Task Force. Cancer 47:1631-1637, 1981.

Combination regimes result in longer survival than radiation alone.[109]

Prognosis

In most series of pancreatic carcinoma, the overall 5-year survival rate has been 2% or less, with over 90% of the patients dying within 1 year of diagnosis.[113,114] Even when the cancer seems confined to the pancreas at the time of surgery, the 5-year survival rate does not exceed 15%.[113,117] The prognosis is directly related to the stage of the tumor[116] (Table 15-1). It has been suggested that there is also a correlation with microscopic grade and size, the better differentiated and smaller tumors having longer median survival times.[115,118]

Anaplastic carcinoma

Anaplastic carcinomas, also known as pleomorphic, sarcomatoid, or undifferentiated carcinomas, are in most cases

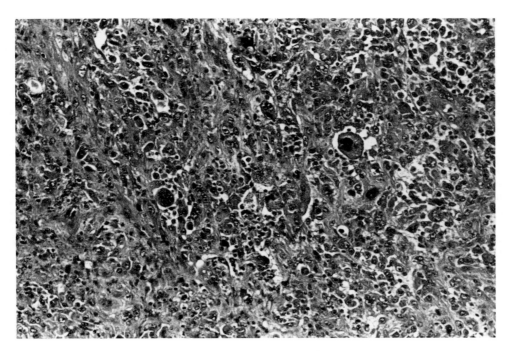

Fig. 15-7 Pleomorphic carcinoma with numerous large bizarre tumor cells. This neoplasm can be confused with sarcoma or metastatic malignant melanoma.

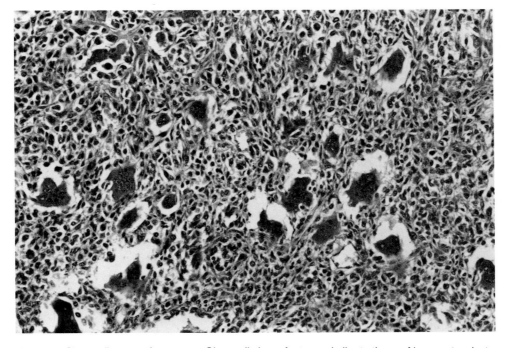

Fig. 15-8 Giant cell tumor of pancreas. Giant cells have features similar to those of bone osteoclasts. There are no areas of epithelial differentiation.

variants of duct-derived carcinomas; however, their appearance is so distinctive and their behavior so aggressive that a distinction from the ordinary ductal adenocarcinoma is warranted.[123] They comprise about 7% of all non-endocrine pancreatic malignancies. Most involve the body or tail of the pancreas rather than the head. Most patients are above the age of 50 at the time of diagnosis, and there is a distinct male predilection. Three morphologic types can be recognized, although they are sometimes seen in combination[119]:

1 Pleomorphic carcinomas that contain a large number of bizarre, multinucleated tumor cells (Fig. 15-7). These can be confused with amelanotic melanoma, liver cell carcinoma, and some types of sarcomas. A high proportion of these tumors occur in the body or tail. Metastases invariably develop, and hematogenous spread is very common.[125]

2 Tumors that are largely composed of spindle-shaped cells and that can be easily confused with sarcomas. Therefore, the diagnosis of primary sarcoma of the pancreas should be regarded with a high degree of skepticism.

3 Tumors that are composed of small, monotonous round cells growing in a solid fashion, somewhat reminiscent of malignant lymphoma. Some of these tumors exhibit features of neuroendocrine differentiation and should be viewed as examples of extrapulmonary small cell carcinomas (see p. 778).

Any of these varieties can be accompanied by areas of clearcut adenocarcinoma. Immunohistochemically, stains for keratin, EMA, and CEA are positive in the obvious epithelial component and sometimes also in the sarcoma-like areas (see Color plate II, *C*).

The prognosis for all of these varieties of anaplastic carcinoma is extremely poor.

Giant cell tumor of the pancreas is included in some series as another variant of anaplastic carcinoma, but it should be kept separate from it because of its better prognosis. Microscopically, the tumor has a dual population: relatively uniform spindle cells of mesenchymal appearance

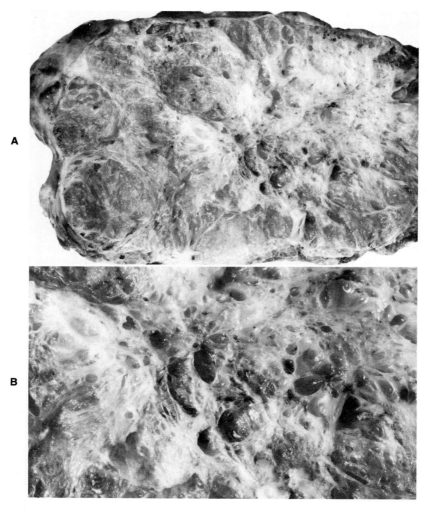

Fig. 15-9 Microcystic (glycogen-rich or serous) cystadenoma of pancreas. Grossly, tumor has spongy appearance due to presence of innumerable small cavities containing clear fluid.

and atypical cytologic features (such as nuclear hyperchromasia and high mitotic activity) alternate with multinucleated giant cells having an appearance and a histochemical profile indistinguishable from that of normal osteoclasts.[120,122] The nuclei of these osteoclast-like cells are uniformly small, and mitoses are absent. Bizarre giant cells with atypical nuclei are not found (Fig. 15-8). In some cases, areas of clearcut epithelial glandular appearance are found, suggesting that giant cell tumor is another variant of carcinoma of ductal derivation.[121,124]

Microcystic cystadenoma

Cystic neoplasms of the pancreas have been traditionally described as a group, the only distinction made among them being whether they are benign or malignant in nature. Compagno and Oertel[127] have made an important contribution to this subject by showing that most of these tumors can be divided into two distinct morphologic types: microcystic and mucinous, each having a remarkably different biologic significance.

Microcystic cystadenoma, also known as glycogen-rich or serous cystadenoma, is invariably benign, usually large, and composed microscopically of many small cysts lined by small, flat, or cuboidal cells containing abundant glycogen but only an insignificant amount of mucin[127,129] (Figs. 15-9 and 15-10). A layer of myoepithelial cells is present beneath this epithelium.[130] Papillae are absent or inconspicuous. Ultrastructural studies have shown prominent microvilli and other features comparable to those of normal centroacinar cells.[126,131] A few cells with dense-core endocrine granules may also be found. Immunohistochemically, there is reactivity for EMA and low molecular weight keratin. The

trabeculae between the locules may contain numerous Langerhans' islets. These trabeculae may also show calcification, which appears in a radiating pattern roentgenographically.[128] The prominent vascularization that is typical of these tumors can be well appreciated by selective angiography.

The patients are usually elderly, and there is no sex predilection. The disease is either discovered incidentally or manifests as an abdominal mass with local discomfort or pain. Some of the cases occur in the context of von Hippel–Lindau disease. Diabetes may be associated with these lesions if sufficient islet cell tissue is destroyed by the tumor. When located in the head of the pancreas, which is often the case, these tumors may result in gastrointestinal or biliary obstruction.[125a]

Mucinous cystic tumors

The mucinous-type cystic tumors of the pancreas are seen in a younger age group than the preceding type, predominate in women, and are characterized by the formation of large multilocular, or, in rare cases, unilocular cysts lined by tall, mucin-producing cells, often forming papillae (Figs. 15-11 and 15-12). Most are found in the body and tail rather than in the head. Calcification in the wall is a common finding. The underlying stroma is often very cellular, its appearance resembling that of ovarian stroma. The clinical presentation is similar to that of the microcystic adenomas and pancreatic pseudocysts. Aspiration of the fluid can be useful in the differential diagnosis. In the mucinous tumors, tall columnar mucin-producing cells are present, and the fluid will contain higher levels of CEA and lower levels of elastase I than the fluid of pseudocysts.[133]

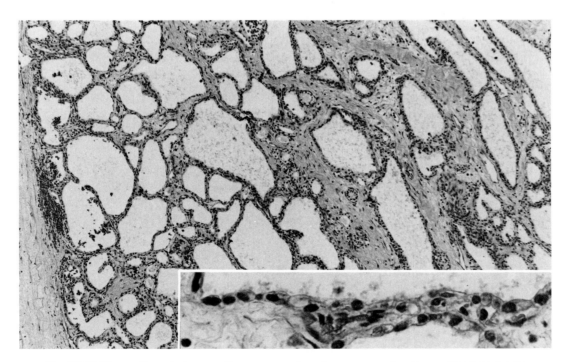

Fig. 15-10 Microcystic cystadenoma. Numerous small cystic spaces are lined by small cuboidal cells with central nucleus and clear cytoplasm, better seen in the **inset.**

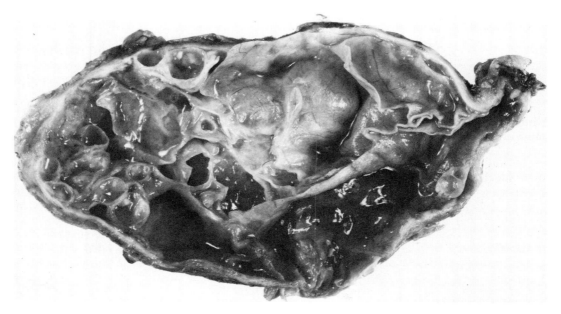

Fig. 15-11 Mucinous cystadenoma. Grossly, tumor contains fewer and larger cavities than microcystic type. These contained a mucous material that was removed before photograph was taken.

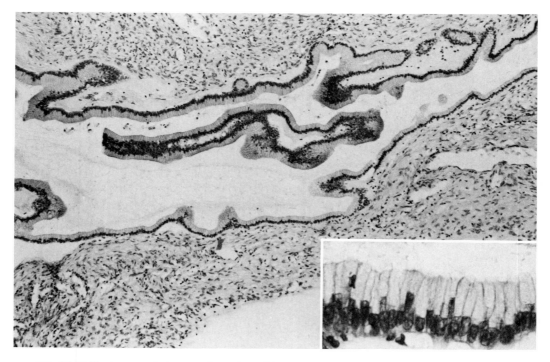

Fig. 15-12 Mucinous cystadenoma. Large branching cystic spaces are lined by tall cylindric cells with basal nuclei and abundant mucin-containing cytoplasm, better seen in the **inset.**

Pancreatic mucinous neoplasms have been divided into a benign (mucinous cystadenoma) and a malignant (mucinous cystadenocarcinoma) category. Actually, if one were to use criteria analogous to those used to assess mucinous tumors of the ovary, these pancreatic tumors could also be divided into benign, borderline, and malignant. The diagnosis of malignancy is based on the presence of invasion of the wall by neoplastic glands or frank anaplasia of the superficial component. The distinction is not always clearcut and requires an extensive sampling of the specimen. Compagno and Oertel[132] regard all of these mucinous cystomas as potentially malignant and recommend total excision (rather than incomplete excision or marsupialization) whenever possible. The evolution of mucinous cystomas is very slow, and metastases, when present, are usually restricted to the abdominal cavity.

In rare cases, these tumors contain a mural nodule with the appearance of a giant cell tumor, a phenomenon analogous to that described in mucinous ovarian neoplasms.

Acinar cell tumors and tumorlike conditions

Acinar cell hyperplasia is a common incidental microscopic finding. On low-power examination, these hyperplastic nodules may be confused with Langerhans' islets.[137] They may exhibit mild atypical changes, and it has been suggested that they might be precursors of acinar cell carcinoma.[139,142]

Acinar cell adenoma is a vanishingly rare lesion, if it exists at all.[144] Some of the cases reported in children blend with the better differentiated forms of pancreatoblastoma.[140]

Acinar cell carcinoma comprises no more than 1% to 2% of all pancreatic cancers.[136] Grossly, it tends to obliterate the architecture of the organ without causing dilatation of the ducts. Rarely, it presents in the form of a multicystic neoplasm (*acinar cell cystadenocarcinoma*) that simulates grossly the appearance of microcystic adenoma.[135,143]

Microscopically, the tumors are made up of nests of cells that in their better differentiated forms closely resemble the appearance of the cells of the normal acini. The cytoplasm is abundant, basophilic, and often distinctly granular (Fig. 15-13).

On ultrastructural examination, numerous zymogen granules are found in the cytoplasm. Immunohistochemically, there is reactivity for lipase, trypsinogen, and chymotrypsinogen.[141]

The main differential diagnosis for the solid form is with islet cell tumors. A point to remember in this regard is that ribbon and festoon formation is not a feature of acinar cell carcinoma.

Several cases have been reported of pancreatic acinar cell carcinoma associated with widespread subcutaneous fat necrosis and arthralgia, as a result of the secretion of lipase by the tumor.[134] It is likely that some of these tumors also secrete amylase. Extrapancreatic neoplasms associated with amylase secretion also have been observed.[138] The prognosis of acinar cell carcinoma is just as poor as that of ductal adenocarcinoma.

Papillary and solid epithelial neoplasm

This distinctive type of low-grade pancreatic malignancy has also been described as papillary-cystic neoplasm and as cystic-solid papillary carcinoma, depending on the proportion of the various components. Most cases are found in

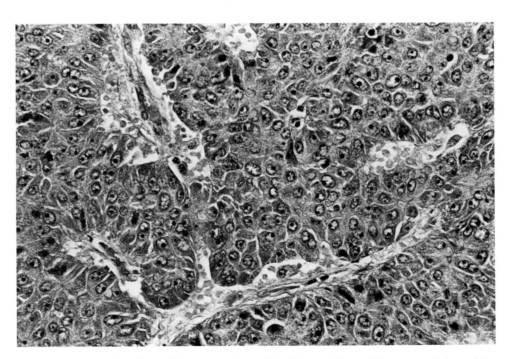

Fig. 15-13 Acinar cell carcinoma. Tumor grows in a solid pattern, and the cells have granular basophilic cytoplasm. Differential diagnosis with islet cell tumors may require special techniques.

young women. Grossly, it is usually large and on cross section contains areas of hemorrhage and necrosis.[145]

Microscopically, it is very cellular and simulates somewhat the appearance of islet cell tumor. Its most distinctive feature is the presence of papillae covered by several layers of epithelial cells. Nuclei are ovoid and folded, with indistinct nucleoli and few mitoses. Hyaline globules and collections of foamy cells may be present.[146,148] The thick fibrovascular core often shows prominent mucinous changes, which is an important diagnostic feature (Fig. 15-14, A). Ultrastructurally, evidence of acinar, ductal, and (sometimes) endocrine cell differentiation has been found.[148] Immunohistochemically, there is reactivity for keratin, desmoplakin, trypsin, chymotrypsin, amylase, and vimentin.[148,149] In addition, focal positivity has been found for neuron-specific enolase,[149,150] and—at least in some studies—for various islet cell hormones, such as insulin and glucagon.[149] These results suggest that papillary and solid epithelial neoplasm is a tumor of primitive pancreatic epithelial cells with predominance of exocrine features, but having the capacity for dual differentiation.[149,151]

The treatment is surgical and the prognosis is excellent, although a few cases resulting in local recurrence and liver metastases have been reported.[147,148]

Infantile pancreatic carcinoma

Infantile pancreatic carcinoma, also known as pancreatoblastoma, is one of the most common forms of pancreatic

neoplasia in childhood.[160] It may attain a large size, extend outside the pancreas, and give rise to hepatic and other distant metastases. Microscopically, it grows in solid nests alternating with well-formed glands, often arranged circumferentially around the nests. The center of the nests may exhibit squamoid features[153,154] (Fig. 15-14, B). Mitoses are relatively rare, and papillae are not formed. The light microscopic appearance is somewhat suggestive of an islet cell tumor or a carcinoid, but electron microscopic examination shows a total absence of secretory granules; instead, features suggestive of acinar cell differentiation have been described.[156] This has been supported by the immunohistochemical demonstration of lipase, trypsinogen, and chymotrypsinogen.[158] Thus pancreatoblastoma could be viewed as a specific type of acinar cell tumor. Alpha-fetoprotein and alpha-1-antitrypsin may be produced by the tumor, in keeping with its primitive nature.[155,159] The prognosis is relatively favorable.[152]

It should be kept in mind that not all pancreatic tumors in childhood are examples of pancreatoblastoma; ductal, ordinary acinar, and islet cell tumors also occur.[157]

Endocrine tumors
General features

Endocrine tumors make up a small fraction of all pancreatic neoplasms. Most occur in adults, although a few have been described in children and even in newborn infants.[163,169]

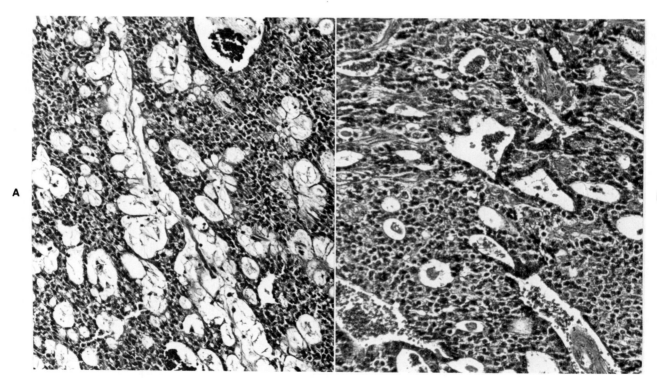

Fig. 15-14 Microscopic appearance of two microscopically similar pancreatic tumors occurring at a young age. **A,** Papillary and solid epithelial neoplasm. Note large expanses of perivascular myxoid degeneration surrounded by solid proliferation of small tumor cells. **B,** Infantile pancreatic carcinoma (pancreatoblastoma). Tumor cells are small and uniform. Pattern of growth is largely solid, but there are several well-formed glands.

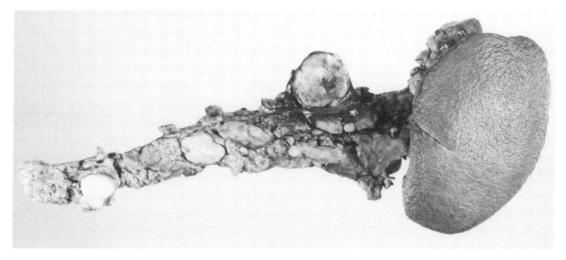

Fig. 15-15 Multiple well-delimited islet cell tumors may be seen in specimen of near-total pancreatec-tomy.

The most common location of islet cell tumors is the body and tail of the organ, correlating with a greater islet concentration in these locations. Grossly, the more cellular tumors have a pinkish cast and may resemble the spleen or a congested lymph node (Fig. 15-15). They do not have a well-defined capsule. Other, presumably longer standing, tumors have a large amount of fibrous tissue and may even contain calcium and bone. A few have a predominantly cystic appearance.[193]

Microscopically, these tumors are usually composed of small, relatively uniform cuboidal cells with centrally located nuclei and acidophilic or amphophilic, finely granular cytoplasm. However, nuclear enlargement and other aberrations are common.

Depending on their pattern of growth, islet cell tumors have been divided into solid, gyriform (with ribbons and festoons), glandular, and nondescript types[173,184,185] (Fig. 15-16). These have been referred to as A, B, C, and D, or as I, II, III, and IV, respectively, and have been related to the various endocrine cell types that may be present. Predominantly gyriform tumors are often of beta or alpha cell type, and glandular tumors are often composed of G or VIP cells; solid tumors, which are the majority, can be of any cell type.

The stroma of pancreatic endocrine tumors is highly vascular. In some cases, an abundant hyaline material separates the tumor cells into scattered nests. Amyloid may be encountered, particularly in insulin-secreting neoplasms,[177,196] and it may have a crystalline configuration.[194] Unusual features of islet cell tumors include mucin production, clear cell changes, oncocytic changes, and psammoma body formation.[174,190,195]

Islet cell tumors may be nonfunctioning, at least at the level of clinical detection.[166,179] Most commonly, they present with an endocrine abnormality resulting from the secretion of one or more hormones.[180] Kahn et al.[178] have shown that many malignant endocrine pancreatic tumors

(but no benign ones) produce chorionic gonadotropin, or its alpha or beta subunits, in conjunction with other hormones.

Study of these tumors with immunocytochemical techniques has shown that multihormonal islet cell tumors are common and that various manifestations of this phenomenon occur: a single tumor with multiple cell types; multiple tumors, each being of a single cell type; and multiple tumors, each of multiple cell types.[162]

The nature of the predominant cell determines the type of clinical syndrome and the name given to the tumor.[180,181] Tumors associated with multihormone production of a type that can be detected clinically or by serum determinations are often malignant.[175] It is important to emphasize at this point that for a proper evaluation of these neoplasms, immunocytochemical and ultrastructural studies are mandatory.

Examination of hematoxylin-eosin sections simply allows the generic diagnosis of islet cell tumor. As previously stated, some correlations can be made between the pattern of growth and the cell type, but this is far from accurate. Traditional special stains for islet cells, including silver techniques, give consistent results in normal tissue but are notoriously unpredictable when applied to neoplasms.[197] Instead, electron microscopy will readily and consistently demonstrate cytoplasmic secretory granules of endocrine type in all but the most undifferentiated members of this group. This will identify the tumor as of endocrine nature and it may also allow the identification of the specific cell type involved (Fig. 15-17). However, the latter is not always the case, because in some tumors the tumor cell granules have a nondescript appearance. This is where immunocytochemistry plays a key role, in view of its high sensitivity and specificity (Figs. 15-18 and 15-19). The markers can be divided into two types: those that stain most or all of the endocrine cells and their tumors, and those specific for the various peptide hormones. The former include neuron-specific enolase, chromogranin, synaptophysin, neurofila-

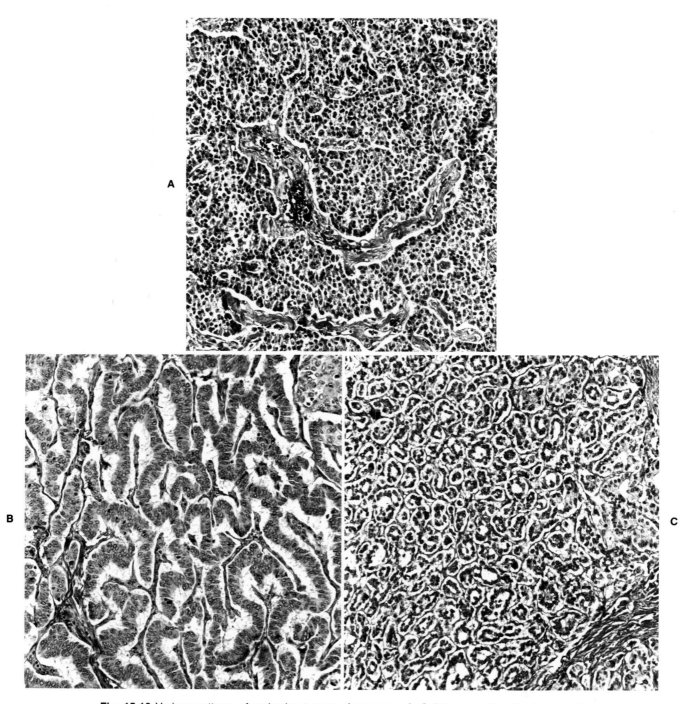

Fig. 15-16 Various patterns of endocrine tumors of pancreas. **A,** Solid pattern. Ill-defined nests of small uniform tumor cells are separated by highly vascularized stroma. There is no evidence of glandular or trabecular differentiation. **B,** Gyriform pattern. Ribbons and festoons of tumor cells are present throughout neoplasm, separated by delicate vascular stroma. **C,** Glandular pattern. Small regular glands showing artifactual retraction from stroma are present throughout. Tumors not fulfilling any of these three patterns are referred to as nondescript.

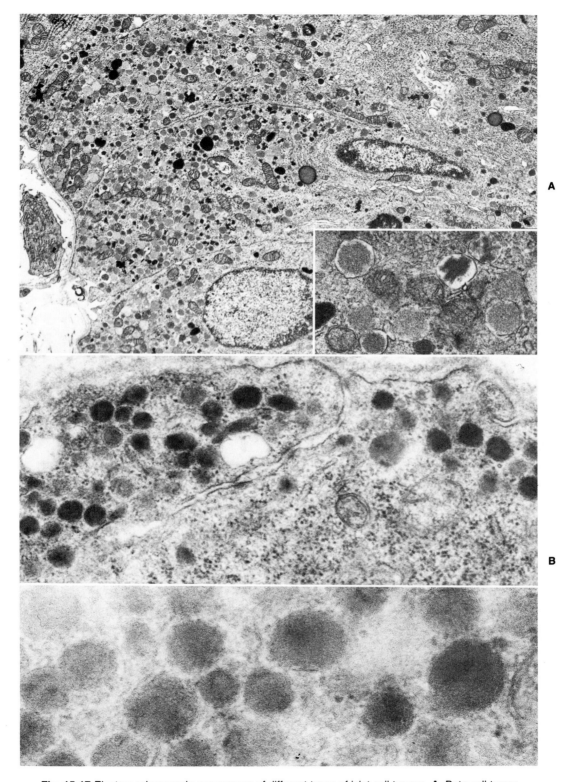

Fig. 15-17 Electron microscopic appearance of different types of islet cell tumors. **A,** Beta cell tumor. Many of granules have irregular or crystalline content. **B,** Alpha cell tumor. Granules are large and have dense peripheral nucleoid. *Continued.*

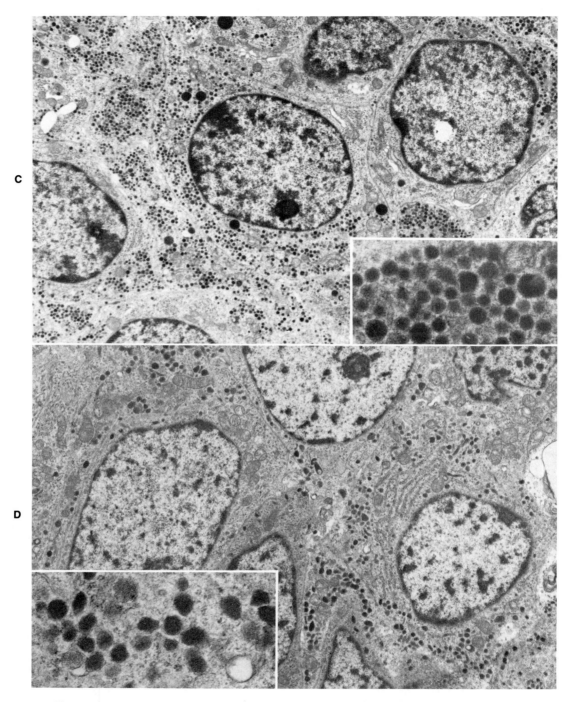

Fig. 15-17, cont'd C, G-cell tumor. Granules are similar to those of VIP-producing tumor and of normal gastrin cells. Most tumors from patients with Zollinger-Ellison syndrome have this appearance. **D,** VIP-producing tumor having larger and more pleomorphic granules. This variety is uncommon in our experience. (Courtesy Dr. M. Greider, St. Louis, MO., and Dr. M.H. McGavran, Houston, TX.)

ments, and opioid peptides.[164,170,182,191] Positivity for chromogranin, which is seen in some tumor types but not in others, seems to correlate with the presence of argyrophilia.[182] Production of chromogranin and other substances by these tumors can result in a corresponding serum level elevation, a feature that is of diagnostic importance.[186,189] Other substances found in many of these tumors are alpha-1-antitrypsin[187] and prealbumin.[167]

The second group of markers has allowed mapping of the endocrine population of the pancreas and correlation with endocrine tumors of this organ.[176,183,192] The endocrine cells recognized in the normal human pancreas are alpha cells (producing glucagon), beta cells (insulin), delta cells (somatostatin), PP cells (pancreatic polypeptide), P cells (of unknown function), and EC cells (5-hydroxytryptamine).

Pancreatic endocrine tumors have been found secreting each of these substances and also gastrin, vasoactive intestinal peptide (VIP), ACTH, ADH, MSH, calcitonin, neurotensin, parathormone, growth hormone, and growth hormone–releasing factor.*

It has been pointed out that the term *islet cell tumor* is properly applied only to tumors composed of cells that are normally present in the pancreatic islets and that a more generic term such as *pancreatic endocrine neoplasm* is therefore preferable.[168] Actually, it is possible that all of these neoplasms arise from primitive multipotential cells located within ducts rather than from the islets themselves.[188]

---

*See references 161, 165, 171, 172, 176, 183, 184, and 192.

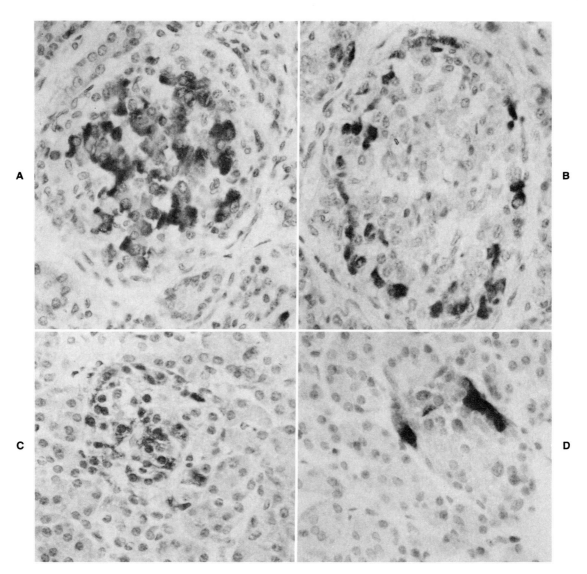

Fig. 15-18 Normal composition of pancreatic islets as shown by immunoperoxidase. **A,** Insulin. **B,** Glucagon. **C,** Somatostatin. **D,** Pancreatic polypeptide.

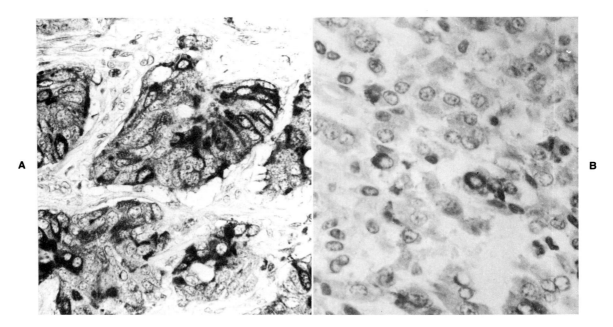

Fig. 15-19 A, Chromogranin staining of pancreatic endocrine tumor. There is strong positivity in nearly all tumor cells. **B,** G-cell tumor of pancreas stained for gastrin. Scattered strong positivity is present.

Specific types

Beta cell tumors (insulinomas) constitute the most common and best known variety of functioning islet cell tumors. The Whipple triad thought to be characteristic of this tumor consists of (1) mental confusion, weakness, fatigue, and convulsions; (2) fasting blood sugar levels below 50 mg%; and (3) relief of symptoms by the administration of glucose.[245] Intravenous tolbutamide tests and determinations of circulating insulin levels are useful tests for the diagnosis of insulinomas.[233] Circulating proinsulin-like material can be detected in the serum.[220] Celiac arteriography has proved extremely useful in the localization of these neoplasms, which may otherwise prove quite elusive at surgical exploration.[201] The reported success rate of angiographic localization is between 60% and 75%.

Over 90% of beta cell tumors are solitary.[227] About 70% of them measure 1.5 cm or less, sometimes as little as 3 or 4 mm. Microscopically, the tumor may grow in a solid or gyriform pattern; glands are almost always absent. Ultrastructurally, dense-core secretory granules are invariably present, but they do not always have the crystalline material that identifies them as being of beta cell type in the normal islets.[242] Immunohistochemically, there is reactivity for insulin, although this is usually of a lesser degree than in the normal beta cells.[229] Beta cell tumors show a lesser degree of reactivity for chromogranin than other islet cell neoplasms.[231]

In children with beta cell tumors, there may be evidence of direct transformation of ductal epithelium into neoplastic islet tissue in the form of nesidioblastosis.[204,210] In some cases of neonatal hypoglycemia, there is diffuse hyperplasia of Langerhans' islets (islet adenomatosis) or nesidioblastosis

without tumor formation.[212,230] Rarely, a similar process is found in adult hypoglycemic patients.[253]

Only 10% of beta cell tumors are malignant if the criteria of infiltration and/or metastases are adhered to. In general, the malignant variety is associated with a shorter history and more pronounced hypoglycemia.[211]

The treatment of beta cell tumors is surgical. If the diagnosis of hyperinsulinism is reasonably certain and surgical exploration fails to reveal a neoplasm, a subtotal pancreatectomy is justified. Of thirty-three patients reported by Laroche et al.[227] in whom this operation was performed, the tumor was found in the resected specimen in fifteen. In about 2% of the cases, insulin-producing islet cell tumors are found outside the pancreas, usually in the duodenal wall.

Extrapancreatic neoplasms may rarely be associated with hypoglycemia that disappears on removal of the tumor. The secretion of an insulin-like hormone has been implicated. Approximately 50% of the lesions have been liver cell carcinomas or mesenchymal tumors, and approximately 53% have been found in the liver or retroperitoneum. Most of them have been extremely large.[246]

Alpha cell tumors (glucagonomas) can be divided into two distinct types. Those associated with the glucagonoma syndrome are usually solitary, large, with a nondescript microscopic pattern, atypical granules ultrastructurally, few cells positive for glucagon immunohistochemically, and high incidence of malignancy[221] (Fig. 15-20). Those unassociated with the glucagonoma syndrome are often multiple, small, have a gyriform pattern of growth, are strongly immunoreactive for glucagon, exhibit typical alpha cell granules ultrastructurally, and are nearly always benign. Argyrophilia can be demonstrated with the Grimelius tech-

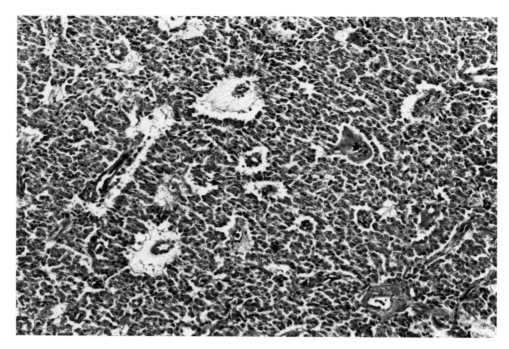

Fig. 15-20 Endocrine tumor of pancreas composed of alpha cells and secreting glucagon (so-called glucagonoma).

nique. The glucagonoma syndrome, seen mainly in adult females, is thought to be the direct or indirect result of the hypersecretion of glucagon.[232,251] Its components are an abnormal glucose tolerance test, normocytic normochromic anemia, a skin rash known as necrolytic migratory erythema, sore red tongue, angular stomatitis, severe weight loss, depression, deep-vein thrombosis, and tendency to develop overwhelming infection. The skin rash involves mainly the legs, perineum, and groin; it starts as erythema, progresses to superficial blisters, and gradually spreads with central clearing.[200] It heals without scarring but with hyperpigmentation in 7 to 14 days. Microscopically, the main features are epidermal necrolysis with liquefaction necrosis of the granular cell layer, and subcorneal clefting or blister formation.[200,226]

G-cell tumors (gastrinomas) lead to the Zollinger-Ellison syndrome as a result of excessive production of gastrin.[225,257,259] The tumors are most often found in the pancreas; in about 23% of the cases they are located in the duodenal wall,[219] and very rarely they occur in the gastric antrum (see Chapter 11; Stomach). This distribution pattern is most peculiar, because it is exactly the opposite of what one would expect to find on the basis of G-cell distribution in the normal tissues. Cases of Zollinger-Ellison syndrome have also been reported in association with tumors of the ovary, mesentery, and intra-abdominal (usually peripancreatic) lymph nodes.[199,248,256] It is not clear whether the latter arise in ectopic islet tissue in the lymph nodes or whether they represent metastases from undetected small primary neoplasms.

The Zollinger-Ellison syndrome is characterized by gastric hyperacidity with gastric, duodenal, or jejunal ulcers.[207,215] Diarrhea is seen in one third of the patients as a result of the excessive gastric secretion. Although the original reports emphasized the atypical location of the ulcers, this has not been substantiated in subsequent series. Radioimmunoassay of gastrin is the most useful test to confirm the diagnosis.[234]

When the G-cell tumor is unaccompanied by other endocrine abnormalities, it is nearly always solitary and often malignant; when it is seen as a component of MEA type I, it is often multiple and less likely to be malignant.[198,254,258]

Some authors claim to obtain positivity in the majority of these tumors with the Grimelius argyrophilic stain,[209] but others have found it very difficult to duplicate these results. Gastrin production by the neoplastic cells is readily demonstrable by immunoperoxidase. The immunocytochemical and electron-microscopic features of the neoplastic cells correlate better not with any of the known normal human islet cells but rather with those of the gastrin-producing G-cells of the gastric antrum.[205,209,218,219]

The non-neoplastic pancreas in patients with G-cell tumors often shows large islets and nesidioblastosis. Immunohistochemically, there is an hyperplasia of all islet cell types.[228]

The classic therapy for G-cell tumor associated with the Zollinger-Ellison syndrome has been the removal of the target organ through the performance of a total gastrectomy. In some instances, this is said to have led to a regression of the tumor.[236] This therapy is still advocated for patients whose tumors are not amenable to resection (undetectable, multicentric, or metastatic) and in whom medical therapy with H_2-receptor blocking agents is unsuccessful.[202,257] In cases of solitary nonmetastasizing tumors, total excision is the treatment of choice.[213,222]

VIP-producing tumors (vipomas) are associated with a diarrheogenic or cholera-like syndrome in the absence of gastric hypersecretion.[206,216,247] This is caused by the secretion of vasoactive intestinal peptide (VIP).[235,244]

The morphologic, histochemical, and fine-structural features of these tumors are indistinguishable from those of G-cell tumors[219]; however, immunocytochemical techniques will show absence of gastrin production by the tumor cells. In addition to VIP, many of these tumors also contain PP, calcitonin, and the alpha chain of HCG.[203,238]

Delta cell tumors (somatostatinomas) seem generally nonfunctioning at the clinical level because of the fact that somatostatin is an inhibitory hormone.[243,252] However, as a result of these inhibitory properties, patients may present with diabetes, cholecystolithiasis, steatorrhea, indigestion, hypochlorydria, and occasionally anemia.[217,241] Some delta cell tumors are located in the duodenal wall instead of in the pancreas. Psammoma bodies are commonly found among the tumor cells.

PP cell tumors are rare if one restricts the definition of the term to neoplasms composed exclusively or predominantly of this cell type.[237,249] On the other hand, a secondary and minor component of PP cells is found in a high proportion of islet cell neoplasms of other cell types, including their metastases.[223,250] Sometimes, the non-neoplastic islets of pancreases with islet cell tumor show a prominent hyperplasia of PP cells.[228]

Carcinoid tumors analogous in every way to those more commonly seen in the gastrointestinal tract can occur in the pancreas.[238a,239,255] They probably arise from Kultschitsky's cells, which are normally present in this organ in connection with the exocrine ducts. In contrast with all other types of pancreatic endocrine neoplasms, they exhibit strong argentaffinity. Some have been associated with the carcinoid syndrome, sometimes in association with hyperinsulinism.[214,240]

Small cell carcinoma also occurs in the pancreas. It is morphologically similar to its more common pulmonary counterpart and is sometimes associated with ectopic ACTH secretion[208] or hypercalcemia.[224]

Malignancy

The correlation between morphologic features as seen in routinely stained sections of pancreatic endocrine tumors and their clinical malignancy is poor. Nuclear pleomorphism is a particularly unreliable criterion, and mitotic activity is only slightly better. Features that correlate with a greater metastatic potential are definite stromal invasion, tumor emboli in pancreatic vessels, and a glandular or solid rather than gyriform pattern of growth. The latter features depend upon the tumor cell type, which is perhaps the best predictor of behavior. Beta cell tumors are malignant in about 10% of the cases, whereas almost all the other types (including nonfunctioning tumors) are malignant in the large majority of cases.

Islet cell carcinomas are slow-growing tumors. In the first reported case of nonfunctioning islet cell tumor, liver metastases were first detected 5 years after the original oper-

ation, and the patient lived another 5 years following this discovery.[261] Metastases are restricted to peripancreatic lymph nodes and liver in the majority of the cases. Resection is justified even in incurable cases because of the long-term symptomatic relief that can be achieved.[260] Specific chemotherapeutic agents, such as streptozocin, have resulted in long-term palliation in several instances.[260]

Multiple endocrine adenomatosis

Multiple endocrine adenomatosis (MEA) syndromes are inherited in an autosomal dominant fashion and are characterized by hyperplastic or neoplastic proliferation of more than one endocrine gland.[274] Three distinct types have been described, although they sometimes seem to overlap.[269]

MEA type I (Werner's syndrome)[263] is characterized by involvement of the pituitary gland (adenomas), pancreas, and parathyroid glands (chief cell hyperplasia). The pancreatic pathology is represented by G-cell tumors in 50% of the cases, beta cell tumors in 30%, VIP cell tumors in 12%, and alpha cell tumors in less than 5%.[271]

Thus the main clinical manifestations are primary hyperparathyroidism, the Zollinger-Ellison syndrome, and acromegaly or hypopituitarism. Other abnormalities, although less constant, involve the adrenal cortex and thyroid gland (in the form of nodular hyperplasia or adenomas), carcinoid tumors of various locations but mainly of foregut derivatives (lung, thymus, and gastrointestinal tract), multiple soft tissue lipomas, and giant rugal hypertrophy of the stomach (Menetrier's disease). We have seen several cases of MEA type I with thymic carcinoid tumors[273] and two associated with Menetrier's disease and multiple carcinoid tumors of the gastric fundus.[262]

MEA type II (Sipple's syndrome; also known as type IIA)[276] is characterized by C-cell hyperplasia and medullary carcinoma of the thyroid gland (often multiple and/or bilateral), pheochromocytoma of the adrenal glands (often bilateral and accompanied by adrenal medullary hyperplasia), and parathyroid chief cell hyperplasia. Thus the overlap between MEA types I and II is represented by the parathyroid involvement, which is morphologically and functionally similar in both disorders.

MEA type III (Gorlin's syndrome; also known as type IIB) comprises medullary carcinoma of the thyroid, adrenal pheochromocytoma, so-called mucosal neuromas (resulting in hypertrophied corneal nerves, bumpy lips, and an enlarged nodular tongue), skeletal abnormalities, and a marfanoid habitus.[265,267,270] Mucosal neuromas (which Carney et al.[266] prefer to designate as mucosal ganglioneuromas or ganglioneuromatosis) represent the most constant feature of this syndrome. In many cases, there is extensive ganglioneuromatosis of the digestive tract, which may result in constipation, diarrhea, and even the production of megacolon.[264] Sometimes the gastrointestinal manifestations represent the initial manifestation of the disease. Some patients with MEA type III also have polyposis coli.[272] Gorlin et al.[267] have emphasized, on the basis of careful clinical and genetic studies, that MEA type III is not merely a variant of MEA type II but rather a well-defined nosologic entity. Parathyroid disease is distinctly unusual in MEA type III.

Other combinations have also been found, suggesting the

existence of additional types or varieties of multiple endocrine adenomatosis. These include the co-existence of islet cell tumors and paraganglioma, paraganglioma and thyroid papillary carcinoma, and others.[268,275,277]

Lymphoid tumors and tumorlike conditions

Most *malignant lymphomas* involving the pancreas originate in peripancreatic or retroperitoneal lymph nodes. Cases have been reported of pancreatic *plasmacytoma*[279] and *plasma cell granuloma.*[278]

Mesenchymal and other primary tumors

Benign mesenchymal tumors of pancreas, all extremely rare, include lymphangioma (not to be confused with microcystic cystadenoma), hemangioma, and neurilemoma.[282,284]

Primary *sarcomas* of the pancreas are also rare, most malignant tumors of sarcomatous appearance involving this organ being anaplastic carcinomas or pancreatic extensions of retroperitoneal sarcomas. Primary liposarcomas, leiomyosarcomas, and malignant fibrous histiocytomas of pancreas have been described.[281,283]

A care of primary *choriocarcinoma* of the pancreas has been reported.[280]

Metastatic tumors

Most tumors metastatic to the pancreas involve the organ by direct extension. Blood-borne metastases are sometimes found at autopsy in carcinomatosis, but a pancreatic metastasis will only exceptionally manifest itself clinically.[285]

Periampullary region
AMPULLARY CARCINOMA AND VILLOUS ADENOMA

Ampullary carcinoma is a malignant epithelial tumor centered in the ampulla of Vater. Although originally defined on topographic grounds, the term ampullary carcinoma also carries a histogenetic significance, in the sense that it implies origin from the intestinal-type mucosa of the ampulla or immediate adjacent duodenal mucosa, often on the basis of a pre-existing villous adenoma or villoglandular polyp.[286,289,293] It should, therefore, be distinguished from carcinomas of pancreas, terminal third of common bile duct, and other portions of duodenal mucosa with secondary involvement of the ampulla. Such a distinction may not be possible in advanced cases, in which the only diagnosis that can be rendered is that of "carcinoma of the pancreatobiliary region."

Grossly, ampullary carcinoma usually bulges into the duodenal lumen. On duodenostomy, the duodenal mucosa appears stretched but otherwise normal if the entire tumor is confined to the ampullary lumen (intra-ampullary carcinoma). In other instances, the tumor presents mainly as a circumferential growth around the ampulla (periampullary carcinoma) (Fig. 15-21). In still others, a combined intra- and periampullary pattern of growth exists (mixed carci-

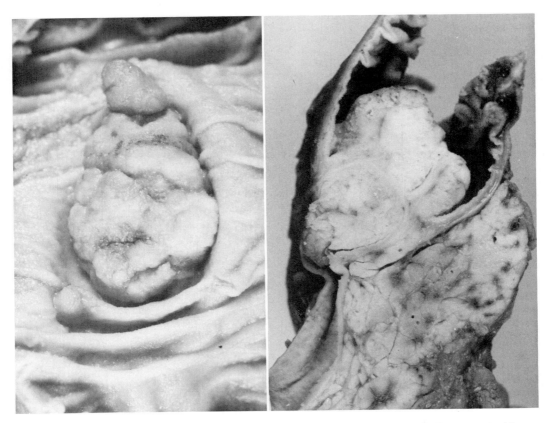

Fig. 15-21 Papillary adenocarcinoma of periampullary area in 67-year-old woman. Tumor resulted in obstructive jaundice and partial duodenal obstruction.

noma).[287] Those tumors with a prominent component of residual villous adenoma present as soft, sessile, papillary masses projecting into the duodenal lumen, which may not be felt through the unopened duodenum because of their softness.

Microscopically, nearly all ampullary carcinomas are adenocarcinomas, often poorly differentiated. Many of them have a superficial papillary component with the appearance of villous adenoma (Fig. 15-22). In the past, by the time exploration was carried out, an invasive carcinoma was almost invariably present at the base. As a result, the whole lesion was regarded as malignant, the superficial portion being interpreted as a better differentiated component. With the increased use of endoscopic procedures for the early detection of these lesions, it has become obvious that a papillary lesion can exist in this area in the absence of stromal invasion.[291] This lesion has morphologic and biologic characteristics akin to those of colorectal *villous adenoma* and less commonly of a villoglandular polyp, including a high propensity for malignant transformation. This tendency is of particularly ominous significance in the ampulla because of difficulties in detection in the period preceding the malignant change.

Ampullary carcinoma may invade by direct extension the adjacent duodenal mucosa, duodenal wall, pancreas, and common bile duct. Perineurial invasion may also be present.

Regional lymph node metastases are found in 35% to 50% of the cases; in general, they are restricted to one adjacent periampullary group.[288.292]

As already stated, the differential diagnosis of ampullary carcinoma includes several other types of carcinoma of this region. Carcinoma of the terminal third of the *common bile duct* shows great longitudinal thickening of this structure and a granular appearance of the mucosa; it may infiltrate deeply and extend upward beneath the bile duct mucosa and downward into the ampullary region. Microscopically, it is usually a well-differentiated adenocarcinoma formed by small glands, with or without a papillary component, and often accompanied by an intense desmoplastic reaction (see Chapter 14). *Nonampullary duodenal carcinomas* do not differ microscopically a great deal from those that originate in the ampulla; like the latter, they often arise on the basis of a lesion that has the features of villous adenoma (see Chapter 11, Small bowel).[290]

The diagnosis of ampullary carcinoma may be made by cytologic examination (see p. 761), endoscopic biopsy, or transduodenal biopsy. The latter is often examined as a frozen section procedure. The biopsy should not be too superficial, or else areas of malignant change may be missed.

The treatment of choice of ampullary carcinoma is the Whipple's procedure. Transduodenal resection may be ad-

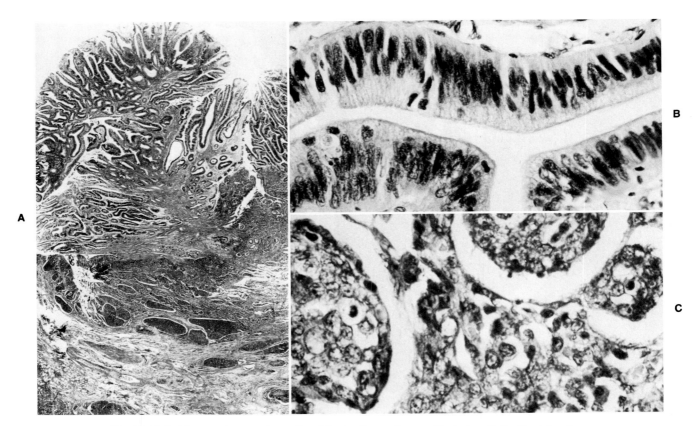

Fig. 15-22 A, Adenocarcinoma of ampulla arising in villous adenoma-like lesion. **B,** Section taken from surface to tumor illustrated in **A,** showing features comparable to those of villous adenoma. **C,** Sections from deepest portion of tumor shown in **A,** illustrating obvious adenocarcinoma.

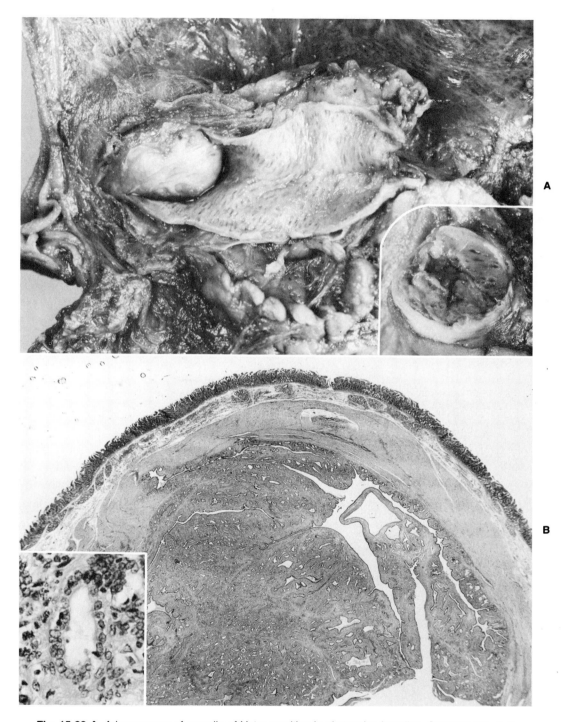

Fig. 15-23 A, Adenomyoma of ampulla of Vater resulting in obstructive jaundice. Common bile duct shows marked dilatation. **Inset,** Cross section of lesion demonstrating its well-encapsulated nature. It could have been easily enucleated. Instead, Whipple's procedure was carried out under clinical impression of malignant neoplasm. **B,** Photomicrograph of same specimen. Glands and stroma intermingle in manner reminiscent of breast fibroadenoma. **Inset** demonstrates benign appearance of glands.

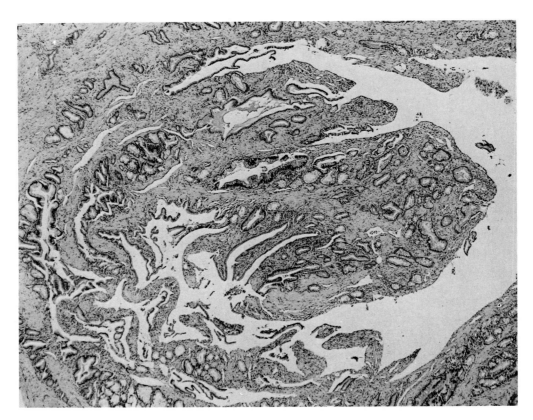

Fig. 15-24 Inflammatory polyp of ampulla producing almost complete obstructive jaundice. Removal resulted in complete relief of symptoms.

equate for the noninvasive papillary or villoglandular lesions, but not when an invasive component has developed.

The prognosis of ampullary carcinoma is significantly better than for pancreatic carcinoma and bile duct carcinoma, hence the importance of the separation. The overall 5-year survival rate is about 25% and twice as good for the cases with negative lymph nodes.[292] It is also directly related to the local extent of the disease, as determined grossly and microscopically.[287,291a,293] In one series, patients with tumors restricted to within the muscle of Oddi (defined as stage I lesions) had a 5-year survival rate of 85%.[293]

The prognosis of ampullary villous adenoma or villoglandular polyp without malignant transformation is excellent if complete excision has been carried out.

OTHER LESIONS

The diagnosis of *fibrosis* of the papilla of Vater is sometimes made in patients with right upper abdominal pain in whom a "pinpoint ampullary opening" is found at surgery.[294,296] More often than not, the microscopic sections show no significant abnormalities. In our experience, clearcut inflammatory or fibrotic changes in the papilla of Vater have always been associated with chronic gallbladder or pancreatic disease.

Benign tumors of the ampulla are extremely rare. A few instances of *adenoma* have been described.[295,299] We have

seen an *adenomyoma* (Fig. 15-23) and a few *inflammatory polyps*[298] (Fig. 15-24) causing partial biliary obstruction; all of these lesions can be treated by local resection. *Gangliocytic paraganglioma* is discussed in Chapter 11 (section on small bowel). *Carcinoid tumors* can also occur in this location.[297]

REFERENCES
Pancreas
ANNULAR PANCREAS

1 Kiernan PD, ReMine SG, Kiernan PC, ReMine WH: Annular pancreas. Mayo Clinic experience from 1957 to 1976 with review of the literature. Arch Surg **115:**46-50, 1980.

2 Sessa F, Fiocca R, Tenti P, Solcia E, Tavani E, Pliteri S: Pancreatic polypeptide rich tissue in the annular pancreas. A distinctive feature of ventral primordium derivatives. Virchows Arch [Pathol Anat] **399:**227-232, 1983.

3 Tendler MJ, Ciuti A: The surgery of annular pancreas. A summary of sixty patients operated upon. Surgery **38:**298-310, 1955.

HETEROTOPIC PANCREAS

4 Busard JM, Walters W: Heterotopic pancreatic tissue. Arch Surg **60:**674-682, 1950.

5 de Castro Barbosa JJ, Dockerty MB, Waugh JM: Pancreatic heterotopia. Surg Gynecol Obstet **82:**527-542, 1946.

6 Dolan RV, ReMine WH, Dockerty MB: The fate of heterotopic pancreatic tissue. A study of 212 cases. Arch Surg **109:**762-765, 1974.

7 Hara M, Tsutsumi Y: Immunohistochemical studies of endocrine cells in heterotopic pancreas. Virchows Arch [Pathol Anat] **408:**385-394, 1986.

PANCREATITIS
Acute pancreatitis

8 Acosta JM, Ledesma CL: Gallstone migration as a cause of acute pancreatitis. N Engl J Med **290:**484-488, 1974.

9 Adams JT, Libertino JA, Schwartz SI: Significance of an elevated serum amylase. Surgery **63:**877-884, 1968.

10 Corfield AP, Cooper MJ, Williamson RCN: Acute pancreatitis. A lethal disease of increasing incidence. Gut **26:**724-729, 1985.

11 Cubilla AL, Fitzgerald PJ: Morphological lesions associated with human primary invasive nonendocrine pancreas cancer. Cancer Res **36:**2690-2698, 1976.

12 Doubilet H: Pancreatic reflux deliberately produced. Surg Gynecol Obstet **84:**710-715, 1947.

13 Dragstedt LR, Haymond HE, Ellis JC: Pathogenesis of acute pancreatitis (acute pancreatic necrosis). Arch Surg **28:**232-291, 1934.

14 Dressel TD, Goodale RL Jr, Arneson MA, Borner JW: Pancreatitis as a complication of anticholinesterase insecticide intoxication. Ann Surg **189:**199-204, 1979.

15 Dressel TD, Goodale RL Jr, Hunninghake DB, Borner JW: Sensitivity of the canine pancreatic intraductal pressure to subclinical reduction in cholinesterase activity. Ann Surg **190:**6-12, 1979.

16 Howard J, Jones R: The anatomy of the pancreatic ducts. The etiology of acute pancreatitis. Am J Med Sci **214:**617-622, 1947.

17 Kukora JS: Extensive colonic necrosis complicating acute pancreatitis. Surgery **97:**290-294, 1985.

18 Longnecker DS: Pathology and pathogenesis of diseases of the pancreas. Am J Pathol **107:**103-121, 1982.

19 Martin JK, VanHeerden JA, Bess MA: Surgical management of acute pancreatitis. Mayo Clin Proc **59:**259-267, 1984.

20 McCutcheon AD: A fresh approach to the pathogenesis of pancreatitis. Gut **9:**296-310, 1968.

21 Opie EL: The etiology of acute hemorrhagic pancreatitis. Bull Hopkins Hosp **12:**182-188, 1901.

22 Paloyan D (ed): Pancreatitis. New Hyde Park, N.Y., 1983, Medical Examination Publishing.

23 Phat VN, Guerrieri MT, Alexandre JH, Camilleri JP: Early histological changes in acute necrotizing hemorrhagic pancreatitis. A retrospective pathological study of 20 total pancreatectomy specimens. Pathol Res Pract **178:**273-279, 1984.

24 Rich AR, Duff GL: Experimental and pathologic studies on the pathogenesis of acute hemorrhagic pancreatitis. Bull Hopkins Hosp **58:**212-260, 1936.

25 Steer ML, Meldolesi J: The cell biology of experimental pancreatitis. N Engl J Med **316:**144-150, 1987.

26 White TT, Morgan A, Hopton D: Postoperative pancreatitis. A study of seventy cases. Am J Surg **120:**132-137, 1970.

Chronic pancreatitis

27 Bartow S, Mukai K, Rosai J: Pseudoneoplastic proliferation of endocrine cells in pancreatic fibrosis. Cancer **47:**2627-2633, 1981.

28 Brown M, Smiley RK: Chronic pancreatitis with steatorrhea following mumps with acute pancreatitis. Am J Dig Dis **17:**280-282, 1950.

29 Comfort MW, Steinberg AG: Pedigree of a family with hereditary chronic relapsing pancreatitis. Gastroenterology **21:**54-63, 1952.

30 Edmondson HA, Bullock WK, Mehl JW: Chronic pancreatitis and lithiasis. Am J Pathol **26:**37-55, 1950.

31 Klöppel G, Bommer G, Commandeur G, Heitz P: The endocrine pancreas in chronic pancreatitis. Virchows Arch [Pathol Anat] **377:**157-174, 1978.

32 Mixter CG Jr, Keynes M, Cope O: Further experience with pancreatitis as a diagnostic clue to hyperparathyroidism. N Engl J Med **266:**265-272, 1962.

33 Morrow CE, Cohen JI, Sutherland DER, Najarian JS: Chronic pancreatitis. Long-term surgical results of pancreatic duct drainage, pancreatic resection, and near-total pancreatectomy and islet autotransplantation. Surgery **96:**608-616, 1984.

34 Mullin GT, Caperton EM Jr, Crespin SR, Williams RC Jr: Arthritis and skin lesions resembling erythema nodosum in pancreatic disease. Ann Intern Med **68:**75-87, 1968.

35 Niederau C, Grendell JH: Diagnosis of chronic pancreatitis. Gastroenterology **88:**1973-1995, 1985.

36 Sarles H: Chronic calcifying pancreatitis—chronic alcoholic pancreatitis. Gastroenterology **66:**604-616, 1974.

37 Sarner M, Cotton PB: Classification of pancreatitis. Gut **25:**756-759, 1984.

38 Stambler JB, Klibaner MI, Bliss CM, LaMont JT: Tuberculous abscess of the pancreas. Gastroenterology **83:**922-925, 1982.

39 Stobbe KC, ReMine WH, Baggenstoss AH: Pancreatic lithiasis. Surg Gynecol Obstet **131:**1090-1099, 1970.

40 Stolte M, Schwabe H, Prestele H: Relationship between diseases of the pancreas and hyperplasia of Brunner's glands. Virchows Arch [Pathol Anat] **394:**75-87, 1981.

41 Strum WB, Spiro HM: Chronic pancreatitis. Ann Intern Med **74:**264-277, 1971.

42 Volkholz H, Stolte M, Becker V: Epithelial dysplasias in chronic pancreatitis. Virchows Arch [Pathol Anat] **396:**331-349, 1982.

Abscess

43 Warshaw AL: Pancreatic abscesses. Current concepts. N Engl J Med **287:**1234-1236, 1972.

Pseudocysts

44 Goulet RJ, Goodman J, Schaffer R, Dallemand S, Andersen DK: Multiple pancreatic pseudocyst disease. Ann Surg **199:**6-13, 1984.

45 Greenstein A, DeMaio E, Nabsetch DC: Acute hemorrhage associated with pancreatic pseudocysts. Surgery **69:**56-62, 1971.

TRUE CYSTS

46 Truong LD, Rangdaeng S, Jordan PH Jr: Lymphoepithelial cyst of the pancreas. Am J Surg Pathol **11:**899-903, 1987.

TUMORS
Ductal adenocarcinoma
General features

47 Bowlby LS: Pancreatic adenocarcinoma in an adolescent male with Peutz-Jeghers syndrome. Hum Pathol **17:**97-99, 1986.

48 Chung YS, Ho JJL, Kim YS, Tanaka H, Nakata B, Hiura A, Motoyoshi H, Satake K, Umeyama K: The detection of human pancreatic cancer–associated antigen in the serum of cancer patients. Cancer **60:**1636-1643, 1987.

49 Cubilla AL, Fitzgerald PJ: Cancer of the exocrine pancreas. The pathologic aspects, Cancer **35:**2-18, 1985.

50 DelFavero G, Fabris C, Plebani M, Panucci A, Piccoli A, Perobelli L, Pedrazzoli S, Baccaglini U, Burlina A, Naccarato R: CA 19-9 and carcinoembryonic antigen in pancreatic cancer diagnosis. Cancer **57:**1576-1579, 1986.

51 DiMagno EP, Shorter RG, Taylor WF, Go VLW: Relationships between pancreaticobiliary ductal anatomy and pancreatic ductal and parenchymal histology. Cancer **49:**361-368, 1982.

52 Ehrenthal D, Haeger L, Griffin T, Compton C: Familial pancreatic adenocarcinoma in three generations. A case report and a review of the literature. Cancer **59:**1661-1664, 1987.

53 Fitzgerald PJ, Fortner JG, Watson RC, Schwartz MK, Sherlock P, Benua RS, Cubilla AL, Schottenfeld D, Miller D, Winawer SJ, Lightdale CJ, Leidner SD, Nisselbaum JS, Menendez-Botet CJ, Poleski MH: The value of diagnostic aids in detecting pancreas cancer. Cancer **41:**868-879, 1978.

53a Hayakawa T, Kondo T, Shibata T, Hamano H, Kitagawa M, Sakai Y, Ono H: Sensitive serum markers for detecting pancreatic cancer. Cancer **61:**1827-1831, 1988.

54 Lafler CJ, Hinerman DL: A morphologic study of pancreatic carcinoma with reference to multiple thrombi. Cancer **14:**944-952, 1961.

55 Levison DA: Carcinoma of the pancreas. J Pathol **129:**203-223, 1979.

56 Longnecker DS: Pathology and pathogenesis of diseases of the pancreas. Am J Pathol **107:**103-121, 1982.

57 MacMahon B: Risk factors for cancer of the pancreas. Cancer **50:**2676-2680, 1982.

58 Morohoshi T, Held G, Klöppel G: Exocrine pancreatic tumours and their histological classification. A study based on 167 autopsy and 97 surgical cases. Histopathology **7:**645-661, 1983.

59 Safi F, Berger HG, Bittner R, Büchler M, Krautzberger W: CA 19-9 and pancreatic adenocarcinoma. Cancer **57:**779-783, 1986.

Location and gross features

60 Cubilla AL, Fitzgerald PJ: Morphological patterns of primary nonendocrine human pancreas carcinoma. Cancer Res **35:**2234-2248, 1975.

Microscopic features

61 Bartow S, Mukai K, Rosai J: Pseudoneoplastic proliferation of endocrine cells in pancreatic fibrosis. Cancer **47:**2627-2633, 1981.

62 Bätge B, Bosslet K, Sedlacek HH, Kern HF, Klöppel G: Monoclonal antibodies against CEA-related components discriminate between pancreatic duct type carcinomas and nonneoplastic duct lesions as well as nonduct type neoplasias. Virchows Arch [Pathol Anat] **408:**361-374, 1986.

63 Chen J, Baithun SI: Morphological study of 391 cases of exocrine pancreatic

tumours with special reference to the classification of exocrine pancreatic carcinoma. J Pathol **146:**17-29, 1985.

64 Chen J, Baithun SI, Ramsay MA: Histogenesis of pancreatic carcinomas. A study based on 248 cases. J Pathol **146:**65-76, 1985.

65 Costa J: Benign epithelial inclusions in pancreatic nerves. Am J Clin Pathol **67:**306-307, 1977.

66 Cubilla AL, Fitzgerald PJ: Morphological lesions associated with human primary invasive nonendocrine pancreas cancer. Cancer Res **36:**2690-2698, 1976.

67 Edis AJ, Kiernan PD, Taylor WF: Attempted curative resection of ductal carcinoma of the pancreas. Review of Mayo Clinic experience, 1951-1975. Mayo Clin Proc **55:**531-540, 1980.

68 Eusebi V, Capella C, Bondi A, Sessa F, Vezzadini P, Mancini AM: Endocrine-paracrine cells in pancreatic exocrine carcinomas. Histopathology **5:**599-613, 1981.

69 Gambill EE: Pancreatitis associated with pancreatic carcinoma. A study of 26 cases. Mayo Clin Proc **46:**173-177, 1971.

70 Haglund C, Roberts PJ, Nordling S, Ekblom P: Expression of laminin in pancreatic neoplasms and in chronic pancreatitis. Am J Surg Pathol **8:**669-676, 1984.

71 Hyland C, Kheir SM, Kashlan NB: An evaluation of pancreatic biopsy with the Vim-Silverman needle. Am J Surg Pathol **5:**179-191, 1981.

72 Ichihara T, Nagura H, Nakao A, Sakamoto J, Watanabe T, Takagi H: Immunohistochemical localization of CA 19-9 and CEA in pancreatic carcinoma and associated diseases. Cancer **61:**324-333, 1988.

73 Kodama T, Mori W: Morphological behavior of carcinoma of the pancreas. II. Argyrophil cells and Langerhans' islets in the carcinomatous tissues. Acta Pathol Jpn **33:**483-493, 1983.

74 Kodama T, Mori W: Morphological lesions of the pancreatic ducts. Significance of pyloric gland metaplasia in carcinogenesis of exocrine and endocrine pancreas. Acta Pathol Jpn **33:**645-660, 1983.

75 Kozuka S, Sassa R, Taki T, Masamoto K, Nagasawa S, Saga S, Hasegawa K, Takeuchi M: Relation of pancreatic duct hyperplasia to carcinoma. Cancer **43:**1418-1428, 1979.

76 Pour PM, Sayed S, Sayed G: Hyperplastic, preneoplastic and neoplastic lesions found in 83 human pancreases. Am J Clin Pathol **77:**137-152, 1982.

77 Reid JD, Yuh S-L, Petrelli M, Jaffe R: Ductuloinsular tumors of the pancreas. A light, electron microscopic and immunohistochemical study. Cancer **49:**908-915, 1982.

78 Schron DS, Mendelsohn G: Pancreatic carcinoma with duct, endocrine, and acinar differentiation. A histologic, immunocytochemical, and ultrastructural study. Cancer **54:**1766-1770, 1984.

79 Tryka AF, Brooks JR: Histopathology in the evaluation of total pancreatectomy for ductal carcinoma. Ann Surg **190:**373-381, 1979.

80 Tsutsumi Y, Nagura H, Watanabe K: Immunohistochemical observations of carcinoembryonic antigen (CEA) and CEA-related substances in normal and neoplastic pancreas. Am J Clin Pathol **82:**535-542, 1984.

Other microscopic types

81 Brayko CM, Doll DC: Squamous cell carcinoma of the pancreas associated with hypercalcemia. Gastroenterology **83:**1297-1299, 1982.

82 Chejfec G, Rieker WJ, Jablokow VR, Gould VE: Pseudomyxoma peritonei associated with colloid carcinoma of the pancreas. Gastroenterology **90:**202-205, 1986.

83 Cubilla AL, Fitzgerald PJ: Morphological patterns of primary nonendocrine human pancreas carcinoma. Cancer Res **35:**2234-2248, 1975.

84 Huntrakoon M: Oncocytic carcinoma of the pancreas. Cancer **51:**332-336, 1983.

85 Ishikawa O, Matsui Y, Aoki I, Iwanaga T, Terasawa T, Wada A: Adenosquamous carcinoma of the pancreas. A clinicopathologic study and report of three cases. Cancer **46:**1192-1196, 1980.

85a Kanai N, Nagaki S, Tanaka T: Clear cell carcinoma of the pancreas. Acta Pathol Jpn **37:**1521-1526, 1987.

Metastases

86 Cubilla AL, Fortner J, Fitzgerald PJ: Lymph node involvement in carcinoma of the head of the pancreas area. Cancer **41:**880-887, 1978.

87 Lee Y-TN, Tatter D: Carcinoma of the pancreas and periampullary structures. Pattern of metastasis at autopsy. Arch Pathol Lab Med **108:**584-587, 1984.

88 Nagai H, Kuroda A, Morioka Y: Lymphatic and local spread of T1 and T2 pancreatic cancer. A study of autopsy material. Ann Surg **204:**65-71, 1986.

89 Tsuchiya R, Oribe T, Noda T: Size of the tumor and other factors influencing prognosis of carcinoma of the head of the pancreas. Am J Gastroenterol **80:**459-462, 1985.

Cytology

90 Goodale RL, Gajl-Peczalska K, Dressel T, Samuelson J: Cytologic studies for the diagnosis of pancreatic cancer. Cancer **47:**1652-1655, 1981.

91 Hajdu EO, Kumari-Subaiya S, Phillips G: Ultrasonically guided percutaneous aspiration biopsy of the pancreas. Semin Diagn Pathol **3:**166-175, 1986.

92 Kline TS, Joshi LP, Goldstein F: Preoperative diagnosis of pancreatic malignancy by the cytologic examination of duodenal secretions. Am J Clin Pathol **70:**851-854, 1978.

93 Nguyen G-k: Percutaneous fine-needle aspiration cytology of the pancreas. Pathol Annu **20**(Pt 1):221-238, 1985.

94 Nieburgs HE, Dreiling DA, Rubio C, Reisman H: The morphology of cells in duodenal-drainage smears. Histologic origin and pathologic significance. Am J Dig Dis **7:**489-505, 1962.

95 Smith EH, Bartrum RJ Jr, Chang YC, Orsi CJ, Lokich J, Abbruzzese A, Dantono J: Percutaneous aspiration biopsy of the pancreas under ultrasonic guidance. N Engl J Med **292:**825-828, 1975.

96 Smithies A, Hatfield ARW, Brown BE: The cytodiagnostic aspects of pure pancreatic juice obtained at the time of endoscopic retrograde cholangiopancreatography (ERCP). Acta Cytol [Baltimore] **21:**191-195, 1977.

97 Tao L-C, Ho C-S, McLoughlin MJ, McHattie J: Percutaneous fine needle aspiration biopsy of the pancreas. Cytodiagnosis of pancreatic carcinoma. Acta Cytol [Baltimore] **22:**215-220, 1978.

98 Tylen U, Arnesjo B, Lindberg LG, Lunderquist A, Akerman M: Percutaneous biopsy of carcinoma of the pancreas guided by angiography. Surg Gynecol Obstet **142:**737-739, 1976.

Exploration and frozen section

99 Beazley RM: Needle biopsy diagnosis of pancreatic cancer. Cancer **47:**1685-1687, 1981.

100 Cote, J, Dockerty MB, Priestly JT: An evaluation of pancreatic biopsy with the Vim-Silverman needle. Arch Surg **79:**588-596, 1959.

101 Forsgren L, Orell S: Aspiration cytology in carcinoma of the pancreas. Surgery **73:**38-42, 1973.

102 Hyland C, Kheir SM, Kashlan MB: Frozen section diagnosis of pancreatic carcinoma. A prospective study of 64 biopsies. Am J Surg Pathol **5:**179-191, 1981.

103 Loquvam GS, Russell WO: Accessory pancreatic ducts of the major duodenal papilla. Am J Clin Pathol **20:**305-313, 1950.

104 Spjut HJ, Ramos AJ: An evaluation of biopsy-frozen section of the ampullary region and pancreas. A report of 68 consecutive patients. Ann Surg **146:**923-930, 1957.

105 Weiland LH: Frozen section diagnosis in tumors of the pancreas. Semin Diagn Pathol **1:**54-58, 1984.

Treatment

106 Fortner JG: Surgical principles for pancreatic cancer. Regional total and subtotal pancreatectomy. Cancer **47:**1712-1718, 1981.

107 Holyoke ED: New surgical approaches to pancreatic cancer. Cancer **47:**1719-1723, 1981.

108 Longmire WP Jr, Traverso LW: The Whipple procedure and other standard operative approaches to pancreatic cancer. Cancer **47:**1706-1711, 1981.

109 Moertel CG, Frytak S, Hahn RF, O'Connell MJ, Reitemeier RJ, Rubin J, Schutt AJ, Weiland LH, Childs DS, Holbrook MA, Lavin PT, Livstone E, Spiro H, Knowlton A, Kalser M, Barkin J, Lessner H, Mann-Kaplan R, Ramming K, Douglas HO Jr, Thomas P, Nave H, Bateman J, Lokich J, Brooks J, Chaffey J, Corson JM, Zamcheck N, Novak JW: Therapy of locally unresectable pancreatic carcinoma. A randomized comparison of high dose (6000 rad) radiation alone, moderate dose radiation (4000 rad + 5-fluorouracil), and high dose radiation + 5-fluorouracil. The Gastrointestinal Tumor Study Group. Cancer **48:**1705-1710, 1981.

110 Newton WT: Mortality and morbidity associated with resection of pancreaticoduodenal cancers. Am Surg **27:**74-79, 1961.

111 Nishimura A, Nakano M, Otsu H, Nakano K, Iida K, Sakata S, Iwabuchi K, Maruyama K, Kihara M, Okamura T, Todoroki T, Iwaski Y: Intraoperative radiotherapy for advanced carcinoma of the pancreas. Cancer **54:**2375-2384, 1984.

112 Tepper J, Nardi G, Suit H: Carcinoma of the pancreas. Review of MGH experience from 1963 to 1973. Analysis of surgical failure and implications for radiation therapy. Cancer **37:**1519-1524, 1976.

Prognosis

113 Baylor SM, Berg JW: Cross-classification and survival characteristics of 5,000 cases of cancer of the pancreas. J Surg Oncol **5:**335-358, 1973.

114 Gudjonsson B: Cancer of the pancreas. 50 years of surgery. Cancer **60**:2284-2303, 1987.

115 Klöppel G, Lingenthal G, Von Bülow M, Kern HF: Histological and fine structural features of pancreatic ductal adenocarcinomas in relation to growth and prognosis. Studies in xenografted tumours and clinico-histopathological correlation in a series of 75 cases. Histopathology **9**:841-856, 1985.

116 Pollard HM, Anderson WAD, Brooks FP, Cohn I Jr, Copeland MM, Connelly RR, Fortner JG, Kissane JM, Lemon HM, Palmer PES, Thomas LB, Webster PD III, Carter S: Staging of cancer of the pancreas. Cancer **47**:1631-1637, 1981.

117 Tepper J, Nardi G, Suit H: Carcinoma of the pancreas. Review of MGH experience from 1963 to 1973. Analysis of surgical failure and implications for radiation therapy. Cancer **37**:1519-1524, 1976.

118 Tsuchiya R, Oribe T, Noda T: Size of the tumor and other factors influencing prognosis of carcinoma of the head of the pancreas. Am J Gastroenterol **80**:459-462, 1985.

Anaplastic carcinoma

119 Alguacil-Garcia A, Weiland LH: The histologic spectrum, prognosis, and histogenesis of the sarcomatoid carcinoma of the pancreas. Cancer **39**:1181-1189, 1977.

120 Berendt RC, Shnitka TK, Wiens E, Manickavel V, Jewell LD: The osteoclast-type giant cell tumor of the pancreas. Arch Pathol Lab Med **111**:43-48, 1987.

121 Posen JA: Giant cell tumor of the pancreas of the osteoclastic type associated with a mucous secreting cystadenocarcinoma. Hum Pathol **12**:944-947, 1981.

122 Rosai J: Carcinoma of pancreas simulating giant cell tumor of bone. Electron microscopic evidence of its acinar cell origin. Cancer **22**:333-344, 1968.

123 Sommers SC, Meissner WA: Unusual carcinomas of the pancreas. Arch Pathol **58**:101-111, 1954.

124 Trepeta RW, Mathur B, Lagin S, LiVolsi VA: Giant cell tumor ("osteoclastoma") of the pancreas. A tumor of epithelial origin. Cancer **48**:2022-2028, 1981.

125 Tschang T, Garza-Garza R, Kissane JM: Pleomorphic carcinoma of the pancreas. An analysis of 15 cases. Cancer **39**:2114-2126, 1977.

Microcystic cystadenoma

125a Alpert LC, Truong LD, Bossart MI, Spjut HJ: Microcystic adenoma (serous cystadenoma) of the pancreas. A study of 14 cases with immunohistochemical and electron-microscopic correlation. Am J Surg Pathol **12**:251-263, 1988.

126 Bogomoletz WV, Adnet JJ, Widgren S, Stavrou M, McLaughlin JE: Cystadenoma of the pancreas. A histological, histochemical and ultrastructural study of seven cases. Histopathology **4**:309-320, 1980.

127 Compagno J, Oertel JE: Microcystic adenomas of the pancreas (glycogen-rich cystadenomas). A clinicopathologic study of 34 cases. Am J Clin Pathol **69**:289-298, 1978.

128 Haukohl RS, Melamed A: Cystadenoma of pancreas. Am J Roentgenol Radium Ther Nucl Med **63**:234-245, 1950.

129 Hodgkinson DJ, ReMine WH, Weiland LH: Pancreatic cystadenoma. A clinicopathologic study of 45 cases. Arch Surg **113**:512-519, 1978.

130 Nyongo A, Huntrakoon M: Microcystic adenoma of the pancreas with myoepithelial cells. Am J Clin Pathol **84**:114-120, 1985.

131 Shorten SD, Hart WR, Petras RE: Microcystic adenomas (serous cystadenomas) of pancreas. A clinicopathologic investigation of eight cases with immunohistochemical and ultrastructural studies. Am J Surg Pathol **10**:365-372, 1986.

Mucinous cystic tumors

132 Compagno J, Oertel JE: Mucinous cystic neoplasms of the pancreas with overt and latent malignancy (cystadenocarcinoma and cystadenoma). A clinicopathologic study of 41 cases. Am J Clin Pathol **69**:573-580, 1978.

133 Tatsuta M, Iishi H, Ichii M, Noguchi S, Yamamoto R, Yamamura H, Okuda S: Values of carcinoembryonic antigen, elastase 1, and carbohydrate antigen determinant in aspirated pancreatic cystic fluid in the diagnosis of cysts of the pancreas. Cancer **57**:1836-1839, 1986.

Acinar cell tumors and tumorlike conditions

134 Burns WA, Matthews MJ, Hamosh M, vander Weider G, Blum R, Johnson FB: Lipase-secreting acinar cell carcinoma of the pancreas with polyarthropathy. A light and electron microscopic, histochemical, and biochemical study. Cancer **33**:1002-1009, 1974.

135 Cantrell BB, Cubilla AL, Erlandson RA, Fortner J, Fitzgerald PJ: Acinar cell cystadenocarcinoma of human pancreas. Cancer **47**:410-416, 1981.

136 Cubilla AL, Fitzgerald PJ: Morphological patterns of primary nonendocrine human pancreas carcinoma. Cancer Res **35**:2234-2248, 1975.

137 Glenner GG, Mallory GK: The cystadenoma and related non-functional tumors of the pancreas. Pathogenesis, classification and significance. Cancer **9**:980-996, 1956.

138 Gomi K, Kameya T, Tsumuraya M, Shimosato Y, Zeze F, Abe K, Yoneyama T: Ultrastructural, histochemical, and biochemical studies of two cases with amylase, ACTH, and β-MSH producing tumor. Cancer **38**:1645-1654, 1976.

139 Kodama T, Mori W: Atypical acinar cell nodules of the human pancreas. Acta Pathol Jpn **33**:701-714, 1983.

140 Lack EE, Cassady JR, Levey R, Vawter GF: Tumors of the exocrine pancreas in children and adolescents. A clinical and pathologic study of eight cases. Am J Surg Pathol **7**:319-327, 1983.

141 Morohoshi T, Kanda M, Horie A, Chott A, Dreyer T, Klöppel G, Heitz PU: Immunocytochemical markers of uncommon pancreatic tumors. Acinar cell carcinoma, pancreatoblastoma, and solid cystic (papillary-cystic) tumor. Cancer **59**:739-747, 1987.

142 Shinozuka H, Lee RE, Dunn JL, Longnecker DS: Multiple atypical acinar cell nodules of the pancreas. Hum Pathol **11**:389-391, 1980.

143 Stamm B, Burger H, Hollinger A: Acinar cell cystadenocarcinoma of the pancreas. Cancer **60**:2542-2547, 1987.

144 Webb JN: Acinar cell neoplasms of the exocrine pancreas. J Clin Pathol **30**:103-112, 1977.

Papillary and solid epithelial neoplasm

145 Boor PJ, Swanson MR: Papillary-cystic neoplasm of the pancreas. Am J Surg Pathol **3**:69-75, 1979.

146 Klöppel G, Morohoshi T, John HD, Oehmichen W, Opitz K, Angelkort A, Lietz H, Rückert K: Solid and cystic acinar cell tumour of the pancreas. A tumour in young women with favourable prognosis. Virchows Arch [Pathol Anat] **392**:171-183, 1981.

147 Kuo T-t, Su I-j, Chien C-h: Solid and papillary neoplasm of the pancreas. Report of three cases from Taiwan. Cancer **54**:1469-1474, 1984.

148 Lieber MR, Lack EE, Roberts JR Jr, Merino MJ, Patterson K, Restrepo C, Solomon D, Chandra R, Triche TJ: Solid and papillary epithelial neoplasm of the pancreas. An ultrastructural and immunocytochemical study of six cases. Am J Surg Pathol **11**:85-93, 1987.

149 Miettinen M, Partanen S, Fräki O, Kivilaakso E: Papillary cystic tumor of the pancreas. An analysis of cellular differentiation by electron microscopy and immunohistochemistry. Am J Surg Pathol **11**:885-865, 1987.

150 Morohoshi T, Kanda M, Horie A, Chott A, Dreyer T, Klöppel G, Heitz PU: Immunocytochemical markers of uncommon pancreatic tumors. Acinar cell carcinoma, pancreatoblastoma, and solid cystic (papillary-cystic) tumor. Cancer **59**:739-747, 1987.

151 Morrison DM, Jewell LD, McCaughey WTE, Danyluk J, Shnitka TK, Manickavel V: Papillary cystic tumor of the pancreas. Arch Pathol Lab Med **108**:723-727, 1984.

Infantile pancreatic carcinoma

152 Buchino JJ, Castello FM, Nagaraj HS: Pancreatoblastoma. A histochemical and ultrastructural analysis. Cancer **53**:963-969, 1984.

153 Frable WJ, Still WJS, Kay S: Carcinoma of the pancreas, infantile type. A light and electron microscopic study. Cancer **27**:667-673, 1971.

154 Horie A, Yano Y, Kotoo Y, Miwa A: Morphogenesis of pancreatoblastoma, infantile carcinoma of the pancreas. Report of two cases. Cancer **39**:247-254, 1977.

155 Iseki M, Suzuki T, Koizumi Y, Hirose M, Laskin WB, Nakazawa S, Ohaki Y: Alpha-fetoprotein–producing pancreatoblastoma. A case report. Cancer **57**:1833-1835, 1986.

156 Kakudo K, Sakurai M, Miyaji T, Ikeda Y, Satani M, Manabe H: Pancreatic carcinoma in infancy. An electron microscopic study. Acta Pathol Jpn **26**:719-726, 1976.

157 Lack EE, Cassady JR, Levey R, Vawter GF: Tumors of the exocrine pancreas in children and adolescents. A clinical and pathologic study of eight cases. Am J Surg Pathol **7**:319-327, 1983.

158 Morohoshi T, Kanda M, Horie A, Chott A, Dreyer T, Klöppel G, Heitz PU: Immunocytochemical markers of uncommon pancreatic tumors. Acinar cell carcinoma, pancreatoblastoma, and solid cystic (papillary-cystic) tumor. Cancer **59**:739-747, 1987.

159 Ohaki Y, Misugi K, Fukuda J, Okudaira M, Hirose M: Immunohistochemical study of pancreatoblastoma. Acta Pathol Jpn **37**:1581-1590, 1987.

160 Taxy JB: Adenocarcinoma of the pancreas in childhood. Report of a case and a review of the English language literature. Cancer **37**:1508-1518, 1976.

Endocrine tumors
General features

161 Berger G, Trouillas J, Bloch B, Sassolas G, Berger F, Partensky C, Chayvialle J-A, Brazeau P, Claustrat B, Lesbros F, Girod C: Multihormonal carcinoid tumor of the pancreas. Secreting growth hormone–releasing factor as a cause of acromegaly. Cancer 54:2097-2108, 1984.

162 Bordi C, De Vita O, Pilato FP, Carfagna G, D'Adda T, Missale G, Peracchia A: Multiple islet cell tumors with predominance of glucagon-producing cells and ulcer disease. Am J Clin Pathol 88:153-161, 1987.

163 Bordi C, Ravazzola M, Pollak A, Lubec G, Orci L: Neonatal islet cell adenoma. A distinct type of islet cell tumor? Diabetes Care 5:122-125, 1982.

164 Bostwick DG, Null WE, Holmes D, Weber E, Barchas JD, Bensch KG: Expression of opioid peptides in tumors. N Engl J Med 317:1439-1443, 1987.

165 Bostwick DG, Quan R, Hoffman AR, Webber RJ, Chang JK, Bensch KG: Growth-hormone–releasing factor immunoreactivity in human endocrine tumors. Am J Pathol 117:167-170, 1984.

166 Broughan TA, Leslie JD, Soto JM, Hermann RE: Pancreatic islet cell tumors. Surgery 99:671-678, 1986.

167 Bussolati G, Papotti M, Sapino A: Binding of antibodies to human prealbumin to intestinal and bronchial carcinoids and to pancreatic endocrine tumours. Virchows Arch [Cell Pathol] (In press.)

168 Capella C, Solcia E, Frigerio B, Buffa R, Usellini L, Fontana P: The endocrine cells of the pancreas and related tumours. Ultrastructural study and classification. Virchows Arch [Pathol Anat] 373:327-352, 1977.

169 Carney CN: Congenital insulinoma (nesidioblastoma). Ultrastructural evidence for histogenesis from pancreatic ductal epithelium. Arch Pathol Lab Med 100:352-356, 1976.

170 Chejfec G, Falkmer S, Grimelius L, Jacobsson B, Rodensjö M, Wiedenmann B, Franke WW, Lee I, Gould VE: Synaptophysin. A new marker for pancreatic neuroendocrine tumors. Am J Surg Pathol 11:241-247, 1987.

171 Clark ES, Carney JA: Pancreatic islet cell tumor associated with Cushing's syndrome. Am J Surg Pathol 8:917-924, 1984.

172 Dayal Y, Lin HD, Tallberg K, Reichlin S, DeLellis RA, Wolfe HJ: Immunocytochemical demonstration of growth hormone–releasing factor in gastrointestinal and pancreatic endocrine tumors. Am J Clin Pathol 85:13-20, 1986.

173 Greider MH, Rosai J, McGuigan JE: The human pancreatic islet cells and their tumors. II. Ulcerogenic and diarrheogenic tumors. Cancer 33:1423-1443, 1974.

174 Guarda LA, Silva EG, Ordóñez NG, Mackay B, Ibanez ML: Clear cell islet cell tumor. Am J Clin Pathol 79:512-517, 1983.

175 Hammar S, Sale G: Multiple hormone producing islet cell carcinomas of the pancreas. A morphological and biochemical investigation. Hum Pathol 6:349-362, 1975.

176 Heitz PU, Kasper M, Polak JM, Klöppel G: Pancreatic endocrine tumors. Immunocytochemical analysis of 125 tumors. Hum Pathol 13:263-271, 1982.

177 Heitz PU, Steiner H, Halter F: Multihormonal, amyloid-producing tumor of the islets of Langerhans in a twelve-year-old boy. Clinical, morphological and biochemical data and review of the literature. Virchows Arch [Pathol Anat] 353:312-324, 1971.

178 Kahn CR, Rosen SW, Weintraub BD, Fajans SS, Gorden P: Ectopic production of chorionic gonadotropin and its sub-units by islet cell tumors. N Engl J Med 297:565-569, 1977.

179 Kent RB III, Van Heerden JA, Weiland LH: Nonfunctioning islet cell tumors. Ann Surg 193:185-190, 1981.

180 Larsson LI: Endocrine pancreatic tumors. Hum Pathol 9:401-416, 1978.

181 Larsson LI, Grimelius L, Hakanson R, Rehfeld JF, Stadil F, Holst J, Angervall L, Sundler F: Mixed endocrine pancreatic tumors producing several peptide hormones. Am J Pathol 79:271-284, 1975.

182 Lloyd RV, Mervak T, Schmidt K, Warner TFCS, Wilson BS: Immunohistochemical detection of chromogranin and neuron-specific enolase in pancreatic endocrine neoplasms. Am J Surg Pathol 8:607-614, 1984.

183 Mukai K: Functional pathology of pancreatic islets. Immunocytochemical exploration. Pathol Annu 18(Pt 2):87-107, 1983.

184 Mukai K, Grotting JC, Greider MH, Rosai J: Retrospective study of 77 pancreatic endocrine tumors using the immunoperoxidase method. Am J Surg Pathol 6:387-399, 1982.

185 Nieuwenhuijzen Kruseman AC, Knijnenburg G, Brutel de la Riviere G, Bosman FT: Morphology and immunohistochemically-defined endocrine function of pancreatic islet cell tumours. Histopathology 2:389-399, 1978.

186 O'Connor DT, Deftos LJ: Secretion of chromogranin A by peptide-producing endocrine neoplasms. N Engl J Med 314:1145-1151, 1986.

187 Ordóñez NG, Manning JT, Hanssen G: Alpha-1-antitrypsin in islet cell tumors of the pancreas. Am J Clin Pathol 80:277-282, 1983.

188 Pour P: Islet cells as a component of pancreatic ductal neoplasms. I. Experimental study. Ductular cells, including islet cell precursors, as primary progenitor cells of tumors. Am J Pathol 90:295-316, 1978.

189 Prinz RA, Bermes EW Jr, Kimmel JR, Marangos PJ: Serum markers for pancreatic islet cell and intestinal carcinoid tumors. A comparison of neuron-specific enolase β-human chorionic gonadotropin and pancreatic polypeptide. Surgery 94:1019-1023, 1983.

190 Radi MJ, Fenoglio-Preiser CM, Chiffelle T: Functioning oncocytic islet-cell carcinoma. Report of a case with electron-microscopic and immunohistochemical confirmation. Am J Surg Pathol 9:517-524, 1985.

191 Simpson S, Vinik AI, Marangos PJ, Lloyd RV: Immunohistochemical localization of neuron-specific enolase in gastroenteropancreatic neuroendocrine tumors. Correlation with tissue and serum levels of neuron-specific enolase. Cancer 54:1364-1369, 1984.

192 Solcia E, Capella C, Buffa R, Usellini L, Fiocca R, Sessa F, Tortora O: The contribution of immunohistochemistry to the diagnosis of neuroendocrine tumors. Semin Diagn Pathol 1:285-296, 1984.

193 Thompson NW, Eckhauser FE, Vinik AI, Lloyd RV, Fiddian-Green RG, Strodel WE: Cystic neuroendocrine neoplasms of the pancreas and liver. Ann Surg 199:158-164, 1985.

194 Tischler AS, Compagno J: Crystal-like deposits of amyloid in pancreatic islet cell tumors. Arch Pathol Lab Med 103:247-251, 1979.

195 Tomita T, Bhatia P, Gourley W: Mucin producing islet cell adenoma. Hum Pathol 12:850-853, 1981.

196 Westermark P, Grimelius L, Polak JM, Larsson LT, van Noorden S, Wilander E, Pearse AGE: Amyloid in polypeptide hormone-producing tumors. Lab Invest 37:212-215, 1977.

197 Woodtli W, Hedinger C: Histologic characteristics of insulinomas and gastrinomas. Value of argyrophilia, metachromasia, immunohistology, and electron microscopy for the identification of gastrointestinal and pancreatic endocrine cells and their tumors. Virchows Arch [Pathol Anat] 371:331-350, 1976.

Specific types

198 Ballard HS, Frame B, Hartsock RJ: Familial multiple endocrine adenoma–peptic ulcer complex. Medicine [Baltimore] 43:481-516, 1964.

199 Bhagavan BS, Slavin RE, Goldberg J, Rao RN: Ectopic gastrinoma and Zollinger-Ellison syndrome. Hum Pathol 17:584-592, 1986.

200 Binnick AN, Spencer SK, Dennison WL, Horton ES: Glucagonoma syndrome. Report of two cases and literature review. Arch Dermatol 113:749-754, 1977.

201 Boden G: Insulinoma and glucagonoma. Semin Oncol 14:253-262, 1987.

202 Bonfils S, Landor JH, Mignon M, Hervoir P: Results of surgical management of 92 consecutive patients with Zollinger-Ellison syndrome. Ann Surg 194:692-697, 1981.

203 Capella C, Polak JM, Buffa R, Tapia FJ, Heitz P, Usellini L, Bloom SR, Solcia E: Morphologic patterns and diagnostic criteria of VIP-producing endocrine tumors. A histologic, histochemical, ultrastructural, and biochemical study of 32 cases. Cancer 52:1860-1874, 1983.

204 Carney CN: Congenital insulinoma (nesidioblastoma). Ultrastructural evidence for histogenesis from pancreatic ductal epithelium. Arch Pathol Lab Med 100:352-356, 1976.

205 Cavallero C, Solcia E, Sampietro R: Cytology of islet tumours and hyperplasias associated with the Zollinger-Ellison syndrome. Gut 8:172-177, 1967.

206 Cerda JJ, Raffensberger EC, Rawnsley HM: Cholera-like syndrome and pancreatic islet cell tumors. Med Clin North Am 54:567-575, 1970.

207 Christlieb AR, Schuster MM: Zollinger-Ellison syndrome. A clinical appraisal based on a review of the literature. Arch Intern Med 114:381-388, 1964.

208 Corrin B, Gilby ED, Jones NF, Patrick J: Oat cell carcinoma of the pancreas with ectopic ACTH secretion. Cancer 31:1523-1527, 1973.

209 Creutzfeldt W, Arnold R, Creutzfeldt C, Track NS: Pathomorphologic, biochemical, and diagnostic aspects of gastrinomas (Zollinger-Ellison syndrome). Hum Pathol 6:47-76, 1975.

210 Dahms BB, Lippe BM, Dakake C, Fonkalsrud EW, Mirra JM: The occurrence in a neonate of a pancreatic adenoma with nesidioblastosis in the tumor. Am J Clin Pathol 65:462-466, 1976.

211 Danforth DN Jr, Gorden P, Brennan MF: Metastatic insulin-secreting carcinoma of the pancreas. Clinical course and the role of surgery. Surgery 96:1027-1037, 1984.

212 Davidson DC, Blackwood MJ, Fox EG: Neonatal hypoglycemia with congenital malformation of the pancreatic islets. Arch Dis Child 49:151-154, 1974.

213 Deveney CW, Deveney KE, Stark D, Moss A, Stein S, Way LW: Resection of gastrinomas. Ann Surg 198:546-553, 1983.

214 Dollinger MR, Ratner LH, Shamoian CA, Blackbourne BD: Carcinoid syndrome associated with pancreatic tumors. Arch Intern Med 120:575-580, 1967.

215 Ellison EH, Wilson SD: The Zollinger-Ellison syndrome updated. Surg Clin North Am **47**:1115-1124, 1967.

216 Field M, Chang EB: Pancreatic cholera. N Engl J Med **309**:1513-1515, 1983.

217 Freisen SR: Tumors of the endocrine pancreas. N Engl J Med **306**:580-590, 1982.

218 Greider MU, McGuigan JE: Electron microscopic identification of the gastrin cell of the human antral mucosa by means of immunocytochemistry. Gastroenterology **63**:572-583, 1972.

219 Greider MH, Rosai J, McGuigan JE: The human pancreatic islet cells and their tumors. II. Ulcerogenic and diarrheogenic tumors. Cancer **33**:1423-1443, 1974.

220 Gutman RA, Lazarus NR, Penhos JC, Fajans S, Recant L: Circulating proinsulin-like material in patients with functioning insulinomas. N Engl J Med **284**:1003-1008, 1971.

221 Hamid QA, Bishop AE, Sikri KL, Varndell IM, Bloom SR, Polak JM: Immunocytochemical characterization of 10 pancreatic tumours, associated with the glucagonoma syndrome, using antibodies to separate regions of the proglucagon molecule and other neuroendocrine markers. Histopathology **10**:119-133, 1986.

222 Harmon JW, Norton JA, Collin MJ, Krudy AG, Shawker TH, Doppman JL, D'Avis J, Jensen RT: Removal of gastrinomas for control of Zollinger-Ellison syndrome. Ann Surg **200**:396-404, 1984.

223 Heitz P, Polak JM, Bloom SR, Adrian TE, Pearse AGE: Cellular origin of human pancreatic polypeptide (HPP) in endocrine tumours of the pancreas. Virchows Arch [Cell Pathol] **21**:259-265, 1976.

224 Hobbs RD, Stewart AF, Ravin ND, Carter D: Hypercalcemia in small cell carcinoma of the pancreas. Cancer **53**:1552-1554, 1984.

225 Isenberg JI, Walsh JH, Grossman MI: Zollinger-Ellison syndrome. Gastroenterology **65**:140-165, 1973.

226 Kheir SM, Omura EF, Grizzle WE, Herrera GA, Lee I: Histologic variation in the skin lesions of the glucagonoma syndrome. Am J Surg Pathol **10**:445-453, 1986.

227 Laroche GP, Ferris DO, Priestley JT, Scholz DA, Dockerty MB: Hyperinsulinism. Surgical results and management of occult functioning islet cell tumor. Review of 154 cases. Arch Surg **96**:763-771, 1968.

228 Larsson L: Two distinct types of islet abnormalities associated with endocrine pancreatic tumours. Virchows Arch [Pathol Anat] **376**:209-219, 1977.

229 Liu T-h, Tseng H-c, Zhu Y, Zhong S-x, Chen J, Cui Q-c: Insulinoma. An immunocytochemical and morphologic analysis of 95 cases. Cancer **56**:1420-1429, 1985.

230 Lloyd RV, Caceres V, Warner TFCS, Gilbert EF: Islet cell adenomatosis. A report of two cases and review of the literature. Arch Pathol Lab Med **105**:198-202, 1981.

231 Lloyd RV, Mervak T, Schmidt K, Warner TFCS, Wilson BS: Immunohistochemical detection of chromogranin and neuron-specific enolase in pancreatic endocrine neoplasms. Am J Surg Pathol **8**:607-614, 1984.

232 Mallinson CM, Bloom SR, Warin AP, Salmon PR, Cox B: A glucagonoma syndrome. Lancet **2**:1-5, 1974.

233 Marks V: Diagnosis of insulinoma. Gut **12**:835-843, 1971.

234 McGuigan JE, Trudeau WL: Immunochemical measurement of elevated levels of gastrin in the serum of patients with pancreatic tumors of the Zollinger-Ellison variety. N Engl J Med **278**:1308-1313, 1968.

235 Mekhjian HS, O'Dorisio TM: VIPoma syndrome. Semin Oncol **14**:282-291, 1987.

236 Morowitz DA, Levine AE: Malignant Zollinger-Ellison syndrome. Remission of primary and metastatic pancreatic tumor after gastrectomy. Report of a case and review of the literature. Am J Gastroenterol **81**:471-473, 1986.

237 Nobin A, Berg M, Ericsson M, Ingemansson S, Olsson E, Sundler F: Pancreatic polypeptide-producing tumors. Report on two cases. Cancer **53**:2688-2691, 1984.

238 Ooi A, Kameya T, Tsumuraya M, Yamaguchi K, Abe K, Shimosato Y, Yanaihara N: Pancreatic endocrine tumours associated with WDHA syndrome. An immunohistochemical and electron microscopic study. Virchows Arch [Pathol Anat] **405**:311-323, 1985.

238a Ordóñez NG, Manning JT Jr, Raymond AK: Argentaffin endocrine carcinoma (carcinoid) of the pancreas with concomitant breast metastasis. An immunohistochemical and electron microscopic study. Hum Pathol **16**:746-751, 1985.

239 Patchefsky AS, Gordon G, Harrer WV, Hoch WS: Carcinoid tumor of the pancreas. Ultrastructural observations of a lymph note metastasis and comparison with bronchial carcinoid. Cancer **33**:1349-1354, 1974.

240 Patchefsky AS, Solit R, Phillips LD, Craddock M, Harrer WV, Cohn HE, Kowlessar OD: Hydroxyindole-producing tumors of the pancreas. Carcinoid-islet cell tumor and oat cell carcinoma. Ann Intern Med **77**:53-61, 1972.

241 Pipeleers D, Couturier E, Gepts W, Reynders J, Somers G: Five cases of somatostatinoma. Clinical heterogeneity and diagnostic usefulness of basal and tolbutamide-induced hypersomatostatinemia. J Clin Endocrinol Metab **56**:1236-1242, 1983.

242 Rawlinson DG, Christiansen RO: Light and electron microscopic observations on a congenital insulinoma. Cancer **32**:1470-1476, 1973.

243 Reichlin S: Somatostatin. N Engl J Med **309**:1495-1563, 1983.

244 Said SI, Faloona GR: Elevated plasma and tissue levels of vasoactive intestinal polypeptide in the watery-diarrhea syndrome due to pancreatic, bronchogenic and other tumors. N Engl J Med **293**:155-160, 1975.

245 Shetty MR, Boghossian HM, Duffell D, Freel R, Gonzales JC: Tumor-induced hypoglycemia. A result of ectopic insulin production. Cancer **49**:1920-1923, 1982.

246 Silverstein MN: Tumor hypoglycemia. Cancer **23**:142-144, 1969.

247 Stoker DJ, Wynn V: Pancreatic islet cell tumour with watery diarrhea and hypokalaemia. Gut **11**:911-920, 1970.

248 Thompson NW, Vinik AI, Eckhauser FE, Strodel WE: Extrapancreatic gastrinomas. Surgery **98**:1113-1120, 1985.

249 Tomita T, Friesen SR, Kimmel JR, Doull V, Pollock HG: Pancreatic polypeptide-secreting islet-cell tumors. Am J Pathol **113**:134-142, 1983.

250 Tomita T, Kimmel JR, Friesen SR, Doull V, Pollock HG: Pancreatic polypeptide in islet cell tumors. Morphologic and functional correlations. Cancer **56**:1649-1657, 1985.

251 Unger RH, Orci L: Glucagon and the A cell. Physiology and pathophysiology. N Engl J Med **304**:1518-1524, 1981.

252 Vinik AI, Strodel WE, Eckhauser FE, Moattari AR, Lloyd R: Somatostatinomas, PPomas, neurotensinomas. Semin Oncol **14**:263-281, 1987.

253 Weidenheim KM, Hinchey WW, Campbell WG: Hyperinsulinemic hypoglycemia in adults with islet-cell hyperplasia and degranulation of exocrine cells of the pancreas. Am J Clin Pathol **79**:14-24, 1983.

254 Wermer P: Duality of pancreatogenous peptic ulcer. N Engl J Med **278**:397-398, 1968.

255 Wilander E, El-Salhy M, Willén R, Grimelius L: Immunocytochemistry and electron microscopy of an argentaffin endocrine tumour of the pancreas. Virchows Arch [Pathol Anat] **392**:263-269, 1981.

256 Wolfe MM, Alexander RW, McGuigan JE: Extrapancreatic, extraintestinal gastrinoma. Effective treatment by surgery. N Engl J Med **306**:1533-1536, 1982.

257 Wolfe MM, Jensen RT: Zollinger-Ellison syndrome. Current concepts in diagnosis and management. N Engl J Med **317**:1200-1209, 1987.

258 Zollinger RM: Gastrinoma. Factors influencing prognosis. Surgery **97**:49-54, 1985.

259 Zollinger RM: Gastrinoma. The Zollinger-Ellison syndrome. Semin Oncol **14**:247-252, 1987.

Malignancy

260 Freisen SR: Tumors of the endocrine pancreas. N Engl J Med **306**:580-590, 1982.

261 Whipple AO: Pancreatoduodenectomy for islet cell carcinoma. Ann Surg **121**:847-852, 1945.

Multiple endocrine adenomatosis

262 Balasa RW, Erlandsen SL, Martinson EJ, Dedecker KL, Delaney JP, Dehner LP, Rosai J: Multiple primary gastrin-secreting tumors of the stomach associated with Menetrier's disease. Histologic, ultrastructural, and immunohistochemical findings (abstract). Lab Invest **34**:308, 1976.

263 Ballard HS, Frame B, Hartsock RJ: Familial multiple endocrine adenoma-peptic ulcer complex. Medicine [Baltimore] **43**:481-516, 1964.

264 Carney JA, Go VLW, Sizemore GW, Hayles AB: Alimentary-tract ganglioneuromatosis. A major component of the syndrome of multiple endocrine neoplasia, type 2b. N Engl J Med **295**:1287-1291, 1976.

265 Carney JA, Sizemore GW, Hayles AB: Multiple endocrine neoplasia, type 2b. Pathobiol Ann **8**:105-153, 1978.

266 Carney JA, Sizemore GW, Lovestedt SA: Mucosal ganglioneuromatosis, medullary thyroid carcinoma, and pheochromocytoma. Multiple endocrine neoplasia, type 2b. Oral Surg **41**:739-752, 1976.

267 Gorlin RJ, Sedano HO, Vickers RA, Cervenka J: Multiple mucosal neuromas, pheochromocytoma and medullary carcinoma of thyroid. A syndrome. Cancer **22**:293-299, 1968.

268 Gould E, Albores-Saavedra J, Shuman J: Pituitary prolactinoma, pancreatic glucagonomas, and aldosterone-producing adrenal cortical adenoma. A suggested variant of multiple endocrine neoplasia type I. Hum Pathol **18**:1290-1293, 1987.

269 Hansen OP, Hansen M, Hansen HH, Rose B: Multiple endocrine adenomatosis of mixed type. Acta Med Scand **200:**327-331, 1976.

270 Khairi MRA, Dexter RN, Burzynski NJ, Johnson CC Jr: Mucosal neuroma, pheochromocytoma and medullary thyroid carcinoma. Multiple endocrine neoplasia type 3. Medicine [Baltimore] **54:**89-112, 1975.

271 Klöppel G, Willemer S, Stamm B, Häcki WH, Heitz PU: Pancreatic lesions and hormonal profile of pancreatic tumors in multiple endocrine neoplasia type I. An immunocytochemical study of nine patients. Cancer **57:**1824-1832, 1986.

272 Perkins JT, Blackstone MO, Riddell RH: Adenomatous polyposis coli and multiple endocrine neoplasia type 2b. A pathogenetic relationship. Cancer **55:**375-381, 1985.

273 Rosai J, Higa E, Davie J: Mediastinal endocrine neoplasm in patients with multiple endocrine adenomatosis. A previously unrecognized association. Cancer **29:**1075-1083, 1972.

274 Schimke RN: Multiple endocrine adenomatosis syndromes. Adv Intern Med **21:**249-265, 1976.

275 Schneider NR, Cubilla AL, Chaganti RSK: Association of endocrine neoplasia with multiple polyposis of the colon. Cancer **51:**1171-1175, 1983.

276 Steiner AL, Goodman AD, Powers SR: Study of a kindred with pheochromocytoma, medullary thyroid carcinoma, hyperparathyroidism and Cushing's disease. Multiple endocrine neoplasia, type 2. Medicine [Baltimore] **47:**371-409, 1968.

277 Tateishi R, Wada A, Ishiguro S, Ehara M, Sakamoto H, Miki T, Mori Y, Matsui Y, Ishikawa O: Coexistence of bilateral pheochromocytoma and pancreatic islet cell tumor. Cancer **42:**2928-2934, 1978.

Lymphoid tumors and tumorlike conditions

278 Abrebanel P, Sarfaty S, Gal R, Chaimoff C, Kessler E: Plasma cell granuloma of the pancreas. Arch Pathol Lab Med **108:**531-532, 1984.

279 Borgia G, Ciampi R, Nappa S, Iovinella V, Crowell J: Pancreatic plasmacytoma. An unusual cause of obstructive jaundice. Arch Pathol Lab Med **108:**773-774, 1984.

Mesenchymal and other primary tumors

280 Childs CC, Korsten MA, Choi H-SH, Schwarz R, Fisse RD: Pancreatic choriocarcinoma presenting as inflammatory pseudocyst. Gastroenterology **89:**426-431, 1985.

281 Elliott TE, Albertazzi VJ, Danto LA: Pancreatic liposarcoma. Case report with review of retroperitoneal liposarcomas. Cancer **45:**1720-1723, 1980.

282 Horie H, Iwasaki I, Iida H, Takizawa J, Itoh F, Kohda S: Benign hemangioendothelioma of the pancreas with obstructive jaundice. Acta Pathol Jpn **35:**975-979, 1985.

283 Ishikawa O, Matsui Y, Aoki Y, Iwanaga T, Terasawa T, Wada A: Leiomyosarcoma of the pancreas. Report of a case and review of the literature. Am J Surg Pathol **5:**597-602, 1981.

284 Murao T, Toda K, Tomiyama Y: Lymphangioma of the pancreas. A case report with electron microscopic observations. Acta Pathol Jpn **37:**503-510, 1987.

Metastatic tumors

285 Tanabe S-i, Soeda S, Mukai T, Oki S, Yun K, Miyahara S-i: A case report of pancreatic metastasis of an intracranial angioblastic meningioma (hemangiopericytoma) and a review of metastatic tumor to the pancreas. J Surg Oncol **26:**63-68, 1984.

Periampullary region
AMPULLARY CARCINOMA AND VILLOUS ADENOMA

286 Baczako K, Büchler M, Beger H-G, Kirkpatrick CJ, Haferkamp O: Morphogenesis and possible precursor lesions of invasive carcinoma of the papilla of Vater. Epithelial dysplasia and adenoma. Hum Pathol **16:**305-310, 1985.

287 Cubilla AL, Fitzgerald PJ: Cancer of the exocrine pancreas. The pathologic aspects. Cancer **35:**2-18, 1985.

288 Cubilla AL, Fortner J, Fitzgerald PJ: Lymph node involvement in carcinoma of the head of the pancreas area. Cancer **41:**880-887, 1978.

289 Kozuka S, Tsubone M, Yamaguchi A, Hachisuka K: Adenomatous residue in cancerous papilla of Vater. Gut **22:**1031-1034, 1981.

290 Lynch ML, Cleary KR: Non-ampullary adenocarcinoma of the duodenum (abstract). Lab Invest **58:**58A, 1988.

291 Rosenberg J, Welch JP, Pyrtek LJ, Walker M, Trowbridge P: Benign villous adenomas of the ampulla of Vater. Cancer **58:**1563-1568, 1986.

291a Talbot IC, Neoptolemos JP, Shaw DE, Carr-Locke D: The histopathology and staging of carcinoma of the ampulla of Vater. Histopathology **12:**155-165, 1988.

292 Wise L, Pizzimbono C, Dehner LP: Periampullary cancer. A clinicopathologic study of sixty-two patients. Am J Surg **131:**141-148, 1976.

293 Yamaguchi K, Enjoji M: Carcinoma of the ampulla of Vater. A clinicopathologic study and pathologic staging of 109 cases of carcinoma and 5 cases of adenoma. Cancer **59:**506-515, 1987.

OTHER LESIONS

294 Acosta JM, Civantos F, Nardi GL, Castleman B: Fibrosis of the papilla of Vater. Surg Gynecol Obstet **124:**787-794, 1967.

295 Cattell RB, Prytek LJ: Premalignant lesions of the ampulla of Vater. Surg Gynecol Obstet **90:**21-30, 1950.

296 Shingleton WW, Gamburg D: Stenosis of the sphincter of Oddi. Am J Surg **119:**35-37, 1970.

297 Stamm B, Hedinger Chr E, Saremaslani P: Duodenal and ampullary carcinoid tumors. A report of 12 cases with pathological characteristics, polypeptide content and relation to the MEN I syndrome and von Recklinghausen's disease (neurofibromatosis). Virchows Arch [Pathol Anat] **408:**475-489, 1986.

298 Ulich TR, Kollin M, Simmons GE, Wilczynski SP, Waxman K: Adenomyoma of the papilla of Vater. Arch Pathol Lab Med **111:**388-390, 1987.

299 Yamaguchi K, Enjoji M: Carcinoma of the ampulla of Vater. A clinicopathologic study and pathologic staging of 109 cases of carcinoma and 5 cases of adenoma. Cancer **59:**506-515, 1987.

16 Adrenal gland and other paraganglia

INTRODUCTION

The cortex and the medulla of the adrenal gland have entirely different origins.[3,4] The cortex arises from mesoderm, whereas the medulla arises from neuroectodermal tissue. Except for cases of heterotopia, cortical tissue is seen only within the anatomic confines of the adrenal gland. Instead, islands of chromaffin tissue morphologically identical to that composing the adrenal medulla are normally found all along the paravertebral sympathetic chain, particularly in the retroperitoneal region.

The specimens received in the Laboratory usually consist of the entire adrenal gland, but in selected cases the diagnosis can be achieved through the performance of a CT-guided biopsy[1] or fine needle aspiration cytology.[2]

LESIONS OF ADRENAL CORTEX
Heterotopia

Heterotopic adrenal cortical tissue has been reported in numerous locations. The most common site is the retroperitoneum, particularly the area adjacent to the adrenal gland. Other described sites include the region of the celiac plexus, kidney, along the course of the spermatic and ovarian veins, testis, adjacent to the tail of the epididymis, broad ligament near the ovary, the ovary itself (but only exceptionally), canal of Nuck, hernial and hydrocele sacs, mesoappendix, liver, lung, and brain.[5,6,8,9]

These nests may undergo marked hyperplasia in patients with Nelson's syndrome or other conditions associated with increased ACTH production[7] and occasionally may give rise to a neoplastic process.

Cortical nodule

Small nodules composed of cortical tissue and located in the periadrenal region are common. Commons and Callaway[10] found nodules greater than 3 mm in 216 (3%) of 7,437 consecutive autopsies. These nodules do not have clinical significance.[11] They increase in number with age but are not correlated with hypertension, diabetes, or cardiovascular disease.

Congenital hyperplasia

Congenital hyperplasia, an inborn error of metabolism, occurs with equal frequency in males and females and is transmitted by an autosomal recessive gene.[15,16] It is responsible for the large majority of cases of adrenogenital syndrome developing within the first year of life, but it can also first present clinically during adulthood.[12] The inherited defect may be in any of the five enzymatic steps required to synthesize cortisol from cholesterol.[19]

In approximately 95% of the cases, the basic defect is an absence of the enzyme 21-hydroxylase, which results in the accumulation of 17OH-progesterone and its catabolite pregnanetriol and in a deficiency of cortisol. The clinical picture is usually that of a pure virilizing syndrome, although in approximately 30% of the patients electrolyte disturbances occur.[17] The second most frequent form is due to a deficiency of 11-beta-hydroxylase and is characterized by virilization and hypertension. Several other variants, all exceptionally rare, have been described.[13,18] The pathologic change is the same in all types and is characterized by diffuse cortical hyperplasia, especially of the zona reticularis. The treatment consists of replacement with cortisol and surgical correction of the external sex organs.[14]

Acquired hyperplasia

Acquired hyperplasia, which is always bilateral, may result in a diffuse or in a nodular ("adenomatous") enlargement of the adrenal gland. An adrenal gland in an adult can be regarded as hyperplastic if it weighs over 6 g provided a careful dissection of the fat has been carried out. Cases of *diffuse* cortical hyperplasia can be ascribed in some cases to pituitary hyperfunction and in others to the presence of an ACTH-producing neoplasm in the lung or some other organ. In many cases, however, the pathogenesis remains obscure.

Microscopically, an increased thickness of the zona reticularis and fasciculata is observed, the relative proportions varying from case to case. Occasionally, cells with large hyperchromatic nuclei are seen in some of the nodules (Fig. 16-1).

Most cases of *nodular* cortical hyperplasia seem to be unrelated to ACTH production, but others may represent a later stage of diffuse hyperplasia.[20a]

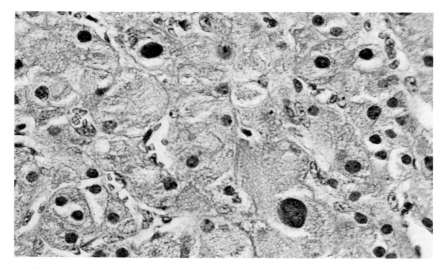

Fig. 16-1 Adrenal cortical hyperplasia in patient with Cushing's syndrome. Note large cells with bizarre nuclei. Mitoses are absent.

A morphologically distinct *primary pigmented nodular adrenal cortical hyperplasia (dysplasia)* has been described as part of a complex syndrome clinically characterized by Cushing's disease and which also includes spotty cutaneous pigmentation, cutaneous and cardiac myxomas, multiple myxoid fibroadenomas of the breast, pituitary tumors, and large-cell calcifying Sertoli cell tumors of the testis[20,21,22] (Fig. 16-2).

Adenoma

Adenomas are usually solitary and well encapsulated. On section, most of them show a solid homogeneous yellow surface (Fig. 16-3, *A*). Foci of necrosis and hemorrhage are rare. Occasionally, adenomas or hyperplastic nodules have a dark brown or even black color because of the presence of pigment, thought to represent either lipofuscin[26] or neuromelanin.[23] Most of these "black adenomas" or "black nod-

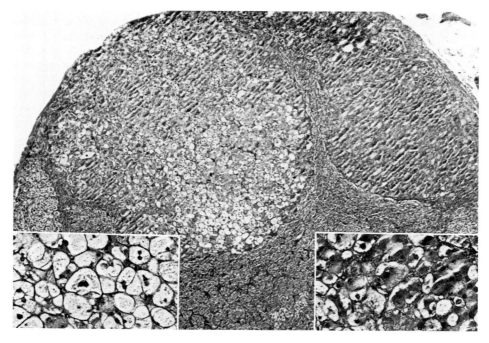

Fig. 16-2 Primary pigmented nodular adrenal cortical hyperplasia. Sharply circumscribed nodules are present, composed of cortical cells of varying appearances. Some of these cells have large vacuolated cytoplasm, whereas in others cytoplasm is darker and pigmented **(insets).** (Courtesy Dr. J.A. Carney, Rochester, MN.)

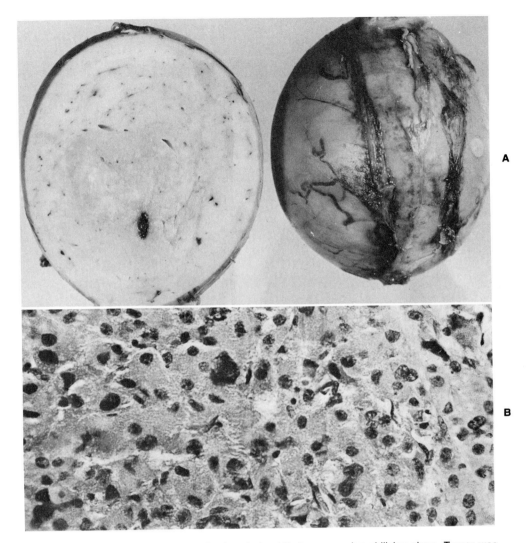

Fig. 16-3 A, Small cortical adenoma of adrenal gland that was causing virilizing signs. Tumor was identified by perirenal air insufflation. **B,** Same tumor illustrated in **A** showing large cells and atypical nuclei. Virilizing signs and symptoms rapidly regressed. Patient has remained well for over 10 years.

ules" are nonfunctioning and are found incidentally at autopsy but on occasion they have been associated with primary aldosteronism[28] or Cushing's syndrome.[25] These nodules have a higher radiologic density than the ordinary yellow cortical tumor.[25]

Adenomas are characteristically small neoplasms that rarely exceed 5 cm or 50 g, a point to remember in the differential diagnosis with carcinoma.[27] In our experience, most large (over 5 cm or 50 g) adrenal cortical tumors have behaved like carcinomas, even if their malignant nature was not apparent on microscopic examination. It is wise never to use the term "adenoma" for large adrenal cortical tumors. Lesions under 50 g are generally cured by excision and, as such, can be safely diagnosed as adenomas; however, exceptions occur.[24]

Microscopically, adenomas may resemble the appearance of the zona fasciculata, the zona glomerulosa, or, more commonly, a combination of both. Occasional bizarre nuclear forms can be seen, as in most other endocrine neoplasms (Fig. 16-3, *B*). However, *mitoses are exceptionally rare or absent.* Immunohistochemically, various steroid hormones and enzymes involved in their synthesis (such as cytochrome $P-450_{C21}$) can be demonstrated.[26a]

Cases of cortical adenoma containing foci of myelolipoma within them have been described.[29]

Carcinoma

Adrenal cortical carcinoma shows an equal sex distribution and presents at an average age of 48 years.[33,43] Pediatric cases are uncommon.[38] The tumor usually weighs over 100 g and sometimes reaches 1,000 g or more before discovery. About half of the cases are accompanied by hormonal manifestations.[33,44a] A palpable adrenal cortical neoplasm is malignant in practically every instance. The cut

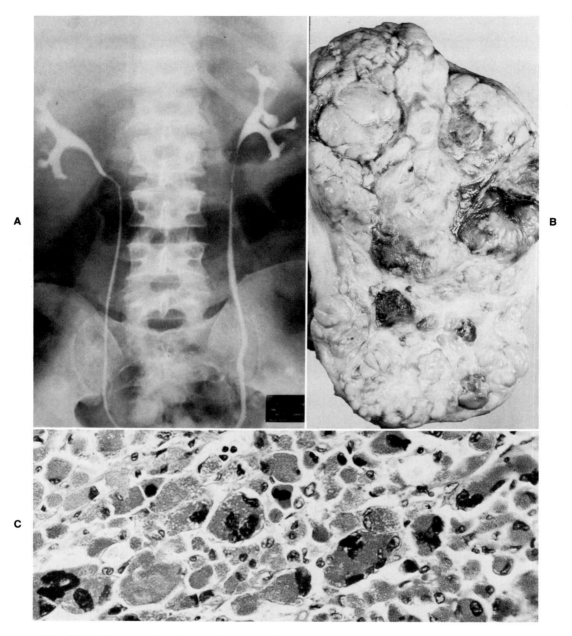

Fig. 16-4 A, Retrograde pyelogram of 47-year-old man with large asymptomatic cortical carcinoma of right adrenal gland displacing right kidney. **B,** Same lesion illustrated in **A** showing large, bright yellow tumor (weight, 900 g), encapsulated, with areas of necrosis. **C,** Same tumor shown in **A** and **B** demonstrating large cells with considerable variations in size and with many bizarre nuclei. There were tumor cells lying free within veins. This finding was significant, for 2 years after surgical removal patient developed pulmonary metastases.

surface shows a variegated pattern, and many of the individual nodules are soft and friable. Areas of necrosis and hemorrhage are frequent (Fig. 16-4, *A* and *B*); they may result in fever and simulate clinically an infectious disease.[51] A capsule may be present but is often infiltrated by tumor. Invasion of major veins is a frequent finding and often leads to total occlusion, thrombosis, and embolism.

Microscopically, a wide range of differentiation exists in these tumors, both at the light and electron microscopic level.[45] In some, the tumor cells closely resemble normal adrenal cortical cells, whereas others are totally undifferentiated. Giant cells with abundant acidophilic cytoplasm and bizarre hyperchromatic nuclei may be present, together with multinucleated forms[36] (Fig. 16-4, *C*). In some instances, a large number of neutrophils is seen within the cytoplasm of the tumor giant cells.

The differential diagnosis between cortical adenomas and well-differentiated cortical carcinomas can be very difficult. Size and weight are of great importance, as already pointed out.[46] Microscopically, mitotic activity (especially if accompanied by atypical forms) and venous invasion correlate best with recurrence or metastasis.[46,47,49] Weiss[49] listed the following microscopic criteria as suggestive of malignancy in an adrenal cortical tumor (particularly when seen together): nuclear grade III or IV, mitotic rate greater than five per fifty high-power fields, atypical mitoses, paucity or absence of clear cells, diffuse architecture, necrosis, capsular invasion, and vascular (venous or sinusoidal) invasion. Another feature suggestive of malignancy is spindling of the tumor cells.[39] Nearly all studies done on the subject have shown that no single parameter short of detection of metastases discriminates sharply between benign and malignant tumors, particularly in pediatric cases[31]; a combined evaluation of clinical features, size or weight, and microscopic appearance is necessary.[35,44,46,49] It appears from preliminary reports that flow cytometric DNA analysis may become an effective predictor of clinical outcome in these tumors[30,48]

Adrenal cortical cancer is generally a highly malignant neoplasm.[30a] It often recurs following surgery and its radiosensitivity is poor. One half of the thirty-eight patients studied by Lipsett et al.[40] died within 2 years of the onset of symptoms. A correlation exists between microscopic degree of differentiation and survival.[37] The most common sites of metastatic involvement are liver (60%), regional lymph nodes (40%), lungs (40%), peritoneal and pleural surfaces, and bone.[32,36,43] Poorly differentiated ("anaplastic") tumors also tend to metastasize to skin.[34] Some of these may masquerade as primary tumors in these sites.[41]

Adrenal cortical carcinomas can directly invade the kidney, whereas renal cell carcinomas can directly invade or metastasize into the adrenal glands. Microscopically, these two tumors resemble each other a great deal, so that the differential diagnosis may become very difficult. Two features favoring the diagnosis of renal cell carcinoma are the presence of glands (particularly if they contain numerous red blood cells) and abundant glycogen, but neither is pathognomonic. Immunohistochemically, strong positivity for cytokeratin, epithelial membrane antigen, and blood group isoantigen favor renal cell carcinoma, whereas positivity for vimentin is more in keeping with adrenal cortical tumor.[50] However, the degree of heterogeneity that exists among these tumors calls for caution in the interpretation of these results.[42]

Clinicopathologic correlation

Acquired hyperplasia, adenoma, and carcinoma may be "nonfunctioning," at least at a clinical level, or be the cause of a variety of syndromes resulting from the secretion of excessive amounts of corticosteroid hormones.[53]

Sometimes, an adrenal lesion, initially silent, may later on clinically result in hormonal manifestations.[52] A fairly accurate prediction regarding the morphologic type of abnormality in the adrenal gland can be made by knowing the clinical syndrome plus the age and sex of the patient.

Nonfunctioning lesions

Whereas instances of cortical hyperplasia and adenomas are found commonly at postmortem examination of asymptomatic individuals,[54] most of the nonfunctioning adrenal cortical lesions seen as surgical specimens are carcinomas.[56] This is explained by the fact that the malignant process often

is accompanied by a deletion in some of the enzymes required for cortisol synthesis. It results in production and release of steroid precursors such as dehydroepiandrosterone and 11-deoxycortisol (compound S). The presence of the latter is a consequence of a deficiency of the 11-beta-hydroxylase enzyme, which is a characteristic feature of adrenal carcinoma.[53a,57] The majority of these carcinomas occur in the older age groups.[55]

The finding of a cortical adenoma in a hypertensive patient does not, in itself, imply any causal relationship.

Aldosteronism

In primary aldosteronism, the excessive amount of secreted aldosterone results in urinary loss of potassium, retention of sodium, suppressed renin levels, hypertension, and muscle weakness.[61,62] The adrenal lesion is an adenoma in over 70% of the cases, cortical hyperplasia being responsible for most of the remaining and carcinoma for exceedingly few.[71] The adenomas can usually be distinguished from the hyperplasia by a combination of clinical and laboratory parameters, but sometimes the morphologic features of one are associated with the biochemical features of the other.[60] Adrenal surgery is more likely to be beneficial in patients with adenoma than in those with hyperplasia. The adenoma is usually unilateral, solitary (91%), and small. In the series of eighteen cases reported by Neville and Symington,[67] 60% of the tumors weighed less than 6 g. The cut surface had a homogenous golden yellow or yellow-brown color.

Microscopically, one would expect these adenomas to have an appearance similar to that of the zona glomerulosa, since this is the area in which aldosterone is produced in the normal adrenal gland. Although this is sometimes the case, most of the tumor cells resemble those of the zona fasciculata or have characteristics intermediate between zona glomerulosa and zona fasciculata cells (so-called hybrid cells). Ultrastructurally, most of the mitochondria in the tumor cells have lamellar cristae (characteristic of the zona glomerulosa),[65] but mitochondria with cristae of the tubulovesicular type (as in the normal zona fasciculata) also can be found.[69] The zona glomerulosa of the nontumoral gland is often atrophic, although it may be normal or even hyperplastic.[68] In patients who have been treated with spironolactone, a characteristic cytoplasmic structure may appear in the tumor cells, as well as in the cells of the adjacent zona glomerulosa. It is a whorled, multilaminar collection of membranes, as large as 20 μm in diameter, and is thought to derive from the smooth endoplasmic reticulum.[58,70] Immunohistochemical positivity in these bodies for aldosterone has been found, suggesting that the hormone is bound to them.[64]

In most of the reported cases where a cortical adrenal carcinoma has resulted in increased aldosterone production, secretion of other steroid hormones was also found, thus excluding them as cases of pure primary aldosteronism.[59,71]

Proper evaluation of a patient suspected of having primary aldosteronism includes pharmacologic exploration of the renin-angiotensin-aldosterone system[62,66] and roentgenographic examination of the adrenal glands, especially arteriography, in order to distinguish primary aldosteronism from cases of renovascular and essential hypertension. A

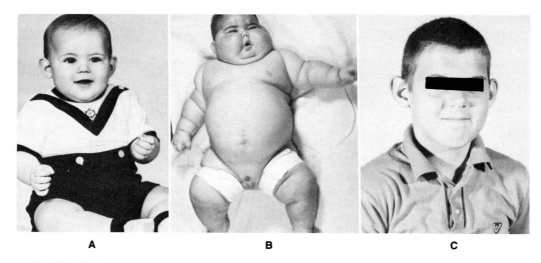

A   **B**   **C**

Fig. 16-5 Child with Cushing's syndrome 7 months before development of tumor, **A,** with tumor at 17 months of age, **B,** and 10 years later, **C.** (**A** and **B,** from Heinbecker P, O'Neal LW, Ackerman LV: Functioning and nonfunctioning adrenal cortical tumors. Surg Gynecol Obstet **105:**21-33, 1957, by permission of Surgery, Gynecology & Obstetrics; **C,** courtesy Dr. L.W. O'Neal, St. Louis, MO.)

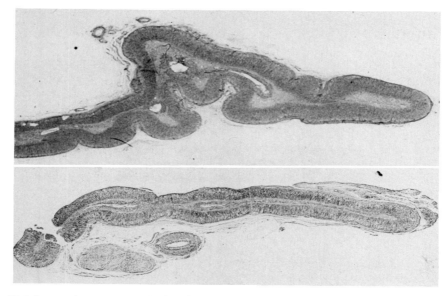

Fig. 16-6 Contrast between normal adrenal gland from 5-month-old girl and markedly atrophic adrenal gland that was contralateral to functioning carcinoma in 7-month-old girl.

radioisotopic technique has been devised for visualization of the adrenal glands. It is based on the uptake and esterification of ^{131}I-19-iodocholesterol by the adrenal glands and has led to the successful localization of aldosterone-producing adenomas.[63]

Cushing's syndrome

Approximately 80% of patients with Cushing's syndrome are females, and a similar proportion are adults. In 20%, the syndrome occurs before puberty (Fig. 16-5). The abnormality encountered in the adrenal gland in cases of Cushing's syndrome may be hyperplasia, adenoma, or carcinoma (in that order of frequency), both in adults and children (see

Fig. 16-1).[74,76-78,83] In cases of adrenal cortical tumor, the remaining adrenal cortex often shows signs of atrophy (Fig. 16-6). The presence of a large adrenal mass in a patient with Cushing's syndrome is practically always indicative of carcinoma. Similarly, cases of Cushing's syndrome associated with obvious changes of virilization ("mixed" type) and markedly increased excretion of 17-ketosteroids are most always due to cortical carcinoma.[77] Schteingart et al.[80] consider the latter finding to be the most reliable biochemical sign of malignancy.

Most carcinomas are easily demonstrated by routine intravenous pyelography because of their large size. In contrast, adenomas usually require a CT scan, NMR, or arteriography for their demonstration. CT is currently the most accurate imaging modality for the preoperative localization of these tumors.[81]

Most of the cases of *diffuse* cortical hyperplasia associated with Cushing's syndrome are due to pituitary hyperfunction (ACTH-dependent), and these are referred to as *Cushing's disease.*[72] Other cases of diffuse cortical hyperplasia are secondary to the presence of nonpituitary ACTH-producing neoplasms. An excellent critical review of the pathology of these neoplasms has been made by Azzopardi and Williams.[73] In contrast to the prevailing opinion that almost any type of tumor may result in the production of Cushing's syndrome, these authors have shown that nearly all acceptable cases fall into four main categories: (1) small cell carcinoma of lung; (2) endocrine tumors of foregut origin, such as carcinoid tumor of the lung, medullary carcinoma of the thyroid gland, and carcinoid tumor of the thymus; (3) pheochromocytoma and related tumors; and (4) certain ovarian tumors. The first two account for more than 90% of the acceptable cases. In this group of patients, hypokalemic alkalosis, very high urinary excretion of free cortisol, skin pigmentation, edema, and severe diabetes mellitus occur more frequently than in the cases due to a primary adrenal lesion. Confirmation that the tumor is related to the Cushing's syndrome requires remission of the syndrome after tumor resection and demonstration of an ACTH-like substance by immunocytochemistry or biochemical assay. Upton and Amatruda[84] have demonstrated that some of these tumors secrete not only ectopic ACTH but also a group of tumor peptides that stimulate the secretion of ACTH from the pituitary gland, thus contributing to the ectopic ACTH syndrome.

Cases of *nodular* adrenal hyperplasia are independent of ACTH production[75,82]; some of these are a component of a peculiar complex syndrome (see p. 790).

Electron microscopic studies of cells from hyperplastic adrenal glands associated with Cushing's syndrome have shown mitochondria with tubulovesicular configuration of the cristae, consistent with elements of the zona fasciculata.[79]

In a patient with Cushing's syndrome without identifiable tumor, adrenal exploration should be transabdominal. If one adrenal gland is found to be atrophic, there is probably a tumor on the opposite side (Fig. 16-6). However, if one adrenal gland is normal or hyperplastic, the other gland may still contain a tumor. We have not found frozen sections helpful in determining whether a given adrenal gland is normal or atrophic.

Adrenogenital syndrome

Excess androgens secreted by an adrenal lesion bring about changes toward adult masculinity in male or female children and toward masculinity in female adults (Fig. 16-7). About 50% of the cases occur before puberty, and 80% of the patients are female.[87] Patterson[89] devised a simple chemical test that is helpful in differentiating virilizing adrenal tumors from cases of adrenal hyperplasia, interstitial cell tumor of the testis, and Sertoli–Leydig cell tumor of the ovary. It is based on the finding of the 17-ketosteroid hormone, dehydroisoandrosterone. The rarest form of endocrine abnormality caused by an adrenal cortical lesion is

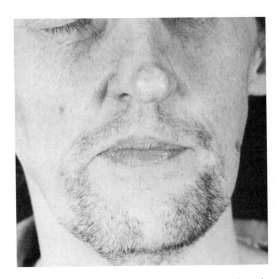

Fig. 16-7 Virilizing changes in woman with huge adrenal cortical tumor weighing over 1,000 g. Microscopically, tumor appeared similar to one shown in Fig. 16-4, **C.** Patient remained free from recurrence for 5 years but in sixth year died of recurrent disease.

feminization in a male adult accompanied by increased output of 17-ketosteroids.

The most common cause of virilization in childhood is congenital adrenal hyperplasia. However, if an adrenal neoplasm is present, it will be a carcinoma in the majority of instances.[85,88] Virilization of adrenal origin in female adults is more often the result of a benign tumor than a malignant one (see Fig. 16-3). If the features of virilization are accompanied by those of Cushing's syndrome, there is a high probability that the lesion is a carcinoma. Practically all the feminizing adrenal tumors in adult males are carcinomas.[86] Young patients succumb rapidly to the disease; older individuals survive slightly longer.

Other manifestations of carcinoma

Less common manifestations of adrenal cortical lesions (particularly carcinomas) include hypoglycemia,[92] polycythemia,[91] and inappropriate secretion of antidiuretic hormone.[90]

LESIONS OF ADRENAL MEDULLA
Tumors of sympathetic nervous system

Tumors of the sympathetic nervous system can be found anywhere along the sympathetic chain, including the neck, mediastinum, and retroperitoneum. They are discussed here because many of them, particularly the poorly differentiated members of this family, arise within or in close proximity to the adrenal gland. The better differentiated the tumor and the older the patient, the less likely the lesion will be located in the adrenal gland.

Neuroblastomas usually are seen in young children, over 70% being detected in those under the age of 4 years. Typical examples occurring in adults are exceptional.[93,120] Neuroblastomas can exhibit familial incidence,[121] be associated with the Beckwith-Wiedermann syndrome[104] and other congenital abnormalities (especially if the tumor itself is congenital[94,144]), present in patients with neurofibromatosis,[151] or occur as a complication of fetal hydantoin syndrome.[137a] Structural rearrangements of chromosome 1p or other chromosomal abnormalities have been detected in over 70% of the cases.[110]

Neuroblastomas are only occasionally bilateral.[143]

Grossly, they are large, soft, gray, and relatively well circumscribed; areas of hemorrhage, necrosis, and calcification are often present (Fig. 16-8). Microscopically, there are collections of small regular cells with round, deeply staining nuclei slightly larger than lymphocytes. There is

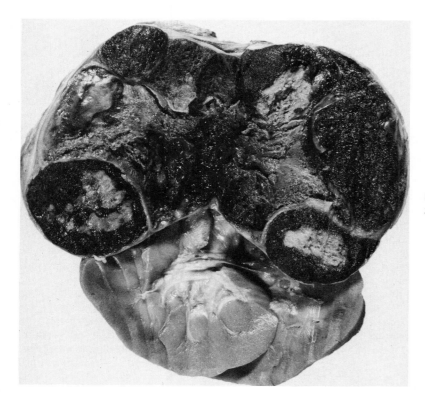

Fig. 16-8 Hemorrhagic neuroblastoma with zones of necrosis.

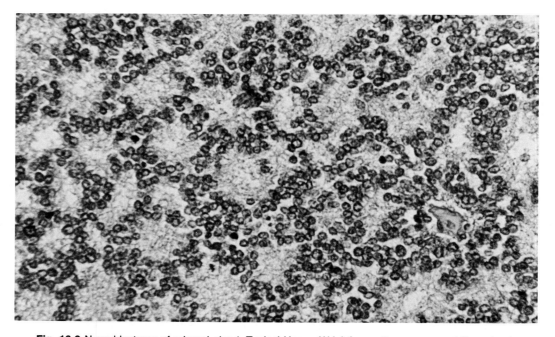

Fig. 16-9 Neuroblastoma of adrenal gland. Typical Homer Wright's rosettes are present throughout. Area encircled by nuclei contains fine network of neurofibrillary material.

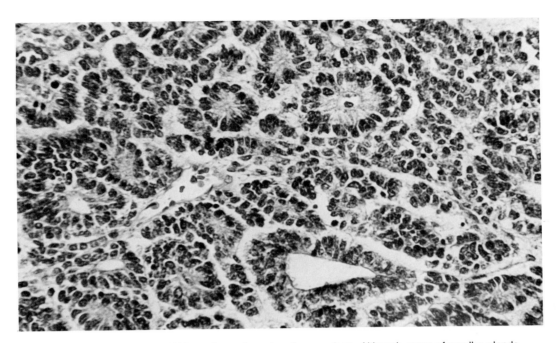

Fig. 16-10 Wilms' tumor of kidney shown for sake of comparison. Although some of smaller glands resemble neuroblastic rosettes, they can be distinguished by presence of central lumen with clear-cut cytoplasmic border.

little cytoplasm and cytoplasmic outlines are poorly defined. Necrosis is usually present, leaving viable tumor cells grouped around blood vessels. Homer Wright's rosettes are present in about a fourth to a third of the cases; they are characterized by a collection of tumor cells not related to blood vessels arranged around a central area filled with a fibrillary material (Figs. 16-9 and 16-10). The latter is composed of a tangled mass of neurites as revealed by silver stains (with some difficulty) and electron microscopy (with relative ease). Ultrastructural examination will show, in addition, neurosecretory granules and synaptic endings.[119,138]

In vitro maturation of neuroblastoma is a well-documented phenomenon, which has been used sometimes as a diagnostic aid. Neurites may develop spontaneously within 24 hours (Fig. 16-11)[127,132] or may be induced with chemical agents such as retinoic acid.[133,147a] Neuroblastomas can also be maintained in a functional state when xenotransplanted in nude mice.[114]

Neuroblastomas produce catecholamines, which can be demonstrated in sections or touch preparations by the technique of formaldehyde-induced fluorescence.[102,131] Immunohistochemically, neuroblastoma cells express neuron-specific enolase, neurofilaments, vasoactive intestinal peptide, microtubule-associated proteins, and other neural-

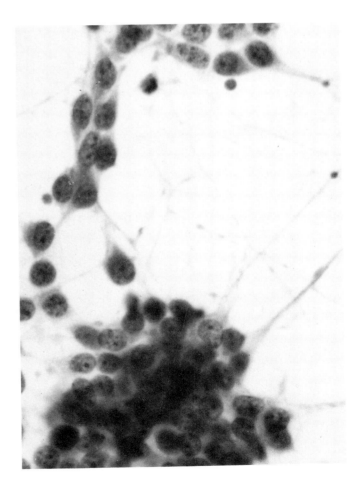

Fig. 16-11 Neuroblastoma cells, in continuous culture for 354 days, explanted from involved lymph node of 2-year-old girl from tissue obtained 1 hour postmortem. Note small nuclei, sparse cytoplasm, and many unipolar beaded neurites extending from cell bodies. (Courtesy Dr. M. Goldstein, St. Louis, MO.)

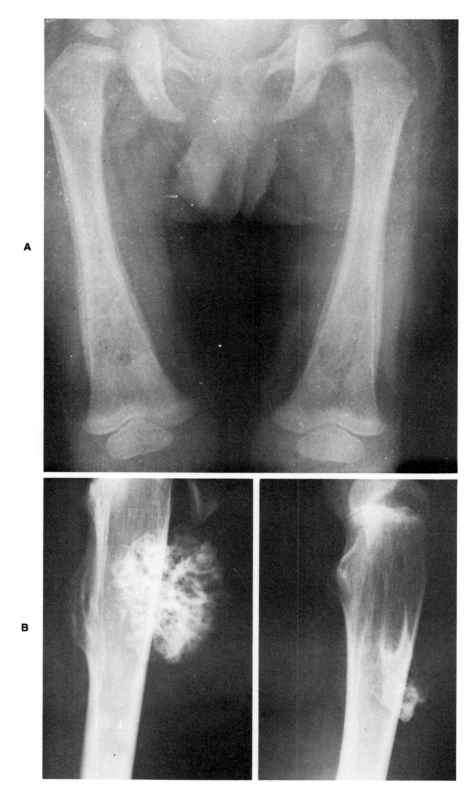

Fig. 16-12 In 1951, 13-month-old boy had neuroblastoma of right posterior mediastinum with numerous metastases to skull and long bones. X-ray films of both femurs showed periosteal bone proliferation with involvement of medullary canal. Patient received 2,000 R to mediastinum, 1,000 R to femurs, and 800 R to both tibias, left arm, and forearm. **B,** In 1964, 12 years after therapy, osteochondroma can be seen in distal portion of right femur and questionable low-grade chondrosarcoma in distal segment of left femur. Patient is alive and well 18 years after therapy and 5 years following removal of cartilaginous tumors. (**A** and **B,** from Perez CA, Vietti T, Ackerman LV, Eagleton MD, Powers WE: Tumors of the sympathetic nervous system in children. An appraisal of treatment and results. Radiology **88:**750-760, 1967.)

related antigens.* These, together with electron microscopy, are of great utility in the differential diagnosis between neuroblastoma and other small cell (blue cell, round cell) tumors of infancy, such as rhabdomyosarcoma, Ewing's sarcoma, and malignant lymphoma.[128,146] Caution should be exercised in the interpretation of results obtained using polyclonal antibodies against neuron-specific enolase[103]; we have obtained more specific results with a set of monoclonal antibodies against this marker.[137] Production of neuron-specific enolase by the tumor may result in increased serum levels in advanced stages of the disease, a finding of prognostic significance.[154]

Adrenal neuroblastomas locally invade the surrounding tissues. They may show intraspinal (dumbbell) extension[115] or spread into the kidney. The most common sites of distant metastases are liver, skeletal system (particularly skull and orbit), and lymph nodes. Bone metastases are usually multiple and sometimes symmetric, a point to remember in the differential diagnosis with Ewing's sarcoma (Fig. 16-12). Most recurrences and metastases develop within 2 years following excision of the primary tumor, but occasional instances of very late recurrences are on record.[100] The pattern of tumor metastases is altered by the therapy.[101]

Very often, collections of neuroblasts resembling small neuroblastomas are seen as incidental findings at autopsy[112,117]; the fact that in most reported cases the infants were less than 3 months of age suggests either that the process was not neoplastic,[148] or, if it was, that it resolved spontaneously. In some instances, typical symptomatic neuroblastomas, even accompanied by metastatic disease, are seen to undergo complete maturation that results in a spontaneous cure.

The overall 3-year survival rate for patients with neuroblastoma is around 30%[106,145]; this has changed relatively little during the past two decades.[111,130,150] The prognosis is related to several factors[98,105,130,134]:

1 *Age of the patient.* Children under 2 years have the best prognosis.[118]
2 *Location of the tumor.* Extra-adrenal tumors have a better outlook; this is probably related to the fact that they tend to be better differentiated.
3 *Surgical staging* (Table 16-1). The prognosis is directly related to the stage of the disease. It decreases from 90% in stage I to 2.4% in stage IV, except for a subtype of stage IV known as *S* (for *special*). This subtype, which apparently lacks the chromosomal abnormalities of other stage IV neuroblastomas, is associated with frequent spontaneous remissions and a 60% to 90% survival rate.[141,142,150]
4 *Microscopic differentiation.* In the typical neuroblastoma, differentiation as judged by standard light microscopic features is either absent or limited to less than 5% of the tumor. This neoplasm has been variously designated as classic, undifferentiated, grades III-IV, or stroma-poor neuroblastoma.[139] In other neuroblastomas, the tumor cells are larger, the chromatin pattern is finer, there is more abundant and better-defined cytoplasm, and an S-100 protein-positive Schwann cell component appears.[139,140] This pattern, which is referred to by some as *differentiating neuroblastoma* and which merges with that of ganglioneuroblastoma (see following), is associated with a

better prognosis.[107,116,122,140] For the undifferentiated neuroblastoma, it would seem that presence of nuclear abnormalities (in the form of mitotic activity and karyorrhexis) and total absence of S-100 protein-positive cells are indicators of a worsened prognosis.[139]
5 *Lymphocytic infiltration.* An infiltration by mature lymphocytes around the tumor is a seemingly favorable prognostic sign.
6 *Low urinary VMA/HVA ratio.* A VMA/HVA ratio of less than 1 is an unfavorable prognostic sign. This is related to a reported relative deficiency of dopamine B-hydroxylase activity in the more primitive and aggressive neoplasms.
7 *Ganglioside composition.* The absence of a particular ganglioside known as Gt1b seems to be indicative of a poor prognosis.[135,152]
8 *Flow cytometric DNA pattern.* A favorable clinical outcome has been found in association with an aneuploid stem line and a low percentage of tumor cells in the S, G2, and M phases of the cell cycle.[109]
9 *Genomic amplification.* Amplification of the N-myc oncogene is associated with rapid clinical progression.[96,136,147b]
10 Factors that do not significantly influence prognosis are sex of the patient, nodal status at diagnosis, or individual treatment modalities.[145]

Ganglioneuroblastomas (malignant ganglioneuromas) are tumors exhibiting a degree of differentiation that is intermediate between neuroblastoma and ganglioneuroma. Most of them are seen in young children, but typical examples in adults are on record. In contrast to neuroblastomas, most of the neoplasms are located in the retroperitoneum or mediastinum rather than in the adrenal gland; thus, their distribution approaches that of ganglioneuroma (Fig. 16-13). Their gross appearance varies depending on the subtype and extent of differentiation; in general, they have a more homogeneous appearance and firmer consistency than neuroblastomas (Fig. 16-14). Calcification is very common (Fig. 16-15).

Microscopically, two distinct varieties can be recognized. In one, sometimes designated as *imperfect,* there are all stages of neuronal differentiation throughout the neoplasm. This may lead to the formation of collections of ganglion cells, many of them immature, multinucleated, or otherwise abnormal. A fine, fibrillary, cobwebby network is seen between masses of cells (Fig. 16-16); this material, which represents an important diagnostic feature of ganglioneuro-

Table 16-1 Staging for neuroblastoma

Stage	Description
I	Tumor confined to the organ or structure of origin
II	Tumors extending in continuity beyond the organ or structure of origin but not crossing the midline
III	Tumors extending in continuity beyond the midline
IV	Remote disease involving skeleton, organs, soft tissues, or distant lymph node groups, etc.
IV-S	Patients who would otherwise be stage I or II but who have remote disease confined to one or more of the following sites: liver, skin or bone marrow and who have lack of radiographic evidence of bone involvement

From Evans AE, D'Angio GY, Randolph Y: A proposed staging for children with neuroblastoma. Cancer **27**:374-378, 1971.

---

*See references 95, 125, 128, 129, 146, 147, and 149.

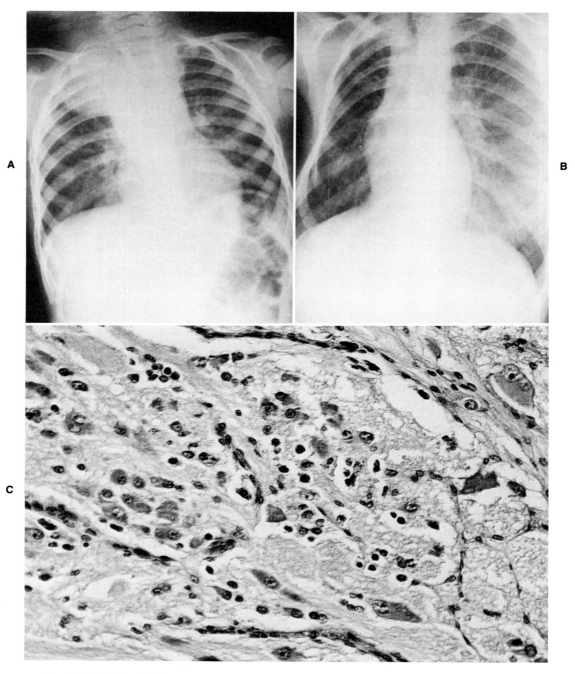

Fig. 16-13 A, Female infant, 17 months old, had tumor of right superior mediastinum. At exploratory thoracotomy, tumor was unresectable. Postoperatively, 2,800 R was given to neoplasm and adjacent mediastinum, **B,** Follow-up x-ray film of chest demonstrates decreased volume of right lung with shifting of mediastinum. Bony structures are not as well developed as on left side. **C,** Photomicrograph of ganglioneuroblastoma shows admixture of ganglion cells and neuroblasts. Patient remains well 15 years later. (**A** to **C,** from Perez CA, Vietti T, Ackerman LV, Eagleton MD, Powers WE: Tumors of the sympathetic nervous system in children. An appraisal of treatment and results. Radiology **88:**750-760, 1967.)

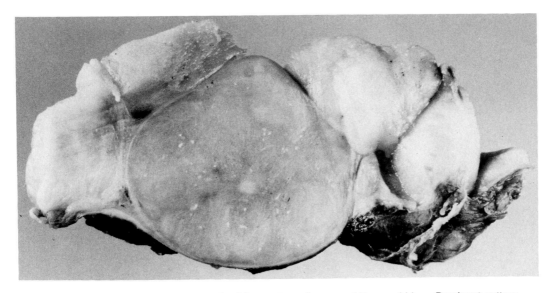

Fig. 16-14 Ganglioneuroblastoma excised from retroperitoneum of 5-year-old boy. Dominant pattern was that of well-differentiated ganglion and Schwann cells, with only few clumps of neuroblasts being identified.

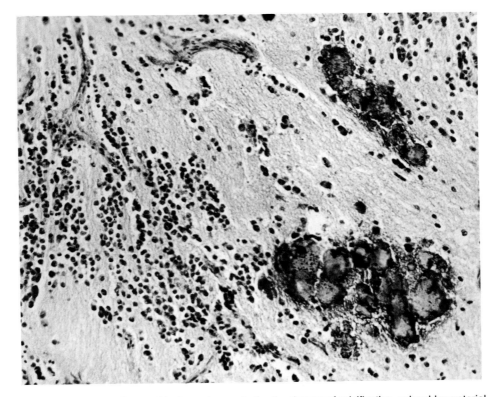

Fig. 16-15 Typical ganglioneuroblastoma demonstrating focal areas of calcification, cobwebby material, and collections of cells with deep-staining nuclei.

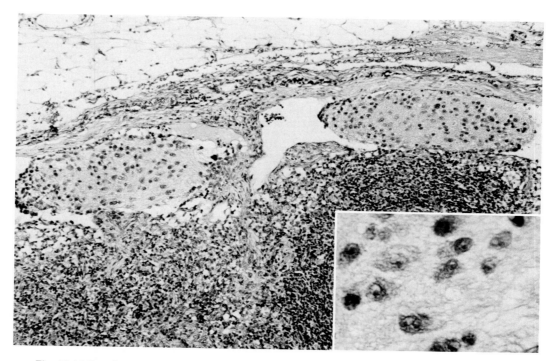

Fig. 16-16 Ganglioneuroblastoma metastatic in retroperitoneal lymph node. Two tumor nodules distend peripheral sinus. Primary tumor was located in adrenal gland. **Inset,** Higher magnification of tumor cells. Weblike material interposed between nuclei is important diagnostic feature.

blastomas, is made of large numbers of neurites emanating from the tumor cells, with occasional formation of synaptic junctions[124] (Fig. 16-17). It seems likely that this variety of ganglioneuroblastoma and the previously mentioned "differentiating neuroblastoma" are identical or, at the most, they simply represent slightly different stages of the maturing process undergone by some neuroblastomas.

The second variety of ganglioneuroblastoma (known to some as *immature* or *composite*) is easier to define and recognize. Basically, it has the gross and microscopic appearance of a ganglioneuroma except for the presence of well-defined, highly cellular areas of neuroblastoma. One should be careful not to confuse perivascular collections of lymphocytes (often present in these neoplasms) with foci of neuroblasts. The boundaries between the two patterns tend to be quite sharp. The difference between these two varieties could be expressed by saying that the first is overwhelmingly formed by cells of intermediate differentiation, whereas the second is made up of the two extremes of the differentiation sequence.

Ultrastructural studies of ganglioneuroblastomas confirm the better differentiated nature of this tumor as compared with neuroblastoma. Tangled unmyelinated cell processes are seen running through a maze of Schwann cells; neurosecretory granules and neurotubules are easily found in the cytoplasm and in extensions of the tumor cells.[124]

The prognosis for ganglioneuroblastoma is appreciably better than that for neuroblastoma. Among the ganglioneuroblastomas, the prognosis is worse for the immature (composite) than for the imperfect variety, especially when the neuroblastoma component is in the form of nodular aggregates.[94a]

Ganglioneuromas represent the fully differentiated members of the group and are invariably benign. They are seen in an older age group than the preceding tumors and constitute the most common neoplasm of the sympathetic nervous system in adults. They can be multiple and/or associated with other independent types of neurogenous neoplasms, such as neuroblastoma and pheochromocytoma. They are only rarely found in the adrenal gland, their most common location being the posterior mediastinum and retroperitoneum. Grossly, they are large, encapsulated masses of firm consistency with a homogeneous, solid, grayish-white cut surface having a focally edematous appearance. Thorough sampling for microscopic examination is crucial; areas of different color or consistency, especially if friable or hemorrhagic, are particularly suspicious of harboring less differentiated foci. Microscopically, the overall appearance resembles that of a neurofibroma except for the presence of numerous collections of abnormal but fully mature ganglion cells, often having more than one nucleus. Ultrastructurally, the resemblance to normal sympathetic ganglion cells is striking[153] (Fig. 16-18, *A* and *B*).

Occasionally the Schwann cell component of the ganglioneuroma may show features of a malignant nerve sheath tumor.[99]

Catecholamine synthesis is an almost constant feature of all the tumors in this series. It very rarely leads to hypertension but has provided very sensitive tests for their detection. Most of the biochemical production is in the form of catecholamine precursors, leading to the excretion of vanilmandelic acid, homovanilic acid, and other products in the urine. There is considerable variation in the relative amount of these products by a given tumor, but in over 95%

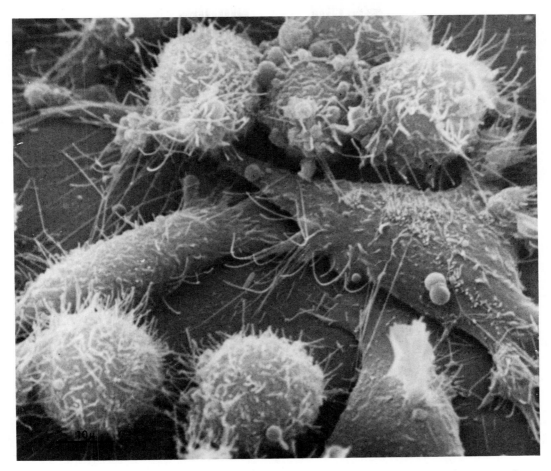

Fig. 16-17 Scanning electron micrograph of established line of mouse neuroblastoma that first appeared in sympathetic ganglion of A/J mouse. Spherical cells are probably in G_1 phase of cell cycle. Others are in late G_1 or S. Filiform cytoplasmic prolongations are extremely numerous. Some probably correspond to dendrites and axons. ($\times$3,000; Courtesy Dr. V. Fonte and Dr. K. Porter, Boulder, CO.)

of the patients, some abnormality will be detected.[106] Occasionally, severe diarrhea is found in association with these tumors, which disappears on their removal[113]; it is more commonly seen with ganglioneuroma than with either ganglioneuroblastoma or neuroblastoma and is due to secretion of vasoactive intestinal peptide.[97] This product can be identified by immunohistochemistry in the differentiating and mature ganglion cells.[123]

Primary **_malignant melanocytic tumors_** arising from cervical, posterior mediastinal, and lumbar sympathetic ganglia have been reviewed by Fu et al.[108] Some of the patients died with metastatic disease. These tumors are thought to arise from neural crest derivatives that have the capacity to produce melanin pigment, in a manner equivalent to that sometimes exhibited by neurofibroma, neurilemoma, malignant schwannoma, neuroblastoma,[126] ganlglioneuroblastoma,[110a] and "melanotic meningioma."

Adrenal medullary hyperplasia

Hyperplasia of the adrenal medulla is a distinct entity, which may result in symptoms similar to those of pheochromocytoma.[159] It may be nodular or diffuse and is always

bilateral. Ultrastructurally and immunohistochemically, the features are similar to those of normal medullary cells: chromogranin, neuron-specific enolase, and Leu-enkephalin reactivity can be demonstrated consistently.[156]

Advanced cases of medullary hyperplasia are easy to recognize, but earlier phases may need morphometric studies to detect minor increases in medullary volume and weight, inasmuch as random sectioning techniques are grossly inadequate for this purpose.[157,158] In most cases, the medullary hyperplasia is a component of multiple endocrine adenomatosis Type IIb (also known as MEA III), together with medullary thyroid carcinoma and parathyroid chief cell hyperplasia, and is the background from which both benign and malignant pheochromocytomas (sometimes multiple and bilateral) develop in these patients (Fig. 16-19).[155]

Pheochromocytoma

Pheochromocytoma can be defined as a paraganglioma of the adrenal medulla (see p. 809). As such, it is the better known and more common tumor of the adrenal medulla. It may secrete norepinephrine, epinephrine, or both. Pheochromocytoma has been called *the 10% tumor*—approximately 10% are malignant, 10% are bilateral (Fig. 16-20), 10% are extra-adrenal, and 10% occur in children. Pheochromocytomas in children are less likely to be malignant but more likely to be extra-adrenal, bilateral, or associated with multiple endocrine adenomatosis (MEA).[170] Series of pheochromocytomas in adults with long-term follow-up suggest that the real incidence of malignancy is much higher than 10%.[193a] When extra-adrenal, pheochromocytomas usually secrete only norepinephrine since the adrenal cortex seems necessary for the methylation of this hormone to epinephrine. The most common locations of extra-adrenal functioning pheochromocytomas (better designated as *paragangliomas*) are the retroperitoneal area (including the region of the Zuckerkandl's body), mediastinum, and urinary bladder.[166] They also have been described in the region of the carotid body and glomus jugulare[188] (see p. 809).

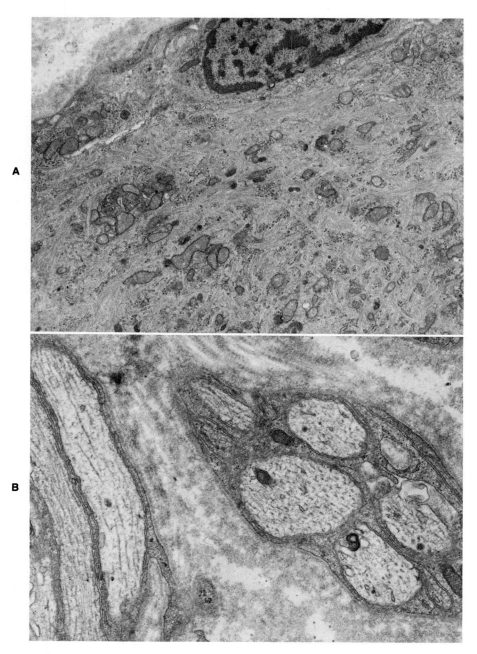

Fig. 16-18 Ganglioneuroma of retroperitoneum. **A,** Huge ganglion cell with eccentrically placed nucleus containing large numbers of cytoplasmic organelles, including microfilaments. This cell is separated from surrounding stroma by basal lamina. **B,** Neural bundles are surrounded by basal lamina; they contain numerous microtubules and other cytoplasmic organelles. (**A,** 7,450; **B,** ×16,850.)

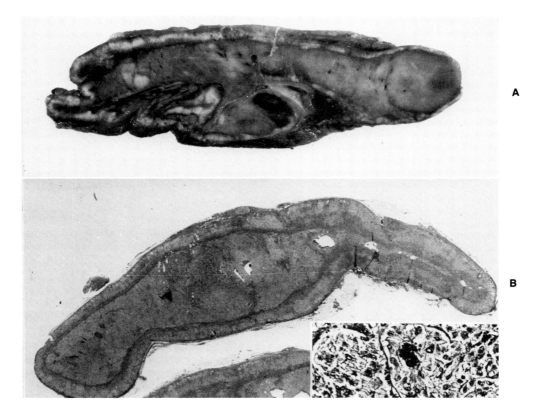

Fig. 16-19 A, Adrenal medullary hyperplasia in patient with MEA, 2B. Several pheochromocytomas have arisen in this background, largest being evident on right pole of specimen. **B,** Microscopic appearance of adrenal medullary hyperplasia. **Inset** shows nesting appearance of medullary cells. (**A,** Courtesy Dr. J. Costa, Lausanne, Switzerland. **B,** Courtesy Dr. J.A. Carney, Rochester, MN.)

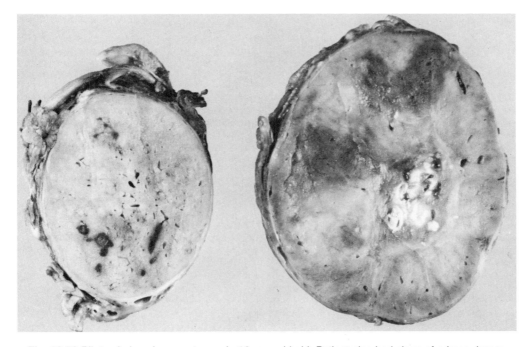

Fig. 16-20 Bilateral pheochromocytomas in 12-year-old girl. Patient also had signs of primary hyperparathyroidism.

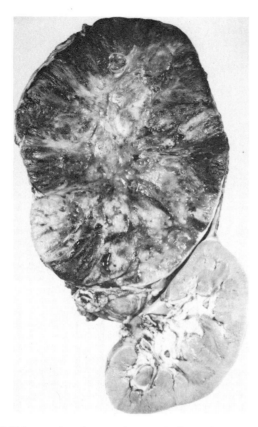

Fig. 16-21 Large pheochromocytoma replacing entire adrenal gland and displacing kidney. Tumor is encapsulated, or variegated in appearance, and focally hemorrhagic.

Pheochromocytomas may be associated with neurofibromatosis,[173] renal artery stenosis due to dysplasia,[164,182] paragangliomas of other sites,[167] adrenal cortical tumors,[195] or cerebellar hemangioblastomas.[185] Many familial cases have been described.[169] When compared to the sporadic examples, they tend to occur in a younger age group, are more commonly bilateral, and are more frequently associated with other primary neoplasms.[198] Familial cases of pheochromocytoma may be seen as a component of MEA, type IIA (Sipple's syndrome) or type IIB or III (Gorlin's syndrome)[162,192] (see Chapter 15). The weight of these tumors ranges from a few grams to 2,000 g. They are encapsulated, usually soft, and, on section, yellowish white to reddish brown (Fig. 16-21). They are extremely well vascularized and can be well demonstrated by selective arteriography (Fig. 16-22). The larger tumors often have areas of necrosis, hemorrhage, and cyst formation. The adrenal gland usually is compressed or incorporated within the tumor.

Microscopically, the tumor cells are characteristically arranged in well-defined nests ("zellballen") bound by a delicate fibrovascular stroma, which may contain amyloid.[195a] The cells vary considerably in size and shape and have a finely granular and basophilic or eosinophilic cytoplasm. The nuclei are usually round or oval with prominent nucleoli and may contain inclusion-like structures resulting from deep cytoplasmic invaginations[163] (Fig. 16-23). Lipid accumulation may develop in the cytoplasm and lead to confusion with an adrenal cortical tumor both on gross and light microscopic examination.[189] Nuclear gigantism and hyper-

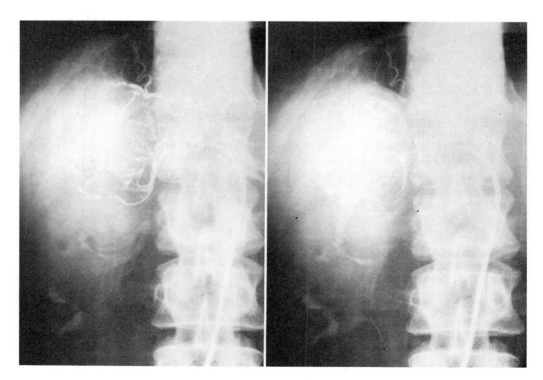

Fig. 16-22 Arteriographic demonstration of adrenal pheochromocytoma, early and late arterial phases. Latter shows typical "tumor stain." (From Meaney TF, Buonocore E: Selective arteriography as a localizing and provocative test in the diagnosis of pheochromocytoma. Radiology **87**:309-314, 1966.)

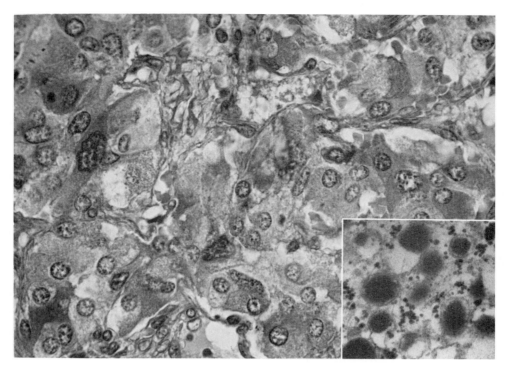

Fig. 16-23 Pheochromocytoma composed of nests of large tumor cells separated by well-vascularized stroma. Some of cells have huge hyperchromatic nuclei. Prominent cytoplasmic granularity is present due to positive reaction to chromate salts. **Inset** shows dense-core granules as seen within cytoplasm of tumor cells on ultrastructural examination.

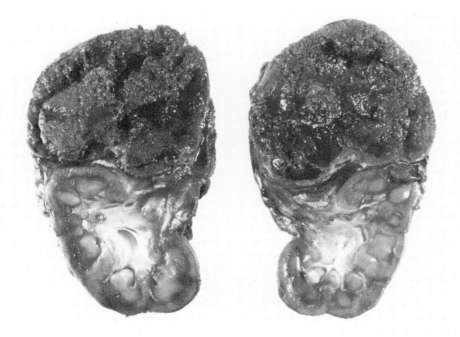

Fig. 16-24 Massive adrenal hemorrhage in newborn. It is possible that at least some of these lesions represent neuroblastomas that have undergone massive hemorrhagic necrosis. (Courtesy Dr. J. Costa, Lausanne, Switzerland.)

chromasia are common and *are not* an expression of malignancy. As a matter of fact, we know of no reliable morphologic markers of malignancy for this tumor other than the presence of metastases. As a group, however, malignant pheochromocytomas are usually larger, have more necrosis, and are composed of smaller cells than their benign counterparts.[181] Flow cytometric determination of DNA promises to provide extremely useful prognostic information.[168]

When pheochromocytoma is immersed in dichromate solution, it takes on a characteristic dark-brown appearance. This is the base of the chromaffin reaction. It should be emphasized that in order to obtain consistent results, the tumor tissue should be fresh and the pH of the dichromate solution kept between 5 and 6.[171] By electron microscopic study, granules of norepinephrine and epinephrine type are present.[161,196] Adipose tissue of the brown (hibernating) type is often found surrounding the tumor capsule,[182] but there is some question as to whether the two processes are related.[180]

Isolated ganglion cells are sometimes found in pheochromocytoma. More rarely, a tumor will be found composed of a mixture of pheochromocytoma and ganglioneuroma or ganglioneuroblastoma, a finding not surprising in view of the close histogenetic relationship of the cell lines.[184] The immunohistochemical features correspond to those of the respective cell types.[196a]

Immunohistochemically, pheochromocytoma cells are always reactive for catecholamines, catecholamine-synthesizing enzymes, neuron-specific enolase, chromogranins, synaptophysin, and opioid peptides (met-enkephalin, leu-enkephalin, beta-endorphin, dynosphin B, and others).[161a,182a] They can also show positivity for neurofilaments, serotonin, somatostatin, calcitonin, gastrin, substance P, vasoactive intestinal peptide, growth hormone–releasing factor, and other neuron-related markers.* Occasionally, the tumor may secrete ACTH and result in Cushing's syndrome[174] or produce parathormone and result in hypercalcemia.[194] A second cell component of pheochromocytoma is represented by the sustentacular cells, which form a peripheral coat around the "zellballen" and which are strongly reactive for S-100 protein. These cells are more numerous in the pheochromocytomas associated with MEA than in the sporadic examples of this tumor.[177]

The previously mentioned chromogranin comprises a group of acidic polypeptides of various sizes that form a major part of the soluble proteins in the secretory granules of the adrenal medulla: A, B, and C (also known as secretogranin II).[193] The largest of these polypeptides is chromogranin A[199]; the plasma concentration of this substance is usually elevated in pheochromocytoma and other peptide-producing neoplasms, a feature of great diagnostic utility.[186] The clinical signs and symptoms of the hormonally active pheochromocytoma derive from the catecholamines they secrete (predominantly epinephrine) and on their relative stimulation of alpha- or beta-adrenergic receptors. Hypertensive attacks are usually intermittent but at times may be sustained, particularly in children.[183] They may be precip-

itated by drugs, anesthetic agents, parturition, surgery for an unrelated condition, or massaging of the tumor.[162] The symptomatic triad of sweating attacks, tachycardia, and headaches is virtually diagnostic of pheochromocytoma. Confirmation of the diagnosis is usually obtained by measuring urinary catecholamines or their catabolites, vanilmandelic acid, and total metanephrines.[190] Provocative pharmacologic tests are used only when the biochemical results are equivocal.[162] The localization of the tumor is currently best achieved by CT scanning, which is highly sensitive and has all but eliminated the need for arteriography in most cases. The high secretion of catecholamines by these tumors may result in myocarditis and noncardiac pulmonary edema.[172] Malignant pheochromocytomas have a marked tendency to metastasize to the skeletal system, particularly ribs and spine, often to the exclusion of other organs. Because of this, a preoperative bone scan is recommended in all patients suspected of having a pheochromocytoma. Most patients with metastatic pheochromocytoma die within 1 year of diagnosis, but long-term relapse-free survival is possible for the locally invasive neoplasms.[176,181]

OTHER ADRENAL LESIONS

Massive *adrenal hemorrhage* can occur in infants within the first few days after delivery; it may present as an abdominal or retroperitoneal mass, septicemia, or adrenal insufficiency.[209] In the first instance, surgery is indicated to rule out the possibility of neuroblastoma.[212] This differential diagnosis also applies to the surgical and pathologic findings, since neuroblastoma can undergo marked hemorrhagic necrosis (Fig. 16-24). Massive adrenal hemorrhage also must be distinguished from renal vein thrombosis. This hemorrhage can be unilateral (especially on the right side) or affect both glands; if the patient survives, calcification rapidly develops around its periphery.[204] The postulated causes include fetal hypoxia, septicemia, thrombocytopenia, coagulopathies, and disseminated thromboembolic disease.

Cysts arising in the adrenal gland can be clinically confused with a retroperitoneal neoplasm because of their occasionally large size (up to 30 cm in diameter.)[207] They are sometimes bilateral. Microscopically, the wall is composed of partially calcified fibrous tissue without an epithelial lining. The content may be cloudy or blood-colored fluid. The mechanism of formation remains controversial. Massive adrenal hemorrhage, vascular malformation or tumor, and cystic degeneration of a primary adrenal neoplasm have been postulated.[200,211,213]

Adrenal cytomegaly refers to the presence in the adrenal cortex of foci of bizarre polyhedral cells with eosinophilic granular cytoplasm and large hyperchromatic nuclei with pseudoinclusions. This condition is usually detected in infancy, often as a component of Beckwith's syndrome; it is not likely to be seen as a surgical specimen.[217]

Presence of *foreign tissue* in the adrenal gland is very unusual. This includes *liver tissue* (usually resulting from adrenohepatic fusion but sometimes as a separate nodule)[214] and stromal spindle-cell foci resembling *ovarian stroma* or *theca*. The latter appear as multiple, often bilateral, wedge-shaped microscopic and occasionally grossly visible nodules

---

*See references 160, 165, 175, 178, 179, 187, 190a, 191, and 197.

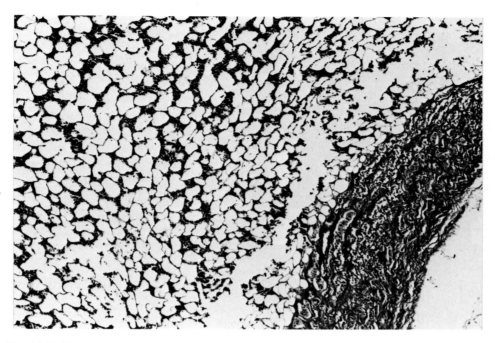

Fig. 16-25 Myelolipoma of adrenal gland. Lesion is largely composed of fat, but it also contains hematopoietic elements.

in the adrenal cortex.[206a] Most patients are postmenopausal women, and no clinical significance is attributed to the nodules,[210] except for their possible role in the genesis of a questionable theca–granulosa cell tumor.[220] *Leydig cells* containing Reinke's crystalloids have also been described in several adrenal disorders,[214] and a few cases of adrenal *Leydig cell tumor* accompanied by virilization are on record.[221]

Tuberculosis of the adrenals is one of the classic causes of Addison's disease; the glands are enlarged, calcified, and massively replaced by granulomatous inflammation.[215]

A case of **malakoplakia** involving the adrenal gland and colon was reported in a 6-week old infant[224] and another was seen in an adult woman with *E. coli* infection.[202]

Myelolipoma is a lesion characterized by the presence within the adrenal gland of adult fat containing active bone marrow elements[219] (Fig. 16-25). Most cases are found incidentally, either at autopsy or through CT scanning done for other reasons. Only occasionally will the lesion attain a size large enough to become clinically apparent.[205,218,225] It is usually unilateral and hormonally inactive, most of the patients being obese adults. Traumatic rupture leading to retroperitoneum may supervene.[216] Myelolipoma has been seen in association with adrenal cortical tumors accompanied by Cushing's syndrome[203] (see p. 791) and with congenital adrenal hyperplasia.[208] A case of pure adrenal myelolipoma associated with Cushing's disease has been reported by Bennett et al.[203] In contrast to other extramedullary foci of hematopoiesis in adults (which are usually an expression of a hematologic disease), adrenal myelolipoma is practically always accompanied by a normal bone marrow.

Rare benign tumors of the adrenal gland include lipoma, angioma, and schwannoma.[201]

Malignant lymphoma involving the adrenal gland is usually a manifestation of widespread disease; exceptionally, it may result in adrenal insufficiency.[206,222]

Metastatic tumors to the adrenal glands are very common at autopsy but sometimes also present as surgical specimens simulating a primary adrenal neoplasm. Bilaterality is the rule. CT scanning is the method of choice for their detection. If extensive enough, they will lead to Addison's disease.[223] The most common sites of the primary tumor are lung, breast, skin (melanoma), and kidney.

TUMORS OF OTHER PARAGANGLIA

The paraganglion system is formed by numerous collections of neuroepithelial cells scattered throughout the body,[235,295,299] their common morphologic denominator being the presence in their cytoplasm of numerous neurosecretory granules containing catecholamines.[232] The most conspicuous member of the group is the adrenal medulla, a neuroeffector system connected with the orthosympathetic systems. Extra-adrenal paraganglia can be divided in two broad categories: those related to the parasympathetic system (ninth, tenth, and possibly third and fifth nerves) and those connected with the orthosympathetic system. The former are usually nonchromaffin, are concentrated in the head, neck, and mediastinum, and seem to have a chemoreceptor function. The latter are chromaffin, predominate in the retroperitoneum along the thoracolumbar para-aortic region, and probably represent lesser homologues of the adrenal medulla. Sometimes, small nests of paraganglion cells are

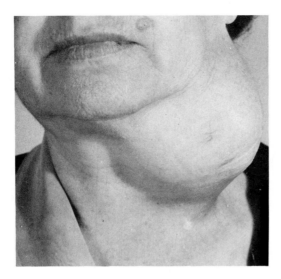

Fig. 16-26 Large, pulsating paraganglioma (carotid body tumor) in neck that had been present for many years. There were symptoms of obstruction. (Courtesy Dr. J.B. Brown, St. Louis, MO.)

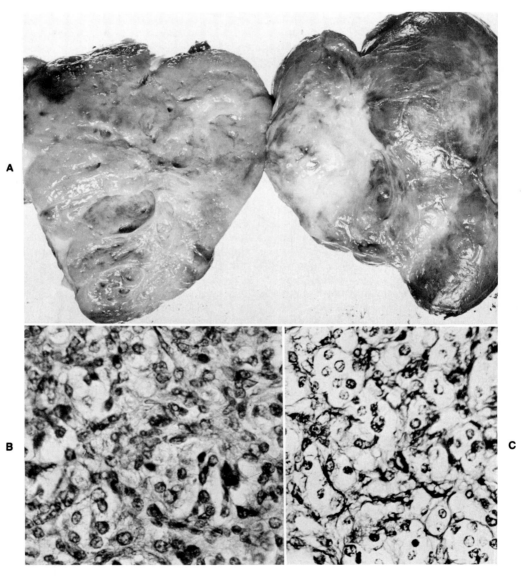

Fig. 16-27 Tumor shown in Fig. 16-26 was resected, and it was found necessary to remove segment of carotid artery. Gross specimen illustrated encapsulated neoplasm. It had vascular, grayish pink color and weighed 140 g. **B,** Same tumor illustrated in **A** showing its cellularity, organoid pattern, and lack of mitotic activity. **C,** Same tumor illustrated in **A** stained with Wilder reticulin stain. Note that nests of tumor cells are encircled by reticulin fibers.

found incidentally in sites such as the bladder, prostate, gallbladder, splenic capsule, and mesosigmoid.[240] Special care should be exercised not to confuse them with metastatic carcinoma.[265]

Tumors arising from these structures are best called *paragangliomas*.[226] The term *chemodectoma* is too restrictive since it can be properly applied only to carotid and aortic body tumors. Paragangliomas that are obviously chromaffin and are associated with clinical evidence of norepinephrine and/or epinephrine secretion also have been designated as *extra-adrenal pheochromocytomas*. It is likely that most of the latter arise from orthosympathetic-related paraganglia, whereas most of the nonchromaffin, nonfunctioning tumors probably originate from parasympathetic-related organs. Unfortunately, it is often impossible on morphologic grounds to distinguish between these two types or to predict whether a tumor is functioning or not.[242,264]

Paragangliomas have been found in practically every site in which normal paraganglia are known to occur, their description sometimes preceding that of the corresponding normal structure (Fig. 16-26). Paragangliomas of the head and neck (particularly carotid body tumors) are about ten times more frequent in persons living at high altitudes than at sea level[280,284]; these have been invariably benign and may actually represent exaggerated examples of the well-known hyperplastic changes that consistently occur in these organs when they are exposed to prolonged and severe hypoxic stimulation.[228,258] A definite familial incidence has been detected.[234] Paragangliomas occurring bilaterally, affecting two or more paraganglia simultaneously, involving a given area in a diffuse or multicentric fashion ("paragangliomatosis") associated with von Hippel–Lindau disease, or as a component of multiple endocrine adenomatosis have been reported.[252,256] Carney et al.[233] have identified a syndrome characterized by the exotic association of extra-adrenal paraganglioma, gastric leiomyosarcoma, and pulmonary chondroma. Most of the cases have occurred in young females.[276]

The gross and microscopic appearance of paragangliomas is practically the same regardless of location and indistinguishable from that of adrenal pheochromocytoma (Fig. 16-27). Well-defined nests of cuboidal cells ("zellballen") are separated by highly vascularized fibrous septa. The individual cells have a moderately abundant granular cytoplasm. As with many other endocrine tumors, bizarre nuclei and vascular invasion are sometimes found. They should not be taken as evidence of malignancy. Mitoses are exceptional. Argentaffin cells can be regularly demonstrated by the del Rio Hortega techniques,[229] but only rarely with the Fontana-Masson or Masson-Hamperl methods as applied to paraffin-embedded material. Argyrophilia is more easily demonstrable in routinely processed material.[261] Treatment of freeze-dried preparations or tumor imprints with formaldehyde vapors or glyoxylic acid induces a bright fluorescence indicative of catecholamines.[237,278]

Ultrastructurally, the tumor cells contain large numbers of cytoplasmic neurosecretory granules of similar appearance to those seen in normal paraganglia[231,244,296] (Fig. 16-28, *A*). A second cell type is the sustentacular cell, which

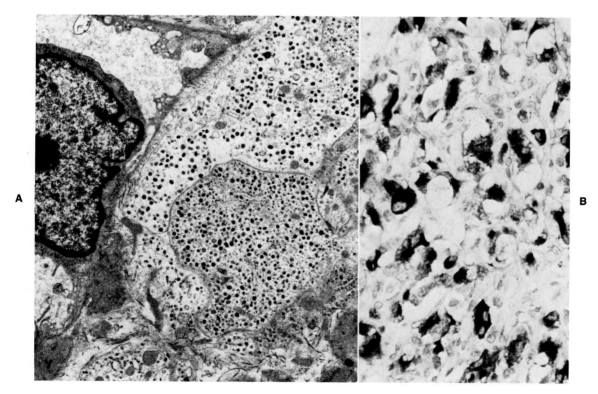

Fig. 16-28 A, Electron microscopic appearance of retroperitoneal paraganglioma, characterized by tumor cells with uniform, small, dense-core granules. Tumor cells are in close proximity to capillary vessels. **B,** Intense immunocytochemical positivity for chromogranin in chief cells of paraganglioma.

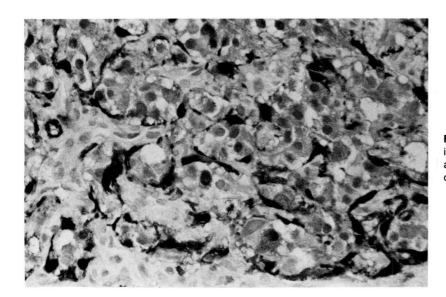

Fig. 16-29 Immunoperoxidase stain for S-100 protein in paraganglioma of glomus jugulare. The "zellballen" are surrounded by S-100 protein-positive sustentacular cells.

wraps around the chief cells and lacks dense-core granules. Biochemical assays of the tumor have confirmed the presence of norepinephrine and sometimes also of epinephrine and dopamine.[236,275] Immunohistochemically, positivity has been found for neuron-specific enolase, chromogranin, synaptophysin, neurofilaments, opioid peptides, serotonin, somatostatin, and a variety of other peptide hormones (Fig. 16-28, *B*).[246a,283,296] Occasional positivity for keratin has also been encountered.[254] The sustentacular cells can be demonstrated with a stain for S-100 protein, a feature of importance in the differential diagnosis from other endocrine neoplasms (Fig. 16-29).[285]

Most paragangliomas follow a benign clinical course. The quoted incidence of malignancy is in the range of 10% — i.e., similar to that of adrenal pheochromocytomas.[246,297] However, as in the latter, long-term follow-up studies suggest that the real incidence of malignancy may be higher, at least for some locations.[272] There are no reliable morphologic criteria by which to separate microscopically the benign from the malignant forms, although high mitotic activity and decreased immunohistochemical reactivity for neuropeptides correlates with clinical malignancy.[261,264a]

Carotid body paragangliomas constitute the most common and important group of extra-adrenal paragangliomas.[239,259,271,286] They are located at the bifurcation of the common carotid artery and become closely adherent to it (see Figs. 16-26 and 16-27). This firm adherence is often misinterpreted by the surgeon as a sign of malignancy. Arteriography demonstrates them particularly well because of their rich vascularity. Often the clinical diagnosis is not made until the paraganglioma's characteristic location is determined at surgery. The high operative risk and high morbidity formerly associated with the removal of a carotid body tumor have been markedly reduced as a result of improved surgical techniques and the use of arterial substitutes.[267] Consequently, early surgical resection is now advocated.[269a]

About 10% of these tumors have behaved in a malignant fashion. This may be manifested as local invasion or met-

astatic spread, particularly to lymph nodes and lung.[266,277,279] The possibility of multicentric paragangliomas should always be considered before concluding that a given tumor has metastasized.[293]

Jugulotympanic paragangliomas are often referred to as *glomus jugulare tumors*. It is better to avoid the term *glomus tumor* in order to prevent confusion with the totally unrelated neoplasm that goes by this name and that arises from specialized smooth muscle cells of the blood vessel wall. Jugulotympanic paragangliomas usually arise laterally in the temporal bones and, through erosion of the floor of the hypotympanum, present as a mass in the middle ear or the external auditory canal.[263,282,287] In other instances, they are located in the adventitia of the jugular bulb and present as a mass at the base of the skull, causing enlargement of the jugular foramen. Rarely, these tumors appear as pedunculated middle ear polyps arising from the cochlear promontory. Extension into the cranial cavity occurs in about 40% of the cases. Most cases occur in adults. There is a striking predilection for females, a fact not apparent for paragangliomas in other locations. Angiographic examination is of great diagnostic value; at surgery, marked bleeding may be encountered. Microscopically, the appearance is similar to that of other paragangliomas, but since these tumors are often removed in small fragments, the artifacts present may render the diagnosis difficult or even impossible. We have seen several cases misdiagnosed as hemangiomas. The recommended treatment is surgical removal followed by external megavoltage radiation.[247] Radiation therapy alone is often inadequate.[290]

Vagal (intravagal) paragangliomas are characteristically located in the anterolateral portion of the neck, near the jugular foramen, and are thought to arise from the paraganglion intravagale, adjacent to the ganglion nodosum.[248,254a,256,269,291] They also can occur at other points along the peripheral distribution of the vagus nerve. The majority are well circumscribed and easily removable, but others may invade locally and even result in intracranial infiltration through the jugular foramen. Hyalinized fibrous septa, continuous with the perineurium of the vagus nerve, are often prominent. A few cases with regional lymph node and/or distant metastases have been observed.[289]

Mediastinal paragangliomas, for the most part, originate in the supra-aortic or aorticopulmonary bodies and are therefore found in the anterosuperior portion of the mediastinum, in the area of the aortic arch.[262,274,298] Others originate from aorticosympathetic paraganglia and are located in the costovertebral sulcus. Olson and Salyer[272] reviewed the literature on aortic body tumors and found a high incidence of aggressive tumor growth in the mediastinum, with resultant important morbidity or death in sixteen of thirty-five cases. Supporting this contention, a patient with aortic body tumor whom we reported in 1965[281] presented with recurrent, highly aggressive, and histologically malignant tumor 15 years following excision.

Retroperitoneal paragangliomas can occur anywhere along the paravertebral chain, sometimes in close proximity to the adrenal gland.[261,273]

Paragangliomas of Zuckerkandl's body are found in the normal location of this structure, i.e., close to the angle formed by the anterior wall of the aorta and the origin of the inferior mesenteric artery.[227,241,270]

Other locations where paragangliomas have been described include cavernous sinus,[250] orbit,[292] tongue,[230] nose and paranasal cavities,[260,294] larynx and trachea,[260,301] thyroid,[245] heart,[238,253] gallbladder,[268] urinary bladder,[243] uterus,[300] and cauda equina.[251] Some of these are discussed with their respective organs. Paragangliomas have also been described in the duodenum,[255] lung,[249,257] and pineal gland,[288] but the placement of these tumors in this category is questionable. Alveolar soft part sarcoma, a tumor once designated as malignant nonchromaffin paraganglioma, is probably unrelated to this group of tumors (see Chapter 25).

REFERENCES
INTRODUCTION

1 Berkman WA, Bernardino ME, Sewell CW, Price RB, Sones PJ Jr: The computed tomography–guided adrenal biopsy. An alternative to surgery in adrenal mass diagnosis. Cancer 53:2098-2103, 1984.

2 Katz RL, Patel S, Mackay B, Zornoza J: Fine needle aspiration cytology of the adrenal gland. Acta Cytol [Baltimore] 28:269-282: 1984.

3 O'Neal LW: Surgery of the adrenal glands. St. Louis, 1968, The C.V. Mosby Co.

4 Symington T: Functional pathology of the human adrenal gland, Baltimore, 1969, The Williams & Wilkins Co.

LESIONS OF ADRENAL CORTEX
Heterotopia

5 Dahl EV, Bahn RC: Aberrant adrenal cortical tissue near the testis in human infants. Am J Pathol 40:587-598, 1962.

6 Grhama LS: Celiac accessory adrenal glands. Cancer 6:149-152, 1953.

7 Johnson RE, Scheithauer B: Massive hyperplasia of testicular adrenal rests in a patient with Nelson's syndrome. Am J Clin Pathol 77:501-507, 1982.

8 Nelson AA: Accessory adrenal cortical tissue. Arch Pathol 27:955-965, 1939.

9 Vestfrid MA: Ectopic adrenal cortex in neonatal liver. Histopathology 4:669-672, 1980.

Cortical nodule

10 Commons, RR, Callaway, CP: Adenomas of the adrenal cortex. Arch Intern Med 81:37-41, 1948.

11 Nevile A: The nodular adrenal. Invest Cell Pathol 1:99-111, 1978.

Congenital hyperplasia

12 Georgitis WJ: Clinically silent congenital adrenal hyperplasia masquerading as ectopic adrenocorticotropic hormone syndrome. Am J Med 80:703-708, 1986.

13 Hsia D Y-Y: Inborn errors of metabolism. I. Clinical aspects. Chicago, 1966, Year Book Medical Publishers, Inc., pp. 245-255.

14 Jones HW Jr, Verkauf BS: Surgical treatment in congenital adrenal hyperplasia. Age at operation and other prognostic factors. Obstet Gynecol 36:1-10, 1970.

15 Mininberg DT, Levine LS, New MI: Current concepts in congenital adrenal hyperplasia. Invest Urol 17:169-175, 1979.

16 Mininberg DT, Levine LS, New MI: Current concepts in congenital hyperplasia. Pathol Annu 17(Pt 2):179-195, 1982.

17 New MI: Congenital adrenal hyperplasia. Pediatr Clin North Am 15:395-407, 1968.

18 Sasano H, Masuda T, Ojima M, Fukuchi S, Sasano N: Congenital 17 β-hydroxylase deficiency. A clinicopathologic study. Hum Pathol 18:1002-1007, 1987.

19 White PC, New MI, Dupont B: Congenital adrenal hyperplasia. N Engl J Med 316:1519-1586, 1987.

Acquired hyperplasia

20 Carney JA, Hruska LS, Beauchamp GD, Gordon H: Dominant inheritance of the complex of myxomas, spotty pigmentation, and endocrine overactivity. Mayo Clin Proc 61:165-172, 1986.

20a Hermus AR, Pieters GF, Smals AG, Pesman GJ, Lamberts SW, Benraad TJ, van Haelst UJ, Kloppenborg PW: Transition from pituitary-dependent to adrenal-dependent Cushing's syndrome. N Engl J Med 38:966-970, 1988.

21 Iseli BE, Hedinger Chr E: Histopathology and ultrastructure of primary adrenocortical nodular dysplasia with Cushing's syndrome. Histopathology 9:1171-1193, 1985.

22 Shenoy BV, Carpenter PC, Carney JA: Bilateral primary pigmented nodular adrenocortical disease. Rare cause of the Cushing syndrome. Am J Surg Pathol 8:335-344, 1984.

Adenoma

23 Damron TA, Schelper RL, Sorensen L: Cytochemical demonstration of neuromelanin in black pigmented adrenal nodules. Am J Clin Pathol 87:334-341, 1987.

24 Gandour MJ, Grizzle WE: A small adrenocortical carcinoma with aggressive behavior. An evaluation of criteria for malignancy. Arch Pathol Lab Med 110:1076-1079, 1986.

25 Komiya I, Takasu N, Aizawa T, Yamada T, Koizumi Y, Hashizume K, Ishihara M, Hiramatsu K, Ichikawa K, Katakura M, Kobayashi M, Yamauchi K, Yanagisawa K, Naka M, Miyamoto T: Black (or brown) adrenal cortical adenoma. Its characteristic features on computed tomography and endocrine data. J Clin Endocrinol Metab 61:711-717, 1985.

26 Macadam RF: Black adenoma of the human adrenal cortex. Cancer 27:116-119, 1971.

26a Sasano H, White PC, New MI, Sasano N: Immunohistochemical localization of cytochrome P-450$_{C21}$ in human adrenal cortex and its relation to endocrine function. Hum Pathol 19:181-185, 1988.

27 Schtenigart DE, Oberman HA, Friedman BA, Conn JW: Adrenal cortical neoplasms producing Cushing's syndrome. A clinicopathologic study. Cancer 22:1105-1013, 1968.

28 Sienkowski IK, Watkins RM, Anderson VER: Primary tumorous aldosteronism due to a black adrenal adenoma. A light and electron microscopic study. J Clin Pathol 37:143-149, 1984.

29 Vyberg M, Sestoft L: Combined adrenal myelolipoma and adenoma associated with Cushing's syndrome. Am J Clin Pathol 86:541-545, 1986.

Carcinoma

30 Amberson JB, Vaughan ED, Gray CF, Naus GJ: Flow cytometric analysis of nuclear DNA from adrenocortical neoplasm. A retrospective study using paraffin-embedded tissue. Cancer 59:2091-2095, 1987.

30a Brennan MF: Adrenocortical carcinoma. CA 37:348-365, 1988.

31 Cagle PT, Hough AJ, Pysher TJ, Page DL, Johnson EH, Kirkland RT, Holcombe JH, Hawkins EP: Comparison of adrenal cortical tumors in children and adults. Cancer 57:2235-2237, 1986.

32 Didolkar MS, Bescher RA, Elias EG, Moore RH: Natural history of adrenal cortical carcinoma. A clinicopathologic study of 42 patients. Cancer 47:2153-2161, 1981.

33 Henley DJ, van Heerden JA, Grant CS, Carney JA, Carpenter PC: Adrenal cortical carcinoma—a continuing challenge. Surgery 94:926-931, 1983.

34 Hogan TF, Gilchrist KW, Westring DW, Citrin DL: A clinical and pathological study of adrenocortical carcinoma. Cancer 45:2880-2883, 1980.

35 Hough AJ, Hollifield HW, Page DL, Hartmann WH: Prognostic factors in adrenal cortical tumors. Am J Clin Pathol 72:390-399, 1979.

36 Huvos AG, Hajdu SI, Brasfield RD, Foote FW Jr: Adrenal cortical carcinoma. Clinicopathologic study of 34 cases. Cancer 25:354-361, 1970.

37 Karakousis CP, Rao U, Moore R: Adrenal adenocarcinomas. Histologic grading and survival. J Surg Oncol **29**:105-111, 1985.

38 Kay R, Schumacher OP, Tank ES: Adrenocortical carcinoma in children. J Urol **130**:1130-1132, 1983.

39 Kay S: Hyperplasia and neoplasia of the adrenal gland. Pathol Annu **11**:103-139, 1976.

40 Lipsett MB, Hertz R, Ross GT: Clinical and pathophysiologic aspects of adrenocortical carcinoma. Am J Med **35**:374-383, 1963.

41 McCartney ACE: Metastatic adrenal carcinoma masquerading as primary bronchial carcinoma. Report of two cases. Thorax **39**:315-316, 1984.

42 Miettinen M, Lehto V-P, Virtanen I: Immunofluorescence microscopic evaluation of the intermediate filament expression of the adrenal cortex and medulla and their tumors. Am J Pathol **118**:360-36(, 1985.

43 Nader S, Hickey RC, Sellin RV, Samaan NA: Adrenal cortical carcinoma. A study of 77 cases. Cancer **52**:707-711, 1983.

44 Page DL, Hough AJ, Gray GF: Diagnosis and prognosis of adrenocortical neoplasm. Arch Pathol Lab Med **110**:993-994, 1986.

44a Samaan NA, Hickey RC: Adrenal cortical carcinoma. Semin Oncol **14**:292-296, 1987.

45 Silva EG, Mackay B, Samaan NA, Hickey RC: Adrenocortical carcinomas. An ultrastructural study of 22 cases. Ultrastruct Pathol **3**:1-7, 1982.

46 Slooten HV, Schaberg A, Smeenk D, Moolenaar AJ: Morphologic characteristics of benign and malignant adrenocortical tumors. Cancer **55**:766-773, 1985.

47 Tang CL, Gray GF: Adrenocortical neoplasms. Prognosis and morphology. Urology **5**:691-695, 1975.

48 Taylor SR, Roederer M, Murphy RF: Flow cytometric DNA analysis of adrenocortical tumors in children. Cancer **59**:2059-2063, 1987.

49 Weiss LM: Comparative histologic study of 43 metastasizing and nonmetastasizing adrenocortical tumors. Am J Surg Pathol **8**:163-169, 1984.

50 Wick MR, Cherwitz DL, McGlennen RC, Dehner LP: Adrenocortical carcinoma. An immunohistochemical comparison with renal cell carcinoma. Am J Pathol **122**:343-352, 1986.

51 Wood KF, Lus F, Rosenthal FD: Carcinoma of the adrenal cortex without endocrine effects. Br J Surg **45**:41-50, 1957.

Clinicopathologic correlation

52 Grunberg SM: Development of Cushing's syndrome and virilization after presentation of a nonfunctioning adrenocortical carcinoma. Cancer **50**:815-816, 1982.

53 O'Hare MJ, Monaghan P, Neville A: The pathology of adrenocortical neoplasia. A correlated structural and functional approach to the diagnosis of malignant disease. Hum Pathol **10**:137-154, 1979.

Nonfunctioning lesions

53a Doerr HG, Sippell WG, Drop SLS, Bidlingmaier F, Knorr D: Evidence of 11 beta-hydroxylase deficiency in childhood adrenocortical tumors. The plasma corticosterone / 11-deoxycorticosterone ratio as a possible marker for malignancy. Cancer **60**:1625-1629, 1987.

54 Hedeland H, Östberg G, Hokfelt B: On the prevalence of adrenocortical adenomas in an autopsy material in relation to hypertension and diabetes. Acta Med Scand **184**:211-214, 1968.

55 Huvos AG, Hajdu SI, Brasfield RD, and Foote FW Jr: Adrenal cortical carcinoma. Clinicopathologic study of 34 cases. Cancer **25**:354-361, 1970.

56 Lewinsky BS, Grigor KM, Symington T, Neville AM: The clinical and pathologic features of "nonhormonal" adrenocortical tumors. Report of twenty new cases and review of the literature. Cancer **33**:778-790, 1974.

57 Nicolis GL, Gabrilove JL: Studies on the efficiency of adrenocortical 11 β-hydroxylation in the human subject. J Clin Endocrinol Metab **29**:831-836, 1969.

Aldosteronism

58 Aiba M, Suzuki H, Kageyama K, Murai M, Tazaki H, Abe O, Saruta T: Spironolactone bodies in aldosteromas and in the attached adrenals. Enzyme histochemical study of 19 cases of primary aldosteronism and a case of aldosteronism due to bilateral diffuse hyperplasia of the zona glomerulosa. Am J Pathol **103**:404-410, 1981.

59 Alterman SL, Dominguez C, Lopez-Gomez A, Lieber AL: Primary adrenocortical carcinoma causing aldosteronism. Cancer **24**:602-609, 1969.

60 Banks WA, Kastin AJ, Biglieri EG, Ruiz AE: Primary adrenal hyperplasia. A new subset of primary hyperaldosteronism. J Clin Endocrinol Metab **58**:783-785, 1984.

61 Ganguly A, Donohue JP: Primary aldosteronism. Pathophysiology, diagnosis and treatment. J Urol **129**:241-247, 1983.

62 George JM, Wright L, Bell NH, Bartter FC, Brown R: The syndrome of primary aldosteronism. Am J Med **48**:343-356, 1970.

63 Hogan MJ, McRae J, Schambelan M, Biglieri EG: Location of aldosterone-producing adenomas with ^{131}I-19-iodocholesterol. N Engl J Med **294**:410-414, 1976.

64 Hsu S-M, Raine L, Martin HF: Spironolactone bodies. An immunoperoxidase study with biochemical correlation. Am J Clin Pathol **75**:92-95, 1981.

65 Kano K, Sato S, Hama H: Adrenal adenomata causing primary aldosteronism. An ultrastructural study of twenty-five cases. Virchows Arch [Pathol Anat] **384**:93-102, 1979.

66 Luetscher JA, Weinberger MH, Dowdy AJ, Nokes TW: Effects of sodium loading, sodium depletion and posture on plasma aldosterone concentration and renin activity in hypertensive patients. J Clin Endocrinol Metab **29**:1310-1318, 1969.

67 Neville AM, Symington T: Pathology of primary aldosteronism. Cancer **19**:1854-1868, 1966.

68 O'Neal LW, Kissane JM, Hartroft PM: The kidney in endocrine hypertension. Cushing's syndrome, pheochromocytoma and aldosteronism. Arch Surg **100**:498-505, 1970.

69 Reidbord H, Fisher ER: Aldosteronoma and nonfunctioning adrenal cortical adenoma. Comparative ultrastructural study. Arch Pathol **88**:155-161, 1969.

70 Shrago SS, Waisman J, Cooper PH: Spironolactone bodies in an adrenal adenoma. Arch Pathol **99**:416-420, 1975.

71 Slee PHTHJ, Schaberg A, Van Brummelen P: Carcinoma of the adrenal cortex causing primary hyperaldosteronism. A case report and review of the literature. Cancer **51**:2341-2345, 1983.

Cushing's syndrome

72 Aron DC, Tyrrell JB, Fitzgerald PA, Findling JW, Forsham PH: Cushing's syndrome. Problems in diagnosis. Medicine [Baltimore] **60**:25-33, 1981.

73 Azzopardi JG, Williams ED: Pathology of "nonendocrine" tumors associated with Cushing's syndrome. Cancer **22**:274-286, 1968.

74 Gilbert MG, Cleveland WW: Cushing's syndrome in infancy. Pediatrics **46**:217-229, 1970.

75 Joffe SN, Brown C: Nodular adrenal hyperplasia and Cushing's syndrome. Surgery **17**:919-925, 1983.

76 Loridan L, Senior B: Cushing's syndrome in infancy. J Pediatr **75**:349-359, 1969.

77 Neville AM, Symington T: The pathology of the adrenal gland in Cushing's syndrome. J Pathol Bacteriol **93**:19-35, 1967.

78 Neville AM, Symington T: Bilateral adrenocortical hyperplasia in children with Cushing's syndrome. J Pathol **107**:95-106, 1972.

79 Reidbord H, Fisher ER: Electron microscopic study of adrenal cortical hyperplasia in Cushing's syndrome. Arch Pathol **86**:419-426, 1968.

80 Schteingart DE, Oberman HA, Friedman BA, Conn JW: Adrenal cortical neoplasms producing Cushing's syndrome. A clinicopathologic study. Cancer **22**:1005-1013, 1968.

81 Scott HW, Abumrad NN, Orth DN: Tumors of the adrenal cortex and Cushing's syndrome. Ann Surg **201**:586-594, 1985.

82 Smals AGH, Pieters GFFM, Van Haelst UJG, Kloppenborg PWC: Macronodular adrenocortical hyperplasia on long-standing Cushing's disease. J Clin Endocrinol Metab **58**:25-31, 1984.

83 Thomas CG Jr, Smith AT, Griffith JM, Askin FB: Hyperadrenalism in childhood and adolescence. Ann Surg **199**:538-548, 1984.

84 Upton GV, Amatruda TT Jr: Evidence for the presence of tumor peptides with corticotropin-releasing-factor-like activity in the ectopic ACTH syndrome. N Engl J Med **285**:419-424, 1971.

Adrenogenital syndrome

85 Burrington JD, Stephens CA: Virilizing tumors of the adrenal gland in childhood. Report of eight cases. J Pediatr Surg **4**:291-302, 1969.

86 Gabrilove JL, Sharma DC, Wotiz HH, Dorfman RI: Feminizing adrenocortical tumors in the male. A review of 52 cases including a case report. Medicine (Baltimore) **44**:37-79, 1965.

87 Heinbecker P, O'Neal LW, Ackerman LV: Functioning and nonfunctioning adrenal cortical tumors. Surg Gynecol Obstet **105**:21-33, 1957.

88 Kenny FM, Hashida Y, Askari HA, Sieber WH, Fetterman GH: Virilizing tumors of the adrenal cortex. Am J Dis Child **115**:445-458, 1968.

89 Patterson J: Diagnosis of adrenal tumours. A new chemical test. Lancet **2**:580-581, 1947.

Other manifestations of carcinoma

90 Falchuk KR: Inappropriate antidiuretic hormone–like syndrome associated with an adrenal carcinoma. Am J Med Sci **266**:393-395, 1973.

91 Lipsett MB, Hertz R, Ross GT: Clinical and pathophysiologic aspects of adrenocortical carcinoma. Am J Med **35**:374-383, 1963.

92 Williams R, Kellie AE, Wade AP, Williams ED, Chalmers TM: Hypoglycaemia and abnormal steroid metabolism in adrenal tumours. Q J Med **30**:269-284, 1961.

LESIONS OF ADRENAL MEDULLA
Tumors of sympathetic nervous system

93 Allan SG, Cornbleet MA, Carmichael J, Arnott SJ, Smyth JF: Adult neuroblastoma. Report of three cases and review of the literature. Cancer **57**:2419-2421, 1986.

94 Anderson HJ, Hariri J: Congenital neuroblastoma in a fetus with multiple malformations. Metastasis in the umbilical cord as a cause of intrauterine death. Virchows Arch [Pathol Anat] **400**:219-222, 1983.

94a Aoyama C, Qualman SJ, Shimada H, Newton WA: Composite ganglioneuroblastoma (C-GNB). Immunohistochemical distinction of stromal components correlates with prognosis (abstract). Lab Invest **58**:5A, 1988.

95 Artlieb U, Krepler R, Wiche G: Expression of microtubule-associated proteins, Map-1 and Map-2, in human neuroblastomas and differential diagnosis of immature neuroblasts. Lab Invest **53**:684-691, 1985.

96 Brodeur GM, Seeger RC, Sather H, Dalton A, Siegel SE, Wong KY, Hammond D: Clinical implications on oncogene activation in human neuroblastomas. Cancer **58**:541-545, 1986.

97 Bunnett N, Reeve JR, Dimaline R, Shively JE, Hawke D, Walsh JH, The isolation and sequence analysis of vasoactive intestinal peptide from a ganglioneuroblastoma. J Clin Endocrinol Metab **59**:1133-1137, 1984.

98 Carlsen NLT, Christensen IJ, Schroeder H, Bro PV, Erichsen G, Hamborg-Pedersen B, Jensen KB, Nielsen OH: Prognostic factors in neuroblastomas treated in Denmark from 1943 to 1980. A statistical estimate of prognosis based on 253 cases. Cancer **58**:2726-2735, 1986.

99 Chandrasoma P, Shibata D, Radin R, Brown LP, Koss M: Malignant peripheral nerve sheath tumor arising in an adrenal ganglioneuroma in an adult male homosexual. Cancer **57**:2022-2025, 1986.

100 Dannecker G, Leidig F, Treuner J, Niethammer D: Late recurrence of neuroblastoma. A reason for prolonged follow-up? Am J Pediatr Hematol Oncol **5**:271-274, 1983.

101 De La Monte SM, Moore GW, Hutchins GM: Nonrandom distribution of metastases in neuroblastic tumors. Cancer **52**:915-925, 1983.

102 DeLellis RA: Formaldehyde-induced fluorescence technique for the demonstration of biogenic amines in diagnostic histopathology. Cancer **28**:1704-1710, 1971.

103 Dranoff G, Bigner DD: A word of caution in the use of neuron-specific enolase expression in tumor diagnosis. Arch Pathol Lab Med **108**:535, 1984.

104 Emery LG, Shields M, Shah NR, Garbes A: Neuroblastoma associated with Beckwith-Wiedemann syndrome. Cancer **52**:176-179, 1983.

105 Evans AE, D'Angio GJ, Koop CE: Diagnosis and treatment of neuroblastoma. Pediatr Clin North Am **23**:161-170, 1976.

106 Fernbach DJ, Williams TE, Donaldson MH: Neuroblastoma. In Sutow WW, Vietti TJ, Fernbach DJ (eds): Clinical pediatric oncology, ed. 2. St. Louis, 1977, The C.V. Mosby Co., pp. 506-537.

107 Fortner J, Nicastri A, Murphy ML: Neuroblastoma. Natural history and results of treating 133 cases. Ann Surg **167**:132-142, 1968.

108 Fu Y, Kaye GI, Lattes R: Primary malignant melanocytic tumors of the sympathetic ganglia, with an ultrastructural study of one. Cancer **36**:2029-2041, 1975.

109 Gansler T, Chatten J, Varello M, Bunin GR, Atkinson B: Flow cytometric DNA analysis of neuroblastoma. Correlation with histology and clinical outcome. Cancer **58**:2453-2458, 1986.

110 Gilbert F, Feder M, Balaban G, Brangman D, Lurie DK, Podolsky R, Rinaldt V, Vinikoor N, Weisband J: Human neuroblastomas and abnormalities of chromosomes 1 and 17. Cancer Res **44**:5444-5449, 1984.

110a Gonzalez-Crussi F, Hsueh W: Bilateral adrenal ganglioneuroblastoma with neuromelanin. Clinical and pathologic observations. Cancer **61**:1159-1166, 1988.

111 Gross RE, Farber S, Martin LW: Neuroblastoma sympatheticum. A study and report of 217 cases. Pediatrics **23**:1179-1191, 1959.

112 Guin GH, Gilbert EF, Jones B: Incidental neuroblastoma in infants. Am J Clin Pathol **51**:126-136, 1969.

113 Hamilton JR, Radde IC, Johnson G: Diarrhea associated with adrenal ganglioneuroma. New findings related to the pathogenesis of diarrhea. Am J Med **44**:453-463, 1968.

114 Hata J-I, Ueyama Y, Nozi H, Tamaoki N, Akatsuka A, Shimizu K, Morikawa Y, Sato K: Morphology and function of human neuroblastoma xenotransplanted in nude mice. Cancer **53**:2497-2506, 1984.

115 Holgersen LO, Santulli TV, Schullinger JN, Berdon WE: Neuroblastoma with intraspinal (dumbbell) extension. J Pediatr Surg **18**:406-411, 1983.

116 Hughes M, Marsden HB, Palmer MK: Histologic patterns of neuroblastoma related to prognosis and clinical staging. Cancer **34**:1706-1711, 1974.

117 Ikeda Y, Lister J, Bouton JM, Buyukpamukcu M: Congenital neuroblastoma, neuroblastoma in situ, and the normal fetal development of the adrenal. J Pediatr Surg **16**:636-644, 1981.

118 Jereb B, Bretsky SS, Vogel R, Helson L: Age and prognosis in neuroblastoma. Review of 112 patients younger than 2 years. Am J Pediatr Hematol Oncol **6**:233-243, 1984.

119 Kay S: Hyperplasia and neoplasia of the adrenal gland. Pathol Annu **11**:103-139, 1976.

120 Kaye JA, Warhol MJ, Kretschmar C, Landsberg L, Frei E III: Neuroblastoma in adults. Three case reports and a review of the literature. Cancer **58**:1149-1157, 1986.

121 Kushner BH, Gilbert F, Helson L: Familial neuroblastoma. Case reports, literature review, and etiologic considerations. Cancer **57**:1887-1893, 1986.

122 Mäkinen J: Microscopic patterns as a guide to prognosis of neuroblastoma in childhood. Cancer **29**:219-228, 1972.

123 Mendelsohn G, Eggleston JC, Olson JL, Said SI, Baylin SB: Vasoactive intestinal peptide and its relationship to ganglion cell differentiation in neuroblastic tumors. Lab Invest **41**:144-149, 1979.

124 Misugi K, Misugi N, Newton WA Jr: Fine structural study of neuroblastoma, ganglioneuroblastoma and pheochromocytoma. Arch Pathol **86**:160-170, 1968.

125 Mukai M, Torikata C, Iri H, Morikawa Y, Shimizu K, Shimoda T, Nukina N, Ihara Y, Kageyama K: Expression of neurofilament triplet proteins in human neural tumors. Am J Pathol **122**:28-35, 1986.

126 Mullins JD: A pigmented differentiating neuroblastoma. A light and ultrastructural study. Cancer **46**:522-528, 1980.

127 Murray MR, Stout AP: Distinctive characteristics of the sympathicoblastoma cultivated in vitro. Am J Pathol **23**:429-442, 1947.

128 Oppedal BR, Brandtzaeg P, Kemshead T: Immunohistochemical differentiation of neuroblastomas from other small round cell neoplasms of childhood using a panel of mono- and polyclonal antibodies. Histopathology **11**:363-374, 1987.

129 Osborn M, Dirk T, Kaser H, Weber K, Altmannsberger M: Immunohistochemical localization of neurofilaments and neuron-specific enolase in 29 cases of neuroblastoma. Am J Pathol **122**:433-442, 1986.

130 Perez CA, Vietti TJ, Ackerman LV, Kulapongs P, Powers WE: Treatment of malignant sympathetic tumors in children. Clinicopathological correlation. Pediatrics **41**:452-462, 1968.

131 Reynolds CP, German DC, Weinberg AG, Smith RG: Catecholamine fluorescence and tissue culture morphology. Am J Clin Pathol **75**:275-282, 1981.

132 Reynolds CP, Smith RG, Frenkel EP: The diagnostic dilemma of the "small round cell neoplasm." Catecholamine fluorescence and tissue culture morphology as markers for neuroblastoma. Cancer **48**:2088-2094, 1981.

133 Robson JA, Sidell N: Ultrastructural features of a human neuroblastoma cell line treated with retinoic acid. Neuroscience **14**:1149-1162, 1985.

134 Sandstedt B, Jereb B, Eklund G: Prognostic factors in neuroblastomas. Acta Pathol Microbiol Immunol Scand [A] **91**:365-371, 1983.

135 Schengrund C-L, Repman MA, Shochat SJ: Ganglioside composition of human neuroblastomas. Correlation with prognosis. A pediatric oncology group study. Cancer **56**:2640-2646, 1985.

136 Seeger RC, Brodeur GM, Sather H, Dalton A, Siegel SE, Wong KY, Hammond D: Association of multiple copies of the N-myc oncogene with rapid progression of neuroblastomas. N Engl J Med **313**:1111-1116, 1985.

137 Seshi B, True L, Carter D, Rosai J: Immunohistochemical characterization of a set of monoclonal antibodies to human neuron-specific enolase. Am J Pathol **131**:258-269, 1988.

137a Sherman S, Roizen N: Fetal hydantoin syndrome and neuroblastoma. Lancet **2**:517, 1976.

138 Shimada H: Transmission and scanning electron microscopic studies on the tumors of neuroblastoma group. Acta Pathol Jpn **32**:415-426, 1982.

139 Shimada H, Aoyama C, Chiba T, Newton WA Jr: Prognostic surgroups for undifferentiated neuroblastoma. Immunohistochemical study with anti-S-100. Hum Pathol **16**:471-476, 1985.

140 Shimada H, Chatten J, Newton JA Jr, Sachs N, Hamoudi AB, Chiba T, Marsden HB, Misugi K: Histopathologic prognostic factors in neuroblastic tumors. Definition of subtypes of ganglioneuroblastoma and an age-linked classification of neuroblastomas. J Natl Cancer Inst **73**:405-416, 1984.

141 Stephenson SR, Cook BA, Mease AD, Ruymann FB: The prognostic significance of age and pattern of metastases in stage IV-S neuroblastoma. Cancer **58**:372-375, 1986.

142 Stokes SH, Thomas PRM, Perez CA, Vietti TJ: Stage IV-S neuroblastoma. Results with definitive therapy. Cancer **53**:2083-2086, 1984.

143 Suzuki H, Honzumi M, Funada M, Tomiyama H: Metachronous bilateral adrenal neuroblastoma. Cancer **56**:1490-1492, 1985.

144 Sy WM, Edmonson JH: The developmental defects associated with neuroblastoma. Etiologic implications. Cancer **22**:234-238, 1968.

145 Thomas PRM, Lee JY, Fineberg BB, Razek AA, Perez CA, Land VJ, Vietti TJ: An analysis of neuroblastoma at a single institution. Cancer **53**:2079-2082, 1984.

146 Triche TJ, Askin FB: Neuroblastoma and the differential diagnosis of small-, round-, blue-cell tumors. Hum Pathol **14**:569-595, 1983.

147 Tsokos M, Linnoila RI, Chandra RS, Triche TJ: Neuron-specific enolase in the diagnosis of neuroblastoma and other small, round-cell tumors in children. Hum Pathol **15**:575-584, 1984.

147a Tsokos M, Scarpa S, Ross RA, Triche TJ: Differentiation of human neuroblastoma recapitulates neural crest development. Study of morphology, neurotransmitter enzymes, and extracellular matrix proteins. Am J Pathol **128**:484-496, 1987.

147b Tsuda T, Obara M, Hirano H, Gotoh S, Kubomura S, Higashi K, Kuroiwa A, Nakagawara A, Nagahara N, Shimizu K: Analysis of N-myc amplification in relation to disease stage and histologic types in human neuroblastomas. Cancer **60**:820-826, 1987.

148 Turkel SB, Itabashi HH: The natural history of neuroblastic cells in the fetal adrenal gland. Am J Pathol **76**:225-244, 1974.

149 Vinores SA, Bonnin YM, Rubinstein LY, Marangos PY: Immunohistochemical demonstration of neuron-specific enolase in neoplasms of the CNS and other tissues. Arch Pathol Lab Med **108**:536-540, 1984.

150 Wilson LMK, Draper GJ: Neuroblastoma, its natural history and prognosis. A study of 487 cases. Br Med J **2**:301-307, 1974.

151 Witzleben CL, Landy RA: Disseminated neuroblastoma in a child with von Recklinghausen's disease. Cancer **34**:786-790, 1974.

152 Wu Z-L, Schwartz E, Seeger R, Ladisch S: Expression of G$_{D2}$ ganglioside by untreated primary human neuroblastomas. Cancer Res **46**:440-443, 1986.

153 Yokoyama M, Okada K, Tokue A, Takayesu H: Ultrastructural and biochemical study of benign ganglioneuroma. Virchows Arch [Pathol Anat] **361**:195-209, 1973.

154 Zeltzer PM, Marangos PJ, Evans AE, Schneider SL: Serum neuron-specific enolase in children with neuroblastoma. Relationship to stage and disease course. Cancer **57**:1230-1234, 1986.

Adrenal medullary hyperplasia

155 Carney JA, Sizemore GW, Sheps SG: Adrenal medullary disease in multiple endocrine neoplasia, type 2. Pheochromocytoma and its precursors. Am J Clin Pathol **66**:279-290, 1976.

156 DeLellis RA, Tischler AS, Lee AK, Blount M, Wolfe HJ: Leu-enkephalin–like immunoreactivity in proliferative lesions of the human adrenal medulla and extra-adrenal paraganglia. Am J Surg Pathol **7**:29-37, 1983.

157 DeLellis RA, Wolfe HJ, Gagel RF, Feldman ZT, Miller HH, Gang DL, Reichlin S: Adrenal medullary hyperplasia. A morphometric analysis in patients with familial medullary thyroid carcinoma. Am J Pathol **83**:117-196, 1976.

158 Kreiner E: Weight and shape of the human adrenal medulla in various age groups. Virchows Arch [Pathol Anat] **397**:7-15, 1982.

159 Visser JW, Axt R: Bilateral adrenal medullary hyperplasia. A clinicopathological entity. J Clin Pathol **28**:298-304, 1975.

Pheochromocytoma

160 Berelowitz M, Szabo M, Barowsky H, Arbel ER, Frohman LA: Somatostatin-like immunoactivity and biological activity is present in a human pheochromocytoma. J Clin Endocrinol Metab **56**:134-138, 1983.

161 Bloom FE: Electron microscopy of catecholamine-containing structures. In Blaschko H, Muschall E (sub eds): Handbook of experimental pharmacology, vol 33, Catecholamines. New York, 1972, Springer-Verlag, New York, Inc., chap. 3, pp. 46-78.

161a Bostwick DG, Null WE, Holmes D, Weber E, Barchas JD, Bensch KG: Expression of opioid peptides in tumors. N Engl J Med **317**:1439-1443, 1987.

162 Bravo EL, Gifford RW: Pheochromocytoma. Diagnosis, localization and management. N Engl J Med **311**:1298-1303, 1984.

163 DeLellis RA, Suchow E, Wolfe HJ: Ultrastructure of nuclear "inclusions" in pheochromocytoma and paraganglioma. Hum Pathol **11**:205-207, 1980.

164 de Mendonca WC, Espat PA: Pheochromocytoma associated with arterial fibromuscular dysplasia. Am J Clin Pathol **75**:749-754, 1981.

165 Hassoun J, Monges G, Giraud P, Henry JF, Charpin C, Payan H, Toga M: Immunohistochemical study of pheochromocytomas. An investigation of methionine-enkephalin, vasoactive intestinal peptide, somatostatin, corticotropin, β-endorphin, and calcitonin in 16 tumors. Am J Pathol **114**:56-63, 1984.

166 Fries JG, Chamberlin JA: Extra-adrenal pheochromocytomas. Literature review and report of cervical pheochromocytoma. Surgery **63**:268-279, 1968.

167 Ganem EJ, Cahill GF: Pheochromocytomas coexisting in adrenal gland and retroperitoneal space, with sustained hypertension. N Engl J Med **238**:692-697, 1948.

168 Hosaka Y, Rainwater LM, Grant CS, Farrow GM, van Heerden JA, Lieber MM: Pheochromocytoma. Nuclear deoxyribonucleic acid patterns studied by flow cytometry. Surgery **10**:1003-1009, 1986.

169 Irvin GL III, Fishman LM, Sher JA: Familial pheochromocytoma. Surgery **96**:938-940, 1984.

170 Kaufman BH, Telander RL, van Heerden JA, Zimmerman D, Sheps SG, Dawson B: Pheochromocytoma in the pediatric age group. Current status. J Pediatr Surg **18**:879-884, 1983.

171 Kennedy JS, Symington T, Woodger BA: Chemical and histochemical observations in benign and malignant phaeochromocytoma. J Pathol Bacteriol **81**:409-418, 1961.

172 Kline IK: Myocardial alterations associated with pheochromocytomas. Am J Pathol **38**:539-551, 1961.

173 Knudson AG Jr, Amromin GD: Neuroblastoma and ganglioneuroma in a child with multiple neurofibromatosis. Implications for the mutational origin of neuroblastoma. Cancer **19**:1032-1037, 1966.

174 Lamovec J, Memoli VA, Terzakis JA, Sommers SC, Gould VE: Pheochromocytoma producing immunoreactive ACTH with Cushing's syndrome. Ultrastruct Pathol **7**:41-48, 1984.

175 Lehto V-P, Virtanen I, Miettinen M, Dahl D, Kahri A: Neurofilaments in adrenal and extra-adrenal pheochromocytoma. Arch Pathol Lab Med **107**:492-494, 1983.

176 Lewi HJE, Reid R, Mucci B, Davidson JK, Kyle KF, MacPherson SG, Semple P, Kaye S: Malignant pheochromocytoma. Brit J Urol **57**:394-398, 1985.

177 Lloyd RV, Blaivas M, Wilson BS: Distribution of chromogranin and S 100 protein in normal and abnormal adrenal medullary tissues. Arch Pathol Lab Med **109**:633-635, 1985.

178 Lloyd RV, Shapiro B, Sisson JC, Kalff V, Thompson NW, Beierwaltes WA: An immunohistochemical study of pheochromocytomas. Arch Pathol Lab Med **108**:541-544, 1984.

179 Lloyd RV, Shapiro B, Sisson JC, Verhofstad AAJ: Immunohistochemical localization of epinephrine, norepinephrine, catecholamine-synthesizing enzymes, and chromogranin in neuroendocrine cells and tumors. Am J Pathol **125**:45-54, 1986.

180 Medeiros LJ, Katsas GG, Balogh K: Brown fat and adrenal pheochromocytoma. Association or coincidence? Hum Pathol **16**:970-972, 1985.

181 Medeiros LJ, Wolf BC, Balogh K, Federman M: Adrenal pheochromocytoma. A clinicopathologic review of 60 cases. Hum Pathol **16**:580-589, 1985.

182 Melicow MM: One hundred cases of pheochromocytoma (107 tumors) at the Columbia-Presbyterian Medical Center, 1926-1976. A clinicopathological analysis. Cancer **40**:1987-2004, 1977.

182a Miettinen M: Synaptophysin and neurofilament proteins as markers for neuroendocrine tumors. Arch Pathol Lab Med **111**:813-818, 1987.

183 Moore TC, Shumacker HB: Adrenalin-producing tumors in childhood. Ann Surg **143**:256-265, 1956.

184 Nakagawara A, Ikeda K, Tsuneyoshi M, Daimaru Y, Enjoji M: Malignant pheochromocytoma with ganglioneuroblastomatous elements in a patient with von Recklinghausen's disease. Cancer **55**:2794-2798, 1985.

185 Nibbelink DW, Peters BH, McCormick WF: On the association of pheochromocytoma and cerebellar hemangioblastoma. Neurology **19**:455-460, 1969.

186 O'Connor DT, Deftos LJ: Secretion of chromogranin A by peptide-producing endocrine neoplasms. N Engl J Med **314**:1145-1151, 1986.

187 O'Connor DT, Frigon RP, Deftos LJ: Immunoreactive calcitonin in catecholamine storage vesicles of human pheochromocytoma. J Clin Endocrinol Metab **56**:582-585, 1983.

188 Parkinson D: Intracranial pheochromocytomas (active glomus jugulare). Case report. J Neurosurg **31**:94-100, 1969.

189 Ramsay JA, Asa SL, van Nostrand AWP, Hassaram ST, de Harven EP: Lipid degeneration in pheochromocytomas mimicking adrenal cortical tumors. Am J Surg Pathol **11**:480-486, 1987.

190 Samaan NA, Hickey RC: Pheochromocytoma. Semin Oncol **14**:297-305, 1987.

190a Sano T, Saito H, Inaba H, Hizawa K, Saito S, Yamanoi A, Mizunuma Y, Matsumura M, Yuasa M, Hiraishi K: Immunoreactive somatostatin and vasoactive intestinal polypeptide in adrenal pheochromocytoma. Cancer **52**:282-289, 1983.

191 Sano T, Saito H, Yamasaki R, Hosoi E, Kameyama K, Saito S, Hirose T, Hizawa K: Production and secretion of immunoreactive growth hormone–releasing factor by pheochromocytomas. Cancer **57**:1788-1793, 1986.

192 Sarosi G, Doe RP: Familial occurrence of parathyroid adenomas, pheochromocytoma, and medullary carcinoma of the thyroid with amyloid stroma (Sipple's syndrome). Ann Intern Med **68**:1305-1309, 1968.

193 Schober M, Fischer-Colbrie R, Schmid KW, Bussolati G, O'Connor DT, Winkler H: Comparison of chromogranins A, B, and secretogranin II in human adrenal medulla and pheochromocytoma. Lab Invest 57:385-391, 1987.

193a Scott HW, Halter SA: Oncologic aspects of pheochromocytoma. The importance of follow-up. Surgery 96:1061-1066, 1984.

194 Shanberg AM, Baghdassarian R, Tansey LA, Bacon D, Greenberg P, Perley M: Pheochromocytoma with hypercalcemia. Case report and review of literature. J Urol 133:258-259, 1985.

195 Sparagana M, Feldman JM, Molnar Z: An unusual pheochromocytoma associated with an androgen-secreting adrenocortical adenoma. Evaluation of its polypeptide hormone, catecholamine, and enzyme characteristics. Cancer 60:223-231, 1987.

195a Steinhoff MM, Wells SA Jr, DeSchryver-Kecskemeti K: Interstitial amyloid in pheochromocytomas (abstract). Lab Invest 58:87A, 1988.

196 Tannenbaum M: Ultrastructural pathology of adrenal medullary tumors. In Sommers SC (ed): Pathology annual, New York, 1970, Appleton-Century-Crofts, pp. 145-172.

196a Tischler AS, Dayal Y, Balogh K, Cohen RB, Connolly JL, Tallberg K: The distribution of immunoreactive chromogranins, S-100 protein, and vasoactive intestinal peptide in compound tumors of the adrenal medulla. Hum Pathol 18:909-917, 1987.

197 Trojanowski JQ, Lee VM-Y: Expression of neurofilament antigens by normal and neoplastic human adrenal chromaffin cells. N Engl J Med 313:101-104, 1985.

198 Wilson RA, Ibanez ML: A comparative study of 14 cases of familial and non-familial pheochromocytomas. Hum Pathol 9:181-188, 1978.

199 Wilson BS, Lloyd RV: Detection of chromogranin in neuroendocrine cells with a monoclonal antibody. Am J Pathol 115:458-468, 1984.

OTHER ADRENAL LESIONS

200 Abell MR, Hart WR, Olson JR: Tumors of the peripheral nervous system. Hum Pathol 1:503-551, 1970.

201 Bedard YC, Horvath E, Kovacs K: Adrenal schwannoma with apparent uptake of immunoglobulins. Ultrastruct Pathol 10:505-513, 1986.

202 Benjamin E, Fox H: Malakoplakia of the adrenal gland. J Clin Pathol 34:606-611, 1981.

203 Bennett BD, McKenna TJ, Hough AJ, Dean R, Page DL: Adrenal myelolipoma associated with Cushing's disease. Am J Clin Pathol 73:443-447, 1980.

204 Black J, Williams DI: Natural history of adrenal haemorrhage in the newborn. Arch Dis Child 48:183-190, 1973.

205 Boudreaux D, Waisman J, Skinner DG, and Low R: Giant adrenal myelolipoma and testicular interstitial cell tumor in a man with congenital 21-hydroxylase deficiency. Am J Surg Pathol 3:109-123, 1979.

206 Carey RW, Harris N, Kliman B: Addison's disease secondary to lymphomatous infiltration of the adrenal glands. Cancer 59:1087-1090, 1987.

206a Carney JA: Unusual tumefactive spindle-cell lesions in the adrenal glands. Hum Pathol 18:980-985, 1987.

207 Cheema P, Cartagena R, Staubitz W: Adrenal cysts. Diagnosis and treatment. J Urol 126:396-399, 1981.

208 Condom E, Villabona CM, Gomez JM, Carrera M: Adrenal myelolipoma in a woman with congenital 17-hydroxylase deficiency. Arch Pathol Lab Med 109:1116-1118, 1985.

209 Desa DJ, Nicholls S: Haemorrhagic necrosis of the adrenal gland in perinatal infants. A clinico-pathological study. J Pathol 106:133-149, 1972.

210 Fidler WJ: Ovarian thecal metaplasia in adrenal glands. Am J Clin Pathol 67:318-323, 1977.

211 Groben PA, Roberson JB Jr, Anger SR, Askin FB, Price WG, Siegal GP: Immunohistochemical evidence for the vascular origin of primary adrenal pseudocysts. Arch Pathol Lab Med 110:121-123, 1986.

212 Gross M, Kottmeier PK, Waterhouse K: Diagnosis and treatment of neonatal adrenal hemorrhage. J Pediatr Surg 2:308-312, 1967.

213 Hodges FV, Ellis FR: Cystic lesions of the adrenal glands. Arch Pathol 66:53-58, 1958.

214 Honore LH: Intra-adrenal hepatic heterotopia. J Urol 133:652-654, 1985.

215 McMurry JF Jr, Long D, McClure R, Kotchen T: Addison's disease with adrenal enlargement on computed tomographic scanning (report of two cases of tuberculosis and review of the literature). Am J Med 77:365-368, 1984.

216 Medeiros LJ, Wolf BC: Traumatic rupture of an adrenal myelolipoma. (Letter to the editor.) Arch Pathol Lab Med 107:500, 1983.

217 Nakamura Y, Yano H, Nakashima T: False intranuclear inclusions in adrenal cytomegaly. Arch Pathol Lab Med 105:358-360, 1981.

218 Newman PH, Silen W: Myelolipoma of the adrenal gland. Report of the third case of a symptomatic tumor and review of the literature. Arch Surg 97:637-639, 1968.

219 Noble MJ, Montague DK, Levin HS: Myelolipoma. An unusual surgical lesion of the adrenal gland. Cancer 49:952-958, 1982.

220 Orselli R, Bassler TJ: Theca granulosa cell tumor arising in adrenal. Cancer 31:474-477, 1973.

221 Pollock WJ, McConnell CF, Hilton C, Lavine RL: Virilizing Leydig cell adenoma of adrenal gland. Am J Surg Pathol 10:816-822, 1986.

222 Schnitzer B, Smid D, Lloyd RV: Primary T-cell lymphoma of the adrenal glands with adrenal insufficiency. Hum Pathol 17:634-636, 1986.

223 Seidenwurm DJ, Elmer EB, Kaplan LM, Williams EK, Morris DG, Hoffman AR: Metastases to the adrenal glands and the development of Addison's disease. Cancer 54:552-557, 1984.

224 Sinclair-Smith C, Kahn LB, Cywes S: Malacoplakia in childhood. Arch Pathol 99:198-203, 1975.

225 Wilhelmus JL, Schrodt R, Alberhasky MT, Alcorn MO: Giant adrenal myelolipoma. Arch Pathol Lab Med 105:532-535, 1981.

TUMORS OF OTHER PARAGANGLIA

226 Abell MR, Hart WR, Olson JR: Tumors of the peripheral nervous system. Hum Pathol 1:503-551, 1970.

227 Altergott R, Barbato A, Lawrence A, Paloyan E, Freeark RJ, Prinz RA: Spectrum of catecholamine-secreting tumors of the organ of Zuckerkandl. Surgery 98:1121-1126, 1985.

228 Arias-Stella J, Valcarcel J: Chief cell hyperplasia in the human carotid body at high altitudes. Physiologic and pathologic significance. Hum Pathol 7:361-373, 1976.

229 Barroso-Moguel R, Costero I: Argentaffin cells of the carotid body tumor. Am J Pathol 41:389-402, 1962.

230 Bertogalli D, Calearo C, Pignataro O: Les paragangliomes non-cromatophiles à siège rare; a propos de deux observations personnelles (paragangliome du pneumogastrique cervical et paragangliome de la base de la langue). Ann d'Otolaryngol (Paris) 76:688-699, 1959.

231 Biscoe TJ, Stehbens WE: Ultrastructure of the carotid body. J Cell Biol 30:563-578, 1966.

232 Bloom FE: Electron microscopy of catecholamine-containing structures. In Blaschko H, Muschall E (sub eds): Handbook of experimental pharmacology, vol. 33, Catecholamines. New York, 1972, Springer-Verlag, New York, Inc., chap. 3, pp. 46-78.

233 Carney JA, Sheps SG, Co VLW, Gordon H: The triad of gastric leiomyosarcoma, functioning extraadrenal paraganglioma and pulmonary chondroma. N Engl J Med 296:1517-1518, 1977.

234 Chedid A, Jao W: Hereditary tumors of the carotid bodies and chronic obstructive pulmonary disease. Cancer 33:1635-1641, 1974.

235 Coupland RE: The chromaffin system. In Blaschko H, Muschall E (sub eds): Handbook of experimental pharmacology. vol. 33, Catecholamines. New York, 1972, Springer-Verlag, New York, Inc.

236 Crowell WT, Grizzle WE, Siegel AL: Functional carotid paragangliomas. Arch Pathol Lab Med 106:599-603, 1982.

237 DeLellis RA, Roth JA: Norepinephrine in a glomus jugulare tumor. Histochemical demonstration. Arch Pathol 92:73-75, 1971.

238 Del Fante FM, Watkins E Jr: Chemodectoma of the heart in a patient with multiple chemodectomas and familial history. Case report and survey of literature. Lahey Clin Found Bull 16:224-229, 1967.

239 Farr HW: Carotid body tumors. A 30 year experience at Memorial Hospital. Am J Surg 114:614-619, 1967.

240 Freedman SR, Goldman RL: Normal paraganglion in the mesosigmoid. Hum Pathol 12:1037-1038, 1981.

241 Glenn F, Gray GF: Functional tumors of the organ of Zuckerkandl. Ann Surg 9:578-585, 1976.

242 Glenner GG, Crout JR, Roberts WC: A functional carotid-body-like tumor. Arch Pathol 73:230-240, 1962.

243 Glucksman MA, Persinger CP: Malignant non-chromaffin paraganglioma of the bladder. J Urol 89:822-825, 1963.

244 Grimley PM, Glenner GG: Histology and ultrastructure of carotid body paragangliomas. Comparison with the normal gland. Cancer 20:1473-1488, 1967.

245 Haegert DG, Wang NS, Farrer PA, Seemayer TA, Thelmo W: Non-chromaffin paragangliomatosis manifesting as a cold thyroid nodule. Am J Clin Pathol 61:561-570, 1974.

246 Hamberger C-A, Hamberger CB, Wersäll J, Wågermark J: Malignant catecholamine-producing tumour of the carotid body. Acta Pathol Microbiol Scand [A] 69:489-492, 1967.

246a Hamid Q, Varndell IM, Ibrahim NB, Mingazzini P, Polak JM: Extraadrenal paragangliomas. An immunocytochemical and ultrastructural report. Cancer 60:1776-1781, 1987.

247 Hatfield PM, James AE, Schulz MD: Chemodectomas of the glomus jugulare. Cancer **30**:1164-1168, 1972.

248 Heinrich MC, Harris AE, Bell WR: Metastatic intravagal paraganglioma. Case report and review of the literature. Am J Med **78**:1017-1024, 1985.

249 Heppleston AG: A carotid-body-like tumour in the lung. J Pathol Bacteriol **75**:461-464, 1958.

250 Ho K-C, Meyer G, Garancis J, Hanna J: Chemodectoma involving the cavernous sinus and semilunar ganglion. Hum Pathol **13**:942-943, 1982.

251 Horoupian DS, Kerson LA, Saiontz H, Valsamis M: Paraganglioma of cauda equina. Clinicopathologic and ultrastructural studies of an unusual case. Cancer **33**:1337-1348, 1974.

252 Hull MT, Roth LM, Glover JL, Walker PD: Metastatic carotid body paraganglioma in von Hippel-Lindau disease. Arch Pathol Lab Med **106**:235-239, 1982.

253 Johnson TL, Shapiro B, Beierwaltes WH, Orringer MB, Lloyd RV, Sisson JC, Thompson NW: Cardiac paragangliomas. A clinicopathologic and immunohistochemical study of four cases. Am J Surg Pathol **9**:827-834, 1985.

254 Johnson TL, Zarbo RJ, Lloyd RV, Crissman JD: Paragangliomas of the head and neck. Neuroendocrine and intermediate filament typing (abstract). Lab Invest **58**:43A, 1988.

254a Kahn LB: Vagal body tumor (nonchromaffin paraganglioma, chemodectoma, and carotid body-like tumor) with cervical node metastasis and familial association. Ultrastructural study and review. Cancer **38**:2367-2377, 1976.

255 Kepes JJ, Zacharias DL: Gangliocytic paragangliomas of the duodenum. Report of two cases with light and electron microscopy examination. Cancer **27**:61-70, 1971.

256 Kipkie GF: Simultaneous chromaffin tumors of the carotid body and the glomus jugularis. Arch Pathol **44**:113-118, 1947.

257 Korn D, Bensch K, Liebow AA, Castleman B: Multiple minute pulmonary tumors resembling chemodectomas. Am J Pathol **37**:641-672, 1960.

258 Lack EE: Hyperplasia of vagal and carotid body paraganglia in patients with chronic hypoxemia. Am J Pathol **91**:497-516, 1978.

259 Lack EE, Cubilla AL, Woodruff JM: Paragangliomas of the head and neck region. A pathologic study of tumors from 71 patients. Hum Pathol **10**:191-218, 1979.

260 Lack EE, Cubilla AL, Woodruff JM, Farr HW: Paragangliomas of the head and neck region. A clinical study of 69 patients. Cancer **39**:397-409, 1977.

261 Lack EE, Cubilla AL, Woodruff JM, Lieberman PH: Extra-adrenal paragangliomas of the retroperitoneum. A clinicopathologic study of 12 tumors. Am J Surg Pathol **4**:109-120, 1980.

262 Lattes R: Nonchromaffin paraganglioma of ganglion nodosum, carotid body and aortic arch bodies. Cancer **3**:667-694, 1950.

263 Lattes R, Waltner JG: Non-chromaffin paraganglioma of the middle ear (carotid-body-like tumor glomus-jugulare tumor). Cancer **2**:447-468, 1949.

264 Levit SA, Sheps SG, Espinosa RE, Remine WH, Harrison EG: Catecholamine-secreting paraganglioma of glomus jugulare region resembling pheochromocytoma. N Engl J Med **281**:805-812, 1969.

264a Linnoila RI, Lack EE, Steinberg SM, Keiser HR: Decreased expression of neuropeptides in malignant paragangliomas. An immunohistochemical study. Hum Pathol **19**:41-50, 1988.

265 Mäkinen J, Nickels J: Paraganglion cells mimicking metastatic clear cell carcinoma. Histopathology **3**:459-465, 1979.

266 Merino MJ, Livolsi VA: Malignant carotid body tumors. Report of two cases and review of the literature. Cancer **47**:1403-1414, 1981.

267 Meyer FB, Sundt TM Jr, Pearson BW: Carotid body tumors. A subject review and suggested surgical approach. J Neurosurg **64**:377-385, 1986.

268 Miller TA, Weber TR, Appelman HD: Paraganglioma of the gallbladder. Arch Surg **105**:637-639, 1972.

269 Murphy TE, Huvos AG, Frazell EL: Chemodectomas of the glomus intravagale. Vagal body tumors, nonchromaffin paragangliomas of the nodose ganglion of the vagus nerve. Ann Surg **172**:246-255, 1970.

269a Nora JD, Hallett JW Jr, O'Brien PC, Naessens JM, Cherry KJ Jr, Pairolero PC: Surgical resection of carotid body tumors. Long-term survival, recurrence, and metastasis. Mayo Clin Proc **63**:348-352, 1988.

270 Ober WB: Emil Zuckerkandl and his delightful little organ. Pathol Annu **18**(Pt 1):103-119, 1983.

271 Oberman HA, Holtz F, Sheffer LA, Magielski JE: Chemodectomas (nonchromaffin paragangliomas) of the head and neck. A clinicopathologic study. Cancer **21**:838-851, 1968.

272 Olson JL, Salyer WR: Mediastinal paragangliomas (aortic body tumor). A report of four cases and a review of the literature. Cancer **41**:2405-2412, 1978.

273 Olson JR, Abell MR: Nonfunctional, nonchromaffin paragangliomas of the retroperitoneum. Cancer **23**:1358-1367, 1969.

274 Pachter MR: Mediastinal nonchromaffin paraganglioma. A clinicopathological study based on 8 cases. J Thorac Cardiovasc Surg **45**:152-160, 1963.

275 Pryse-Davies J, Dawson IMP, Westbury G: Some morphologic, histochemical and chemical observations on chemodectomas and the normal carotid body, including a study of the chromaffin reaction and possible ganglion cell elements. Cancer **17**:185-202, 1964.

276 Raafat F, Salman WD, Roberts K, Ingram L, Rees R, Mann JR: Carney's triad. Gastric leiomyosarcoma, pulmonary chondroma and extra-adrenal paraganglioma in young females. Histopathology **10**:1325-1333, 1986.

277 Rangwala AF, Sylvia LC, Becker SM: Soft tissue metastasis of a chemodectoma. Cancer **42**:2865-2869, 1978.

278 Reynolds CP, German DC, Weinberg AG, Smith RG: Catecholamine fluorescence and tissue culture morphology. Technics in the diagnosis of neuroblastoma. Am J Clin Pathol **75**:275-282, 1981.

279 Robertson DI, Cooney TP: Malignant carotid body paraganglioma. Light and electron microscopic study of the tumor and its metastases. Cancer **46**:2623-2633, 1980.

280 Rodriguez-Cuevas H, Lau I, Rodriguez HP: High-altitude paragangliomas. Diagnostic and therapeutic considerations. Cancer **57**:672-676, 1986.

281 Rosai J, Mettler EA: Quimiodectoma de mediastino. Rev Asoc Med Arg **79**:242-246, 1965.

282 Rosenwasser H: Glomus jugulare tumors. Arch Otolaryngol **88**:1-40, 1968.

283 Saito H, Saito S, Sano T, Kagawa N, Hizawa K, Tatara K: Immunoreactive somatostatin in catecholamine-producing extra-adrenal paraganglioma. Cancer **50**:560-565, 1982.

284 Saldana MJ, Salem LE, Travezan R: High altitude hypoxia and chemodectomas. Hum Pathol **4**:251-263, 1973.

285 Schroder HD, Johannsen L: Demonstration of S-100 protein in sustentacular cells of phaeochromocytomas and paragangliomas. Histopathology **10**:1023-1033, 1986.

286 Shamblin WR, ReMine WH, Sheps SG, Harrison EG: Carotid body tumor (chemodectoma). Clinicopathologic analysis of 90 cases. Am J Surg **122**:732-739, 1971.

287 Shermer KL, Pantius EE, Dziabis MD, McQuistan RJ: Tumors of the glomus jugulare and glomus tympanicum. Cancer **19**:1273-1280, 1966.

288 Smith WT, Hughes B, Ermocilla R: Chemodectoma of the pineal region, with observations of the pineal body and chemoreceptor tissue. J Pathol Bacteriol **92**:69-76, 1966.

289 Someren A, Karcioglu Z: Malignant vagal paraganglioma. Report of a case and review of the literature. Am J Clin Pathol **68**:400-408, 1977.

290 Spector GJ, Compagno J, Perez CA, Maisel RH, Ogura JH: Glomus jugulare tumors. Effects of radiotherapy. Cancer **35**:1316-13221, 1975.

291 Tannir NM, Cortas N, Allam C: A functioning catecholamine-secreting vagal body tumor. A case report and review of the literature. Cancer **52**:932-935, 1983.

292 Thacker WC, and Duckworth JK: Chemodectoma of the orbit. Cancer **23**:1233-1238, 1969.

293 Tu H, Bottomley RH: Malignant chemodectoma presenting as a miliary pulmonary infiltrate. Cancer **33**:244-249, 1974.

294 Ueda N, Yoshida A, Fukunishi R, Fujita H, Yanagihara N: Nonchromaffin paraganglioma in the nose and paranasal sinuses. Acta Pathol Jpn **35**:489-495, 1985.

295 Walters G: Catecholamine-secreting tumours. In Dyke SC (ed): Recent advances in clinical pathology. Series 5, Boston, 1968, Little, Brown & Co.

296 Warren WH, Lee I, Gould VE, Memoli VA, Jao W: Paragangliomas of the head and neck. Ultrastructural and immunohistochemical analysis. Ultrastruct Pathol **8**:333-343, 1985.

297 Whimster WF, Masson AF: Malignant carotid body tumor with extradural metastases. Cancer **26**:239-244, 1970.

298 Wilkinson R, Forgan-Smith R: Chemodectoma in relation to the aortic arch (aortic body tumour). Thorax **24**:488-491, 1969.

299 Winkler H, Smith AD: Phaeochromocytoma and other catecholamine-producing tumours. In Blaschko H, Muschall E (sub eds): Handbook of experimental pharmacology, vol. 33, Catecholamines. New York, 1972, Springer-Verlag, New York, Inc.

300 Young TW, Thrasher TV: Nonchromaffin paraganglioma of the uterus. A case report. Arch Pathol Lab Med **106**:608-609, 1982.

301 Zeman MS: Carotid body tumor of the trachea, glomus jugularis tumor, tympanic body tumor, nonchromaffin paraganglioma. Ann Otol Rhinol Laryngol **65**:960-962, 1956.

17 Urinary tract

Kidney, renal pelvis, and ureter

Michael Kashgarian, M.D.,* and Juan Rosai, M.D.

Bladder and urethra

Kidney, renal pelvis, and ureter

Michael Kashgarian, M.D.,* and Juan Rosai, M.D.

*Professor and Vice Chairman of the Department of Pathology, Yale University School of Medicine; author of "Non-neoplastic conditions."

Non-neoplastic conditions
ROLE OF RENAL BIOPSY

Since its introduction nearly 50 years ago, the use of needle biopsy of the kidney as an important adjunct to the management of patients with renal disease has become widespread. Needle biopsy technique has evolved so that renal tissue can be obtained with ease and safety from patients at various stages during the course of their illness, and the use of electron microscopic and immunochemical techniques has increased the accuracy of diagnosis. Such diagnoses have proved to be of great importance in the clinical management of patients with renal disease in terms of determining therapy and predicting prognosis.[1-5] The renal pathologist, therefore, has become an integral part of the clinical team and thus must be aware not only of the pathogenesis and morbid anatomy of renal disease but also of the nephrologist's approach to the diagnosis and clinical management of these patients.

The importance of the role of renal biopsy in clinical nephrology is underscored by the fact that there are a large number of histopathologic entities that can lead to a limited number of clinical presentations. The clinical syndromes recognized by the nephrologist include the nephrotic syndrome, persistent proteinuria, acute nephritis, persistent or recurrent hematuria, hypertension, urinary tract infections, acute renal failure, and chronic renal failure. The problem is illustrated in Table 17-1, which compares the clinical presentations of acute glomerulonephritis, recurrent hematuria, persistent proteinuria, and nephrotic syndrome with the spectrum of histologic appearances seen in each of those presentations. It is obvious that in the majority of instances one cannot predict with certainty the specific histopathologic diagnosis. Despite this lack of strict correlation, it is convenient to classify the various histopathologic entities in groupings that relate to their more common clinical presentations.[4,6] Thus glomerular lesions will be categorized in this text as primary lesions associated with the nephrotic syndrome or persistent proteinuria, as primary glomerular lesions associated with acute nephritis or hematuria, and as glomerular lesions associated with systemic diseases such

as lupus and systemic vasculitis. Tubulointerstitial lesions, renal vascular lesions, and congenital cystic diseases of the kidneys will be treated separately as will the interpretation of renal biopsies performed in renal transplants.

PATHOLOGIC EXAMINATION

The advances made in the study of the pathogenesis of renal disease in experimental animals has led to a more accurate description of the immunologic events involved in many forms of glomerular and interstitial disease. Although our knowledge is as yet incomplete, the correlation of these experimental studies with clinical pathologic studies in patients has led to a more detailed description of the morphologic changes of specific disease categories.

The complex anatomy of the kidneys and the small amount of tissue available for study in percutaneous needle biopsies require that biopsies be routinely examined by light, immunofluorescence, and electron microscopy in every case. Light microscopic examination is best performed on thin (3 to 4 μm) serial sections using multiple stains including hematoxylin-eosin, PAS, Masson trichrome, and silver methenamine. This extensive examination is needed to permit an accurate evaluation of lesions, especially those that may be focal and segmental in distribution or minor in degree. Terminology is also important.[7,8,9] *Focal* is taken to mean disease affecting some but not all glomeruli as contrasted to *diffuse,* which means disease affecting all or nearly all glomeruli. *Segmental* refers to a lesion involving only a portion of a glomerulus, whereas *global* describes lesions involving the entire glomerulus. Lesions that can be identified by light microscopy include mesangial, endothelial, and epithelial proliferation; sclerosis; hyalinosis; thrombosis; necrosis; and leukocytic infiltration.

Immunofluorescence microscopy should be performed to evaluate the presence or absence of immunoglobulins in glomerular lesions. Routine staining for IgG, IgM, IgA, C3, C1, or C4, fibrinogen, and albumin should be performed. In special instances other antigens should also be investigated including IgE, kappa and lambda chains, properdin and hepatitis antigens. The major patterns that can

Table 17-1 Clinical presentation versus histologic appearance in glomerular disease

Histological appearance	Clinical presentations (% of cases)			
	AGN*	RH*	PP*	NS*
Minor or absent glomerular proliferation				
Minimal changes	0	6	10	84
Membranous nephropathy	2	0	21	77
Focal (segmental) glomerulosclerosis	1	6	42	51
Obvious glomerular proliferation				
Proliferative and exudative (endocapillary)	76	4	5	15
Mesangial proliferative	30	18	14	38
Predominant extracapillary proliferative (>80% crescents)	74	1	5	20
Mesangiocapillary glomerulonephritis	2	8	25	45
Focal proliferative and/or necrotizing glomerulonephritis	4	26	40	30
Chronic glomerulonephritis	6	8	41	45

*AGN—Acute glomerulonephritis; RH—Recurrent hematuria; PP—Persistent symptomless proteinuria; NS—Nephrotic syndrome.

Table 17-2 Glomerular lesions associated with the nephrotic syndrome

Disease	Light microscopy	Electron microscopy	Immunofluorescence microscopy	Clinical features
Minimal change lesion and variants				
Lipoid nephrosis, minimal change disease, foot process disease	Minimal change: mild segmental mesangial proliferation	Extensive foot process fusion	Negative; occasionally focal fibrin	Nephrotic syndrome, usually in younger age group; usually steroid responsive; selective proteinuria
Mild lesions				
Mesangial proliferative glomerulonephritis	Mild, diffuse; mesangial widening	Mesangial sclerosis; occasionally mesangial deposits	Occasionally mesangial IgM, C3	Similar to minimal change; sometimes progresses to focal sclerosis
Focal and segmental glomerulosclerosis (FGS)	Focal and segmental; mesangial sclerosis, begins in J-M nephrons; focal tubular atrophy	Extensive foot process fusion with mesangial sclerosis	Occasional focal IgM, C3 ("nonspecific trapping")	Nephrotic syndrome with progression to renal failure, usually steroid resistant; nonselective proteinuria
FGS in AIDS and/or IV drug abuse	FGS with mesangial proliferation and epithelial hypertrophy; interstitial nephritis	Extensive foot process fusion with mesangial sclerosis; intraendothelial tuboloreticular structures (viroids)	Inconsistent	Proteinuria or nephrotic syndrome; rapid progression to renal insufficiency
Membranous lesions				
Membranous; epimembranous glomerulonephropathy	Uniform, diffuse capillary wall thickening without significant proliferation; "spike and dome" on silver (Jones) stain	Four stages of epi- and intramembranous deposits	Confluent granular deposits; IgG, >IgM, >IgA, occasionally C3	Persistent proteinuria or nephrotic syndrome, steroid resistant; usually in adults
Diabetes mellitus				
Kimmelsteil-Wilson	Mesangial nodules and/or diffuse membranous thickening; insudative lesions	Increased mesangial matrix and diffuse membranous thickening	Linear albumin and/or Ig	Hypertension, proteinuria; occasionally nephrotic syndrome
Amyloidosis	Mesangial vascular and interstitial deposition of crystal violet– and congo red–positive material with green birefringence	Accumulation of 75-80 "A" fibrils	Monoclonal kappa or lambda light type chain	Nephrotic syndrome, normotension; associated with myeloma, chronic diseases, or hereditary forms
Light chain disease	Mesangial widening and hypercellularity	Granular, dense deposit along basement membranes	Linear kappa or lambda light chain	Proteinuria; azotemia associated with myeloma
Hereditary nephritis				
Alport's	Mesangial proliferation and focal sclerosis	Lamination of basement membrane with focal thickening and thinning	Does not stain with anti-GBM serum	Hematuria, proteinuria, renal insufficiency, deafness
Benign hematuria	Minor changes	Attenuation of basement membrane	Negative	Hematuria
Nail-patella	Similar to Alport's	Thickening of basement membrane with fibrillar collagen	Negative	Similar to Alport's; bone and nail changes
Congenital nephritis				
Nephrotic syndrome				
Finnish type	Microcysts; glomerular sclerosis	Glomerular sclerosis	Ig and C3, nonspecific trapping	Nephrotic syndrome; renal failure in first year
French type	Global glomerular sclerosis	Irregular basement membranes; sclerosis	Negative	Nephrotic syndrome; later onset renal failure (2-4 years)

From Textbook of surgery. The biological basis of modern surgical practice, ed. 13, edited by David C. Sabiston, Jr., M.D., WB Saunders Co, 1986, p. 1666.

be described are continuous linear deposits in glomerular and/or tubular basement membranes, granular deposits in the peripheral capillary loops, granular deposits in the mesangial regions, and granular deposits in tubular and vascular structures.

Electron microscopic studies should be performed to carefully assess glomerular stuctures, in particular epithelial cell morphology, mesangial morphology, and the localization of electron-dense deposits. The latter can be seen in three major patterns including mesangial, subendothelial, and subepithelial localizations. By using all three morphologic modalities, an extremely precise diagnostic categorization can be made; it is this precision of diagnosis and classification that enhances the clinical utility of this procedure.

GLOMERULAR LESIONS ASSOCIATED WITH THE NEPHROTIC SYNDROME

Nephrotic syndrome (Table 17-2) is a clinical syndrome referring to the presence of massive proteinuria, hypoproteinemia, edema, and hyperlipidemia. It is the result of a major pathophysiologic abnormality of the glomerulus that allows proteins, in particular albumin, to be filtered into the urine, resulting in the excretion of greater than 3.5 g of protein in a 24-hour period. While a spectrum of renal histologic findings have been correlated with this defect, many are characterized by an absence of a significant inflammatory or proliferative response within the glomerulus. These include primary nephrotic syndrome with minimal glomerular change; membranous glomerular nephropathy; diabetes mellitus; amyloidosis; and various forms of hereditary and congenital nephritis. The major histologic, electron microscopic, and immunofluorescence findings in each of these categories are summarized in Table 17-2.

Minimal change glomerulonephropathy and its variants

Minimal change disease has been variously called lipoid nephrosis, nil disease, minimal change disease, foot process disease, visceral epithelial cell disease, and primary nephrotic syndrome. The term *lipoid nephrosis* was used by pathologists before the advent of electron microscopic examination since the most prominent feature by light microscopy was vacuolization of the tubular epithelium by abundant lipid resorption droplets. Minimal change disease is ten to fifteen times more common in children than in adults. Over 80% of children with nephrosis[11,13,15] have minimal change diseases whereas only 20% to 30% of adults with the nephrotic syndrome fall into this category.[10,12] In the vast majority of cases, the lesion does not progress to renal insufficiency although the patients do exhibit a relapsing or polycyclic course. They are generally responsive to glucocorticoid therapy, and a few patients who are not responsive may respond to other forms of immunosuppression including cytotoxic agents and cyclosporin.

Light microscopic examination generally reveals essentially normal-appearing glomeruli[10-13,15] (Fig. 17-1). Subtle abnormalities can sometimes be identified including swelling of the visceral epithelial cells and a proteinaceous precipitate in Bowman's capsule. In some patients there may be mild mesangial prominence caused by mild increases in mesangial cellularity or matrix. In some instances the mesangial widening is prominent enough to warrant the term *mesangial proliferative glomerulonephritis*. Proximal tubular epithelial cells may be vacuolated or show prominent hyalin droplets or lipid resorption droplets. Colloidal iron and Alcian blue stains reveal a loss of staining in the glomerulus, reflecting loss of negatively charged glomerular

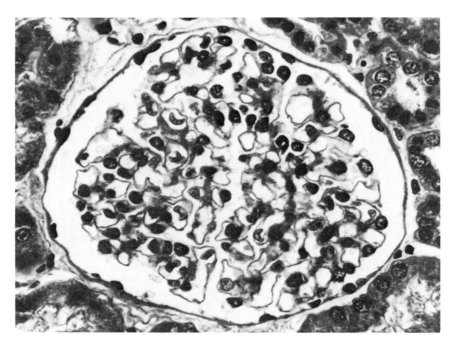

Fig. 17-1 Normal glomerulus from 11-year-old boy with steroid-responsive but dependent minimal change (nil lesion) nephrotic syndrome.

glycoproteins. In the majority of cases immunofluorescence examination is usually completely negative.[14] Small amounts of complement and fibrinogen may be found in the peripheral capillary walls. In some patients with mesangial prominence, IgM and complement may be found. Electron microscopic changes are most prominent in the visceral epithelial cells.[10-12] There is generally a loss of the normal epithelial cell foot processes on the external side of the glomerular basement membrane (so-called foot process fusion) with basal condensation of the cytoplasmic microfilaments and microvillus transformation of the epithelial cells in Bowman's space (Fig. 17-2). It should be noted, however, that although epithelial cell changes are characteristic of this entity, the diagnosis is essentially a diagnosis of exclusion. The etiology of the disease is unknown as is the mechanism of the glomerular permeability defect, although it has been suggested that lymphokine production by T-cells may be involved.

Diffuse mesangial hypercellularity with nephrotic syndrome

Several histologic variants of the primary nephrotic syndrome deserve discussion. In some patients there is a more pronounced degree of mesangial hypercellularity and sclerosis, which is associated with immunofluorescent staining for IgM and C3 and the presence of small mesangial electron-dense deposits.[16,20] Since these patients generally do not behave significantly differently from those with very minimal changes, it is likely that this group of patients represents only a variant in the spectrum of the same disease. It has been suggested that the accumulation of IgM and C3 is merely the result of an overload of the capability of the glomerulus to clear unfiltered macromolecules.[17] Thus, although the presence of these mesangial abnormalities must be described, they do not alter the clinical approach to such a patient in terms of therapy or prognosis.[17-19,21]

Focal and segmental glomerulosclerosis

A more important variant in this spectrum of disease is the presence of focal and segmental glomerular sclerosis.[32,41] Numerous studies have described the association of this lesion with steroid resistance and a higher incidence of nonselective proteinuria, hematuria, and hypertension complicating the nephrotic syndrome. Patients with this lesion early in the course of the disease have a rather distinctive clinical picture.[39] Most patients have a poorly selective proteinuria accompanied by microscopic hematuria and hypertension and frequently do not respond to steroid or cytotoxic therapy. The prognosis of such patients is poor, with progression to renal insufficiency and possible recurrence of the disease in renal transplants.[30,36] It appears, therefore, that when focal sclerosis is present early in the course of the disease it is likely to be associated with therapeutic unresponsiveness and a guarded prognosis. In other cases, however, focal sclerosis may evolve from a minimal lesion.[42] Patients whose initial biopsies indicate minimal changes have shown, after many relapses, the development of focal sclerotic lesions late in the course of their disease. Presence of focal sclerosis late in the disease, however, is not necessarily accompanied by a lack of response to steroids or immunosuppression nor does it necessarily have the same prognostic significance in terms of progression to renal failure that early focal sclerosis demonstrates.

By light microscopy the lesions consist of glomerulosclerosis involving only portions of the glomerular tuft (segmental) of a limited number of glomeruli (focal) (Fig.

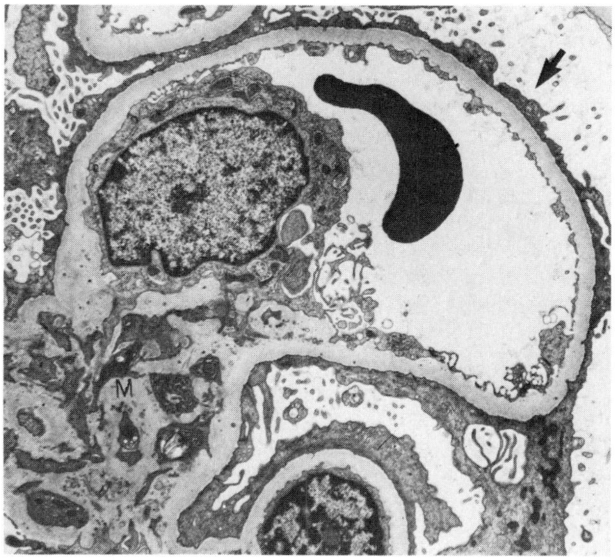

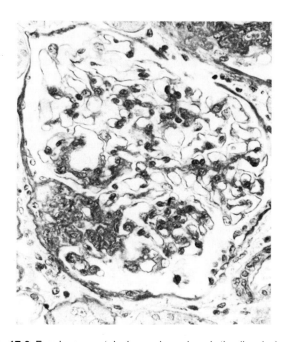

Fig. 17-2 Minimal change (nil lesion) nephrotic syndrome in adult. Diffuse obliteration of epithelial cell foot processes (arrow) with microvillus transformation in glomerulus. Note mild increase in mesangial matrix, *M*. (×4,700.)

Fig. 17-3 Focal segmental glomerular sclerosis/hyalinosis in 15-year-old boy with steroid-resistant nephrotic syndrome. Sclerotic lobule is adherent to Bowman's capsule.

17-3). The sclerotic lesions are generally more common in juxtamedullary glomeruli.[40] Hyaline material is frequently seen in the vascular pole of the glomerulus and in the afferent arterioles. Occasionally synechiae are present between the segmental sclerotic lesions and Bowman's capsule. Uninvolved portions of the glomerulus may show mild mesangial hypercellularity and widening. Interstitial fibrosis and tubular atrophy are often prominent and may be the only finding present in some cases. Immunofluorescence is variable but frequently reveals the presence of IgM and C3. By electron microscopy the sclerotic lesions contain abundant matrix material associated with wrinkled and collapsed glomerular capillary loops.[24,28] The hyaline deposits seen are sometimes electron dense but do not have the typical characteristics of an immune complex. The epithelial cells show changes very similar to those seen in minimal change disease, but they occasionally also show more severe alterations, including detachment from the basement membrane.

The etiology and pathogenesis of the focal and segmental sclerosis are unclear, and morphologically similar lesions are seen in a wide variety of other glomerular lesions, as follows: reflux and obstructive nephropathy, hypertension, solitary kidney (segmental hypoplasia), healed focal glomerulonephritis, radiation nephritis, and aging. Most recently it has been suggested that local glomerular hemodynamic alterations that produce hyperfiltration, increased hydraulic flow through the mesangium, and increased mesangial uptake of macromolecules may be the stimulus for the segmental glomerulosclerosis.[22,31]

A particular form of focal and segmental glomerulosclerosis has recently been described in patients with acquired immune deficiency disease (AIDS).[27,34,38] The lesion has been implicated as a cause of chronic renal failure in some patients with AIDS but not in others.[35] There appears to be a predilection for focal and segmental glomerular sclerosis among black heroin abusers with AIDS but an apparent absence of the lesion in white patients with homosexuality as the only risk factor. The lesion appears to have several distinct clinical and pathologic characteristics, and there is a relatively rapid clinical progression of the lesion to renal failure. By light microscopy, focal and segmental sclerosis in all stages of evolution is present in many of the glomeruli.[37] The segmental sclerosis is characterized by localized hyperplasia and vacuolization of the visceral epithelial cells overlying the sclerotic segment. In addition, the tubules display striking alterations, including the presence of large hyaline casts in many tubules, as well as the presence of degenerative changes and necrosis of the tubular epithelial cells. An active interstitial nephritis is frequent. Immunofluorescence findings are variable, but once again IgM and C3 are frequently found in an amorphous granular pattern and segmental distribution. Less frequently other immunoglobulin classes may also be localized. By electron microscopy the changes are not dissimilar from those of focal and segmental sclerosis seen in the absence of AIDS. The endothelial cells, however, are frequently filled with numerous and prominent tubular reticular structures[23,33] (Fig. 17-4). These structures most recently have been thought to be associated with interferon activity,[29,41] although a more

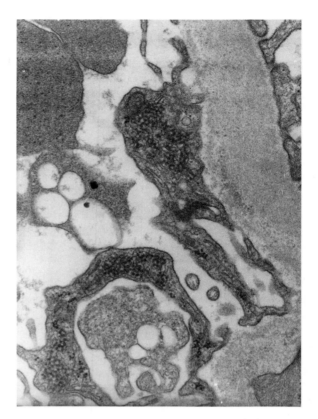

Fig. 17-4 AIDS nephropathy. Numerous tubuloreticular structures are present in endothelial cell cytoplasm. These are thought to be directly or indirectly induced by alpha interferon. (×32,000.)

direct relation to viral infection has also been suggested. Similar lesions have also been seen in patients with a history of intravenous drug abuse without concurrent AIDS.[25,26]

Membranous glomerulonephropathy

Membranous glomerulonephropathy (also termed membranous nephropathy, membranous glomerulonephritis, extramembranous glomerulonephritis, and epimembranous nephropathy) is similar to primary nephrotic syndrome in that it is characterized clinically by massive proteinuria and the nephrotic syndrome. In contrast to the primary nephrotic syndrome, however, there is an increased permeability of the glomerular capillaries to serum proteins of high- and low-molecular weight, and in the majority of instances there is a gradual but progressive reduction in surface area for ultrafiltration leading to renal insufficiency.[44] In most series of adults with the nephrotic syndrome, membranous nephropathy is the most common diagnosis occurring in approximately 25% of such patients.[46,53,57] However, the percentage and incidence of membranous nephropathy in different populations appears to vary. There is an unusually high incidence in Japanese children[47] and in some specific populations in Africa.[50,68,69] This is likely related to a high incidence of hepatitis B infection and parasitic infestations in these various populations. Membranous nephropathy is much less common in other children, accounting for less than 10% of children with nephrosis, but incidence increases

DISEASES ASSOCIATED WITH MEMBRANOUS NEPHROPATHY

Malignancy
Lung, GI tract, breast, lymphomas
Infections
Hepatitis, malaria, parasites, leprosy, syphilis
Drugs
Gold, penicillamine, captopril, nonsteroidals
Toxins
Mercury, heavy metals
Autoimmune diseases
Rheumatoid arthritis, Hashimoto's thyroiditis, myasthenia gravis, Guillain-Barré syndrome
Lupus erythematosus

with age, forming a continuum with young adults.[56] Although not completely characteristic, remission of proteinuria is not uncommon in membranous nephropathy, and even in the absence of complete remission disappearance of the nephrotic syndrome is quite common.[46,55] The long-term clinical course of such patients is not that unfavorable, although in groups of patients followed up to 10 to 15 years, approximately 50% will have developed renal failure while the other half will be in remission or have mild proteinuria. At the present time it is thought that corticosteroid therapy may benefit the long-term prognosis, and it is generally used in most patients.[45] Although the majority of patients identified with membranous nephropathy and the nephrotic syn-

drome are idiopathic, individual patients may have an associated systemic disease or exposure to drugs or toxins. Perhaps the most interesting association is with malignancy (see box, opposite). A variety of malignancies have been reported connected with the nephrotic syndrome, including carcinoma of the lung, esophagus, stomach, breast, and certain lymphomas.[61,64,65] In some cases carcinoembryonic antigen (CEA) has been identified as present in the immune complexes of the glomerular capillary walls, as well as in patients' serum.[47] It has also been reported that the nephrotic syndrome has abated and glomerular lesions have regressed after resection and treatment of the carcinoma. Although a wide variety of glomerular lesions have been reported in patients with lymphoma, membranous glomerulonephropathy has been seen both in Hodgkin's and in non-Hodgkin's lymphoma.[54]

A variety of other identifiable antigens have also been reported. Infections, including malaria, a variety of parasites, leprosy, and syphilis, are all commonly associated with membranous nephropathy. Perhaps of greatest interest is the frequent association of hepatitis virus carrier states with membranous nephropathy.[49,59,63,66] This has been particularly observed among children and in those geographic populations with a high incidence of both membranous nephropathy and hepatitis such as in the Far East and Africa.[67] A wide variety of drugs have also been implicated, including gold therapy in association with rheumatoid arthritis,[52] penicillamine,[58] captopril,[60] and nonsteroidal prostaglandin inhibitors.[43] Of the toxins, exposure to mercury has been the best described as an associated cause of membranous nephropathy. A variety of other diseases—in which an immune response is thought to be involved in the pathogenesis, such as rheumatoid arthritis, Hashimoto's thyroiditis, my-

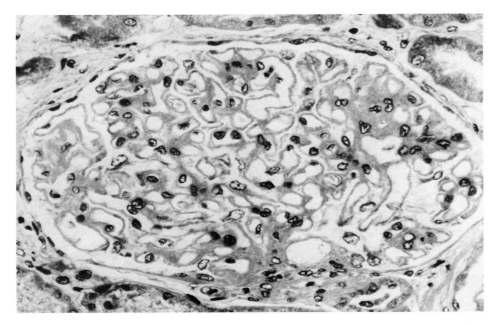

Fig. 17-5 Membranous glomerulonephritis in 54-year-old man with 3-year history of nephrotic syndrome that initially responded to steroid therapy. Capillary walls are uniformly thickened, and there is mild mesangial matrix and cellular increase.

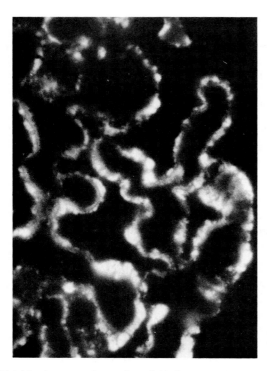

Fig. 17-6 Membranous glomerulonephritis in 4-year-old girl with nephrotic syndrome. Characteristic, diffuse, finely granular subepithelial deposits of IgG. Note outline of lamina densa.

asthenia gravis, and Guillain-Barré syndrome—have also been implicated. Membranous nephropathy also is part of the wide spectrum of renal lesions seen in lupus erythematosus, which will be discussed more thoroughly later.

By light microscopy, the glomeruli usually appear somewhat moderately enlarged and associated with a mild-to-moderate degree of mesangial prominence (Fig. 17-5). The peripheral capillary walls are thickened, varying from a minimal increase to striking thickening. Where the change is minimal, a "stiffness" to the appearance of the glomerular capillary loops is apparent. Silver methenamine stains are particularly useful in evaluating membranous nephropathy as they reveal a "spike and dome" pattern and vacuolization of the thickened peripheral capillary walls.[51] The interstitium may show varying degrees of interstitial scarring and tubular atrophy, and recent studies have suggested that the degree of tubulointerstitial alteration may be the best predictor of progression to renal insufficiency.

Immunofluorescence staining generally reveals a granular peripheral capillary staining for immunoglobulins (Fig. 17-6). The extent of the granularity may be so great as to give a pseudolinear appearance. The immunoglobulin involved most commonly is IgG, followed by IgM and finally IgA.[44] It is of interest that where IgG subtypes have been looked for, the IgG seen in membranous glomerulonephropathy was most commonly IgG 4.[48] A granular deposition of C3 is also commonly seen, but other complement compo-

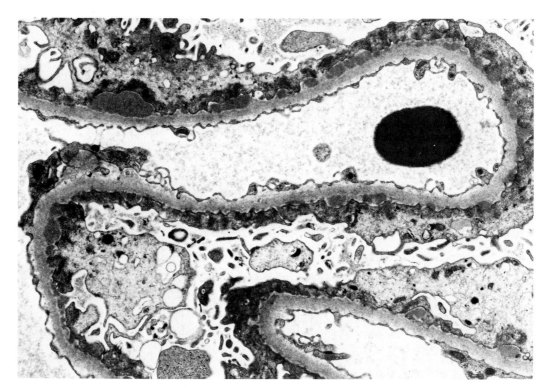

Fig. 17-7 Membranous glomerulonephritis in 69-year-old man with insidious onset of ankle edema who was found to have nephrotic syndrome. Normal glomeruli were seen by light microscopy. Electron photomicrograph demonstrates stage I disease with variably sized subepithelial deposits and normal lamina densa. (×7,620.)

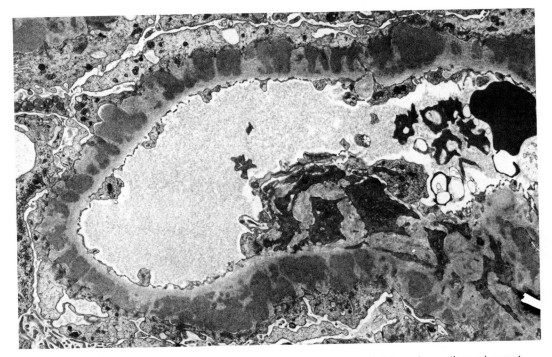

Fig. 17-8 Membranous glomerulonephritis in 46-year-old woman with hilar adenopathy and recent onset of nephrotic syndrome. Electron photomicrograph demonstrates stage II disease with thickened capillary wall secondary to subepithelial deposits and "spikes" of basement membrane. (×8,320.)

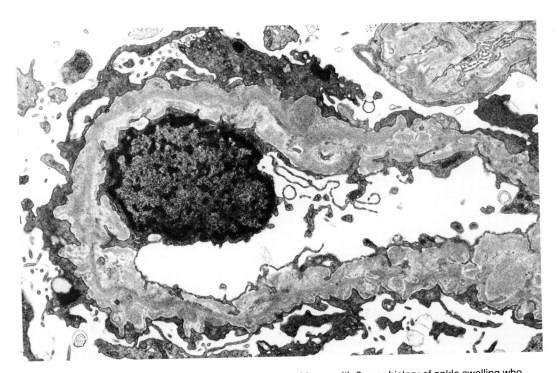

Fig. 17-9 Membranous glomerulonephritis in 55-year-old man with 2-year history of ankle swelling who was found to have nephrotic syndrome, mild hypertension, and mild renal insufficiency. Electron photomicrograph demonstrates stage III disease with subepithelial and intramembranous deposits of variable size, shape, and electron density. (×7,060.)

nents have also been demonstrated to occur in a granular pattern. Mesangial deposits may be present in a minority of cases. The presence of mesangial deposits is frequently associated with an identifiable antigen such as hepatitis antigen.

Electron microscopic studies have described four stages of development of the membranous lesion.[51] While these stages may be useful for descriptive purposes, it is likely that there is a continuum of changes representing initial immune complex formation to incorporation into the basement membrane and dissolution. In stage I, scattered electron-dense deposits are noted on the subepithelial aspect of a normal-appearing glomerular basement membrane. Foot process effacement is generally seen in relationship to the presence of these deposits. The number of deposits is usually small, and the deposits are scattered along different portions of the capillary loops (Fig. 17-7). In stage II, the subepithelial deposits are more abundant and there appears to be a deposition of basement membrane–like material in between the deposits, giving rise to the "spike and dome" appearance (Fig. 17-8). In stage III, the apical portions of the spikes have formed an enclosed basement membrane–like structure so that deposits are now completely surrounded by basement membrane material and are now intramembranous rather than epimembranous (Fig. 17-9). In stage IV, there is usually dissolution of the deposits with rarification and evidence of glomerular basement membrane repair within irregular thickening. It is thought that the immune complexes seen by immunofluorescence and electron microscopy are the result of the in situ formation of immune complexes at specific sites, perhaps related to the presence of a specific glycoprotein (GP330) that has been associated with coated endocytic pits and vesicles of the epithelial cell.[48,62]

Diabetic nephropathy

Diabetes mellitus is a common cause of the nephrotic syndrome, associated with what has been termed diabetic nephropathy. This term encompasses a variety of renal lesions and includes diffuse membranous glomerulosclerosis, nodular glomerulosclerosis, insudative changes or fibrin caps, and arteriolar nephrosclerosis.[70,71] In general, it is found that the incidence of glomerulosclerosis and the degree of severity increases with the duration of diabetes, particularly if the diabetes is poorly controlled.[75,76] These observations have led to the speculation that nonenzymatic glycosylation of basement membrane proteins may contribute to its pathogenesis.[73] The lesion is more common in patients with an early onset of diabetes, and in most patients the renal involvement first appears some 10 or more years after the diagnosis of carbohydrate intolerance is made.[78] The abnormality is a diffuse microangiopathy that involves multiple peripheral small vessels, retinal vessels being of particular clinical importance.[72] Proteinuria is usually accompanied by some degree of renal insufficiency and, as might be expected, is not improved by glucosteroid or cytotoxic therapy.

By light microscopy, the diffuse diabetic glomerulosclerotic lesion is characterized by a diffuse thickening of the glomerular capillary wall and a generalized increase in

mesangial matrix in all mesangial regions of all glomeruli (Fig. 17-10, A). In early stages, the changes may be minimal and not readily observed by light microscopy except perhaps with the use of silver methenamine staining. Nodular diabetic glomerulosclerotic lesions as described by Kimmelstiel and Wilson may be variably present.[77] These consist of sclerotic nodules in one or more intercapillary or mesangial regions of the glomerular tuft. Silver staining reveals these nodules to be laminated and to consist of material with the same staining properties as mesangial matrix and glomerular basement membrane. This material is generally acellular and consists predominantly of matrix. Occasionally, exudative or insudative or fibrin cap lesions are present. These consist of eosinophilic accumulations of the plasma protein on Bowman's capsule or on the peripheral capillary wall.[79] The arterioles show marked hyaline arteriosclerosis, which may involve both afferent and efferent arterioles. The tubules occasionally show vacuolization and increased glycogen deposition in the S3 segment of the proximal tubules.

Immunofluorescence demonstrates an interesting finding that may be related to a nonspecific accumulation of plasma proteins within the abnormal glomerular capillary wall. A diffuse linear staining, which mimics that of anti-GBM disease, may be seen in immunofluorescent stains for albumin and IgG.[70,79] The staining is thin and delicate, not as intense as that seen with antiglomerular basement membrane disease, and the complement is usually absent.

Electron microscopy reveals diffuse and even thickening of the basement membrane (Fig. 17-10, B). This occurs very early and may be identified even when the glomeruli appear normal by light microscopy. Thickening progresses with the disease attaining five to ten times normal thickness in some instances.[74] The mesangium shows an increase in matrix material and occasionally a slight increase in cellularity. "Exudative" and "hyaline" deposits appear as granular electron-dense deposits in the subendothelial and mesangial regions, as well as in arterioles and Bowman's capsule.

Amyloidosis

Amyloid involvement of the kidney frequently causes heavy proteinuria, renal insufficiency, and the nephrotic syndrome. Although the single term amyloidosis describes a histopathologic entity characterized by the deposition of a hyaline material, the disease process itself is diverse in terms of its clinical manifestations, pathogenesis, biochemical and immunologic aspects.[81] The primary fibrillar protein that is seen by electron microscopy and that stains with Congo red is amyloid protein A. This is the predominant protein in secondary amyloidosis associated with conditions such as rheumatoid arthritis or chronic infection. In so-called primary amyloidosis, when there is no evidence of coexisting disease or when there is association with multiple myeloma, the amyloid A protein is associated with immunoglobulin light chains.[82] Numerous familial forms of amyloidosis have also been described, and in these cases the A protein may be either the predominant protein or may be associated with a subset-specific protein and pre-albumin. Clinically these patients may present with massive proteinuria sometimes in excess of 12 to 20 g in a 24-hour period.

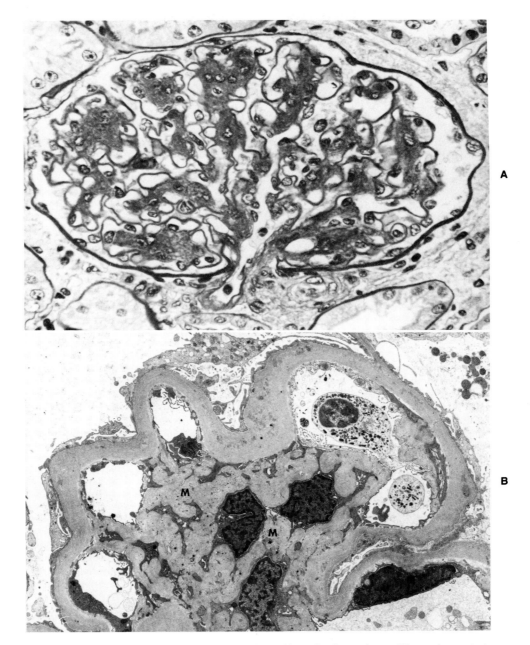

Fig. 17-10 A, Diabetes mellitus in 17-year-old patient with nephrotic syndrome. Biopsy demonstrates diffuse intercapillary glomerulosclerosis and capillary wall thickening. **B,** Same case as in **A.** Portion of glomerular lobule showing diffuse capillary wall thickening and mesangial widening secondary to increase in mesangial matrix, *M,* and cells. ($\times$2,900.)

Treatment with glucocorticoids is not useful and the overall outlook is generally poor, although occasional patients have been reported with prolonged survival.

Amyloid is an amorphous, homogeneous-appearing substance with a characteristic fibrillar structure by electron microscopy and a beta-pleated structure by x-ray diffraction. This structural characteristic makes amyloid resistant to proteolysis and is undoubtedly responsible for its accumulation and persistence in tissues. Amyloid deposits usually predominate in the glomeruli and appear as an amorphous eo-

sinophilic material[80] (Fig. 17-11). Congo red stains display an apple-green birefringence when examined with polarized light. Amyloid deposits also are prominent in tubular basement membranes and vessel walls. The interstitial tissue particularly in the medulla may also be a site of deposition.

Immunofluorescence may reveal the accumulation of immunoglobulins in deposits in a nonspecific pattern. Patients with primary amyloidosis may show the specific deposition of monoclonal kappa or lambda light chains.

Electron microscopy reveals amyloid fibrils that are reg-

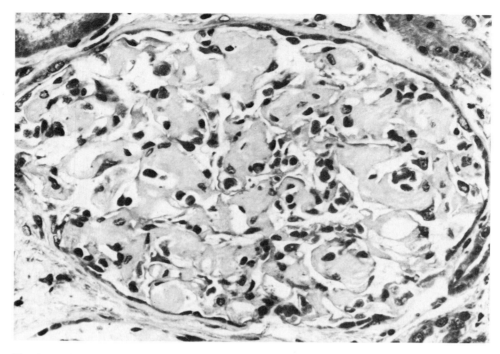

Fig. 17-11 Amyloidosis in 56-year-old alcoholic with hepatomegaly and nephrotic syndrome. Biopsy demonstrates acellular mesangial widening and capillary loop thickening related to deposits of amyloid.

ular nonbranching fibrils, ranging from 70 to 120 Å in width and of variable length (Fig. 17-12). They are generally seen deposited in the mesangium and peripheral capillary basement membrane and may be present as large masses of fibrils that have traversed the glomerular capillary wall resulting in spikes of basement membrane and amyloid.

Light chain disease

In approximately 7% to 10% of patients with multiple myeloma there may be an extracellular deposition of light chains in the blood vessels of many organs in a manner similar to amyloidosis (AL). The glomerulus is a particular site of deposition giving rise to significant proteinuria and occasionally the nephrotic syndrome.[83-86] By light microscopy the glomeruli show capillary wall thickening and a nodular glomerular sclerosis that resembles diabetic glomerular sclerosis. Immunofluorescence microscopy demonstrates a linear deposition of monoclonal light chains of either kappa or lambda type. Electron microscopy shows a granular electron-dense deposit in glomerular and tubular basement membranes in a diffuse linear pattern.

Hereditary and familial nephropathies

Proteinuria is a prominent feature in some types of hereditary nephropathy and in some instances is severe enough to be associated with the nephrotic syndrome. Three types that have been best described include Alport's syndrome,[92] thin basement membrane syndrome,[91] and nail-patella syndrome.[87]

Alport's syndrome covers several different hereditary nephritic syndromes that vary in their clinical presentation and in genetic transmission.[90] Type I Alport's syndrome is the classic form that is dominantly inherited and associated with deafness. Affected males have no offspring. Other types of Alport's syndrome may be X-linked dominant or autosomal dominant and may or may not be associated with deafness, thrombocytopathia, eye defects, or varying combinations depending on the kindred studied. It has been suggested that a glomerular basement membrane component is absent in Alport's syndrome since the glomerular basement membrane of some patients does not stain with anti-GBM serum or antibodies directed against a noncollagenous fragment of type IV collagen.[89] These patients present with hematuria and proteinuria that may be severe enough to be associated with the nephrotic syndrome. Progression to renal insufficiency is variable and is in some cases sex- and type-linked.

Early in the disease the glomeruli and tubules may not show any significant abnormalities by light microscopy. As the lesion progresses, glomerulosclerosis associated with interstitial scarring and tubular atrophy is present. Not infrequently collections of foam cells may be seen in the interstitium. Immunofluorescence examination generally does not reveal specific abnormalities. Electron microscopy reveals a characteristic lesion in the glomeruli, which consists of thickening and splitting of the basement membrane in an irregular pattern[88] (Fig. 17-13). Between the laminations of the basement membrane, small dense granules may be present. Similar lamination and splitting also occurs in tubular basement membranes and focal attenuation of the basement membrane may be present. The lesion may not be uniform in all cases and may affect some capillary loops more severely than others.

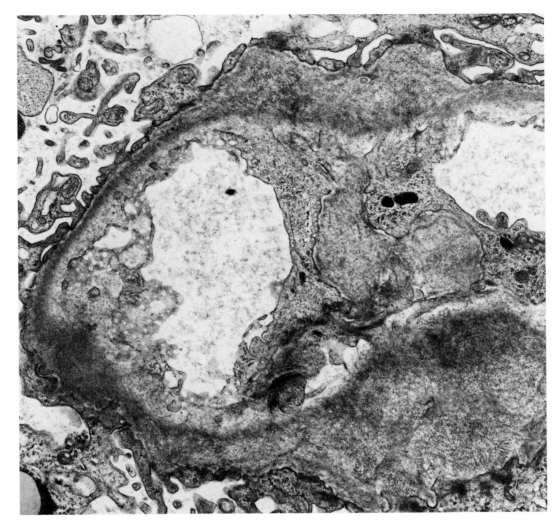

Fig. 17-12 Amyloidosis in 73-year-old woman with congestive heart failure and nephrotic syndrome. Lamina densa is focally thickened and replaced by haphazardly arranged fibrils of amyloid. (×13,140.)

Congenital nephrotic syndrome

Nephrotic syndrome occurring before the age of 1 is rare and often fatal. There are two major types of primary congenital nephrotic syndrome and both appear to be inherited as an autosomal recessive characteristic. They are generally referred to as the Finnish type[94-96] and the French type,[93] relating to the initial reports of pedigrees. In both types there is evidence of significant glomerulosclerosis with rapid progression to renal insufficiency.

In the Finnish type the infants are usually premature and of low birth weight. The placenta is enlarged, weighing approximately one third of the fetal body weight. The nephrotic syndrome may be present at birth or develops during the first 3 months of life. It is not responsive to corticosteroid therapy. By light microscopy many glomeruli are immature and others show varying degrees of mesangial proliferation and sclerosis. There is evidence of tubular cyst formation in the cortex predominantly at the cortical medullary junction, giving rise to the term *microcystic disease*. Arteriolar medial hypertrophy is frequently striking. Immunofluorescence microscopy is generally negative. Electron microscopy shows diffuse obliteration of the epithelial foot processes and other changes similar to that seen in minimal change disease. Basement membranes are thin but no other structural abnormalities are noted.

In the French type the nephrotic syndrome develops during the first year of life, as early as the first week after birth but usually after 3 months. There is generally a relatively rapid progression to renal insufficiency within 1 to 3 years. By light microscopy the glomeruli show mesangial and later global sclerosis without significant cellular proliferation. The lesion is usually uniform and corresponding tubular atrophy with interstitial fibrosis is present. Immunofluorescence microscopy is negative. Electron microscopy reveals glomerular changes typical of the nephrotic syndrome with obliteration of the foot processes and edema of the podocytes. The basement membrane is irregularly thickened and there is a marked increase in mesangial matrix.

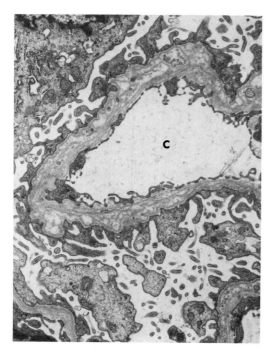

Fig. 17-13 Alport's syndrome in which lamina densa is thickened and transformed into heterogeneous network of strands and lucent zones. This change is characteristic of Alport's syndrome but may be seen focally in other disease processes. Capillary lumen, C. (×8,200.)

GLOMERULAR LESIONS ASSOCIATED WITH THE SYNDROME OF ACUTE NEPHRITIS

Another major clinical presentation of patients with glomerular lesions is the acute nephritis syndrome (Table 17-3). The patient with nephritis presents with hematuria, azotemia, oliguria, and mild to moderate hypertension; urinalysis reveals an "active" sediment. An active sediment consists of the presence of red blood cells, leukocytes, and red blood cell casts. Proteinuria is generally present but is rarely in the nephrotic range. Edema, when present, is usually mild and frequently is noted as facial puffiness. Variants of the clinical syndrome include the fulminant form of rapidly progressive glomerulonephritis and milder forms identified by the presence of microscopic hematuria and nonnephrotic proteinuria, occasionally associated with mild hypertension and clinical symptoms. Gross hematuria and microscopic hematuria alone form yet another variant. As with the nephrotic syndrome, the histopathologic lesions that can give rise to this presentation are varied.

Acute post-infectious glomerulonephritis

The pathogenesis and natural history of acute post-infectious glomerulonephritis is better understood than any other form of renal disease. Although it has been known for a long time that acute glomerulonephritis followed certain acute infections, studies have established the most common cause to be associated with infections of group A hemolytic streptococci of specific types, including types 12, 3, 1 and

49.[99] Less commonly, a variety of other infectious agents including viruses, protozoa, spirochetes, mycobacteria, and bacteria other than streptococcus—including staphylococcus, salmonella, and enterococcus—have all been implicated. On the basis of experimental observations in animals with immunologically induced renal disease and studies of human biopsy material, it is generally thought that the immunohistopathologic lesion is an immune complex–mediated inflammatory response within the glomeruli.[104]

Post-streptococcal glomerulonephritis is the prototypic form of acute nephritis and can vary in the severity of both the clinical and pathologic changes seen.* Clinically, the onset of renal symptoms occurs after a latent period of 1 to 4 weeks. In the typical case the patient notices darkening of the urine, reduced urine volume, generalized malaise, and a gradual onset of edema. In most instances, the streptococcal infection is upper respiratory but skin infections with nephritogenic streptococci are also important. Since the clinical syndrome may be quite distinctive and since the general prognosis is excellent, biopsies generally are not performed on patients with this syndrome unless some atypical features complicate the presentation such as the nephrotic syndrome, anuria, persistent or severe hypertension, and failure to show recovery within 4 to 6 weeks.

Light microscopy biopsies performed within the first few weeks after the onset of nephritis show a diffuse glomerular hypercellularity with partial obliteration of the capillary lumina caused by proliferation of endocapillary cells and leukocytic infiltration (Fig. 17-14). The severity of the proliferative response varies in individual cases but generally involves all of the glomeruli equally. Segmental necrosis and thrombosis associated with crescent formation are usually not seen although they may occur rarely. A necrotizing arteritis has also been reported in unusual instances.[101]

Immunofluorescent microscopy shows the deposition of IgG and complement in a peripheral granular and mesangial pattern[97] (Fig. 17-15). Other immunoglobulins are generally not present. C1 or C4 is usually not seen. Fibrinogen may be present in a mesangial pattern. Electron microscopy of very early biopsies occasionally demonstrates the presence of small subendothelial deposits. The most characteristic finding, however, is the presence of subepithelial electron-dense deposits ("humps")[103] (Fig. 17-16). These deposits vary in size and number and are often inhomogeneous in density. There is foot process effacement, evidence of endothelial cell swelling, and prominent mesangial widening caused by proliferation of mesangial cells, infiltration of mononuclear leukocytes, and some increase in mesangial matrix.

Serial studies have shown that a gradual resolution of the histopathologic changes[107] takes place. Cellularity is decreased, and a disappearance of deposits and complete restoration to normal histology may be seen as early as 6 months and certainly by 2 to 3 years. Only a small percentage appear to have residual changes, which include persistent mesangial hypercellularity and the presence of mesangial deposits by immunofluorescence and electron microscopy.

*See references 97, 98, 100, 102, 105, 106, and 108.

Table 17-3 Primary glomerular lesions associated with the nephrotic syndrome

Disease	Light microscopy	Electron microscopy	Immunofluorescence microscopy	Clinical features
Proliferative lesions				
Acute poststreptococcal; postinfectious; endocapillary glomerulonephritis	Endocapillary proliferation and exudation	Subepithelial "humps"	Granular IgG, C3 mesangial fibrin	Hematuria, proteinuria, cylinduria, azotemia hypertension; occasionally nephrotic syndrome, usually with evidence for preceding streptococcal infection
		Three groups by electron and immunofluorescence microscopy		
Rapidly progressive; subacute; crescentic; extracapillary glomerulonephritis	Endo- and extracapillary proliferation; necrosis, fibrin exudation, and epithelial crescents or fibrous crescents	Subepithelial "humps" and mesangial deposits; GBM gaps; fibrin tactoids	Granular IgG, IgM, C3	Post-infectious; hematuria, proteinuria and rapid reduction in renal function usually with evidence for preceding streptococcal infection
		GBM gaps; fibrin tactoids; no deposits	Linear IgG or IgM and C3; fibrin	Two clinical subgroups without evidence of streptococcal infection 1. Without lung involvement 2. With lung involvement (Goodpasture's syndrome)
		GBM gaps; fibrin tactoids; no deposits	Negative for Ig	"Idiopathic" has similar clinical presentation; sometimes associated with systemic vasculitis
		Two types by electron and immunofluorescence microscopy		
Chronic hypocomplementic; membranoproliferative; lobular; mesangiocapillary glomerulonephritis	Lobular accentuation with mesangial proliferation and/or hyalinization "tram track" on silver stain occasionally crescents	Type I—mesangial, subendothelial, subepithelial deposits	Type I—lumpy bumpy IgG, C3, IgM granular fibrin	Type I—persistent proteinuria, nephrotic syndrome or may resemble acute glomerulonephritis without evidence of preceding streptococcal infection; hypertension, frequent "nephritic nephrotic"
		Type II—fibrin tactoids, linear dense intramembranous deposits	Type II—granular C3, fibrin in capillary and mesangium	Type II—"dense deposit disease" associated with C3 NEF, lipodystrophy, and poorer prognosis
Mesangial proliferative; focal glomerulitis (Berger's disease, IgA); latent glomerulonephritis	Segmental mesangial widening	Focal mesangial hypercellularity	Mesangial IgA, IgG; sometimes negative	Recurrent gross hematuria or persistent microscopic hematuria
Chronic (irreversible) lesions				
Chronic glomerulonephritis; end stage kidney	Generalized glomerular sclerosis; vascular sclerosis	Mesangial sclerosis and capillary collapse "exudative lesions"	No consistent pattern; may reflect original lesion	Variable; mild persistent hematuria/proteinuria to nephrotic syndrome; renal function may be moderate to markedly reduced

Diffuse crescentic glomerulonephritis

Rapidly progressive glomerulonephritis is a variant of the acute nephritic syndrome in which patients initially present with acute glomerulonephritis associated with the rapid onset of severe acute renal failure. The clinical course is not only rapid but also generally not reversible.[110,114] The onset of the disease is characterized by oliguria or anuria, advancing azotemia, proteinuria of varying amounts, hematuria with cellular casts, and hypertension, which is sometimes in the malignant range. The nephrotic syndrome, when present, is unresponsive to therapy and persists until oliguria and renal insufficiency supervene. In a few patients renal

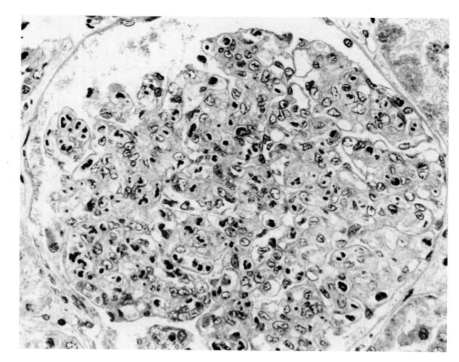

Fig. 17-14 Acute poststreptococcal glomerulonephritis in 10-year-old boy. Note obliteration of capillary lumina by endocapillary proliferation and exudation.

function eventually stabilizes at an impaired level after several weeks, but in most patients progression to end stage renal insufficiency occurs. A variety of therapeutic modalities have been suggested, which include pulse steroids, pulse cyclophosphamide, various anticoagulation protocols, and plasmapheresis, but no uniform results have been observed. The clinicopathologic entity can be divided into three subgroups.[112,113] The first are patients with post—infectious glomerulonephritis of a severe nature. The second are patients in which an antibody to glomerular basement membrane can be identified; the third are "idiopathic" in that no definite relationship to infection exists and no immune complexes are identified. The prognosis is apparently better in crescentic glomerulonephritis associated with post-infectious processes than in anti-GBM and idiopathic varieties.

By light microscopy, the most characteristic feature is the presence of glomerular crescents[111,116-119,121] (Fig. 17-17). The crescents may be cellular or fibrous depending on the state of evolution of the glomerular lesion. In the early stages the crescents consist of accumulation of cells derived from the parietal epithelium and infiltrating monocytes in Bowman's space. Occasional tubule-like structures are formed by the proliferating cells. They are associated with the presence of fibrin in Bowman's space as detected by trichrome stains, and gaps or disruptive lesions of the glomerular capillary wall as determined by silver methenamine and PAS stains. As the crescents develop, collagen is deposited and fibroepithelial and then finally fibrous crescents are formed. Segmental areas of necrosis are usually seen, as well as areas of glomerular capillary collapse and focal increases in mesangial matrix. The tubules may appear atrophic, and a leukocytic interstitial infiltrate is frequently identified. The light microscopic picture is similar in all three subtypes, which are subcategorized on the basis of immunofluorescence and electron microscopy.

By immunofluorescence the findings are variable and fall into three groups.[115] In those cases that are probably post-infectious in etiology, granular IgG and C3 are seen in a pattern similar to that of acute glomerulonephritis. In pa-

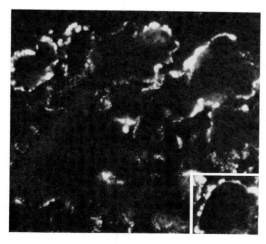

Fig. 17-15 Acute poststreptococcal glomerulonephritis. Note large granular capillary wall deposits of IgG and, **inset,** subepithelial granular deposits of IgG. Basement membrane is also clearly visible.

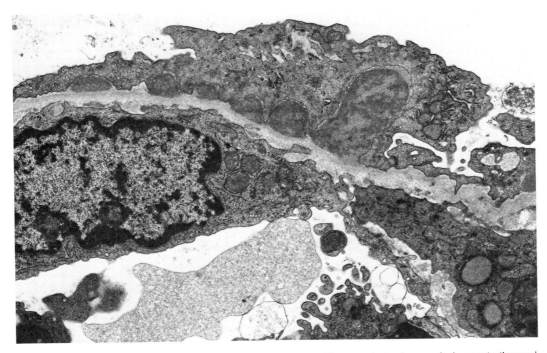

Fig. 17-16 Acute poststreptococcal glomerulonephritis. Electron photomicrograph demonstrating variably sized subepithelial "humps." Note variegated density of deposits. (×10,520.)

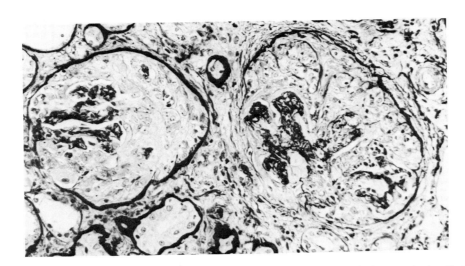

Fig. 17-17 Idiopathic crescentic glomerulonephritis. Two glomeruli illustrated show marked epithelial proliferation, resulting in compression and obliteration of glomerular tufts. (Jones' silver methenamine.)

tients with anti-glomerular basement membrane disease there is a diffuse linear staining of the basement membranes usually with IgG (Fig. 17-18) but occasionally with IgM or IgA antibodies.[109,122] An associated granular deposition of complement components occurs. Fibrinogen is usually seen deposited focally within glomerular capillary loops and in Bowman's space associated with crescents. Linear staining for immunoglobulins may also be found along tubular basement membranes as well. Anti-glomerular basement

membrane disease associated with pulmonary hemorrhage is identified as "Goodpasture's syndrome."[120] In the third group no immunoglobulin deposits are identified. Complement components and fibrinogen may be present and are usually seen in association with the crescents.

Electron microscopy also is variable but falls into two subgroups: patients with granular deposition of IgG by immunofluorescence where subepithelial humps, mesangial deposits, and occasionally subendothelial electron-dense de-

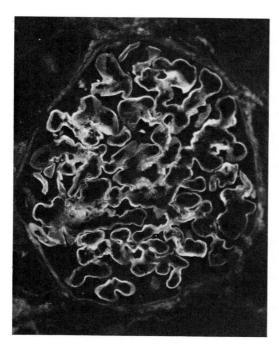

Fig. 17-18 Goodpasture's syndrome in 23-year-old man with acute renal failure and hemoptysis. Antiglomerular basement membrane antibodies were demonstrable in serum. Linear IgG along capillary walls is evident.

posits are seen, and patients with anti-GBM disease or with no specific immunofluorescence where no electron-dense deposits are seen. In most instances fibrin deposition is prominent and is often associated with breaks within the capillary wall in the basement membrane. The crescents consist of two types of cells. One cell type is often connected by desmosomes, contains relatively few organelles, and may show surface specialization consistent with epithelial cells. The second cell type demonstrates lysosomes and rough endoplasmic reticulum and has characteristics suggestive of monocyte-macrophage–type cells. Occasionally multinucleated giant cells may also be identified.

Mesangiocapillary glomerulonephritis

Mesangiocapillary glomerulonephritis is known by a variety of synonyms. These include membranoproliferative glomerulonephritis, hypocomplementic glomerulonephritis, and lobular glomerulonephritis. This entity is defined more by its morphology than by a specific clinical presentation. The clinical presentation varies, but in the classic case it consists of a combination of acute nephritis, the nephrotic syndrome, and hypertension. It primarily affects children and young adults but has been reported in all age groups.[123,127-129,131,132] The history of infection preceding the onset is not uncommon, but a causal or even temporal relationship has not been confirmed. The clinical course is variable but generally is characterized by a progressive course with intermittent remissions and gradual loss of renal function. A variety of different therapeutic modalities have been used; these include steroids, cytotoxic drugs, and most recently dipyridamole and aspirin.[124,126,133,134]

By light microscopy, the most prominent finding is glomerular enlargement and accentuation of the lobular architecture (Fig. 17-19). Mesangial areas are expanded by increased numbers of mesangial cells and matrix. In some instances a nodular accumulation of matrix exists within the lobule, giving rise to what has been termed "lobular" glomerulonephritis. The hypercellularity is predominantly mesangial, but infiltration with leukocytes is common and may be extensive. Another characteristic feature is thickening of the capillary wall. This is the result of extension of mesangial cells and matrix around the peripheral capillary and thus results in a double contour or "tram track" appearance with special stains such as silver methenamine–Masson. Necrosis is uncommon, but crescents may be seen in approximately one fifth of cases. Rarely, focal forms in which only a portion of the glomeruli are involved are found. Two subtypes are defined by immunofluorescence and electron microscopy.

Type I immunofluorescence reveals deposition of immunoglobulins, most frequently IgG and IgM but also occasionally IgA (Fig. 17-20). It is accompanied by abundant deposition of C3, as well as the early complement components C1, C4, and C2. Fibrin is occasionally seen. Electron microscopy reveals electron-dense deposits in the subendothelial and mesangial regions (Figs. 17-21 and 17-22). Occasionally subepithelial humps are also present. The mesangium is significantly expanded, and it contains increased numbers of cells and abundant matrix. The peripheral capillary basement membrane is usually identifiable as a distinct basement membrane but is separated from the endothelial cells by mesangial cells and matrix continuous with the mesangial area, thus giving rise to the "tram track" or double contour appearance (Fig. 17-23). The electron-dense deposits may lie in this subendothelial mesangial matrix. The epithelial cells show foot process effacement.

Type II is also known as dense deposit glomerulonephritis. In addition to the other clinical features, patients with type II will have the presence of C3 Nef in the serum. There is an apparent familial incidence of this type, which is associated with the occurrence of partial peripheral lipodystrophy.[125,130]

Immunofluorescence microscopy shows extensive deposition of C3 in the mesangium and occasionally in the peripheral capillary walls in an interrupted double track linear pattern (Fig. 17-24). Immunoglobulins are usually absent, but fibrin is occasionally seen. The most striking change is seen by electron microscopy. A very electron-dense material is present within the lamina densa of the glomerular capillary basement membranes, which is often widened by the presence of the deposit (Fig. 17-25). The deposit forms a long ribbon of hazy electron-dense material. In some instances the ribbon is discontinuous and the electron density has a sausage-like appearance.

Diffuse mesangial proliferative glomerulonephritis

Diffuse mesangial proliferation may occur in a variety of conditions including systemic diseases such as lupus erythematosus and Henoch-Schönlein purpura (to be discussed later) or as part of the spectrum of the primary nephrotic

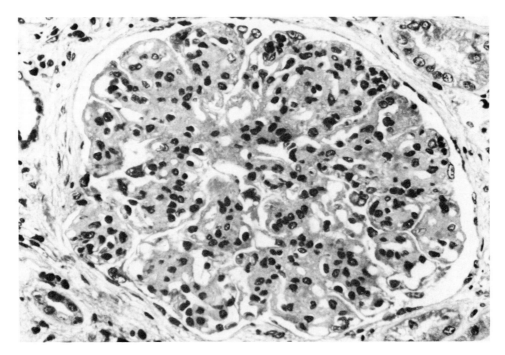

Fig. 17-19 Membranoproliferative glomerulonephritis in 17-year-old girl who presented with nephritic syndrome during pregnancy. There are marked lobular accentuation secondary to mesangial proliferation and irregular capillary wall thickening.

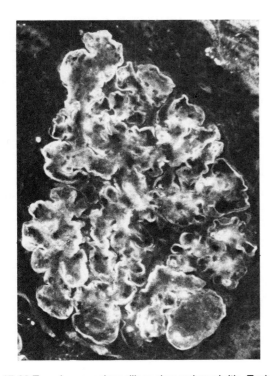

Fig. 17-20 Type I mesangiocapillary glomerulonephritis. Typical peripheral lobular staining of capillary wall for IgG.

syndrome (as discussed earlier). There is a distinct group of patients without evidence of systemic disease who present with gross or microscopic hematuria, proteinuria or combined proteinuria and hematuria, and on biopsy show mild mesangial proliferation.[138,139,144,146] A portion of these patients have mild resolving or persistent post-infectious glomerulonephritis and are said to have latent glomerulonephritis. Patients in another group have elevated serum IgA levels and deposition of IgA immune complexes in the mesangium; their condition has been termed IgA nephropathy or Berger's disease.[135] As a group, these patients generally have a favorable prognosis although a small percentage have been reported to progress rapidly to chronic renal failure.

The clinical presentation of patients with IgA nephropathy consists of a history of episodes of recurrent gross and microscopic hematuria often preceded by upper respiratory tract infections and mimicking recurrent episodes of acute glomerulonephritis.[137,142,143,145] Although proteinuria may be present, it is usually of minor degree and rarely in the nephrotic range. Some patients have only hematuria and proteinuria of unexplained origin.[140] Although frequent and sometimes prolonged remissions occur between episodes, the disease has a chronic and persistent course.[137]

Light microscopy shows expansion of the mesangial areas by an increase in mesangial cells and mesangial matrix. The endothelial cells are neither swollen nor is there evidence of proliferation and the capillary lumina are patent. The expansion of the mesangium may be mild with only small clusters of four or more cells per area or more diffuse and prominent with numerous cells and a marked increase in

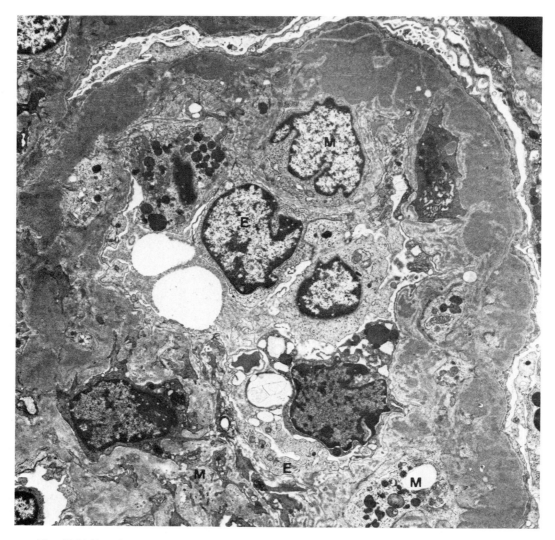

Fig. 17-21 Type I mesangiocapillary glomerulonephritis (same case as shown in Fig. 17-19). Lamina densa is markedly widened and is replaced by granular deposits. Endothelial proliferation and mesangial interposition are evident. Endothelium, *E*. Mesangium, *M*. (×4,600.)

matrix. Immunofluorescence microscopy correlates closely with the clinical picture. The presence of IgG and C3 alone is consistent with a post-infectious origin or latent glomerulonephritis. The presence of IgA and C3 is consistent with the category of Berger's disease or IgA nephropathy. It should be noted that marked similarities exist between the morphologic findings in Berger's disease and Henoch-Schönlein purpura and that the separation of these two categories is predominantly on the basis of the clinical presentation.[136,141] Electron microscopy shows mesangial changes that consist of an increase in mesangial matrix cells and the presence of electron-dense deposits. Occasionally the electron-dense deposits are also seen in the paramesangial subendothelial location, but there is no evidence of involvement of the peripheral capillary loops. In rare instances small subepithelial humps have been observed.

Lupus nephritis

Lupus erythematosus is a systemic autoimmune disease that affects both adults and children and has a wide variety of clinical manifestations. In 1971 the American Rheumatism Association set forth criteria for the diagnosis of systemic lupus erythematosus; the criteria include both clinical manifestations and laboratory findings.[152,164] Based on clinical signs of renal disease, the incidence of renal involvement in adult patients ranges from 50% to 80%. Clinicopathologic correlations have demonstrated a significant relationship between the underlying histopathology of the renal disease and the subsequent clinical course.[149,153,162] In patients with mild mesangial hypercellularity and membranous nephropathy, renal function is preserved for long periods although patients with the membranous lesion commonly exhibit heavy proteinuria and the nephrotic syn-

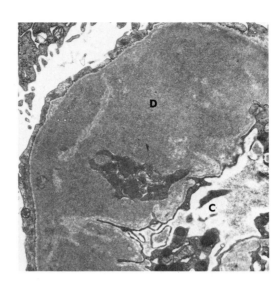

Fig. 17-22 Type I mesangiocapillary glomerulonephritis (same case as shown in Fig. 17-19). Lamina densa is widened, replaced by granular deposits, *D,* difficult to discern and best demonstrated with silver-stained sections. Capillary lumen, *C.* (× 16,400.)

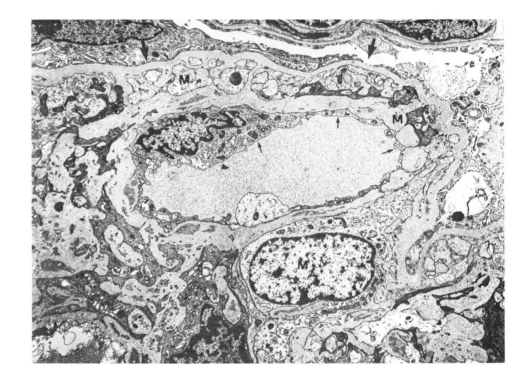

Fig. 17-23 Type I membranoproliferative glomerulonephritis. Mesangial cytoplasm and matrix, *M,* are interposed between endothelial cell (small arrows) and intact basal lamina (large arrows). This change is responsible for capillary wall thickening evident by light microscopy. (× 4,500.)

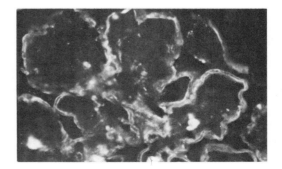

Fig. 17-24 Dense intramembranous deposit disease. Double-contour pattern for C3 along capillary walls is characteristic of this disease. Note mesangial globs and "rings."

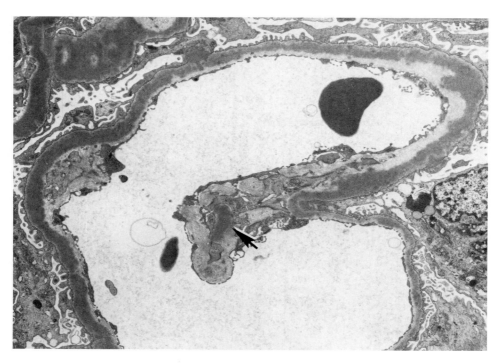

Fig. 17-25 Dense intramembranous deposit disease. Widening and partial replacement of lamina densa by electron-dense material in 6-year-old girl who presented with acute nephritic syndrome. Capillary wall thickening was evident by light microscopy. Several subepithelial deposits also are evident. Mesangial deposit (arrow) may correspond with "mesangial rings" seen by immunofluorescence. (×4,900.)

drome. In contrast, the clinical course of patients with diffuse proliferative glomerulonephritis is usually hectic and the 2-year patient survival has been less than 30% despite the use of high-dose steroid therapy. A variety of reports have emphasized that the presence and location of electron-dense deposits is an important index of the clinical course in addition to the pattern of injury as observed by light microscopy. Based on the analysis of clinical series, the presence of subendothelial electron-dense deposits[153] correlates with a high incidence of heavy proteinuria and renal insufficiency. In addition to the proliferative changes within the glomerulus, other reports have emphasized that glomerulosclerosis and interstitial fibrosis represent a significant indicator for progression to renal failure. Thus evidence from analysis of clinical series suggests that a histologic pattern of renal injury is important in determining the long-term prognosis of renal disease in lupus nephropathy and is an important adjunct in determining the therapeutic management of such patients.[165]

The pathogenesis of lupus nephritis is thought to be similar to that of experimental chronic immune complex glomerulonephritis.[154,155,160] The major immunologic problem appears to be a faulty regulation of the immune response system resulting in an autoimmune disease with antibodies directed to nuclear proteins, cytoplasmic and plasma membrane constituents, and to specific plasma proteins. The presence of antibodies to nuclear proteins forms an important part of the clinical diagnosis of lupus. The variety of

lesions seen in lupus can thus be attributed to individual differences in the immune response in different patients or in the same individual patients during the course of time.

Because of the broad spectrum of lesions that have been seen in patients with lupus erythematosus, the World Health Organization created a classification of lupus nephritis to combine all morphologic modalities of biopsy interpretation and added a semiquantitative assessment of severity as well[161] (Table 17-4). It is now in general use and has been widely accepted by clinical nephrologists and renal pathologists alike. It provides a significant improvement over previous classifications since it includes immunofluorescence and electron microscopic evaluation as well as light microscopic evaluation and therefore can differentiate patients with mild, purely mesangial forms from those with significant peripheral capillary involvement and subendothelial deposits on electron microscopy who generally have a more severe clinical course.[159]

Class I is essentially the absence of a specific microscopic lesion. Renal biopsy generally reveals essentially a normal kidney by light, electron, and immunofluorescence microscopy; there is no clinical evidence of significant renal involvement. Focal thickening of the basement membrane by electron microscopy and a segmental linear deposition of immunoglobulin by immunofluorescence has been observed occasionally. Since this class is really an absence of significant morphologic evidence of glomerular damage, it may not really represent a true class of renal disease.

Table 17-4 WHO classification of lupus nephritis

Disease	Light microscopy	Electron microscopy	Immunofluorescence microscopy	Clinical features
Lupus nephritis				
WHO class I (normal)	No lesion	No lesion	No deposits	Negative, normal urine
WHO class II (mesangial)	Mild mesangial	Mesangial deposits	Mesangial IgG, C3; hypercellularity	Moderate proteinuria, occasionally active sediment
WHO class III (focal segmental)	Focal and segmental necrosis and proliferation	Mesangial and subendothelial deposits	Granular capillary and mesangial Ig, C3	Proteinuria, active sediment
WHO class IV (diffuse)	Mesangial proliferation; membranoproliferative and/or crescentic pattern	Endothelial and marked mesangial proliferation; sometimes subepithelial deposits; viroids; fingerprint deposits	Same as class III "full house pattern"	Acute nephritis with active sediment and/or nephrotic syndrome
WHO class V	Diffuse membranous thickening	Epi- and intramembranous deposits; frequently mesangial deposits	Peripheral granular IgG, C3	Nephrotic syndrome or severe proteinuria

Class II is confined to glomerular lesions that are purely mesangial. It is subdivided into class IIA and class IIB. In class IIA minimal or no significant changes are shown by light microscopy although there may be immunofluorescence and electron microscopic evidence of immune deposits confined to the mesangium (Fig. 17-26). Class IIB shows definite glomerular mesangial hypercellularity by light microscopy, which is in the center of tubules away from the vascular pole. No significant changes exist in the peripheral capillary walls. Immune deposits are present by

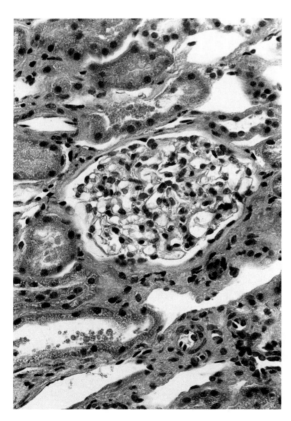

Fig. 17-26 Lupus nephritis, WHO class II. There is mild diffuse mesangial hypercellularity and increase in matrix. Mesangial deposits may be identified by immunofluorescence and electron microscopy.

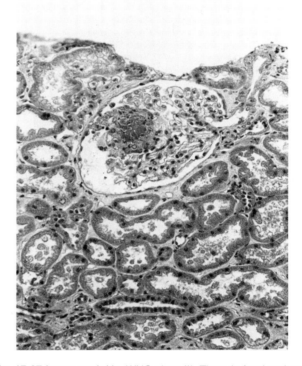

Fig. 17-27 Lupus nephritis, WHO class III. There is focal and segmental glomerulonephritis characterized by segmental necrosis, adhesions to Bowman's capsule, and leukocytic infiltration.

immunofluorescence but are confined to the mesangial region. Electron microscopy reveals mesangial dense deposits, which occasionally may extend to the paramesangial subendothelial space. Tubular, interstitial, or vascular changes are insignificant. Clinically, the majority of these patients have mild to moderate evidence of renal involvement and in general have a good prognosis.

Class III is represented by light microscopic findings of a focal and segmental glomerulonephritis (Fig. 17-27). The changes may be proliferative, necrotizing, or sclerosing. A combination of these changes may be seen scattered in different glomeruli. The lesions are usually superimposed on a mild diffuse mesangial prominence such as seen in class II. Segmental intra- and extracapillary proliferation with obliteration of the capillary lumina is often found. The presence of necrosis with fibrinoid material, necrotic debris, and leukocytic infiltration may also be seen. The segmental necrotic lesions may occasionally be associated with focal crescents. In advanced stages segmental sclerotic scars with focal capsular adhesions may be seen. Less than 50% of the glomeruli are involved, and the glomeruli show only focal damage, occupying less than 50% of the glomerular surface. Despite the focal nature of the lesions by light microscopy, immunofluorescence generally reveals a more diffuse and irregular peripheral granular deposition of immunoglobulins and complement. Electron microscopy reveals the presence of subendothelial deposits in addition to mesangial deposits. Subepithelial deposits are variably found. Interstitial and tubular changes are frequently encountered but are usually focal in distribution. The similarity of immunofluorescence and electron microscopic findings

in class III disease with those in class IV suggest that the two may actually be portions of a continuum of morphologic change. Clinically, the disease in these patients tends to behave aggressively, with a natural history similar to patients of class IV.

Class IV is the most common form of renal involvement and is characterized by a diffuse proliferative glomerulonephritis (Fig. 17-28). The majority or all of the glomeruli are involved and each glomerulus shows a diffuse hypercellularity. In addition focal areas of necrosis and crescent formation may be present. The presence of condensed nuclear debris has been given the term hematoxyphil body. Some areas of the peripheral capillary loop may be thickened to form wire loop lesions. The range of glomerular lesions may extend from only diffuse mesangial hypercellularity without necrosis, sclerosis, or wire loops to a severe necrotizing and crescentic glomerulonephritis. Approximately 25% of this class of patients show lobular accentuation and mesangial extension into the peripheral capillary loops in a pattern similar to membranoproliferative glomerulonephritis. By immunofluorescence, immunoglobulins are present in a coarsely granular pattern in both the mesangium and the peripheral capillary wall. The pattern is often irregular in density and distribution. Complement components, fibrinogen, and properdin may also be identified. Electron microscopy reveals the presence of large subendothelial electron-dense deposits, which are accompanied by mesangial and frequently subepithelial and intramembranous deposits (Fig. 17-29). Mesangial hypercellularity with circumferential mesangial interposition is also seen and may incorporate the subendothelial deposits. The electron-dense

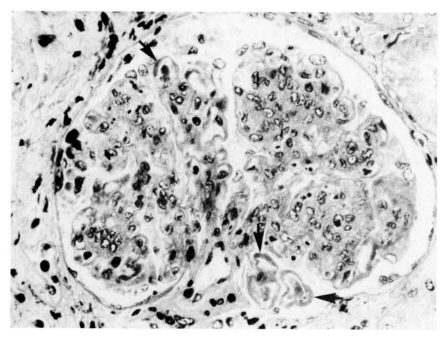

Fig. 17-28 Systemic lupus erythematosus in young woman with hematuria and nephrotic syndrome. Biopsy revealed generalized diffuse proliferative glomerulonephritis, WHO class IV. Note karyorrhectic debris and numerous "wire loops" (arrows).

deposits may also show a distinctive crystalline structure, which has been termed a "fingerprint" pattern (Fig. 17-30). Endothelial cell swelling and proliferation are present. The endothelial cells may contain tubulovesicular structures that resemble myxovirus-like particles (Fig. 17-31). These structures are similar to those seen in the endothelial cells of patients with AIDS. Patients with class IV lesions generally have a relatively severe clinical picture with nephrotic range proteinuria and an active sediment. Without therapy these patients are considered to have the worst prognosis since a high percentage of patients with this lesion progress on to renal failure rapidly if left untreated.

Class V is represented by a diffuse membranous glomerulonephropathy. This is essentially identical to that seen with idiopathic membranous glomerulonephropathy. By light microscopy, there is a generalized diffuse thickening of the peripheral capillary walls, which with silver methenamine–Masson stain exhibits the so-called "spike and dome" pattern. The degree of mesangial widening with both cells and matrix is variable. Immunofluorescence demonstrates a confluent peripheral granular deposition of immunoglobulin, which is usually accompanied by mesangial granular deposits. Electron microscopy reveals numerous epimembranous and intramembranous deposits and frequently mesangial deposits. The mesangial deposits are usually prominent and may help distinguish this lesion from that of idiopathic membranous glomerulonephropathy. Clinically these patients generally tend to have proteinuria that can be in the nephrotic range, but this lesion tends to progress in a relatively indolent fashion similar to that of idiopathic disease.

The immunofluorescence findings in lupus are of special interest. The so-called "full house" pattern, or multiple immunoglobulin deposition, is quite characteristic of lupus.[147,150,151,158] IgG and IgM are the classes of immunoglobulin most commonly deposited. IgA, though frequently found, is not as common nor is its distribution as extensive or impressive as the other two immunoglobulins. IgE deposition is infrequently found and is thought to be associated with a poorer prognosis. Complement components including the membrane attack complex, fibrinogen, and properdin are usually associated with the presence of immunoglobulins, particularly in class IV. Occasionally a pure linear pattern similar to that seen with antiglomerular basement membrane antibody is present, but no clear clinical or pathologic implication of this type of deposition exists.

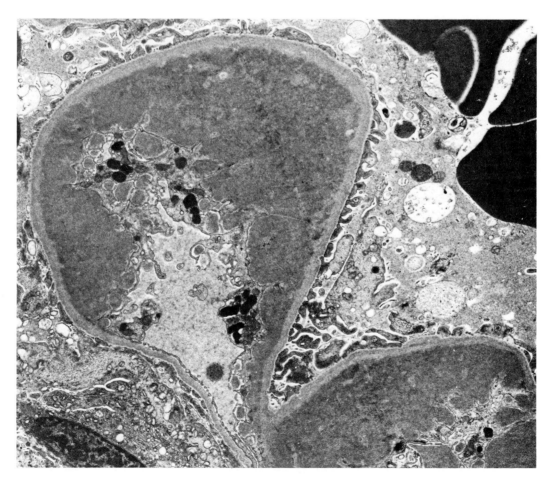

Fig. 17-29 Systemic lupus erythematosus, WHO class IV (same case as shown in Fig. 17-28). Large subendothelial deposit, which corresponds to "wire loops" seen by light microscopy, is evident. (×7,350.)

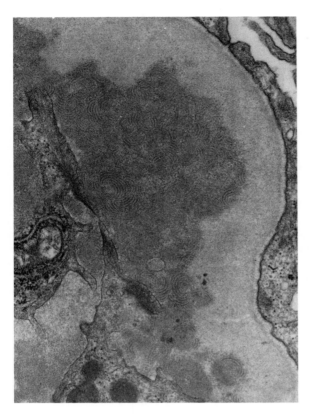

Fig. 17-30 Lupus nephritis, WHO class IV. Mesangial deposit demonstrates well-defined "fingerprint" pattern. (×36,000.)

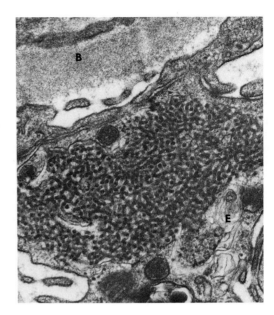

Fig. 17-31 Systemic lupus erythematosus. Tubuloreticular structures are demonstrated in nearly all cases of systemic lupus erythematosus but are not pathognomonic of this disorder. Particles are found in cytoplasm of endothelial cells. Basal lamina, *B.* Endothelial cell, *E.* (×34,250.)

Tubulointerstitial disease is also frequently encountered in all classes of lupus nephritis. Severe active tubulointerstitial nephritis is most commonly seen in patients with class III or IV glomerular lesions and is comprised of an infiltrate of lymphocytes, plasma cells, and granulocytes, sometimes including eosinophils. Immunofluorescence occasionally reveals peritubular deposits and, very rarely, the presence of a linear immunoglobulin deposit. Electron microscopy in those instances where there is granular immunofluorescence demonstrates electron-dense deposits in the tubular basement membrane. Of interest is the observation that tubulointerstitial disease may progress independently of the glomerular disease in some patients.[163]

Necrotizing vasculitis with vascular necrosis and leukocytic infiltration is a rare finding in the kidney of lupus patients; when it occurs it is associated with a severe necrotizing glomerular lesion and malignant hypertension. More commonly, evidence of venulitis is seen with a perivenular leukocytic infiltration, which is generally found in association with severe tubulointerstitial nephritis. Immunofluorescence examination will occasionally demonstrate granular immune deposits and complement in the vessels. Recently attention has been drawn to a group of patients in which prominent evidence exists of intravascular coagulation with multiple capillary thrombi containing fibrinogen.[156,157] It is thought that this may be related to the presence of lupus antibodies acting as plasminogen inactivators and

that this may contribute independently to the progression of renal disease.

Some studies have suggested the use of semiquantitative analysis of lupus biopsies to assess chronicity and severity.[147,148] Activity has been related to the presence of necrosis, crescent formation, endocapillary and mesangial cellular proliferation, glomerular leukocytic infiltration, and the presence of hyaline thrombi in the glomeruli. Chronicity has been graded on the degree of glomerulosclerosis and fibrosis, as well as the amount of interstitial scarring, chronic inflammation, and tubular atrophy. The predictive value of quantification in an individual case appears best correlated with the degree of interstitial disease rather than with that of glomerular disease. The severity of the glomerular disease appears to be more related to the systemic activity and the need for aggressive immunosuppressive therapy.

GLOMERULONEPHRITIS ASSOCIATED WITH SYSTEMIC VASCULITIS
Hypersensitivity angiitis and periarteritis nodosa

The renal lesions found in cases of hypersensitivity angiitis caused by exogenous antigens, such as drugs as well as those associated with several different clinical syndromes in which a small vessel angiitis occurs, bear a close resemblance to each other.[166-169] It is important to point out that all the clinical syndromes are manifested by a widespread vasculitis that includes renal involvement, and distinction of one type from another is based on the pattern of organ involvement, associated pathologic lesions, and the severity of the disease process (Table 17-5). A useful classification of systemic vasculitis or periarteritis was provided by

Table 17-5 Systemic diseases with renal involvement

Disease	Light microscopy	Electron microscopy	Immunofluorescence microscopy	Clinical features
Glomerulonephritis associated with systemic disease				
Systemic vasculitis, i.e., periarteritis nodosa, hypersensitivity angiitis, Wegener's granulomatosis	Focal or diffuse segmental or global necrotizing and proliferative, sometimes granulomatous, crescents	Fibrin deposition with mesangial proliferation; usually no deposits; rarely mesangial and paramesangial deposits	Mesangial and subendothelial fibrin occasionally, IgG, C3	Multisystem involvement including skin, lung, bowel and visceral organs; hematuria, proteinuria, azotemia
Henoch-Schonlein purpura	Variable from mesangial proliferation to membranoproliferative to crescentic pattern	Mesangial and occasionally subendothelial deposits	Mesangial IgA, IgG, C3, fibrin	Abdominal pain, arthritis rash, guiac and stools hematuria, proteinuria
Cryoglobulinemia	Hyaline thrombi, membranoproliferative pattern	Intraluminal finely granular material; crystalline subendothelial deposits	Granular IgM, IgG or IgA, or mixed	Systemic manifestations of paraproteinemia, nephrotic syndrome
Glomerular diseases associated with disseminated intravascular coagulation				
Hemolytic uremic syndrome; toxemia of pregnancy; thrombotic thrombocytopenic purpura; postpartum nephrosclerosis	Early—intracapillary fibrin and platelet thrombi Late—marked endothelial and mesangial hyperplasia and swelling, ± necrosis End—glomerular hyalinization and tubular atrophy, varies from minimal to marked Deposition of fibrin	Early—fibrin thrombi in capillaries with subendothelial fibrin Late—fibrin and/or fluffy subendomaterial, endothelial swelling End—glomerular sclerosis	Mesangial and capillary fibrin	Varied—acute renal failure to progressive renal failure, hypertension, eclampsia, fibrin split products, schistocytes; depletion of coagulation factor; hemolytic anemia
Toxemia of pregnancy	Endothelial cell swelling with capillary narrowing	Endothelial cell swelling and separation from basement membrane	Fibrin, occasionally Ig	Proteinuria, hypertension

Zeek.[170] Two forms of periarteritis nodosa have been described based on the size of the vessel involved. In the classic or macroscopic form of periarteritis nodosa the renal lesion is characterized by necrotizing arteritis involving medium-size arteries such as the renal artery, interlobular arteries, or arcuate arteries. The lesions are quite focal, occurring frequently at branch points with aneurysm formation. The inflammatory process may involve several or all layers of the vessel wall and is characterized by leukocytic infiltration associated with fibrinoid necrosis and focal intraluminal thrombosis. Electron microscopy reveals evidence of endothelial cell swelling, rupture of the internal elastic lamina, and infiltration by leukocytes. Because of the focal nature of the large vessel lesions, active vasculitis may not be found in needle biopsies. Areas of scarring secondary to ischemia may be the only lesion seen or may be accompanied by healed lesions in the vessels characterized by medial fibrosis and disruption of the elastic lamina. The microscopic form of periarteritis nodosa involves smaller arteries, which include the cortical and perforating radial arteries and the arterioles. In addition, there usually is evidence of glomerular involvement ranging from a focal and segmental necrotizing glomerulonephritis to a severe

diffuse crescentic glomerulonephritis. Immunofluorescent stains occasionally reveal the deposition of immunoglobulins IgG or IgM with C3, and electron microscopy may show mesangial deposits, as well as prominent intracapillary fibrin deposits, endothelial cell swelling, and rupture of the peripheral glomerular capillary wall. Healed and healing lesions are seen as focal and segmental areas of glomerular sclerosis. A tubulointerstitial infiltrate including eosinophils is frequently seen.

Wegener's granulomatosis

In Wegener's granulomatosis there is a necrotizing granulomatous vasculitis that involves multiple organ systems.[171] Microscopically, there is a necrotizing and granulomatous inflammation of both arteries and veins with frequent involvement of the upper and lower respiratory tract associated with a glomerulonephritis. The glomerulonephritis may range from a focal and segmental endocapillary and extracapillary proliferative and necrotizing glomerulonephritis to a granulomatous form of crescentic glomerulonephritis in which the inflammatory process extends through Bowman's capsule into the interstitium[172-174] (Fig. 17-32). Necrotizing arteritis in the kidney is unusual but has been described.

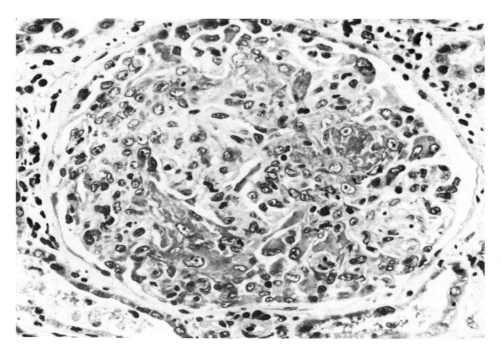

Fig. 17-32 Wegener's granulomatosis in 39-year-old woman with sinusitis, necrotizing granulomatous pulmonary lesions, and acute renal failure. Glomerulus demonstrates foci or fibrinoid necrosis, epithelial proliferation, and formation of multinucleated giant cells. Similar morphology may be seen in Goodpasture's syndrome, idiopathic crescentic glomerulonephritis, and polyarteritis nodosa.

Interstitial granulomas are rare and are often found to represent destroyed glomeruli. Occasionally mesangial or subepithelial electron-dense deposits are seen by means of electron microscopy, and there is a corresponding deposition of immunoglobulin by immunofluorescence.

Henoch-Schönlein purpura

Henoch-Schönlein purpura is a clinical syndrome characterized by the presence of skin, joint, and gastrointestinal symptoms that may be episodic.[175-178,180] Renal involvement occurs in approximately 25% of cases and in many instances presents as acute nephritis but in others may be symptomless hematuria and proteinuria. The renal involvement is probably the major cause of morbidity and mortality in this syndrome, but the overall prognosis, particularly in children, is generally good with the disease being a self-limited one in most instances.

A wide spectrum of renal lesions is seen by light microscopy, and the overall pattern is similar to that seen in idiopathic IgA nephropathy.[175,176,178] Glomeruli may show lesions ranging from a mild mesangial hypercellularity to a focal and segmental glomerulonephritis to a severe, diffuse crescentic glomerulonephritis. Healed lesions may also be found because of the episodic nature of the disease; they consist of capsular adhesions, fibrous crescents, and focal and segmental glomerulosclerosis. Immunofluorescence reveals the presence of IgA frequently associated with IgG and C3. IgM and properdin are also found occasionally. Electron microscopy[179] reveals prominent mesangial deposits with occasional subendothelial and subepithelial deposits

as well. Clinical pathologic studies have shown that the prognosis depends on the severity of the glomerular lesions. Overall, the larger the number of glomeruli affected by the presence of crescents or necrosis, the poorer the prognosis. In addition, the final outcome also seems to be related to the number of recurrent episodes.

Glomerulonephritis of cryoglobulinemia

Cryoglobulinemia has been demonstrated in patients with a variety of infectious processes and in individuals with primary or essential cryoglobulinemia associated with a dysproteinemia.[181] Up to a half of patients with cryoglobulins in their serum may demonstrate renal manifestations. A distinct syndrome characterized by the combination of purpura, arthralgias, weakness, and glomerulonephritis has been described in patients with mixed cryoglobulinemia. Three subtypes have been characterized on the basis of the nature of the cryoglobulins. In type I, a monoclonal immunoglobulin is mixed with isolated immunoglobulins of other classes. In type II, the monoclonal component is an antibody to the second component of the cryoprecipitate, and in type III the cryoglobulins represent circulating immune complexes without a monoclonal component. In type II cryoglobulinemia, a distinct histopathologic picture is present.

By light microscopy there is a diffuse proliferative glomerulonephritis with lobular accentuation associated with infiltration by neutrophils. Intraluminal eosinophilic occlusive thrombi are also present.[182,183] In some instances, particularly in chronic cases, the picture is similar to that seen

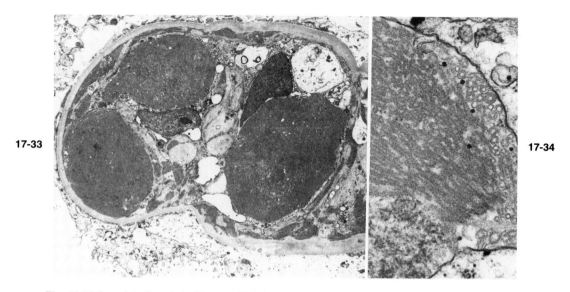

17-33

17-34

Fig. 17-33 Cryoglobulinemia in 42-year-old diabetic patient who developed acute renal failure following episode of acute pyelonephritis. In addition to diabetic changes, note subendothelial and mesangial deposits and capillary thrombi. (×3,100.)

Fig. 17-34 Longitudinal and cross-sectional tubular deposits characteristic of cryoglobulinemia. (×42,000.)

in membranoproliferative glomerulonephritis. Crescents are also often present.

Immunofluorescence shows characteristic large peripheral capillary deposits containing both IgG and IgM. C3, C1, and C4 are present in a granular fashion along the capillary walls.

By electron microscopy, subendothelial deposits and mesangial deposits are prominent and are associated with capillary thrombi (Fig. 17-33). The deposits have a distinctive organized appearance composed of parallel arrays of fibrils or tubules (Fig. 17-34). In some instances, protein crystals are seen and may be found in the epithelial and endothelial cells. Cylindric or annular bodies are also found.

GLOMERULAR DISEASE ASSOCIATED WITH DISSEMINATED INTRAVASCULAR COAGULATION
Hemolytic uremic syndrome

The hemolytic uremic syndrome is a clinical syndrome in which microangiopathic hemolytic anemia, thrombocytopenia, and acute renal failure occur simultaneously.[184,185] The disorder is more common in young children but occurs in all age groups. In children it has been associated with gastrointestinal and upper respiratory tract infections of both bacterial or viral origin. In adults, mainly women in the postpartum period or those using oral contraceptives have been affected. The prognosis appears to be better in children than in adults and may be related to the extent of the renal lesions.

The pathologic lesion has been described as a thrombotic microangiopathy.[187,188] The initial findings are numerous thrombi within the glomerular capillaries. They may be associated with focal areas of necrosis, which may appear bland because of the lack of leukocytic infiltration. Frag-

mented red blood cells may also be entrapped within the glomeruli. The arterioles may also be involved by the thrombotic process. As the lesions develop, the capillary walls thicken with a prominent double contour (Fig. 17-35). The small arteries and arterioles will show myointimal proliferation with accumulation of a mucoid material and focal areas of thrombosis. Some arterioles, particularly at the hilus of the glomerulus, develop aneurysms with thrombosis, organization, and re-endothelialization forming so-called glomeruloid structures.[189] The acute lesions subsequently result in evidence of glomerulosclerosis and ischemic damage. Malignant nephrosclerosis develops in some patients.

Immunofluorescence microscopy generally reveals the presence of fibrinogen or fibrin-related antigens within the capillary wall and within the mesangium. Occasionally, immunoglobulins are also nonspecifically trapped. Similar changes are seen within the walls of the arteries and arterioles. By electron microscopy a characteristic separation of the endothelium from the basement membrane and the accumulation of a granular material in the new subendothelial space are seen (Fig. 17-36). Occasionally, fibrin tactoids and fragments of red blood cells and platelets are also entrapped. A thin layer of basement membrane–like substance may be identified following the outline of the endothelial cells in giving rise to double contour appearance by light microscopy. Endothelial separation and granular material are also found in the walls of small arteries.[186]

Thrombotic thrombocytopenic purpura

Whether thrombotic thrombocytopenic purpura and hemolytic uremic syndrome should be considered two distinct diseases or two different expressions of the same dis-

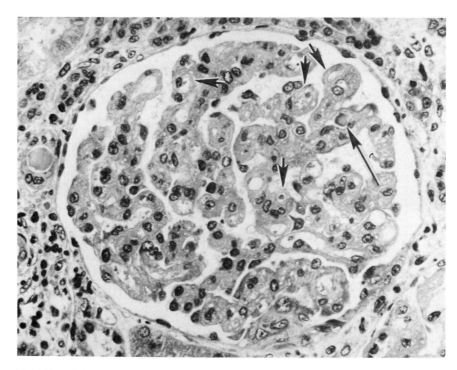

Fig. 17-35 Hemolytic-uremic syndrome in 4-year-old girl with microangiopathic hemolytic anemia and acute nephritis. Glomerulus demonstrates membranoproliferative glomerulonephritis-like pattern that may be seen in this syndrome. Note capillary wall double contours (short arrows) and fibrin thrombus (long arrow).

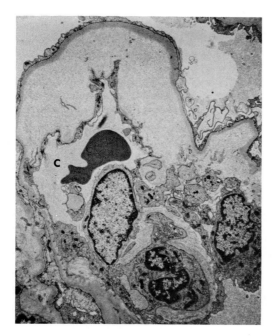

Fig. 17-36 Hemolytic-uremic syndrome in 24-year-old woman. Subendothelial widening secondary to accumulation of flocculent material is typically seen in diseases associated with fibrin deposition within glomerular loops. Capillary lumen C. (×3,000.)

ease is not clear. Because of the similarity of the clinical and pathologic presentations it seems likely that they may form variants within a spectrum of disease processes involving spontaneous intravascular coagulation.[190,191] Although thrombocytopenic purpura and hemolytic uremic syndrome share the common features of microangiopathic hemolytic anemia, thrombocytopenia, and renal failure, renal failure predominates in hemolytic uremic syndrome whereas in thrombocytopenic purpura other organ involvement, especially central nervous system involvement, appears to be more prominent. The course is also somewhat more chronic and less fulminant. The pathology of the lesions is essentially identical, although platelets may appear more prominently in thrombotic thrombocytopenic purpura. Immunofluorescence and electron microscopy do not help in distinguishing these two nosologic entities.

Toxemia of pregnancy

The triad of hypertension, proteinuria, and edema is characteristic of pre-eclampsia or toxemia of pregnancy.[194] The clinical syndrome, however, encompasses at least three different major disease groups: primary renal disease in pregnancy, hypertensive cardiovascular disease in pregnancy, and so-called pre-eclampsia syndrome. Pre-eclampsia is more common in first pregnancies. Its etiology is at present still unclear. Hereditary and familial influences, hormonal influences, and immunologic factors have all been implicated in possibly playing an active role in the pathogenesis. Most recently, antibodies to laminin have been found in

Table 17-6 Renal allograft pathology

Terminology	Lesion	Time course	Putative mechanism
Hyperacute (peracute)	Glomerular capillary thrombosis	1-2 days	Preformed antibodies
Acute imminent	Tubular necrosis with or without acute infiltrate	First month	Preservation injury
Acute rejection			
Interstitial (cellular)	Interstitial lymphoblasts, plasma cells, phagocytes, occasional eosinophils	Anytime after 7 days	Delayed type immunity (predominantly cellular)
Vascular (humoral)	Vasculitis with lymphoid cells, glomerular endothelial swelling, vascular thrombosis, interstitial hemorrhage		Combined cellular and humoral
Combined	Interstitial and vascular lesions		
Chronic rejection			
Vasculopathy	Myointimal proliferation of vessels, interstitial scarring	Late, after several months	Unknown
Glomerulopathy	Glomerular hypercellularity and sclerosis; electron microscopy shows basement membrane thickening		
Acute and interactive cyclosporin toxicity	Absence of lesion in most cases, occasionally tubular and vascular changes	Early in course	Tubulotoxic vs. vasospastic; interactive with ischemic injury
Chronic cyclosporin toxicity	Streak fibrosis	Late, with long-term use	Vascular constriction

some patients.[192] Some form of endothelial injury in association with the normal hypercoagulable state seen in pregnancy is likely to be the cause of the renal lesions.[193] If severe hypertension or convulsions occur, treatment requires the termination of pregnancy or death may occur as a result of cerebral hemorrhage and renal failure. By light microscopy, the glomeruli are enlarged because of swelling of the endothelial cells, and the capillary lumina are narrowed and appear bloodless. Mesangial hypercellularity is also present. Occasionally, a picture similar to that seen in the hemolytic uremic syndrome is present with intracapillary thrombi. Immunofluorescence reveals substantial deposition of fibrinogen and IgM, but other immunoglobulins in complement components are also present. Electron microscopy shows extensive endothelial cell swelling and separation of the endothelial cells from the basement membrane, similar to that seen in hemolytic uremic syndrome.

RENAL TRANSPLANT REJECTION

Whereas evaluation of the renal biopsy for glomerular disease is usually referred to the nephropathology specialist, the general surgical pathologist is frequently called upon to evaluate renal transplant biopsies for rejection. The renal biopsy in the evaluation of allograft rejection is used to answer two major questions: (1) is the failure of the graft caused by rejection or some other unrelated lesion? (2) if rejection is present, is the lesion potentially reversible using available therapeutic approaches? In evaluating the biopsy to answer the first question, if rejection is not present, it

should be ascertained if the cause of the graft failure results from acute tubular necrosis, acute infectious pyelonephritis, obstruction of the vasculature or urinary outflow tract, the presence of recurrent or *de novo* glomerular disease, or toxicity associated with the therapy. In assessing whether or not the rejection lesions are potentially reversible, it is necessary to evaluate not only the intensity but also the nature of the rejection episode. Rejection has been classified as hyperacute, acute, or chronic (Table 17-6).

Hyperacute rejection

Hyperacute rejection refers to allograft failure that occurs within minutes or hours after transplantation.[197] It is thought to be the result of pre-existing circulating antibodies of the recipient, which are directed against antigens present in the grafted endothelium. Presensitization of the recipient is often related to previous pregnancies, blood transfusions, or previous cross-match testing. The occurrence of hyperacute rejections is extremely rare. However, hyperacute rejections may be related to endothelial damage that is not immunologic in nature. A separate form of acute graft failure that is not immunologic has been termed acute imminent transplant nephropathy and has been related to injury occurring in the graft during the preservation phase.[195,196]

Microscopically, fibrin thrombi are seen in all renal vessels, including the glomerular capillaries and peritubular venules. The vascular thrombosis is associated with infarction and tubular necrosis. Immunofluorescence may show linear staining for immunoglobulin along the capillary walls of the peritubular venules, but this is not a constant finding. Electron microscopy demonstrates platelets, fibrillar fibrin, sludged red blood cells, and necrosis of glomerular capillaries and other vascular structures.

Acute rejection

Acute rejection, despite its terminology, can occur at any time during the course of transplantation. It is most frequently seen during the initial months after grafting. The type of reaction that occurs falls into two patterns.

Acute interstitial allograft rejection has also been called cellular rejection, or acute reversible rejection.[206-211] Light microscopy reveals edema and infiltration of the interstitium by immunoblasts, lymphocytes, plasma cells, macrophages, and a scattering of polymorphonuclear leukocytes and eosinophils. The infiltrate is generally diffuse but appears somewhat more concentrated around vessels and glomeruli. Identification of the lymphocytes in the infiltrate demonstrates a large population of T-cells identifiable by the CD3 antigen and a greater number of cytotoxic T-cells identified by the antigen CD8 than helper-inducer cells identified by the presence of the antigen CD4.* Very high levels of CD8-positive cells have been associated with a poor therapeutic response. Immunofluorescence is generally negative. Electron microscopy will reveal evidence of tubular damage and regeneration as well as interstitial cellular infiltration. Glomerular and vascular changes are invariably present but may be mild. Predominantly cellular rejection is thought to be easily reversible with a variety of therapeutic approaches.

Acute predominantly vascular rejection has also been termed acute humoral rejection or acute irreversible rejection.[211] Histologically, it is characterized by prominent vascular involvement. There is evidence of endothelial cell swelling of arteries and arterioles and infiltration of the vascular wall predominantly in the subendothelial space with macrophages, lymphocytes, and immunoblasts. In more severe cases, a necrotizing arteritis will be present with fibrinoid necrosis and thrombosis and more generalized infiltration of vessel walls with a mixed inflammatory infiltrate. The glomeruli show endothelial cell swelling, increase in cellularity, and occasionally glomerular thrombosis.[210] Interstitial hemorrhage, as well as tubular necrosis and infarctions, is also seen. Immunofluorescence microscopy will occasionally demonstrate the presence of complement components in vascular walls and in the glomeruli and, rarely, the presence of immunoglobulins. Electron microscopy demonstrates endothelial cell swelling associated with separation of the endothelium from the basement membrane by fluffy fibrillar material, which occasionally contains fibrin tactoids and platelet fragments.

Although it is convenient to describe the two types of allograft rejection reactions independently, every case of allograft rejection is really a combination of both interstitial and vascular changes. Since the interstitial component of allograft rejection appears to be more responsive to some forms of therapy than the vascular form, it is essential to identify and to semiquantify the relative degree of involvement of both types.[201] This is essential in assisting the cli-

nician in determining whether or not the rejection episode should be treated with steroids, monoclonal antibodies, or a complete change in the immunosuppressive approach. It is also of importance in studying follow-up biopsies after therapy, particularly where the therapeutic response has not been favorable.

Chronic rejection occurs anywhere from several months to several years after transplantation. Clinically, it is associated with a slow and gradual decrease in renal function in contrast to the more acute, explosive loss of renal function seen in acute rejection. Microscopically, the picture is similar to nephrosclerosis. There is arterial and arteriolar narrowing of the interlobar arcuate and radial arteries by a myointimal hyperplasia and medial hypertrophy.[206] The vascular lesions are associated with a diffuse interstitial fibrosis and tubular atrophy.[200] The glomerular lesions consist of ischemic glomerular capillary collapse, thickening of the capillary walls, and segmental and global sclerosis.[204,209] Immunofluorescent studies are unrevealing. By electron microscopy the glomeruli show varying degrees of glomerulosclerosis with an increase in mesangial matrix, mesangial interposition, and irregular thickening of the basement membrane. Occasionally, there is separation of the endothelial cells from the basement membrane with the accumulation of a granular material in the subendothelial space. Immunofluorescent studies show occasionally linear and sometimes granular deposition of IgM, IgG, and complement components.

Cyclosporin toxicity

One of the most important innovations in the field of organ transplantation has been the introduction of the drug cyclosporin.[213,214,217] Immunosuppression has been revolutionized by the ability of this drug to control allograft rejection with increased graft survival and reduced morbidity. The drug, however, is not without its disadvantages. Indeed, nephrotoxicity is one of the special hazards present and further confounds the interpretation of the renal transplant biopsy. The nephrotoxicity can be divided into three groups: early interactive nephrotoxicity characterized by the interaction of cyclosporin with other factors such as ischemia,[215,216] acute direct nephrotoxicity usually associated with very high blood levels of cyclosporin,[220,222] and chronic nephrotoxicity seen only after long-term usage of the drug.[218,220,223]

Interactive nephrotoxicity does not show changes that are specific for cyclosporin, but rather changes that would be associated with the complicating factor such as acute tubular necrosis. Changes that may be identified initially are evidence of tubular vacuolization and peritubular capillary congestion. With prolonged graft failure, biopsies will show a diffuse nonspecific interstitial fibrosis associated with tubular atrophy, suggestive of recovering acute tubular necrosis. Acute toxic tubulopathy, which is associated with high blood levels of cyclosporin, may show changes similar to that of acute tubular necrosis by light microscopy. These include tubular epithelial vacuolization, eosinophilic inclusion bodies within the tubular epithelium, and peritubular congestion. Electron microscopy may be helpful with the demonstration of giant mitochondria.

*See references 198, 199, 202, 203, 205, 207, and 208.

Chronic cyclosporin nephrotoxicity has a distinctive appearance of having stripes of interstitial fibrosis and atrophic tubules within the renal cortex. Tubules in other areas appear essentially normal and mononuclear cell infiltration, though present, is not specific. A vascular arteriolopathy has also been described in which there is mucoid thickening of the subintimal region with myocyte necrosis and narrowing of the vascular lumen. With the advent of better control of cyclosporin therapeutic levels, overt changes of cyclosporin nephrotoxicity are infrequent. The renal biopsy of a patient with graft failure and acute cyclosporin toxicity is essentially one of absence of significant pathologic findings rather than of an identifiable specific pathologic lesion. Since a mild interstitial infiltrate may persist in some allografts, the degree of interstitial infiltrates should be correlated with the severity of the graft failure, and a mild interstitial infiltrate in the face of significant graft failure is strongly suggestive of cyclosporin nephrotoxicity.[212,219,221] Analysis of the lymphocyte population in these instances often reveals greater numbers of lymphocytes with CD4 markers than those with CD8 markers.

TUBULOINTERSTITIAL NEPHRITIS

Tubulointerstitial nephritis describes a group of diverse renal diseases with involvement of the renal tubules and interstitium. The various etiologies include infection, obstruction, and immune-mediated and toxic-tubulointerstitial diseases (see box opposite). Despite diverse etiology, the clinical presentation usually has great similarities. The functional manifestations include impaired concentrating ability, impaired ability to secrete acid, diminished reabsorption of sodium, hyperkalemia, and azotemia. Symptoms may be acute or chronic with corresponding morphologic changes.

Acute and chronic pyelonephritis

Infectious tubulointerstitial nephritis is generally designated as pyelonephritis, implying that there is involvement of the collecting system, as well as the renal parenchyma, by the inflammatory process.[224,231] There are three peaks of incidence: infancy and early childhood, women of childbearing age, and both men and women older than 60. Both acute and chronic pyelonephritis are frequently associated with congenital or acquired obstructive lesions of the lower urinary tract or are associated with conditions resulting in residual retention of urine in the bladder.[229] In infancy and young childhood, congenital lesions are often the cause, whereas in the older groups obstruction by nodular hyperplasia of the prostate gland in men and the development of cystoceles in women are of importance. In addition, cancer of the cervix and stones are also commonly associated with infection. In acute pyelonephritis, which is associated with an ascending infection, an acute inflammatory infiltrate involving both the medullary and cortical portions of the kidney is present (Fig. 17-37). Infiltration occurs with polymorphonuclear leukocytes both in the interstitium and within the tubular lumina. In the cortex, areas of necrosis and abscess formation may be seen. Infection of the kidney can also occur via a hematogenous route and results in the presence of numerous small cortical abscesses without significant medullary involvement. A variety of pathogens may

---

CLASSIFICATION OF TUBULOINTERSTITIAL DISEASES

Infections
  Acute pyelonephritis
    Ascending vs. hematogenous
    Bacterial; fungal; other
  Chronic pyelonephritis
    Nonobstructive (reflux associated)
    Obstructive
    Xanthogranulomatous
    Malakoplakia
Obstructive uropathy
  Hydronephrosis without infection
  Hydronephrosis with infection
  Reflux-associated nephropathy
Allergic tubulointerstitial nephritis
  Drug induced (antibiotics, diuretics, nonsteroidals)
  Associated with systemic vasculitis
  Lupus associated
  Anti-tubular basement membrane
Toxic tubulointerstitial nephritis
  Drug induced
    Aminoglycosides
    Cyclosporin
    Lithium
    Analgesics
  Heavy metal toxicity
    Cisplatin
    Lead, mercury, and others
Other
  Radiation
  Sarcoid
  Idiopathic

---

be identified by using special staining techniques. Generally speaking, ascending infections are usually associated with gram negative organisms, in particular *Escherichia coli*.[230] Hematogenous infections are most frequently caused by *Staphylococcus aureus* or fungal organisms, including *Candida* and *Aspergillus,* especially in immunosuppressed individuals.

Chronic pyelonephritis results in a coarse renal scarring, which is characteristically focal in its distribution.[228] The cortical and papillary scars overlie dilatated, blunted, and deformed calyces. The medulla is distorted, and the papilla may be flattened. Microscopically, the findings consist of tubular damage, interstitial inflammation, and scarring. The tubules are either atrophic or dilatated, lined by a flattened epithelium, and filled with colloid casts. This latter pattern has been termed thyroidization. The inflammatory infiltrate is quite variable but tends to predominate with lymphocytes and mononuclear cells, as well as plasma cells. In chronic pyelonephritis associated with reflux or obstruction, Tamm-Horsfall protein can be localized in the interstitium by the presence of strongly PAS-positive amorphous fibrillar material. Inflammatory infiltrate frequently surrounds these

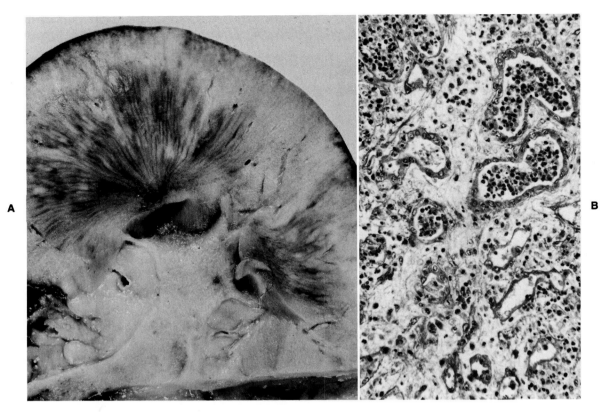

Fig. 17-37 A, Surgical specimen of kidney from patient with slight hydronephrosis and acute pyelonephritis. Note linear streaks in medulla due to pus within tubules. **B,** Acute pyelonephritis in renal transplant patient presenting with fever and elevated creatinine. Biopsy revealed acute inflammatory infiltrate in interstitium and tubular lumina.

masses of protein. Although the glomeruli are not primarily involved, they are frequently secondarily involved by periglomerular fibrosis. Ischemic changes consisting of focal and segmental sclerosis and hyalinosis may also be seen.

The histopathologic changes associated with chronic pyelonephritis have also been described with vesicoureteral reflux and chronic urinary obstruction. An extreme form of the focal scarring is seen in the so-called Ask-Upmark kidney.[226] In these kidneys scarring of a lobule of the kidney is total, resulting in an appearance of segmental hypoplasia.

Xanthogranulomatous pyelonephritis is a distinct type of infectious pyelonephritis characterized by the appearance of yellow, lobulated masses replacing the normal renal architecture[225] (Fig. 17-38). The mass-occupying nature of this lesion frequently mimics that of renal cell carcinoma, resulting in nephrectomies. A correct pre-operative diagnosis is rarely made. Microscopically, there is a diffuse granulomatous, inflammatory infiltrate, which includes large numbers of foamy histiocytes and occasional multinucleated giant cells in addition to lymphocytes, plasma cells, and neutrophils. The lesion is destructive and renal parenchyma may not be identified within the affected areas. *Escherichia coli* is frequently the etiologic agent, but *Proteus mirabilis* and *Staphylococcus aureus* have also been reported.

Malakoplakia has a similar gross and microscopic appearance. Confluent nodules of a homogenous yellow-tan tissue are seen to replace large areas of renal parenchyma. Microscopically, there is an inflammatory infiltrate, which consists of histiocytes with relatively few lymphocytes and plasma cells. Characteristic Michaelis-Gutmann bodies are found both within cells and extracellularly in the stroma.[227] The calcospherites stain positively with PAS. Fibroblastic proliferation and scarring are also prominent.

Acute allergic tubulointerstitial nephritis

It is now widely recognized that a large variety of drugs including beta lactam antibiotics, nonsteroidal anti-inflammatory drugs, diuretics, and an increasingly diverse group of other drugs can be associated with an acute tubulointerstitial nephritis.[232] Although the clinical manifestations may be variable, they are usually heralded by fever and hematuria, as well as azotemia. Eosinophilia occurs in a majority of cases. Urinalysis reveals hematuria, sterile pyuria, and moderate proteinuria. Eosinophils may be detected in the urine sediment.[234] A skin rash is seen in some patients, lending additional support to the concept that the disease may be immunologically mediated. The azotemia may be severe and may mimic that of acute renal failure, leading to the use of the renal biopsy as a diagnostic procedure.

Light microscopy reveals generalized interstitial ede-

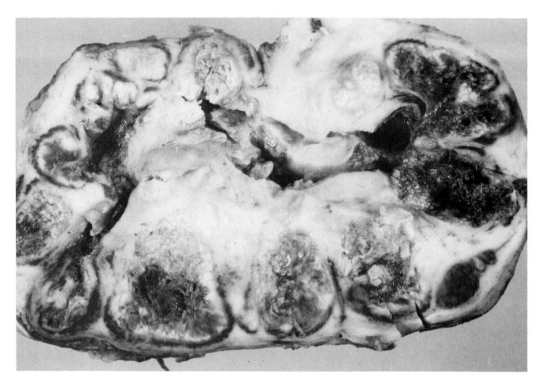

Fig. 17-38 Extreme hydronephrosis with wide areas of cortical destruction simulating tuberculosis. This is classic pyelonephritis with xanthogranulomatous changes.

ma and infiltration of the interstitium by mononuclear cells, principally lymphocytes, macrophages, and plasma cells.[233,236-238] Neutrophils are seen and eosinophils are present, often in large numbers. Variable degrees of tubular epithelial cell damage with evidence of regeneration are always found. Leukocytes can be present within the tubular lumina. The glomeruli are generally not affected and evidence of vasculitis is generally not seen. Occasionally, granulomata with giant cells may be found.[239]

Although bacterial infection and drugs are the most common causes of acute interstitial nephritis, a similar picture can be found in patients with lupus and, rarely, in association with antitubular basement membrane antibodies. Both the clinical and pathologic findings are similar to those seen with allergic tubulointerstitial nephritis. Biopsy-proven instances of acute oliguric tubulointerstitial nephritis have also been reported without any apparent associated cause. One special group includes the association of acute interstitial nephritis with anterior uveitis and bone marrow and lymph node granulomata, which occurs predominantly in adolescent and young adult women.[235]

Renal papillary necrosis

Papillary necrosis occurs as a complication of pyelonephritis and in a variety of other situations. Infection associated with obstruction and diabetes mellitus, alcoholism, vascular thrombosis, sickle cell disease, and analgesic abuse have all been reported. Development of papillary necrosis occurs in three stages. In the early stage, the kidneys are of normal weight, but the papillae are firmer than normal

and show gray streaks. Microscopically, there is interstitial homogenization and thickening of the basement membranes of the loops of Henle and the peritubular capillaries. Foci of necrotic epithelial, endothelial, and interstitial cells are associated with fine calcification. In this stage, the cortex remains normal. In the second stage, the papillae are shrunken and grossly brown. Microscopically, confluent zones of necrosis within the inner medulla are evident, again involving the loops of Henle, peritubular capillaries, and the vasa recta.[240] The cortex may have foci of tubular atrophy, interstitial fibrosis, and patches of chronic inflammation. In the third stage, the kidneys are reduced in weight and show gross changes that are typically seen in chronic pyelonephritis. Total papillary necrosis occurs, extensive calcification is usually present, and rarely metaplastic bone formation occurs. If the necrotic papillae have not been sloughed, the overlying cortex will show marked degrees of tubular atrophy, interstitial fibrosis and inflammation, and glomerular sclerosis thought to be secondary to obstruction of the urine flow. If the papillae are sloughed, minor cortical changes similar to the second stage are found. Retrograde pyelograms show ragged calyces, ring shadows, and clubbing and are of definite value in making the diagnosis of papillary necrosis.

Causes of renal papillary necrosis include sickle cell anemia, diabetes mellitus, obstruction with acute pyelonephritis, transplant rejection, and vascular thrombosis. As in analgesic abuse, the necrotic papillae may be passed and identified in the urinary sediment.

Pyelitis and ureteritis cystica

Hinman and Cordonnier[241] demonstrated that pyelitis and ureteritis cystica are the result of chronic inflammation of variable etiology. They believe that their development is caused by chronic inflammation of the mucous membrane followed by downward proliferation of the surface epithelium. These buds of epithelium become pinched off possibly by the upgrowing connective tissue and form epithelial cell nests. Degeneration occurs centrally, and a cystic structure forms. This lesion may be diagnosed by identifying peculiar mottled bubble-like defects in the ureterogram.

Pelvic lipomatosis

Pelvic lipomatosis must be differentiated from a true lipoma of the kidney. The former consists of fatty replacement of normal tissue and an increase of fat in the hilus of the kidney. This replacement occurs whenever atrophy of the kidney occurs. It is present quite frequently in association with chronic pyelonephritis and renal lithiasis.[242,243]

Grossly, there is diffusely distributed fat in the region of the hilus, and the remaining kidney is atrophic. Microscopically, mature fat is present. Clinically, extensive lipomatosis associated with lithiasis may simulate renal neoplasm because of the filling defects usually seen pyelographically.

Nephrolithiasis and nephrocalcinosis

Primary renal stones are defined as those occurring in the absence of renal abnormality, persistent infection, or metabolic disease. Practically all renal stones develop within the renal pelvis, often in a major or minor calyx. About 65% of the stones are composed of combination of calcium oxalate and calcium phosphate. Uric acid, xanthine, and cystine stones comprise 20%, and 15% are composed of magnesium ammonium phosphate. The latter usually are associated with urea-splitting bacterial infections. Numerous theories exist concerning the pathogenesis of stone formation. In short, stones may begin as a nidus, which, according to Boyce,[244] is composed of an organic substance identified as a mucoprotein. There is also evidence to the contrary, suggesting that the nidus of most calcium containing stones consists of calcium phosphate.[245]

In Randall's study[250] of 1,154 pairs of kidneys, 227 (19.6%) showed calcium salt deposition in one or more renal papillae, and 65% showed a renal calculus attached to a renal papilla. These calculi were subepithelial and represented a plaque of calcium salt in the interstitial tissue. Randall postulated that ulceration of the surface of the papilla acted as the nidus upon which urinary salts crystallized.[250,251] Actually, Randall's plaque is infrequently found in kidneys removed for lithiasis.[249] Once a nidus is formed, however, further growth of the nidus depends on the appropriate pH and supersaturated urine with respect to the constituents of the stone.

The formation of renal stones within the pelvic calyceal system can result in gross and microscopic changes in the renal parenchyma that are identical to those seen in chronic pyelonephritis and hydronephrosis.

The presence of calcium within the renal parenchyma is known as nephrocalcinosis. Characteristically, the calcium deposition occurs on the tubular basement membranes and in the interstitium. It is accompanied by tubular atrophy, interstitial fibrosis, and periglomerular fibrosis. Varying numbers of glomeruli may also be sclerosed.

Several conditions are related to nephrocalcinosis and to the formation of stones. Calcium phosphate and oxalate stones occur in hyperparathyroidism, sarcoidosis, the milk-alkali syndrome, excessive dietary intake of vitamin D, multiple myeloma, and renal tubular acidosis. However, some patients may be normocalciuric.

Uric acid stone formation occurs in an acid urine and is associated with hyperuricosuria, which may result from an inborn error of metabolism such as gout or the Lesch-Nyhan syndrome, glycogen storage disease following treatment of hematopoietic malignancies, overindulgence in dietary proteins, and the use of uricosuric drugs.[248,252] Uric acid stones are usually radiolucent, often small and thus may be passed, but larger ones may develop in the renal pelvis, sometimes forming staghorn calculi. Uric acid crystals also may be deposited within the renal parenchyma. They may be demonstrated within the collecting tubules as elongated or rectangular crystals or within the interstitium with a surrounding giant cell reaction. The latter collections are doubly refractile under polarized light.

Cystinuria is expressed clinically as urinary tract calculus disease. These stones are radiopaque and are formed in an acid urine. The disorder is characterized by the defective transport of cystine, lysine, arginine, and ornithine by epithelial cells of the renal tubules and the gastrointestinal tract; it is transmitted as an autosomal recessive trait.[246] Complications of calculi formation include urinary tract obstruction and infection, which may result in renal failure.

Hyperoxaluria is characterized by recurrent calcium oxalate nephrolithiasis and/or nephrocalcinosis, often terminating in chronic renal failure. Type 1 and type 2 hyperoxaluria are two rare genetic disorders of glycoxalate metabolism resulting in hyperoxaluria. Ethylene glycol poisoning, methoxyflurane anesthesia, pyridoxine deficiency, and a variety of chronic gastrointestinal disorders (including Crohn's disease, chronic pancreatitis, and status post-jejunoileal bypass procedure) have been associated with oxalosis.[247] Parenchymal damage is characterized by the deposition of oxalate crystals having radial striations that can be demonstrated particularly well with polarized light. The crystals are deposited in the tubules, interstitium, and rarely, in the glomeruli. Tubular atrophy, interstitial fibrosis and inflammation, and glomerular sclerosis are the end result.

RENAL VASCULAR DISEASE
Renal arteriolar disease

The kidney plays an essential role in hypertension, and the vessels of the kidney are susceptible to a variety of pathologic changes directly related to increased pressure.[253,254] The vessels most susceptible are small arteries and arterioles with pre-glomerular vessels being more prominently affected. The vascular pathology of the small vessels of the kidney falls into three general categories: hyaline arteriolar sclerosis, myointimal hypertrophy and hyperplasia, and fibrinoid necrosis.[255]

Hyaline is derived from the Greek term *hyalos* meaning "glass." Hyaline arteriolosclerosis is so-called because the walls of the vessels are thickened by a deposition of a homogeneous glassy material, which is eosinophilic. Ultrastructurally, the deposition of hyaline is associated with atrophy of the smooth muscles and by a regular thickening of the basement membrane collagen. Mild hyaline arteriolosclerosis is often encountered with increasing age but is most prominently seen in patients with hypertension and diabetes. The lesion in hypertension is the most traumatic with the hyaline material causing marked narrowing of the lumen of the arteriole. The exact nature of the hyaline is not understood.[257] Hyaline stains positively with PAS, and it is thought to be composed largely of glycoproteins mixed with various collagen types.

The second type of vascular abnormality seen in hypertension is myointimal hyperplasia. Hyperplastic lesions are not unique to the arterioles and occur in small and large arteries as well. A uniform concentric thickening of the vessel by proliferating myointimal cells has led to the descriptive term "onion skinning." The hyperplasia causes marked narrowing of the lumen, and there is also an increase in basement membrane–like material within the vessel wall.

The third and perhaps most dramatic lesion associated with hypertension is necrotizing arteriolitis.[256] Fibrinoid necrosis of the arterioles is considered by some to be the hallmark of malignant or accelerated hypertension. The lesion is generally superimposed on existing hyperplastic or hyaline lesions but is also occasionally seen as the first event in young patients presenting with severe acute malignant hypertension. The lesion consists of obliteration of the normal medial architecture by necrosis, with the deposition of deep eosinophilic granular, fibrin-like material. Ultrastructural examination reveals the fibrillar material embedded in hyaline to have a periodicity considered to be characteristic of fibrin. Immunofluorescence shows the presence of fibrin or fibrinogen within the walls.[258] The fibrin is sometimes accompanied by extravasation of red blood cells and intraluminal thrombosis. Occasionally leukocytes may be present in the wall, suggesting an inflammatory arteriolitis.

Renal arterial disease

The larger renal arteries are also subject to pathologic change. Atheromatous disease of the major renal arteries is accelerated in patients with hypertension and can perpetuate the disease by creating renal artery stenosis (Fig. 17-39). In addition, it may also be the source of atheromatous embolization contributing to distal renal parenchymal infarc-

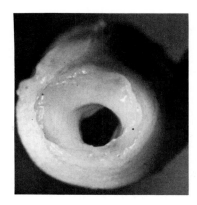

Fig. 17-39 Eccentric arteriosclerotic plaque in renal artery causing almost complete obstruction and hypertension. This was resected and arterial continuity reestablished.

tion. Arteries down to the arcuate size can show arteriosclerotic change, but smaller vessels are more commonly involved by intimal thickening of the hyperplastic type, similar to that seen in the small arteries. Disease of the major arteries becomes particularly important when it involves a main renal artery and causes significant stenosis, resulting in secondary hypertension.[259,262] The lesions involving the main renal artery can be broken down into three categories: arteriosclerosis, dysplastic diseases of the fibromuscular vessels, and a miscellaneous group that includes congenital anomalies, Takayasu's aortitis, and radiation injury.

The most common cause of renal artery stenosis is obstruction by an atheromatous plaque involving the orifice of the main renal artery. It is usually associated with severe atheromatous disease of the aorta and as such is seen more frequently in males and patients with diabetes mellitus. The lesion is frequently associated with aneurysmal dilatation of the aorta distal to the renal arteries and with neurothrombosis.

The second group of lesions leading to stenosis are the so-called dysplastic lesions of the renal artery[260] (Table 17-7). The dysplastic lesions can involve other systemic vessels, suggesting that there may be an underlying basic defect in vessel structure. The dysplastic lesions become clinically important when they cause obstruction of a major renal artery, thereby initiating severe hypertension, which is not responsive to medical antihypertensive therapy. The lesions can be subdivided into six separate groups: intimal fibro-

Table 17-7 Dysplastic lesions of the renal artery

Diagnosis	Age and sex incidence		Relative frequency	Lesion
Intimal fibroplasia	1-50%	M = F	1-2%	Narrowing by intimal proliferation without lipid
Medial fibroplasia with aneurysms	30-60%	F > M	60-70%	"String of beads," alternating stenosis and mural thinning
Medial hyperplasia	30-60%	F > M	5-15%	Smooth muscle hyperplasia and thickening
Perimedial fibroplasia	30-60%	F > M	15-24%	Fibrosis of outer media, occasionally aneurysms
Medial dissection	30-60%	F > M	5-15%	Fibrosis of media with dissecting aneurysms
Periarterial fibroplasia	15-50%	F > M	1%	Perivascular fibrosis and inflammation

plasia, medial fibroplasia, medial hyperplasia, perimedial fibroplasia, medial dissection, and periarterial fibroplasia. The term fibromuscular dysplasia has been used to encompass several of the separate categories but it appears useful to subclassify them as they may affect different patient populations.

In intimal fibroplasia the lesion consists of hyperplasia of the intima that is essentially indistinguishable from the proliferative stage of atherosclerosis. It is not associated with an increased deposition of lipids, however. The elastica and media are preserved, maintaining a relatively normal architecture except for the intimal hyperplastic lesion. The lesion has been reported in individuals as young as 1 year but is most common in the third and fourth decades. The most common of the dysplastic lesions is medial fibroplasia. Grossly, this results in a multifocal stenotic lesion alternating with microaneurysms, which produces a characteristic "string of beads" appearance[261] (Fig. 17-40). Microscopically, there is atrophy of the muscle and fibrosis of the media in the regions of small aneurysms, alternating with medial muscular hypertrophy and fibrosis in the stenotic regions. The second most frequently encountered variation is perimedial fibroplasia (Fig. 17-41). In contrast to medial hyperplasia, segmental aneurysmal dilatation is not present. Microscopically, the outer half of the media thickens where the medial muscle is distorted and fibrous tissue increases. The inner portion of the media, elastica, and intima maintain a relatively normal architecture. Less commonly seen is medial hyperplasia. This is characterized by a hyperplasia of the muscle that results in a circumferential uniform thickening of the vessel wall and a narrowing of the lumen. Periarterial fibroplasia is a rare lesion in which fibrosis of the adventitia is present. This extends into the surrounding adipose and connective tissue, resulting in constriction of the vessel from without rather than from within the structure of the vessel wall.

Of the miscellaneous causes of renal artery stenosis, radiation injury is of particular interest. The lesion is char-

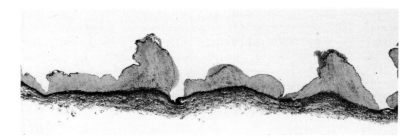

Fig. 17-40 Fibromuscular dysplasia in young woman with hypertension. Note aneurysmal formations in this longitudinally sectioned artery demonstrating medial fibrodysplasia with mural aneurysms.

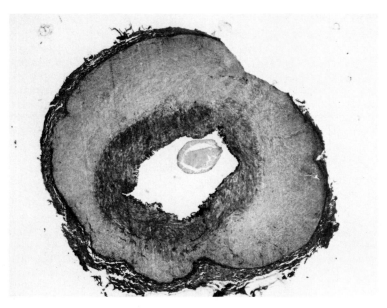

Fig. 17-41 Fibromuscular dysplasia in 23-year-old woman with hypertension. Segmental resection revealed artery with perimedial variety of fibrodysplasia.

acterized by a loss of muscle and an intense fibrosis in all layers of the vessel. It usually occurs as a distant event after radiation therapy usually for a malignant lesion in which the radiation port included the main renal artery. Takayasu's aortitis or pulseless disease is a chronic sclerosing aortitis of unknown etiology that can cause renal artery stenosis, resulting from narrowing of the ostium. An inflammatory infiltrate is present frequently, suggesting a possible immunologic mechanism.

Regardless of the cause of the renal artery stenosis, the ischemic kidney is generally smaller than the contralateral kidney. The glomeruli are small, and the tubules are collapsed. Interstitial fibrosis is present. The juxtaglomerular apparatus is hyperplastic, and increased granulation can be seen with special stains. The small vessels are protected from the hypertension in contrast to the contralateral kidney where biopsy may show hypertensive microvascular disease.

CYSTIC DISEASES OF THE KIDNEY

Although a variety of classification systems for cystic renal diseases have been developed, none are universally satisfactory, and they are not based on a defined etiologic or pathogenetic basis. The most useful classification is one based on the overall gross appearance of the kidney, which has some correlation with both the clinical presentation and the putative hereditary transmission (Table 17-8). Variants of these forms continue to be reported, but the basic classification does have significant usefulness both clinically and pathologically.

Renal dysplasia

Renal dysplasia is characterized by an abnormal disorganized development of the renal parenchyma caused by anomalous differentiation of metanephric tissue (Fig. 17-42). Multicystic renal dysplasia is the most common cause of cystic renal disease in the newborn period; it presents as an abdominal mass. The dysplasia can be unilateral, bilateral, segmental, or focal.[263] It is frequently associated with abnormalities of the collecting system including obstruction of the ureteral pelvic junction, ureteral atresia, or urethral obstruction. Grossly, the dysplastic kidney initially presents as a large reniform mass of cysts of various sizes with no obvious renal parenchyma. In focal and segmental dysplasia, the dysplastic change with cysts may occupy only a portion of the kidney. Microscopically, the findings are quite characteristic.[264,265] The cysts are lined by cuboidal epithelial cells and are surrounded by immature stromal elements. Primitive tubules and glomerular structures may also be present, as well as islands of dysplastic connective tissue that include cartilage and fibromuscular tissue.

Adult-type polycystic disease

Polycystic disease of the adult type is an inherited autosomal dominant disorder that has been mapped to chromosome 16.[266,269] It is extremely common, occurring at a rate of 1 to 2 per 1,000 population. The clinical presentation is variable but tends to be similar within individual pedigrees. It can present at any time during life but most frequently it becomes symptomatic during the fourth to fifth decade with a gradual onset of renal failure. Flank pain and hematuria are occasionally the presenting symptoms. The disease is bilateral. Grossly, the kidneys are markedly enlarged and have a bosselated outer cortical surface produced by multiple cysts of varying sizes[267] (Fig. 17-43). When fully developed, normal renal parenchyma is apparent only microscopically. Microscopically, the cysts are lined by a flattened epithelium, and hyperplastic polypoid foci are often found. Intervening renal parenchyma appears relatively normal although foci of interstitial scarring, tubular atrophy, and pyelonephritis are common. The cysts occur in all nephron segments.

Approximately one third of the patients with adult onset polycystic renal disease have cysts involving other organs

Table 17-8 Cystic diseases of the kidney

Name	Prevalence	Heredity	Age at presentation	Clinical features
Renal dysplasia	Common	None in majority, rarely familial	Infancy	Unilateral, bilateral segmental, focally irregular cystic kidneys, immature mesenchyme, associated with obstruction
Adult type polycystic disease	Common 1-2/1000 of population	Autosomal dominant, mapped to chromosome 16	Usually adult	Large bilateral bosselated kidneys, intact functional nephrons, cysts in liver, pancreas, lung; cerebral berry aneurysms
Infantile polycystic disease	Uncommon	Autosomal recessive	Neonatal	Huge kidneys, bilateral cylindric cysts in cortex and medulla; aberrant ductules in liver
Medullary sponge kidney	Common	Unknown	Adult	Bilateral; dilatated ducts of Bellini; Calculi; concentrating defect
Uremic medullary cystic disease	Rare	Familial	Young adults	Bilateral cysts at corticomedullary junction; severe interstitial fibrosis; Functional tubular defects; Fanconi's syndrome, uremia

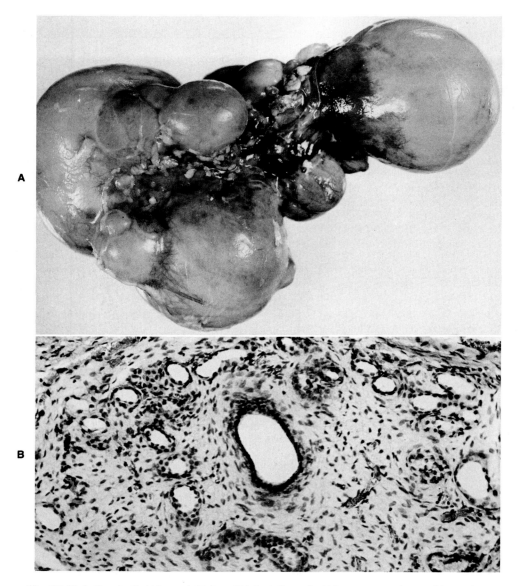

Fig. 17-42 A, Dysplastic kidney of 17-day-old infant. Opposite kidney appeared normal by pyelogram.
B, Same kidney illustrated in **A** showing embryonic-like connective tissue and tubules.

including the liver, pancreas, spleen, and lungs. Another well-documented association is the presence of cerebral artery aneurysms.[268]

Infantile polycystic renal disease

Infantile polycystic renal disease is the spectrum of diseases inherited as an autosomal recessive trait.[270] The disease usually manifests itself in the neonatal period and is rarely seen in older children and adults. When seen later in life it is frequently associated with a variety of hepatic abnormalities including congenital diffuse hepatic fibrosis. The kidneys are enlarged bilaterally but retain their reniform configuration. The cysts consist of dilatated tubular structures lined by a flattened epithelium. The cysts tend to be linear and radiate from the medulla to the outer cortex.

Microscopically, the cysts are lined by a flattened epithelium and the intervening tissue may contain uninvolved nephrons, but this depends on the severity of the disorder.

Medullary sponge kidney

Medullary sponge kidney is a disorder that is usually discovered during adulthood during the course of radiologic examination in patients who present with nephrolithiasis or pyelonephritis.[271] The disorder is regarded as a developmental defect of the collecting tubules that exhibit dilatation and a characteristic radiologic appearance on intravenous and retrograde urography. Intravenous urography demonstrates multiple ectatic or cystic dilatations of the papillary collecting ducts. Microscopically, the cysts are multiple, small cysts that are limited to the renal medulla and have

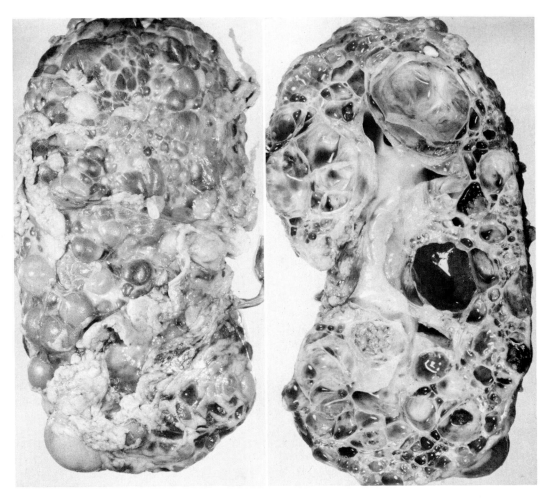

Fig. 17-43 External and cut surface of surgically excised kidney with adult polycystic disease. It weighed 3,850 g. Patient, 32-year-old woman on chronic dialysis, developed left flank pain, dysuria, and fever.

the appearance of dilatated ducts of Bellini. Multiple papillae may be involved. In instances where there is nephrolithiasis and pyelonephritis, the cortex may show significant cortical scarring.

Medullary cystic disease

Medullary cystic disease is a complex of several different clinical syndromes that may present as functional tubular defects and Fanconi syndrome associated with azotemia and uremia.[272] The disease is genetically transmitted but is variable in mechanism and may range from autosomal recessive to an autosomal dominant trait. The syndrome in children has been termed juvenile nephronopthisis. In a second group the presentation occurs during the third and fourth decade of life and has been termed uremic medullary cystic disease. It appears to be transmitted as an autosomal dominant trait. Renal failure occurs within 3 to 5 years after the clinical onset. Pathologically the cysts are localized to the cortical medullary junction and may vary from microscopic cysts to large cysts of up to 1 to 2 cm in diameter. The cortex of the kidney is commonly focally scarred. The cysts are lined by flattened epithelium and interstitial fibrosis is present, with a chronic inflammatory infiltrate in the intervening tissue.

Acquired cysts in renal dialysis patients

The kidneys of patients who have been on long-term dialysis may develop cysts that in the most florid instance resemble adult polycystic disease.[273,274] The mean duration of such patients on dialysis is between 3 and 4 years, and 79% of patients on dialysis longer than 3 years may present with some cystic change. Pathologically, the kidneys are modestly enlarged and have a bosselated appearance resulting from multiple cysts involving both cortex and medulla. Microscopically, the cysts are lined by flattened epithelium, but foci of papillary hyperplasia of the tubular epithelium is common. Cytologic atypia is often seen, and overt renal cell carcinoma may be associated with the proliferative change.

Tumors and tumorlike conditions
WILMS' TUMOR
General features

Wilms' tumor is also known as nephroblastoma, embryoma, carcinosarcoma, adenosarcoma, and adenomyosarcoma. It is seen primarily in infants, 50% of the cases occurring before the age of 3 years and 90% before the age of 10 years. However, Wilms' tumor is only exceptionally seen as a congenital neoplasm, a point of great importance in the differential diagnosis with mesoblastic nephroma.[280] There are also well-documented cases of Wilms' tumors in adolescents[286] and adults.[278] The latter should be investigated and treated according to the same guidelines used for the pediatric neoplasms.[276]

The classic location for Wilms' tumor is the kidney, the incidence of synchronous or metachronous bilateral involvement being 5% to 10%.[289] However, cases with the typical morphologic features of Wilms' tumor have been recorded in extrarenal sites, including retroperitoneum, sacrococcygeal region, testis, inguinal canal, and mediastinum.[275,279,283,296] Some of them have arisen within a teratoma, and even those in which this was not evident could be viewed as teratomas with a predominant or exclusive nephroblastic component.

Wilms' tumor has been reported in monozygous twins and other familial settings[281] and in patients with Recklinghausen's disease,[294] hemihypertrophy, genitourinary tract malformations,[277,284,290] the omphalocele-macroglossia (Beckwith-Wiedemann's) syndrome,[293] and aniridia.[287] The incidence of congenital abnormalities is particularly high for Wilms' tumors occurring during the first year of life and/or involving both kidneys. Individuals with the Wilms' tumor/aniridia syndrome have been found to have a specific deletion in the short arm of chromosome 11.[292] Other types of chromosomal abnormalities have been found in a few of the sporadic cases.[282] Maurer et al.[285] have suggested that the development of Wilms' tumor requires the occurrence of two successive mutational events, one of which may be a germinal mutation. Wilms' tumor has also been encountered in association with other malignancies, such as osteosarcoma, botryoid rhabdomyosarcoma, and retinoblastoma.[288] Type I insulinlike growth factor receptors have been found in Wilms' tumor, which may be responsible for increased proliferation and inhibition of differentiation.[278a]

The classic clinical presentation of Wilms' tumor is in the form of an abdominal mass felt by the mother when handling the child. Hematuria is rare. Hypertension, present in a minority of the cases, has been shown to be caused by renin secretion by the tumor.[291] Proteinuria may be caused by the presence of tumor-associated glomerular disease in the non-neoplastic kidney.[295]

Intravenous pyelogram shows an intrarenal mass that displaces and distorts the pelvis. Ultrasonography and CT scan are used to further define the tumor extent.

Morphologic features

Grossly, most Wilms' tumors are large, relatively well circumscribed, and of firm consistency. The cut section is predominantly solid and often exhibits areas of necrosis and hemorrhage (Fig. 17-44).

Microscopically, three major components are identified: undifferentiated blastema, mesenchymal tissue, and epithelial tissue.[298,302,312] Most Wilms' tumors show a representation of all three components in various proportions. However, some tumors are biphasic and still others are monophasic (monomorphous). The blastematous areas are extremely cellular, composed of small round-to-oval primitive cells; the cytoplasm is usually very scanty but sometimes it exhibits an oncocytoid appearance. Wilms' tumors in which the blastematous component predominates can be confused with any of the small round cell tumors, including neuroblastoma. The mesenchymal elements usually have a spindle-cell fibroblast-like configuration but may also exhibit differentiation toward various cell types, particularly smooth muscle and skeletal muscle.[301] Sometimes this mesenchymal component predominates almost to the exclusion of others.[318] Wilms' tumors with an extensive skeletal muscle component are invariably seen in young children and are bilateral in over one half of the cases.[303] Predominantly rhabdomyosarcomatous Wilms' tumors involving the renal pelvis acquire morphologic features very similar to those of botryoid rhabdomyosarcoma.[311,317] In some instances, these largely mesenchymal neoplasms are seen in the opposite kidney of patients with typical Wilms' tumor.[307]

The epithelial component is characterized by the formation of embryonic tubular (and sometimes glomerular) structures that closely recapitulate the appearance of normal developing metanephric tubules (and glomeruli) at the light microscopic, ultrastructural, and lectin histochemistry levels[297,299,314,319] (Fig. 17-45). The differentiation can be so pronounced that tumor analogs of nearly all segments of the normal nephron can be formed.[305] These tubular structures can acquire papillary and fibroadenoma-like features.[300,308] They can also be small and round, thus simulating the rosettes of neuroblastoma. Features favoring tubules over rosettes are presence of lumen, single cell layer, distinct basal lamina, and surrounding fibromyxoid stroma.[298] The differential diagnosis of predominantly epithelial Wilms' tumors also includes multicystic nephroma and renal cell carcinoma.[298,308]

Anaplastic features may be present focally or extensively in Wilms' tumors; they are discussed in the section on prognosis.

Additional morphologic features that can be encountered in Wilms' tumor include ciliated, mucinous, squamous, or transitional epithelium[298,306]; endocrine cells of various types[306]; renin-producing cells[309]; neuroepithelium, neuroblasts and mature ganglion cells[304,313]; adipose tissue; cartilage, bone, and hematopoietic cells.[306] Sometimes the variety of tissues present is such that the distinction between Wilms' tumor and teratoma becomes blurred[298]; the term teratoid Wilms' tumor is sometimes used for these cases.[316]

Immunohistochemically, the blastematous elements show only focal positivity for vimentin; the epithelial elements react for keratin, EMA, various lectins, and the various components of the basement membrane[315]; the mesenchymal elements show a reactivity pattern consonant with their mor-

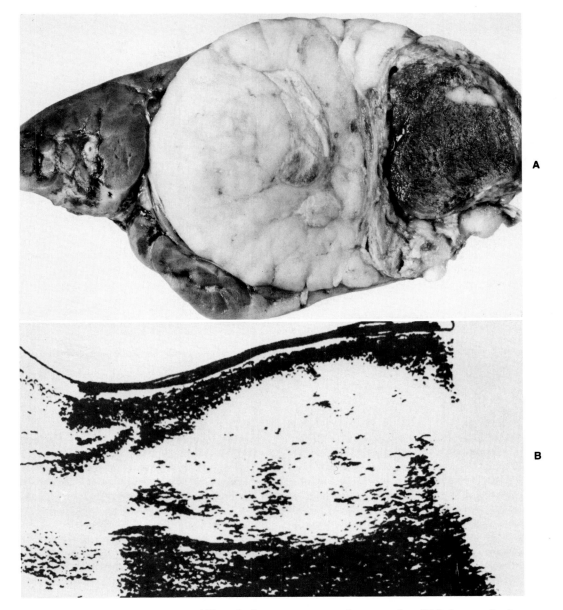

Fig. 17-44 Wilms' tumor in 3-year-old boy. **A,** Gross appearance of cross section. Well-circumscribed solid white mass replaces most of renal parenchyma. Several foci of hemorrhage and necrosis are present. **B,** Ultrasound scan of kidney shown in **A.** Lower pole appears normal. Tumor appears as large solid mass with scattered irregular echoes corresponding to areas of necrosis. (**B,** Courtesy Dr. E. Cubilla, St. Louis, MO.)

phologic appearance (i.e., positivity for myoglobin and desmin in rhabdomyoblastomatous foci); and the neural elements—when present—exhibit reactivity for neuron-specific enolase, glial fibrillary acidic protein, and S-100 protein.[310]

Spread and metastases

In advanced cases, local spread occurs in the perirenal soft tissues. From here, the tumor may involve adrenal glands, bowel, liver, or vertebrae. Direct invasion of renal pelvis or ureter is a rare and late event. Metastases in re-gional lymph nodes are found in 15% of the cases. The most common sites of distant metastases are lungs, liver, and peritoneum. Presence of lung metastases in a child with a retroperitoneal neoplasm strongly favors a diagnosis of Wilms' tumor over that of neuroblastoma. Conversely, presence of bone metastases suggests a diagnosis other than Wilms' tumor.

Therapy

The therapy for Wilms' tumor has quickly evolved over the past few years, largely through the results of the National

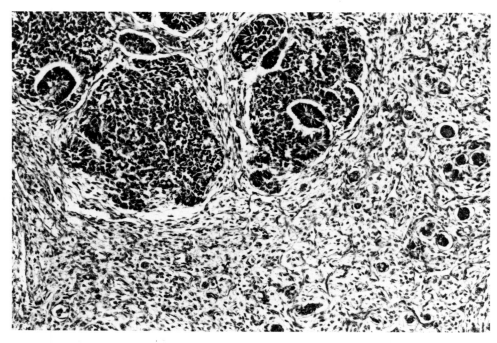

Fig. 17-45 Typical Wilms' tumor showing the three components of this neoplasm: undifferentiated blastema, stroma, and epithelial tubular formations.

Wilms' Tumor Study instituted in 1969.[321,322] The current choice of therapy depends on surgical and pathologic staging. Stage I tumors with "favorable histology" (i.e., without anaplastic features) are treated with nephrectomy and two-agent chemotherapy (actinomycin D and vincristine) for no longer than 6 months without radiation therapy.[321] Other chemotherapeutic agents and radiation therapy are added to tumors of higher surgical and/or pathologic grading. The nephrectomy is done via a wide transperitoneal route, which allows visualization of the opposite kidney and regional lymph nodes. During the operation, it is important to examine the contralateral kidney, examine and sample suspicious lymph nodes, and carefully explore the other infradiaphragmatic structures.

The effects of chemotherapy and radiation therapy are more pronounced in the blastematous component than in the mesenchymal or epithelial areas.[320] The incidence of anaplasia does not seem to be affected by this treatment modality.[324]

It remains essential to obtain a histologic diagnosis through laparotomy before embarking on radiation therapy or chemotherapy, inasmuch as the percentage of incorrect clinicoroentgenographic diagnoses is as high as 5%.[323]

Prognosis

An overall cure rate of 80% to 90% in unilateral Wilms' tumor has been achieved.[330,332,333] A small percentage of long-term survivors of Wilms' tumor develop a second malignant neoplasm, either because of a genetic predisposition to neoplasia or secondarily to therapy.[325]

Listed below are the prognostic connotations of various clinical and morphologic parameters.

1 *Age.* Patients under 2 years of age have significantly fewer metastases and a better 5-year survival rate than those over 2 years.[329,337,338]

2 *Stage.* Clinicopathologic staging of Wilms' tumor is the most important prognostic determinator (Table 17-9). Capsular invasion, rupture at surgery, extrarenal vein invasion, tumor implants, lymph node metastases, distant metastases, and bilaterality are the main criteria used.[334]

3 *Anaplasia.* In order for a case of Wilms' tumor to be placed into the anaplastic category, it should meet the following three criteria: (1) marked enlargement of nuclei within the blastemal, epithelial, or stromal cell lines (excepting skeletal muscle cells) to at least three times the diameter of adjacent nuclei of the same cell type: (2) obvious hyperchromasia of the enlarged nuclei; and (3) multipolar mitotic figures. (Fig. 17-46).

Anaplasia thus defined is present in about 4% of the cases, the incidence being higher in blacks and in older patients.[328] It is very uncommon in tumors from patients under 2 years of age; this is probably the reason for the better prognosis exhibited by this age group. Sometimes it is found in the metastases and not in the primary tumor. It can be extensive or very focal, indicating the need for thorough tumor sampling (one section for each centimeter of tumor diameter). The finding of anaplasia carries very important prognostic connotations regard-

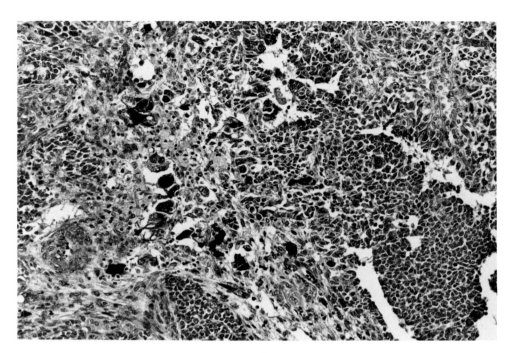

Fig. 17-46 Wilms' tumor with areas of anaplasia. Clusters of tumor cells with huge hyperchromatic nuclei are seen surrounded by more typical components of this neoplasm.

Table 17-9 Clinicopathologic staging of Wilms' tumor*

Stage	Characteristics	Stage	Characteristics
I	Tumor limited to the kidney and completely excised. The surface of the renal capsule is intact. The tumor was not ruptured before or during removal. There is no residual tumor apparent beyond the margins of excision.		b. There has been diffuse peritoneal contamination by the tumor such as by spillage of tumor beyond the flank before or during surgery or by tumor growth that has penetrated through the peritoneal surfaces. c. Implants are found on the peritoneal surfaces. d. The tumor extends beyond the surgical margins either microscopically or grossly. e. The tumor is not completely resectable because of local infiltration into vital structures.
II	Tumor extends beyond the kidney, but is completely excised. There is regional extension of the tumor, i.e., penetration through the outer surface of the renal capsule into the perirenal soft tissues. Vessels outside the kidney substance are infiltrated or contain tumor thrombus. The tumor may have been biopsied or there has been local spillage of tumor confined to the flank. There is no residual tumor apparent at or beyond the margins of excision.	IV	Hematogenous metastases. Deposits beyond stage III, e.g., lung, liver, bone, and brain.
III	Residual nonhematogenous tumor confined to the abdomen. Any of the following may occur: a. Lymph nodes on biopsy are found to be involved in the hilus, the periaortic chains, or beyond.	V	Bilateral renal involvement at diagnosis. An attempt should be made to stage each side according to the above criteria on the basis of extent of disease prior to biopsy.

From Belasco J, D'Angio GJ: Wilms' tumor. CA **31**:258-270, copyright, 1981, American Cancer Society, Inc.

*This staging, which is done on the basis of gross and microscopic tumor distribution, is the same for tumors with favorable and with unfavorable histologic features. The patient should be characterized, however, by a statement of both criteria, e.g., stage II, favorable histology, or stage II, unfavorable histology.

less of its amount.[327] Wilms' tumors with this feature are referred to as having an "unfavorable histology," and they are grouped for prognostic purposes with rhabdoid tumor (see p. 869) and clear cell sarcoma (see p. 867).

4 *Extensive tubular differentiation.* This is said to be a good prognostic sign. According to some authors, this also applies to cases with extensive glomerular differentiation.[335,336,338]

5 *Skeletal muscle differentiation.* This feature does not seem to have a significant effect on prognosis except when present in massive amounts. In the latter instance, it is said to be associated with a better prognosis.[331,340]

6 *Mucin production.* It has been suggested that the rare patients with Wilms' tumors in whom mucin is detected in the serum have a poor prognosis.[326]

7 *DNA ploidy.* Preliminary observations suggest that evaluation of DNA ploidy may give information of prognostic utility.[339]

OTHER PEDIATRIC RENAL TUMORS
Mesoblastic nephroma

Mesoblastic nephroma, also known as fetal, mesenchymal, or leiomyomatous hamartoma, is a congenital renal neoplasm that is usually discovered before the patient reaches 6 months of age. Grossly, it is solid, yellowish gray to tan, with a whorled configuration reminiscent of uterine leiomyoma (Fig. 17-47). It usually is well circumscribed, but it may be seen infiltrating the renal parenchyma. Areas of hemorrhage and necrosis are usually absent. A cystic variant of this tumor has been described.[344]

Microscopically, a variably cellular growth of spindle cells is the predominant feature.[351] Wigger[352] believes that these cells have the features of secondary mesenchyme, which, in contrast with those of the primary mesenchyme or mesoblast, lack the capacity to form epithelial structures. Instead, the proliferating cells acquire the features of fibroblasts, myofibroblasts, or smooth muscle cells.[342] As such, they contain vimentin, fibronectin, and sometimes actin,

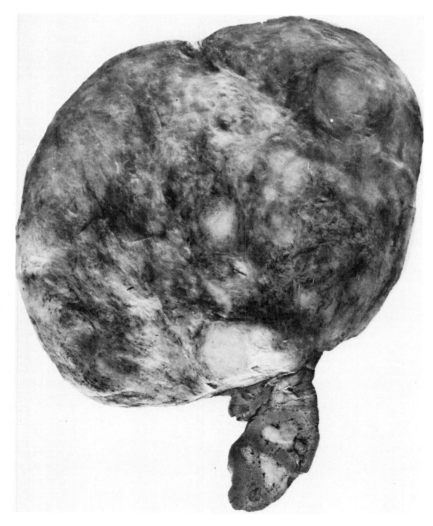

Fig. 17-47 Mesoblastic nephroma involving upper pole of kidney. This lesion is more solid, firm, and homogeneous than Wilms' tumor. (Courtesy Dr. H. Rodriguez, Mexico City, Mexico.)

but not keratin or laminin.[349] Some tubules and glomeruli are seen surrounded by the spindle cells. Most of them are at the periphery and are probably the result of entrapment; others, more centrally located and with a complex and variegated appearance, may be a component of the tumor.[343] No capsule separates the tumor from the uninvolved parenchyma. Some of these tumors are very cellular and mitotically active; these have a tendency to infiltrate the renal pelvis or perirenal tissue and may contain areas of hemorrhage and necrosis.[350] These tumors have been referred to as *atypical mesoblastic nephromas.*[348]

The large majority of mesoblastic nephromas behave in a benign fashion following nephrectomy.[347] Radiation therapy or chemotherapy are not indicated. Exceptionally, recurrence with local invasion of retroperitoneum will occur and may prove fatal.[346,348] Cases associated with distant metastases have also been reported; all of these aggressive tumors have had atypical morphologic features, as previously defined.[345,348] However, Beckwith and Weeks[341] have pointed out that in all but one of the recurrent mesoblastic nephromas the patients were over 3 months of age at the time of the original nephrectomy; they believe that age at diagnosis and adequacy of excision may be more important prognostic factors than morphologic features.

Multicystic nephroma

Multicystic nephroma (multilocular cystic nephroma, multilocular cyst) is an uncommon but distinctive lesion that arises in early infancy but that may present clinically at any age. It is nearly always unilateral. Clinical manifestations result from the presence of a mass or, not uncommonly, from ureteral obstruction by one of the daughter locules.

Grossly, the lesion is sharply delineated from the uninvolved renal parenchyma.[354] The usual size range is between 5 and 15 cm, and the outer surface is coarsely nodular. The cut surface shows a multilocular appearance, the individual cysts measuring from 1 mm to 3 cm or more (Fig. 17-48). The wall of these cysts is thin, sometimes translucent, and lacks papillary projections. The fluid within the cavity is usually serous. The cysts do not communicate with each other or with the pelvis. The remaining renal parenchyma is normal.

Microscopically, the cysts are lined by tubular epithelium, which ranges in height from columnar to extremely flat, resembling endothelium and simulating the appearance of lymphangioma. Ultrastructurally, this epithelium resembles collecting tubule cells.[358] The stroma between the cysts usually has a fibroblastic nondescript nature, but it may contain smooth muscle, skeletal muscle, or cartilage[355] (Fig. 17-49). Sometimes it also contains immature nephroblastomatous tissue with an appearance indistinguishable from that of Wilms' tumor. Some authors prefer to designate this entity as *multilocular cyst* when nephroblastomatous tissue is absent and as *multicystic nephroma* when it is present.[356] It has been further suggested that this entity represents the end of a spectrum of differentiation of Wilms' tumor and that it could be viewed as a fully differentiated variant of this tumor.[356] The occasional co-existence of Wilms' tumor

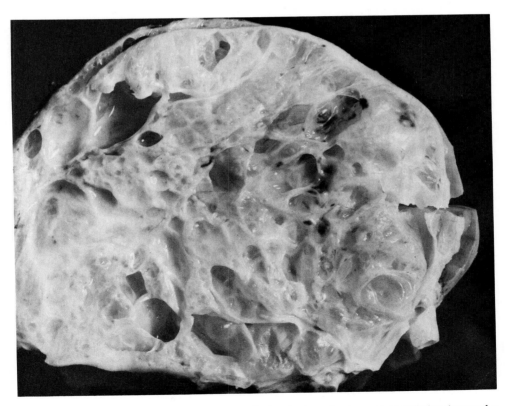

Fig. 17-48 Multicystic nephroma from young girl. Patient had received course of radiation therapy for presumed Wilms' tumor. When mass failed to regress, nephrectomy disclosed this lesion.

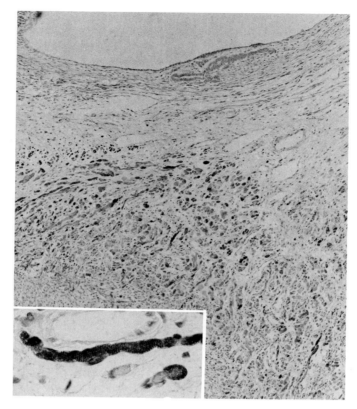

Fig. 17-49 Multicystic nephroma with prominent skeletal muscle component stained for myoglobin with immunoperoxidase technique. **Inset,** Skeletal muscle fiber showing diffuse cytoplasm positively as well as accentuation of cross sections.

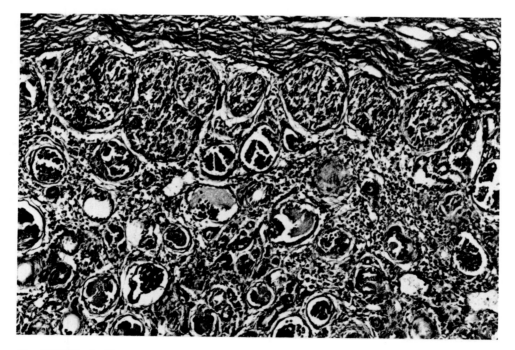

Fig. 17-50 Nephroblastomatosis. Solid nests of renal blastema are seen beneath renal capsule, contiguous to normally developing glomeruli.

and multicystic nephroma would seem to support this concept.[353] From a practical standpoint, however, it is important for these entities to be kept separate because of the fact that multicystic nephroma/multilocular cyst is a benign process that can be cured by nephrectomy alone.

A few cases of this lesion have been reported in adult patients to contain clusters of clear cells with the appearance of renal cell carcinoma, suggesting that this entity may have a potential for malignant degeneration. However, no metastases have so far been encountered in any of these cases.[357,359]

Nephroblastomatosis

Nephroblastomatosis is a congenital dysontogenetic rather than neoplastic disorder, but it is discussed here because of its frequent confusion and possible histogenetic relationship with Wilms' tumor.[362,364,367] It appears as single or multifocal, unilateral or bilateral subcapsular aggregates of primitive metanephric epithelium (Fig. 17-50). When microscopic in size, these aggregates are referred to as (persistent) nodular renal blastema, nephrogenic rests, or metanephric hamartomas; when massive, they are designated as nephroblastomatosis, but a morphologic continuum exists.[368] The presence of a sclerotic background probably indicates that the lesion is regressing.

Foci of neuroblastomatosis are found in 1% of neonatal kidneys and in 30% of kidneys containing Wilms' tumors.[362] In its most florid form, the process is often associated with a variety of congenital anomalies and with hypertension.[366]

Arteriography is highly characteristic. Grossly, the most exuberant examples of this disease can be distinguished from Wilms' tumor because of the diffuse nature of the process and the involvement of the entire subcapsular region. Microscopically, the mass is composed of tightly packed nephrogenic epithelial cells that have a primitive but not anaplastic appearance. Stromal tissue is scanty; cartilage, striated cells, and primitive mesenchyme are absent. The natural history and significance of this process are still poorly understood. On the basis of present evidence, a conservative therapeutic approach is indicated.[363]

Recently, some authors[360,361,365] have proposed a division of nephroblastomatosis into a more common, peripherally located *perilobular* form and an *intralobular* form; the latter occurs randomly in cortex or medulla and has irregular, often indistinct margins. These authors believe that the intralobular form is much more commonly associated with Wilms' tumor than the perilobular variety.[365]

Intrarenal neuroblastoma

Neuroblastomas can invade the kidney secondarily from an adrenal or some other retroperitoneal site, or they may initially present as a primary intrarenal tumor. When the latter occurs, a misdiagnosis of Wilms' tumor is likely. This issue is further complicated by the fact that the embryonal tubules of Wilms' tumor can simulate rosettes and that true neuroblastic elements can occur in Wilms' tumor. Ultrastructural examination, immunohistochemical studies, oncogene assays, and determination of catecholamines in serum and urine are of help in this differential diagnosis.[369,369a]

Clear cell sarcoma

Clear cell sarcoma, also known as bone-metastasizing renal tumor, is a distinctive renal malignancy formerly regarded as a morphologic variant of Wilms' tumor.[371,372,376] It comprises about 4% of childhood renal tumors. Grossly, the margins are infiltrative. The cut surface is homogeneous and tan or gray-tan; cystic formations are common. Microscopically, the most common pattern is that of a diffuse growth of relatively small cells with round normochromatic nuclei, inconspicuous nucleoli, light-staining (sometimes vacuolated) cytoplasm, and indistinct cell margins (Fig. 17-51). Despite the tumor name, clear cytoplasm is a prominent feature in only 20% of the cases.[373] Mitoses are infrequent. The fibrovascular stroma may result in arrangements of the tumor cells in nests, palisades, cords, or trabeculae. The latter should not be confused with the tubules of Wilms' tumor (Fig. 17-52). Myxoid changes, fibrosis, and hyalinization may be present, the appearance of the hyalinized tissue sometimes simulating osteoid. Cysts may result from dilatation of entrapped tubules or from stromal degeneration. It has been remarked that the distinctive alveolar and arborizing vascular stroma is a more reliable diagnostic feature than the clear cells or the sclerosis.[374]

Ultrastructurally, there are scanty organelles, generally sparse cytoplasmic filaments, primitive cell junctions, and complex cytoplasmic processes.[370] Immunohistochemically, only focal reactivity for vimentin has been encountered.[377]

The origin of this neoplasm remains uncertain. It probably

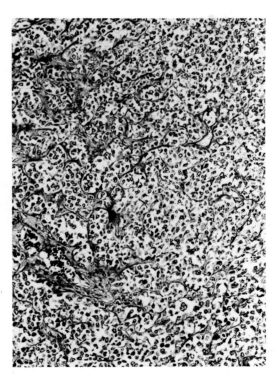

Fig. 17-51 Clear cell sarcoma of kidney. Tumor grows in ill-defined nests separated by prominent fibrovascular stroma. Cytoplasm is clear and nuclei are centrally located.

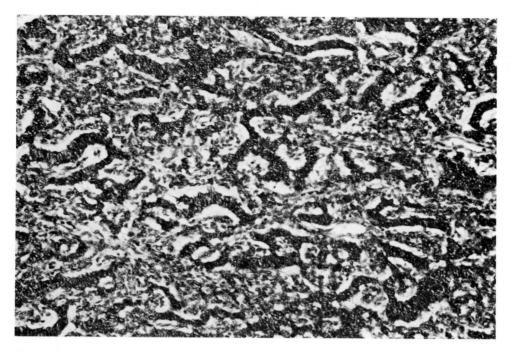

Fig. 17-52 Clear cell sarcoma with trabecular pattern of growth that simulates tubules of Wilms' tumor.

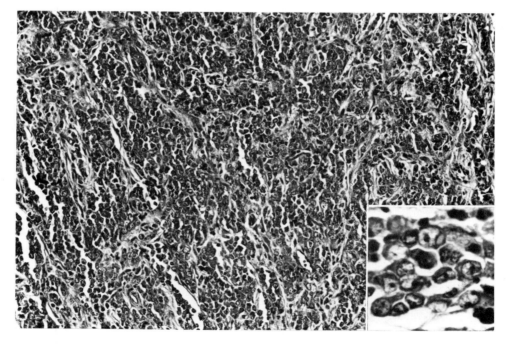

Fig. 17-53 Rhabdoid tumor. Neoplasm is growing in solid pattern and is composed of monotonous small round cells. **Inset** shows characteristic perinuclear hyaline globule deforming nucleus in some of the tumor cells.

is histogenetically related to Wilms' tumor,[374,375] but it should be kept in a separate category because of its substantially different natural history. Clear cell sarcoma is a very malignant tumor, with a high tendency for relapse and a striking propensity for skeletal metastases, particularly skull.[376] In this regard, it should be noted that skeletal metastases are extraordinarily rare in conventional Wilms' tumors. The reported mortality rate was over 50%, but substantially better results have recently been obtained with the administration of adriamycin.[373]

Rhabdoid tumor

Rhabdoid tumor was regarded for many years as a solid, monophasic, or rhabdomyosarcomatoid variant of Wilms' tumor but is now thought of as a separate tumor type. Most cases occur in young infants, the median age at diagnosis being 18 months.[385] Some of the cases have been associated with hypercalcemia.[382] Grossly, it is solid and soft, with infiltrative features. Microscopically, it is a monomorphic neoplasm that always involves the medullary region and has a generally diffuse but sometimes alveolar or trabecular pattern of growth. The tumor cells are medium sized and generally round or oval in shape. However, they can also be spindle, prompting the possibility of confusion with mesoblastic nephroma. The most characteristic feature is the presence of a large cytoplasmic eosinophilic hyaline globule that displaces the nucleus laterally to result in a plasmacytoid appearance (Fig. 17-53). Ultrastructurally, this globule is made up of a tangle of intermediate filaments.[380] Immunohistochemically, there is strong reactivity for vimentin and usually also for keratin but not for desmin, myoglobin, or other skeletal muscle markers. The histogenesis remains controversial; an origin from multipotential cells located in the renal medulla seems the most likely. The behavior is extremely aggressive, even when occurring in young infants. The death rate is over 75%. High tumor stage and male sex are unfavorable prognostic signs.[385]

Tumors morphologically indistinguishable from rhabdoid tumor of kidney have been reported in several other sites, including soft tissue, pelvis, bladder, and thymus.[379,383,384] Renal rhabdoid tumor has been seen in association with primary embryonal tumors in the midline posterior fossa, particularly medulloblastoma.[378,381]

Other sarcomas

The existence in children of malignant renal tumors having a sarcomatous appearance but not belonging to any of the tumor types previously described has been proposed.[386,387] Such tumors probably exist, but their nosologic position as independent entities is still controversial both conceptually and practically.

RENAL CELL CARCINOMA
General features

Renal cell carcinoma is generally a tumor of adults (average age at diagnosis: 55 to 60 years); the male to female ratio is about 2:1. It is bilateral in 1% of the cases. The rare renal cell carcinomas occurring in children have an appearance and behavior equivalent to those developing in adults.[395,402,408]

A familial form of the disease has been described associated with a chromosomal defect[389]; chromosomal abnormalities have also been detected in some sporadic cases.[415] Conditions that may be complicated by renal cell carcinoma are the following:

1 *von Hippel–Lindau's disease.* The tumors in these patients tend to be multiple and cystic.[405,409]
2 *Acquired cystic disease.* Half of the patients on long-term dialysis develop an acquired form of polycystic renal disease, which in a few cases has been complicated by the appearance of renal cell adenomas and carcinomas. The tumors tend to be small, multiple, and bilateral, with a metastatic rate of 5% to 7%.[391,393] They have also been described in the kidneys with acquired cystic disease of patients who have not had dialysis. Papillary hyperplasia of the epithelium of the cysts is a consistent feature in these cases and the likely pathogenetic basis for tumor development.[404]
3 *Adult form of polycystic renal disease* (p. 857) and *multicystic nephroma (multilocular cyst)* (p. 865). As with the preceding entity, the carcinoma is accompanied and probably preceded by foci of papillary hyperplasia.[390]

Renal carcinoma usually presents with hematuria (59%), flank pain (41%), and abdominal mass (45%). However, the combination of these three features, classically regarded as the diagnostic triad of renal cell carcinoma, occurs in only 9% of the patients.[414] Other manifestations are weight loss (28%), anemia (21%), fever (7%), and symptoms caused by a metastatic deposit (10%). Rare systemic manifestations include leukemoid reaction, systemic amyloidosis,[394,416] polyneuromyopathy, gastrointestinal disturbances, hepatosplenomegaly, and hepatic dysfunction.[398,412] It also can produce hypercalcemia as a result of the production of a parathormone-like hormone or some other substance,[397,400] hypertension caused by renin secretion,[403] polycythemia secondary to the secretion of an erythropoietic-stimulating substance,[411] gynecomastia as a result of gonadotropin and placental lactogen production,[401] and Cushing's syndrome due to the secretion of an ACTH-like substance.[410] Secretion of prolactin, enteroglucagon, insulin-like substance, and prostaglandin A have also been reported.[388]

In general, the investigation of a suspected renal mass begins with intravenous pyelography and is followed by ultrasonography and CT scan.[399] If a solid mass is revealed, renal arteriography and/or inferior vena cavogram may be carried out to further determine the extent of the tumor. With the increasing use of these modalities, the number of incidentally found renal cell carcinomas is increasing.[407]

One of the many peculiarities of renal cell cancer is its occasional regression in the absence of all treatment, a phenomenon found also with gestational choriocarcinoma, malignant melanoma, neuroblastoma, and—in lesser proportion—with several other tumors.[396,406]

Renal cell carcinoma is the most common "recipient" of the curious phenomenon of metastasis of a cancer into another cancer. Lung carcinoma is the most common "donor," the resulting microscopic appearance leading to interesting problems of interpretation.[392,413]

Morphologic features

Grossly, most renal cell carcinomas are well delineated and centered on the cortex. On occasion, only a small portion is connected with the cortex, the bulk of the tumor appearing as an extrarenal mass. Extension to the renal pelvis occurs only late in the course of the disease. In about 5% of the cases, multiple tumor nodules are seen scattered throughout the organ. In a typical case, the cut surface shows a solid golden-yellow tumor sharply separated from the surrounding tissues by a fibrous pseudocapsule. The common occurrences of hemorrhage, necrosis, calcification, and cystic change result in the variegated appearance that is so characteristic of this neoplasm (Fig. 17-54). A remarkable range of color may be seen; however, in the presence of a white granular tumor in the kidney, the diagnosis is likely to be something other than renal cell carcinoma. Sometimes, the cystic degeneration is so advanced that a mural nodule remains as the only evidence of the real nature of the lesion (Fig. 17-55). Sometimes even this disappears, and the diagnosis is made only on microscopic examination. Cortical cysts composed of a thick fibrous (often partially calcified) capsule and containing a grumous, yellow, necrotic material represent, in most cases, necrotic renal cell carcinomas. Predominantly cystic renal cell carcinomas are designated by some as *cystadenocarcinomas,* but they should not be viewed as a special tumor type.[431]

Microscopically, the tumor cells are large, the appearance of the cytoplasm ranging from optically clear, with sharply outlined boundaries ("vegetable cells"), to deeply granular, with many transitional forms[435] (Fig. 17-56). The cytoplasm may also contain hyaline droplets, phagocytosed blood pigment, and, exceptionally, Mallory-like bodies.[425] The clear cell appearance results from the accumulation of glycogen and also of fat, which can be easily demonstrated with PAS and Oil red O stains, respectively. Cytoplasmic mucin is nearly always absent. Tubular, papillary, and cystic formations may be present (Fig. 17-57). The nuclei are generally centrally located; their size, chromatin pattern, and nucleolar appearance vary notably from case to case, this constituting the main basis for microscopic grading (see p. 874).

Architecturally, most renal cell carcinomas show evidence of glandular differentiation, hence their alternative designation as renal adenocarcinomas. In the usual case, however, the pattern of growth is predominantly solid, with formation of large nests of tumor cells separated by a stroma that is characteristically endowed with prominent sinusoid-like vessels. Some renal cell carcinomas are predominantly *papillary;* these are often found to be hypovascular or avascular on angiography, tend to be localized to the kidney, are often necrotic, and may show prominent stromal infiltration by neutrophils or foamy macrophages.[428] Large sections or mul-

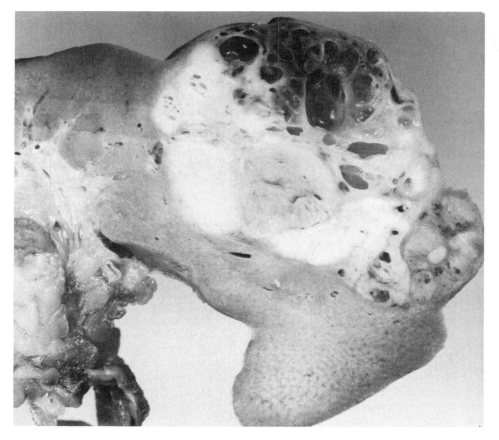

Fig. 17-54 Small circumscribed renal cell carcinoma extending through capsule. Lesion was bright yellow in color, hemorrhagic, and did not involve renal pelvis. There was no hematuria.

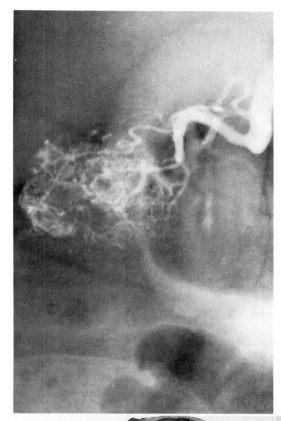

Fig. 17-55 Renal cell carcinoma illustrating phenomenon of massive necrosis not uncommonly seen with this neoplasm. Mural nodule of residual cancer was clearly demonstrated by arteriography.

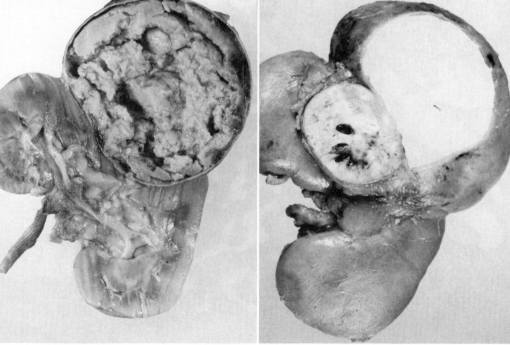

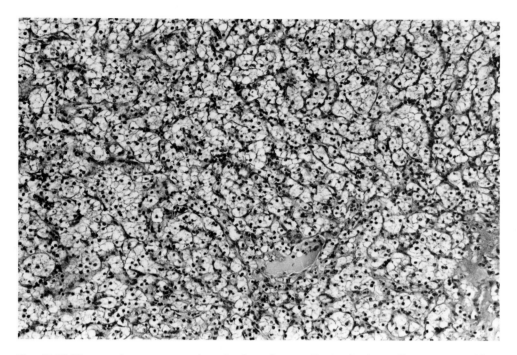

Fig. 17-56 Microscopic appearance of renal cell carcinoma with classic clear cell pattern resembling that of vegetable cells.

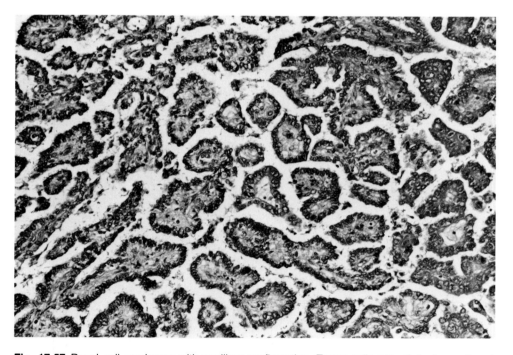

Fig. 17-57 Renal cell carcinoma with papillary configuration. Tumor cells are relatively small and cuboidal; papillae are well-formed and have branching configuration.

tiple sections usually show diverse patterns in the same tumor, a feature that renders subclassifications based on morphologic pattern of little significance, except for the types described in the following discussion.

Ultrastructurally, the clear cells are seen to contain abundant glycogen, variable amounts of fat, scanty organelles, well-defined microvilli on the apical surface, and numerous cell junctions.[427] In the granular cells, organelles are more numerous and glycogen and fat are scantier. Rarely, myelinoid lamellated cytoplasmic inclusions are found.[424,427] Variable numbers of mitochondria are seen, reaching their highest concentration in oncocytic tumors.[427]

Immunohistochemically, renal cell carcinoma shows reactivity for epithelial markers such as keratin, EMA, and CEA.[420,430,432] The keratins expressed by the conventional clear cell carcinoma are 8 and 18 (i.e., of simple epithelial type). In the other tumor types there is often also expression of keratins 7 and 19.[430] Co-expression of keratins and vimentin is the rule, a feature not present in normal tubular

cells.[423,437] Other antigens detected in the cells of renal cell carcinoma are brush border membrane/villin,[421,423,438] alpha-1-antitrypsin and alpha-1-antichymotrypsin,[419] S-100 protein (particularly the α subunit)[434] two forms of enolase isozymes,[422] and angiotensin-converting enzyme.[433] The lectin-binding pattern has been found to be similar to that of normal proximal tubules.[436] In addition, a variety of monoclonal antibodies against various defined and undefined epitopes of renal cell carcinomas are being currently evaluated for their potential diagnostic utility.[417,426,429] In general, the application of these various markers to renal cell carcinoma has supported the long-held impression that most examples of this tumor differentiate in the direction of proximal renal tubules.[418,427]

Cytology

Cytologic examination of voided urine or bladder washing is an inefficient method for the diagnosis of renal cell carcinoma, the detection rate in most series being no higher

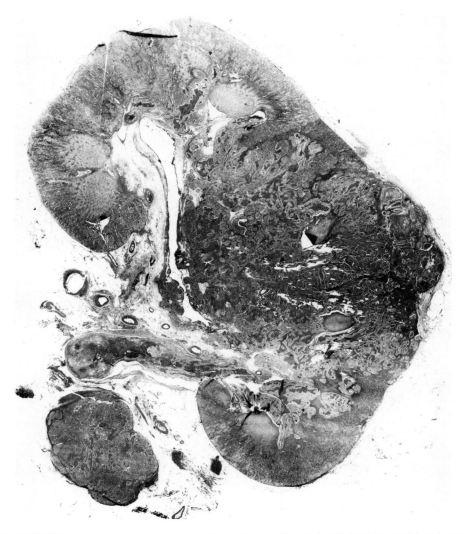

Fig. 17-58 Whole-mount section of renal cell carcinoma with renal vein invasion and lymph node metastasis. (Courtesy Dr. C. Perez-Mesa, Columbia, MO.)

than 25%. Better results have been obtained by using retrograde brushing cytology in pyelocalyceal carcinomas and renal cell carcinomas that have invaded the collecting system.[439]

Percutaneous fine needle aspiration is a safe and relatively accurate technique.[440] Its main use is in the differential diagnosis between a renal cyst and an avascular or hypovascular renal tumor and in confirmation of tumor recurrence in the renal fossa after nephrectomy.[440]

Spread and metastases

Approximately one third of renal cell carcinomas are found to invade perinephric fat and/or regional lymph nodes at the time of operation[449] (Fig. 17-58). Similarly, one third of the patients already have distant metastases at the time they seek medical attention.[445] The most common sites of distant metastases are lung and bones (particularly the pelvis and femur), but they can appear in adrenal gland, liver, thyroid, skin, soft tissue, central nervous system, and almost any other site. These metastases are often solitary, at least at the clinical level. Even at autopsy, 8% of the patients have metastatic involvement of only one or two organs.[448] Because of this and the fact that the primary tumor is often clinically silent, these metastases tend to be confused with primary tumors of the organs in which they lodge. That is certainly the case when renal cell carcinoma metastasizes to the *contralateral* adrenal gland, a phenomenon documented by several observers.[443,447] In these instances, EMA positivity favors a diagnosis of renal cell carcinoma.[450] An additional source of misinterpretation stems from the fact that sometimes these metastases develop years or decades after the removal of the primary tumor.[446] Several cases have been documented in which these metastases have undergone spontaneous regression.[442,444]

Metastases are extremely rare in tumors that measure 3 cm or less, but they can certainly occur.[441]

Therapy

The primary treatment of renal cell carcinoma is surgical excision. The preferred approach is a transabdominal or thoracoabdominal radical nephrectomy, with removal of the entire kidney, surrounding fat, Gerota's fascia, and adrenal gland.[452,453,459,461] Some authors advocate node dissection in continuity with the nephrectomy or after the renal mass has been removed. The dissection should include a minimum distance of 4 to 6 cm above and below the renal vessel; however, the indication for the performance of this regional lymphadenectomy remains controversial.[455,457] No benefits have yet been demonstrated for the administration of adjunctive radiation therapy or chemotherapy.[457]

Renal cell carcinomas that are bilateral or that occur in a solitary kidney are treated with partial nephrectomy, if technically feasible.[456,458,460]

Limited surgical resection of the lung is justified in patients with unilateral pulmonary metastases. A relatively long survival can be expected if the metastasis is found to be solitary on pathologic examination, if it shows extensive necrosis, and if the hilar lymph nodes are negative.[451,454]

Prognosis

The overall 5-year survival rate for renal cell carcinoma is about 70%. The prognosis is related to several clinicopathologic parameters.

1 *Sex and race.* These factors carry little if any prognostic connotation by themselves.

2 *Age.* The relationship between age and prognosis is minimal.[470] Even the rare renal cancers occurring in patients below the age of 40 years seem to follow the same course as in older patients.[465]

3 *Staging.* Patients who do not have distant metastases at diagnosis are given a stage on the basis of surgical findings. There are four stages: stage I, confined to the kidney; stage II, extension to perirenal fat but within Gerota's fascia; stage III, renal vein or vena caval involvement or regional lymph node metastases; and stage IV, extension to adjacent organs other than adrenal or distant metastases.

The 5-year survival rate following nephrectomy is 60% to 80% in stage I, 40% to 70% in stage II, 10% to 40% in stage III, and 5% or less in stage IV.

4 *Distant metastases.* Presence of distant metastatic disease at the time of operation is, not surprisingly, the single most important prognostic parameter.[470,471]

5 *Tumor size.* Size of the primary tumor relates to prognosis for the very small (less than 3 cm) and the very large (over 12 cm) tumors but not for those in between these extremes, which represent the large majority.[463,464]

6 *Renal vein invasion.* Traditionally, gross invasion of the renal vein has been regarded as a poor prognostic sign and has therefore constituted a criterion for the surgical staging (see preceding discussion). However, some recent series have shown that this factor has little prognostic significance by itself,[468,470] or that it affects outcome only in the high-grade tumors.[467a]

7 *Invasion of renal pelvis.* This feature does not seem to be of prognostic significance.[467]

8 *Microscopic grade.* Nuclear grade of the tumor as determined in microscopic sections is an important predictor of survival. It is strongly correlated with surgical staging, but it also maintains statistical validity independently from it. Four grades are generally used. In one series, the incidence of metastases was 0% for grade I tumors and 50% for the others.[463] In other series, the incidence of metastases for low-grade tumors has been higher.[472] It would seem that the most marked prognostic difference is between grades I and II tumors on one side and grades III and IV on the other.[467,467a,470] It is possible that the use of nuclear morphometry may further refine the criteria for nuclear grading.[473]

9 *Oncocytic appearance.* As indicated on p. 875, tumors with an exclusively oncocytic appearance metastasize very rarely.[467a,470] This is in part related to the fact that most of them are low-grade tumors.[463,467]

10 *Sarcomatoid appearance.* Sarcomatoid carcinomas have an extremely poor prognosis. This may again be viewed as related to tumor grade since these neoplasms belong by definition to the grade IV category.[469]

11 *Clear versus granular cytoplasm.* Clear cell tumors are, as a group, less aggressive than granular cell tumors, but this is largely a function of the nuclear grade.[463,470]

12 *DNA ploidy.* A close correlation has been found between DNA ploidy and morphologic nuclear grading, and therefore flow cytometry evaluation of these tumors could prove to be of prognostic use.[462,466]

RENAL CELL CARCINOMA–RELATED TUMORS
Adenoma

Renal adenomas, defined as minute cortical foci of tubular or papillary epithelium, are present in about 20% of adult kidneys; most of them measure 1 to 3 mm in diameter and rarely exceed 6 mm. Their ultrastructural appearance does not indicate an origin from a special segment of the nephron.[476] These tumors seem to be associated with arteriolonephrosclerosis and other forms of renal scarring,[475] and are particularly common in end stage kidneys in patients on long-term dialysis.[477] They probably are not true neoplasms but rather foci of nodular hyperplasia.

In the past, some authors have designated as adenoma

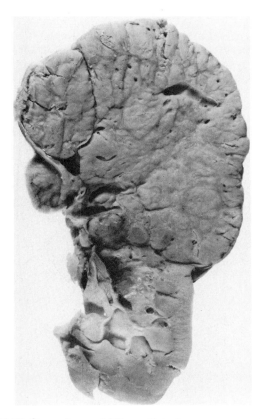

Fig. 17-59 Oncocytoma of kidney. Note homogeneous solid appearance of tumor, nodularity, and absence of hemorrhage and necrosis. Tumor measured 8 cm and had uniform brown color.

any renal epithelial neoplasm measuring 3 cm or less. We do not agree with this practice and regard renal tumors having a solid pattern of growth and/or predominantly composed of clear cells as carcinomas regardless of their size. Distant metastases from tumors as small as 1 cm have been documented.[474]

Oncocytoma

Renal oncocytomas are typically mahogany-brown and solid (Fig. 17-59). A central stellate scar is often present. They can reach extremely huge sizes.[480] Some are multicentric,[488] and a few are bilateral.[490] Invasion of the renal capsule or renal vein may be encountered. Microscopically, they are composed entirely of cells with abundant acidophilic granular cytoplasm (Fig. 17-60). The nuclei are usually small, round, and regular, and therefore most of these tumors qualify as grade I lesions.[484] Focal nuclear pleomorphism can occur, but the typical case of oncocytoma should not contain prominent papillary formations, clear cells, or necrosis.[479,486] If strict morphologic criteria are employed, it will be found that the large majority of the tumors will behave in a benign fashion regardless of size.[478,482,484,485,489] Immunohistochemically, these cells express keratins 8 and 18 but, in contrast to the conventional renal cell carcinomas, do not show reactivity for vimentin.[487] Ultrastructurally, packing of the cytoplasm by mitochondria is the most striking feature.[481]

We like to view oncocytoma as a distinct morphologic type of renal cell carcinoma associated with a particularly good prognosis, which depends at least in part on the fact that most of them are grade I tumors. Oncocytic tumors of higher nuclear grade are associated with a significant risk of metastases.[483,484] Consequently, we designate renal oncocytomas as renal cell carcinomas of oncocytic type.

Collecting duct carcinoma

Collecting duct carcinoma is the name given to a form of renal cell carcinoma that, in contrast to the usual type, is thought to arise from or differentiate toward collecting (Bellini's) ducts. These tumors are centered in the medulla, have a tubulopapillary architecture, and are surrounded by a desmoplastic reaction[492] (Fig. 17-61). Atypical changes in the adjacent ducts are common. The ultrastructural appearance, lectin-binding pattern, and expression of high molecular weight keratins recapitulate those of the lower nephron.[491,493,494] It is estimated that this tumor variant constitutes only 1% to 2% of all renal cell carcinomas. The number of cases so far identified is too small to know whether their behavior is significantly different from the usual type. It is likely that some of the cases formerly described as papillary renal cell carcinomas belong to this category.[495]

Sarcomatoid carcinoma

Sarcomatoid renal cell carcinoma (also known as spindle cell carcinoma, anaplastic carcinoma, or carcinosarcoma) makes up about 1% of all renal tumors in adults.[499] It is largely composed of spindle and/or pleomorphic tumor giant cells, which simulate the appearance of a sarcoma[497,498] (Figs. 17-62 and 17-63). Numerous sections

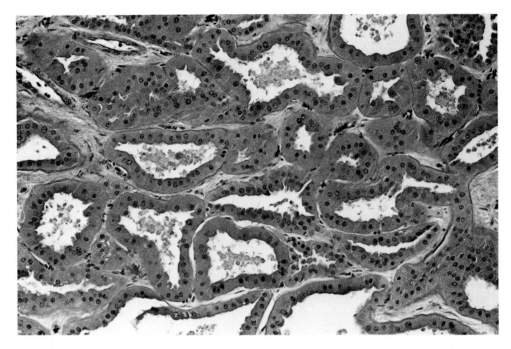

Fig. 17-60 Microscopic appearance of renal oncocytoma. Well-formed tubules are lined by cells with abundant granular acidophilic cytoplasm.

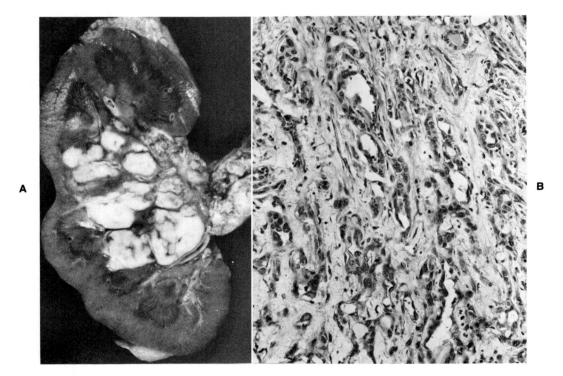

Fig. 17-61 Collecting duct carcinoma. **A,** Gross appearance of tumor, which is centered in medullary portion of kidney and extends into renal pelvis. **B,** Microscopic appearance is characterized by irregular neoplastic ducts lined by flattened cells, separated by abundant desmoplastic stroma.

may be necessary to find areas of recognizable carcinoma. The sarcomatoid component may differentiate in the direction of cartilage or bone. By immunohistochemistry and electron microscopy, epithelial markers may still be found in the sarcomatoid cells.[496]

The behavior of sarcomatoid carcinoma is extremely aggressive, in keeping with its grade IV cytology (p. 874). Extrarenal invasion is usually present at operation.[499] Multiple metastases of this tumor in the skeletal system have been known to simulate the entity of multicentric osseous fibrosarcoma. When a sarcomatoid pattern is found in a metastatic site, this will also be present in the primary renal tumor in nearly every instance.

Small cell carcinoma

Small cell carcinoma of the kidney with features similar to those of the homonymous pulmonary tumor has been described.[500] Evidence of neuroendocrine differentiation has been found in it ultrastructurally and immunohistochemically.[500,501] Some of the cases have appeared to arise from pelvic epithelium.[500a] The behavior of the few reported cases has been rather aggressive.

ANGIOMYOLIPOMA

Angiomyolipoma is a rare renal neoplasm composed of an intimate mixture of fat, blood vessels, and smooth muscle. The appearance on ultrasonography and CT scan is highly characteristic.[505] Grossly, this tumor may show a striking resemblance to renal cell carcinoma because of its yellow color, intratumoral hemorrhages, and frequent extrarenal growth[508] (Fig. 17-64). Multiple tumors are found

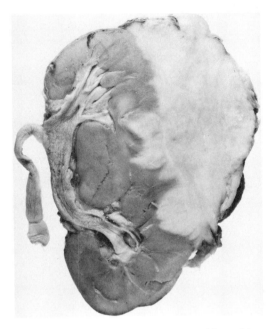

Fig. 17-62 Sarcomatoid renal cell carcinoma. Most of tumor had appearance of spindle cell sarcoma. Its epithelial nature was evident only focally.

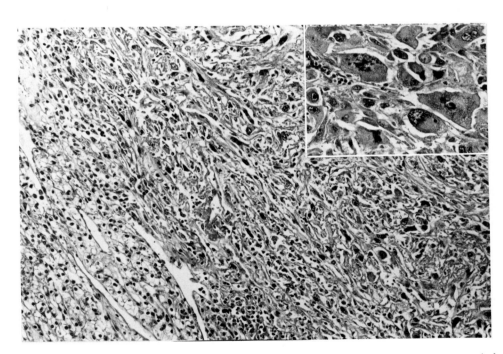

Fig. 17-63 Sarcomatoid carcinoma of kidney. Area of characteristic renal cell carcinoma composed of clear cells (left lower corner) merges with component having highly pleomorphic sarcoma-like appearance. Bizarre look of tumor cells can be clearly appreciated in **inset**.

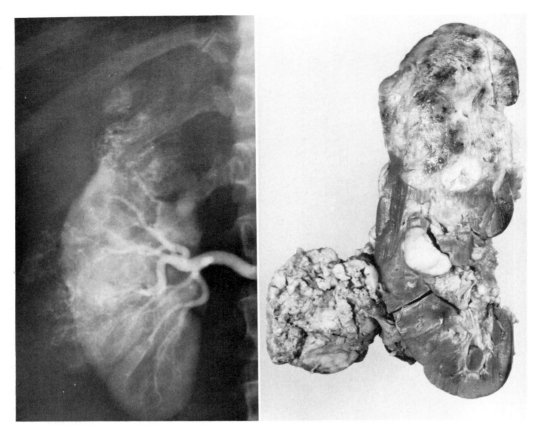

Fig. 17-64 Multiple angiomyolipoma. Contralateral kidney of patient, 51-year-old woman, also was affected. Lesion was confused clinically and roentgenographically with renal cell carcinoma.

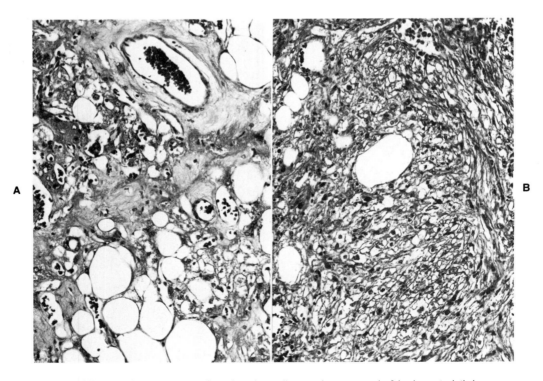

Fig. 17-65 Microscopic appearance of renal angiomyolipoma. Appearance in **A** is characteristic because of admixture of large blood vessels, mature adipose tissue, and some smooth muscle cells. Appearance in **B,** in which very cellular pattern of smooth muscle elements predominates, can be confused with retroperitoneal soft tissue sarcoma.

in about one third of the cases and bilateral tumors in 15%.[506] The regional lymph nodes may be involved, but this is regarded as an expression of multicentricity rather than true metastases.[503,504] Microscopically, the vascular component is composed of tortuous, thick-walled blood vessels that frequently lack an elastic tissue lamina.[512] The adipose tissue is of mature type. The smooth muscle component is troublesome because it may exhibit hypercellularity, marked pleomorphism, and moderate mitotic activity; these features may prompt a mistaken diagnosis of leiomyosarcoma[502] (Fig. 17-65). In addition, many cases show bizarre, sometimes multinucleated, cells with plump acidophilic or clear cytoplasm that may contain abundant glycogen; these cells, which are actin-positive and probably of smooth muscle nature, may result in confusion with renal cell carcinoma.

Neurologic and/or cutaneous findings diagnostic or suggestive of tuberous sclerosis are found in approximately one third of the patients with renal angiomyolipoma. The incidence is higher in cases of multiple or bilateral tumors. It has been estimated that about 80% of the patients with the complete or severe form of tuberous sclerosis have renal tumors of this type.[502] Renal angiomyolipomas have also been found in association with the lymphangiomyomatosis syndrome, supporting the concept that the latter represents a forme frustre of tuberous sclerosis.[510]

Renal angiomyolipoma may cause massive and sometimes fatal hemorrhage. Capsular invasion is present in a fourth of the cases, and occasionally there is massive local recurrence, which may result in death.[509] However, there are no well-documented instances of distant metastases. The treatment is surgical.[511]

Several cases have been reported of angiomyolipoma coexisting with renal cell carcinoma.[507] In some of the examples we have seen of this combination, the carcinomatous component arose in intimate connection and apparently within the angiomyolipoma (Fig. 17-66). Co-existence with renal oncocytoma has also been recorded.[513]

JUXTAGLOMERULAR CELL TUMOR

Patients with juxtaglomerular cell tumor present clinically with hypertension because of excessive renin production.[515] The light microscopic appearance is reminiscent of hemangiopericytoma.[516] Renin can be demonstrated by bioassay or immunohistochemistry.[514,515] Ultrastructurally, adrenergic nerve terminals are seen in contact with the tumor cells, which have various types of secretory granules, some of them containing a rhomboid crystalline material[514,518,520] (Fig. 17-67). All of the reported cases have behaved in a benign nature, but some patients have remained hypertensive following nephrectomy.[520]

It should be noted that renin secretion can be associated with other renal and extrarenal neoplasms, such as renal cell carcinoma, Wilms' tumor, and pancreatic adenocarcinoma.[517,519,521]

OTHER BENIGN TUMORS AND TUMORLIKE CONDITIONS

Hematomas can develop in the kidney or perirenal tissues as a result of trauma, from rupture of hemangiomas (see

following discussion), and sometimes for no apparent cause. A few of the perirenal hematomas have been found to contain peculiar periodic structures with radial striations that can simulate parasites.[529]

Teratoma of the kidney is exceptionally rare.[528] Most cases in which this diagnosis has been considered represent either retroperitoneal teratomas with renal extension or Wilms' tumors with teratoid features.[522,523]

Lipomas, leiomyomas, and *fibromas* are found frequently at autopsy as small incidental nodules. It is very rare for any of them to become clinically apparent.[524-527] Most of the lipomas are cortical or even capsular,[530] whereas the fibromas are characteristically medullary. It should be remembered that renal angiomyolipomas can be predominantly fatty and that the perirenal region is the most common location of retroperitoneal liposarcomas, many of which are very well differentiated and lipoma-like.

Hemangioma is frequently located in the medullary portion, where it can give rise to copious hematuria (see p. 881).

OTHER MALIGNANT PRIMARY TUMORS

Carcinoid tumor has been reported in the kidney in a few occasions, both in a pure form[547,548] and as a component of cystic teratoma.[534,536] Some of these tumors have exhibited an oncocytic appearance.[534a]

Sarcomas of various types can arise in the adult kidney.[533,546] These include leiomyosarcoma, fibrosarcoma, rhabdomyosarcoma, malignant fibrous histiocytoma,[545] liposarcoma, malignant hemangiopericytoma, angiosarcoma,[531] osteosarcoma,[539] chondrosarcoma[540] and malignant mesenchymoma.[538] Some of the chondrosarcomas have been of the mesenchymal variety.[537] A few of these sarcomas have been seen to arise from the renal capsule.[541] Before a diagnosis of primary sarcoma of the kidney is made, the more common possibilities of sarcomatoid renal cell carcinoma and primary retroperitoneal soft tissue sarcoma (particularly liposarcoma) with secondary renal invasion should be considered.

Malignant lymphoma of the kidney is usually the expression of generalized disease,[544] but sometimes the kidney is the only site of tumor.[542] Renal failure may result from diffuse involvement of the organ.[532,543] The majority of the cases are of large cell type. Two varieties of lymphoma with a predilection for secondary renal involvement are thymic large cell lymphoma with sclerosis (see Chapter 8) and lymphomatoid granulomatosis (see Chapter 7).

Plasmacytomas may be found within the kidney, usually as a result of dissemination in multiple myeloma but sometimes as an expression of extramedullary tumor.[535]

METASTATIC TUMORS

Metastatic carcinoma can affect the kidney as a part of a disseminated process, but the renal involvement is only rarely of clinical significance.[550] The metastasis may appear years or decades after the removal of the primary tumor.[551] Out of 295 malignant tumors presenting in the kidney, Mazeman et al.[552] found that only eight were metastatic. In contrast to renal cell carcinoma, metastatic tumors are bilateral in over 50% of the cases.[554] Thirty-one percent of

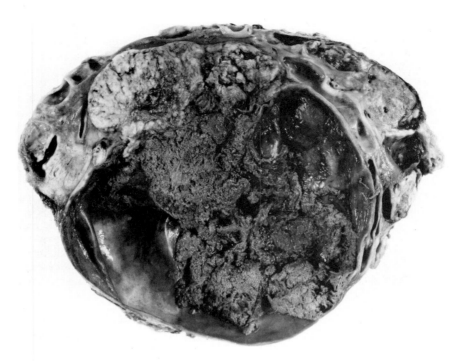

Fig. 17-66 Cut surface of kidney largely replaced by huge tumor mass exhibiting cystic, necrotic, and hemorrhagic changes. This case represents example of rare combination of angiomyolipoma and renal cell carcinoma.

the eighty-one patients reported by Wagle et al.[554] had microscopic hematuria. Sometimes, the metastases are exclusively limited to the renal glomeruli, in an intra- or extracapillary fashion, and may be diagnosable by needle biopsy.[549,553]

TUMORS OF RENAL PELVIS AND URETER
Transitional cell carcinoma

Most transitional cell carcinomas of the renal pelvis occur in adults, but pediatric cases also have been documented.[566] There is a history of analgesic abuse and/or co-existence of renal papillary necrosis in about one fourth of the cases.[563,564] Cases have been seen following administration of Thorotrast for radiographic purposes,[578] and, more recently, following cyclophosphamide therapy.[569] These tumors have also been reported in horseshoe kidneys; their incidence may actually be increased in this abnormality.[572] Hematuria is the most common clinical presentation.[576] Synchronous or metachronous tumors elsewhere in the urinary tract are found in almost 40% of the patients[563]; exceptionally, an independent renal cell carcinoma may be found in the same kidney.[582]

Grossly, these tumors form soft grayish red masses with smooth, glistening surfaces that resemble the transitional cell tumors of the bladder (Fig. 17-68, *A*).[564] They often diffusely involve the entire renal pelvis and form arborescent masses that may extend down the ureter. Grade III and grade IV lesions can spread massively into the renal parenchyma and even reach the renal capsule. They can be distinguished from renal cell carcinoma because of their whitish or gray color, granular appearance, and extensive pelvic involvement.

Transitional cell carcinomas of the ureter may be located anywhere along the length of the organ and usually result in dilatation of the proximal portion[559,570] (Fig. 17-68, *B*).

The microscopic appearance of these transitional carcinomas, whether located in the renal pelvis or ureter, is identical to that of their more common homologues in the bladder. The majority are grade II or grade III neoplasms. The pelvic neoplasms sometimes extend proximally along the collecting tubules, a pattern that should not be confused with adenocarcinoma[557] (Fig. 17-69). The adjacent urothelium is often abnormal, the changes ranging from hyperplasia to carcinoma in situ.[567] The presence of fibrous thickening of small stromal vessels has been found to correlate with a history of a long-term analgesic ingestion.[574]

Rarely, these tumors acquire a *sarcomatoid* appearance, with prominent spindling of the tumor cells.[581] In other instances, a neoplasm with features analogous to those of giant cell tumor of bone is seen in the pelvis in association with papillary or in situ transitional cell carcinoma.[560,565] In still others, a transitional cell carcinoma pattern is seen associated with small cell carcinoma (see p. 877).[571a]

The standard treatment of pyeloureteral transitional cell carcinoma is nephroureterectomy. Segmental resection has sometimes been employed for mid-ureteral lesions,[561] and endoscopic removal has been done for low-grade noninvasive lesions,[562] but the high incidence of multicentricity and co-existent dysplasia (particularly with the high-grade tumors) indicates that radical surgery is the treatment of choice for the large majority of the cases.[556,568] Furthermore, these tumors have a tendency to implant along the ureter, especially in its terminal (intramural) portion. Therefore it is important for a resection of the bladder cuff to be performed to avoid tumor recurrence.[577,579] For tumors occurring in solitary kidneys or for bilateral tumors, nephroureterectomy with renal autotransplantation and pyelocystostomy has been advocated.[575] The overall 5-year survival rate in the surgically resected cases is about 50%.[563] The prognosis is largely determined by the stage of the lesion for both the pelvic and ureteral lesions.[555,558,571,580]

Carcinoma in situ of the renal pelvis and ureter also occurs, but its detection at this stage is very difficult.[573]

Adenocarcinoma

As in the urinary bladder, it is not rare for transitional cell carcinomas of the pelvis or ureter to have small pools of mucin admixed with the tumor cells. These tumors should not be called adenocarcinomas. The term *adenocarcinoma* should be reserved for the rare neoplasms that not only secrete abundant mucin but also form unquestionable glandular structures.[583] This tumor may present in a pure form or be admixed with ordinary transitional cell carcinoma. The histogenesis of primary adenocarcinoma of the renal pelvis is closely related to glandular metaplasia of transitional epithelium (pyelitis glandularis and pyelitis cystica) induced by long-standing chronic inflammation, sometimes related to renal stones.[584]

Epidermoid carcinoma

Epidermoid carcinoma of the renal pelvis is often associated with squamous metaplasia ("leukoplakia"), renal calculi, and infection[585] (Fig. 17-70). Cases have also been reported many years following retrograde pyelography in which Thorotrast was used.[587] Grossly, the tumor is usually large, necrotic, and ulcerated (Fig. 17-71). Renal stones and features of pyelonephritis are often found. Invasion of the renal parenchyma and retroperitoneal soft tissues is common. The prognosis is very poor.[586]

Other tumors and tumorlike conditions

Fibroepithelial polyp[591,598] (Fig. 17-72) and *hypertrophic infundibular stenosis of the calyces*[599] are two rare tumorlike masses of the pelvic region. Excessive proliferation of peripelvic fat, known as *pelvic lipomatosis* or *fibrolipomatosis*, may simulate radiographically a neoplasm.[596] *Amyloidosis* can present as a localized nodule in the wall of one or both ureters (so-called amyloid tumor).[593] *Malakoplakia* of the pelvis or ureter may result in obstruction and hydronephrosis.[601,604]

Benign pyeloureteral tumors include inverted papilloma,[594] so-called nephrogenic adenoma,[605] hemangioma,[588,590] leiomyoma,[608] and neurofibroma.[588] The hemangiomas are often located at the tips of the papillae, are multiple in about 10% of the cases, and may result in recurrent episodes of hemorrhage.[589,592] Owing to their small size, extensive sectioning may be needed to find the lesion.

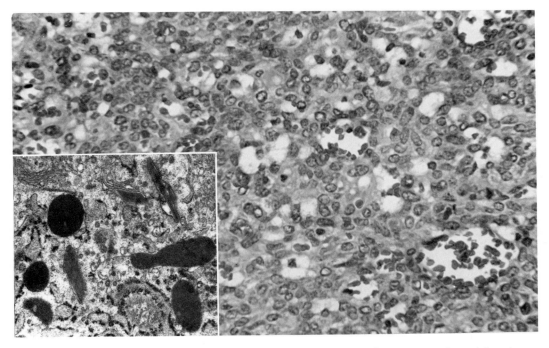

Fig. 17-67 Renin-producing juxtaglomerular cell tumor. Light microscopic appearance is reminiscent of hemangiopericytoma. Inset shows secretory granules as seen ultrastructurally. Some of them are diamond shaped, identical to those seen in normal juxtaglomerular cells. This case has been reported by Conn, et al.[515] (Courtesy Dr. M.R. Abell, Ann Arbor, MI.)

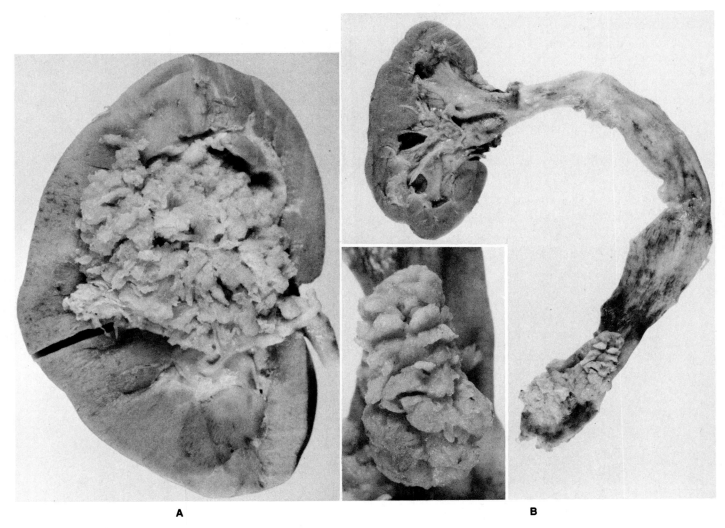

A   **B**

Fig. 17-68 A, Typical gross appearance of low-grade transitional cell carcinoma of renal pelvis in 49-year-old woman with gross painless hematuria. Only minimal stromal invasion was present. **B,** Transitional cell carcinoma of distal end of ureter. Note papillary configuration of tumor (better appreciated in **inset**) and proximal dilatation.

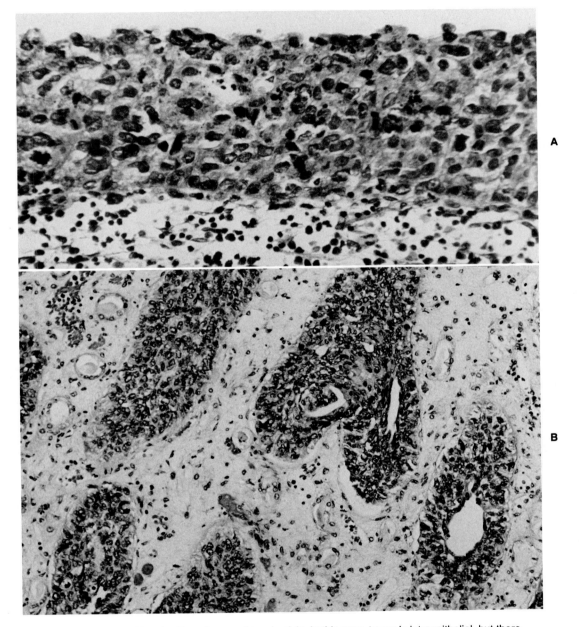

Fig. 17-69 A, Transitional cell carcinoma of renal pelvis. In this area, tumor is intraepithelial, but there were foci of stromal invasion elsewhere. **B,** Extension of tumor shown in **A** into collecting tubules reminiscent of extension into endocervical glands by in situ carcinoma of uterine cervix.

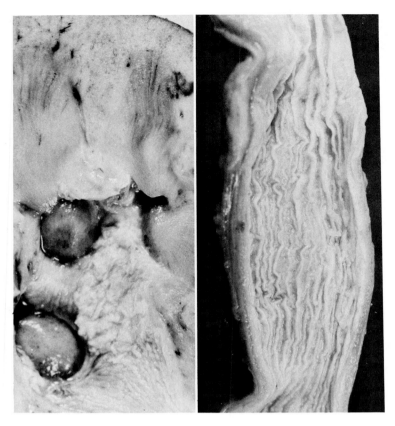

Fig. 17-70 Extensive leukoplakia of renal pelvis and ureter without stones.

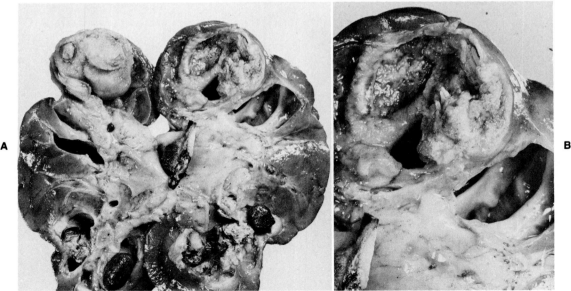

Fig. 17-71 A, Kidney with hydronephrosis, chronic pyelonephritis, leukoplakia, stone formation, and keratinizing epidermoid carcinoma. **B,** Epidermoid carcinoma can be seen clearly but was not suspected prior to pathologic examination.

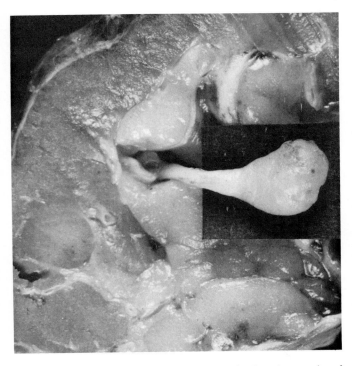

Fig. 17-72 Benign fibroepithelial polyp emerging from lower calyx of left kidney in 61-year-old woman. Tumor caused hematuria, and total nephrectomy was done.

Malignant tumors of nonepithelial type are exceptional. A few cases of leiomyosarcoma have been reported.[609] Non-Hodgkin's malignant lymphoma of the retroperitoneum can involve the ureter secondarily.[606] A case of primary malignant lymphoma has been reported in the pelvis of a transplanted kidney.[600]

Ureterosigmoidoscopy, an operation no longer practiced, can be complicated by the appearance of a tumor at the site of anastomosis many years following the operation.[603] The tumor is usually an *adenocarcinoma*, and it develops on the colonic side, usually on a background of hyperplastic mucosa of the so-called transitional type.[607] A few cases of benign and malignant tumors have been reported in uretero-ileal conduits.[597,602]

Carcinomas *metastatic* to the retroperitoneum can invade the ureteral wall and result in obstruction; breast and lung are the most common sites for the primary tumors.[595,602a]

REFERENCES
Non-neoplastic conditions
ROLE OF RENAL BIOPSY

1 Bohle A, Eichenseher N, Fischbach H, Neild GH, Wehner H, Edel HH, Losse H, Renner E, Reichel W, Schütterle G: The different forms of glomerulonephritis. Morphologic and clinical aspects analyzed in 2,500 patients. Klin Wochenschr **55**:59-73, 1973.
2 Cohen AH, Nast CC, Adler SG, Kopple JD: The clinical usefulness of kidney biopsy in the diagnosis and management of renal disease (abstract). Kidney Int **27**:135, 1985.

3 Dische FE, Parsons V: Experience in the diagnosis of glomerulonephritis using combined light microscopical, ultrastructural and immunofluorescence techniques. An analysis of 134 cases. Histopathology **1**:331-362, 1977.
4 Kashgarian M, Hayslett JP, Spargo BH: Renal disease. Am J Pathol **89**:187-272, 1977.
5 Morel-Maroger L: The value of renal biopsy. Am J Kidney Dis **4**:244-248, 1982.
6 Pirani CL, Salinas-Madrigal L, Koss M: Evaluation of percutaneous renal biopsy. In Sommers S (ed): Kidney Pathology Decennial, 1966-1975. New York, 1975, Appleton-Century-Crofts, pp. 109-163.

PATHOLOGIC EXAMINATION

7 Churg J, Sobin LH: Renal disease. Classification and atlas of glomerular diseases. New York, 1982, Igaku-Shoin.
8 Pirani CL: Interpretation of renal biopsy. In Tisher CC, Brenner BM (eds): Renal pathology. Philadelphia, 1988, J.B. Lippincott Co. (In press.)
9 Zollinger HU, Mihatsch NJ: Renal pathology and biopsy. Light, electron and immunofluorescent microscopy and clinical aspects. Berlin, 1978, Springer-Verlag.

GLOMERULAR LESIONS ASSOCIATED WITH THE NEPHROTIC SYNDROME
Minimal change glomerulonephropathy and its variants

10 Cameron JS, Turner DR, Ogg CS, Sharpstone P, Brown CB: The nephrotic syndrome in adults with "minimal change" glomerular lesions. Q J Med **43**:461-488, 1974.
11 Churg J, Habib R, White RHR: Pathology of the nephrotic syndrome in children. A report for the International Study of Kidney Disease in Children. Lancet **1**:1299-1302, 1970.
12 Coggins CH: Minimal change nephrosis in adults. In Proceedings of the 8th International Congress of Nephrology. Basel, 1981, S Karger, p. 336.
13 Habib R, Kleinknecht C: The primary nephrotic syndrome of children. Classification and clinicopathologic study of 406 cases. In Sommers SC (ed): Kidney Pathology Decennial, 1966-1975. New York, 1975, Appleton-Century-Crofts, pp. 165-224.
14 Prasad D, Zimmerman S, Burkholder P: Immunohistologic features of minimal-change nephrotic syndrome. Arch Pathol Lab Med **101**:345-349, 1977.
15 Report of the International Study of Kidney Disease in Children: Nephrotic syndrome in children. Prediction of histopathology from clinical and laboratory characteristics at time of diagnosis. Kidney Int **13**:159-165, 1978.

Diffuse mesangial hypercellularity with nephrotic syndrome

16 Cohen AH, Border WA, Glassock RJ: Nephrotic syndrome with glomerular mesangial IgM deposits. Lab Invest **38**:610-619, 1978.
17 Ji-Yun Y, Melvin T, Sibley R, Michael AF: No evidence for a specific role of IgM in mesangial proliferation of idiopathic nephrotic syndrome. Kidney Int **25**:100-106, 1984.
18 Report of the International Study of Kidney Disease in Children: Primary nephrotic syndrome in children. Clinical significance of histopathologic variants of minimal change and of diffuse mesangial hypercellularity. Kidney Int **20**:765-771, 1981.
19 Report of the Southwest Pediatric Nephrology Study Group: Childhood nephrotic syndrome associated with diffuse mesangial hypercellularity. Kidney Int **23**:87-94, 1983.
20 Tejani A, Nicastri M: Mesangial IgM nephropathy (editorial). Nephron **35**:1-5, 1983.
21 Waldherr R, Gubler MC, Levy M, Broyer M, Habib R: The significance of pure diffuse mesangial proliferation in idiopathic nephrotic syndrome. Clin Nephrol **10**:171-179, 1978.

Focal and segmental glomerulosclerosis

22 Brenner BM, Meyer TW, Hostetter TH: Dietary protein intake and the progressive nature of renal disease. N Engl J Med **307**:652-659, 1982.
23 Chawder P, Soni A, Suri A, Bhagwat R, Yoo J, Treser G: Renal ultrastructural markers in AIDS associated nephropathy. Am J Pathol **126**:513-526, 1987.
24 Cohen AH, Mampaso F, Zamboni L: Glomerular podocyte degeneration in human renal disease. An ultrastructural study. Lab Invest **37**:20-42, 1976.
25 Eknoyan G, Gyorkey F, Dichoso C, Hyde SE, Gyorkey P, Suki W, Maldonado MM: Renal involvement in drug abuse. Arch Intern Med **132**:801-806, 1973.
26 Friedman EA, Rao TKS, Nicastri AD: Heroin associated nephropathy. Nephron **13**:421-426, 1974.

27 Gardenswartz MH, Lerner CW, Seligson GR, Zabetakis PM, Rotterdam H, Tapper ML, Michelis MF, Bruno MS: Renal disease in patients with AIDS. A clinicopathologic study. Clin Nephrol 21:197-204, 1984.

28 Grishman E, Churg J: Focal glomerular sclerosis in nephrotic patients. An electron microscopic study of glomerular podocytes. Kidney Int 7:111-122, 1975.

29 Grimley PM, Kang Y-H, Silverman RH, Davis G, Hoofnagle JH: Blood lymphocyte inclusions associated with alpha interferon. Lab Invest 48:30A-31A, 1983.

30 Hoyer J: Focal segmental glomerulosclerosis, Semin Nephrol 2:253-263, 1982.

31 Kanwar YS: Biophysiology of glomerular filtration and proteinuria. Lab Invest 51:7-21, 1984.

32 Kashgarian M: Lipoid nephrosis and focal sclerosis. Distinct entities on spectrum of disease. Nephron 13:105-108, 1974.

33 Orenstein JM, Schulob RS, Simon GL: Ultrastructural markers in the acquired immune deficiency syndrome (letter to the editor). Arch Pathol Lab Med 108:857-858, 1984.

34 Pardo V, Aldana M, Colton RM, Fischl MA, Jaffe D, Moskowitz L, Hensley GT, Bourgoignie JJ: Glomerular lesions in the acquired immunodeficiency syndrome. Ann Intern Med 101:429-434, 1984.

35 Pardo V, Meneses R, Ossa L, Jaffe DJ, Strauss J, Roth D, Bourgoignie JJ: AIDS-related glomerulopathy. Occurrence in specific risk groups. Kidney Int 31:1167-1173, 1987.

36 Pinto J, Lacerda G, Cameron JS: Recurrence of focal segmental glomerulosclerosis in renal allografts. Transplantation 32:83-89, 1981.

37 Rao RKS, Friedman EA, Nicastri AD: The types of renal disease in the acquired immunodeficiency syndrome. N Engl J Med 316:1062-1068, 1987.

38 Rao TKS, Filippone EJ, Nicastri AD, Landesman SH, Frank E, Chen CK, Friedman EA: Associated focal and segmental glomerulosclerosis in the acquired immunodeficiency syndrome. N Engl J Med 310:669-673, 1984.

39 Report of the Southwest Pediatric Nephrology Study Group: Focal segmental glomerulosclerosis in children with idiopathic nephrotic syndrome. Kidney Int 27:442-449, 1985.

40 Rich AR: A hitherto undescribed vulnerability of the juxtamedullary glomeruli in lipoid nephrosis. Bull Johns Hopkins Hosp 100:173-186, 1957.

41 Rich SA: Human lupus inclusions and interferons. Science 213:772-775, 1981.

42 Siegel NJ, Kashgarian M, Spargo BH, Hayslett JP: Minimal change and focal sclerotic lesions in lipoid nephrosis. Nephron 13:125-137, 1974.

Membranous glomerulonephropathy

43 Barr RD, Rees PH, Cordy PE: Nephrotic syndrome in adult Africans in Nairobi. Br Med J 2:131-134, 1972.

44 Cameron JS: Histology, protein clearances and response to treatment in the nephrotic syndrome. Br Med J 427:352-356, 1968.

45 Coggins CH: Is membranous nephropathy treatable? Am J Nephrol 1:219-221, 1981.

46 Collaborative study of the adult idiopathic nephrotic syndrome: A controlled study of short-term prednisone treatment in adults with membranous nephropathy. N Engl J Med 301:1301-1306, 1979.

47 Costanza ME, Pinn VW, Schwartz RS, Nathanson L: Carcinoembryonic antigen-antibody complexes in a patient with colonic carcinoma and nephrotic syndrome. N Engl J Med 289:520-522, 1973.

48 Couser WG, Salant DJ: In situ immune complex formation and glomerular injury. Kidney Int 17:1-13, 1980.

49 Del Vecchio-Blanco C, Polito C, Caporaso N, Del Gado R, Busachi CA, Coltorti M, DiToro R: Membranous glomerulopathy and hepatitis B virus (HBV) infection in children. Int J Pediatr Nephrol 4:35, 1983.

50 Dreyer L: The frequency of hepatitis B surface antigen in membranous nephropathy in black and white South Africans. S Afr Med J 65:166-168, 1984.

51 Ehrenreich T, Churg J: Pathology of membranous nephropathy. Pathol Annu 3:145-186, 1968.

52 Empire Rheumatism Council Research Subcommittee: Gold therapy in rheumatoid arthritis. Report of a multicenter controlled trial. Ann Rheum Dis 19:95-119, 1960.

53 Forland M, Spargo BH: Clinicopathological correlations in idiopathic nephrotic syndrome with membranous nephropathy. Nephron 6:498-525, 1969.

54 Gagliano RG, Costanzi JJ, Beathard GA, Sarles HE, Bell JD: The nephrotic syndrome associated with neoplasia. Am J Med 60:1026-1031, 1976.

55 Groggel GC, Adler S, Rennke HG, Couser WG, Salant DJ: Role of the terminal complement pathway in experimental membranous nephropathy in the rabbit. J Clin Invest 72:1948-1957, 1983.

56 Habib R, Kleinknecht C: The primary nephrotic syndrome of childhood. Classification and clinicopathologic study of 406 cases. Pathol Annu 6:417-474, 1971.

57 Hayslett JP, Kashgarian M, Bensch KG: Clinicopathologic correlations in the nephrotic syndrome due to primary renal disease. Medicine [Baltimore] 52:93-120, 1973.

58 Hill HFH, Hill AGS, Day AT, Brown RM, Golding JR, Lyle WH: Maintenance dose of penicillamine in rheumatoid arthritis. A comparison between a standard and a response-related flexible regimen. Ann Rheum Dis 38:429-433, 1979.

59 Hirose H, Udo K, Kojima M, Takahasi Y, Miyakawa Y, Miyamoto K, Yoshizawa H, Mayumi M: Deposition of hepatitis B antigen in membranous glomerulonephritis. Identification by F(ab')₂ fragments of monoclonal antibody. Kidney Int 26:338-341, 1984.

60 Hoorntje SJ, Donker AJ, Prins EJ, Weening JJ: Membranous glomerulopathy in a patient on captopril. Acta Med Scand 208:325-329, 1980.

61 Kaplan BS, Klassen J, Gault MH: Glomerular injury in patients with neoplasia. Annu Rev Med 27:117-125, 1976.

62 Kerjaschki D, Miettinen A, Farquhar MG: qp330-Anti-qp330 immune complexes form in epithelial coated pits and rapidly become attached to the glomerular basement membrane. J Exp Med 166:109-128, 1987.

63 Kleinknecht C, Levy M, Peix A, Broyer M, Courtecuisse V: Membranous glomerulonephritis and hepatitis B surface antigen in children. J Pediatr 95:946-952, 1979.

64 Lewis MG, Loughridge LW, Phillips TM: Immunological studies in nephrotic syndrome associated with extrarenal malignant disease. Lancet 2:134, 1972.

65 Row PG, Cameron JS, Turner OR, Evans DJ, White RHR, Ogg CS, Chantler C, Brown CB: Membranous nephropathy. Long-term follow-up and association with neoplasia. Q J Med (New Series) 44:207-239, 1975.

66 Slusarcyzk J, Michalak T, Nazarewicz-de Mezer T, Krawczynski K, Nowoslawski A: Membranous glomerulopathy associated with hepatitis B core antigen immune complexes in children. Am J Pathol 98:29-43, 1980.

67 Takekoshi Y, Tanaka M, Shida N, Satake Y, Saheki Y, Matsumoto S: Strong association between membranous nephropathy and hepatitis-B surface antigenaemia in Japanese children. Lancet 2:1065-1068, 1978.

68 Warnhin DM, Rees PH, Barr RD: Nairobi nephrosis. The nephrotic syndrome and skin lightening cream. East Afr Med J 51:953-960, 1974.

69 Wing AJ, Hutt MS, Kibukamusoke JW: Progression and remission in the nephrotic syndrome associated with quartan malaria in Uganda. Q J Med 163:273-289, 1972.

Diabetic nephropathy

70 Ainsworth SK, Hirsch HZ, Brackett NC Jr, Brissie RM, Williams AV Jr, Hennigar GR: Diabetic glomerulonephropathy. Histopathologic, immunofluorescent, and ultrastructural studies of 16 cases. Hum Pathol 13:470-478, 1982.

71 Churg J, Dachs S: Diabetic renal disease. Arteriosclerosis and glomerulosclerosis. In Kidney Pathology Decennial, 1966-1975. New York, 1975, Appleton-Century-Crofts.

72 Friedman EA, L'Esperance FA (eds): Diabetic renal-retinal syndrome, vol. 1, 2. Miami, 1980, 1982, Grune & Stratton, Inc.

73 Ghiggeri GM, Candiano G, Delfino G, Bianchini F, Queirolo C: Glycosyl albumin and diabetic microalbuminuria. Demonstration of an altered renal handling. Kidney Int 25:565-570, 1984.

74 Gundersen JH, Gotzsche O, Hirose K, Droustrup JP, Mogensen CE, Seyer-Hansen K, Osterby R: Early structural changes in glomerular capillaries and their relationship to long-term diabetic nephropathy. Acta Endocrinol 97(Suppl):19-21, 1981.

75 Jones RH, Hayakawa H, Mackay JD, Parsons V, Watkins PJ: Progression of diabetic nephropathy. Lancet 1:1105-1106, 1979.

76 Keen H, Viberti GC: Genesis and evolution of diabetic nephropathy. J Clin Pathol 34:1261-1266, 1981.

77 Kimmelstiel P, Wilson C: Intercapillary lesions in the glomeruli of the kidney. Am J Pathol 1:83-98, 1936.

78 Mauer SM, Steffes MW, Brown DM: The kidney in diabetes. Am J Med 70:603-612, 1981.

79 Salinas-Madrigal L, Pirani CL, Pollak VE: Glomerular and vascular insudative lesions of diabetic nephropathy. Electron microscopic observations. Am J Pathol 59:369-397, 1970.

Amyloidosis

80 Franklin EC, Gorevic PD: The amyloid disease. In Fougerau M, Daussett J (eds): Progress in immunology, vol. 1. London, 1980, Academic Press.

81 Glenner GG, Costa PP, Freitas AF: Amyloid and amyloidosis. In Proceedings of the Third International Symposium on Amyloidosis. Povoa de Varzim, Portugal, Amsterdam, 1980, Excerpta Medica.

82 Kyle RA, Griepp PR: Amyloidosis (AL) clinical and laboratory features in 29 cases. Mayo Clinic Proc **58**:665-683, 1983.

Light chain disease

83 King JT, Valenzuela R, McCormack LJ, Osborne DG: Granular dense deposit disease. Lab Invest **39**:591-596, 1978.

84 Morel-Maroger L, Verroust P: Glomerular lesions in dysproteinemias. Kidney Int **5**:249-252, 1974.

85 Randall RE, Williamson WC, Mullinax F, Tung MY, Still WJS: Manifestations of systemic light chain deposition. Am J Med **60**:293-299, 1976.

86 Verroust P, Mery JP, Morel-Maroger L, Clauvel JP, Richet G: Glomerular lesions in monoclonal gammopathies and mixed essential cryoglobulineminas IgG-IgM. In Hamberger J, Crosnier J, Maxwell MH (eds): Advances in nephrology, vol 1, Chicago, 1971, Year Book Medical Publishers, Inc., pp. 161-194.

Hereditary and familial nephropathies

87 Bennett WM, Musgrave JE, Campbell RA, Elliot D, Cox R, Brooks RE, Lovrien EW, Beacs RK, Porter GA: The nephropathy of the nail-patella syndrome. Clinicopathologic analysis of 11 kindred. Am J Med **54**:304-319, 1973.

88 Churg J, Sherman RL: Pathologic characteristics of hereditary nephritis. Arch Pathol **95**:374-379, 1973.

89 Jenis EH, Valeski JE, Calcagno PL: Variability of anti-GBM binding in hereditary nephritis. Clin Nephrol **15**:111-114, 1981.

90 McKusick VA: Mendelian inheritance in man. Baltimore, 1983, Johns Hopkins University Press.

91 Rogers PW, Kurtzman NA, Bunn SM Jr, White MG: Familial benign essential hematuria. Arch Intern Med **131**:257-262, 1973.

92 Rumpelt HG, Langer KH, Scharer K: Split and extremely thin glomerular basement membranes in hereditary nephropathy (Alport's syndrome). Virchows Arch [Pathol Anat] **364**:225-233, 1974.

Congenital nephrotic syndrome

93 Habib R, Bois E: Heterogeneite des syndromes nephrotiques a debut precoce du nourrisson (syndrome nephrotique "infantile"). Étude anatomoclinique et genêtique de 37 observations. Helv Paediatr Acta **28**:91-107, 1973.

94 Hallman N, Norio R, Rapola J: Congenital nephrotic syndrome. Nephron **11**:101-110, 1973.

95 Huttunen N-P: Congenital nephrotic syndrome of Finnish type. Study of 75 patients. Arch Dis Child **51**:344-348, 1976.

96 Huttunen N-P, Rapola J, Vilska J, Hallman N: Renal pathology in congenital nephrotic syndrome of Finnish type. A quantitative light microscopic study of 50 patients. Int J Pediatr Nephrol **1**:10-16, 1980.

GLOMERULAR LESIONS ASSOCIATED WITH THE SYNDROME OF ACUTE NEPHRITIS
Acute post-infectious glomerulonephritis

97 Berger J, Yaneva H, Hinglais N: Immunohistochemistry of glomerulonephritis. In Hamberger J, Crosnier J, Maxwell MH (eds): Advances in nephrology, vol. 1. Chicago, 1971, Year Book Medical Publishers, Inc., p. 11.

98 Dodge WF, Spargo BH, Bass JA, Travis LB: The relationship between the clinical and pathologic features of poststreptococcal glomerulonephritis. A study of the early natural history. Medicine [Baltimore] **47**:227-267, 1986.

99 Earle DP: Natural history of acute glomerulonephritis in adults. In Metcoff J (ed): Acute glomerulonephritis, Boston, 1967, Little, Brown & Co., pp. 3-14.

100 Edelmann CM Jr, Greifer I, Barnett HL: The nature of kidney disease in children who fail to recover from apparent acute glomerulonephritis. J Pediatr **64**:879-887, 1964.

101 Ingelfinger JR, McClusky RT, Scheeberger EE, Grupe WE: Necrotizing arteritis, acute poststreptococcal glomerulonephritis. J Pediatr **91**:228-232, 1977.

102 Jennings RB, Earle DP: Post-streptococcal glomerulonephritis. Histopathologic and clinical studies of the acute, subsiding acute, and early chronic latent phases. J Clin Invest **40**:1525-1595, 1961.

103 Kobayashi O, Okawa K-I, Kamiyama T, Wada H: Electron microscopic alterations of the glomerular capillaries in children with post-streptococcal glomerulonephritis. Acta Med Biol **19**:79-91, 1971.

104 Michael AF, Drummond KM, Good RA, Vernier RL: Acute post-streptococcal glomerulonephritis. Immune deposit disease. J Clin Invest **45**:237-248, 1966.

105 Morel-Maroger L, Leathem A, Richet G: Glomerular abnormalities in nonsystemic diseases. Relationship between findings by light microscopy and immunofluorescence in 433 renal biopsy specimens. Am J Med **53**:170-184, 1972.

106 Nissenson AR, Mayon-White R, Potter EV, Mayon-White V, Abidh S, Poon-King T, Earle DP: Continued absence of clinical renal disease seven to twelve years after poststreptococcal acute glomerulonephritis in Trinidad. Am J Med **67**:255-262, 1979.

107 Törnroth T: The fate of subepithelial deposits in acute poststreptococcal glomerulonephritis. Lab Invest **35**:461-474, 1976.

108 Travis LB, Dodge WF, Bethard GA, Spargo BH, Lorentz WB, Carvajal HF, Bergen M: Acute glomerulonephritis in children. A review of the natural history with emphasis on prognosis. Clin Nephrol **1**:169-181, 1973.

Diffuse crescentic glomerulonephritis

109 Abuelo JG, Esparza AR, Matarese RA, Endreny RG, Carvalho JS, Allegra SR: Crescentic IgA nephropathy. Medicine [Baltimore] **63**:396-406, 1984.

110 Bacani RG, Valasquez F, Kanter A, Pirani CL, Pollak VE: Rapidly progressive (nonstreptococcal) glomerulonephritis. Ann Intern Med **69**:463-485, 1968.

111 Beirne GJ, Wagnild JP, Zimmerman SW, Macken PD, Burkholder P: Idiopathic crescentic glomerulonephritis. Medicine [Baltimore] **56**:349-381, 1977.

112 Glassock RJ: A clinical and immunopathologic dissection of rapidly progressive glomerulonephritis. Nephron **2**:53-264, 1978.

113 Glassock RM, Bennett CM: The glomerulopathies. In Brenner BM, Rector FC (eds): The kidney, vol. 2, ed. 3. Philadephia, 1986, W.B. Saunders.

114 Leonard CD, Nagle RB, Striker GE, Cutler RE, Schribner BH: Acute glomerulonephritis with prolonged oliguria. An analysis of 29 cases. Ann Intern Med **73**:703-711, 1970.

115 Lewis EJ, Cavallo T, Harrington JT, Cotran RS: An immunopathologic study of rapidly progressive glomerulonephritis in the adult. Hum Pathol **2**:185-208, 1971.

116 Morita T, Suzuki Y, Churg J: Structure and development of the glomerular crescent. Am J Pathol **72**:349-368, 1973.

117 Morrin P, Hinglais N, Habarra B, Kreis H: Rapidly progressive glomerulonephritis. Am J Med **65**:446-460, 1978.

118 Olsen S: Extracapillary glomerulonephritis. Acta Pathol Microbiol Scand [A] **82**(Suppl 249):7-19, 29-54, 1974.

119 Stilmant MM, Bolton WK, Sturgill BC, Schmitt GW, Couser WG: Crescentic glomerulonephritis without immune deposits. Clinicopathologic features. Kidney Int **15**:184-195, 1979.

120 Walker RG, Scheinkestel C, Becker GJ, Owen JE, Dowling JP, Kincaid-Smith P: Clinical and morphological aspects of the management of crescentic anti-glomerular basement membrane antibody (anti-GBM) nephritis/Goodpasture's syndrome. Q J Med **54**:75-89, 1985.

121 Whitworth JA, Morel-Maroger L, Mignin F, Richet G: The significance of extracapillary proliferation. Nephron **16**:1-19, 1976.

122 Wilson CB, Dixon FJ: Anti-glomerular basement membrane antibody induced glomerulonephritis. Kidney Int **3**:74-89, 1973.

Mesangiocapillary glomerulonephritis

123 Cameron JS, Turner DR, Heaton J, Williams DG, Ogg CS, Chantler C, Haycock GB, Hicks J: Idiopathic mesangiocapillary glomerulonephritis. Comparison of types I and II in children and adults and long term prognosis. Am J Med **74**:175-192, 1983.

124 Cattran DC, Cardella CJ, Roscoe JM, Charron RC, Rance PC, Ritchie SM, Corey PN: Results of a controlled trial in membranoproliferative glomerulonephritis. Kidney Int **27**:436-441, 1985.

125 Coleman TH, Forristal J, Kosaka T, West CD: Inherited complement component deficiencies in membranoproliferative glomerulonephritis. Kidney Int **24**:681-690, 1983.

126 Donadio JV, Anderson CFJ, Mitchell JC, Holley KE, Ilstrup DM, Fuster V, Chesebro JH: Membranoproliferative glomerulonephritis. A prospective clinical trial of platelet-inhibitor therapy. N Engl J Med **310**:1421-1426, 1984.

127 Donadio JV, Holley KE: Membranoproliferative glomerulonephritis. Semin Nephrol **2**:214-227, 1982.

128 Habib R, Gubler MC, Loirat C, Ben Maiz H, Levy M: Dense deposit disease. A variant of membranoproliferative GN. Kidney Int **7**:204-215, 1975.

129 Habib R, Kleinknecht C, Gubler MC, Levy M: Idiopathic membranoproliferative GN in children. Report of 105 cases. Clin Nephrol **1**:194-214, 1973.

130 Habib R, Levy M, Gubler MC, Broyer M, Habib M: Lipodystrophie partielle, hypocomplementémie et glomérulonéphrite. Arch Fr Pediatr **34**(Suppl):197-212, 1977.

131 Kin Y, Michael AF: Idiopathic membranoproliferative GN. Annu Rev Med **31**:273-288, 1980.

132 Levy M, Gubler MC, Habib R: New concepts on membranoproliferative GN. In Kincaid Smith P, d'Apice AJP, Atkins RC (eds): Progress in glomerulonephritis, New York, 1979, John Wiley & Sons, pp. 280-316.

133 McEnery P, McAdams AJ, West CD: The effect of prednisone in a high-dose, alternative day regimen on the natural history of idiopathic membranoproliferative glomerulonephritis. Medicine [Baltimore] **64**:401-424, 1986.

134 Zimmerman SW, Moorthy AV, Dreher WH, Friedman A, Varanasi U: Prospective trial of warfarin and dipyridamole in patients with membranoproliferative glomerulonephritis. Am J Med **75**:920-927, 1983.

Diffuse mesangial proliferative glomerulonephritis

135 Berger J, Hinglais N: Les depots intercapillaires d'IgA-IgG. J Urol Nephrol **74**:694-695, 1968.

136 Counahan R, Winterborn MH, White RHR, Heaton JM, Meadow SR, Bluett HH, Swethshin H, Cameron JS, Cantler C: Prognosis of Henoch-Schönlein nephritis in children. Br Med J **2**:11-14, 1977.

137 D'Amico G, Imbasciati E, Barbiano Di Belgioioso G, Bertoli S, Fogazzi G, Ferrario F, Fellin G, Ragni A, Colosanti G, Minetti L, Ponticelli C: Idiopathic IgA mesangial nephropathy. Clinical and histological study of 374 patients. Medicine [Baltimore] **64**:49-60, 1985.

138 Hendler ED, Kashgarian M, Hauslett JP: Clinicopathologic correlations of primary hematuria. Lancet **1**:458-463, 1972.

139 Heptinstall RH, Joekes AM: Focal glomerulonephritis. A study based on renal biopsies. Q J Med **28**:329-346, 1959.

140 Kitajimi T, Murakami M, Sakai O: Clinicopathological features in the Japanese patients with IgA nephropathy. Jpn J Med **22**:219-222, 1983.

141 Levy M, Broyer M, Arsan A, Levy-Bentolila D, Habib R: Anaphylactoid purpura nephritis in childhood. Natural history and immunopathology. Adv Nephrol **6**:183-228, 1976.

142 Levy M, Gonzales-Burchard G, Broyer M, Dommergues JP, Foulard M, Sorez JP, Habib R: Berger's disease in children. Natural history and outcome. Medicine [Baltimore] **64**:157-180, 1985.

143 Nicholls KM, Fairley KF, Dowling JP, Kincaid-Smith P: The clinical course of mesangial IgA nephropathy. Q J Med **53**:227-250, 1984.

144 Pardo V, Berian MG, Levi DF, Strauss L: Benign primary hematuria. Clinicopathologic study of 65 patients. Am J Med **67**:817-822, 1979.

145 Report of the Southwest Pediatric Nephrology Study Group: A multicenter study of IgA nephropathy in children. Kidney Int **2**:643-652, 1982.

146 West CD: Asymptomatic hematuria and proteinuria in children. Causes and appropriate diagnostic studies. J Pediatr **89**:173-182, 1976.

Lupus nephritis

147 Appel GB, Silva FG, Pirani CL, Metzler JI, Estes D: Renal involvement in systemic lupus erythematosus. Medicine [Baltimore] **57**:371-410, 1978.

148 Austin HA, Muenz LR, Joyce KM, Antonovych TT, Balow JE: Diffuse proliferative lupus nephritis. Identification of specific pathologic features affecting renal outcome. Kidney Int **25**:689-695, 1984.

149 Baldwin DS, Lowenstein J, Rothfield NF, Gallo G, McCluskey RT: The clinical causes of the proliferative and membranous forms of lupus nephritis. Ann Intern Med **73**:929-942, 1970.

150 Banfi G, Mazzucco G, Barbranodi B, Belgiosa G, Bestetti Bosisio M, Stratta P, Confalonieri R, Ferrario F, Imbasciati E, Monga G: Morphological parameters in lupus nephritis. Their relevance for classification and relationship with clinical and histological findings and outcome. Q J Med **55**:153-168, 1985.

151 Churg J, Sobin DH: Renal disease. Classification and atlas of glomerular diseases. New York, 1982, Igaku-Shoin. pp. 127-149.

152 Cohen AS, Reynolds WE, Franklin ED, Kulka JP, Ropes MW, Shulman LE, Wallace SL: Preliminary criteria for the classification of systemic lupus erythematosus. Bull Rheum Dis **21**:643-648, 1971.

153 Comerford FR, Cohen AS: The nephropathy of systemic lupus erythematosus. An assessment of clinical, light and electron microscopic criteria. Medicine [Baltimore] **46**:425-473, 1967.

154 Dixon FJ: The pathogenesis of murine systemic lupus erythematosus. Am J Pathol **97**:10-16, 1979.

155 Hayslett JP, Hardin JH (eds): Advances in systemic lupus erythematosus. Am J Kidney Dis **2**(Suppl 1):1-236, 1982.

156 Kant KS, Pollak VE, Dosekun A, Glass-Grenwalt P, Weiss MA, Glueck HI: Lupus nephritis with thrombosis and abnormal fibrinolysis. Effect of ancrod. J Lab Clin Med **105**:77-88, 1985.

157 Kant KS, Pollak VE, Weiss MA, Glueck HI, Miller MA, Hess EV: Glomerular thrombosis in systemic lupus erythematosus. Prevalence and significance. Medicine [Baltimore] **60**:71-86, 1981.

158 Kashgarian M: New approaches to clinical pathological correlation in lupus nephritis. Am J Kidney Dis **2**(Suppl 1):68-73, 1982.

159 Kashgarian M, Hayslett JP: Renal involvement in systemic lupus erythematosus. In Tisher CC, Brenner BM (eds). Renal pathology. Philadelphia, 1988, J.B. Lippincott Co.

160 Kunkel AG: The immunopathology of SLE. Hosp Pract **15**:47-56, 1980.

161 McCluskey RT: Lupus nephritis. In Summers SC(ed): Kidney Pathology Decennial, 1966-1975. New York, 1985, Appleton-Century Crofts, pp. 456-459.

162 Pollak VE, Pirani CL: Renal histologic findings in SLE. Mayo Clin Proc **44**:630-644, 1969.

163 Schwartz MM, Fennel JS, Lewis EJ: Pathology of the renal tubule in systemic lupus erythematosus. Hum Pathol **13**:534-547, 1982.

164 Tan EM, Cohen AS, Fries JF, Masi AT, McShane DJ, Rothfield NF, Schaller JG, Talal N, Winchester RJ: The 1982 revised criteria for the classification of systemic lupus erythematosus. Arthritis Rheum **25**:1271-1277, 1982.

165 Wallace JD, Podell T, Weiner J, Klinenberg JR, Forouzesh S, Dubois EL: Systemic lupus erythematosus—survival patterns. Experience with 609 patients. JAMA **245**:934-938, 1981.

GLOMERULONEPHRITIS ASSOCIATED WITH SYSTEMIC VASCULITIS
Hypersensitivity angiitis and periarteritis nodosa

166 Alarcon-Segovia D: The necrotizing vasculitides. A new pathogenic classification. Med Clin North Am **61**:240-260, 1977.

167 Fauci AS, Haynes BF, Katz P: The spectrum of vasculitis. NIH conference. Ann Intern Med **89**:660-676, 1978.

168 McCluskey RT, Feinberg R: Vasculitis in primary vasculitides, granulomatoses and connective tissue disease. Hum Pathol **14**:305-315, 1983.

169 Pirani CL, Manaligod JR: The kidneys in collagen diseases. In Mostofi FK, Smith DE (eds): The kidney. Baltimore, 1966, Williams & Wilkins Co.

170 Zeek PM: Periarteritis nodosa. A clinical review. Am J Clin Pathol **22**:777-790, 1952.

Wegener's granulomatosis

171 Appel GB, Gee B, Kashgarian M, Hayslett JP: Wegener's granulomatosis. Clinical-pathological correlations and long term course. Am J Kidney Dis **1**:27-38, 1981.

172 Balow JE, Antonovych T, Fauci AS, Wilson CB: The nephritis of Wegener's granulomatosis (abstract). Kidney Int **14**:706, 1978.

173 Horn RG, Fauci AS, Rosenthal AS, Wolff SM: Renal biopsy pathology in Wegener's granulomatosis. Am J Pathol **74**:423-440, 1974.

174 McCluskey RT, Feinberg R: Vasculitis in primary vasculitides, granulomatoses and connective tissue disease. Hum Pathol **14**:305-315, 1983.

Henoch-Schönlein purpura

175 Counahan R, Winterborn MH, White RHR, Heaton JM, Meadow SR, Bluett HH, Swetshin H, Cameron JS, Chantler C: Prognosis of Henoch-Schönlein nephritis in children. Br Med J **2**:11-14, 1977.

176 Levy M, Broyer M, Arsan A, Levy-Bentolila D, Habib R: Anaphylactoid purpura nephritis in childhood. Natural history and immunopathology. Adv Nephrol **6**:183-228, 1976.

177 Levy M, Gonzales-Burchard G, Broyer M, Dommergues JP, Foulard M, Sorez JP, Habib R: Berger's disease in children. Natural history and outcome. Medicine [Baltimore] **64**:157-180, 1985.

178 Niaudet P, Levy M, Broyer M, Habib R: Clinicopathologic correlations in severe forms of Henoch-Schönlein purpura nephritis based on repeat biopsies. Contrib Nephrol **40**:255-263, 1984.

179 Mihatsch MJ, Imbasciati E, Fogazzi G, Giani M, Ghio L, Gaboardi F: Ultrastructural lesions of Henoch-Schönlein syndrome and of IgA nephropathy. Similarities and differences. Contrib Nephrol **40**:255-263, 1984.

180 Report of the Southwest Pediatric Nephrology Study Group: A multicenter study of IgA nephropathy in children. Kidney Int **2**:643-652, 1982.

Glomerulonephritis of cryoglobulinemia

181 Brouet JC, Clauvel JP, Danon F, Klein M, Seligmann M: Biologic and clinical significance of cryoglobulins. A report of 86 cases. Am J Med **57**:775-788, 1974.

182 Morel-Maroger L, Verroust P: Glomerular lesions in dysproteinemias. Kidney Int **5**:249-252, 1974.

183 Verroust P, Mery JP, Morel-Maroger L, Clauvel JP, Richet G: Glomerular lesions in monoclonal gammopathies and mixed essential cryoglobulinemias IgG-IgM. In Hamburger J, Crosnier J, Maxwell MH (eds): Nephrology, vol. 1. Chicago, 1971, Year Book Medical Publishers, Inc., pp. 161-194.

GLOMERULAR DISEASE ASSOCIATED WITH DISSEMINATED INTRAVASCULAR COAGULATION
Hemolytic uremic syndrome

184 Drummond K: Hemolytic-uremic syndrome. Then and now. N Engl J Med **312**:116-118, 1985.

185 Kaplan BS, Drummond KL: The hemolytic-uremic syndrome is a syndrome (editorial). N Engl J Med **298**:964-966, 1978.

186 Linton AL, Gavras H, Gleadle RI, Hutchison HE, Lawson DH, Lever AF, Macadam RF, McNicol GP, Robertson JIS: Microangiopathic haemolytic anaemia and the pathogenesis of malignant hypertension. Lancet **1**:1277-1282, 1969.

187 Morel-Maroger L, Kaufer A, Solez K, Sraer JD, Richet G: Prognostic importance of vascular lesions in acute renal failure with microangiopathic hemolytic anemia. Kidney Int **15**:548-558, 1979.

188 Pirani CL: Coagulation and renal disease. In Bertani R, Remuzzi G (eds): Glomerular injury 300 years after Morgagni, Milan, 1983, Wichtig Editore, pp. 119-138.

189 Umlas J: Glomeruloid structures in thrombohemolytic thrombocytopenic purpura, glomerulonephritis and disseminated intravascular coagulation. Hum Pathol **3**:437-441, 1972.

Thrombotic thrombocytopenic purpura

190 Feldman JD, Mardiney MR, Unanue ER, Cutting H: The vascular pathology of thrombotic thrombocytopenic purpura. An immunohistochemical and ultrastructural study. Lab Invest **15**:927-946, 1966.

191 Kincaid-Smith P: Participation of intravascular coagulation in the pathogenesis of glomerular and vascular lesions. Kidney Int **7**:242-253, 1975.

Toxemia of pregnancy

192 Foidart JM, Nochy D, Nusgens B, Goidart JB, Nahieu PR, Lapiere CM, Lambotte R, Bareity J: Accumulation of several basement membrane proteins in glomeruli of patients with pre-eclampsia and other hypertensive syndromes of pregnancy. Lab Invest **49**:250-259, 1983.

193 Mason R, Sharp D, Chuang HYK, Mohammad SF: The endothelium. Roles in thrombosis and hemostasis. Arch Pathol Lab Med **101**:61-64, 1977.

194 Pirani CL, Pollak VE: Renal involvement in toxemia of pregnancy. In Becker EL (ed): Structural basis of renal disease, New York, 1968, Hoeber Medical Division, Harper & Row, pp. 401, 427.

RENAL TRANSPLANT REJECTION
Hyperacute rejection

195 Gattone VH II, Filo RS, Evan AP, Leapman SB, Smith EJ, Luft FC: Time course of glomerular endothelial injury related to pulsatile perfusion preservation. Transplantation **39**:396-399, 1985.

196 Spector D, Limas C, Frost JL, Zachary JB, Sterioff S, Williams M, Rolley RT, Sadler JH: Perfusion nephropathy in human transplants. N Engl J Med **295**:1217-1221, 1976.

197 Williams GM, Hume DM, Hudson RP, Morris PJ, Kado K, Milgrom F: Hyperacute renal homograft rejection in man. N Engl J Med **279**:611-618, 1968.

Acute rejection

198 Axelsen RA, Seymour AE, Mathew TH, Canny A, Pascoe V: Glomerular transplant rejection. A distinctive pattern of early graft damage. Clin Nephrol **23**:1-11, 1985.

199 Bishop GA, Hall BM, Duggin GG, Horvath JS, Sheil AG, Tiller DJ: Immunopathology of renal allograft rejection analyzed with monoclonal antibodies to mononuclear cell markers. Kidney Int **29**:708-717, 1986.

200 Busch GJ, Galvanek EG, Reynolds ES Jr: Human renal allografts. Analysis of lesions in long-term survivors. Hum Pathol **2**:253-298, 1971.

201 Finkelstein FD, Siegel NJ, Bastl C, Forrest JN, Kashgarian M: The role of the renal biopsy in the diagnosis and management of acute rejection reaction. Kidney Int **10**:171-178, 1976.

202 Hall BM, Bishop GA, Farnsworth A, Dussin GG, Horvath JS, Sheil AG, Tiller DJ: Identification of the cellular subpopulations infiltrating rejecting cadaver renal allografts. Preponderance of the T4 subset of T cells. Transplantation **37**:564-570, 1984.

203 Kolbeck PC, Tatum AH, Sanfilippo F: Relationships among the histologic pattern, intensity, and phenotypes of T cells infiltrating renal allografts. Transplantation **38**:709-713, 1984.

204 Maryniak BK, First MR, Weiss MA: Transplant glomerulopathy. Evolution of morphologically distinct changes. Kidney Int **27**:799-806, 1985.

205 Mason DW, Dallman MJ, Arthur RP, Morris PJ: Mechanisms of allograft rejection. The roles of cytotoxic T cells and delayed-type hypersensitivity. Immunol Rev **77**:167-184, 1984.

206 Olsen S: Pathology of the renal allograft rejection. In Churg J, Spargo BH, Mostofi F (eds): Kidney disease. Present status, Baltimore, 1979, Williams & Wilkins Co., pp. 327-355.

207 Stelzer GT, McLeish KR, Lorden RE, Watson SL: Alterations in T lymphocyte subpopulations associated with renal allograft rejection. Transplantation **37**:261-264, 1984.

208 Vanselista A, Frasca G, Nanni-Costs A, Bonomini V: Detection of lymphocyte subsets in renal graft biopsy by monoclonal antibodies. Proc Eur Dial Transplant Assoc **20**:315-319, 1983.

209 Verani RR, Bergman D, Kerman RH: Glomerulopathy in acute and chronic rejection. Relationship of ultrastructure to graft survival. Am J Nephrol **3**:253-263, 1983.

210 Waush J, Bishop GA, Hall BM, Phillips J, Fraser C, Brown SC, Dussin GG, Horvath JS, Sheil AG, Tiller DJ: T cell subsets in fine needle aspiration biopsies from renal transplant recipients. Transplant Proc **17**:1763-1767, 1985.

211 Zollinger HU, Hatsch MJ: Renal pathology in biopsy. Berlin, Heidelberg, New York, 1978, Springer-Verlag.

Cyclosporin toxicity

212 Bergstrand A, Bohman SO, Farnsworth A, Gokel JM, Krause PH, Lang W, Hihatsch MJ, Oppedal B, Sell S, Sibley RK: Renal histopathology in kidney transplant recipients immunosuppressed with cyclosporin A. Results of an international workshop. Clin Nephrol **24**:107-119, 1985.

213 Calne RY, Rolles K, White DJG, Thiru S, Evans DB, Henderson R, Hamilton DL, Boone N, McMaster P, Gibby O, Williams R: Cyclosporin A in clinical organ-grafting. Transplant Proc **13**:349-358, 1981.

214 Canadian Multicentre Transplant Study Group: A randomized clinical trial of cyclosporin in cadaveric renal transplantation. N Engl J Med **309**:809-815, 1983.

215 Castro LA, Hillebrand G, Land W: Cyclosporine in patients with oligo-anuria after cadaveric kidney transplantation. In Kahan BD (ed): Cyclosporine. Biological activity and clinical applications. A transplantation proceedings reprint of suppl. 1, vol. 15, 1983. New York, 1984, Grune & Stratton, p. 483.

216 Deviveni R, McKenzie N, Duplan J, et al.: Renal effects of cyclosporine. Clinical and experimental observations. In Kahan BD (ed): Cyclosporine. Biological activity and clinical applications. A transplantation proceedings reprint of suppl. 1, vol. 15, 1983. New York, 1984, Grune & Stratton, p. 479.

217 European Multicentre Trial Group: Cyclosporin in cadaveric renal transplantation. One-year follow-up of a multicentre trial. Lancet **2**:986-989, 1983.

218 Klintmalm G, Bohman SO, Sundelin B, Wilczek H: Interstitial fibrosis in renal allografts after 12 to 46 months of cyclosporin treatment. Beneficial effects of lower doses early after transplantation. Lancet **2**:950-954, 1984.

219 Kolbeck PC, Scheinman JI, Sanfilippo F: Acute cellular rejection and cyclosporine nephrotoxicity monitored by biopsy in a renal allograft recipient. Arch Pathol Lab Med **110**:389-393, 1986.

220 Mihatsch MJ, Thiel G, Spichtin HP, Oberholzer M, Brunner FP, Harder F, Olivieri V, Bremer R, Ryffel B, Stöcklin E, Torhost J, Gudat F, Zollinger HU, Lörtscher R: Morphological findings in kidney transplants after treatment with cyclosporine. In Kahan BD (ed): Cyclosporine. Biological activity and clinical applications. A transplantation proceedings reprint of suppl. 1, vol. 15, 1983. New York, 1984, Grune & Stratton, p. 605.

221 Neild GH, Taube DH, Hartley RB, Bignardi L, Cameron JS, Williams DG, Ogg CS, Rudge CJ: Morphological differentiation between rejection and cyclosporin nephrotoxicity in renal allografts. J Clin Pathol **39**:152-159, 1986.

222 Sibley RK, Ferguson RM, Suthrland DER, Simmons RL, Najarian JS: Morphology of cyclosporine nephrotoxicity and of acute rejection in cyclosporine-prednisone immunosuppressed renal allograft recipients. In Kahan BD (ed): Cyclosporine. Biological activity and clinical applications. A transplantation proceedings reprint of suppl. 1, vol. 15, 1983. New York, 1984, Grune & Stratton, p. 620.

223 Thiru S, Maher ER, Hamilton DV, Evans DB, Calne RY: Tubular changes in renal transplant recipients on cyclosporine. In Kahan BD (ed): Cyclosporine. Biological activity and clinical applications. A transplantation proceedings reprint of suppl. 1, vol. 15, 1983. New York, 1984, Grune & Stratton, p. 630.

TUBULOINTERSTITIAL NEPHRITIS
Acute and chronic pyelonephritis

224 Cotran RS, Thiru S, Verani R, Wallace AC, Zollinger HU, Ryffel B, Thiel G, Wonigeit K: Tubulo-interstitial nephropathies. In Brenner BM, Rector FC (eds): The kidney. Philadelphia, 1988, W.B. Saunders Co.

225 Goodman M, Curry T, Russel T: Xanthogranulomatous pyelonephritis (XGP). A local disease with systemic manifestations. Report of 23 patients and review of the literature. Medicine [Baltimore] 58:171-181, 1979.

226 Hodson CJ, Cotran RS: Vesicoureteral reflux, reflux nephropathy and chronic pyelonephritis. In Brenner B, Stein J (series eds), Cotran RS (guest ed): Tubulo-interstitial nephropathies. Contemporary issues in nephrology, vol. 10. New York, 1983, Churchill Livingstone, pp. 83-102.

227 Lambrid PA, Yardley JH: Urinary tract malakoplakia. Johns Hopkins Med J 126:1-14, 1970.

228 Ransley PG, Risdon RA: The renal papilla, intrarenal reflux and chronic pyelonephritis. In Hodson CJ, Kincaid-Smith P (eds): Reflux nephropathy. New York, 1979, Masson Publishing Co., pp. 126-133.

229 Stamey TA: Pathogenesis and treatment of urinary tract infection. Baltimore, 1980, Williams & Wilkins Co.

230 Svanborg-Eden C, Gotschlich EC, Korhonen TK, Leffler H, Schoolnik G: Aspects of structure and funtion of p. 1. on *Escherichia, coli*. Prog Allergy 33:189-195, 1983.

231 Tolkoff-Rubin NE, Rubin RH: Urinary tract infection. In Brenner B, Stein J (series eds), Cotran RS (guest ed): Tubulo-interstitial nephropathies. Contemporary issues in nephrology, vol. 10. New York, 1983, Churchill Livingstone, pp. 49-82.

Acute allergic tubulointerstitial nephritis

232 Appel GB, Kunis CL: Acute tubulo-interstitial nephritis. In Brenner B, Stein J (series eds), Cotran RS (guest ed): Tubulo-interstitial nephropathies. Contemporary issues in nephrology, vol. 10. New York, 1983, Churchill Livingstone Inc.

233 Baldwin DS, Levine BB, McCluskey RT, Gallo GR: Renal failure and interstitial nephritis due to penicillin and methicillin. N Engl J Med 279:1245-1252, 1968.

234 Corwin HL, Korbet SM, Schwartz MM: Clinical correlates of eosinophiluria. Arch Intern Med 145:1097-1099, 1985.

235 Dobrin RS, Vernier RL, Fish AJ: Acute eosinophilic interstitial nephritis and renal failure with bone marrow–lymph node granulomas and anterior uveitis. A new syndrome. Am J Med 59:325-332, 1975.

236 Feinfeld DA, Olesnicky L, Pirani CL, Appel GB: Nephrotic syndrome associated with use of the nonsteroidal anti-inflammatory drug. Nephron 37:174-179, 1984.

237 Heptinstall RA: Interstitial nephritis. A brief review. Am J Pathol 83:214-236, 1976.

238 Laberke HG, Bohle A: Acute interstitial nephritis. Correlations between clinical and morphological findings. Clin Nephrol 14:263-273, 1980.

239 Magil AB: Drug-induced acute interstitial nephritis with granulomas. Hum Pathol 14:36-41, 1983.

Renal papillary necrosis

240 Garrett RA, Norris MS, Vellios F: Renal papillary necrosis. A clinicopathologic study. J Urol 72:609-617, 1954.

Pyelitis and ureteritis cystica

241 Hinman F, Cordonnier J: Cystitis follicularis. J Urol 34:302-308, 1935.

Pelvic lipomatosis

242 Hamm FC, DeVeer JA: Fatty replacement following renal atrophy or destruction. J Urol 41:850-866, 1939.

243 Young HH: Lipomatosis or destructive fat replacement of renal cortex. Report of 11 cases. J Urol 29:631-644, 1933.

Nephrolithiasis and nephrocalcinosis

244 Boyce WH: Organic matrix of human urinary concretions. Am J Med 45:673-683, 1968.

245 Chambers A, Hodgkinson A, Hornung G: Electron probe analysis of small urinary tract calculi. Invest Urol 9:376-384, 1972.

246 Crawhall JC, Purkiss P, Watts RWE, Young EP: The excretion of amino acids by cystinuric patients and their relatives. Ann Hum Genet 33:149-169, 1969.

247 Gelbart GR, Brewer LL, Fajardo LF: Oxalosis and chronic renal failure after intestinal bypass. Arch Intern Med 137:239-243, 1977.

248 Gutman AB, Yu T-F: Uric acid nephrolithiasis. Am J Med 45:756-779, 1968.

249 Heptinstall RH: Pathology of the kidney, ed. 2. Boston, 1974, Little, Brown & Co.

250 Randall A: Origin and growth of renal calculi. Ann Surg 105:1009-1027, 1937.

251 Randall A: The etiology of primary renal calculus. Int Abstr Surg 71:2209-2240, 1940.

252 Talbott JH: Gout. Med Clin North Am 54:431-441, 1970.

RENAL VASCULAR DISEASE
Renal arteriolar disease

253 Bohle A, Ratschek M: The compensated and decompensated form of benign nephrosclerosis. Pathol Res Pract 174:357-367, 1982.

254 Fishberg AM: Anatomic findings in essential hypertension. Arch Intern Med 35:650-668, 1925.

255 Kashgarian M: Pathology of the kidney in hypertension. In Kaplan NM, Brenner BM, Laragh JH (eds): The kidney in hypertension. New York, 1987, Raven Press.

256 Kincaid-Smith P: Malignant hypertension. Mechanisms and management. Pharmacol Ther 9:245-269, 1980.

257 McGee WF, Ashworth CT: Fine structure of chronic hypertensive arteriopathy in the human kidney. Am J Pathol 43:273-299, 1963.

258 Valenzuela R, Gogate PA, Deodar SD, Gifford RW: Hyaline arteriolonephrosclerosis. Immunofluorescent findings in vascular lesions. Lab Invest 43:530-534, 1980.

Renal arterial disease

259 Breslin DJ, Swinton NW, Libertino JA, Zinman L: Renovascular hypertension. Baltimore, 1982, Williams & Wilkins Co.

260 Harrison EG, McCormack LV: Pathologic classification of renal arterial disease in renovascular hypertension. Mayo Clin Proc 46:161-166, 1971.

261 McCormack LJ, Poutasse EF, Meaney TF, Noto TJ, Duston HP: Arteriographic correlations of renal artery disease. Am Heart J 72:188-198, 1966.

262 Stanley JC, Ernst CB, Fry WJ: Renovascular hypertension. Philadelphia, 1984, W.B. Saunders.

CYSTIC DISEASES OF THE KIDNEY
Renal dysplasia

263 Bernstein J: Developmental abnormalities of the renal parenchyma. Renal hypoplasia and dysplasia. Pathol Annu 3:213-247, 1968.

264 Okayasu I, Kaijita A: Histopathological study of congenital cystic kidneys with special reference to the multicystic, dysplastic type. Acta Pathol Jpn 28:427-434, 1978.

265 Risdon RA: Renal dysplasia. Part I. A clinical pathologic study of 76 cases. Part II. A necroscopy study of 41 cases. J Clin Pathol 24:57-71, 1971.

Adult-type polycystic disease

266 Bernstein J: A classification of renal cysts. In Gardner KD Jr (ed): Cystic disease of the kidney. New York, 1976, John Wiley & Sons, Inc., pp. 7-30.

267 Kissane JM: Morphology of renal cystic disease. In Gardner KD Jr (ed): Cystic diseases of the kidney. New York, 1976, John Wiley & Sons, Inc. pp. 31-64.

268 Poutasse EF, Gardner WJ, McCormack LJ: Polycystic kidney disease and intracranial aneurysm. JAMA 154:741-744, 1954.

269 Reeders ST, Breuning MH, Davies KE, Nichols RD, Jarman AP, Higgs DR, Pearson PL, Weatherall DJ: A highly polymorphic DNA marker linked to adult polycystic kidney disease on chromosome 16. Nature 317:542-544, 1985.

Infantile polycystic renal disease

270 Lieberman E, Salinas-Madrigal L, Gwinn JL, Brennan LP, Fine RN, Landing BH: Infantile polycystic disease of the kidneys and liver. Clinical, pathological and radiological correlations and comparison with congenital hepatic fibrosis. Medicine [Baltimore] 50:277-318, 1971.

Medullary sponge kidney

271 Kuiper JJ: Medullary sponge kidney. In Gardner KD Jr (ed): Cystic disease of the kidney. New York, 1976, John Wiley & Sons, Inc., pp. 151-172.

Medullary cystic disease

272 Gardner KD Jr: Evolution of clinical signs in adult-onset cystic disease of the renal medulla. Ann Intern Med 74:47-54, 1971.

Acquired cysts in renal dialysis patients

273 Dunnill MS, Millard PR, Oliver D: Acquired cystic disease of the kidneys. A hazard of long term maintenance hemodialysis. J Clin Pathol 30:818-877, 1977.

274 Grantham JJ, Levine E: Acquired cystic disease. Replacing one kidney disease for another. Kidney Int 28:99-105, 1985.

Tumors and tumorlike conditions
WILMS' TUMOR
General features

275 Akhtar M, Kott E, Brooks B: Extrarenal Wilms' tumor. Report of a case and review of the literature. Cancer **40**:3087-3091, 1977.

276 Babaian RJ, Skinner DG, Waisman J: Wilms' tumor in the adult patient. Diagnosis, management, and review of the world medical literature. Cancer **45**:1713-1719, 1980.

277 Bolande RP: Neoplasia of early life and its relationships to teratogenesis. Perspect Pediatr Pathol **3**:145-183, 1976.

278 Farrow GM, Harrison EG Jr, Utz DC: Sarcomas and sarcomatoid and mixed malignant tumors of the kidney in adults. Cancer **22**:545-563, 1968.

278a Gansler T, Allen KD, Burant CF, Inabnett T, Scott A, Buse MG, Sens DA, Garvin AJ: Detection of type 1 insulinlike growth factor (IGF) receptors in Wilms' tumors. Am J Pathol **130**:431-435, 1988.

279 Ho J, Ma L, Wong KC: An extrarenal Wilms' tumor arising from an undescended testis. Pathology **13**:619-624, 1981.

280 Hrabovsky EE, Othersen HB Jr, deLorimier A, Kelalis P, Beckwith JB, Takashima J: Wilms' tumor in the neonate. A report from the National Wilms' Tumor Study. J Pediatr Surg **21**:385-387, 1986.

281 Juberg RC, St. Martin EC, Hundley JR: Familial occurrence of Wilms' tumor. Nephroblastoma in one of monozygous twins and in other sibling. Am J Hum Genet **27**:155-164, 1975.

282 Kondo K, Chilcote RR, Maurer HS, Rowley JD: Chromosome abnormalities in tumor cells from patients with sporadic Wilms' tumor. Cancer Res **44**:5376-5381, 1984.

283 Luchtrath H, deLeon F, Giesen H, Gök Y: Inguinal nephroblastoma, Virchows Arch [Pathol Anat] **405**:113-118, 1984.

284 Manivel JC, Sibley RK, Dehner LP: Complete and incomplete Drash syndrome. A clinicopathologic study of five cases of a dysontogenetic-neoplastic complex, Hum Pathol **18**:80-89, 1987.

285 Maurer HS, Pendergrass TW, Borges W, Honig GR: The role of genetic factors in the etiology of Wilms' tumor. Two pairs of monozygous twins with congenital abnormalities (aniridia; hemihypertrophy) and discordance for Wilms' tumor. Cancer **43**:205-208, 1979.

286 Merten DF, Yang SS, Bernstein J: Wilms' tumor in adolescence. Cancer **37**:1532-1538, 1976.

287 Miller RW, Fraumeni JF, Manning MD: Association of Wilms' tumor with aniridia, hemihypertrophy and other congenital malformations. N Engl J Med **270**:922-927, 1964.

288 Nakamura Y, Nakashima T, Nakashima H, Hashimoto T: Bilateral cystic nephroblastomas and botryoid sarcoma involving vagina and urinary bladder in a child with microcephaly, arhinencephaly, and bilateral cataracts. Cancer **48**:1012-1015, 1981.

289 Ragab AH, Vietti TJ, Crist W, Perez C, McAllister W: Bilateral Wilms' tumor. A review. Cancer **30**:983-988, 1972.

290 Rajfer J: Association between Wilms' tumor and gonadal dysgenesis. J Urol **125**:388-390, 1981.

291 Sheth KJ, Tang TT, Blaedel ME, Good TA: Polydipsia, polyuria, and hypertension associated with renin-secreting Wilms' tumor. J Pediatr **92**:921-924, 1978.

292 Slater RM, deKraker J: Chromosome number 11 and Wilms' tumor. Cancer Genet Cytogenet **5**:237-246, 1982.

293 Sotelo-Avila C, Gooch WM III: Neoplasms associated with the Beckwith-Wiedemann syndrome. Perspect Pediatr Pathol **3**:255-272, 1976.

294 Stay EJ, Vawter G: The relationship between nephroblastoma and neurofibromatosis (von Recklinghausen's disease). Cancer **39**:2550-2555, 1977.

295 Thorner P, McGraw M, Weitzman S, Balfe JW, Klein M, Baumal R: Wilms' tumor and glomerular disease. Occurrence with features of membranoproliferative glomerulonephritis and secondary focal, segmented glomerulosclerosis. Arch Pathol Lab Med **108**:141-146, 1984.

296 Ward SP, Dehner LP: Sacrococcygeal teratoma with nephroblastoma (Wilms' tumor). A variant of extragonadal teratoma in childhood. A histologic and ultrastructural study. Cancer **33**:1355-1363, 1974.

Morphologic features

297 Balsaver AM, Gibley CW Jr, Tessmer CF: Ultrastructural studies in Wilms' tumor. Cancer **22**:417-427, 1968.

298 Beckwith JB: Wilms' tumor and other renal tumors of childhood. A selective review from the National Wilms' Tumor Study Pathology Center. Hum Pathol **14**:481-492, 1983.

299 Chatten J: Epithelial differentiation in Wilms' tumor. A clinicopathologic appraisal. Perspect Pediatr Pathol **3**:225-254, 1976.

300 Delemarre JFM, Sandstedt B, Tournade MF: Nephroblastoma with fibroadenomatous-like structures. Histopathology **8**:55-62, 1984.

301 Garvin AJ, Surrette F, Hintz DS, Rudisill MT, Sens MA, Sens DA: The in vitro growth and characterization of the skeletal muscle component of Wilms' tumor. Am J Pathol **121**:298-310, 1985.

302 Gonzalez-Crussi F: The pathology of Wilms' tumor. Wilms' tumor (nephroblastoma) and related renal neoplasms of childhood. 1984, Boca Raton, FL, CRC Press, pp. 178-206.

303 Gonzalez-Crussi F, Hsueh W, Ugarte N: Rhabdomyogenesis in renal neoplasia of childhood. Am J Surg Pathol **5**:525-532, 1981.

304 Grimes MM, Wolff M, Wolff JA, Jaretzki A III, Blanc WA: Ganglion cells in metastatic Wilms' tumor. Review of a histogenetic controversy. Am J Surg Pathol **6**:565-571, 1982.

305 Hennigar RA, Spicer SA, Sens DA, Othersen HB Jr, Garvin AJ: Histochemical evidence for tubule segmentation in a case of Wilms' tumor. Am J Clin Pathol **85**:724-731, 1986.

306 Hou LT, Azzopardi JG: Muco-epidermoid metaplasia and argentaffin cells in nephroblastoma. J Pathol Bacteriol **93**:477-481, 1967.

307 Hughson MD, Hennigar GR, Othersen HB Jr: Cyto-differentiated renal tumours occurring with Wilms' tumors of the opposite kidneys. Report of two cases. Am J Clin Pathol **66**:376-389, 1976.

308 Kodet R, Marsden HB: Papillary Wilms' tumour with carcinoma-like foci and renal cell carcinoma in childhood. Histopathology **9**:1091-1102, 1985.

309 Lindop GBM, Fleming S, Gibson AAM: Immunocytochemical localisation of renin in nephroblastoma. J Clin Pathol **37**:738-742, 1984.

310 Magee F, Mah RG, Taylor GP, Dimmick JE: Neural differentiation in Wilms' tumor. Hum Pathol **18**:33-37, 1987.

311 Mahoney JP, Saffos RO: Fetal rhabdomyomatous nephroblastoma with a renal pelvic mass simulating sarcoma botryoides. Am J Surg Pathol **5**:297-306, 1981.

312 Marsden HB: The pathology and natural history of childhood tumours. Recent Results Cancer Res **88**:11-25, 1983.

313 Masson P: The role of the neural crest in the embryonal adenosarcomas of the kidney. Am J Cancer **33**:1-32, 1938.

314 Mierau GW, Beckwith JB, Weeks DA: Ultrastructure and histogenesis of the renal tumors of childhood. An overview. Ultrastruct Pathol **11**:313-333, 1987.

315 Sariola H, Ekblom P, Rapola J, Vaheri A, Timpl R: Extracellular matrix and epithelial differentiation of Wilms' tumor. Am J Pathol **118**:96-107, 1985.

316 Variend S, Spicer RD, Mackinnon AE: Teratoid Wilms' tumor. Cancer **53**:1936-1942, 1984.

317 Weinberg AG, Currarino G, Hurt GE Jr: Botryoid Wilms' tumor of the renal pelvis. Arch Pathol Lab Med **108**:147-148, 1984.

318 Wigger HJ: Fetal rhabdomyomatous nephroblastoma. A variant of Wilms' tumor. Hum Pathol **7**:613-623, 1976.

319 Yeger H, Baumal R, Harason P, Phillips MJ: Lectin histochemistry of Wilms' tumor. Comparison with normal adult and fetal kidney. Am J Clin Pathol **88**:278-285, 1987.

Therapy

320 Becht EW, Rumpelt HJ, Frohneberg D, Gutjahr P, Thoenes W: Angioma-like pseudometamorphosis in Wilms' tumors subjected to preoperative radio- and chemotherapy. Pathol Res Pract **177**:22-31, 1983.

321 D'Angio GJ: Oncology seen through the prism of Wilms' tumor. Med Pediatr Oncol **13**:53-58, 1985.

322 D'Angio GJ, Evans A, Breslow N, Beckwith B, Bishop H, Farewell V, Goodwin W, Leape L, Palmer N, Sinks L, Sutow W, Tefft M, Wolff J: The treatment of Wilms' tumor. Results of the second National Wilms' Tumor Study. Cancer **47**:2302-2311, 1981.

323 Ehrlich RM, Bloomberg SD, Gyepes MT, Levitt SB, Kogan S, Hanna M, Goodwin WE: Wilms' tumor, misdiagnosed preoperatively. A review of 19 National Wilms' Tumor Study I cases. J Urol **122**:790-792, 1979.

324 Zuppan C, Beckwith B: Pretreated anaplastic Wilms' tumor (abstract). Lab Invest **58**:108A, 1988.

Prognosis

325 Antman KH, Ruxer RL Jr, Aisner J, Vawter G: Mesothelioma following Wilms' tumor in childhood. Cancer **54**:367-369, 1984.

326 Ater JL, Gooch WM III, Bybee BL, O'Brien RT: Poor prognosis for mucin-producing Wilms' tumor. Cancer **53**:319-323, 1984.

327 Beckwith JB, Palmer NF: Histopathology and prognosis of Wilms' tumor. Results from the First National Wilms' Tumor Study. Cancer 41:1937-1948, 1978.

328 Bonadio JF, Storer B, Norkool P, Farewell VT, Beckwith JB, D'Angio GJ: Anaplastic Wilms' tumor. Clinical and pathologic studies. J Clin Oncol 3:513-520, 1985.

329 Breslow NE, Palmer NF, Hill LR, Buring J, D'Angio GJ: Wilms' tumor. Prognostic factors for patients without metastases at diagnosis. Results of the National Wilms' Tumor Study. Cancer 41:1577-1589, 1978.

330 D'Angio GJ: Oncology seen through the prism of Wilms' tumor. Med Pediatr Oncol 13:53-58, 1985.

331 Gonzalez-Crussi F, Hsueh W, Ugarte N: Rhabdomyogenesis in renal neoplasia of childhood. Am J Surg Pathol 5:525-532, 1981.

332 Editorial. Wilms' tumour. Br Med J 15:1166-1167, 1976.

333 Jenkin RDT: The treatment of Wilms' tumor. Pediatr Clin North Am 23:147-160, 1976.

334 Jereb B, Tournade MF, Lemerle J, Voute PA, Delemarte JF, Ahstrom L, Flamant R, Gerard-Marchant R, Sandstedt B: Lymph node invasion and prognosis in nephroblastoma. Cancer 45:1632-1636, 1980.

335 Khair S, Pritchett PS, Moreno H, Robinson CA: Histologic grading of Wilms' tumor as a potential prognosis factor. Results of a retrospective study of 26 patients. Cancer 41:1199-1207, 1978.

336 Lawler W, Marsden HB, Palmer MK: Wilms' tumor. Histologic variation and prognosis. Cancer 36:1122-1126, 1975.

337 Leape LL, Breslow NE, Bishop HC: The surgical treatment of Wilms' tumor. Results of the National Wilms' Tumor Study. Ann Surg 187:351-356, 1978.

338 Lemerle J, Tournade MF, Gerard-Marchant R, Flamant R, Sarrazin D, Flamant F, Lemerle M, Jundt S, Zucker JM, Schweisguth O: Wilms' tumor. Natural history and prognostic factors. A retrospective study of 248 cases treated at the Institut Gustave-Roussy 1952-1967. Cancer 37:2557-2566, 1976.

339 Schmidt D, Wiedemann B, Keil W, Sprenger E, Harms D: Flow cytometric analysis of nephroblastomas and related neoplasms. Cancer 58:2494-2500, 1986.

340 Wigger HJ: Fetal rhabdomyomatous nephroblastoma. A variant of Wilms' tumor. Hum Pathol 7:613-623, 1976.

OTHER PEDIATRIC RENAL TUMORS
Mesoblastic nephroma

341 Beckwith JB, Weeks DA: Congenital mesoblastic nephroma. When should we worry? Arch Pathol Lab Med 110:98-99, 1986.

342 Bogdan R, Taylor DEM, Mostofi FK: Leiomyomatous hamartoma of the kidney. A clinical and pathologic analysis of 20 cases from the Kidney Tumor Registry. Cancer 31:462-467, 1973.

343 Bolande R, Bernstein J, Libcke J: Tubulogenesis in mesoblastic nephroma (abstract). Lab Invest 58:2P, 1988.

344 Ganick DJ, Gilbert EF, Beckwith JB, Kiviat N: Congenital cystic mesoblastic nephroma. Hum Pathol 12:1039-1043, 1981.

345 Gonzalez-Crussi F, Sotelo-Avila C, Kidd JM: Malignant mesenchymal nephroma of infancy. Report of a case with pulmonary metastases. Am J Surg Pathol 4:185-190, 1980.

346 Gonzalez-Crussi F, Sotelo-Avila C, Kidd JM: Mesenchymal renal tumors in infancy. A reappraisal. Hum Pathol 12:78-85, 1981.

347 Howell CG, Othersen HB, Kiviat NE, Norkool P, Beckwith JB, D'Angio GJ: Therapy and outcome in 51 children with mesoblastic nephroma. A report of the National Wilms' Tumor Study. J Pediatr Surg 17:826-831, 1982.

348 Joshi VV, Kasznica J, Walters TR: Atypical mesoblastic nephroma. Pathologic characterization of a potentially aggressive variant of conventional congenital mesoblastic nephroma. Arch Pathol Lab Med 110:100-106, 1986.

349 Kumar S, Marsden HB, Carr T, Kodet R: Mesoblastic nephroma contains fibronectin but lacks laminin. J Clin Pathol 38:507-511, 1985.

350 Sandstedt B, Delemarre JFM, Krul EJ, Tournade MF: Mesoblastic nephromas. A study of 29 tumours from the SIOP nephroblastoma file. Histopathology 9:741-750, 1985.

351 Shen SC, Yunis EJ: A study of the cellularity and ultrastructure of congenital mesoblastic nephroma. Cancer 45:306-314, 1980.

352 Wigger HG: Fetal mesenchymal hamartoma of kidney. A tumor of secondary mesenchyme. Cancer 36:1002-1008, 1975.

Multicystic nephroma

353 Andrews MJ Jr, Askin FB, Fried FA, McMillan CW, Mandell J: Cystic partially differentiated nephroblastoma and polycystic Wilms' tumor. A spectrum of related clinical and pathologic entities. J Urol 129:577-580, 1983.

354 Baldauf MC, Schulz DM: Multilocular cyst of the kidney. Report of three cases with review of the literature. Am J Clin Pathol 65:93-102, 1976.

355 Gallo GE, Penchansky L: Cystic nephroma. Cancer 39:1322-1327, 1977.

356 Joshi VV, Banerjee AK, Yadav K, Pathak IC: Cystic partially differentiated nephroblastoma. A clinicopathologic entity in the spectrum of infantile renal neoplasia. Cancer 40:789-795, 1977.

357 Sherman ME, Silverman ML, Balogh K, Tan SS-G: Multilocular renal cyst. A hamartoma with potential for neoplastic transformation? Arch Pathol Lab Med 111:732-736, 1987.

358 Tang TT, Harb JM, Oechler HW, Camitta BM: Multilocular renal cyst. Electron microscopic evidence of pathogenesis. Am J Pediatr Hematol Oncol 6:27-32, 1984.

359 Taxy JB, Marshall FF: Multilocular renal cysts in adults. Possible relationship to renal adenocarcinoma. Arch Pathol Lab Med 107:633-637, 1983.

Nephroblastomatosis

360 Beckwith JB, Kiviat NB: Studies of nephroblastomatosis. Intralobar nephroblastomatosis and related Wilms' tumor. Cancer (In press.)

361 Beckwith JB, Kiviat NB, Bonadio JF: Studies of nephroblastomatosis. I. Introduction and classification. A report of the National Wilms' Tumor Study. Cancer (In press.)

362 Bove KE, McAdams AJ: The nephroblastomatosis complex and its relationship to Wilms' tumor. A clinico-pathologic treatise. Perspect Pediatr Pathol 3:185-223, 1976.

363 de Chadarevian J-P, Fletcher BD, Chatten J, Rabinovitch HH: Massive infantile nephroblastomatosis. A clinical, radiological, and pathological analysis of four cases. Cancer 39:2294-2305, 1977.

364 Heideman RL, Haase GM, Foley CL, Wilson HL, Bailey WC: Nephroblastomatosis and Wilms' tumor. Clinical experience and management of seven patients. Cancer 55:1446-1451, 1985.

365 Machin GA, McCaughey WTE: A new precursor lesion of Wilms' tumor (nephroblastoma): intralobar multifocal nephroblastomatosis. Histopathology 8:35-53, 1984.

366 Perlman M, Levin M, Wittels B: Syndrome of fetal gigantism, renal hamartomas, and nephroblastomatosis with Wilms' tumor. Cancer 35:1212-1217, 1975.

367 Stambolis C: Benign epithelial nephroblastoma. A contribution to its histogenesis. Virchows Arch [Pathol Anat] 376:267-272, 1977.

368 Vogler CA, Sotelo-Avila C, Ramón-García G, Salinas-Madrigal L: Nodular renal blastema and metanephric hamartomas in children with urinary tract malformations. A morphologic spectrum of abnormal metanephric differentiation. Semin Diagn Pathol 5:122-131, 1988.

Intrarenal neuroblastoma

369 Beckwith JB: Wilms' tumor and other renal tumors of childhood. A selective review from the National Wilms' Tumor Study Pathology Center. Hum Pathol 14:481-492, 1983.

369a Nisen PD, Rich MA, Gloster E, Valderrama E, Saric O, Shende A, Lanzkowsky P, Alt FW: N-myc oncogene expression in histopathologically unrelated bilateral pediatric renal tumors. Cancer 61:1821-1826, 1987.

Clear cell sarcoma

370 Haas JE, Bonadio JF, Beckwith JB: Clear cell sarcoma of the kidney with emphasis on ultrastructural studies. Cancer 54:2978-2987, 1984.

371 Marsden HB, Lawler W, Kumar PM: Bone metastasizing renal tumor of childhood. Morphological and clinical features and differences from Wilms' tumor. Cancer 42:1922-1928, 1978.

372 Morgan E, Kidd JM: Undifferentiated sarcoma of the kidney. A tumor of childhood with histopathologic and clinical characteristics distinct from Wilms' tumor. Cancer 42:1916-1921, 1978.

373 Pysher TJ, Beckwith JB: Clear cell sarcoma of the kidney (CCSK). Analysis of 82 cases from the second and third National Wilms' Tumor Studies (NWTS-2 and NWTS-3) (abstract). Lab Invest 58:73A, 1988.

374 Sandstedt BE, Delemarre JFM, Harms D, Tournade MF: Sarcomatous Wilms' tumour with clear cells and hyalinization. A study of 38 tumours in children from the SIOP nephroblastoma file. Histopathology 11:273-285, 1987.

375 Schmidt D, Harms D, Evers KG, Bliesener JA, Beckwith JB: Bone metastasizing renal tumor (clear cell sarcoma) of childhood with epithelioid elements. Cancer 56:609-613, 1985.

376 Sotelo-Avila C, Gonzalez-Crussi F, Sadowinski S, Gooch WM III, Pena R: Clear cell sarcoma of the kidney. A clinicopathologic study of 21 patients with long-term follow-up evaluation. Hum Pathol 16:1219-1230, 1986.

377 Takagi M, Takakuwa T, Ushigome S, Nakata K, Fujioka T, Watanabe A: Sarcomatous variants of Wilms' tumor. Immunohistochemical and ultrastructural comparison with classical Wilms' tumor. Cancer 59:963-971, 1987.

Rhabdoid tumor

378 Bonnin JM, Rubinstein LJ, Palmer NF, Beckwith JB: The association of embryonal tumors originating in the kidney and in the brain. A report of seven cases. Cancer **54**:2137-2146, 1984.

379 Frierson HF Jr, Mills SE, Innes DJ Jr: Malignant rhabdoid tumor of the pelvis. Cancer **55**:1963-1967, 1985.

380 Haas JE, Palmer NF, Weinberg AG, Beckwith JB: Ultrastructure of malignant rhabdoid tumor of the kidney. A distinctive renal tumor of children. Hum Pathol **12**:646-657, 1981.

381 Howat AJ, Gonzales MF, Waters KD, Campbell PE: Primitive neuroectodermal tumour of the central nervous system associated with malignant rhabdoid tumour of the kidney. Report of a case. Histopathology **10**:643-650, 1986.

382 Mayes LC, Kasselberg AG, Roloff JS, Lukens JN: Hypercalcemia associated with immunoreactive parathyroid hormone in a malignant rhabdoid tumor of the kidney (rhabdoid Wilms' tumor). Cancer **54**:882-884, 1984.

383 Sotelo-Avila C, Gonzalez-Crussi F, deMello D, Vogler C, Gooch WM III, Gale G, Pena R: Renal and extrarenal rhabdoid tumors in children. A clinicopathologic study of 14 patients. Semin Diagn Pathol **3**:151-163, 1986.

384 Tsuneyoshi M, Daimaru Y, Hashimoto H, Enjoji M: Malignant soft tissue neoplasms with the histologic features of renal rhabdoid tumors. An ultrastructural and immunohistochemical study. Hum Pathol **16**:1235-1242, 1985.

385 Weeks DA, Beckwith JB, Mierau GA: Rhabdoid tumor of kidney. The National Wilms' Tumor Study experience (abstract). Lab Invest **58**:101A, 1988.

Other sarcomas

386 Gonzalez-Crussi F, Baum ES: Renal sarcomas of childhood. A clinicopathologic and ultrastructural study. Cancer **51**:898-912, 1983.

387 Penchansky L, Gallo G: Rhabdomyosarcoma of the kidney in children. Cancer **44**:285-292, 1979.

RENAL CELL CARCINOMA
General features

388 Altaffer LF III, Chenault DW Jr: Paraneoplastic endocrinopathies associated with renal tumors. J. Urol **122**:573-577, 1979.

389 Berg S, Jacobs SC, Cohen AJ, Li F, Marchetto D, Brown RS: The surgical management of hereditary multifocal renal carcinoma. J Urol **126**:313-315, 1981.

390 Bernstein J, Evan AP, Gardner KD Jr: Epithelial hyperplasia in human polycystic kidney diseases. Its role in pathogenesis and risk of neoplasia. Am J Pathol **129**:92-101, 1987.

391 Bretan PN Jr, Busch MP, Hricak H, Williams RD: Chronic renal failure. A significant risk factor in the development of acquired renal cysts and renal cell carcinoma. Case reports and review of the literature. Cancer **57**:1871-1879, 1986.

392 Campbell LV Jr, Gilbert E, Chamberlain CR Jr, Watne AL: Metastases of cancer to cancer. Cancer **22**:635-643, 1968.

393 Chung-Park M, Ricanati E, Lankerani M, Kedia K: Acquired renal cysts and multiple renal cell and urothelial tumors. Am J Clin Pathol **79**:238-242, 1983.

394 Dalakas MC, Fujihara S, Askanas V, Engel WK, Glenner GG: Nature of amyloid deposits in hypernephroma. Immunocytochemical studies in 2 cases associated with amyloid polyneuropathy. Am J Pathol **116**:447-454, 1984.

395 Dehner LP, Leestma JE, Price EB Jr: Renal cell carcinoma in children. A clinicopathologic study of 15 cases and review of the literature. J Pediatr **76**:358-368, 1970.

396 Everson TC: Spontaneous regression of cancer. Ann NY Acad Sci **114**:721-735, 1964.

397 Fan K, Smith DJ: Hypercalcemia associated with renal cell carcinoma. Probable role of neoplastic stromal cells. Hum Pathol **14**:168-173, 1983.

398 Fletcher MS, Packham DA, Pryor JP, Yates-Bell AJ: Hepatic dysfunction in renal carcinoma. Br J Urol **53**:533-536, 1981.

399 Frohmuller HG, Grups JW, Heller V: Comparative value of ultrasonography, computerized tomography, angiography and excretory urography in the staging of renal cell carcinoma. J Urol **138**:482-484, 1987.

400 Goldberg MF, Tashjian AH Jr, Order SE, Dammin GJ: Renal adenocarcinoma containing a parathyroid hormone-like substance and associated with marked hypercalcemia. Am J Med **36**:805-814, 1964.

401 Golde DW, Schambelan M, Weintraub BD, Rosen SW: Gonadotropin-secreting renal carcinoma. Cancer **33**:1048-1053, 1974.

402 Hartman DS, Davis CJ Jr, Madewell JE, Friedman AC: Primary malignant renal tumors in the second decade of life. Wilms' tumor versus renal cell carcinoma. J Urol **127**:888-891, 1982.

403 Hollifield JW, Page DL, Smith C, Michelakis AM, Staab E, Rhamy R: Reninsecreting clear cell carcinoma of the kidney. Arch Intern Med **135**:859-864, 1975.

404 Hughson MD, Buchwald D, Fox M: Renal neoplasia and acquired cystic kidney disease in patients receiving long-term dialysis. Arch Pathol Lab Med **110**:592-601, 1986.

405 Kaplan C, Sayre GP, Greene LF: Bilateral nephrogenic carcinomas in Lindau-von Hippel disease. J Urol **86**:36-42, 1961.

406 Katz SE, Schapira HE: Spontaneous regression of genitourinary cancer. An update. J Urol **128**:1-4, 1982.

407 Konnak JW, Grossman HB: Renal cell carcinoma as an incidental finding. J Urol **134**:1094-1096, 1985.

408 Lack EE, Cassady R, Sallan SE: Renal cell carcinoma in childhood and adolescence. A clinical and pathological study of 17 cases. J Urol **133**:822-828, 1985.

409 Malek RS, Omess PJ, Benson RC Jr, Zincke H: Renal cell carcinoma in von Hippel-Lindau syndrome. Am J Med **82**:236-238, 1987.

410 Marshall FF, Walsh PC: Extrarenal manifestations of renal cell carcinoma. J Urol **117**:439-440, 1977.

411 Okabe T, Urabe A, Kato T, Chiba S, Takaku F: Production of erythropoietin-like activity by human renal and hepatic carcinomas in cell culture. Cancer **55**:1918-1923, 1985.

412 Ramos CV, Taylor HB: Hepatic dysfunction associated with renal carcinoma. Cancer **29**:1287-1292, 1972.

413 Singh EO, Benson RC Jr, Wold LE: Cancer-to-cancer metastasis. J Urol **132**:340-342, 1984.

414 Skinner DG, Colvin RB, Vermillion CD, Pfister RC, Leadbetter WF: Diagnosis and management of renal cell carcinoma. A clinical and pathologic study of 309 cases. Cancer **28**:1165-1177, 1971.

415 Teyssier JR, Henry I, Dozier C, Ferre D, Adnet JJ, Pluot M: Recurrent deletion of the short arm of chromosome 3 in human renal cell carcinoma. Shift of the c-raf 1 locus. JNCI **77**:1187-1195, 1986.

416 Vanatta PR, Silva FG, Taylor WE, Costa JC: Renal cell carcinoma and systemic amyloidosis. Demonstration of AA protein and review of the literature. Hum Pathol **14**:195-201, 1983.

Morphologic features

417 Borowitz MJ, Weiss MA, Bossen EH, Metzgar RS: Characterization of renal neoplasms with monoclonal antibodies to leukocyte differentiation antigens. Cancer **57**:251-256, 1986.

418 Cordon-Cardo C, Finstad CL, Bander NH, Melamed MR: Immunoanatomic distribution of cytostructural and tissue-associated antigens in the human urinary tract. Am J Pathol **126**:269-284, 1987.

419 Fleming S, Gibson AAM: Proteinase inhibitors in the kidney and its tumours. Histopathology **10**:1303-1313, 1986.

420 Fleming S, Lindop GBM, Gibson AAM: The distribution of epithelial membrane antigen in the kidney and its tumours. Histopathology **9**:729-739, 1985.

421 Gröne H-J, Weber K, Helmchen U, Osborn M: Villin. A marker of brush border differentiation and cellular origin in human renal cell carcinoma. Am J Pathol **124**:294-302, 1986.

422 Haimoto H, Takashi M, Koshikawa T, Asai J, Kato K: Enolase isozymes in renal tubules and renal cell carcinoma. Am J Pathol **124**:488-495, 1986.

423 Holthöfer H, Miettinen A, Paasivuo R, Lehto V-P, Linder E, Alfthan O, Virtanen I: Cellular origin and differentiation of renal carcinomas. A fluorescence microscopic study with kidney-specific antibodies, antiintermediate filament antibodies, and lectins. Lab Invest **49**:317-326, 1983.

424 Hull MT, Eble JN: Myelinoid lamellated cytoplasmic inclusions in human renal adenocarcinomas. An ultrastructural study. Ultrastruct Pathol **12**:41-48, 1988.

425 Jagirdar J, Irie T, French SW, Patil J, Schwarz R, Paronetto F: Globular Mallory-like bodies in renal cell carcinoma. Report of a case and review of cytoplasmic eosinophilic globules. Hum Pathol **16**:949-952, 1985.

426 Liebert M, Jaffe R, Taylor RJ, Ballou BT, Solter D, Hakala TR: Detection of SSEA-1 on human renal tumors. Cancer **59**:1404-1408, 1987.

427 Mackay B, Ordóñez NG, Khoursand J: The ultrastructure and immunocytochemistry of renal cell carcinoma. Ultrastruct Pathol **11**:483-502, 1987.

428 Mancilla-Jimenez R, Stanley RJ, Blath RA: Papillary renal cell carcinoma. A clinical, radiologic, and pathologic study of 34 cases. Cancer **38**:2469-2480, 1976.

429 Oosterwijk E, Ruiter DJ, Wakka JC, Meij JWH-VD, Jonas U, Fleuren G-J, Zwartendijk J, Hoedemaeker P, Warnaar SO: Immunohistochemical analysis of monoclonal antibodies to renal antigens. Application in the diagnosis of renal cell carcinoma. Am J Pathol **123**:301-309, 1986.

430 Pitz S, Moll R, Störkel S, Thoenes W: Expression of intermediate filament proteins in subtypes of renal cell carcinomas and in renal oncocytomas. Distinction of two classes of renal cell tumors. Lab Invest **56**:642-653, 1987.

431 Reznicek SB, Narayana AS, Culp DA: Cystadenocarcinoma of the kidney. A profile of 13 cases. J Urol 134:256-259, 1985.

432 Shazizadeh M, Kagawa S, Kurokawa K: Immunohistochemical studies of human renal cell carcinoma for ABO(H) blood group antigens, T antigen–like substance and carcinoembryonic antigen. J Urol 133:762-766, 1985.

433 Takada Y, Hiwada K, Yokoyama M, Ochi K, Takeuchi M, Kokubu T: Angiotensin converting enzyme. A possible histologic indicator for human renal cell carcinoma. Cancer 56:130-133, 1985.

434 Takashi M, Haimoto H, Murase T, Mitsuya H, Kato K: An immunochemical and immunohistochemical study of S 100 protein in renal cell carcinoma. Cancer 61:889-895, 1988.

435 Thoenes W, Störkel S, Rumpelt HJ: Histopathology and classification of renal cell tumors (adenomas, oncocytomas and carcinomas). The basic cytological and histopathological elements and their use for diagnostics. Pathol Res Pract 181:125-143, 1986.

436 Ulrich W, Horvat R, Krisch K: Lectin histochemistry of kidney tumours and its pathomorphological relevance. Histopathology 9:1037-1050, 1985.

437 Waldherr R, Schwechheimer K: Co-expression of cytokeratin and vimentin intermediate-sized filaments in renal cell carcinomas. Comparative study of the intermediate-sized filament distribution in renal cell carcinomas and normal human kidney. Virchows Arch [Pathol Anat] 408:15-27, 1985.

438 Yoshida SO, Imam A, Olson CA, Taylor CR: Proximal renal tubular surface membrane antigens identified in primary and metastatic renal cell carcinomas. Arch Pathol Lab Med 110:825-832, 1986.

Cytology

439 Bibbo M, Gill WB, Harris MJ, Lu C-T, Thomsen S, Wied GL: Retrograde brushing as a diagnostic procedure of ureteral, renal pelvic and renal calyceal lesions. A preliminary report. Acta Cytol [Baltimore] 18:137-141, 1974.

440 Nguyen G-K: Percutaneous fine-needle aspiration biopsy cytology of the kidney and adrenal. Pathol Annu 22(Pt 1):163-191, 1987.

Spread and metastases

441 Aizawa F, Suzuki M, Kikuchi Y, Nikaido T, Matsumoto K: Clinicopathological study on small renal cell carcinomas with metastases. Acta Pathol Jpn 37:947-954, 1987.

442 Fairlamb DJ: Spontaneous regression of metastases of renal cancer. A report of two cases including the first recorded regression following irradiation of a dominant metastasis and review of the world literature. Cancer 47:2102-2106, 1981.

443 Foucar E, Dehner LP: Renal cell carcinoma occurring with contralateral adrenal metastasis. A clinical and pathological trap. Arch Surg 114:959-963, 1979.

444 Garfield DH, Kennedy BJ: Regression of metastatic renal cell carcinoma following nephrectomy. Cancer 30:190-196, 1972.

445 Holland JM: Cancer of the kidney. Natural history and staging. Cancer 32:1030-1042, 1973.

446 McNichols DW, Segura JW, DeWeerd JH: Renal cell carcinoma. Long-term survival and late recurrence. J Urol 126:17-23, 1981.

447 Previte SR, Willscher MK, Burke CR: Renal cell carcinoma with solitary contralateral adrenal metastasis. Experience with 2 cases. J Urol 128:132-134, 1982.

448 Saitoh H, Hida M, Nakamura K, Takao S, Shiramizu T, Satoh H: Metastatic processes and a potential indication of treatment for metastatic lesions of renal adenocarcinoma. J Urol 128:916-918, 1982.

449 Skinner DG, Colvin RB, Vermillion CD, Pfister RC, Leadbetter WF: Diagnosis and management of renal cell carcinoma. A clinical and pathologic study of 309 cases. Cancer 28:1165-1177, 1971.

450 Wick MR, Cherwitz DL, McGlennen RC, Dehner LP: Adrenocortical carcinoma. An immunohistochemical comparison with renal cell carcinoma. Am J Pathol 122:343-352, 1986.

Therapy

451 Appelqvist P: The role and value of surgery in metastatic renal adenocarcinoma. A retrospective clinical study of 106 nephrectomized cases. J Surg Oncol 26:138-145, 1984.

452 Bissada NK: Renal cell adenocarcinoma. Surg Gynecol Obstet 145:97-104, 1977.

453 DeKernion JB, Berry D: The diagnosis and treatment of renal cell carcinoma. Cancer 45:1947-1956, 1980.

454 Katzenstein A-L, Purvis R Jr, Gmelich J, Askin F: Pulmonary resection for metastatic renal adenocarcinoma. Pathologic findings and therapeutic value. Cancer 41:712-723, 1978.

455 Marshall FF, Powell KC: Lymphadenectomy for renal cell carcinoma. Anatomical and therapeutic considerations. J Urol 128:677-681, 1982.

456 Marshall FF, Walsh PC: In situ management of renal tumors. Renal cell carcinoma and transitional cell carcinoma. J Urol 131:1045-1049, 1984.

457 McDonald MW: Current therapy for renal cell carcinoma. J Urol 127:211-217, 1982.

458 Novick AC: Partial nephrectomy for renal cell carcinoma. Urol Clin North Am 14:419-433, 1987.

459 Robson CJ, Churchill BM, Anderson W: The results of radical nephrectomy for renal cell carcinoma. Trans Am Assoc Genitourin Surg 60:122-126, 1968.

460 Topley M, Novick AC, Montie JE: Long-term results following partial nephrectomy for localized renal adenocarcinoma. J Urol 131:1050-1052, 1984.

461 Waters WB, Richie JP: Aggressive surgical approach to renal cell carcinoma. Review of 130 cases. J Urol 122:306-309, 1979.

Prognosis

462 Ekfors TO, Lipasti J, Nurmi MJ, Eerola E: Flow cytometric analysis of the DNA profile of renal cell carcinoma. Pathol Res Pract 182:58-62, 1987.

463 Fuhrman SA, Lasky LC, Limas C: Prognostic significance of morphologic parameters in renal cell carcinoma. Am J Surg Pathol 6:655-663, 1982.

464 Kay S: Renal carcinoma. A 10-year study. Am J Clin Pathol 50:428-432, 1968.

465 Lieber MM, Tomera FM, Taylor WF, Farrow GM: Renal adenocarcinoma in young adults. Survival and variables affecting prognosis. J Urol 125:164-168, 1981.

466 Ljungberg B, Stenling R, Roos G: DNA content and prognosis in renal cell carcinoma. A comparison between primary tumors and metastases. Cancer 57:2346-2350, 1986.

467 Medeiros LJ, Gelb AB, Weiss LM: Low-grade renal cell carcinoma. A clinicopathologic study of 53 cases. Am J Surg Pathol 11:633-642, 1987.

467a Medeiros LJ, Gelb AB, Weiss LM: Renal cell carcinoma. Prognositc significance of morphologic parameters in 121 cases. Cancer 61:1639-1651, 1988.

468 Nurmi MJ: Prognostic factors in renal carcinoma. An evaluation of operative findings. Br J Urol 56:270-275, 1984.

469 Rafla S: Renal cell carcinoma. Natural history and results of treatment. Cancer 23:26-40, 1970.

470 Selli C, Hinshaw WM, Woodard BH, Paulson DF: Stratification of risk factors in renal cell carcinoma. Cancer 52:899-903, 1983.

471 Siminovitch JMP, Montie JE, Straffon RA: Prognostic indicators in renal adenocarcinoma. J Urol 130:20-23, 1983.

472 Tomera KM, Farrow GM, Lieber MM: Well differentiated (grade 1) clear cell renal carcinoma. J Urol 129:933-937, 1983.

473 Tosi P, Luzi P, Baak JPA, Miracco C, Santopietro R, Vindigni C, Mattei FM, Acconcia A, Massai MR: Nuclear morphometry as an important prognostic factor in stage I renal cell carcinoma. Cancer 58:2512-2518, 1986.

RENAL CELL CARCINOMA–RELATED TUMORS
Adenoma

474 Aizawa S, Suzuki M, Kikuchi Y, Nikaido T, Matsumoto K: Clinicopathological study on small renal cell carcinomas with metastases. Acta Pathol Jpn 37:947-954, 1987.

475 Budin RE, McDonnell PJ: Renal cell neoplasms. Their relationship to arteriolonephrosclerosis. Arch Pathol Lab Med 108:138-140, 1984.

476 Holm-Nielsen P, Olsen TS: Ultrastructure of renal adenoma. Ultrastruct Pathol 12:27-39, 1988.

477 Hughson MD, Hennigar GR, McManus JFA: Atypical cysts, acquired renal cystic disease, and renal cell tumors in end stage dialysis kidneys. Lab Invest 42:475-480, 1980.

Oncocytoma

478 Alanen KA, Ekfors TO, Lipasti JA, Nurmi MJ: Renal oncocytoma. The incidence of 18 surgical and 12 autopsy cases. Histopathology 8:731-737, 1984.

479 Barnes CA, Beckman EN: Renal oncocytoma and its congeners. Am J Clin Pathol 79:312-318, 1983.

480 Choi H, Almagro UA, McManus JT, Norback DH, Jacobs SC: Renal oncocytoma. A clinicopathologic study. Cancer 51:1887-1896, 1983.

481 Eble JN, Hull MT: Morphologic features of renal oncocytoma. A light and electron microscopic study. Hum Pathol 15:1054-1061, 1984.

482 Klein MJ, Valensi QJ: Proximal tubular adenomas of kidney with so-called oncocytic features. A clinicopathologic study of 13 cases of a rarely reported neoplasm. Cancer 38:906-914, 1976.

483 Lewi HJE, Alexander CA, Fleming S: Renal oncocytoma. Br J Urol 58:12-15, 1986.

484 Lieber MM, Tomera KM, Farrow GM: Renal oncocytoma. J Urol 125:481-485, 1981.

485 Medeiros LJ, Gelb AB, Weiss LM: Low-grade renal cell carcinoma. A clinicopathologic study of 53 cases. Am J Surg Pathol **11**:633-642, 1987.

486 Merino MJ, LiVolsi VA: Oncocytomas of the kidney. Cancer **50**:1852-1856, 1982.

487 Pitz S, Moll R, Störkel S, Thoenes W: Expression of intermediate filament proteins in subtypes of renal cell carcinomas and in renal oncocytomas. Distinction of two classes of renal cell tumors. Lab Invest **56**:642-653, 1987.

488 van der Walt JD, Reid HAS, Risdon RA, Shaw JHF: Renal oncocytoma. A review of the literature and report of an unusual multicentric case. Virchows Arch [Pathol Anat] **398**:291-304, 1983.

489 Yu GSM, Rendler S, Herskowitz A, Molnar JJ: Renal oncocytoma. Report of five cases and review of literature. Cancer **45**:1010-1018, 1980.

490 Zhang G, Monda L, Wasserman NF, Fraley EE: Bilateral renal oncocytoma. Report of 2 cases and literature review. J Urol **133**:84-86, 1985.

Collecting duct carcinoma

491 Aizawa S, Kikuchi Y, Suzuki M, Furusato M: Renal cell carcinoma of lower nephron origin. Acta Pathol Jpn **37**:567-574, 1987.

492 Fleming S, Lewi HJE: Collecting duct carcinoma of the kidney. Histopathology **10**:1131-1141, 1986.

493 Fleming S, Symes CE: The distribution of cytokeratin antigens in the kidney and in renal tumours. Histopathology **11**:157-170, 1987.

494 Kennedy S, Robertson C, Merino M: Collecting duct adenocarcinoma (tumors of the duct of Bellini). A pathologic, immuunohistochemical and ultrastructural study of 6 cases (abstract). Lab Invest **58**:47A, 1988.

495 Mancilla-Jimenez R, Stanley RJ, Blath RA: Papillary renal cell carcinoma. A clinical, radiologic and pathologic study of 34 cases. Cancer **38**:2469-2480, 1976.

Sarcomatoid carcinoma

496 Deitchman B, Sidhu GS: Ultrastructural study of a sarcomatoid variant of renal cell carcinoma. Cancer **46**:1152-1157, 1980.

497 Farrow GM, Harrison EG Jr, Utz DC: Sarcomas and sarcomatoid and mixed malignant tumors of the kidney in adults. Cancer **22**:545-563, 1968.

498 Ro JY, Ayala AG, Sella A, Samuels ML, Swanson DA: Sarcomatoid renal cell carcinoma: clinicopathologic. A study of 42 cases. Cancer **59**:516-526, 1987.

499 Tomera KM, Farrow GM, Lieber MM: Sarcomatoid renal carcinoma. J Urol **130**:657-659, 1983.

Small cell carcinoma

500 Capella C, Eusebi V, Rosai J: Primary oat cell carcinoma of the kidney. Am J Surg Pathol **8**:855-861, 1984.

500a Mills SE, Weiss MA, Swanson PE, Wick MR: Small cell undifferentiated carcinoma of the renal pelvis. A light microscopic, immunocytochemical, and ultrastructural study. Surg Pathol **1**:83-88, 1988.

501 Têtu B, Ro JY, Ayala AG, Ordóñez NG, Johnson DE: Small cell carcinoma of the kidney. A clinicopathologic, immunohistochemical, and ultrastructural study. Cancer **60**:1809-1814, 1987.

ANGIOMYOLIPOMA

502 Bernstein J, Robbins TO, Kissane JM: The renal lesions of tuberous sclerosis. Semin Diagn Pathol **3**:97-105, 1986.

503 Brecher ME, Gill WB, Straus FH II: Angiomyolipoma with regional lymph node involvement and long-term follow-up study. Hum Pathol **17**:962-963, 1986.

504 Busch FM, Bark CJ, Clyde HR: Benign renal angiomyolipoma with regional lymph node involvement. J Urol **116**:715-717, 1976.

505 Daughtry JD, Rodan BA: Renal angiomyolipoma. Definitive diagnosis by ultrasonography and computerized tomography. South Med J **78**:195-197, 1985.

506 Farrow GM, Harrison EG Jr, Utz DC, Jones DR: Renal angiomyolipoma. A clinicopathologic study of 32 cases. Cancer **22**:564-570, 1968.

507 Graves N, Barnes WF: Renal cell carcinoma and angiomyolipoma in tuberous sclerosis. Case Report. J Urol **135**:122-123, 1986.

508 Hajdu SI, Foote FW Jr: Angiomyolipoma of the kidney. Report of 27 cases and review of the literature. J Urol **102**:396-401, 1969.

509 Kragel PJ, Toker C: Infiltrating recurrent renal angiomyolipoma with fatal outcome. J Urol **133**:90-91, 1985.

510 Monteforte WJ Jr, Kohnen PW: Angiomyolipomas in a case of lymphangiomyomatosis syndrome. Relationships to tuberous sclerosis. Cancer **34**:317-321, 1974.

511 Oesterling JE, Fishman EK, Goldman SM, Marshall FF: The management of renal angiomyolipoma. J Urol **135**:1121-1124, 1986.

512 Tweeddale DN, Dawe CJ, McDonald JR, Culp OS: Angiolipoleiomyoma of the kidney. Cancer **8**:764-770, 1955.

513 Waters DJ, Holt SA, Andres DF: Unilateral simultaneous renal angiomyolipoma and oncocytoma. J Urol **135**:568-570, 1986.

JUXTAGLOMERULAR CELL TUMOR

514 Camilleri J-P, Hinglais N, Bruneval P, Bariety J, Tricottet V, Rouchon M, Mancilla-Jimenez R, Corvol P, Menard J: Renin storage and cell differentiation in juxtaglomerular cell tumors. An immunohistochemical and ultrastructural study of three cases. Hum Pathol **15**:1069-1079, 1984.

515 Conn JW, Cohen EL, Lucas CP, McDonald WJ, Mayor GH, Blough WM Jr, Eveland WC, Bookstin JJ, Lapides J: Primary reninism. Hypertension, hyper-reninemia, and secondary aldosteronism due to renin-producing juxtaglomerular cell tumors. Arch Intern Med **130**:682-696, 1972.

516 Gherardi GJ, Arya S, Hickler RB: Juxtaglomerular body tumor. A rare occult but curable cause of lethal hypertension. Hum Pathol **5**:236-240, 1974.

517 Lindop GBM, Leckie B, Winearls CG: Malignant hypertension due to a renin-secreting renal cell carcinoma. An ultrastructural and immunocytochemical study. Histopathology **10**:1077-1088, 1986.

518 Lindop GBM, Stewart JA, Downie TT: The immunocytochemical demonstration of renin in a juxtaglomerular cell tumor by light and electron microscopy. Histopathology **7**:421-431, 1983.

519 Ruddy MC, Atlas SA, Salerno FG: Hypertension associated with a renin-secreting adenocarcinoma of the pancreas. N Engl J Med **307**:993-997, 1982.

520 Squires JP, Ulbright TM, DeSchryver-Kecskemeti K, Engleman W: Juxtaglomerular cell tumor of the kidney. Cancer **53**:516-523, 1984.

521 Tomita T, Poisner A, Inagami T: Immunohistochemical localization of renin in renal tumors. Am J Pathol **126**:73-80, 1987.

OTHER BENIGN TUMORS AND TUMORLIKE CONDITIONS

522 Baker WJ, Ragins AB: Pararenal teratoma. J Urol **63**:982-990, 1950.

523 Beckwith JB: Wilms' tumor and other renal tumors of childhood. A selective review from the National Wilms' Tumor Study Pathology Center. Hum Pathol **14**:481-492, 1983.

524 Bennington JL, Beckwith JB: Tumors of the kidney, renal pelvis and ureter. In Atlas of tumor pathology. Second series, Fasc. 12, Washington, D.C., AFIP, 1975.

525 Bossart MI, Spjut HJ, Wright JE, Pranke DW: Multilocular cystic leiomyoma of the kidney. Ultrastruct Pathol **3**:367-374, 1982.

526 Dineen MK, Venable DD, Misra RP: Pure intrarenal lipoma. Report of a case and review of the literature. J Urol **132**:104-107, 1984.

527 Glover SD, Buck AC: Renal medullary fibroma. A case report. J Urol **127**:758-760, 1982.

528 Kojiro M, Ohishi H, Isobe H: Carcinoid tumor occurring in cystic teratoma of the kidney. A case report. Cancer **38**:1636-1640, 1976.

529 Sneige N, Dekmezian RH, Silva EG, Cartwright J Jr, Ayala AG: Pseudoparasitic Liesegang structures in perirenal hemorrhagic cysts. Am Clin Pathol **89**:148-153, 1988.

530 Stone NN, Cherry J: Renal capsular lipoma. J Urol **134**:118-119, 1985.

OTHER MALIGNANT PRIMARY TUMORS

531 Allred CD, Cathey WJ, McDivitt RW: Primary renal angiosarcoma. A case report. Hum Pathol **12**:665-668, 1981.

532 Ellman L, Davis J, Lichtenstein NS: Uremia due to occult lymphomatous infiltration of the kidneys. Cancer **33**:203-205, 1974.

533 Farrow GM, Harrison EG Jr, Utz DC: Sarcomas and sarcomatoid and mixed malignant tumors of the kidney in adults. Cancer **22**:545-563, 1968.

534 Fetissof F, Benatre A, Dubois MP, Lanson Y, Arbeille-Brassart B, Jobard P: Carcinoid tumor occurring in a teratoid malformation of the kidney. An immunohistochemical study. Cancer **54**:2305-2308, 1984.

534a Hannah J, Lippe B, Lai-Goldman M, Bhuta S: Oncocytic carcinoid of the kidney associated with periodic Cushing's syndrome. Cancer **61**:2136-2140, 1988.

535 Kandel LB, Harrison LH, Woodruff RD, Williams CD, Ahl ET Jr: Renal plasmacytoma. A case report and summary of reported cases. J Urol **132**:1167-1169, 1984.

536 Kojiro M, Ohishi H, Isobe H: Carcinoid tumor occurring in cystic teratoma of the kidney. A case report. Cancer **38**:1636-1640, 1976.

537 Malhotra CM, Doolittle CH, Rodil JV, Vezeridis MP: Mesenchymal chondrosarcoma of the kidney. Cancer **54**:2495-2499, 1984.

538 Mead JH, Herrera GA, Kaufman MF, Herz JH: Case report of a primary cystic sarcoma of the kidney, demonstrating fibrohistiocytic, osteoid, and cartilaginous components (malignant mesenchymoma). Cancer **50**:2211-2214, 1982.

539 Micolonghi TS, Liang D, Schwartz S: Primary osteogenic sarcoma of the kidney. J Urol **131**:1164-1166, 1984.

540 Nativ O, Horowitz A, Lindner A, Many M: Primary chondrosarcoma of the kidney. J Urol **134**:120-121, 1985.

541 Ng WD, Chan KW, Chan YT: Primary leiomyosarcoma of renal capsule. J Urol **133**:834-835, 1985.

542 Osborne BM, Brenner M, Weitzmer S, Butler JJ: Malignant lymphoma presenting as a renal mass. Four cases. Am J Surg Pathol **11**:375-382, 1987.

543 Randolph VL, Hall W, Bramson W: Renal failure due to lymphomatous infiltration of the kidneys. Cancer **52**:1120-1121, 1983.

544 Richmond J, Sherman RS, Diamond HD, Craver LF: Renal lesions associated with malignant lymphomas. Am J Med **32**:184-207, 1962.

545 Scriven RR, Thrasher TV, Smith DC, Stewart SC: Primary renal malignant fibrous histiocytoma. A case report and literature review. J Urol **131**:948-949, 1984.

546 Srinivas V, Sogani PC, Hajdu SI, Whitmore WF Jr: Sarcomas of the kidney. J Urol **132**:13-16, 1984.

547 Stahl RE, Sidhu GS: Primary carcinoid of the kidney. Light and electron microscopic study. Cancer **44**:1345-1349, 1979.

548 Zak FG, Jindrak K, Capozzi F: Carcinoidal tumor of the kidney. Ultrastruct Pathol **4**:51-59, 1983.

METASTATIC TUMORS

549 Belghiti D, Hirbec G, Bernaudin JF, Pariente EA, Martin N: Intraglomerular metastases. Report of two cases. Cancer **54**:2309-2312, 1984.

550 Davis RI, Corson JM: Renal metastases from well-differentiated follicular thyroid carcinoma. A case report with light and electron microscopic findings. Cancer **43**:265-268, 1979.

551 Johnson MW, Morettin LB, Sarles HE, Zaharopoulos P: Follicular carcinoma of the thyroid metastatic to the kidney 37 years after resection of the primary tumor. J Urol **127**:114-116, 1982.

552 Mazeman E, Wemeau L, Lemaitre G, Kozyreff P: Les tumeurs secondaires du rein. J Urol Nephrol [Paris] **82**:145-160, 1976.

553 Toth T: Extracapillary tumorous metastatic crescents in glomeruli of the kidney. Pathol Res Pract **182**:240-243, 1987.

554 Wagle DG, Moore RH, Murphy GP: Secondary carcinomas of the kidney. J Urol **114**:30-32, 1975.

TUMORS OF RENAL PELVIS AND URETER
Transitional cell carcinoma

555 Akaza H, Koiso K, Niijima T: Clinical evaluation of urothelial tumors of the renal pelvis and ureter based on a new classification system. Cancer **59**:1369-1375, 1987.

556 Auld D, Grigor KM, Fowler JW: Histopathological review of transitional cell carcinoma of the upper urinary tract. Br J Urol **56**:485-489, 1984.

557 Balslev E, Fischer S: Transitional cell carcinoma of the renal collecting tubules (renal urothelioma). Acta Pathol Microbiol Immunol Scand [A] **91**:419-424, 1983.

558 Batata MA, Whitmore WF Jr, Hilaris BS, Tokita N, Grabstald H: Primary carcinoma of the ureter. A prognostic study. Cancer **35**:1626-1632, 1975.

559 Bloom NA, Vidone RA, Lytton B: Primary carcinoma of the ureter. A report of 102 new cases. J Urol **103**:590-598, 1970.

560 Borg-Grech A, Morris JA, Eyden BP: Malignant osteoclastoma-like giant cell tumor of the renal pelvis. Histopathology **11**:415-425, 1987.

561 Heney NM, Nocks BN, Daly JJ, Blitzer PH, Parkhurst EC: Prognostic factors in carcinoma of the ureter. J Urol **125**:632-636, 1981.

562 Huffman JL, Bagley DH, Lyon ES, Morse MJ, Herr HW, Whitmore WF Jr: Endoscopic diagnosis and treatment of upper-tract urothelial tumors. A preliminary report. Cancer **55**:1422-1428, 1985.

563 Johansson S, Angervall L, Bengtsson U, Wahlqvist L: Uroepithelial tumors of the renal pelvis associated with abuse of phenacetin-containing analgesics. Cancer **33**:743-753, 1974.

564 Johansson S, Angervall L, Bengtsson U, Wahlqvist L: A clinicopathologic and prognostic study of epithelial tumors of the renal pelvis. Cancer **37**:1376-1383, 1976.

565 Kenney RM, Prat J, Tabernero M: Giant-cell tumor-like proliferation associated with a papillary transitional cell carcinoma of the renal pelvis. Am J Surg Pathol **8**:139-144, 1984.

566 Koyanagi T, Sasaki K, Arikado K, Hirano T, Tsuji I: Transitional cell carcinoma of the renal pelvis in an infant. J Urol **113**:114-117, 1975.

567 Mahadevia PS, Karwa GL, Koss LG: Mapping of urothelium in carcinomas of the renal pelvis and ureter. A report of nine cases. Cancer **51**:890-897, 1983.

568 McCarron JP Jr, Chasko SB, Gray GF Jr: Systematic mapping of nephroureterectomy specimens removed for urothelial cancer. Pathological findings and clinical correlations. J Urol **128**:243-246, 1982.

569 McDougal WS, Cramer SF, Miller R: Invasive carcinoma of the renal pelvis

following cyclophosphamide therapy for nonmalignant disease. Cancer **48**:691-695, 1981.

570 McIntyre D, Pyrah LN, Raper FP: Primary ureteric neoplasms. Report of 40 cases. Br J Urol **37**:160-191, 1965.

571 Mills C, Vaughan ED Jr: Carcinoma of the ureter. Natural history, management and 5-year survival. J Urol **129**:275-277, 1983.

571a Mills SE, Weiss MA, Swanson PE, Wick MR: Small cell undifferentiated carcinoma of the renal pelvis. A light microscopic, immunocytochemical, and ultrastructural study. Surg Pathol **1**:83-88, 1988.

572 Murphy DM, Zincke H: Transitional cell carcinoma in the horseshoe kidney. Report of 3 cases and review of the literature. Br J Urol **54**:484-485, 1982.

573 Murphy WM, von Buedingen RP, Poley RW: Primary carcinoma in situ of renal pelvis and ureter. Cancer **34**:1126-1130, 1974.

574 Palvio DHB, Andersen JC, Falk E: Transitional cell tumors of the renal pelvis and ureter associated with capillarosclerosis indicating analgesic abuse. Cancer **59**:972-976, 1987.

575 Pettersson S, Brynger H, Henriksson C, Johansson SL, Nilson AE, Ranch T: Treatment of urothelial tumors of the upper urinary tract by nephroureterectomy, renal autotransplantation, and pyelocystostomy. Cancer **54**:379-386, 1984.

576 Strobel SL, Jasper WS, Gogate SA, Sharma HM: Primary carcinoma of the renal pelvis and ureter. Evaluation of clinical and pathologic features. Arch Pathol Lab Med **108**:697-700, 1984.

577 Strong DW, Pearse HD: Recurrent urothelial tumors following surgery for transitional cell carcinoma of the upper urinary tract. Cancer **38**:2178-2183, 1976.

578 Verhaak RLOM, Harmsen AE, van Unnik AJM: On the frequency of tumor induction in a Thorotrast kidney. Cancer **34**:2061-2068, 1974.

579 Wagle DG, Moore RH, Murphy GP: Primary carcinoma of the renal pelvis. Cancer **33**:1642-1648, 1974.

580 Werth DD, Weigel JW, Mebust WK: Primary neoplasms of the ureter. J Urol **125**:628-631, 1981.

581 Wick MR, Perrone TL, Burke BA: Sarcomatoid transitional cell carcinomas of the renal pelvis. An ultrastructural and immunohistochemical study. Arch Pathol Lab Med **109**:55-58, 1985.

582 Yokoyama I, Berman E, Rickert RR, Bastidas J: Simultaneous occurrence of renal cell adenocarcinoma and urothelial carcinoma of the renal pelvis in the same kidney diagnosed by preoperative angiography. Cancer **48**:2762-2766, 1981.

Adenocarcinoma

583 Aufderheide AC, Streitz JM: Mucinous adenocarcinoma of the renal pelvis. Report of two cases. Cancer **33**:167-173, 1974.

584 Kobayashi S, Ohmori M, Akaeda T, Ohmori H, Miyaji Y: Primary adenocarcinoma of the renal pelvis. Report of two cases and brief review of literature. Acta Pathol Jpn **33**:589-597, 1983.

Epidermoid carcinoma

585 Hertle L, Androulakakis P: Keratinizing desquamative squamous metaplasia of the upper urinary tract. Leukoplakia—cholesteatoma. J Urol **127**:631-635, 1982.

586 Strobel SL, Jasper WS, Gogate SA, Sharma HM: Primary carcinoma of the renal pelvis and ureter. Evaluation of clinical and pathologic features. Arch Pathol Lab Med **108**:697-700, 1984.

587 Verhaak RLOM, Harmsen AE, van Unnik AJM: On the frequency of tumor induction in a Thorotrast kidney. Cancer **34**:2061-2068, 1974.

Other tumors and tumorlike conditions

588 Abeshouse BS: Primary benign and malignant tumors of the ureter. A review of the literatue and report of one benign and twelve malignant tumors. Am J Surg **91**:237-271, 1956.

589 Chabrel CM, Hickey BB, Parkinson C: Pericaliceal haemangioma. A cause of papillary necrosis? Case report and review of 7 similar vascular lesions. Br J Urol **54**:334-340, 1982.

590 Cubilla E, Hesker AE, Stanley RJ: Cavernous hemangioma of the kidney. An angiographic-pathologic correlation. J Can Assoc Radiol **24**:254-256, 1973.

591 Edelman R, Kim ES, Bard RH: Benign fibroepithelial polyp of the renal pelvis. Br J Urol **54**:321-322, 1982.

592 Edward HG, Deweerd JH, Woolner LB: Renal hemangiomas. Proc Staff Meetings Mayo Clin **37**:545-551, 1962.

593 Farrands PA, Tribe CR, Slade N: Localized amyloid of the ureter. Case report and review of the literature. Histopathology **7**:613-622, 1983.

594 Fromowitz FB, Steinbook ML, Lautin EM, Friedman AC, Kahan N, Bennett MJ, Koss LG: Inverted papilloma of the ureter. J Urol **126**:113-116, 1981.

595 Geller SA, Lin C-S: Ureteral obstruction from metastatic breast carcinoma. Arch Pathol **99**:476-478, 1975.

596 Hurwitz RS, Benjamin JA, Cooper JF: Excessive proliferation of peripelvic fat of the kidney. Urology **11**:448-456, 1978.

597 Kochevar J: Adenocarcinoid tumor, goblet cell type, arising in a ureteroileal conduit. A case report. J Urol **131**:957-959, 1984.

598 Macksood MJ, Roth DR, Chang C-H, Perlmutter AD: Benign fibroepithelial polyps as a cause of intermittent ureteropelvic junction obstruction in a child. A case report and review of the literature. J Pathol **134**:951-952, 1985.

599 MacMahon HE: Hypertrophic infundibular stenosis of the calyces of the kidney. Hum Pathol **5**:363-364, 1974.

600 Maeda K, Hawkins ET, Oh HK, Kini SR, Van Dyke DL: Malignant lymphoma in transplanted renal pelvis. Arch Pathol Lab Med **110**:626-629, 1986.

601 Matthews PN, Greenwood RN, Hendry WF, Cattell WR: Extensive pelvis malacoplakia. Observations on management. J Urol **135**:132-134, 1986.

602 Peterson NE: Adenoma of ileal urinary conduit. J Urol **131**:1171-1172, 1984.

602a Recloux P, Weiser M, Piccart M, Sculier J-P: Ureteral obstruction in patients with breast cancer. Cancer **61**:1904-1907, 1988.

603 Rivard JY, Bedard A, Dionne L: Colonic neoplasms following ureterosigmoidostomy. J Urol **113**:781-786, 1975.

604 Rudd EG, Matthews MD: Malacoplakia. An unusual etiology of ureteral obstruction. Obstet Gynecol **60**:134-136, 1982.

605 Satodate R, Koike H, Sasou S, Ohori T, Nagane Y: Nephrogenic adenoma of the ureter. J Urol **131**:332-334, 1984.

606 Scharifker D, Chalasani A: Ureteral involvement by malignant lymphoma. Ten years' experience. Arch Pathol Lab Med **102**:541-542, 1978.

607 Strachan JR, Rees HC, Williams G. Histochemical changes after ureterosigmoidostomies and colonic diversion. Br J Urol **57**:700-702, 1985.

608 Uchida M, Watanabe H, Mishina T, Shimada N: Leiomyoma of the renal pelvis. J Urol **125**:572-574, 1981.

609 Werner JR, Klingersmith W, Denko JV: Leiomyosarcoma of the ureter. Case report and review of literature. J Urol **82**:68-71, 1959.

Bladder and urethra

URACHUS AND URACHAL LESIONS

The urachus is a 5 to 6 cm vestigial structure located between the apex of the bladder and umbilicus. The function of the urachus is to connect the bladder with the allantois during development. At birth the urachus retracts from the bladder, but its lumen may persist within the bladder wall and be continuous with the bladder cavity. The lining may be of transitional or columnar type. Schubert et al.[3] found tubular urachal remnants in 32% of the 122 bladders studied at autopsy.

Anomalies related to urachal remnants include patent urachus through which urine may pass, blind sinuses in the anterior abdominal wall, and granulomatous omphalitis.[4] Tumors may also develop from this structure, of which adenocarcinoma is the most common; others include villous adenoma, "fibroadenoma," transitional cell carcinoma, and epidermoid carcinoma.[1,2] Most of these tumors arise from the intramural portion of the urachus and grow into the wall of the bladder, sometimes in the absence of mucosal involvement. Others occur beneath the peritoneum of the anterior abdominal wall between the umbilicus and the bladder dome.

EXSTROPHY

Bladder exstrophy is a congenital abnormality characterized by absence of the anterior vesicle and lower abdominal wall, with eversion of the posterior bladder wall. These changes may be partial or complete and often are associated with other anomalies of the urogenital tract. Malignant change was found in three (7.5%) of forty-two patients with exstrophic bladder reported by Engel and Wilkinson.[5] All three patients had adenocarcinoma; one also had a epidermoid carcinoma.

DIVERTICULOSIS

Diverticula of the bladder develop because of partial urinary obstruction in the urethra or bladder neck. Long-standing increased muscular contractions required to empty the bladder cause thickening of the wall and mucosal herniation in areas of weakness. The usual cause of urinary obstruction is nodular hyperplasia of the prostate.[8,9] The diverticula are most commonly located in the posterior wall above the trigone, the region of the ureteral orifices, and the dome at the site of an obliterated urachus. The communication into the bladder is usually large, but may be pinpoint in size. The wall of the diverticulum usually consists of fibrous tissue with little or no muscle. Squamous metaplasia of the lining epithelium often occurs if there is associated infection.

Complications of bladder diverticula include lithiasis, free perforation into the peritoneal cavity, and tumor development.[11] The tumors are usually transitional cell carcinomas[6,7,12] but may be of other types.[10] They may grow to a large size before detection because of their hidden location. This complication may be related to the obstruction, chronic inflammation, epithelial hyperplasia, and squamous metaplasia to which these diverticula are prone.

LITHIASIS

Bladder calculi (Fig. 17-73) occur much more often in male than in female individuals; most of the patients are elderly. The majority of these stones are solitary and composed of phosphate salts; others are made up of urate and oxalate salts.[13] The most common associated abnormality is nodular hyperplasia of the prostate gland.

Treatment is removal either via urethra after crushing the stone or by cystotomy. Recurrence develops in about 10% of the patients.

ENDOMETRIOSIS

Endometriosis may involve the bladder, either as an isolated focus or associated with similar lesions in other sites.[14,15] In most instances, there is a history of previous surgery or of some gynecologic disease.[16] In nearly half of the cases, the lesion can be palpated at the base of the bladder. Serosal foci are the most common and are usually asymptomatic; those occurring in the wall, beneath an intact mucosa, result in a bluish cast on cystoscopic examination and may be accompanied by hyperplasia of the muscle.

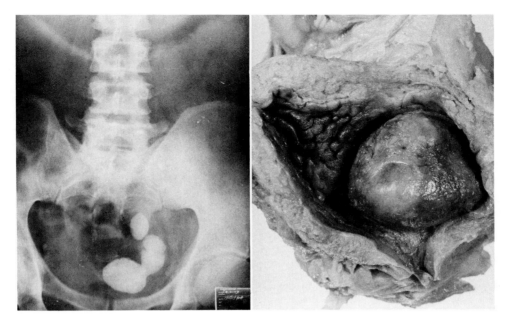

Fig. 17-73 Lithiasis of bladder as seen roentgenographically and after opening of specimen.

AMYLOIDOSIS

Amyloidosis of the bladder may be the expression of a generalized process or present as a nodular localized mass ("amyloid tumor").[19] The few patients with the latter form who have been reported with adequate follow-up have remained free of disease following local excision of the mass. Therefore the presence of an amlyoid tumor should not be necessarily regarded as a manifestation of myeloma.[18] Most cases of bladder amyloidosis are made up of AL protein (immunoglobulin light chain.)[17]

CYSTITIS
Interstitial (Hunner's) cystitis

The classic clinical description of interstitial (Hunner's) cystitis is that of an adult or elderly female with ulceration and marked submucosal edema of the bladder resulting in prominent lower abdominal, suprapubic, or perineal pain and urinary frequency, unresponsive to medical therapy.[20]

The lesion can be located anywhere in the bladder. Microscopically, there is mucosal ulceration covered by fibrin and necrotic material. The underlying lamina propria and muscularis show edema, hemorrhage, granulation tissue, and a mononuclear inflammatory infiltrate that often exhibits a perineurial location.[21,23] Mast cells are numerous; they are found beneath the ulcer, within the detrusor muscle bundles, and between the epithelial cells in the adjacent mucosa.[21,22]

Eosinophilic cystitis

Eosinophilic cystitis can occur in two different clinical settings. The first is seen in women and children and is often associated with allergic disorders and eosinophilia. The second presents in older men and is usually associated with bladder injury related to other conditions of the bladder and prostate.[25]

Clinically, eosinophilic cystitis presents with dramatic and recurrent episodes of dysuria and hematuria.[26] The cystoscopic appearance is that of a diffuse edematous and erythematous mucosa, with broad-based polypoid growths. Microscopically, a dense inflammatory infiltrate rich in eosinophils, often accompanied by fibrosis and muscle necrosis, and sometimes by giant cells, is present.[24] This condition is not related to eosinophilic granuloma (histiocytosis X).

Polypoid cystitis

Polypoid cystitis may simulate a neoplasm grossly, but it is a perfectly benign process of a reactive nature. Most cases are the result of the introduction of a catheter and, consequently, are seen involving the posterior wall. The frequency of this condition increases with increasing use of the catheter and reaches its peak by 3 months. Bullous cystitis is a variant with broad, rounded elevations. Microscopically, stromal edema and congestion are the main features. Inflammation is minimal, and epithelial atypia is absent.[27]

Cystitis emphysematosa

Cystitis emphysematosa is an inflammatory condition caused by gas-forming bacteria and is associated with gas-filled vesicles in the bladder wall. About 50% of the patients are diabetic. Microscopically, multinucleated giant cells are seen partially lining the cysts.[28]

Cystitis glandularis and cystitis cystica

These two related disorders represent metaplastic changes of the transitional epithelium resulting from chronic inflammation or other causes of mucosal irritation, such as ureteral reimplantation, neurogenic bladder, or bladder exstrophy.[31,33] They may regress completely if the underlying path-

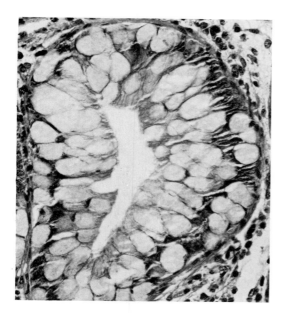

Fig. 17-74 Cystitis glandularis with formation of mucin-producing glands.

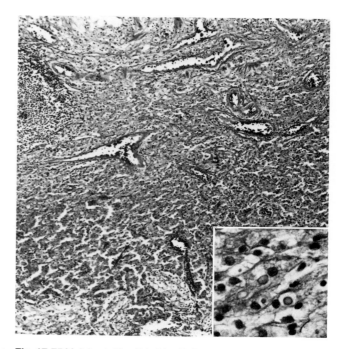

Fig. 17-75 Malakoplakia of bladder. Diffuse histiocytic infiltrate results in marked thickening of bladder wall. **Inset** shows characteristic Michaelis-Gutmann bodies.

ogenetic factor is removed. Grossly, they usually present as irregular mamillated lesions that may be confused cystoscopically with carcinoma. The trigone is the area most commonly affected, but rare instances of involvement of the entire bladder mucosa have been reported.[29] Similar lesions may be present in the ureter and renal pelvis.

Microscopically, the initial change in focal proliferation of the basal layer of the transitional epithelium, which produces buds that later become solid nodules (von Brunn's nests or islands) located within the lamina propria. Some of these nodules develop a central cystic area caused by the accumulation of mucin. When the cells lining the cyst maintain a transitional appearance, the condition is called *cystitis cystica;* when they acquire morphologic features analogous to those of colonic epithelium, they are designated either as *cystitis glandularis* or as *intestinal (glandular, colonic) metaplasia*[30,32,34] (Fig. 17-74). The common occurrence of transitional forms suggests that these represent various stages of manifestations of the same basic process. Patients in whom the intestinal metaplasia is very extensive are at a high risk for the development of adenocarcinoma.[30]

Tuberculosis

Tuberculosis remains the most frequent cause of granulomatous inflammation of the bladder in many parts of the world. It invariably develops from secondary foci, most often in the kidney.[35] Secondary involvement of the prostate can also occur. Most bladder lesions are found in the region of the trigone, especially around the ureteral orifices. Early lesions are superficial and small, with a floor of soft caseous material and a peripheral hyperemic zone. As the disease progresses, multiple ulcers coalesce to form larger ones that produce much fibrosis and involve the underlying musculature.

Malakoplakia

Malakoplakia of the bladder is characterized by the appearance of multiple nodular thickenings of the mucosa and submucosa, usually in the region of the trigone, that may be mistaken for cancer.[37,45,46] It has been associated with immune deficiency states and has been reported on several occasions in renal transplant recipients.[36,47]

Microscopically, collections of histiocytes with granular acidophilic cytoplasm accumulate beneath the surface epithelium. In some of these cells, rounded, concentrically layered intracytoplasmic inclusions known as Michaelis-Guttman bodies or calcospherites are seen (Fig. 17-75); these are basophilic and PAS-positive and stain for iron and calcium.[45] Ultrastructurally and immunohistochemically, intracellular bacteria can be identified.[41,42,44] The presence of transitional forms between these bacteria, lipid inclusions, and Michaelis-Gutmann bodies suggest that the latter represent the end result of bacterial degradation.[40] Accordingly, malakoplakia is presently regarded as a defect in the host macrophage (phagolysosomal) response to a bacterial infection, usually from gram-negative coliform bacilli.[39,40,49] *Xanthogranulomatous cystitis* is morphologically and probably pathogenetically similar to malakoplakia, but it lacks Michaelis-Guttman bodies.[50] Malakoplakia may also involve the renal pelvis and parenchyma, ureter, prostate gland, testis, epididymis, broad ligament, endometrium, retroperitoneal structures, colon, stomach, appendix, lymph nodes, brain, lungs, bones, and skin.[38,43,48,51]

Other forms of cystitis

Other morphologic types of cystitis that have been described are giant cell cystitis, follicular cystitis, radiation cystitis, and encrusted cystitis.[51a]

TUMORLIKE CONDITIONS

Granulomas of necrotizing, palisading (rheumatoid nodule–like) and foreign-body type can occur after bladder surgery, presumably as a local reaction to tissue necrosis caused by surgery or catheterization; these lesions heal by fibrous scarring.[53a,54]

Another post-operative bladder lesion is a *spindle-cell (pseudosarcomatous) nodule* that may microscopically simulate a sarcoma (particularly leiomyosarcoma) because of its marked cellularity and high mitotic activity.[53] It appears a few weeks following a TUR procedure and is characteristically located in the operative area. Cystoscopically, it presents as a small sessile friable nodule that bleeds easily. The fascicular pattern of growth, ulcerated surface, red blood cell extravasation, and lack of significant pleomorphism, together with the history of a recent surgical procedure, distinguish this lesion from true sarcoma.

Polypoid masses of similar pathogenesis have been recently described in the bladder as *inflammatory pseudotumor*,[52] and *pseudosarcoma*[55] (Fig. 17-76). The main differential diagnosis is with embryonal rhabdomyosarcoma.

Condyloma acuminatum can involve the bladder, often in conjunction with similar lesions in the external genitalia and adjacent areas.[51b]

BENIGN TUMORS

Inverted papilloma (brunnian adenoma) is a benign epithelial tumor, more commonly seen in adult and elderly males, and almost always located in the trigone, bladder neck, or prostatic urethra[61,70,73] (Fig. 17-77). It is usually solitary and presents with hematuria and/or obstruction. Cystoscopy reveals a polypoid lesion of smooth contours, usually pedunculated. Microscopically, the most characteristic feature of the lesion is the invagination of the epithelium, which shows no atypical features. Papillae are absent, and connective tissue is very scanty.

In some lesions, there is a distinct trabecular arrangement, with peripheral palisading of the tumor cells; in others there are islands of urothelial cells accompanied by gland-like and mucin-secreting structures.[74] The latter type probably derives from an unduly proliferative form of cystitis glandularis or cystitis cystica.[65,74] There is no evidence that inverted papilloma predisposes to the development of carcinoma, but the occasional co-existence of the two lesions suggests a pathogenetic relationship.[57,75]

Inverted papilloma should be distinguished from transitional cell carcinoma spreading into Brunn's islands and growing in an inverted fashion, a rare but well-documented phenomenon. Simple excision is adequate treatment.

Adenomatoid tumor (nephrogenic adenoma; mesonephric adenoma) of the bladder has been traditionally regarded as a benign neoplasm, but most likely it represents a localized or diffuse metaplastic change of the urothelium in response to chronic infection, calculi, or prolonged catheterization[63,68,79] (Fig. 17-78). As such, it is often associated

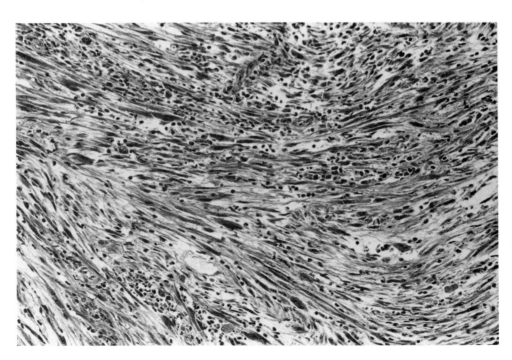

Fig. 17-76 Inflammatory pseudotumor of bladder. Proliferating spindle cells of elongated shape arranged in fascicular pattern are separated by edematous and inflamed tissue.

with cystitis glandularis. Most cases are seen in adults, but children can also be affected.[72] Grossly, these tumors can be papillary, polypoid, or sessile; about 20% are multiple.[83] Their microscopic appearance is that of small tubular formations lined by cuboidal and hobnail cells having a light-

microscopic, ultrastructural, and lectin-binding appearance that is remarkably similar to those of mesonephric tubules.[59,66] The main differential diagnosis is with adenocarcinoma of mesonephroid (clear cell) type (see p. 913).

Paraganglioma (extra-adrenal pheochromocytoma) can

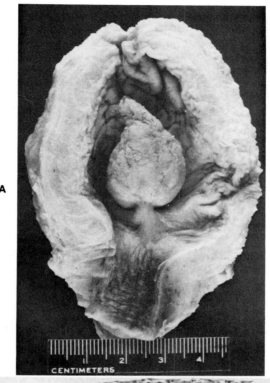

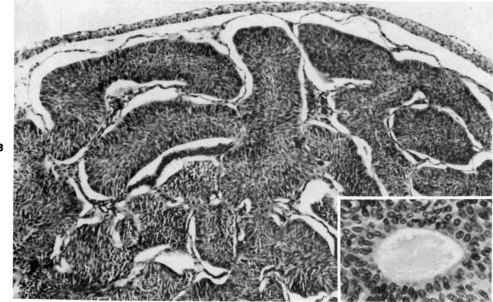

Fig. 17-77 A, Inverted papilloma of bladder. Large polypoid, but not papillary, mass protrudes in trigone. **B,** Complex anastomosing pattern of regular cells is present. Well-defined glandular space is shown in **inset.** (From Kim YH, Reiner L: Brunnian adenoma [inverted papilloma] of the urinary bladder. Report of a case. Hum Pathol **9:**229-231, 1978.)

present as a primary bladder neoplasm localized within the wall.[64] Its histologic appearance and immunohistochemical profile is the same as for paragangliomas in other sites.[77a] Approximately half of the patients reported by Albores-Saavedra et al.[56] had symptoms produced by the excessive secretion of catecholamines, sometimes associated with voiding. Two tumors were multicentric. Local recurrence was found in two patients and metastases in three, an in-

dication that these tumors should be necessarily regarded as benign.

Other rare **benign tumors** of the bladder include villous adenoma (microscopically similar to its colorectal counter-part),[58,77] mucin-secreting "cystadenoma" of possible müllerian origin,[69,81] leiomyoma,[76] hemangioma,[71] arteriovenous malformation,[78] lymphangioma,[60] granular cell tumor,[67] and neurofibroma.[62,82] The hemangiomas are usually

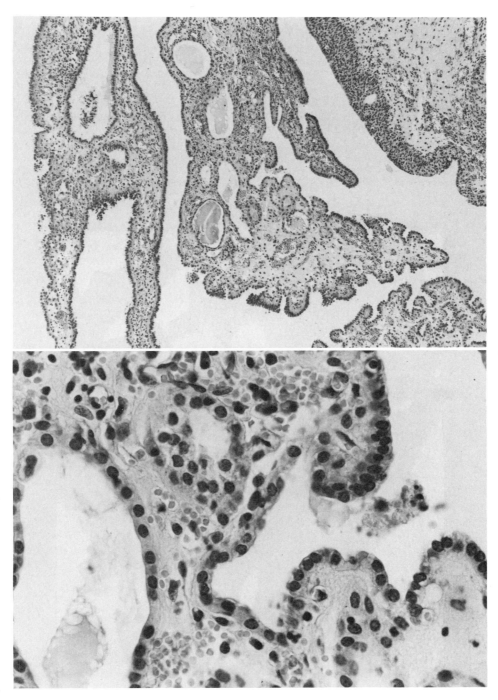

Fig. 17-78 So-called adenomatoid tumor (nephrogenic adenoma) of urinary bladder. Lesion occurred in 12-year-old boy and was very extensive. (Courtesy Dr. F. Algaba, Barcelona, Spain.)

seen in children; they are usually located in the lateral or posterior walls, are sessile, sometimes associated with cutaneous hemangiomas, and may be the cause of gross painless hematuria.[80]

TRANSITIONAL CELL CARCINOMA
General features

Transitional cell carcinoma comprises about 90% of all primary tumors of this organ. Most cases present in patients over the age of 50 years, but they can also occur in younger adults and children.[85,91] A well-known risk factor, which however accounts for only a minority of the cases, is exposure to aniline dyes, particularly benzidine and beta-naphthylamine.[84,86,94,95] It has been postulated that urinary tryptophan metabolites may be the endogenous counterparts of the carcinogenic dyes.[87,93] An increased incidence has also been reported in relation to smoking[88,90,92] and cyclophosphamide ingestion.[89,92a] Schistosomiasis is also a predisposing factor but more for epidermoid carcinoma than for transitional cell carcinoma (see p. 913).

Hematuria is the most common symptom of transitional cell carcinoma, followed by symptoms related to associated urinary tract infection. Dysuria is more often seen with high-grade tumors, perhaps as a result of involvement of the bladder wall.

Morphologic features

About 75% of transitional cell tumors of the bladder arise in the region of the trigone; as a consequence, partial or complete blockage of one or both ureters is frequent, with resulting hydronephrosis and pyelonephritis. These tumors can also be located elsewhere in the bladder mucosa. Some have been seen to arise from urachal remnants at or above the dome (see p. 898), within diverticula (see p. 898), and even from regenerated urothelium over a lyophilized dura patch.[105] Grossly, they can be papillary or nonpapillary and pedunculated or sessile, features that are related to their microscopic grade (Fig. 17-79) (see p. 905). Microscopically, they are made up of transitional cell epithelium, which differs little from the normal in grade I tumors but is hardly recognizable as such in grade IV neoplasms. Some authors sharply divide these tumors into papillary and nonpapillary (solid) types, but a frequent merging and overlap exists between the two patterns of growth.[100,102] Foci of glandular metaplasia are common. Ward[107] found that 25% to 30% had evidence of

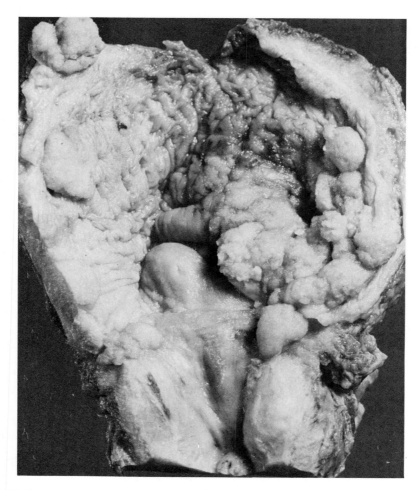

Fig. 17-79 Cystectomy specimen with papillomatous tumor involving entire bladder with area of invasion.

focal mucin production and a similar number (but not necessarily the same cases) showed some glandular formation. These tumors, sometimes designated as "mixed carcinomas," behave as conventional transitional cell cancers. A clear distinction should be made between them and the pure adenocarcinoma of the bladder (see p. 912). Similarly, many otherwise typical transitional cell cancers (especially grade III and grade IV lesions) show foci of squamous differentiation. These tumors should still be regarded as of transitional origin and clearly separated from pure epidermoid cancers (see p. 913).

Lymphocytic infiltration is sometimes seen at the interphase between tumor and stroma. Occasionally, a heavy infiltration by eosinophils is present; this seems to be particularly common in tumors with squamous features.[101]

Ultrastructurally, the high-grade tumors are accompanied by a decrease of specialized junctions;[96] pleomorphic microvilli are apparent by scanning electron microscopy regardless of tumor grade.[98]

Immunohistochemically, transitional cell carcinomas express various keratin types,[103] CEA (particularly in high-grade lesions),[99,106] and Leu-M1.[97] The blood group antigens shown by the normal urothelium may be poorly expressed or deleted in the tumors, particularly the high-grade ones, a feature of prognostic significance (see p. 911).

Biopsy

Bladder tumors should be sampled or removed with a "cold" biopsy instrument. Ideally, the biopsy should include a portion of the underlying muscle. The urologist should not fulgurate a papillary tumor without biopsy simply because it appears benign. It is true that tumors wholly composed of delicate papillary fronds are usually well differentiated, but exceptions may occur. It is recommended that, in addition to the main tumor, biopsies should be taken from apparently normal adjacent mucosa and from three other sites (one lateral to each ureteral orifice and one from the upper posterior wall).[108] These biopsies should be submitted separately and sectioned at various levels. The pathology report of a bladder biopsy that contains a tumor should include the following information:

1. Grade
2. Configuration (papillary or solid)
3. Depth of penetration
4. Presence of muscle
5. Lymphatic invasion
6. Blood vessel invasion
7. Changes in adjacent mucosa if present

Cytology

Exfoliative cytology is of little practical value in the initial evaluation of most bladder tumors because of their accessibility to formal biopsy. Exceptions are the cases associated with extensive chronic inflammation in which the biopsy may be negative because of sampling, in the detection of carcinoma in situ, and for carcinomas hidden in a bladder diverticulum. Specimens obtained from bladder irrigation are superior to those obtained from voided urine.[109]

A drawback of cytology is the fact that well-differentiated (grade I and some grade II) lesions are often overlooked because the cells are very similar to those of normal bladder mucosa.[111,114,117] Esposti et al.[110] recognized cytologically 68% of 124 cases of grade II to grade IV cancers from the first samples of urine and bladder washings. In twenty-two additional cases, "suspicious" cells were identified. The greatest value of urinary bladder cytology is in the follow-up evaluation of patients who have received surgical or radiotherapeutic treatment for bladder carcinoma.[112,118] In some cases, the recurrence may not become clinically apparent until more than a year after the malignant cells have been detected in the urine.[115,116]

Although radiation therapy may result in atypia of normal cells, a pathologist experienced with the morphology of irradiation effect and provided with accurate clinical information is unlikely to confuse these changes with those of recurrent carcinoma.[110]

Flow cytometric techniques have been developed for the evaluation of DNA abnormalities in cytologic specimens from the bladder; these have reached a degree of accuracy equivalent to that of conventional cytologic examination.[109,113]

Grading

Several systems have been proposed for the grading of transitional cell carcinoma. These are primarily based on the *cytologic appearance* of the tumor rather than its architecture or invasiveness, although an obvious correlation exists between these three parameters (Table 17-10 and Figs. 17-80 and 17-83). The most widely used grading system is still the one originally proposed by Ash in 1940.[119] He felt that even the most benign-appearing papillary tumors should be classified as carcinoma because of their great tendency to recur locally and also because the microscopic pattern does not always conform with the clinical behavior, a fact that recent series have confirmed.[122] In his scheme, the tumors are divided into four grades as follows:

Table 17-10 Comparison of three different grading systems

Ash, 1940[119]	Mostofi, 1960[123] (adopted by the American Bladder Tumor Registry)	Bergkvist et al., 1965[120]
Transitional cell carcinoma, grade I	Papilloma	Transitional cell tumor, grade 0 Transitional cell tumor, grade I
Transitional cell carcinoma, grade II	Transitional cell carcinoma, grade I	Transitional cell tumor, grade II
Transitional cell carcinoma, grade III	Transitional cell carcinoma, grade II	Transitional cell tumor, grade III
Transitional cell carcinoma, grade IV	Transitional cell carcinoma, grade III	Transitional cell tumor, grade IV

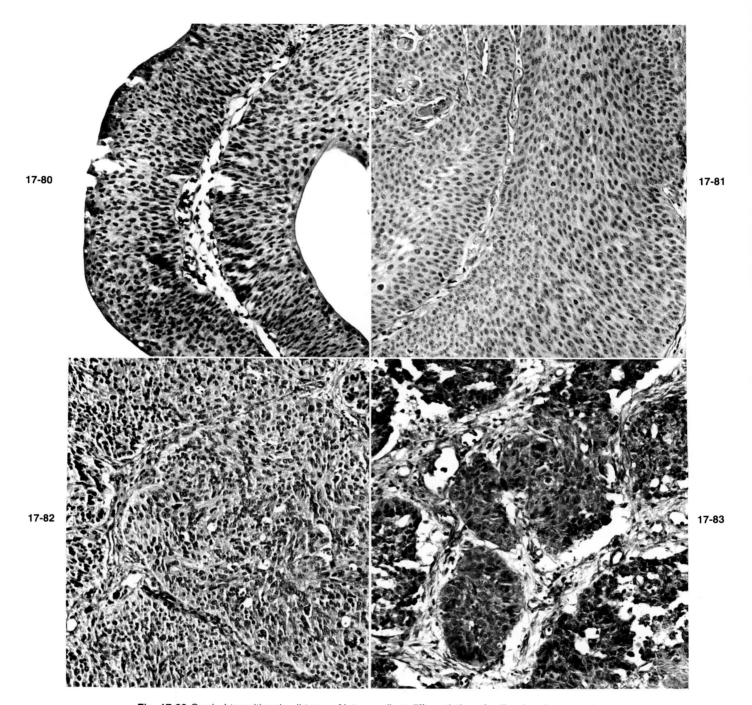

Fig. 17-80 Grade I transitional cell tumor. Note excellent differentiation of cells, abundant cytoplasm, and few mitotic figures.

Fig. 17-81 Grade II transitional cell carcinoma. Note variation in cell size, increase in prominence of cell nuclei, and numerous mitotic figures.

Fig. 17-82 Grade III transitional cell carcinoma. Note loss of any pattern with considerable cell variation.

Fig. 17-83 Grade IV transitional cell carcinoma. There is complete disorganization with extreme variation in size and shape of cells.

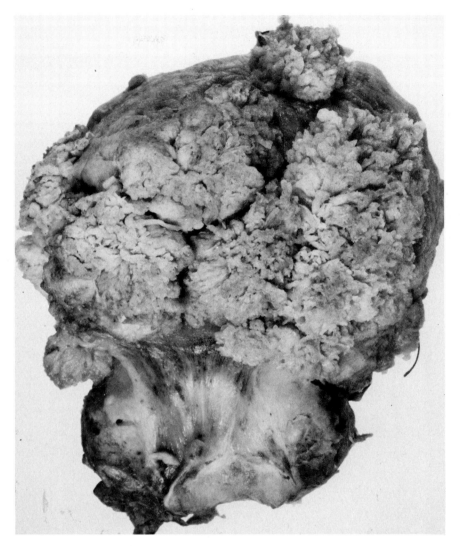

Fig. 17-84 Grade II transitional cell carcinoma involving large portion of bladder. Papillary configuration persists, but some of nodules are more solid than in grade I lesions. This was B$_1$ tumor according to Jewett's classification.

1 *Grade I.* Grossly, these tumors have a soft pink color and delicate frond-like papillary structures that cystoscopically look like ferns suspended by pedicles. The majority are pedunculated, but they may be sessile. Necrosis is extremely rare. Microscopically, regular frond-like papillae are present throughout, composed of a central fibrovascular core that is covered by a few layers of uniform transitional cells practically identical to those in the normal bladder. Mitoses are rare or absent[104] (Fig. 17-80).

2 *Grade II.* Grossly, these tumors may be pedunculated or sessile. Necrosis is rare. They differ from the preceding group by virtue of their more solid appearance and firmer consistency (Fig. 17-84). Microscopically, the papillary configuration persists, but there is more crowding and layering of cells, enlargement and hy-

perchromasia of nuclei, and more than an occasional mitotic figure (Fig. 17-81).

3 *Grade III.* Grossly, a high percentage of these tumors have a sessile, cauliflower-like appearance. Necrosis and ulceration are frequent. Microscopically, papillary areas may still be present but are irregularly distributed. The cell masses are in smaller groups, and mitotic figures are easily found (Fig. 17-82).

4 *Grade IV.* Grossly, most of these lesions are sessile, cauliflower-like, necrotic, and ulcerated (Fig. 17-85). Microscopically, papillary areas are scanty or absent. Cellular atypia and pleomorphism is so marked that the transitional cell nature of the tumor may be obscured (Fig. 17-83). Mitotic figures are frequent and often atypical. These tumors are usually widely invasive (Fig. 17-86).

In the alternative terminology proposed by Mostofi[123] and adopted by the American Bladder Tumor Registry, the better differentiated papillary tumors are designated as papillomas. Bergqvist et al.[120] wisely avoided drawing a sharp distinction between benign and malignant categories by using the designation of *transitional cell tumor* and grading them from 0 to IV. We, like them and others,[121a] prefer not to designate the grade I lesions as carcinomas.

The grading of transitional cell tumors of the bladder by any of these schemes is of great prognostic significance; however, some cautionary comments are in order. The differentiation of a given neoplasm may vary from area to area, and biopsies often show a lower degree of malignancy than

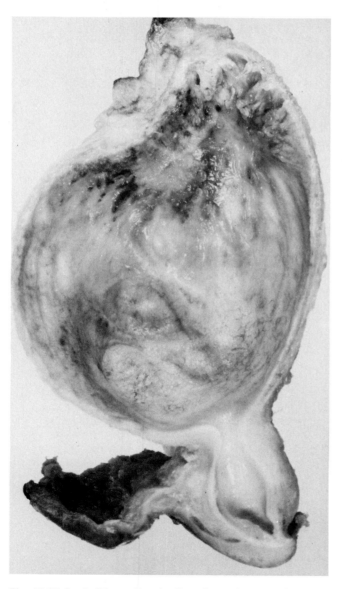

Fig. 17-85 Grade IV transitional cell carcinoma in dome of bladder. Tumor is ulcerated and deeply invasive.

is present in the surgical specimen. Obviously, if the biopsy shows a very poorly differentiated tumor, the prognosis will be poor. If, on the other hand, the tumor is well differentiated in the biopsy, it may still be poorly differentiated in other areas.[121] Whether quantitative morphometric grading will prove superior to the subjective methods currently used remains to be seen.[124]

Local spread and metastases

Invasive bladder cancers (especially high-grade tumors) are often associated with zones of atypical proliferation, carcinoma in situ, and early invasive carcinomas in areas remote from the main tumor mass (Fig. 17-87). In some instances, this atypical proliferation extends into the ureters. Thus Sharma et al.[132] detected ureteral lesions that they interpreted as carcinoma in situ in seventeen (8.5%) of 205 patients undergoing cystectomy for bladder carcinoma. The incidence was highest in patients with multifocal tumors and in those with high-stage and high-grade neoplasms. In a similar study, Schade et al.[131] found ureteral changes varying from mild atypia to early invasive carcinoma in many of the cases. Bladder carcinoma also may extend into the neck of the bladder, urethra, prostatic ducts, and seminal vesicle, perhaps even more commonly than to the ureters.[125,128,130,130a] This is responsible for the occasional instances of urethral recurrence following cystectomy for carcinoma of the bladder.[126] In view of this fact, a routine diagnostic transurethral biopsy has been recommended in the work-up of patients with in situ and high-grade bladder carcinoma.[130]

Lymph node metastases in the pelvic chains are found in 25% of the invasive tumors.[127] The most common sites of distant metastases are lungs, liver, and bone.[129]

Carcinoma in situ and dysplasia

Most cases of *carcinoma in situ* and *dysplasia* of the bladder are seen in association with conventional transitional cell carcinoma and are especially common in high-grade lesions[137,140,144,146]; in these instances, the invasive component tends to be multifocal.[134,147] In a study using giant histologic sections, Soto et al.[147] found that almost two thirds of forty-five patients with invasive cancer had adjacent carcinoma in situ.

Sometimes, carcinoma in situ is found in the bladder in the absence of an invasive component, nearly always associated with various degrees of hyperplasia and dysplasia.[135,136,141,142,148] The lesion may be asymptomatic but often presents with irritative bladder symptoms. Grossly, it has a slightly raised, granular or cobblestone appearance, and it may be accompanied by marked hyperemia. The diagnosis is made through urinary cytology and/or multiple random cold biopsies.

The microscopic criteria are essentially the same as for carcinoma in situ of other locations, notably the uterine cervix. The process is nonpapillary and is characterized by full-thickness changes (Fig. 17-88).

Sometimes the tumor cells spread along the basement membrane and lift up the normal transitional cells, resulting in a pagetoid pattern of growth.[139] The cancer cells have a great tendency to detach from the stroma; this results in a

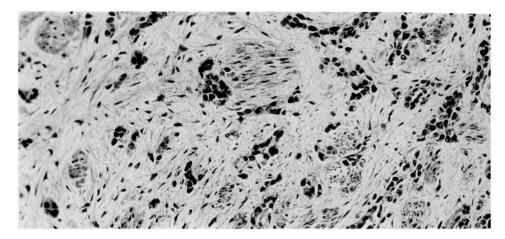

Fig. 17-86 Extensive growth of bladder carcinoma within lymphatics of bladder musculature.

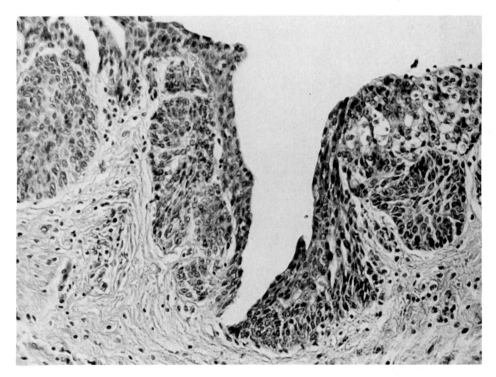

Fig. 17-87 Apparently normal bladder epithelium taken at distance from invasive carcinoma. These changes represent early carcinoma and suggest multiple foci of origin.

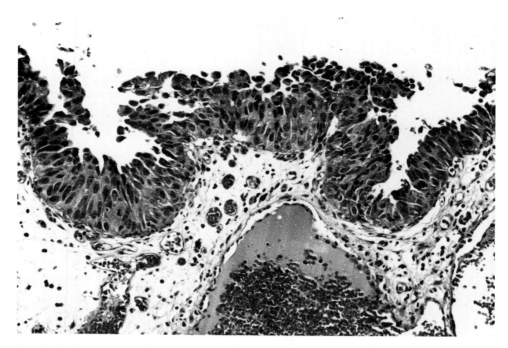

Fig. 17-88 Carcinoma in situ of bladder. Full thickness atypia is present in transitional epithelium. Underlying stroma shows marked hyperemia and edema and some degree of chronic inflammation.

typical cystoscopic appearance ("denuding cystitis") and is also the cause of false negative biopsies.[143] If the clinical suspicion is high, multiple repeat biopsies are imperative.

Of twenty-five cases of carcinoma in situ of the bladder studied by Melamed et al.,[141] eight patients subsequently developed invasive carcinoma after intervals ranging from 8 to 67 months. Seemayer et al.[145] have shown that a high proportion of patients with carcinoma in situ of the bladder have extensive intraductal prostatic involvement, a feature with obvious prognostic and therapeutic implications.

The abnormalities of blood group antigen expression[133] and DNA ploidy[138] that exist in invasive bladder carcinoma have also been documented in in situ carcinoma.

Treatment

The therapy of bladder carcinoma needs to be individualized, taking into account the age of the patient and the surgical risk; the extent, stage, and microscopic grade of the tumor; and the presence of dysplasia or carcinoma in situ elsewhere in the bladder.[160]

The recommended treatment for carcinoma in situ is total cystectomy except for small and apparently localized lesions; for these, intravesical chemotherapy may induce temporary and sometimes complete remission[152,158,165]; however, in 40% to 70% of the cases, new tumors will develop, usually within a 6-month to 12-month period.[163]

Grade I and grade II transitional cell tumors without muscle invasion usually are treated with transurethral resection; this is sometimes supplemented with intravesical chemo-

therapy or radiation therapy, especially in cases of multiple or recurrent tumors.[149,153a,159,164] Grades III and IV transitional cell tumors and tumors with muscle invasion irrespective of grade are best treated by radical cystectomy, with or without preoperative radiation therapy or chemotherapy.[156,161,162] In a few centers, they have also been treated by radiation alone.[166] The radiation tends to obliterate the superficial papillary component of the tumor but has little discernable effect in the invasive component; it also leads to an increased nuclear pleomorphism and induces metaplastic squamous changes.[157]

Radical cystectomy in the male includes the bladder, prostate, seminal vesicles, and the adjacent perivesical tissues; in the female, it includes the bladder, uterus, tubes, ovaries, anterior vagina, and urethra. At present, operative mortality for this procedure is low, and pyelonephritis is no longer a frequent complication if conduit ureteral diversion is accomplished by implantation of the ureters into an isolated segment of the ileum.[150,153]

Segmental (partial) cystectomy has fallen into disfavor because of the high rate of recurrence in the residual bladder. There is no convincing evidence that adding a pelvic lymphadenectomy to the cystectomy procedure improves survival, and argument persists as to whether an urethrectomy should be part of the procedure.[151] Another controversial form of treatment is intravesical immunotherapy with the Calmette-Guerin bacillus, which in some series has shown remarkable reduction of the tumor recurrence rate[155]; microscopically, this therapy results in superficial mucosal erosion, submu-

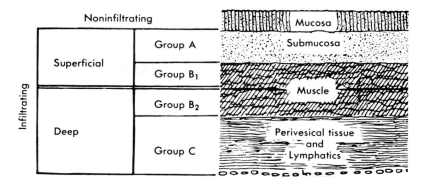

Fig. 17-89 Schematic representation of depth of invasion of bladder cancer. More superficial the tumor, better the prognosis. (From Jewett HJ: Carcinoma of the bladder. Influence of depth of infiltration of the five-year results following complete extirpation of the primary growth. J Urol **67**:672-680, 1952.)

cosal granulomatous inflammation, and reactive epithelial atypia.[154]

Prognosis

The prognosis of bladder carcinoma is related to many parameters:

1 *Stage* is by far the most important prognostic determinator, as the pioneer studies of Jewett, among others, have demonstrated[168,184,185,202] (Fig. 17-89). Several staging systems have been proposed as modifications of his original scheme. The sharp decrease in survival associated with invasion of the muscle wall is possibly a result of the access that the tumor thus gains into the rich vascular network present at this level. The importance of this feature makes it imperative for the pathologist to state whether there is muscle in a biopsy specimen and, if so, whether it is invaded by tumor.[178] It should be realized that smooth muscle bundles may be present in the lamina propria, occasionally forming a veritable muscularis mucosae.[202a] Although extension of tumor in perivesical tissues is a very poor prognostic sign, long-term cures have been achieved in some of these patients.[174] The current overall 5-year survival rate for deeply invasive bladder cancer (B_2 and C) is between 45% and 55%.[204]

2 *Lymph node involvement*, which is actually incorporated into the staging scheme, is an ominous prognostic sign. The long-term survival rate of these patients is nearly zero.[174]

3 *Microscopic grade* is related to the stage, in the sense that most grade I and II tumors are superficial, whereas many grade III and IV tumors are deeply invasive[190]; however, grading has prognostic value within a given stage.[179,181,186,200] For the grade I lesions ("papillomas"), the recurrence rate following local excision is about 30% to 35% if tumors are solitary and 65% to 75% if they are multiple.[192,197] In about 10% of the cases, the recurrence shows a higher grade than the original lesion. These "recurrences," which may be the result of implantation or multicentric growth, are particularly common in the bladder vault.[170] It should be pointed out that, important as

these low-grade noninvasive tumors are in the development of invasive high-grade neoplasms, the large majority of the latter do not have a history of preceding noninvasive malignancy.[171,189]

4 *Patient's age*. The few tumors presenting during the first two decades of life are usually well differentiated and noninvasive and are therefore associated with an excellent prognosis.[183]

5 *Location*. Tumors located in the dome or anterior surface of the bladder have a worse prognosis than those located at the base.

6 *Abnormalities in the remaining bladder mucosa*. Presence of smaller, independent tumors or dysplastic changes away from the main tumor mass are related to a high recurrence rate.*

7 *Vascular invasion*, as determined microscopically in either lymph vessels or blood vessels, is associated with an increased rate of recurrence.[169,182]

8 Type of *tumor margin* and *inflammatory response*. Tumors with pushing margins associated with lymphocytic reaction have a better prognosis.[203]

9 *Status of blood group antigens*. ABH and Lewis antigens are normally expressed by the urothelial mucosa but may be markedly reduced or absent in tumors, particularly high-grade ones.[188,194,196,200a] This deletion can be evaluated by the red cell adherence test, immunofluorescence, or immunoperoxidase.[173,196,208] It appears to correlate with an aggressive clinical course, in the form of increased probability of recurrence and the acquisition of invasive features.[187,196,206] Some of the conflicting results among different series may be attributed to methodologic factors.[193] Radiation therapy has been found to induce false-positive results.[167,210] Along related lines, expression of T (Thomsen-Friedenreich) antigen as a result of unmasking has been found to correlate with the presence of invasion and a higher risk of lymph node involvement.[191,195,207]

10 *DNA distribution* as determined by flow cytometry promises to become a powerful tool for the prognostic

---

*See references 176, 181, 197, 201, 205, and 209.

evaluation and perhaps the diagnosis of bladder cancer, judging from preliminary results obtained in recent years.[172,177,180,198] A high degree of correlation between DNA ploidy, microscopic grade, and clinical outcome has been observed.[199] Flow cytometry has also been used for the detection of Ca antigen, a cell surface determinant associated with invasive bladder tumors.[175]

OTHER PRIMARY CARCINOMAS
Adenocarcinoma

Bladder adenocarcinomas constitute about 2% of the malignant tumors of this organ. Most develop from sequential changes initiated by chronic inflammation—from Brunn's islands, to cystitis glandularis and cystica, and, finally, to adenocarcinoma, which is usually mucin-secreting.[225] The tumors arising on this basis are usually located in the trigone area.[216] Other adenocarcinomas arise in bladders with exstrophy[214] (Figs. 17-90 to 17-92) or at the dome of the bladder from urachal remnants[217] (see p. 898) (Fig. 17-93).

Seventeen of the forty-four cases of bladder adenocarcinoma reported by Mostofi et al.[216] were thought to arise from the latter.

Grossly, advanced cases appear as fungating masses that ulcerate the mucosa and invade the bladder wall. The surface or the mucin-producing tumors is covered with thick, slimy, gelatinous material.[224] Microscopically, there is a wide range of glandular differentiation.[212] Deep invasion of the muscle is the rule, but very superficial examples of this tumor have been observed.[218] The mucin histochemical profile is similar to that of colorectal adenocarcinoma.[211,226] Some tumors have been found to contain Paneth cells and endocrine cells.[219,222] Focal positivity for prostatic acid phosphatase has been found in a few cases (perhaps as the result of cross reactivity) but not for prostate-specific antigen.[215]

It should be pointed out that focal mucin positivity is not an uncommon finding in transitional cell carcinoma of the bladder; the term *adenocarcinoma* should be reserved for those malignant tumors in which the glandular component predominates.[212] The overall prognosis is poor: in one series

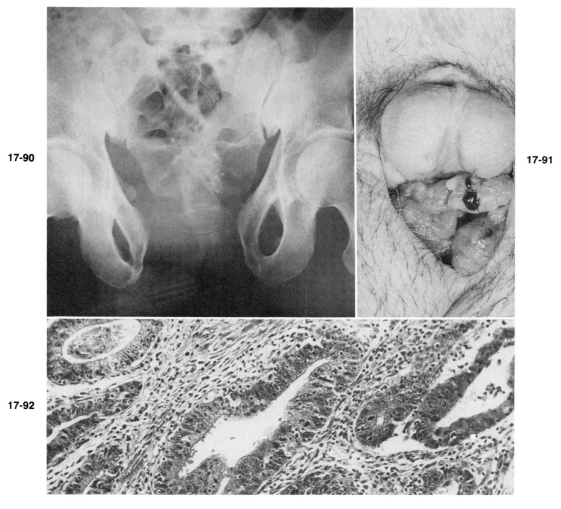

17-90

17-91

17-92

Fig. 17-90 Pelvis in patient with exstrophy of bladder showing typical separation of symphysis pubis.
Fig. 17-91 Exstrophy of bladder with carcinoma arising from it.
Fig. 17-92 Same tumor shown in Fig. 17-91. It is well-differentiated adenocarcioma.

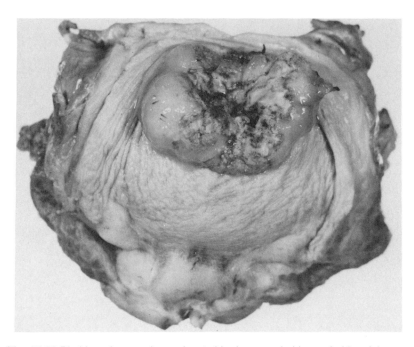

Fig. 17-93 Bladder adenocarcinoma located in dome, probably urachal in origin.

of sixty-four cases, the 5-year survival was only 18%.[212] The pattern and frequency of metastases are similar to those of high-grade, conventional transitional cell carcinoma.

A distinct variant of bladder adenocarcinoma is the *clear cell (mesonephric, mesonephroid) type*, which can also occur in the urethra.[227] The tumor is usually papillary and is characterized microscopically by a mixture of tubular glands, papillae, cysts, and areas of solid growth. Two of its most distinguishing features are hobnail cells and abundant cytoplasmic glycogen.[227] This lesion is distinguished from the more common adenomatoid tumor (nephrogenic adenoma) on the basis of clinical, gross, and microscopic features; sheets of clear cells, marked pleomorphism, and mitotic activity favor a diagnosis of malignancy.[227,228]

Another distinct type of adenocarcinoma is *signet ring carcinoma*.[221,223] The pattern of infiltration of the bladder wall is diffuse, similar to that seen in signet ring carcinoma (linitis plastica) of the stomach.[220] The clinical course of the disease has been rapidly progressive and fatal in nearly all the reported cases with follow-up information.[213]

Small cell carcinoma and related "neuroendocrine" tumors

Like most other organs, the urinary bladder can be the site of tumors exhibiting various degrees of endocrine differentiation. The most common manifestation is the presence of scattered endocrine cells in what is otherwise a typical adenocarcinoma; these tumors behave like other adenocarcinomas and should be labeled as such. Another is an exceptionally rare *carcinoid tumor* of the bladder, which exhibits typical architectural features and numerous dense core granules on ultrastructural examination.[230] Yet another is the highly malignant bladder tumor known as *small cell carcinoma*, which is morphologically sim-

ilar to its homonyms in the lung and other organs (Fig. 17-94). This may be seen in a pure form or combined with in situ or invasive transitional cell carcinoma, adenocarcinoma, epidermoid carcinoma, or sarcomatoid carcinoma.[229,232,233] Microscopically, small cells with very hyperchromatic nuclei and extremely scanty cytoplasm are seen growing in a predominantly solid fashion, sometimes associated with occasional rosette formation. Dense-core granules can be demonstrated ultrastructurally but usually in small numbers and with some difficulty.[231,233] Staining for neuron-specific enolase may be positive.[233] Some of these cases have been associated with hypercalcemia[235] or ectopic ACTH production.[234] The behavior is extremely aggressive.[232]

Epidermoid carcinoma

Epidermoid carcinoma comprises approximately 5% of all bladder tumors. Some of these tumors arise on a background of chronic cystitis with marked squamous metaplasia, a condition sometimes designated as *leukoplakia*[237,242,243] (Figs. 17-95 to 17-97). Some cases have been reported in patients who had received cyclophosphamide for prolonged periods.[245] A well-known but still controversial association, reported from Egypt and other countries, is with schistosomiasis.[238,240] Some epidermoid carcinomas of the bladder probably represent squamous metaplastic changes in tumors that were originally of transitional cell type.

Since focal squamous cell changes are common in high-grade transitional cell tumors, the term *epidermoid carcinoma* should be reserved for those tumors that are squamous throughout.

Grossly, these tumors are usually large, ulcerated, and necrotic. Microscopically, most are poorly differentiated

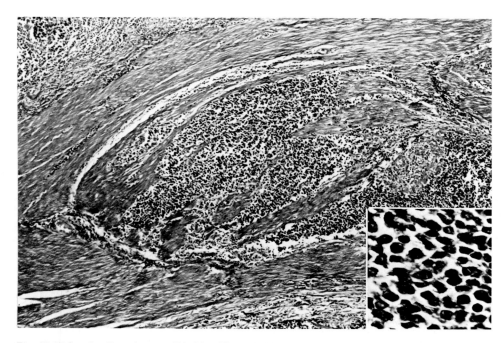

Fig. 17-94 Small cell carcinoma of bladder diffusely infiltrating muscle wall. Inset shows cellular features of tumor, which are identical to those of small cell carcinoma of lung.

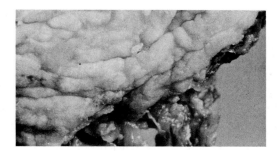

Fig. 17-95 Prominent squamous metaplasia of bladder. Note plaque-like areas of piled-up epithelium. This is lesion often referred to as "leukoplakia."

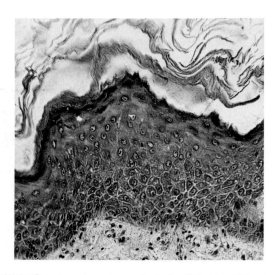

Fig. 17-96 Extreme squamous metaplasia of bladder. Lining is made of stratified squamous epithelium.

(Fig. 17-98) and have nearly always invaded the muscle at the time of diagnosis.[241,244] The prognosis is very poor regardless of the degree of differentiation.[236] Death within the first year occurred in 59% of the patients reviewed by Newman et al.[241]; in another series, the 5-year survival rate was 37% for patients with submucosal or muscular invasion and 13% for those with perivesical invasion.[239]

Sarcomatoid carcinoma

Sarcomatoid carcinoma (also known as spindle cell carcinoma and carcinosarcoma) is a high-grade malignancy of the bladder in which a malignant epithelial component (of transitional, glandular, squamous, or undifferentiated type) coexists with areas having a sarcomatous appearance[248,254] (Figs. 17-99 and 17-100). The latter may have a nonspecific spindle-cell or pleomorphic look (sometimes with osteoclast-like giant cells)[251] or may exhibit specific features of differentiation, such as rhabdomyosarcoma, chondrosarcoma, or osteosarcoma.[252,257] Transitions are sometimes seen between the two components, suggesting that the sarcoma-like areas are also of epithelial nature, hence the synonym "carcinoma with sarcoma-like stroma," which is sometimes applied to them.[249] Further evidence of the epithelial nature of these proliferations is provided by the immunoreactivity for keratin often detected in them.[256a]

Grossly, these tumors are often large and polypoid. They are equivalent in every respect to the more common ones located in the upper aerodigestive tract[249]; as in those, the obvious epithelial component is sometimes present only in the form of carcinoma in situ on the surface and at the periphery of the invasive sarcoma-like tumor.[247] Most patients are elderly males and the death rate is about 50%.[257]

Metastases occur in regional lymph nodes and distantly; they may consist of only the epithelial or the sarcoma-like component.[256]

A bladder malignancy somewhat analogous to carcinosarcoma is the rare transitional cell carcinoma with areas having morphologic and immunohistochemical features of *choriocarcinoma* and which is sometimes accompanied by

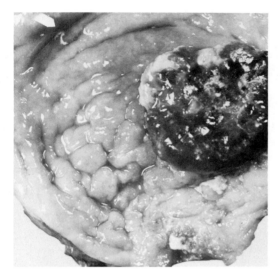

Fig. 17-97 Epidermoid carcinoma of bladder with leukoplakia.

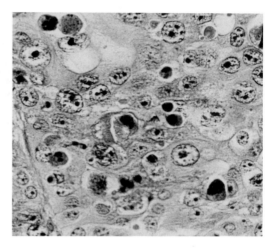

Fig. 17-98 Poorly differentiated epidermoid carcinoma of bladder.

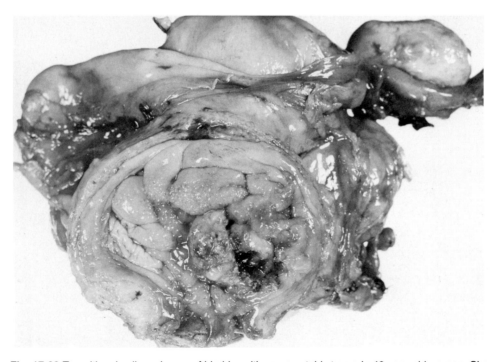

Fig. 17-99 Transitional cell carcinoma of bladder with sarcomatoid stroma in 40-year-old woman. She was alive and well 10 years later.

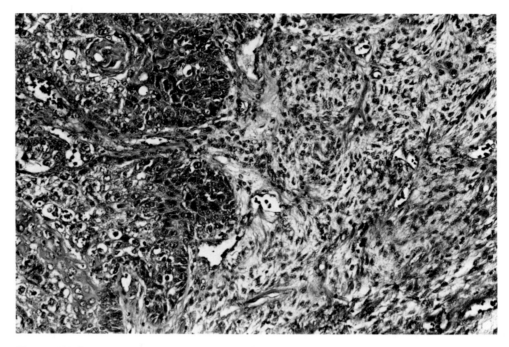

Fig. 17-100 Sarcomatoid carcinoma of bladder. Sharp separation exists between clearly identifiable epithelial component and sarcoma-like elements.

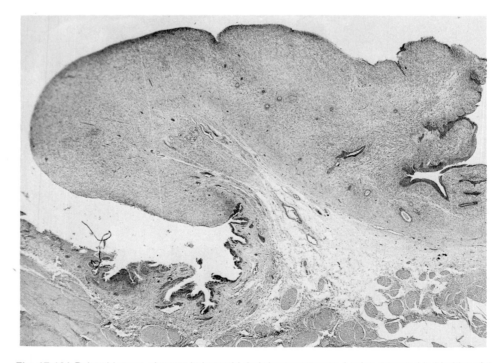

Fig. 17-101 Polypoid mass of tumor in botryoid rhabdomyosarcoma. Lesion occurred in bladder of 4-year-old boy.

serum elevations of HCG.[246,253,255] Some transitional cell cancers are associated with immunohistochemical reactivity for this marker and other placental glycoproteins even if they lack identifiable foci of choriocarcinoma.[250]

OTHER MALIGNANT TUMORS

Embryonal rhabdomyosarcoma (particularly the botryoid subtype) is the most common malignant tumor of the bladder in children.[269] Sporadic cases have been seen in association with Wilms' tumor; one such case was reported in a child with Dandy-Walker syndrome.[266] The trigone is the most common location. Grossly, it has a mucoid, polypoid appearance. It infiltrates surrounding tissues, but distant metastases are rare. Microscopically, it shows myxomatous tissue in which small malignant cells are seen (Fig. 17-101). These are characteristically grouped beneath the epithelium (the "cambium layer"). Cross striations may or may not be present. Traditionally, the prognosis has been poor, with isolated cures being achieved with radical cystectomy or radiation therapy.[268] The addition of multidrug chemotherapy to these modalities has notably increased the survival rates, even when the surgical resection was incomplete.[264]

Sarcomas of the adult prostate include leiomyosarcoma,[273] the myxoid variant of this tumor,[277] rhabdomyosarcoma,[267] rhabdoid tumor,[263a] malignant fibrous histiocytoma[262] and its inflammatory variant,[265] osteosarcoma,[260,278] and malignant mesenchymoma.[274a] Care should be exercised to rule out by appropriate sampling and immunohistochemical testing the alternative possibility of a sarcomatoid carcinoma (carcinosarcoma)[265] (see p. 914).

Primary *malignant melanoma* can occur in the bladder,[258,259] although not so commonly as in the urethra or as metastases in the bladder from a melanoma arisen elsewhere.[270]

Cases of primary *malignant lymphoma* have been described.[275] The lesions may be solitary or multiple; they are covered by a normal mucosa and tend to remain localized for a long period of time. The bladder also can be involved by *leukemia*,[271] *plasmacytoma*,[276] and *Hodgkin's disease*.[261]

A case of *yolk sac tumor* (endodermal sinus tumor) of the bladder has been described in a 1-year-old child.[274]

Most cases of *metastatic tumors* in the bladder are from breast carcinoma[263,272] and malignant melanoma.[270]

REFERENCES

Urachus and urachal lesions

1 Eble JN, Hull MT, Rowland RG, Hostetter M: Villous adenoma of the urachus with mucusuria. A light and electron microscopic study. J Urol 135:1240-1244, 1986.
2 Jimi A, Munaoka H, Sato S, Iwata Y: Squamous cell carcinoma of the urachus. A case report and review of literature. Acta Pathol Jpn 36:945-952, 1986.
3 Schubert GE, Pavkovic MB, Bethke-Bedürftig BA: Tubular urachal remnants in adult bladders. J Urol 127:40-42, 1982.
4 Steck WD, Helwig EB: Umbilical granulomas, pilonidal disease, and the urachus. Surg Gynecol Obstet 120:1043-1057, 1965.

EXSTROPHY

5 Engel RM, Wilkinson HA: Bladder exstrophy. J Urol 104:699-704, 1970.

DIVERTICULOSIS

6 Abeshouse BS, Goldstein AE: Primary carcinoma in a diverticulum of the bladder. A report of four cases and a review of the literature. J Urol 49:534-557, 1943.

7 Faysal MH, Freiha FS: Primary neoplasm in vesical diverticula. A report of 12 cases. Br J Urol 53:141-143, 1981.
8 Fox M, Power RF, Bruce AW: Diverticulum of the bladder. Presentation and evaluation of treatment of 115 cases. Br J Urol 34:286-298, 1962.
9 Kretschmer HL: Diverticula of the urinary bladder. A clinical study of 236 cases. Surg Gynecol Obstet 71:491-503, 1940.
10 McCormick SR, Dodds PR, Kraus PA, Lowell DM: Nonepithelial neoplasms arising within vesical diverticula. Urology 25:405-408, 1985.
11 Mitchell RJ, Hamilton SG: Spontaneous perforation of bladder diverticula. Br J Surg 58:712, 1971.
12 Shirai T, Arai M, Sakata T, Fukushima S, Ito N: Primary carcinomas of urinary bladder diverticula. Acta Pathol Jpn 34:417-424, 1984.

LITHIASIS

13 Wishard WN, Nourse MH: Vesical calculus with report of a gigantic stone in the female bladder. J Urol 63:794-801, 1950.

ENDOMETRIOSIS

14 Fein RL, Horton BF: Vesical endometriosis. A case report and review of the literature. J Urol 95:45-50, 1966.
15 Lichtenheld FR, McCauley RT, Staples PP: Endometriosis involving the urinary tract. A collective review. Obstet Gynecol 17:762-768, 1961.
16 Vermesh M, Zbella EA, Menchaca A, Confino E, Lipshitz S: Vesical endometriosis following bladder injury. Am J Obstet Gynecol 153:894-895, 1985.

AMYLOIDOSIS

17 Fujihara S, Glenner GG: Primary localized amyloidosis of the genitourinary tract. Immunohistochemical study on eleven cases. Lab Invest 44:55-60, 1981.
18 Lipper S, Kahn LB: Amyloid tumor. A clinicopathologic study of four cases. Am J Surg Pathol 2:141-145, 1978.
19 Malek RS, Greene LF, Farrow GM: Amyloidosis of the urinary bladder. Br J Urol 43:189-200, 1971.

CYSTITIS
Interstitial (Hunner's) cystitis

20 Hunner GL: A rare type of bladder ulcer in women. Report of cases. Trans South Surg Gynecol Assoc 27:247-288, 1914.
21 Johansson SL, Fall M: The spectrum of light microscopic changes in the bladders of patients with interstitial cystitis (abstract). Lab Invest 58:43A, 1988.
22 Larsen S, Thompson SA, Hald T, Barnard RJ, Gilpin CJ, Dixon JS, Gosling JA: Mast cells in interstitial cystitis. Br J Urol 54:283-286, 1982.
23 Smith BH, Dehner LP: Chronic ulcerating interstitial cystitis (Hunner's ulcer). A study of 28 cases. Arch Pathol 93:76-81, 1972.

Eosinophilic cystitis

24 Antonakopoulos GN, Newman J: Eosinophilic cystitis with giant cells. A light microscopic and ultrastructural study. Arch Pathol Lab Med 108:728-731, 1984.
25 Hellstrom HR, David BK, Shonnard JW: Eosinophilic cystitis. A study of 16 cases. Am J Clin Pathol 72:777-784, 1979.
26 Marshall FF, Middleton AW Jr: Eosinophilic cystitis. J Urol 112:335-337, 1974.

Polypoid cystitis

27 Ekelund P, Johansson S: Polypoid cystitis. A catheter associated lesion of the human bladder. Acta Pathol Microbiol Scand [A] 87:179-184, 1979.

Cystitis emphysematosa

28 Rocca JM, McClure J: Cystitis emphysematosa. Br J Urol 57:585-596, 1985.

Cystitis glandularis and cystitis cystica

29 Bell TE, Wendel RG: Cystitis glandularis. Benign or malignant? J Urol 100:462-465, 1968.
30 Bullock PS, Thoni DE, Murphy WM: The significance of colonic mucosa (intestinal metaplasia) involving the urinary tract. Cancer 59:2086-2090, 1987.
31 Kroovand RL, Chang C-H, Broecker BH, Perrin EV, Oldford J, Perlmutter AD: Epithelial lesions of bladder mucosa following ureteral reimplantation. J Urol 126:822-823, 1981.
32 Lapertosa G, Baracchini P, Fulcheri E, Tanzi R: O-acetylated sialic acid variants in intestinal glandular metaplasia of the urinary tract. Histopathology 10:707-712, 1986.
33 Walther MM, Campbell WG Jr, O'Brien DP III, Wheatley JK, Graham SD Jr: Cystitis cystica. An electron and immunofluorescence microscopic study. J Urol 137:764-768, 1987.
34 Wiener DP, Koss LG, Sablay B, Freed SZ: The prevalence and significance of Brunn's nests, cystitis cystica and squamous metaplasia in normal bladders. J Urol 122:317-321, 1979.

Tuberculosis

35 Auerbach O: The pathology of urogenital tuberculosis. Int Clin **3:**21-61, 1940.

Malakoplakia

36 Biggar WD, Crawford L, Cardella C, Bear RA, Gladman D, Reynolds WJ: Malakoplakia and immunosuppressive therapy. Reversal of clinical and leukocyte abnormalities after withdrawal of prednisone and azathioprine. Am J Pathol **119:**5-11, 1985.

37 Bleisch VR, Konikov NF: Malakoplakia of urinary bladder. Report of four cases and discussion of etiology. Arch Pathol **54:**388-397, 1952.

38 Brown RC, Smith BH: Malakoplakia of the testis. Am J Clin Pathol **47:**135-147, 1967.

39 Lewin KJ, Fair WR, Steigbigel RT, Winberg CD, Drolier MJ: Clinical and laboratory studies into the pathogenesis of malacoplakia. J Clin Pathol **29:**354-363, 1976.

40 Lou TY, Teplitz C: Malakoplakia: pathogenesis and ultrastructural morphogenesis. A problem of altered macrophage (phagolysosomal) response. Hum Pathol **5:**191-207, 1974.

41 McClure J, Cameron CHS, Garrett R: The ultrastructural features of malakoplakia. J Pathol **134:**13-25, 1981.

42 McClurg FV, D'Agostino AN, Martin JH, Race GJ: Ultrastructural demonstration of intracellular bacteria in three cases of malakoplakia of the bladder. Am J Clin Pathol **60:**780-788, 1973.

43 Moore WM III, Stokes TL, Cabanas VY: Malakoplakia of the skin. Report of a case. Am J Clin Pathol **59:**218-221, 1973.

44 Qualman SJ, Gupta PK, Mendelsohn G: Intracellular *Escherichia coli* in urinary malakoplakia. A reservoir of infection and its therapeutic implications. Am J Clin Pathol **81:**35-42, 1984.

45 Smith BH: Malacoplakia of the urinary tract. Am J Clin Pathol **43:**409-417, 1965.

46 Stanton MJ, Maxted W: Malacoplakia. A study of the literature and current concepts of pathogenesis, diagnosis and treatment. J Urol **125:**139-146, 1981.

47 Streem SB: Genitourinary malacoplakia in renal transplant recipients: pathogenic, prognostic and therapeutic considerations. J Urol **132:**10-12, 1984.

48 Terner JH, Lattes R: Malakoplakia of the colon and retroperitoneum. Am J Clin Pathol **44:**20-31, 1965.

49 Thorning D, Vracko R: Malakoplakia. Defect in digestion of phagocytized material due to impaired vacuolar acidification? Arch Pathol **99:**456-460, 1975.

50 Walther M, Glenn JF, Vellinos F: Xanthogranulomatous cystitis. J Urol **134:**745-746, 1985.

51 Yunis EJ, Estevez J, Pinzon GJ, Moran TJ: Malakoplakia. Discussion of pathogenesis and report of three cases including one of fatal gastric and colonic involvement. Arch Pathol **83:**180-187, 1967.

Other forms of cystitis

51a Young RH: Pseudoneoplastic lesions of the urinary bladder. Pathol Annu **23**(Pt 1):67-104, 1988.

TUMOR-LIKE CONDITIONS

51b Del Mistro A, Koss LG, Braunstein J, Bennett B, Saccomano G, Simons KM: Condylomata acuminata of the urinary bladder. Natural history, viral typing, and DNA content. Am J Surg Pathol **12:**205-215, 1988.

52 Nochomovitz LE, Orenstein JM: Inflammatory pseudotumor of the urinary bladder. Possible relationship to nodular fasciitis. Two case reports, cytologic observations, and ultrastructural observations. Am J Surg Pathol **9:**366-373, 1985.

53 Proppe KH, Scully RE, Rosai J: Postoperative spindle cell nodules of genitourinary tract resembling sarcomas. A report of eight cases. Am J Surg Pathol **8:**101-108, 1984.

53a Sørensen FB, Marcussen N: Iatrogenic granulomas of the prostate and the urinary bladder. Pathol Res Pract **182:**822-830, 1987.

54 Spagnolo DV, Waring PM: Bladder granulomata after bladder surgery. Am J Clin Pathol **86:**430-437, 1986.

55 Young RH, Scully RE: Pseudosarcomatous lesions of the urinary bladder, prostate gland, and urethra. A report of three cases and review of the literature. Arch Pathol Lab Med **111:**354-358, 1987.

BENIGN TUMORS

56 Albores-Saavedra J, Maldonado ME, Ibarra J, Rodriguez H: Pheochromocytoma of the urinary bladder. Cancer **23:**1110-1118, 1969.

57 Anderström C, Johansson S, Pettersson S: Inverted papilloma of the urinary tract. J Urol **127:**1132-1134, 1982.

58 Assor D: A villous tumor of the bladder. J Urol **119:**287-288, 1978.

59 Bhagavan BS, Tiamson EM, Wenk RE, Berger BW, Hamamoto G, Eggleston JC: Nephrogenic adenoma of the urinary bladder and urethra. Hum Pathol **12:**907-916, 1981.

60 Bolkier M, Ginesin Y, Lichtig C, Levin DR: Lymphangioma of bladder. J Urol **129:**1049-1050, 1983.

61 Caro DJ, Tessler A: Inverted papilloma of the bladder. A distinct urological lesion. Cancer **42:**708-713, 1978.

62 Charron JW, Gariepy G: Neurofibromatosis of bladder. Case report and review of literature. Can J Surg **13:**303-306, 1970.

63 Christoffersen J, Møller JE: Adenomatoid tumours of the urinary bladder. Scand J Urol Nephrol **6:**295-298, 1972.

64 Davaris P, Petraki K, Arvanitis D, Papacharalammpous N, Morakis A, Zorzos S: Urinary bladder paraganglioma (U.B.P.). Pathol Res Pract **181:**101-105, 1986.

65 DeMeester L, Farrow GH, Utz DS: Inverted papilloma of the urinary bladder. Cancer **36:**505-513, 1975.

66 Devine P, Ucci AA, Krain H, Gavris VE, Bhagavan BS, Heaney JA, Alroy J: Nephrogenic adenoma and embryonic kidney tubules share PNA receptor sites. Am J Clin Pathol **81:**728-732, 1984.

67 Fletcher MS, Aker M, Hill JT, Pryor JP, Whimster WF: Granular cell myoblastoma of the bladder. Br J Urol **57:**109-110, 1985.

68 Ford TF, Watson GM, Cameron KM: Adenomatous metaplasia (nephrogenic adenoma) of urothelium. An analysis of 70 cases. J Urol **57:**427-433, 1985.

69 Goven ADT: A case of solitary mucus-secreting cystadenoma of the urinary bladder. J Pathol Bacteriol **58:**293-295, 1946.

70 Henderson DW, Allen PW, Bourne AJ: Inverted urinary papilloma. Report of five cases and review of the literature. Virchows Arch [Pathol Anat] **336:**177-186, 1975.

71 Hendry WF, Vinnicombe J: Haemangioma of bladder in children and young adults. Br J Urol **43:**209-216, 1971.

72 Kay R, Lattanzi C: Nephrogenic adenoma in children. J Urol **133:**99-101, 1985.

73 Kim YH, Reiner L: Brunnian adenoma (inverted papilloma) of the urinary bladder. Report of a case. Hum Pathol **9:**229-231, 1978.

74 Kunze E, Schauer A, Schmitt M: Histology and histogenesis of two different types of inverted urothelial papillomas. Cancer **51:**348-358, 1983.

75 Lazarevic B, Garret R: Inverted papilloma and papillary transitional cell carcinoma of urinary bladder. Report of four cases of inverted papilloma, one showing papillary malignant transformation and review of the literature. Cancer **42:**1904-1911, 1978.

76 McLucas B, Stein JJ: Bladder leiomyoma. A rare cause of pelvic pain. Am J Obstet Gynecol **153:**896, 1985.

77 Miller DC, Gang DL, Gavris V, Alroy J, Ucci AA, Parkhurst EC: Villous adenoma of the urinary bladder. A morphologic or biologic entity? Am J Clin Pathol **79:**728-731, 1983.

77a Moyana TN, Kontozoglou T: Urinary bladder paragangliomas. An immunohistochemical study. Arch Pathol Lab Med **112:**70-72, 1988.

78 Nuovo GJ, Nagler HM, Fenoglio JJ Jr: Arteriovenous malformation of the bladder presenting as gross hematuria. Hum Pathol **17:**94-97, 1986.

78a Paulson J, Metwalli N, Wu P, Nochomovitz L: Transitional cell carcinoma of bladder with features of inverted papilloma (abstract). Lab Invest **58:**71A, 1988.

79 Ritchey ML, Novicki DE, Schultenover SJ: Nephrogenic adenoma of bladder. A report of 8 cases. J Urol **131:**537-539, 1984.

80 Sarma DP, Weiner M: Hemangioma of the urinary bladder. J Surg Oncol **24:**142-144, 1983.

81 Steele AA, Byrne AJ: Paramesonephric (müllerian) sinus of urinary bladder. Am J Surg Pathol **6:**173-176, 1982.

82 Winfield HN, Catalona WJ: An isolated plexiform neurofibroma of the bladder. J Urol **134:**542-543, 1985.

83 Young RH, Scully RE: Nephrogenic adenoma. A report of 15 cases, review of the literature, and comparison with clear cell adenocarcinoma of the urinary tract. Am J Surg Pathol **10:**268-275, 1986.

TRANSITIONAL CELL CARCINOMA
General features

84 Anthony HM, Thomas GA: Tumors of the urinary bladder. An analysis of the occupations of 1,030 patients in Leeds, England. J Natl Cancer Inst **45:**879-895, 1970.

85 Benson RC Jr, Tomera KM, Kelalis PP: Transitional cell carcinoma of the bladder in children and adolescents. J Urol **130:**54-55, 1983.

86 Bonser GM, Faulds JS, Stewart MJ: Occupational cancer of the urinary bladder in dyestuffs operatives and of the lung in asbestos textile workers and iron-ore miners. Am J Clin Pathol **25:**126-134, 1955.

87 Bryan GT: The role of urinary tryptophan metabolites in the etiology of bladder cancer. Am J Clin Nutr **24:**841-847, 1971.

88 Friedell GH: National bladder cancer conference. Cancer Res **37:**2737-2969, 1977.

89 Fuchs EF, Kay R, Poole R, Barry JM, Pearse HD: Uroepithelial carcinoma in association with cyclophosphamide ingestion. J Urol **126**:544, 1981.

90 Glashan RW, Cartwright RA: Occupational bladder cancer and cigarette smoking in West Yorkshire. Br J Urol **53**:602-604, 1981.

91 Javadpour N, Mostofi FK: Primary epithelial tumors of the bladder in the first two decades of life. J Urol **101**:706-710, 1969.

92 Morrison AS, Buring JE, Verhoek WG, Aoki K, Leck I, Ohno Y, Obata K: An international study of smoking and bladder cancer. J Urol **131**:650-654, 1984.

92a Pedersen-Bjergaard J, Ersbøll J, Hansen VL, Sørensen BL, Christoffersen K, Hou-Jensen K, Nissen NI, Knudsen JB, Hansen MM: Carcinoma of the urinary bladder after treatment with cyclophosphamide for nonHodgkin's lymphoma. N Engl J Med **318**:1028-1032, 1988.

93 Price JM, Wear JB, Brown RR, Satter EJ, Olson C: Studies on etiology of carcinoma of urinary bladder. J Urol **83**:376-382, 1960.

94 Schulte PA, Ringen K, Hemstreet GP, Altekruse EB, Gullen WH, Tillett S, Allsbrook WC Jr, Crosby JH, Witherington R, Stringer W, Brubaker MM: Risk factors for bladder cancer in a cohort exposed to aromatic amines. Cancer **58**:2156-2162, 1986.

95 Vineis P, Magnani C: Occupation and bladder cancer in males. A case-control study. Int J Cancer **35**:599-606, 1985.

Morphologic features

96 Alroy J, Pauli BU, Weinstein RS: Correlation between numbers of desmosomes and the aggressiveness of transitional cell carcinoma in human urinary bladder. Cancer **47**:104-112, 1981.

97 Hoshi S, Orikasa S, Numata I, Nose M: Expression of Leu-M1 antigens in carcinoma of the urinary bladder. J Urol **135**:1075-1077, 1986.

98 Jacobs JB, Cohen SM, Farrow GM, Friedell GH: Scanning electron microscopic features of human urinary bladder cancer. Cancer **48**:1399-1409, 1981.

99 Jautzke G, Altenaehr E: Immunohistochemical demonstration of carcinoembryonic antigen (CEA) and its correlation with grading and staging on tissue sections of urinary bladder carcinomas. Cancer **50**:2052-2056, 1982.

100 Kakizoe T, Matsumoto K, Nishio Y, Kishi K: Analysis of 90 step-sectioned cystectomized specimens of bladder cancer. J Urol **131**:467-472, 1984.

101 Lowe D, Fletcher CDM, Gower RL: Tumour-associated eosinophilia in the bladder. J Clin Pathol **37**:500-502, 1984.

102 Murphy WM: Current topics in the pathology of bladder cancer. Pathol Annu **18**(Pt 1):1-25, 1983.

103 Ramaekers F, Huysmans A, Moesker O, Schaart G, Herman C, Vooijs P: Cytokeratin expression during neoplastic progression of human transitional cell carcinomas as detected by a monoclonal and a polyclonal antibody. Lab Invest **52**:31-38, 1985.

104 Royce RK, Spjut HJ: Transitional cell carcinoma of the bladder, grade 1. (So-called papilloma.) J Urol **82**:486-489, 1959.

105 Selli C, Carcangiu ML, Carini M: Bladder carcinoma arising from regenerated urothelium over lyophilized dura patch. Urology **27**:53-55, 1986.

106 Shevchuk MM, Fenoglio CM, Richart RM: Carcinoembryonic antigen localization in benign and malignant transitional epithelium. Cancer **47**:899-905, 1981.

107 Ward AM: Glandular metaplasia and mucin production in transitional cell carcinomas of bladder. J Clin Pathol **24**:481, 1971.

Biopsy

108 National Bladder Cancer Collaborative Group A: Development of a strategy for a longitudinal study of patients with bladder cancer. Cancer Res **37**:2898-2906, 1977.

Cytology

109 Badalament RA, Kimmel M, Gay H, Cibas ES, Whitmore WF Jr, Herr HW, Fair WR, Melamed MR: The sensitivity of flow cytometry compared with conventional cytology in the detection of superficial bladder carcinoma. Cancer **59**:2078-2085, 1987.

110 Esposti PL, Moberger G, Zajicek J: The cytologic diagnosis of transitional cell tumors of the urinary bladder and its histologic basis. Acta Cytol (Baltimore) **14**:145-155, 1970.

111 Koss LG, Deitch D, Ramanathan R, Sherman AB: Diagnostic value of cytology of voided urine. Acta Cytol (Baltimore) **29**:810-816, 1985.

112 MacFarlane EWE, Ceelen GH, Taylor JN: Urine cytology after treatment of bladder tumors. Acta Cytol (Baltimore) **8**:288-292, 1964.

113 Melamed MR, Klein FA: Flow cytometry of urinary bladder irrigation specimens. Hum Pathol **15**:302-305, 1984.

114 National Bladder Cancer Collaborative Group A: Cytology and histopathology of bladder cancer cases in a prospective longitudinal study. Cancer Res **37**:2911-2915, 1977.

115 Orell SR: Transitional cell epithelioma of the bladder. Correlation of cytologic and histologic diagnosis. Scand J Urol Nephrol **3**:93-98, 1969.

116 Reichborn-Kjennerud S, Hoeg K: The value of urine cytology in the diagnosis of recurrent bladder tumors. Acta Cytol (Baltimore) **16**:269-272, 1972.

117 Wolinska WH, Melamed MR, Klein FA: Cytology of bladder papilloma. Acta Cytol (Baltimore) **29**:817-822, 1985.

118 Wolinska WH, Melamed MR, Schellhammer PF, Whitmore WF Jr: Urethral cytology following cystectomy for bladder carcinoma. Am J Surg Pathol **1**:225-233, 1977.

Grading

119 Ash JE: Epithelial tumors of the bladder. J Urol **44**:135-145, 1940.

120 Bergkvist A, Ljungqvist A, Moberger G: Classification of bladder tumours based on the cellular pattern. Acta Chir Scand **130**:371-378, 1965.

121 Jewett HJ, Blackman SS: Infiltrating carcinoma of the bladder. Histologic pattern and degree of cellular differentiation in 97 autopsy cases. J Urol **56**:200-210, 1946.

121a Jordan AM, Weingarten J, Murphy WM: Transitional cell neoplasms of the urinary bladder. Can biologic potential be predicted from histologic grading? Cancer **60**:2766-2774, 1984.

122 Matthews PN, Madden M, Bidgood KA, Fisher C: The clinicopathological features of metastatic superficial papillary bladder cancer. J Urol **132**:904-906, 1984.

123 Mostofi FK: Standardization of nomenclature and criteria for diagnosis of epithelial tumors of urinary bladder. Acta Unio Int Contra Cancr **16**:310-314, 1960.

124 Ooms ECM, Kurver PHJ, Veldhuizen RW, Alons CL, Boon ME: Morphometric grading of bladder tumors in comparison with histologic grading by pathologists. Hum Pathol **14**:144-150, 1983.

Local spread and metastases

125 Chibber PJ, McIntyre MA, Hindmarsh JR, Hargreave TB, Newsam JE, Chisholm GD: Transitional cell carcinoma involving the prostate. Br J Urol **53**:605-609, 1981.

126 Cordonnier JJ: Cystectomy for carcinoma of the bladder. J Urol **99**:172-173, 1968.

127 Hopkins SC, Ford KS, Soloway MS: Invasive bladder cancer. Support for screening. J Urol **130**:61-64, 1983.

128 Kirk D, Savage A, Makepeace AR, Gostelow BE: Transitional cell carcinoma involving the prostate. An unfavourable prognostic sign in the management of bladder cancer? Br J Urol **53**:610-612, 1981.

129 Kishi K, Hirota T, Matsumoto K, Kakizoe T, Murase T, Fujita J: Carcinoma of the bladder. A clinical and pathological analysis of 87 autopsy cases. J Urol **125**:36-39, 1981.

130 Mahadevia PS, Koss LG, Tar IJ: Prostatic involvement in bladder cancer. Prostate mapping in 20 cystoprostatectomy specimens. Cancer **58**:2096-2102, 1986.

130a Ro JY, Ayala AG, el-Naggar A, Wishnow KI: Seminal vesicle involvement by in situ and invasive transitional cell carcinoma of the bladder. Am J Surg Pathol **11**:951-958, 1987.

131 Schade ROK, Serek-Hanssen A, Swinney J: Morphological changes in the ureter in cases of bladder carcinoma. Cancer **27**:1267-1272, 1971.

132 Sharma TC, Melamed MR, Whitmore WF Jr: Carcinoma in situ of the ureter in patients with bladder carcinoma treated by cystectomy. Cancer **26**:583-587, 1970.

Carcinoma in situ and dysplasia

133 Coon JS, McCall A, Miller AW III, Farrow GM, Weinstein RS: Expression of blood-group-related antigens in carcinoma *in situ* of the urinary bladder. Cancer **56**:797-804, 1985.

134 Farrow GM, Utz DC, Rife CC: Morphological and clinical observations of patients with early bladder cancer treated with total cystectomy. Cancer Res **36**:2495-2501, 1976.

135 Friedell GH, Jacobs JB, Nagy GK, Cohen SM: The pathogenesis of bladder cancer. Am J Pathol **89**:431-440, 1977.

136 Friedell GH, Soloway MS, Hilgar AG, Farrow GM: Summary of workshop on carcinoma in situ of the bladder. J Urol **136**:1047-1048, 1986.

137 Fukui I, Yokokawa M, Sekine H, Yamada T, Hosoda K, Ishiwata D, Oka K, Sarada T, Tohma T, Yamada T, Oshima H: Carcinoma in situ of the urinary bladder. Effect of associated neoplastic lesions on clinical course and treatment. Cancer **59**:164-173, 1987.

138 Hofstädter F, Delgado R, Jakse G, Judmaier W: Urothelial dysplasia and carcinoma in situ of the bladder. Cancer **57**:356-361, 1986.

139 Iwasaki H, Enjoji M, Kano M: Nonpapillary carcinoma in situ of the urinary bladder. A histopathologic study and mapping of the urothelial lesions. Acta Pathol Jpn **29**:623-633, 1979.

140 Kakizoe T, Matumoto K, Nishio Y, Ohtani M, Kishi K: Significance of carcinoma in situ and dysplasia in association with bladder cancer. J Urol **133**:395-398, 1985.

141 Melamed MD, Voutsa NG, Grabstald H: Natural history and clinical behavior of in situ carcinoma of the human urinary bladder. Cancer **17**:1533-1545, 1964.

142 Murphy WM, Soloway MS: Urothelial dysplasia. J Urol **127**:849-854, 1982.

143 Ooms ECM, Blomjous CEM, Zwartendijk J, Veldhuizen RW, Blok APR, Heinhuis RJ, Boon ME: Connective tissue stroma in bladder papillary transitional cell carcinoma, carcinoma in situ and benign cystitis. Histopathology **10**:613-619, 1986.

144 Prout GR Jr, Griffin PP, Daly JJ, Heney NM: Carcinoma in situ of the urinary bladder with and without associated vesical neoplasms. Cancer **52**:524-532, 1983.

145 Seemayer TA, Knaack J, Thelmo WL, Wang N-S, Ahmed MN: Further observations on carcinoma in situ of the urinary bladder. Silent but extensive intraprostatic involvement. Cancer **36**:514-520, 1975.

146 Skinner DG, Richie JP, Cooper PH, Waisman J, Kaufman JJ: The clinical significance of carcinoma in situ of the bladder and its association with overt carcinoma. J Urol **112**:68-71, 1974.

147 Soto EA, Friedell GH, Tiltman AJ: Bladder cancer as seen in giant histologic sections. Cancer **39**:447-455, 1977.

148 Utz DC, Farrow GM, Rife CC, Segura JW, Zincke H: Carcinoma in situ of the bladder. Cancer **45**:1842-1848, 1980.

Treatment

149 BLINST Italian Cooperative Group: Intravesical doxorubicin for the prophylaxis of superficial bladder tumors. A multicenter study. Cancer **54**:756-761, 1984.

150 Cordonnier JJ: Cystectomy for carcinoma of the bladder. J Urol **99**:172-173, 1968.

151 Coutts AG, Grigor KM, Fowler JW: Urethral dysplasia and bladder cancer in cystectomy specimens. Br J Urol **57**:535-541, 1985.

152 Fukui I, Yokokawa M, Sekine H, Yamada T, Hosoda K, Ishiwata D, Oka K, Sarada T, Tohma T, Yamada T, Oshima H: Carcinoma in situ of the urinary bladder. Effect of associated neoplastic lesions on clinical course and treatment. Cancer **59**:164-173, 1987.

153 Grossman H: Current therapy of bladder carcinoma. J Urol **121**:1-7, 1979.

153a Huland H, Otto U, Droese M, Klöppel G: Long-term mitomycin C instillation after transurethral resection of superficial bladder carcinoma. Influence on recurrence, progression and survival. J Urol **132**:27-29, 1984.

154 Lage JM, Bauer WC, Kelley DR, Ratliff TL, Catalona WJ: Histological parameters and pitfalls in the interpretation of bladder biopsies in bacillus Calmette-Guerin treatment of superficial bladder cancer. J Urol **135**:916-919, 1986.

155 Lamm DL: Bacillus Calmette-Guerin immunotherapy for bladder cancer. J Urol **134**:40-47, 1985.

156 Montie JE, Strasson RA, Stewart BH: Radical cystectomy without radiation therapy for carcinoma of the bladder. J Urol **131**:477-482, 1984.

157 Neumann MP, Limas C: Transitional cell carcinomas of the urinary bladder. Effects of preoperative irradiation on morphology. Cancer **58**:2758-2763, 1986.

158 Pavone-Macaluso M, Tripi M, Ingargiola GD: Cooperative studies of chemoprophylaxis after transurethral resection of bladder tumors. Cancer Chemother Pharmacol **11**(Suppl):S16-S21, 1983.

159 Quilty PM, Duncan W: Treatment of superficial (T_1) tumours of the bladder by radical radiotherapy. Br J Urol **58**:147-152, 1986.

160 Royce RK, Ackerman LV: Carcinoma of the bladder. Clinical, therapeutic and pathologic aspects of 135 cases. J Urol **65**:66-86, 1951.

161 Skinner DG: Current perspectives in the management of high-grade invasive bladder cancer. Cancer **45**:1866-1874, 1980.

162 Smith JA Jr, Batata M, Grabstald H, Sogani PC, Herr H, Whitmore WF Jr: Preoperative irradiation and cystectomy for bladder cancer. Cancer **49**:869-873, 1982.

163 Soloway MS: Rationale for intensive intravesical chemotherapy for superficial bladder cancer. J Urol **123**:461-466, 1980.

164 Soloway MS: The management of superficial bladder cancer. Cancer **45**:1856-1865, 1980.

165 Utz DC, Farrow GM, Rife CC, Segura JW, Zincke H: Carcinoma in situ of the bladder. Cancer **45**:1842-1848, 1980.

166 Yu WS, Sagerman RH, Chung CT, Dalal PS, King GA: Bladder carcinoma. Experience with radical and preoperative radiotherapy in 421 patients. Cancer **56**:1293-1299, 1985.

Prognosis

167 Alroy J, Teramura K, Miller AW III, Pauli BU, Gottesman JE, Flanagan M, Davidsohn I, Weinstein RS: Isoantigens A, B and H in urinary bladder carcinomas following radiotherapy. Cancer **41**:1739-1745, 1978.

168 Baker R: Pitfalls of clinical versus microscopic staging of cancer of the bladder in relationship to potential curability. Am Surg **36**:269-275, 1970.

169 Bell JT, Burney SW, Friedell GH: Blood vessel invasion in human bladder cancer. J Urol **105**:675-678, 1971.

170 Boyd PJR, Burnand KG: Site of bladder-tumour recurrence. Lancet **2**:1290-1292, 1974.

171 Brawn PN: The origin of invasive carcinoma of the bladder. Cancer **50**:515-519, 1982.

172 Coon JS, Schwartz D, Summers JL, Miller AW III, Weinstein RS: Flow cytometric analysis of deparaffinized nuclei in urinary bladder carcinoma. Comparison with cytogenetic analysis. Cancer **57**:1594-1601, 1986.

173 Coon JS, Weinstein RS: Detection of ABH tissue isoantigens by immunoperoxidase methods in normal and neoplastic urothelium. Comparison with the erythrocyte adherence method. Am J Clin Pathol **8**:163-171, 1981.

174 Cordonnier JJ: Cystectomy for carcinoma of the bladder. J Urol **99**:172-173, 1968.

175 Czerniak B, Koss LG: Expression of Ca antigen on human urinary bladder tumors. Cancer **55**:2380-2383, 1985.

176 Dalesio O, Schulman CC, Sylvester R, De Pauw M, Robinson M, Denis L, Smith P, Viggiano G, and Members of the European Organization for Research on Treatment of Cancer, Genitourinary Tract Cancer Cooperative Group: Prognostic factors in superficial bladder tumors. A study of the European Organization for Research on Treatment of Cancer, Genitourinary Tract Cancer Cooperative Group. J Urol **129**:730-733, 1983.

177 Farsund T, Hoestmark JG, Laerum OD: Relation between flow cytometric DNA distribution and pathology in human bladder cancer. A report on 69 cases. Cancer **54**:1771-1777, 1984.

178 Friedell GH, Parija GC, Nagy GK, Soto EA: The pathology of human bladder cancer. Cancer **45**:1823-1831, 1980.

179 Gilbert HA, Logan JL, Kagan AR, Friedman HA, Cove JK, Fox M, Muldoon TM, Lonni YW, Rowe JH, Cooper JF, Nussbaum H, Chan P, Rao A, Starr A: The natural history of papillary transitional cell carcinoma of the bladder and its treatment in an unselected population on the basis of histologic grading. J Urol **119**:488-492, 1978.

180 Hadjissotiriou GG, Green DK, McIntyre MA, Hargreave TB, Chisholm GD: DNA/RNA ratio in bladder cancer. A factor indicating the recurrence rate? Br J Urol **57**:668-675, 1985.

181 Heney NM, Ahmed S, Flanagan MJ, Frable W, Corder MP, Hafermann MD, Hawkins IR for National Bladder Cancer Collaborative Group A: Superficial bladder cancer. Progression and recurrence. J Urol **130**:1083-1086, 1983.

182 Heney NM, Proppe K, Prout GR Jr, Griffin PP, Shipley WU: Invasive bladder cancer. Tumor configuration, lymphatic invasion and survival. J Urol **130**:895-897, 1983.

183 Javadpour N, Mostofi FK: Primary epithelial tumors of the bladder in the first two decades of life. J Urol **101**:706-710, 1969.

184 Jewett HJ: Carcinoma of the bladder. Influence of depth of infiltration on the five-year results following complete extirpation of the primary growth. J Urol **67**:672-680, 1952.

185 Jewett HJ, King LR, Shelley WM: A study of 365 cases of infiltrating bladder cancer. Relation of certain pathological characteristics to prognosis after extirpation. J Urol **92**:668-678, 1964.

186 Jordan AM, Weingarten J, Murphy WM: Transitional cell neoplasms of the urinary bladder. Can biologic potential be predicted from histologic grading? Cancer **60**:2766-2774, 1987.

187 Juhl BR, Hartzen SH, Hainau B: A, B, H antigen expression in transitional cell carcinomas of the urinary bladder. Cancer **57**:1768-1775, 1986.

188 Juhl BR, Hartzen SH, Hainau B: Lewis a antigen in transitional cell tumors of the urinary bladder. Cancer **58**:222-228, 1986.

189 Kaye KW, Lange PH: Mode of presentation of invasive bladder cancer. Reassessment of the problem. J Urol **128**:31-33, 1982.

190 Kern WH: The grade and pathologic stage of bladder cancer. Cancer **53**:1185-1189, 1984.

191 Lehman TP, Cooper HS, Mulholland SG: Peanut lectin binding sites in transitional cell carcinoma of the urinary bladder. Cancer **53**:272-277, 1984.

192 Lerman RI, Hutter RVP, Whitmore WF Jr: Papilloma of the urinary bladder. Cancer **25**:333-342, 1970.

193 Limas C, Lange P: A, B, H antigen detectability in normal and neoplastic urothelium. Influence of methodologic factors. Cancer **49**:2476-2484, 1982.

194 Limas C, Lange PH: Lewis antigens in normal and neoplastic urothelium. Am J Pathol **121**:176-183, 1985.

195 Limas C, Lange P: T-antigen in normal and neoplastic urothelium. Cancer **58**:1236-1245, 1986.

196 Limas C, Lange P, Fraley EE, Vessella RL: A, B, H antigens in transitional cell tumors of the urinary bladder. Correlation with the clinical course. Cancer **44**:2099-2107, 1979.

197 Lund F, Lundwall F: Papillomas of the urinary bladder. Acta Pathol Microbiol Scand **105**[Suppl]:118-134, 1955.

198 Murphy WM: DNA flow cytometry in diagnostic pathology of the urinary tract. Hum Pathol **18**:317-319, 1987.

199 Murphy WM, Chandler RW, Trafford RM: Flow cytometry of deparaffinized nuclei compared to histological grading for the pathological evaluation of transitional cell carcinomas. J Urol **135**:694-697, 1986.

200 Narayana AS, Loening SA, Slymen DJ, Culp DA: Bladder cancer. Factors affecting survival. J Urol **130**:56-60, 1983.

200a Ørntoft TF, Nielsen MJS, Wolf H, Olsen S, Clausen H, Hakomori S-I, Dabelsteen E: Blood group antigen ABO and Lewis antigen expression during neoplastic progression of human urothelium. Immunohistochemical study of type 1 chain structures. Cancer **60**:2641-2648, 1987.

201 Pocock RD, Ponder BAJ, O'Sullivan JP, Ibrahim SK, Easton DF, Shearer RJ: Prognostic factors in non-infiltrating carcinoma of the bladder. A preliminary report. Br J Urol **54**:711-715, 1982.

202 Prout GR Jr: Classification and staging of bladder carcinoma. Cancer **45**:1832-1841, 1980.

202a Ro JY, Ayala AG, el-Naggar A: Muscularis mucosa of urinary bladder. Importance for staging and treatment. Am J Surg Pathol **11**:668-673, 1987.

203 Sarma KP: The role of lymphoid reaction in bladder cancer. J Urol **104**:843-849, 1970.

204 Skinner DG: Current perspectives in the management of high-grade invasive bladder cancer. Cancer **45**:1866-1874, 1980.

205 Smith G, Elton RA, Beynon LL, Newsam JE, Chisholm GD, Hargreave TB: Prognostic significance of biopsy results of normal-looking mucosa in cases of superficial bladder cancer. Br J Urol **55**:665-669, 1983.

206 Srinivas M, Orihuela E, Lloyd KO, Old LJ, Whitmore WF Jr: Estimation of ABO(H) isoantigen expression in bladder tumors. J Urol **133**:25-28, 1985.

207 Summers JL, Coon JS, Ward RM, Falor WH, Miller AW III, Weinstein RS: Prognosis in carcinoma of the urinary bladder based upon tissue blood group ABH and Thomsen-Friedenreich antigen status and karyotype of the initial tumor. Cancer Res **43**:934-939, 1983.

208 Vallancien G, Rouger Ph, LeClerc JP, Kuss R: Immunofluorescence study of the distribution of A, B, and H cell surface antigens in bladder tumors. J Urol **130**:67-70, 1983.

209 Wolf H, Højgaard K: Prognostic factors in local surgical treatment of invasive bladder cancer, with special reference to the presence of urothelial dysplasia. Cancer **51**:1710-1715, 1983.

210 Wolk FN, Bishop MC: The specific red cell adherence test in transitional cell carcinoma of the bladder before and after radiotherapy in patients with blood group A. J Urol **130**:71-73, 1983.

OTHER PRIMARY CARCINOMAS
Adenocarcinoma

211 Alroy J, Roganovic D, Banner BF, Jacobs JB, Merk FB, Ucci AA, Kwan PWL, Coon JS IV, Miller AW III: Primary adenocarcinomas of the human urinary bladder. Histochemical, immunological, and ultrastructural studies. Virchows Arch [Pathol Anat] **393**:165-181, 1981.

212 Anderström C, Johansson SL, von Schultz L: Primary adenocarcinoma of the urinary bladder. A clinicopathologic and prognostic study. Cancer **52**:1273-1280, 1983.

213 Choi H, Lamb S, Pintar K, Jacobs SC: Primary signet-ring cell carcinoma of the urinary bladder. Cancer **53**:1985-1990, 1984.

214 Engel RM, Wilkinson HA: Bladder exstrophy. J Urol **104**:699-704, 1974.

215 Epstein JI, Kuhajda FP, Lieberman PH: Prostate-specific acid phosphatase immunoreactivity in adenocarcinomas of the urinary bladder. Hum Pathol **17**:939-942, 1986.

216 Mostofi FK, Thomson RV, Dean AL Jr: Mucous adenocarcinoma of the urinary bladder. Cancer **8**:741-758, 1955.

217 Nocks BN, Heney NM, Daly JJ: Primary adenocarcinoma of urinary bladder. Urology **21**:26-29, 1983.

218 O'Brien AME, Urbanski SJ: Papillary adenocarcinoma in situ of bladder. J Urol **134**:544-546, 1985.

219 Pallesen G: Neoplastic Paneth cells in adenocarcinoma of the urinary bladder. A first case report. Cancer **47**:1834-1837, 1981.

220 Poore TE, Egbert B, Jahnke R, Kraft JK: Signet ring cell adenocarcinoma of the bladder. Linitis plastica variant. Arch Pathol Lab Med **105**:203-204, 1981.

221 Rosas-Uribe A, Luna MA: Primary signet ring cell carcinoma of the urinary bladder. Arch Pathol **88**:294-297, 1969.

222 Satake T, Takeda A, Matsuyama M: Argyrophil cells in the urachal epithelium and urachal adenocarcinoma. Acta Pathol Jpn **34**:1193-1199, 1984.

223 Tanaka T, Kanai N, Sugie S, Nakamura A, Hayashi H, Fujimoto Y, Takeuchi T: Primary signet-ring cell carcinoma of the urinary bladder. Pathol Res Pract **182**:130-132, 1987.

224 Thomas DG: A study of 52 cases of adenocarcinoma of the bladder. Br J Urol **43**:4-15, 1971.

225 Ward AM: Glandular neoplasia within the urinary tract. The aetiology of adenocarcinoma of the urothelium with a review of the literature. I. Introduction. The origin of glandular epithelium in the renal pelvis, ureter, and bladder. Virchows Arch [Pathol Anat] **352**:296-311, 1971.

226 Wells M, Anderson K: Mucin histochemistry of cystitis glandularis and primary adenocarcinoma of the urinary bladder. Arch Pathol Lab Med **109**:59-61, 1985.

227 Young RH, Scully RE: Clear cell adenocarcinoma of the bladder and urethra. A report of three cases and review of the literature. Am J Surg Pathol **9**:816-826, 1985.

228 Young RH, Scully RE: Nephrogenic adenoma. A report of 15 cases, review of the literature, and comparison with clear cell adenocarcinoma of the urinary tract. Am J Surg Pathol **10**:268-275, 1986.

Small cell carcinoma and related "neuroendocrine" tumors

229 Abenoza P, Manivel C, Sibley RK: Adenocarcinoma with neuroendocrine differentiation of the urinary bladder. Clinicopathologic, immunohistochemical, and ultrastructural study. Arch Pathol Lab Med **110**:1062-1066, 1986.

230 Colby TV: Carcinoid tumor of the bladder. A case report. Arch Pathol Lab Med **104**:199-200, 1980.

231 Cramer SF, Aikawa M, Cebelin M: Neurosecretory granules in small cell invasive carcinoma of the urinary bladder. Cancer **47**:724-730, 1981.

232 Mills SE, Wolfe JT III, Weiss MA, Swanson PE, Wick MR, Fowler JE Jr, Young RH: Small cell undifferentiated carcinoma of the urinary bladder. A light-microscopic, immunocytochemical, and ultrastructural study of 12 cases. Am J Surg Pathol **11**:606-617, 1987.

233 Ordóñez NG, Khorsand J, Ayala AG, Sneige N: Oat cell carcinoma of the urinary tract. An immunohistochemical and electron microscopic study. Cancer **58**:2519-2530, 1986.

234 Partanen S, Asikainen U: Oat cell carcinoma of the urinary bladder with ectopic adrenocorticotropic hormone production. Hum Pathol **16**:313-315, 1985.

235 Reyes CV, Soneru I: Small cell carcinoma of the urinary bladder with hypercalcemia. Cancer **56**:2530-2533, 1985.

Epidermoid carcinoma

236 Bessette PL, Abell MR, Herwig KR: A clinicopathologic study of squamous cell carcinoma of the bladder. J Urol **112**:66-67, 1974.

237 DeKock MLS, Anderson CK, Clark PB: Vesical leukoplakia progressing to squamous cell carcinoma in women. Br J Urol **53**:316-317, 1981.

238 El-Bolkainy MN, Mokhtar NM, Ghoneim MA, Hussein MH: The impact of schistosomiasis on the pathology of bladder carcinoma. Cancer **48**:2643-2648, 1981.

239 Faysal MH: Squamous cell carcinoma of the bladder. J Urol **126**:598-599, 1981.

240 Ghoneim MA, Ashamalla A, Gaballa MA, Ibrahim EI: Cystectomy for carcinoma of the bilharzial bladder. 126 patients 10 years later. Br J Urol **57**:303-305, 1985.

241 Newman DM, Brown JR, Jay AC, Pontius EE: Squamous cell carcinoma of the bladder. J Urol **100**:470-473, 1968.

242 O'Flynn JD, Mullaney J: Leukoplakia of the bladder. A report on 20 cases, including 2 cases progressing to squamous cell carcinoma. Br J Urol **39**:461-471, 1967.

243 Royce RK, Ackerman LV: Carcinoma of the bladder. J Urol **65**:66-86, 1951.

244 Rundle JSH, Hart AJL, McGeorge A, Smith JS, Malcolm AJ, Smith PM: Squamous cell carcinoma of bladder. A review of 114 patients. Br J Urol **54**:522-526, 1982.

245 Wall RL, Clausen KP: Carcinoma of the urinary bladder in patients receiving cyclophosphamide. N Engl J Med **293**:271-273, 1975.

Sarcomatoid carcinoma

246 Dennis PM, Turner AG: Primary choriocarcinoma of the bladder evolving from a transitional cell carcinoma. J Clin Pathol 37:503-505, 1984.

247 Fromowitz FB, Bard RH, Koss LG: The epithelial origin of a malignant mixed tumor of the bladder. Report of a case with long-term survival. J Urol 132:978-981, 1984.

248 Holtz F, Fox JE, Abell MR: Carcinosarcoma of the urinary bladder. Cancer 29:294-304, 1972.

249 Jao W, Soto JM, Gould VE: Squamous carcinoma of bladder with pseudosarcomatous stroma. Arch Pathol 99:461-466, 1975.

250 Kawamura J, Machida S, Yoshida O, Osek F, Imura H, Hattori M: Bladder carcinoma associated with ectopic production of gonadotropin. Cancer 42:2773-2780, 1978.

251 Kitazawa M, Kobayashi H, Ohnishi Y, Kimura K, Sakurai S, Sekine S: Giant cell tumor of the bladder associated with transitional cell carcinoma. J Urol 133:472-475, 1985.

251a Mostofi FK, Sesterhenn IA, Davis CJ Jr: Human chorionic gonadotropin and other placental glycoprotein production in nongerminal tumors of genitourinary tract (abstract). Lab Invest 58:65A, 1988.

252 Murao T, Tanahashi T: Carcinosarcoma of the urinary bladder. Report of a case with electron microscopy and review of the literature. Acta Pathol Jpn 35:981-988, 1985.

253 Obe JA, Rosen N, Koss LG: Primary choriocarcinoma of the urinary bladder. Report of a case with probable epithelial origin. Cancer 52:1405-1409, 1983.

254 Sen SE, Malek RS, Farrow GM, Lieber MM: Sarcoma and carcinosarcoma of the bladder in adults. J Urol 133:29-30, 1985.

255 Shah VM, Newman J, Crocker J, Chapple CR, Collard MJ, O'Brien JM, Considine J: Ectopic β-human chorionic gonadotropin production by bladder urothelial neoplasia. Arch Pathol Lab Med 110:107-111, 1986.

256 Smith JA Jr, Herr HW, Middleton RG: Bladder carcinosarcoma. Histologic variation in metastatic lesions. J Urol 129:829-831, 1983.

256a Wick MR, Brown BA, Young RH, Mills SE: Spindle-cell proliferations of the urinary tract. An immunohistochemical study. Am J Surg Pathol 12:379-389, 1988.

257 Young RH: Carcinosarcoma of the urinary bladder. Cancer 59:1333-1339, 1987.

OTHER MALIGNANT TUMORS

258 Ainsworth AM, Clark WH Jr, Mastrangelo M, Conger KB: Primary malignant melanoma of the urinary bladder. Cancer 37:1928-1936, 1976.

259 Anichkov NM, Nikonov AA: Primary malignant melanomas of the bladder. J Urol 128:813-815, 1982.

260 Berenson RJ, Flynn S, Freiha FS, Kempson RL, Torti FM: Primary osteogenic sarcoma of the bladder. Case report and review of the literature. Cancer 57:350-355, 1986.

261 Bocian JJ, Flam MS, Mendoza CA: Hodgkin's disease involving the urinary bladder diagnosed by urinary cytology. A case report. Cancer 50:2482-2485, 1982.

262 Goodman AJ, Greaney MG: Malignant fibrous histiocytoma of the bladder. Br J Urol 57:106-107, 1985.

263 Haid M, Ignatoff J, Khandekar JD, Graham J, Holland J: Urinary bladder metastases from breast carcinoma. Cancer 46:229-232, 1980.

263a Harris M, Eyden BP, Joglekar VM: Rhabdoid tumour of the bladder. A histological, ultrastructural and immunohistochemical study. Histopathology 11:1083-1092, 1987.

264 Hays DM, Raney RB, Lawrence W, Soule EH, Gehan EA, Tefft M: Bladder and prostatic tumors in the Intergroup Rhabdomyosarcoma Study (IRS-1). Results of therapy. Cancer 50:1472-1482, 1982.

265 Henriksen OB, Mogensen P, Engelholm AJ: Inflammatory fibrous histiocytoma of the urinary bladder. Clinicopathological report of a case. Acta Pathol Microbiol Immunol Scand [A] 90:333-337, 1982.

266 Kinoshita T, Nakamura Y, Kinoshita M, Fukuda S, Nakashima H, Hashimoto T: Bilateral cystic nephroblastomas and botryoid sarcoma in a child with Dandy-Walker syndrome. Arch Pathol Lab Med 110:150-152, 1986.

267 Krumerman MS, Katatikarn V: Rhabdomyosarcoma of the urinary bladder with intraepithelial spread in an adult. Arch Pathol Lab Med 100:395-397, 1976.

268 Mackenzie AR, Sharma TC, Whitmore WF Jr, Melamed MR: Non-extirpative treatment of myosarcomas of the bladder and prostate. Cancer 28:329-334, 1971.

269 Mackenzie AR, Whitmore WF Jr, Melamed MR: Myosarcomas of the bladder and prostate. Cancer 22:833-844, 1968.

270 Meyer JE: Metastatic melanoma of the urinary bladder. Cancer 34:1822-1824, 1974.

271 Pentecost CL, Pizzolato P: Involvement of the genitourinary tract in leukemia. J Urol 53:725-731, 1945.

272 Perez-Mesa C, Pickren JW, Woodruff MN, Mohallatee A: Metastatic carcinoma of the urinary bladder from primary tumors in the mammary gland of female patients. Surg Gynecol Obstet 121:813-818, 1965.

273 Swartz DA, Johnson DE, Ayala AG, Watkins DL: Bladder leiomyosarcoma. A review of 10 cases with 5-year followup. J Urol 133:200-202, 1985.

274 Taylor G, Jordan M, Churchill B, Mancer K: Yolk sac tumor of the bladder. J Urol 129:591-594, 1983.

274a Terada Y, Saito I, Morohoshi T, Niijima T: Malignant mesenchymoma of the bladder. Cancer 60:858-863, 1987.

275 Wang CC, Scully RE, Leadbetter WF: Primary malignant lymphoma of the urinary bladder. Cancer 24:772-776, 1969.

276 Yang C, Motteram R, Sandeman TF: Extramedullary plasmacytoma of the bladder. A case report and review of literature. Cancer 50:146-149, 1982.

277 Young RH, Proppe KH, Dickersin GR, Scully RE: Myxoid leiomyosarcoma of the urinary bladder. Arch Pathol Lab Med 111:359-362, 1987.

278 Young RH, Rosenberg AE: Osteosarcoma of the urinary bladder. Report of a case and review of the literature. Cancer 59:174-178, 1987.

Index

A

AAT; *see* Alpha-1-antitrypsin
Aberrant thyroid, 434
Abeta-lipoproteinemia of small bowel, 527
Abnormal localization of immature precursors, 1402
Abortion
  placenta and, 1174
  specimen from, 1889-1890
Abscess
  Bartholin's gland, 997
  breast, 1197
  Dubois', 349
  liver, 704
  lung, 273-275
  Pautrier's, 154, 156
  pericecal, 575
  pericolic, 575
  prostate, 926
  spleen, 1363
  tubo-ovarian, 1098
Acanthocytosis of small bowel, 527
Acantholysis, 54, 79
  epidermoid carcinoma and, 181, 1237
    adenoid variant of, 93, 94
Acanthoma, clear cell, 103-104
Acanthosis, 54
  psoriasis and, 63
  verrucous carcinoma and, 183
Acanthosis nigricans, 83
Accessory spleen, 1362
Accessory tragi of external ear, 1849
Accessory urethral canal, 988
Acetaminophen lesion of liver, 683
Acetylcholine receptor, 360
Acetylcholinesterase, 33
  Hirschsprung's disease and, 573
Achalasia of esophagus, 469, 470
Acid fastness, 31
Acidophil stem cell adenoma, 1779, 1784
Acinar cell adenoma, 769
Acinar cell carcinoma, 769
Acinar cell cystadenocarcinoma, 769
Acinar cell hyperplasia, 769
Acinar cell tumors, 769
Acinic cell carcinoma of salivary glands, 658-659
  gingiva and, 186
Acinic cell tumor, 326
Ackerman LV, 1
Acoustic neurofibromas, 1754
Acoustic neuroma of middle and inner ear, 1854
Acquired arteriovenous fistula, 1694-1695
Acquired cysts, 270
  in renal dialysis patient, 859
Acquired hemolytic anemia of spleen, 1366, 1367

Acquired immune deficiency syndrome, 321, 824
  bone marrow, 1389, 1391-1394
  cryptosporidiosis and, 533
  glomerular lesions and, 821
  Kaposi's sarcoma and, 151
  lymphadenopathy and, 1288-1290
  lymphomas and, 679, 1337
  nephropathy and, 824
  serous degeneration and, 1385
Acquired melanosis
  conjunctiva, 1813
  eyelid, 1796
Acquired myopathies, 1776
Acquired progressive lymphangioma, 146
Acquired tufted angioma, 146
Acral arteriovenous tumor, 146
Acral melanoma, 128
Acrochordon, 90
  trichofolliculomas and, 111
Acrospiroma, 100
ACTH cell adenoma, 1782-1783
Actin, 37
  rhabdomyosarcoma and, 1600
Actinic keratoacanthomas, 112
Actinic keratosis
  epidermis, 90-91
  external ear, 1851
Actinic melanosis, 126
Actinomycosis, 281
  breast, 1198
  cervix, 1023
  ovary, 1117
  prostate, 926
  uterus, 1053
Acute appendicitis, 557-560
Acute cholecystitis, 740-742
Acute cyclosporin toxicity, 849
Acute epiglottitis, 246
Acute fatty liver of pregnancy, 694
Acute focal appendicitis, 558
Acute gastric ulcer, 490
Acute gastritis, 490
Acute imminent renal allograft rejection, 849
Acute infectious nonbacterial gastroenteritis, 490
Acute infectious-type colitis, 586
Acute interstitial pneumonia, 282
Acute jaundice, 676
Acute jejunitis, 532
Acute leukemia, 1394-1397
Acute megakaryoblastic leukemia, 1394, 1395
  acute myelofibrosis and, 1398-1399
Acute myelodysplasia with myelofibrosis, 1397
Acute myelofibrosis, 1397-1400
Acute myelogenous leukemia, 1394-1397
Acute myelosclerosis, 1397

Acute necrotizing arteritis of appendix, 561
Acute nephritis, 832-844
Acute pancreatitis, 757-760
Acute rejection in renal allograft pathology, 849
Acute self-limited colitis, 586
Acute suppurative appendicitis, 558
Acute thyroiditis, 394
Acute vanishing bile duct syndrome, 704
Acute viral hepatitis, 676-679
Adamantinomas
  long bones, 1509
  pituitary, 1785
Adenoacanthoma, 762
  endometrium, 1068, 1070
  gallbladder, 750
Adenoameloblastoma, 209-213
Adenocarcinoid
  appendix, 567
  small bowel, 541
Adenocarcinoma
  anus, 633
  appendix, 566
  bladder, 912
  cervix, 1034-1041
  Cowper's gland, 943
  ear, 1852, 1853, 1855
  endometrium, 1063, 1075
  esophagus, 479
  eyelid, 1795, 1796
  fallopian tube, 1104
  fetal type, 321
  gallbladder, 748, 750-751
  larynx, 255, 256
  lung, 297-300
  male urethra, 992
  nasal cavity, 232-233, 235
  prostate, 933
  renal pelvis and ureter, 881, 885
  rete testis, 985
  salivary gland, 187-189, 661-663
  small bowel, 538, 540
  stomach, 498, 503
  trachea, 260
  uterus, 1143
  vagina, 1015, 1016
Adenocystic carcinoma, 105
Adenofibroma
  fallopian tube, 1105
  uterine, 1082, 1083
Adenoid basal carcinoma
  cervix, 1040
  prostate, 935
Adenoid cystic carcinoma
  breast, 1245-1246
  cervix, 1037-1040
  lacrimal gland, 1800